The Dental Assistant

FIFTH EDITION

Richard E. Richardson, D.D.S.
Professor of Oral Diagnosis
School of Dentistry
University of North Carolina at
Chapel Hill

Roger E. Barton, D.D.S.
Professor of Ecology and
Associate Dean for Administration
School of Dentistry
University of North Carolina at
Chapel Hill

McGraw-Hill Book Company

New York • St. Louis • San Francisco • Auckland • Bogotá
Düsseldorf • Johannesburg • London • Madrid • Mexico
Montreal • New Delhi • Panama • Paris • São Paulo
Singapore • Sydney • Tokyo • Toronto

THE DENTAL ASSISTANT

Copyright © 1978, 1970, 1964, 1960, 1955 by McGraw-Hill, Inc. All rights reserved. Printed in the United States of America. No part of this publication may be reproduced, stored in a retrieval system, or transmitted, in any form or by any means, electronic, mechanical, photocopying, recording, or otherwise, without the prior written permission of the publisher.

4567890 VHVH 8321

This book was set in Souvenir Light by Progressive Typographers. The editors were Stuart D. Boynton and Henry C. De Leo; the designer was Judith Michael; the production supervisor was Angela Kardovich.
Von Hoffmann Press, Inc., was printer and binder.

Library of Congress Cataloging in Publication Data

Richardson, Richard Edgeworth.
    The dental assistant.

    Includes bibliographies and index.
    1. Dental assistants. I. Barton, Roger E., joint author. II. Title. [DNLM: 1. Dental assistants. WU90 D412]
RK60.5.R53   1978   617'.6   77-23958
ISBN 0-07-052301-0

Contents

List of Contributors **v**
Preface **vii**

1 The Dental Profession **1**
Richard E. Richardson

2 Practice Administration **38**
Ethel M. Earl

3 Applied Psychology **61**
Benjamin R. Baker

4 Dental Anatomy and Physiology **81**
R. Jack Shankle

5 Oral Histology **106**
Walter T. McFall, Jr.

6 Microbiology **117**
James J. Crawford

7 Sterilization and Disinfection **135**
James J. Crawford

8 Oral Pathology **151**
Grover C. Hunter, Jr.

9 Pharmacology **166**
Cecil R. Lupton

10 Dental Materials: Gypsum Products **181**
James E. Overberger

11 Impression Materials, Dental Waxes, and Synthetic Resin Materials **197**
Roger E. Barton

12 Dental Cements and Resin Restorative Materials **215**
Roger E. Barton

13 Amalgam **234**
James E. Overberger

14 Golds and Gold Alloys **244**
Roger E. Barton

15 Investments and Casting Procedures **260**
Karl F. Leinfelder

16 Instruments, Equipment, and Their Care **273**
    Roger E. Barton
17 Oral Diagnosis **320**
    Richard E. Richardson
18 Dental Radiology **341**
    Stephen R. Matteson
19 Preventive Dentistry **375**
    William R. Stanmeyer
20 Nutrition **399**
    William R. Stanmeyer
21 First Aid **420**
    Matthew T. Wood
22 Anesthesia and Pain Control **445**
    Cecil R. Lupton
23 Oral Surgery **457**
    Cecil R. Lupton
24 Endodontics **467**
    R. Jack Shankle
25 Periodontics **482**
    Grover C. Hunter, Jr.
26 Pedodontics **501**
    Benjamin R. Baker
27 Orthodontics **527**
    Robert M. Nelson
28 Operative Dentistry **552**
    William D. Strickland
29 Fixed Prosthodontics **614**
    Gene A. Holland
30 Removable Prosthodontics **644**
    David P. Dobson

Appendix **686**
Glossary **701**
Index **740**

List of Contributors

Benjamin Rives Baker, B.A., M.Ed., D.D.S., M.S.
Private Practice of Pedodontics

Roger Evans Barton, D.D.S.
Professor of Ecology and Associate Dean for Administration, School of Dentistry, University of North Carolina at Chapel Hill

James Joseph Crawford, B.A., M.A., Ph.D.
Associate Professor of Oral Biology and Endodontics, School of Dentistry; Lecturer in Microbiology, School of Medicine, University of North Carolina at Chapel Hill

David Phillip Dobson, D.D.S., M.S.
Professor of Removable Prosthodontics, School of Dentistry, University of North Carolina at Chapel Hill

Ethel McKee Earl, B.S., C.D.A.
Clinical Associate Professor of Dental Ecology and Director, Dental Assistant Program, School of Dentistry, University of North Carolina at Chapel Hill

Gene Allen Holland, A.A., D.D.S., M.S.
Associate Professor of Fixed Prosthodontics, School of Dentistry, University of North Carolina at Chapel Hill

Grover Cleveland Hunter, Jr., A.B., D.D.S., M.S.
Professor of Periodontics, School of Dentistry, University of North Carolina at Chapel Hill

Karl Francis Leinfelder, D.D.S., M.S.
Professor of Operative Dentistry, School of Dentistry, University of North Carolina at Chapel Hill

Cecil Rhodes Lupton, D.D.S.
Professor of Oral Surgery, School of Dentistry, University of North Carolina at Chapel Hill

Walter Thompson McFall, Jr., B.S., D.D.S., M.S.D.
Professor of Periodontics, School of Dentistry, University of North Carolina at Chapel Hill

Stephen Robert Matteson, D.D.S.
Assistant Professor of Oral Diagnosis, School of Dentistry, University of North Carolina at Chapel Hill

Robert Mellinger Nelson, B.A., D.D.S., M.S.
Professor of Orthodontics, School of Dentistry, University of North Carolina at Chapel Hill

James Edwin Overberger, B.S., D.D.S., M.S.
Associate Dean, School of Dentistry, West Virginia University

Richard Edgeworth Richardson, D.D.S.
Professor of Oral Diagnosis, School of Dentistry, University of North Carolina at Chapel Hill

Robert Jack Shankle, D.D.S.
Professor of Endodontics and Director of Public Relations and Development, School of Dentistry, University of North Carolina at Chapel Hill

William Robert Stanmeyer, D.D.S.
Associate Professor of Oral Diagnosis, School of Dentistry, University of North Carolina at Chapel Hill

William Douglas Strickland, B.S., D.D.S.
Professor of Operative Dentistry, School of Dentistry, University of North Carolina at Chapel Hill

Matthew Thomas Wood, A.B., D.D.S., M.S. (Pros.)
Professor and Chairman, Department of Removable Prosthodontics, School of Dentistry, University of North Carolina at Chapel Hill

Preface

Dentistry is changing rapidly and so is the position of the dental assistant. Since the last edition of this book, the opportunities and responsibilities of the dental assistant have increased remarkably. The extent to which the assistant may become involved in the delivery of dental care is being considered by virtually everyone concerned with planning for dentistry and its future: governments, professional organizations, and legislative and administrative bodies. Although precise parameters cannot be defined, general trends seem to be developing, and the probable position of the assistant can be anticipated. Undoubtedly, the dental assistant of the future will have more formal training, the position will require higher skills, and there will be greater latitude in positional levels that the assistant may achieve.

In view of this changing situation, it would be impractical to attempt to include in a basic textbook everything that a well trained assistant should know. Such a book would be enormous in size, prohibitive in cost, and almost immediately out of date. From its beginning 4 editions and about 25 years ago, *The Dental Assistant* has been written on the assumption that a broad, general coverage of dentistry and specifics about some fundamental procedures form the best foundation for the dental assistant, who must then learn and grow as the field itself does. We still think this is the best approach, although the number of fundamental procedures described has increased. Once again we have also included broad perspectives of dental practice so that an assistant may have a feeling for and some knowledge of modern dentistry's role in society.

The editors of this book hope that it will continue to be a valuable tool in formal teaching programs and in all modes of learning for dental assistants: universities, colleges, technical schools, extension courses, and on-the-job training. Teachers in formal programs and practicing dentists should find it useful in the development of effective dental assisting.

There are many changes in the fifth edition. A number of new authors appear, and although basic subject coverage is essentially the same, many of the subjects have been entirely or extensively redeveloped and expanded. Much of the material has been rearranged. New chapters on oral diagnosis and periodontics have been included. The first two chapters and those on anesthesia, fixed prosthodontics, investments and casting, microbiology, nutrition, oral surgery, orthodontics, pharmacology, preventive dentistry, and radiology are handled by new authors or the material is entirely new. All other chapters have had critical review with updating and new material added where appropriate. All of the best and enduring has been retained from the previous edition and there has been no attempt to make changes merely for changes' sake; a sincere effort has been made to present as much relevant material as is practical.

Dedicated efforts of a considerable number of people are necessary for making a good book and there is no way that due recognition can be included for all who worked hard to produce this edition. The editors are indebted to the contributors for their diligence in preparing and revising their manuscripts; to the families of all who had to use personal time to get the job done; to the secretaries for their careful work; to many outside sources for permission to use valuable material; to those who so kindly posed for illustrative material; and to the publishing staff for their cooperation, technical skill, and counseling. Special appreciation is acknowledged for the staff of the Learning Resources Center, University of North Carolina at Chapel Hill, School of Dentistry, and its Director, Mr. Thomas Edwards, for their fine work in producing the new illustrations. Thanks to Dr. Murry Holland for the use of his office in photographing some of the illustrations that appear in Chapter 1.

Many years ago there were dentists who envisioned the development of the dental assistant in an increasingly critical role in the delivery of dental care. There were some who promoted such ideas. One such man who did something about it was Dr. John Charles Brauer. As early as 1950 Dr. Bauer worked toward the goal of a properly trained assistant who would do many of the things in a dental office formerly thought of as requiring the personal attention of the dentist. A tangible effort in this direction was the publication of *The Dental Assistant,* which Dr. Brauer saw through four editions since 1955, three as editor. Dr. Brauer has deceased since publication of the fourth edition and his name and personality will be sincerely missed in this edition. He gave a great deal to dentistry during his illustrious career, and he especially was a leader and friend of the cause of the dental assistant. The chapters in the fourth edition that Dr. Brauer wrote have been completely rewritten or revised by new authors.

Those who are familiar with previous editions will sadly note the passing of Drs. Marvin Evans and Monte Miska and Mr. Kent Davis who were contributors to previous editions; to these dedicated men humble tribute is offered.

Richard E. Richardson
Roger E. Barton

Creed for Dental Assistants

To be loyal to my employer, my calling and myself.

To develop initiative—having the courage to assume responsibility and the imagination to create ideas and develop them.

To be prepared to visualize, take advantage of and fulfill the opportunities of my calling.

To be a co-worker—creating a spirit of co-operation and friendliness rather than one of fault-finding and criticism.

To be enthusiastic—for therein lies the easiest way to accomplishment.

To be generous, not alone of my name but of my praise and my time.

To be tolerant with my associates, for at times I too make mistakes.

To be friendly, realizing that friendship bestows and receives happiness.

To be respectful of the other person's viewpoint and condition.

To be systematic, believing that system makes for efficiency.

To know the value of time for both my employer and myself.

To safeguard my health, for good health is necessary for the achievement of a successful career.

To be tactful—always doing the right thing at the right time.

To be courteous—for this is the badge of good breeding.

To walk on the sunny side of the street, seeing the beautiful things in life rather than fearing the shadows.

To keep smiling always.

Juliette A. Southard

To The Dental Assistant
Whose service is dedicated to the health and welfare of people everywhere, and whose service to the profession lends dignity and value to the practice of dentistry

1

Richard E. Richardson
The Dental Profession

INTRODUCTION

A National Center for Health Statistics survey (1965) indicated that in the early 1960s one-half the teeth of the average American had become carious by the age of 25 to 34 years. In the 45- to 54-year-old group, only about 10 or 11 teeth per person remained undamaged, and approximately one-half of 55- to 65-year-old persons had no remaining teeth. Only 26.1 percent of the adult population of the United States was free from some degree of periodontal disease. About 20 percent of all adults at ages 18 to 79 years had lost all their permanent teeth (Pelton, 1969).

Sognnaes (1959) estimated that it would take 10 years' work by $2^1/_2$ times as many dentists

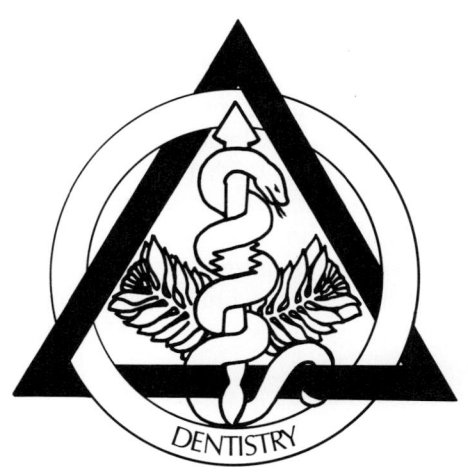

as then existed in the United States just to repair existing ordinary dental defects.

Tooth decay is the most prevalent chronic disease affecting the American people; it affects nearly everyone, except for those who resided in areas where adequate fluorides were received at the time of tooth formation and maturation and who received good preventive management. Dental caries has its greatest incidence in youths and young people, but it can and does affect people of all ages as long as they have any natural teeth. Periodontal disease has a greater incidence in adults and at older ages, but it can and does affect the young. Malocclusion is found frequently in children and adults, and cleft palate occurs in about 1 out of every 750 live births in the United States (Pelton, 1955).

Undoubtedly there has been some improvement over the years in the statistics cited, because there has been improvement in the nature of dental treatment; the utilization of fluorides has increased; dental care has become more available; and the principles of prevention have become more generally understood. However, the problems have not disappeared and are not likely to in the foreseeable future. The control of these human needs lies in the hands of the profession of dentistry, which includes all of those persons who work together to assure quality dental care for all people.

Role of the Dental Assistant

The dental assistant is profoundly concerned with every aspect of dental practice as, indeed, are all persons who work together within this health-science field. Those who have, or are planning, careers in dentistry would do well to try to understand dentistry in its broadest sense; to master not just its techniques and economics but also the implications of its heritage, its mission, and its future.

No one should think exclusively of the assistant, the hygienist, the laboratory technician, or others in the office as working *for* the dentist, but surely as working *with* the dentist. The *team* concept has existed for a long, long time among smart practitioners, but now the word has a much broader concept; it must be accepted by all. Whatever any individual serving in the field of dentistry does, says, or thinks has some effect on the status and effectiveness of dental practice within that person's sphere of activity. One person's success may be materially affected by all others in the same professional field.

To be included in this high level of mutual participation and its rewards, each individual must share responsibility for team effectiveness. A feeling for dentistry and its service, as well as for its material benefits, demands more than just being technically great and personally attractive.

The assistant will need to be a part of developing dental programs; will want to associate with organizational interests; should know what changes in the field are being proposed; will need to participate in continuing education; will work toward a more humane service; and, in short, will need to be a professional person.

Health is defined in the World Health Organization's basic charter as a state of complete physical, mental, and social well-being, not merely the absence of disease. The goal of all health professionals, the public, and the government is to ensure the right to health for everyone. We are concerned with dental and oral health, and the trends have always been to make it more available or more possible. In recent times there has been a greatly intensified concern and effort by legislators and health professionals toward this important end.

All of this should be a clear indication that the dental assistant is involved in an important career, which should provide a continuing opportunity to participate in an important activity and in service to a large segment of human need. There is ample opportunity to satisfy personal desires for inner satisfaction and for material gains.

HISTORY

Origins

Just where dentistry was first practiced is rather uncertain, but probably some special attention has been given to ailments of the teeth ever since ancient times. Taylor (1922) has stated that considerable fragmentary evidence still exists as to the general methods used by ancients.

Early dental treatment was rendered by the priesthood as a part of medicine and has been referred to as sacerdotal medicine. This practice was evidently based on early belief that illness was imposed as divine punishment for some wrongdoing.

The first physician of record was I-Em-Hetep who lived about 4000 B.C. in Egypt. The earliest record of treatment of toothache occurs in the Papyrus of Ebers, discovered by Professor George Ebers at Thebes in 1872. This document covers the period from 3500 to 1500 B.C. and gives remedies for toothache but does not mention dental surgery (Taylor, 1922).

Hwang-ti, referred to as the Chinese Father of Medicine, lived about 2700 B.C. Medical works of China of this period refer to toothache as *Ya-tong* and describe various forms of this ailment and gum diseases; 26 acupuncture sites were used for the relief of toothache.

Evidence exists which shows that the Etruscans, early Italians living in Etruria about 1000 to 200 B.C., made bridges to replace lost teeth. The Romans also made prosthetic devices for missing teeth, specimens of which are preserved in museums.

Hippocrates, known as the Father of Medicine, was born on the Greek island of Cos about 460 B.C. He wrote about dental ailments and their treatment; he also invented crude dental instruments.

Dentistry even has a patron saint, Saint Apollonia, who was canonized by the Church of Rome in 300 A.D. Apollonia was tortured by having her teeth drawn out one by one, was clubbed, and was burned at the stake for her refusal to renounce the Christian faith. Her intercession has been sought ever since by devout believers for relief of dental pain.

Gradually medicine and dentistry came to be practiced by lay people instead of by priests, and for centuries barbers and any persons who so desired performed dental services. History records many individuals who developed dentistry to quite an art, but it did not become a true profession until fairly recent times.

Development of Modern Dentistry

Pierre Fauchard (Brittany, 1678–Paris, 1761) has been called the Founder of Modern Dentistry for his efforts to develop the body of dental knowledge and practice into a learned profession. He was the author of one of the earliest comprehensive works on dental practice, *Le Chirugien Dentiste,* published in 1728, revised in 1746 and in 1786. He was a strong proponent of formal education and examination for qualification to practice.

Evidently numerous individuals practiced dentistry in America to some degree from about 1700, but they often limited their services and had other interests; they also moved about frequently. It is probable that Josiah Flagg (1764–1816) was one of the first, if not the first, native-born, full-time dentists to practice in America. These early dentists certainly had to be ingenious, for they had no formal education, and they performed a wide range of services (Fig. 1-1).

In 1840 the first formal school of dentistry, Baltimore College of Dental Surgery, was established by Horace H. Hayden and Chapin A. Harris. *The American Journal of Dental Science* and the American Society of Dental Surgeons were founded about this same time. Dentistry began to emerge as a true profession. Shortly, more schools were founded, and efforts were

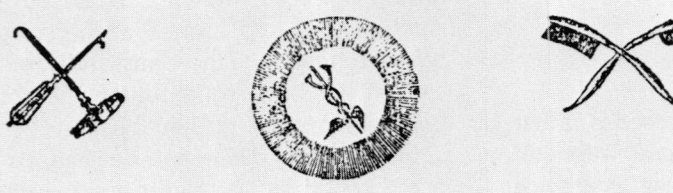

Figure 1-1 | Eighteenth-century dentist's broadside (handbill).

made to formalize dental education and dental practice; specific requirements and laws governing dentistry came into being.

Scientific dentistry was on the horizon, but the name of one man, Greene Vardiman Black (1834–1915), stands out in the coming of age of dentistry as a scientific discipline. Dean of Northwestern University Dental School (1897–1915), he was instrumental in elevating dental education to high standards; he was a pathologist of note; he developed the formula for the first dental silver alloy that was scientifically balanced; and his last published paper (posthumous) was on Colorado brown stain, which was the subject of research that ultimately led to the discovery of the relationship of fluorides to dental defects and the value of fluorides in the prevention of dental caries.

Dentistry claims credit for the discovery of general anesthesia, obviously, one of the greatest boons of all times. On December 11, 1844, in Hartford, Connecticut, Dr. Horace Wells demonstrated the anesthetic properties of nitrous oxide by submitting to its inhalation and having a tooth extracted by Dr. John M. Riggs. Dr. William T. G. Morton, another dentist, successfully administered ether to perform a painless dental extraction on September 30, 1846.

In its first 100 years, formal dental education made rapid advances, and dentistry became an accepted and honored profession. In its second 100 years, so far, dentistry has set its objectives on even higher levels of performance and service to the public. Requirements for qualification of all individuals to participate in dental service are more and more precise and exacting, but the rewards are ever greater.

For further interest in the development of dentistry, bibliographic entrys related to its history are noted (Bremmer; Guerini; Koch; Prinz; Robinson; Taylor; Weinberger).

AREAS OF PRACTICE

Dentistry is a profession. A dentist is one who has been educated and trained in this health science and who has the legal right to treat the hard structures designated as teeth, their supporting bone and soft tissues, and the related tissues of the mouth or oral cavity. Within this field the dentist is the preeminent authority.

General Practice

The practice of dentistry in private life assumes two main forms, the first of which is known as general practice. In this type of practice, the dentist accepts for treatment all patients who present with any form of dental illness or need within the limits of general dental training and ability. The dentist restores teeth which have cavities, removes teeth that must be lost, replaces those which have been extracted or are absent, cleans teeth, and treats their supporting structures. Sometimes the general practitioner rearranges the alignment of the teeth and arches. In some instances, however, the dentist will call upon those practitioners who limit their practices to certain fields to perform procedures that require unusual skill.

Specialty Practice

The second form of private dental practice is the limitation of operations to a specialized field. A specialist is expected and required to have had advanced training and to possess special skill and knowledge in his or her field (see "Principles of Ethics, ADA," Section 18, later in this chapter).

The following areas in dentistry are now recognized as specialties:

Endodontics deals with the diagnosis and treatment of diseases of the dental pulp and periapical tissues.
Orthodontics deals with the alignment of teeth and arches as they relate to function and esthetics.
Oral surgery deals with the surgical procedures in and about the oral cavity, including the extraction of teeth.
Oral pathology deals with abnormal conditions and disease of the hard and soft tissues of the oral cavity.
Pedodontics deals with the practice of dentistry for children but does not include major orthodontic treatment.

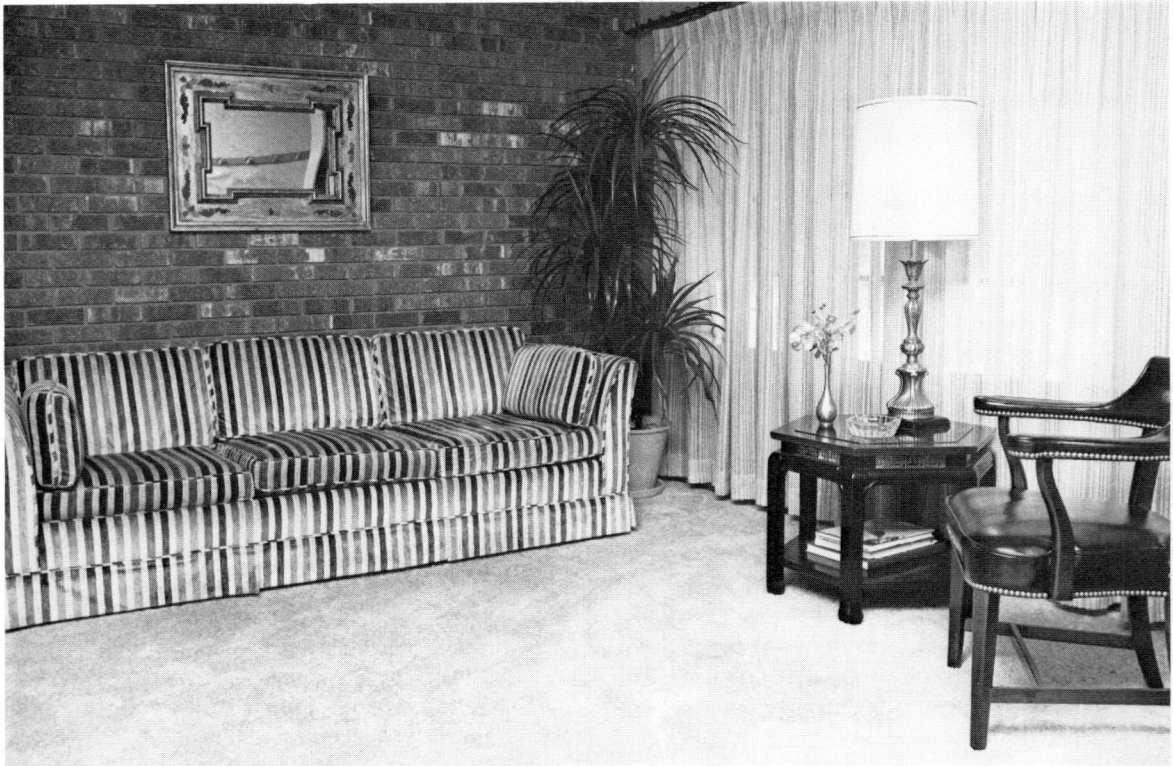

Figure 1-2 | Reception room.

Periodontics deals with the prevention and treatment of diseases and other conditions of the hard and soft tissues surrounding the teeth.

Prosthodontics deals with the replacement of lost or absent natural teeth with artificial teeth.

Public Health Dentistry deals with dental-health problems through education, prevention, and correction on a community, state, or national level.

Each of the eight recognized specialties has an American board, such as the American Board of Orthodontics, which certifies those who have adequately qualified themselves and who have successfully passed the examinations. Some states have laws governing the practice of dental specialties.

The Armed Forces, Federal, and Other Health Services

Aside from private practice, a dentist may serve with one of the armed forces, or he or she may be employed by one of the federal services, by a health department on a state or local level, or by a large corporation to render dental service to its employees.

Army, Air Force, and Navy

Dentists occupy an important place in the armed forces of our country not only during emergency periods under the Selective Service Act but in lifetime careers. The Army, Air Force, and Navy call upon the profession to supply the dental care needed by men and women in service, and dentists are commissioned in various ranks and become a regular part of the defense forces of our nation. These officers may be a part of the regular armed forces or on tours of active duty as reserve officers.

Federal Services

The U.S. Public Health Service affords a lifetime career in various dental health programs. Its research projects cover practically every phase of dental disease in relation to the health of the nation. One of its great contributions in recent years concerns the study and evaluation of fluoridation of communal water supplies.

Another federal service, the Veterans Administration, employs an appreciable number of dentists on a career basis. These dentists render service in veterans' hospitals or clinics, while a small percentage are delegated to administrative duties.

State, County, and Local Departments of Health

Various state, county, and local departments of health have dental-health programs which are most important to the general public health. These programs are planned and guided by dentists who have had special training and experience and who have chosen this work for their professional careers.

The dental divisions or sections of the health departments are concerned with education, prevention, and treatment programs. Some dental departments or divisions also have active research programs in the prevention and control of dental disease.

Auxiliary Personnel

Associated with the practice of dentistry are certain auxiliary personnel who render valuable service to the dentist in performing many important duties in the office. They enable the dentist to function much more effectively than could be done without their services.

In addition to the dental assistant, whose duties are discussed in other chapters, there are the dental hygienist and the laboratory technician.

Dental Hygienist

Not every dental office employs a dental hygienist, but the position and area of service are becoming more widely accepted as being of importance to the dentist. A dental hygienist is licensed by law to clean and polish teeth. In addition to these duties, the hygienist instructs patients in the fundamentals of oral hygiene and preventive dentistry. Not only does this relieve the dentist of these time-consuming operations but it serves to underline the importance of this phase of oral health.

Dental Laboratory Technician

The dental laboratory technician performs the mechanical operations that are necessary to prepare dental appliances and restorations for placement in the mouth—casts inlays, fabricates crowns, prepares models, and processes full and partial dentures. In some offices a full-time technician is employed to do this work. In most instances, however, some of this work is done by the dentist and the dental assistant, and the remainder is sent to commercial dental laboratories.

Support Services

It is probable that no division of human endeavor is totally independent of all other divisions, but that each depends in some way, large or small, upon the others. Usually each business or profession has associated with it certain other enterprises that are vital to its successful operation. This is true of dentistry. There are many areas associated with this profession in which close cooperation with other persons is necessary. It is true that a dental office might be developed to the point at which it is practically independent of all other services, but it would still have to be supplied with basic materials, equipment, and instruments by manufacturers and suppliers. Actually, nearly every practice comes to depend upon others for a good deal of its service.

Dental Supply Company

Probably the most vital of all the support services is the dental supply company. Such companies have developed a very successful and efficient system of providing the dentist with a dependable source of supply for nearly all the products that are necessary to his or her practice. Not only are they in business to sell goods, but their business is based on a line of service that begins with the original office planning and ends, in some cases, with office disposal following termination of practice.

Usually these companies operate from a central or home office, having in strategic areas a network of smaller or local offices which are able to cover given territories in a prompt and regular manner. Representing the supply houses are contact agents or salespeople, who usually are well-qualified individuals. These people are familiar with the supply and maintenance needs of the dentist. Such sales representatives make regular visits to the dental office to present new developments in commercial products and to sell supplies.

The assistant who is well trained and familiar with the office's needs will greet these salespeople with courtesy and consideration. In order that such visits will not interrupt the regular routine of the office, he or she will know beforehand what business must be transacted with each of them and will maintain good relations with these important lines of supply. Usually the dentist will want to speak to the supply representatives, but the assistant can follow through on the necessary business. Lists of office needs should be kept up to date, and provisions for the immediate and long-range future should be planned in advance.

These sales agents render considerable service in the average dental office in the maintenance of equipment and instruments throughout the years of association. On many occasions they play a big part in maintaining the dental office as an efficient service unit.

Commercial Dental Laboratory

Another of the important support services is that provided by the commercial dental laboratory. There are some dental offices that accomplish most of their own dental laboratory procedures when a dental laboratory technician is directly employed. However, the majority of dentists depend upon the commercial dental laboratory for many of the mechanical processes.

Such commercial laboratories are equipped to do most of the laboratory work that is accomplished outside the mouth. In the main they do the finishing of artificial dentures, the repairing of dental appliances, porcelain crownwork and bridgework, the finishing of fixed bridgework, and the construction of removable bridgework and partial dentures. This service is an important adjunct to the busy dental office and permits the dentist to serve many more patients.

The assistant will have a considerable responsibility to manage the flow of laboratory work, which involves such things as forwarding of all necessary items with proper instructions and the dentist's prescription; control of forwarding and return dates to coordinate with appointment plans for delivery to the patient; and maintenance of good communication with the laboratory.

In most instances, laboratories are located conveniently in order to render the maximum and most efficient service. Good relations with a well-established and reputable laboratory are important to the smooth functioning of the average dental practice.

Pathology Laboratory

As the realization grows that the dentist is concerned with the total health of the patients, the need for close cooperation with medical laboratory procedures is increased. The dentist has the opportunity to observe signs of the early stages of the processes of many diseases. The dentist, therefore, on occasion will require medical laboratory studies. Such laboratory procedures may include blood counts, blood tests, urine analyses, metabolism tests, examinations of tissue sections, chest x-rays, etc. The dentist may be trained and qualified to do some of these procedures, but more often they are done by a member of the medical or dental professions in a pathology laboratory.

Matters of general health are referred to the patient's physician for study and report. In some instances when an examination of tissue sections for the determination of the exact nature of lesions is needed, the services of a laboratory are required. In the larger areas of population where there are well-equipped hospitals, such services are readily obtainable. Many of these tests will be done by public health centers and offices.

While the pathology laboratory has not yet come to be a routine line of service to the dental profession at large, it is important to the dentist in the evaluation of a patient's needs and total health picture. Whether these tests are made by a physician, dentist, or laboratory, they are vital to a complete diagnosis.

Pharmacist

The relationship of the dentist to the pharmacist is one in which there is constant association and cooperation. Not only does the dentist depend upon the pharmacist for many medical supplies and much equipment, but for precise care in compounding prescriptions.

With modern developments in drug therapy, prescription writing and drug administration have become routine but complex matters. The use of drugs involves a thorough understanding of the care and handling of them. The dentist will rely upon the pharmacist to procure, maintain, and supply a stock of drugs that will be constantly available and in a perfect state of preparation. Furthermore, the prescription the dentist writes must be filled with painstaking care without substitution or alteration.

Important also is the fact that through the pharmacist's store the dentist may be assured that patients will be able to procure the solutions, preparations, brushes, etc., that they must use.

There should be friendliness and understanding between the dental-office personnal and the pharmacist, for there are many services that can be obtained through this kind of relationship.

STATUS OF DENTAL PRACTICE

Status among one's peers and in society as a whole is of concern to most people, and it is related to one's effectiveness and success. Dentistry has enjoyed a position of respect for a long time and has achieved remarkable goals in a comparatively brief span of history.

The fact that so much dental disease exists demands that the goal of dental health for all be uppermost in the minds of all those who are active in the profession. The question is, How can this be achieved?

In a special supplement to the *New York Times,* the American Dental Association (ADA) (1975) held that we can control dental disease for a relatively small cost; that dental service is available for virtually everyone; and that a minimal personal effort with preventive methods of brushing, flossing, and a reasonable diet is important to this control. Dental care too often is put aside and not sought until the needs are severe. It is an important concept that competent, reasonably priced care must eventually be available to all. But equally important is the fact that people must be educated and motivated to seek such care. Not much more than half of the people in this country seek adequate dental services.

Federal Programs

Greene (1976) has stated that health care is one of this country's most important businesses; that federal government programs exert an important influence on health affairs; some $4^1/_2$ million people are employed in health-related activities; health-related costs are over $100 billion and account for about 8 percent of our gross national product. About one-fourth of the U.S. Department of Health, Education, and Welfare (USDHEW) budget was allocated to health activities, and roughly 1.2 percent, or $330 million, was allocated to dental activities. These statistics are for the year 1974.

Greene further indicated that prevention is an important factor in our dental-health resources but that we have a long way to go in this effort. After 30 years, fluoridation of public water supplies is only about one-half accomplished. The Public Health Service dental-disease prevention program is the responsibility of the Center for Disease Control in Atlanta, including fluoridation and all other preventive dental action programs of the service.

The question is raised as to whether to increase the number of dentists or to emphasize distribution and efficiency of dental service and greater utilization of auxiliary personnel. It is important that demands for dental care be stimulated, because access will do little good if it is not used.

One of the federal programs to meet the problems of maldistribution of dentists is The National Health Service Corps (NHSC). The NHSC assigns dentists (and physicians) to critical-shortage, or underserved, areas. The assignments are for 2 years and are made by the

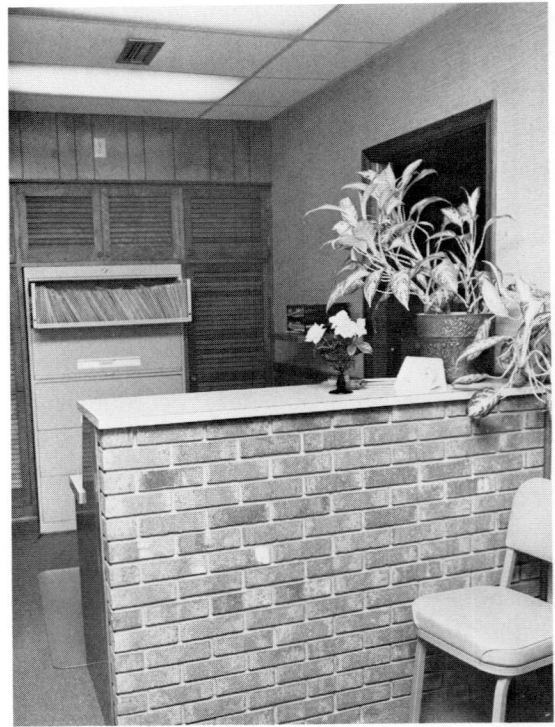

Figure 1-3 | Business secretary's center.

Secretary of Health, Education, and Welfare on approval of the area's application. Usually, the state and district dental societies must certify to the area's need. The dentist is encouraged to stay in that area. As of 1975 the NHSC had supplied 75 dentists to the 736 designated critical-shortage areas.

The USDHEW programs include biologic research, disease prevention and control, planning and development programs in dental manpower, education, and services research, and regulation and compliance functions such as quality assurance. Other programs, such as the Indian Health Service, provide direct dental service to specified groups, and give financial assistance, as does Medicaid.

It seems a certainty that some form of national

health insurance will be adopted and that some dental coverage will be included, probably a children's program (Greene, 1976).

Dental Personnel

For years the United States population grew faster proportionately than the number of professionally active dentists, but now the trend is reversed. Population growth has declined, and the number of dental-school graduates has increased. In the latter part of the 1960s, the population per active dentist was slightly in excess of 2000; in mid 1972 it was 1982; and it is projected to be about 1687 in 1985 (ADA Bureau of Economic Research, 1973).

It is not just the number of dentists that indicates actual availability of dental care, for the effectiveness in delivering dental care depends in large measure upon the training and utilization of dental assistants, dental hygienists, and dental laboratory technicians. The dental assistant, in particular, is looming ever more important in the team concept of dental-care delivery; it is evident that this emerging role is and will be of increasing significance in the solution of the problem of good dental care for everyone who wants it.

In 1973 the ADA's survey of dental practice indicated that independant dentists employed an estimated 187,000 full-time and 63,100 part-time assistants, hygienists, dental technicians, secretaries, and receptionists. Between 1970 and 1972 the number of full-time auxiliaries increased 21 percent and part-time 24 percent. Of independent dentists responding to the survey, 80 percent employed full-time dental assistants, 44 percent employed full-time secretaries and receptionists, 19 percent employed full-time hygienists, and 4 percent employed full-time dental technicians.

It is evident that the numbers of support or allied personnel utilized by dentists is increasing, and it is equally evident that they must be better trained for more duties in the delivery of dental care. It also appears that the dental assistant will be a key person in the developing programs, for effective use of well-trained chairside dental assistants can greatly facilitate the delivery of sufficient dental care.

Cost and Payment of Dental Care

The ADA *New York Times* supplement stated that the annual cost of controlling dental disease is around $70 for most persons. Regardless of the accuracy of that statistic, paying for dental care is a problem for large numbers of people. Most people can afford good dental care if they consider it to be a high priority.

Aside from national health insurance, much thought and effort has been given to many programs to meet the costs of dental care. Federal assistance for dental care is provided to some degree for the needy under Title XIX of the Social Security Act, known as Medicaid. However, most people must have other resources to meet such costs. Many labor unions and corporations have employee benefit programs that include dental insurance, and their numbers are increasing.

It has been estimated that 30 million people in this country were covered by some form of third-party dental prepayment or insurance programs during 1975. More than 60 commercial insurance companies provided dental insurance for about 16 million Americans. There were 43 active corporations of the dental-society-sponsored Delta Dental Plans system, which then covered about 11 million persons. The Blue Cross and Blue Shield Plans had an enrollment of about 3 million. There are also self-insured, self-administered trust funds and group practice prepayment systems (ADA, 1976a). It has been estimated that by 1980, 60 million people may have some form of dental insurance or prepayment program (ADA, 1975).

Many advantages accrue from prepayment programs, the chief of which is that care is rendered earlier and before the problem becomes too serious; regular care is more widely sought, there are less emergency demands, and there is more freedom from budgetary uncertainties and worries.

Delivery of Dental Care

Solo Practice

Traditionally, dental care has been provided by individual dentists in offices that are staffed and operated at the general dentistry or specialist level. This dental office will vary widely in numbers and types of support personnel such as receptionist, business secretary or manager, appointment secretary, assistants, hygienist, laboratory technician, custodian or maid, and janitor. This mode of dental-care delivery has provided the impetus for the development of dentistry to the high levels of quality accepted as the standard of care. Undoubtedly, the solo dentist will continue to provide an important type of practice for a long time to come.

The responsibilities and complexities of delivering dental care are increasing at a rapid rate, and the dental office has become a much more involved operation than it has been in the past. The forces for change in how dental care is delivered to the people have produced a rapidly expanding change in the dentist's involvement.

Jerge (1974) has stated that "there will likely be a major movement toward relatively small (seven to ten practitioner) private dental group practices as well as considerable participation on the part of dentists in community health centers, health maintenance organizations (HMOs), community hospitals, and other health care service and educational institutions."

Group Practice

There has been a growing tendency for dentists to organize into various forms of group practice. This has been brought about by the realization that many of the responsibilities of delivering dental care may be more effectively met by joint

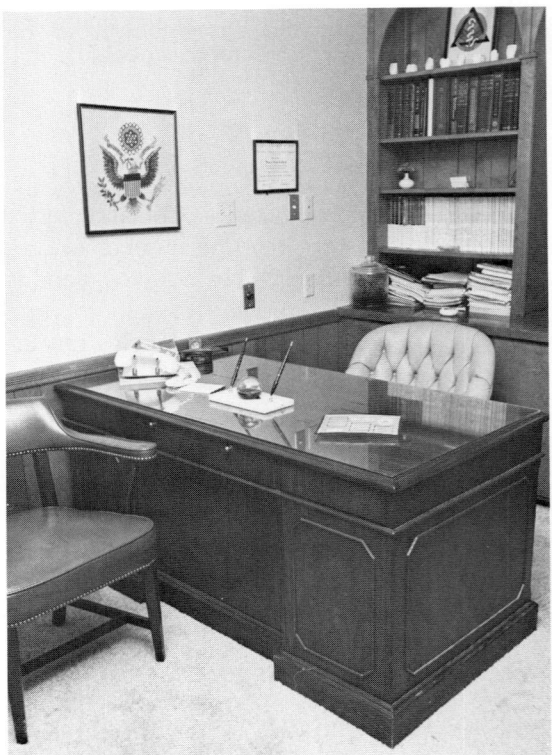

Figure 1-4 | Consultation room.

efforts to produce more efficient office systems and more effective care.

Group practices may vary from as few as three or four dentists to actually unlimited numbers, but probably around six to a dozen. These practices may vary widely in organizational structure. Some dentists are simply grouped together for convenience in locating office space and various other management or operational benefits and are not actually partners. In some instances the groups are planned for the balancing of responsibility for delivery of different types of dental care such as surgery, orthodontics, general care, prosthodontics, etc. Therefore, group practice may be made up of all general practitioners or a varying structure of general practitioners and specialists. The net effect of group practice is not only business advantages but probably the delivering of better dental care.

A fairly recent development is the corporate dental group practice. It has been established that dentists may incorporate to form a business basis that will provide financial advantages for not only the dentist but also auxiliary personnel. The incorporated dental practice gains certain tax advantages, such as retirement annuities, that have been available to commercial enterprises for a long time but not to professional people. A dental corporation may consist of from one to any number of dentists.

With the increasing involvement of third-party payment plans in dentistry (such as insurance and employee benefits plans) individual as well as groups of dentists have become involved in various bases for participation. Under one arrangement a group of dentists agree to provide service for the beneficiaries of a particular plan and benefits are available only from this group; this has come to be known as a *closed panel.* Most dental benefit plans pay for services provided by any qualified dentist; this is referred to as an *open panel.*

Community Health Centers

In 1965 the Office of Economic Opportunity authorized a grant for the formation of "neighborhood health centers." Many such centers have been established in areas where numbers of people are provided health services, including dental care, who would have found it difficult to obtain such care. These centers have been set up primarily to serve the poor, but the concept may work to the advantage of others in the future. The principle of a community health service is to bring together all health services in a convenient location to meet the total health needs of a defined population group (Jerge, 1974).

Health Maintenance Organizations

In the developing efforts to provide a broader base for total health care, there has come into being a government-sponsored system designed to offer a comprehensive health service to an enrolled population on a prepaid capitational basis; this differs from the conventional method of fee for service in that an annual fee per person is established. These systems are known as Health Maintenance Organizations (HMOs). The federal government has made grants of various amounts to enable these systems to become established.

HMOs have developed in an effort to establish some organization and incentives to the delivery of health care; comprehensive health care on a prepaid basis is their aim.

An HMO consists of (1) an organized healthcare delivery system providing or arranging for all the health service a population might require; (2) an enrolled population which contracts for the delivery of health services; (3) a financial plan which is based on costs of agreed-upon services, prenegotiated and prepaid per person or per family; and (4) a managing organization which assures full accountability. All four of these elements must be present in an HMO (Meyers, 1971).

STATUS OF THE DENTAL ASSISTANT

Formal Education and Certification

Traditionally, the dental assistant received training while on the job. That is to say, more assistants have not had formal training for their duties than those who have. These people, who for many years have worked with the dentist so earnestly, have seen that the dental assistant must look to more formal education, more professional attitudes, changing duties, and must be determined to "keep up."

Long ago, dental assistants foresaw the advantages of being organized, and it was Juliette A. Southard who in 1924, together with a few other dedicated dental assistants, provided inspiration and leadership at the first meeting of the

American Dental Assistants Society in Dallas, Texas. This organization, now called the American Dental Assistants Association (ADAA), has grown to a membership of more than 24,000 with a full-time staff and central office in Chicago, Illinois.

The Education Committee of the ADAA provided the first study-course outline for dental assistants in 1940. It listed material that required 104 hours of study. During the 1940s, a number of community and junior colleges and vocational and technical schools began to develop educational programs on a formal basis.

In 1948 a charter was issued to the ADAA which authorized a board to grant certificates to those who had completed a course of study and who had passed satisfactorily the Certification examination (Rowley, 1967; Sullens, 1967). Thus, the first national formal education standards for dental assistants were developed and administered by agencies of the ADAA (Sullens, 1967). It was during this period that evaluation of formal education programs of 1000 or more clock hours of instruction was initiated by the Education Committee of the ADAA in cooperation with the ADA Council on Dental Education (Sullens, 1967).

The ADAA began approving junior college, post-high school, vocational, and technical school courses of 1 to 2 years in duration in the early 1950s. It was planned that such courses would eventually replace the 104-hour course.

Through the efforts of the ADA House of Delegates, the Council on Dental Education, the American Association of Dental Examiners, and the ADAA in meetings and deliberations from 1956 to 1960, there was developed "Requirements for an Accredited Program in Dental Assisting" and "Requirements for Approval of a Certification Board for Dental Assistants." The 1960 ADA House of Delegates approved the requirements, which earned recognition and official sanction of the Certifying Board and served as standards for education of dental assistants. In 1975 there were some 264 accredited schools of dental assisting (Resnick, 1975).

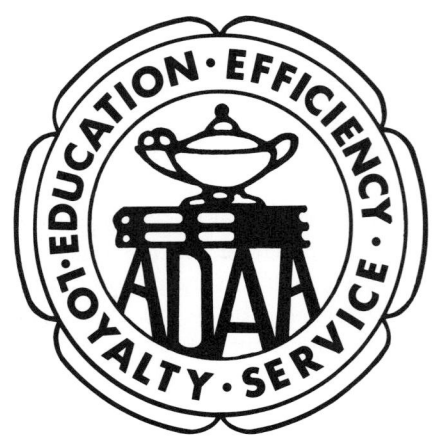

The examination for certification sponsored by the ADAA Certifying Board is not a licensing mechanism, but is taken voluntarily to verify competence. Approximately 6000 dental assistants take the examination each year, and it is given at least once annually in all of the accredited schools (Resnick, 1975). In 1976, there were about 40,000 certified dental assistants in this country.

On passing the examination the assistant receives the title of Certified Dental Assistant. Furthermore, by participating in a program of continuing education requirements, the assistant may achieve the status of currently Certified Dental Assistant on an annual basis; this is further evidence that the assistant is determined to become exceptionally well qualified.

The ADAA was the first dental organization to require continuing education to maintain current status.

Certifying Board Rules and Regulations

Listed below, in part, are the rules and regulations of the board which pertain to Certification for the dental assistants who have completed successfully the 1- or 2-year approved educational programs (excerpted from the 1976 "Cer-

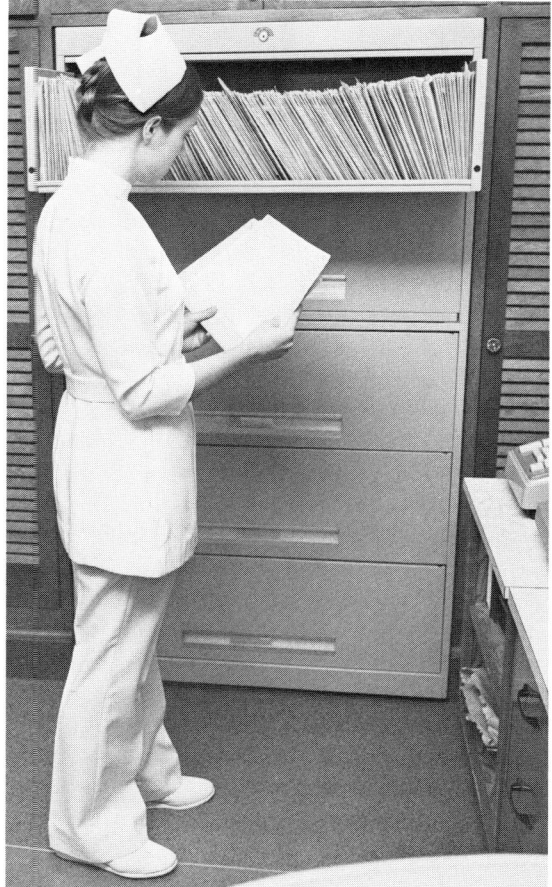

Figure 1-5 | Records storage.

tification Examination" brochure). To become Certified the candidate must

1. Pass the written examination
2. Provide proof of professional ethics
3. Be a graduate of a dental-assisting or dental-hygiene program accredited by the Commission on Accreditation of Dental and Dental Auxiliary Educational Programs

With reference to the annual renewal of certificates (i.e., for the status of currently Certified Dental Assistant), all who were Certified after October 1960 must

1. Provide proof of professional ethics.
2. Pay the annual renewal fee.
3. Provide proof of having obtained a minimum of 12 clock hours of continuing education annually. Credits may be realized by attendance at lectures on education, workshops or seminars, continuing education courses, by preparation and presentation of professional papers or table clinics, by reading educational material, or by participation in community dental projects.

It is evident that the status of currently Certified Dental Assistant can be achieved on an annual basis with a moderate interest and participation on the part of any qualified dental assistant.

In addition to the wearing of the Certification wreath, which is attached to the ADAA emblem pin, the initials CDA should be used after the name of currently Certified Dental Assistants.

A dental assistant may also qualify for Certification by completing the correspondence dental-assisting program conducted by the Extension Division of the University of North Carolina at Chapel Hill (UNC-CH). This post-high school program consists of seven courses and can be completed in a minimum of 64 weeks. Qualification for Certification also can be achieved by those who have been employed as an assistant for at least 4 years by challenging the final examination in each of the seven courses in the UNC-CH program (Resnick, 1975).

Assistants who seek active membership in the ADAA as of 1978 must be currently Certified. As of 1976, Certification was not a legal requirement for employment as a dental assistant, but it is evidence of serious and dedicated effort to achieve a high degree of qualification in the field of dental assisting. The possession of a currently Certified status opens the doors to a high level of employment, responsible position, and professional standing. Furthermore, several states have also established Certification as a requirement for certain expanded functions of dental assistants.

The Board of Trustees of the ADAA (*ADA News,* 1976) has elected to express concern over qualifications of individuals practicing as dental assistants in mandating that each state association

pursue with its state legislature the necessity of establishing in its state dental-practice act regulation of all dental assistants in the state through either registration or licensure and that such registration or licensure be formulated on American Dental Association approved educational standards.

While licensure or registration of all dental assistants in all states may not be in the immediate offing, the development of expanded duty functions may stimulate such action.

Accreditation of Education Programs

From the early 1940s until 1975, the ADA Council on Education was the recognized national accrediting organization for dentistry and related programs. In 1973 the association established an expanded agency, the Commission on Accreditation of Dental and Dental Auxiliary Educational Programs, on recommendation of the Council on Dental Education, to provide representation of groups affected by accreditation activities. On January 1, 1975 the Council on Dental Education's accreditation authority was transferred to the Commission on Accreditation. The Council on Dental Education continues to function as a separate agency of the association and retains its *bylaw* authority in matters not directly associated with accreditation activities (ADA Commission on Accreditation, 1975).

The commission is comprised of 20 members, 12 of whom are members of the Council on Dental Education. Other members include a representative of the ADA, representatives of the other individual disciplines accredited by the commission, and public representatives. This commission is recognized as the accrediting agency for dental-assistant education by the Council on Post-secondary Accreditation and the United States Office of Education. Policies and standards for the accreditation of dental-assistant programs comply with policies of these two agencies (ADA Commission on Accreditation, 1975).

DAU and TEAM

In the 1960s the federal government sponsored and supported the development and operation in dental schools of the program called Dental Auxiliary Utilization (DAU). DAU is designed for the training of dental students to work with auxiliaries at the dental chair; its objective is to maximize efficient utilization of chairside assistants in the delivery of more and better patient care. The DAU program is now included in all dental curriculums and is no longer sponsored by the federal government.

As a continuation or extension of the DAU program, Training in Expanded Auxiliary Management (TEAM) programs were developed in the 1970s. The TEAM concept and programs were developed in dental schools to implement further utilization of auxiliary personnel through more effective team-management training. In addition, the programs involve training of dental assistants and dental hygienists in expanded functions. TEAM programs are funded by the federal government through special grants.

DAU and TEAM training has emphasized the value of maximum use of dental auxiliary personnel for dental graduates and will have an important influence on the delivery of dental care.

EXPANDED FUNCTIONS

Rationale

While there is a difference between need and demand for dental care, it is apparent that demand for dental care has been increasing for a long time. Need for dental care in the United States was underlined by the high rejection rate of early draftees in World War II because of inadequate

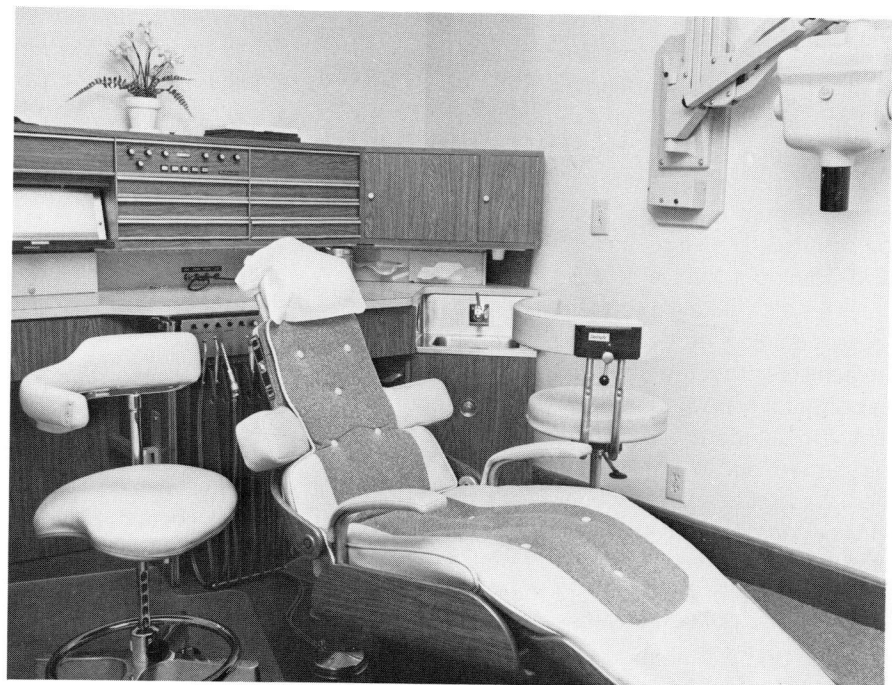

Figure 1-6 | Operatory.

dentition; the requirement of an adequate dentition had to be dropped and treatment provided after induction.

In many quarters it has been held that existing ability to meet demands has been inadequate and that demand has been and will be increasing further. Many countries have developed programs to meet dental needs which embody government supports and departures from the conventional methods of delivering dental care. As early as 1921, New Zealand embarked on a "dental nurse" program of care. Great Britain in 1960 established a program where some dental-care duties are delegated to dental auxiliaries (Brearley and Rosenblum, 1972; Hammons and Jamison, 1967).

No doubt the disparity between demand and professional service has lessened in recent years because there has been an increase in the number of dental graduates and qualified auxiliaries and a lower birthrate, but the problem is far from solved. The determination to provide health care for all who will accept it will undoubtedly create further demands. One solution, or help, appears to be the training and utilization of expanded-function auxiliaries to perform some of the procedures traditionally reserved for the qualified dentist.

In 1950 leaders of the dental profession felt that a survey of dentistry was needed. In 1957 the ADA reached an agreement with the American Council on Education to conduct such a survey. Published in 1961, one of the recommendations of the survey commission was that "the dental profession conduct studies designed to develop and expand the duties of auxiliary personnel" (Hollinshead, 1961).

In 1959 the World Health Organization's Expert Committee on Auxiliary Dental Personnel indicated that "where use is now being made of auxiliary personnel, research should be carried out and a study made of the possibility of their useful employment in additional fields."

The House of Delegates of the ADA in 1960 resolved that the Council on Dental Education be requested to urge accredited dental schools and training activities of the federal dental services to undertake experimentation and research in the training of dental assistants and dental hygienists so that the profession might enlarge its capacity for service to the people of this country. These resolutions directed that such programs be carried out in consultation with constituent dental societies and state boards of examiners to ensure consistency with policies of the profession in concerned areas.

The House of Delegates of the ADA in 1967 voted approval of a resolution asking state dental societies and examining boards to consider recommending revisions of dental practice acts to achieve more effective utilization of the services of dental assistants and dental hygienists and to consider the educational standards established by the ADA in determining their qualifications to perform functions prescribed within rules or regulations of the boards (ADA, 1967a).

Experimental Programs

The first experimental program to investigate the possibilities of expanded functions of dental auxiliaries was a pilot study by Ludwick, Schnoebelen, and Knoedler in 1959. Using many dental technicians trained in expanded functions and working in teams with a dentist, it was reported in 1964 that, without loss of quality, dentist productivity could be increased by 100 percent over conventional methods. Similar findings in a study by the Royal Canadian Dental Corps was reported by Baird, Purdy, and Prothers in 1963.

A study at the University of Alabama by Hammons, Jamison, and Wilson, reported in 1967 and 1971, was most comprehensive and compared well-trained dental assistants with dental students in their abilities to insert amalgam, silicate, and temporary restorations, apply rubber dams, and place matrix bands. The assistants earned higher scores than the dental students in the majority of instances. Common to these and other experiments was the feature that no cutting of tissues or other procedures of an irreversible nature were performed by the assistants (ADA, 1967b).

Many other experimental programs related to expanded functions for dental assistants and hygienists have been developed including those by Abramowitz (1966), Arnold (1969), and Lotzkar, Johnson, and Thompson (1971a, 1971b). All of these studies have shown that such delegation of functions to properly trained and supervised auxiliary personnel can result in increased production of dental care to a substantial degree.

The Teaching of Expanded Functions

The Council on Dental Education of the ADA in 1972 prepared a document in the form of a booklet, *A Compilation of Facts Related to the Teaching of Expanded Functions,* which set forth the status of expanded functions for dental auxiliaries and defined principles of evaluation of education programs that include instruction in expanded functions. The council held that as dental practice and delivery of dental-care concepts change, the roles of auxiliaries will change and that quality of care must be maintained regardless of who provides the care. An overlap of functions of the assistant and hygienist occurs in the expanded functions.

The council felt that curriculums should be restructured and noted that ADA requirements for accredited auxiliary education programs do not prohibit teaching expanded functions; it also expressed the opinion that the present auxiliary education system provides the most effective place for teaching expanded functions. Many different expanded functions have been proposed,

Permitted function	Number of expanded-function states						Percent of expanded-function states permitting the function	
	With function specifically identified		With open provision & function not specifically prohibited		Total permitting the function			
	DA*	DH†	DA	DH	DA	DH	DA	DH
Placing rubber dams	12	13	19	17	31	30	79.5	76.9
Taking impressions for study casts	12	17	13	12	25	29	64.1	74.4
Placing and removing matrices	5	6	19	15	24	21	61.5	53.8
Placing and removing temporary restorations	4	8	12	11	16	19	41.0	48.7
Placing, carving, and finishing amalgam restorations	1	1	5	6	6	7	15.4	17.9
Placing and finishing resin, composite, and silicate restorations	1	1	5	6	6	7	15.4	17.9
Performing preliminary oral examinations	6	21	15	12	21	33	53.8	84.6
Making radiographic exposures	23	24	12	13	35	37	89.7	94.9
Providing oral health instruction	11	19	19	17	30	36	76.9	92.3
Polishing coronal surfaces of teeth	7	35	3	4	10	39	25.6	100.0
Applying topical anticariogenic agents	15	24	12	13	27	37	69.2	94.9
Removing sutures and dressings	12‡	18‡	19	17	31	35	79.5	89.7
Administering local anesthetic agents	0	3	4	6	4	9	10.3	23.1
Removing excess cement from coronal surfaces of teeth	14	13	15	18	29	31	74.4	79.5
Applying topical anesthetic agents	8	11	19	20	27	31	69.2	79.5

* Dental assistant.
† Dental hygienist.
‡ Some states list removal of sutures only.

Figure 1-7 | Adapted from Tables 3 and 4 in *Legal Provisions on Expanded Functions for Dental Hygienists and Assistants* (USDHEW, 1974).

but certain ones have come to be accepted in one or more states for assignment to auxiliaries. The guidelines have been developed by the council for use in structuring on-the-job training and continuing education programs for employed auxiliaries, and for restructuring formal education programs (ADA Council on Dental Education, 1972).

Legal Provisions

Many states authorize dentists to delegate to dental assistants and dental hygienists new and additional tasks of greater skill and responsibility which were formerly performed only by the dentist (Fig. 1-7). These tasks are collectively referred to as "expanded functions," and include such functions as taking impressions for study casts, placement of rubber dams, placement of matrices, and removal of sutures and dressings. Among the more advanced proposals in the dental community is to permit specially trained and qualified auxiliaries to administer local anesthetic agents and to place and carve restorations after the cavity has been prepared by the dentist (USDHEW, 1974).

There is a great variation among the states with regard to the delineation of auxiliary tasks, with no two states being alike. With regard to the assignment of expanded functions, the state laws range from a comparatively extensive authorization of functions to a very minimal authorization. Among the 44 states which had some legal provisions for expanded functions in 1973, 39 states had such functions actually in effect—they were not only authorized but implemented. In 34 of these 39 states, expanded functions might be delegated to both assistants and hygienists, in 3 states to hygienists only, and in another 2 states to assistants only. In the remaining 5 states of the 44, expanded functions were authorized in enabling provisions of the law but would not be in actual effect until the board of dentistry issued the necessary implementing rules and regulations. In some of these states, such rules and regulations were being prepared, but these had not yet been formally issued. Some states listed functions which were specifically prohibited for auxiliaries (Fig. 1-8) (USDHEW, 1974).

No doubt many changes have been and will be made in the data referred to in the preceding paragraphs, for these are concepts that are still being developed. This material has been excerpted from the USDHEW publication *Legal Provisions on Expanded Functions for Dental Hygienists and Assistants,* which also lists detailed information for each of the various states. Since changes in state laws and regulations are occurring and since the states vary so widely, anyone wishing to be advised on the current situation should contact the State Board of Dentistry in their state.

The ADA is so interested in solving the problems of expanded functions for all concerned that the 1975 House of Delegates resolved that the Council on Dental Education should sponsor a national workshop on expanded-duty dental-auxiliary training and utilization. The council considered it essential to include representatives of all groups and agencies directly affected by association decisions on this subject. The workshop was held and the council issued a special report that included a position statement and a resolution presented to the House of Delegates for action. The resolution included principles of dental-auxiliary utilization and education, expanded functions that should not be delegated, those that could be delegated, and those that would require formal education.

Comprehensive policies on expanded auxiliary duties and auxiliary education were adopted by the 1976 House of Delegates.

They are contained in a "Statement on Expanded Function Dental Auxiliary Utilization and Education" (ADA, 1976b). The statement includes the association philosophy that "the purpose of delegating expanded functions to dental auxiliaries is to improve the productivity of the

Prohibited function†	Expanded-function states prohibiting the function	
	Number	Percent
Diagnosis and treatment planning	34	100.0
Prescription of drugs and medications	19	55.9
Administering local anesthetic agents	16	47.1
Administering general (systemic) anesthetic agents	17	50.0
Placing any final (permanent) restoration	15	44.1
Any cutting of hard and/or soft tissues	21	61.8
Surgery on hard and/or soft tissues	16	47.1
Correcting malformations or performing other orthodontic procedures	7	20.6
Laboratory work authorizations for fabrication of prosthetic, orthodontic, or other appliances	8	23.5
Taking of final impressions for intra-oral prostheses, appliances and/or restorations	11	32.4
Any intra-oral procedure leading to fabrication of oral appliances or prostheses	13	38.2
Any irremediable or irreversible procedure which requires the professional knowledge, judgment, and skill of the dentist	9	26.5

* Of the 39 expanded-function states, five do not have a list of functions specifically prohibited to dental auxilliaries. Thus, the percentages in this table are based on 34 of the expanded-function states.

† A task which is deemed to require the special knowledge and skill of the dentist and is therefore reserved for the dentist.

Figure 1-8 | Table 5 from *Legal Provisions on Expanded Functions for Dental Hygienists and Assistants* (USDHEW, 1974).

dentist by assigning those functions which should increase the availability of services at a continuing reasonable cost with assurances of quality control."

Included in the statement are principles for applying that philosophy and a list of functions and procedures that should not be delegated to dental auxiliaries "because effective and safe performance is dependent upon making judgments that require synthesis and application of knowledge acquired in professional dental education."

The statement (ADA, 1976b) lists the functions that are not to be delegated as including, but not limited to,

1. Diagnosis and treatment planning
2. Surgical or cutting procedures on hard or soft tissue
3. Prescribing drugs and medicaments and preparing work authorizations
4. Taking impressions for fabrication of fixed or removable restorations or appliances
5. Making occlusal adjustments
6. Performing pulp capping and pulpotomy procedures

7. Placing and adjusting fixed and removable appliances
8. Intraoral restorative procedures
9. Administering local and/or general anesthesia

STATUS OF THE DENTAL HYGIENIST

History

Dental hygiene, as an organized movement, apparently originated in the United States in New York City, where the Dental Hygiene Council was organized on January 12, 1909 with Dr. H. L. Wheeler as chairman. The dental nurse was prominently mentioned in an editorial in the *Dental Cosmos,* June 1912 (Kirk, 1912), and agitation was begun to give the position legal status (Taylor, 1922). However, in 1905 Dr. Alfred C. Fones of Bridgeport, Connecticut, trained his office assistant Mrs. Irene Newman in prophylactic procedures; the following year she performed prophylaxes for his patients. It was largely through the efforts of Dr. Fones that the first formally organized training course for dental hygienists was established at Bridgeport. In 1916 the first dental-hygiene school with prescribed educational requirements for admission was established at Hunter College in New York. There were only 6 schools by 1920; 10 in 1925; 35 in 1956; and by 1976 there were 181 accredited dental hygiene programs operating in the United States with 3 more planned (Robinson, 1976; Hollinshead, 1961).

The Connecticut Dental Hygienists Association was formed in April 1915 with 46 members; by June 1916 there were 95 members. The American Dental Hygienists' Association (ADHA) was organized in Cleveland, Ohio, on September 12, 1923 by 46 hygienists from 11 states; by May 1976 there were approximately 26,250 members (Robinson, 1976). The first dental law regulating the education and licensing of dental hygienists went into effect in Connecticut on July

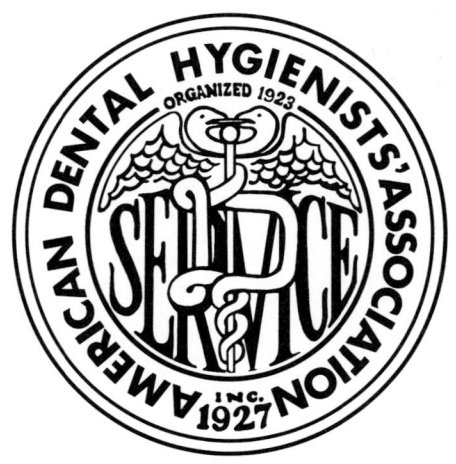

1, 1917. The Forsyth Infirmary and the Eastman Dispensary were pioneers in the teaching of dental hygienists (Taylor, 1922).

Duties

The Council on Dental Education of the ADA, in 1966, set forth guidelines for the dental hygiene curriculums. These guidelines indicated that "the duties and functions assigned to the hygienist by the dental profession are viewed as essentially professional in nature." The duties basically include oral prophylaxis, application of topical fluorides, and providing dental-health education services for patients and community health programs. The council specified that curriculums be offered at the college level, should include biologic and physical sciences as well as the dental sciences, and that a licensed dentist must be available to supervise and direct all clinical phases of dental hygiene training.

The *Survey of Dentistry* in 1961 recommended that "the dental profession conduct studies designed to develop and expand the duties of auxiliary personnel" (Hollinshead, 1961). The developments related to such expansion concern both the hygienist and the assistant and are discussed under the heading "Expanded

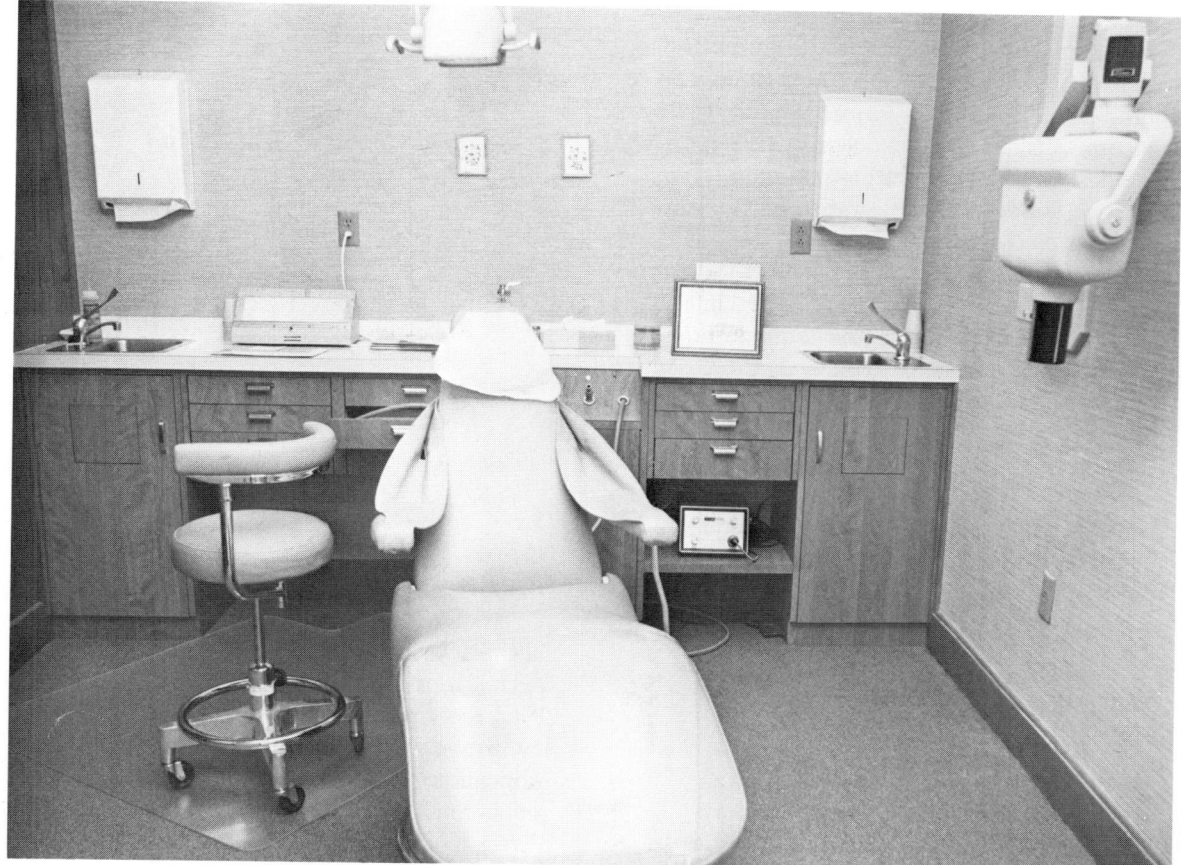

Figure 1-9 | Hygienist's operatory.

Functions." It may be that the functions of the hygienist will be influenced by inclusion of some expanded duties.

The dental hygienist, following graduation from an accredited school, must be licensed by a state board of dental examiners before being permitted to practice.

Education and Training

Admission requirements for dental-hygiene training vary from school to school, as do the teaching programs and credit systems, but they include the same general criteria. A high school diploma with a college preparatory course, with emphasis on math and science, and an above average academic standing are required by all schools. There is an increasing emphasis on college-level work before entering a dental-hygiene program, particularly in 4-year colleges and universities and in programs affiliated with dental schools. One or more of the standard college entrance examinations is required, and the Dental Hygiene Aptitude Test may be required. Some schools require physical and dental examinations and personal interviews (ADHA, 1976).

Certificate or associate degrees require 2 years of post-high school education in an accredited dental hygiene program. These programs are offered by junior and 2-year community colleges and universities and schools of dentistry. They are designed to prepare the graduate for office practice, work in clinics, and some local public health projects (ADHA, 1976).

Post certificate and post bachelor's degrees, bachelor of science degrees, and graduate work leading to a master's degree require additional college and university work and are designed primarily for teaching and administration careers (ADHA, 1976).

There is increasing emphasis on continuing education in all professions, and many dental-hygiene courses are available to enable the hygienist to maintain high levels of competence throughout the years following graduation.

THE DENTAL LABORATORY TECHNICIAN

Status

The dental-laboratory technician performs a most important function in providing dental service for the patient in that this person constructs most of the appliances and prosthetic restorations which constitute a large portion of dental practice. The modern technician has a background of increasingly high qualifications of training and standards of service.

The technician may work in a variety of settings such as private dental offices, commercial laboratories, governmental institutions, hospitals, and schools. Relatively few dental offices have employed full-time dental technicians; in such cases the technician may be considered to be an auxiliary person in dentistry. Far more are employed by or own commercial dental laboratories and as such constitute allied or support persons (National Association of Dental Laboratories, 1975b).

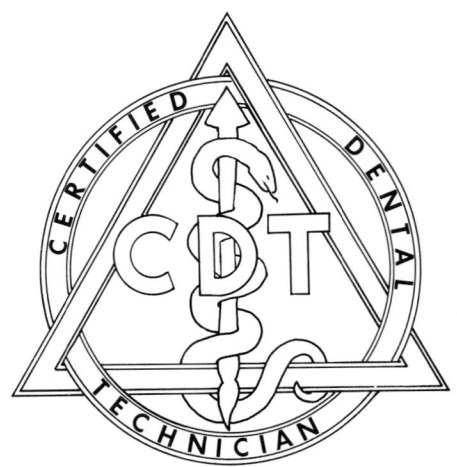

Some states have provisions for licensure or registration of the individual technician or the laboratory owner or manager (Morr, 1976).

The report of the *Survey of Dentistry* in 1961 recommended that dentists be required by law to write prescriptions to technicians for the fabrication of dental appliances and that such regulations be strictly enforced (Hollinshead, 1961). Today such laws are in effect throughout the United States (Morr, 1976).

Training and Certification

Traditionally, the dental technician has been trained in the dental office or in the commercial laboratory and, in fact, this on-the-job training is a common practice. However, for those individuals who elect to pursue formal training, a 2-year curriculum is available. Such programs are generally found in the community or junior colleges and vocational schools or institutes. There have been established "Requirements for an Accredited Dental Laboratory Technology Education Program" approved by the House of Delegates of the ADA (November, 1973). The ADA has for years had an active Council on Dental Laboratory Relations.

In 1956 the National Association of Dental Laboratories (NADL) House of Delegates approved the requirements for the approval of a certification board, the National Board for Certification (NBC); in the following year the ADA House of Delegates adopted the same set of requirements (Morr, 1976).

The NBC administers examinations for Certification and the right to use the letters CDT, for Certified Dental Technician, with the technician's name.

While formal training may not at present be a requirement for Certification, or Certification itself be required, these accomplishments are indications of an individual's determination to achieve higher levels of qualification.

The NBC's Recognized Graduate Program was instituted in 1974 and is open to candidates for graduation from accredited schools of dental technology. Prior to graduation, these students are given opportunity to take an NBC examination at their respective schools. After passing the examination and graduating these persons are enrolled as *Recognized Graduate* and are entitled to all educational services and publications of NBC until such time as they have completed the remaining portion of the NBC's 5-year education and experience requirement to take the Certified Dental Technician Examination (NADL, NBC, 1976).

National Association of Dental Laboratories

The NADL has come to be recognized as the guiding force in the current high quality of dental laboratory service; it has worked closely with organized dentistry at state and national levels.

Figure 1-10 | Preparing instrument tray.

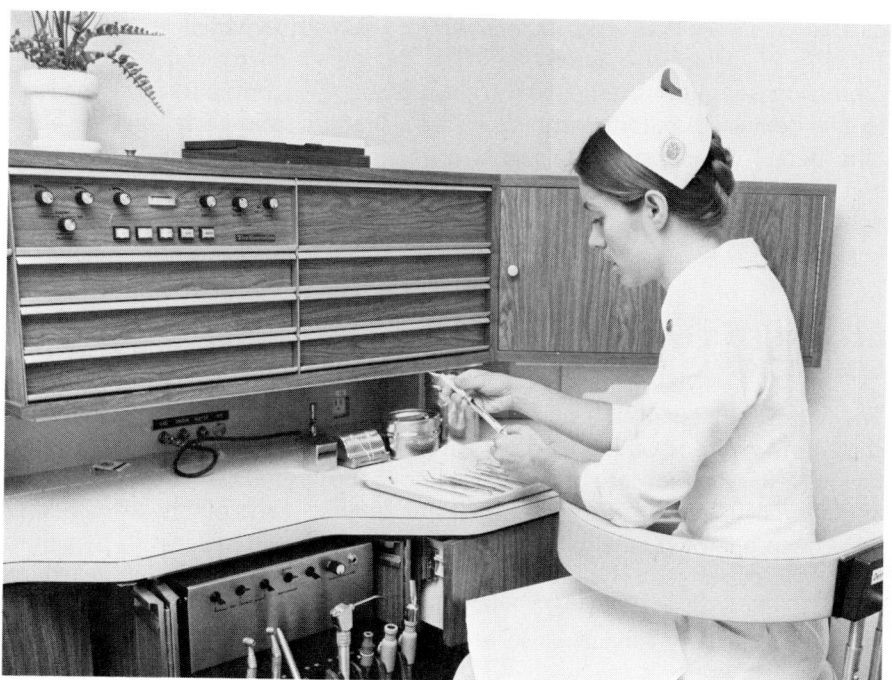

This organization has been responsible for establishing qualifications for standards of conduct and certification and achieved these levels in part by its relationship to the ADA through its Council on Dental Laboratory Relations.

The NADL encourages its members to engage only in ethical and legal practices, and specifically to provide their services to the dental profession in accordance with state laws. There is no national organization for individual laboratory technicians. Except where expressly permitted by law the NADL strongly recommends that no one in the industry engage in any practice that places that person in direct personal contact with the dental patient, including shade-taking and emergency repairs (NADL, 1975a).

The NADL publishes a code of ethics that enjoins its membership to maintain "high standards of business conduct and a harmonious relationship with members of the dental profession." The code of ethics covers standards of advertising, general conduct, and laboratory sanitation and hygiene (NADL, 1976).

The ADA Council on Dental Education has indicated in its *Policies and Guidelines for the Training of Dental Auxiliaries* that "the dental profession does not assign patient contact duties to the dental laboratory technician," and that "the dental laboratory technician is an exceptional and highly qualified craftsman in his own right" (1966).

ADVANCED PLACEMENT IN EDUCATIONAL PROGRAMS

There are dental assistants, laboratory technicians, and perhaps others who are involved in the delivery of dental care but who have not had any formal training. The dental assistant may have been trained on the job in the dental office or in military service. The laboratory technician may have been trained on the job in a dental office, in the military service, or in a commercial

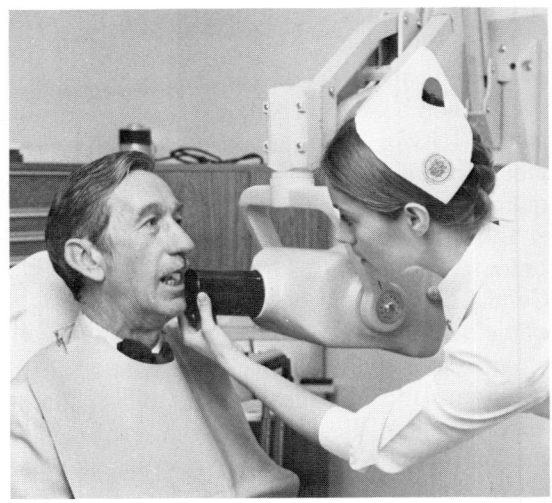

Figure 1-11 | Radiographic examination.

laboratory. Some individuals may have received training in dental-hygiene functions in military service. These people may possess high levels of experience, skills, and knowledge. With the increasing requirements and advantages of formal training, many such persons desire to attain such levels of education, but the time and costs involved make it difficult for them to do so.

Some accredited schools now have, and others are planning to have, advanced placement in the training of dental assistants, dental hygienists, and dental technicians through equivalency tests for individuals who have acquired some previous formal training and/or experience. This procedure can shorten the time and lessen the cost of obtaining accredited training, Certification, or degree status.

Formal education programs are in existence, and others are developing, to prepare dental assistants, dental hygienists, and dental technicians for careers in teaching. There are persons in these fields who would find such careers highly rewarding.

JURISPRUDENCE

Background of Law

Jurisprudence is the philosophy of positive law and its administration—a system of laws. A law is a rule of civil conduct established and enforced by sovereign authority. *Rules of law* or *law* result from the effort of society to avoid frictions by the interposition of various types of regulations binding on and enforceable against its members in relation to each other and in relation to other social groups (Carnahan, 1955).

While the interposition of laws may, at times, seem onerous, unfair, or an unreasonable burden, it is obvious to a thinking person that human relationships would be a hazardous affair without them. It should be recognized that the intent of all laws is to protect the rights of individuals and to maintain an orderly society.

Responsibilities under the law are intricate and complex at best, and there will be no attempt here to be definitive as to all of the ramifications of legal responsibilities on the practice of dentistry and the persons engaged in this activity—there is too much involved to discuss that here. However, it is reasonable that some attention be drawn to the fact that the dental assistant, in such capacity, will exercise considerable responsibility and influence in the proper conduct of the practice.

A very pertinent rule of law, known as *respondent superior,* holds that a superior is responsible for errors committed by an employee while the latter is acting in that capacity. Thus a dentist is liable for the acts of the assistants and other employees while they are exercising the authority to carry out their duties. The implications become immediately obvious, for the assistant performs many duties that, unless properly done, might involve the dentist in untoward incidents of practice. In fact, a dedicated, well-trained, and thinking assistant can support and help protect the dentist from legal liabilities in patient relationships. Obviously the dentist is the one who will have to pay if liabilities occur as a result of wrongs against a patient. However, there is no law that says an employee cannot also be held accountable if the employee's wrongdoing was a factor in injury to a patient. It is the dentist's responsibility to employ only people of sufficient training and capability to carry out the assigned duties.

Another rule of law of considerable importance and interest is *stare decisis* or stability of the law. Much of American law is based on the system of "unwritten" or "common" law which has been developed by principles and judgments handed down from previous legal decisions. The rule states that judges shall "stand by the decided cases." However, law is adaptable to changing standards and times, for judges and legislative bodies have the power to change trends in legal interpretations. The rule does provide protection and a sense of fairness in the application of legal principles.

The *common or unwritten law* is divided into *criminal law,* which concerns action of the state or society against the individual, and *civil law,* which concerns actions between individuals. The *written law* consists of federal and state constitutions, statutes, and legislation, and municipal ordinances.

The supreme law of the land lies in the Constitution of the United States and its amendments. The federal government has power given it by the states, but there are many areas of law in which the states can act individually. Therefore, it must be remembered that law rules or their interpretation may vary from state to state.

Contracts

The dentist is involved in a contractual arrangement with each patient as well as with each employee. The mechanics of these contracts may vary, but, from a legal standpoint, they do exist.

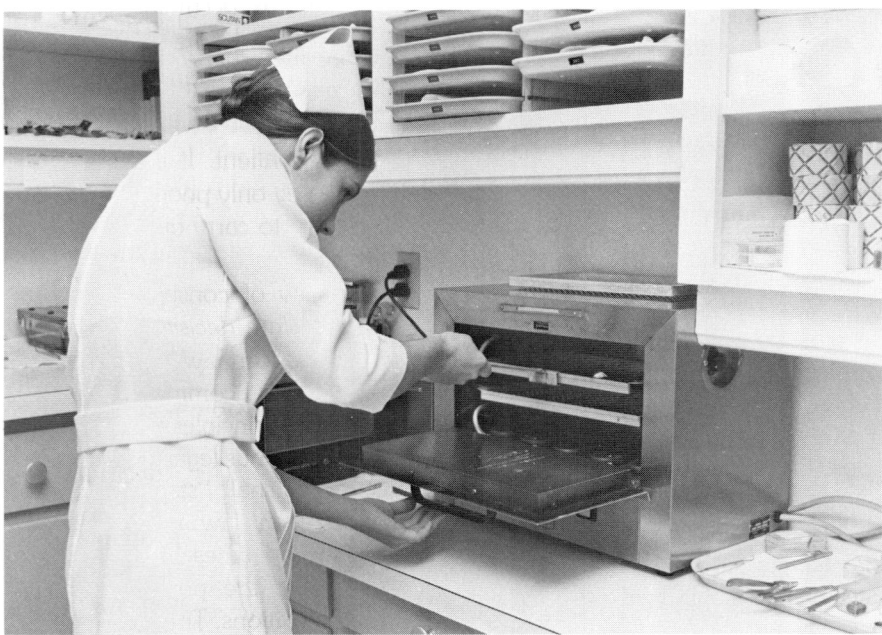

Figure 1-12 | Instrument sterilization.

Express contracts are those that are actually established and expressed by the individuals concerned and clearly state the terms of agreement. Express contracts may be *oral* or *written*. The problem with oral contracts is that memories concerning details fail people, and this makes possible subsequent differences of opinion. Written contracts constitute the wisest method for reaching agreements; they do not have to be in elaborate form or even "all in one piece," but some form of writing or memorandum should indicate the terms of any professional or business agreement.

Implied contracts are often the type of agreement that exists between dentist and patient. The law generally holds that when one person gives or does something for another, in the absence of evidence that this was to be a gift, something is expected in return. In the case of the dentist, he or she is held to "promise" that he or she possesses reasonable skill and learning and will use skill, care, and diligence in treatment. The patient, by accepting treatment, "promises" to make reasonable payment. The dentist is not held to have promised a cure or to have used extraordinary skill.

This implied contract has been a sound basis for dentist-patient relationships where mutual respect and friendly attitudes are maintained; problems may arise if this basis breaks down. Therefore it is best to have some form of written agreement. In fact, there are several instances in which the law requires that contracts, to be valid, be in writing; among those in which a dentist may be involved are promises by third parties to pay patients' fees and and promises to pay while in bankruptcy.

The law stipulates certain requisites for any contract to be valid: that there be an offer and an acceptance, called "a meeting of minds"; that something of value be exchanged; that the individuals be of a legal majority, sane, and sober; and that the subject matter be legal.

Malpractice

The specter that lurks in the background of every dental practice is the fear of disagreements with patients and the possibility of a lawsuit. Not every dentist must face such an experience, but the threat is generally more real if careless practice attitudes and unhappy patient relationships are allowed to exist. Legal questions and actions can develop in any dental practice, but, if sound principles of procedure are followed, such instances, or the threat of them, can be minimized and defenses made more impregnable.

Malpractice is "bad" or "faulty" practice and is defined as failure to comply with standards set by the profession. In a malpractice suit in order for the dentist to be liable for damages, it must be shown that (1) the dentist had a duty to treat the patient; (2) the dentist was negligent in the treatment; (3) injury resulted; (4) the negligence was directly related to the injury. The dentist is not legally required to accept a patient for treatment but, if treatment is begun he or she has a *duty* to complete treatment. *Negligence* involves failure to possess proper skill and learning, failure to use such skill and learning, or failure to use one's best judgement and attention.

A dentist will have malpractice insurance, but this does not provide immunity from lawsuits; it only helps with the costs involved. Obviously, it is best not to have patients bring charges; to this end the assistant can give considerable support by trying to understand the dentist's legal obligations, by being competent, and by helping to maintain good patient relationships.

The dentist has the legal obligation to know something of the patient's physical status; he or she is expected to take an adequate medical history and to do a proper examination prior to treatment and not to render treatment that would be hazardous with the existence of some untoward finding. All employees are expected to treat patients with courteous and solicitous care; the assistant should see that patients are not left unattended when they are in the operating areas, and handicapped persons should be attended in all areas of the office.

It is well to note that legal involvement can result from patient injury on the premises of the office, unrelated to actual treatment.

Some rules for the avoidance of malpractice lawsuits are well within the province of the assistant and associated staff:

1. Make every effort to promote goodwill between doctor and patient and the office as a whole; this is absolutely the best "insurance" of all.
2. Be careful of unthinking conversation related to treatment or personalities—remember *respondeat superior*. Also, keep all knowledge relative to the patient and treatment in absolute confidence.
3. See that accurate records are entered, maintained, and preserved; especial care with radiographs.
4. Be alert to signs of undesirable patient attitudes; patient confidence and cooperation are essential to successful practice.
5. Help to keep patient passageways clear of hazards—rugs, equipment, etc.
6. Take care with dangerous drugs and solutions.
7. Take care in management of handpiece with bur.
8. Do not leave sharp instruments unguarded on operating tray.

The dental assistant should give careful thought as to the possibility of liability if involved in some negligent act. While the rule of *respondeat superior* ordinarily will protect the assistant, there is no reason to believe that the assistant cannot also be sued for such negligence. It would be wise for the assistant to carry individual malpractice insurance. It is to be hoped that the need for such insurance is a remote possibility; however, with the increasing involvement in patient contact through expanded duties, increasing liability is likely to develop. Malpractice insurance at relatively low cost is available to members of the ADAA and to nonmembers from other sources.

Contributory Negligence

Negligence on the part of the patient may result in injury or increased severity of an injury related to some dental treatment and may have some influence on liability of the dentist; this is known as *contributory negligence.* The patient is expected to behave in a reasonable manner, to return for postoperative care if indicated, and to follow home-care instructions as capably as possible.

Consent

Every individual has the right to say what shall be done in terms of professional treatment and the right to have what is going to be done and its possible outcome explained in advance; this is known as *informed consent.* A wife's consent does not require the husband's consent under ordinary circumstances. Consent for a child or minor must be given by the responsible parent or guardian.

While it is not legally required that consent be in writing, under ordinary circumstances, it is wise to have some such written evidence maintained with the patient's file, especially if the treatment may be unusually involved, extensive, or of uncertain outcome.

Fees and Payment

Even if the dentist knows that he or she will not be paid for services rendered, every patient is entitled to the same standard of care as other patients. It is well to have fees clearly understood by the patient in advance of treatment.

Generally speaking, a husband is responsible for payment for treatment of a wife or child, but if such treatment is to exceed what might be considered "ordinary," it probably would be wise to get his consent.

Dissatisfaction with treatment alone is not adequate ground for nonpayment unless some promise or guarantee relative thereto was made; hence, take care in making idle statements!

Ownership of Protheses

It should be understood that once delivery of a prosthetic device has been made, it may not be taken away from the patient without consent.

Sources for Details

Source material has included references from Carnahan, Howard and Parks, Myren, and Sarner, and these may be available for those who wish to study this subject in greater depth or specificity. While legal details tend to become involved, the obligation imposed by all law is to be fair and straightforward in dealings with people.

ETHICS

Ethics is the systematic study of the ultimate problems of human conduct. It is not a positive science, but a normative science; it is not primarily occupied with the actual character of human conduct but with its ideal—not so much with what human conduct is, as with what it ought to be (*Encyclopedia Britannica*). Ethical principles are not laws; they are guides to behavior. Therefore, there may be considerable variation in actual practices. A *code,* or set of principles, is established by a profession or group of individuals to provide a framework of behavioral guidelines which extend beyond purely legal requirements. Thus laws define what an individual *must* do, whereas ethics is concerned with what an individual *should* do.

Tawney stated long ago:

A *profession* is defined most simply as a trade which is organized (incompletely, no doubt) but genuinely, for the performance of function. It is not simply a collec-

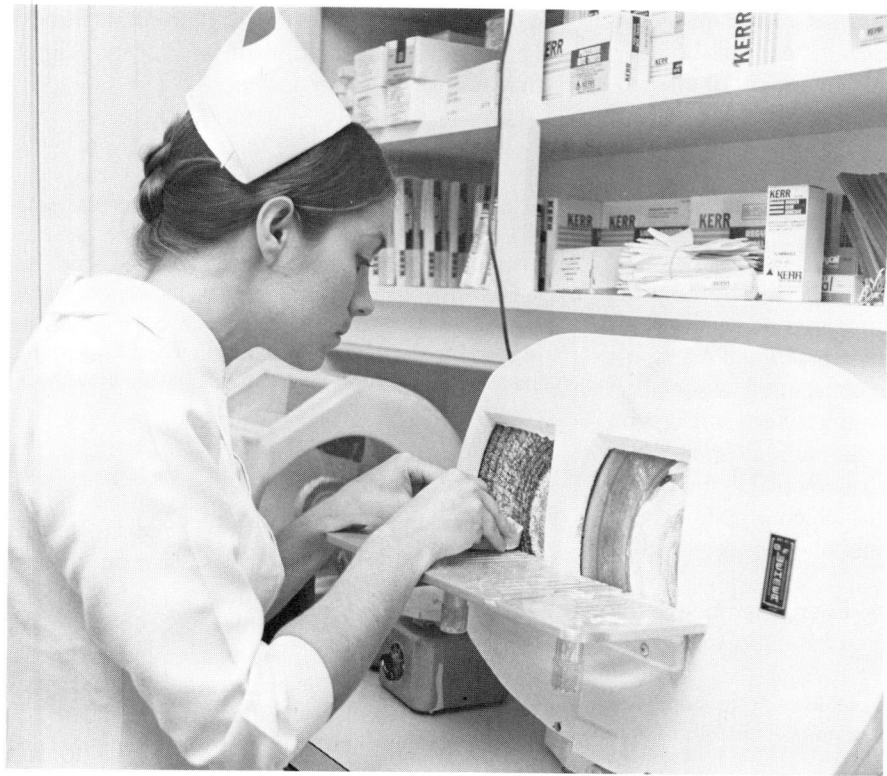

Figure 1-13 | Model trimming.

tion of individuals who get a living for themselves by the same kind of work. Nor is it merely a group which is organized exclusively for the economic protection of its members, though that is normally among its purposes. It is a body of men who carry on their work in accordance with rules designed to enforce certain standards both for the better protection of its members and for better service of the public.

Principles of Ethics and Practice

It is very important that the dental assistant, and all dental-office personnel, have knowledge of the *Principles of Ethics* as formally adopted by the ADAA, the ADHA, and the ADA. The high purpose and obligation designated by these principles provide the standards of conduct for dental office personnel.

Although the *Principles of Ethics* of the ADA is not a legal instrument, it relates to federal and state laws, and has the effect of law in setting forth the standards of conduct in the practice of dentistry. A dentist may lose eligibility for membership in the ADA if it can be shown that there is failure to practice within these guidelines. Without membership a dentist loses many benefits such as information and continuance of education through meetings and publications, information relative to legal rules and public programs, eligibility for professional appointive and elected positions, advantageous insurance programs, and many other direct and indirect benefits. Without ethical principles an individual in a profession is an outsider instead of being a leader or supporter in the betterment of the profession in its efforts to provide a high public service.

Principles of Ethics, ADAA

Section 1. Conduct of Members. The conduct of every member shall be governed by the *Principles of Ethics* of the American Dental Assistants Association and of the constituent association and component society within which jurisdiction the member is located. The member shall maintain honesty in all things, obedience to the dental practice act of the state in which employed and adherence to the professional ethics required by the employer.

Section 2. Obligations. Every member of this Association shall have the obligation to

A. Hold in confidence the details of professional services rendered by any employer and the confidences of any patient.
B. Increase abilities and skills by seeking additional education in the dental assisting field, through services provided by this Association, the constituent associations and component societies.
C. Participate actively in the efforts of this Association and the constituent associations and component societies to improve the educational status of the dental assistant.
D. Refrain from performing any service for patients which requires the professional competence of a dentist, or is prohibited by the dental practice act of the state in which the member is employed.
E. Support these Principles of Ethics and the Pledge.

Section 3. Use of the Title, "Certified Dental Assistant." Those dental assistants who hold certificates issued for the current year, by the Certifying Board of the American Dental Assistants Association, may use the title "Certified Dental Assistant," in connection with employment and Association activities.

Section 4. Dental Assistants Pledge. The following shall be the official pledge of the American Dental Assistants Association, as written by Dr. Charles Nelson Johnson of Chicago, Illinois, first advisor to the association:

I solemnly pledge that, in the practice of my profession, I will always be loyal to the welfare of the patients who come under my care, and to the interest of the practitioner whom I serve. I will be just and generous to the members of my profession, aiding them and lending them encouragement to be loyal, to be just, to be studious. I hereby pledge to devote my best energies to the service of humanity in that relationship of life to which I consecrated myself when I elected to become a dental assistant.

Principles of Ethics, ADHA

Each member of the American Dental Hygienists' Association has the ethical obligation to subscribe to the following principles:

To provide oral health care utilizing highest professional knowledge, judgment, and ability.
To serve all patients without discrimination.
To hold professional patient relationships in confidence.
To utilize every opportunity to increase public understanding of oral health practices.
To generate public confidence in members of the dental health professions.
To cooperate with all health professions in meeting the health needs of the public.
To recognize and uphold the laws and regulations governing this profession.
To participate responsibly in this professional Association and uphold its purpose.
To maintain professional competence through continuing education.
To exchange professional knowledge with other health professions.
To represent dental hygiene with high standards of personal conduct.

Principles of Ethics, ADA

In addition to the published *Principles of Ethics,* the Council on Judicial Procedure of the ADA provides published advisory opinions which should also be consulted in specific instances of ethical questions. The entire *Principles of Ethics* follows (from *Principles of Ethics,* including the "Preambles," copyright of the American Dental Association; reprinted by permission):

The practice of dentistry first achieved the stature of a profession in the United States where, through the heritage bestowed by the efforts of many generations of dentists, it acquired the three unfailing characteristics of a profession: education beyond the usual level, the primary duty of service to the public and the right to self-government.

The maintenance and enrichment of this heritage of professional status places on everyone who practices dentistry an obligation which should be willingly accepted and willingly fulfilled. This obligation cannot be reduced to a changeless series of urgings and prohibitions for, while the basic obligation is constant, its fulfillment may vary with the changing needs of a society composed of the human beings that a profession is dedicated to serve. The spirit and not the letter of the obligation, therefore, must be the guide of conduct for the professional man. In its essence, this obligation has been summarized for all time and for all men in the golden rule which asks only that "whatsoever ye would that men should do to you, do ye even so to them."

The following statements constitute the *Principles of Ethics* of the American Dental Association. The constituent and component societies are urged to adopt additional provisions or interpretations not in conflict with these *Principles of Ethics* which would enable them to serve more faithfully the traditions, customs, and desires of the members of these societies.

Section 1. Education beyond the Usual Level. The right of a dentist to professional status rests in the knowledge, skill, and experience with which he serves his patients and society. Every dentist has the obligation of keeping his knowledge and skill freshened by continuing education through all of his professional life.

Section 2. Service to the Public. The dentist's primary duty of serving the public is discharged by giving the highest type of service of which he is capable and by avoiding any conduct which leads to a lowering of esteem of the profession of which he is a member.

In serving the public, a dentist may exercise reasonable discretion in selecting patients for his practice. However, a dentist may not refuse to accept a patient into his practice or deny dental service to a patient solely because of the patient's race, creed, color, or national origin.

Section 3. Government of a Profession. Every profession receives from society the right to regulate itself, to determine and judge its own members. Such regulation is achieved largely through the influence of the professional societies, and every dentist has the dual obligation of making himself a part of a professional society and of observing its rules of ethics.

Section 4. Leadership. The dentist has the obligation of providing freely of his skills, knowledge, and experience to society in those fields in which his qualifications entitle him to speak with professional competence. The dentist should be a leader in his community, including all efforts leading to the improvement of the dental health of the public.

Section 5. Emergency Service. The dentist has an obligation when consulted in an emergency by the patient of another dentist to attend to the conditions leading to the emergency and to refer the patient to his regular dentist who should be informed of the conditions found and treated.

Section 6. Use of Auxiliary Personnel. The dentist has an obligation to protect the health of his patient by not delegating to a person less qualified any service or operation which requires the professional competence of a dentist. The dentist has a further obligation of prescribing and supervising the work of all auxiliary personnel in the interests of rendering the best service to the patient.

Section 7. Consultation. The dentist has the obligation of seeking consultation whenever the welfare of the patient will be safeguarded or advanced by having recourse to those who have special skills, knowledge and experience. A consultant will hold the details of a consultation in confidence and will not undertake treatment without the consent of the attending practitioner.

Section 8. Justifiable Criticism and Expert Testimony. The dentist has an obligation to report to the appropriate agency of his component or constituent dental society instances of gross and continual faulty treatment by another dentist. If there is evidence of faulty treatment, the welfare of the patient demands that corrective treatment be instituted. The dentist may provide expert testimony when that testimony is essential to a just and fair disposition of a judicial or administrative action. A dentist has the obligation to refrain from commenting disparagingly, without justification, about the services of another dentist.

Section 9. Rebates and Split Fees. The dentist may not accept or tender "rebates" or "split fees."

Section 10. Secret Agents and Exclusive Methods. The dentist has an obligation not to prescribe, dispense or promote the use of drugs or other agents whose complete formulae are not available to the dental profession. He also has the obligation not to prescribe or dispense, except for limited investigative purposes, any therapeutic agent, the value of which is not supported by scientific evidence. The dentist has the further obligation of not holding out as exclusive, any agent, method or technic.

Section 11. Patents and Copyrights. The dentist has the obligation of making the fruits of his discoveries and labors available to all when they are useful in safeguarding or promoting the health of the public. Patents and copyrights may be secured by a dentist provided that they and the remuneration derived from them are not used to restrict research, practice or the benefits of the patented or copyrighted material.

Section 12. Advertising. Advertising reflects adversely on the dentist who employs it and lowers the public esteem of the dental profession. The dentist has the obligation of advancing his reputation for fidelity, judgment and skill solely through his professional services to his patients and to society. The use of advertising in any form to solicit patients is inconsistent with this obligation.

Section 13. Cards, Letterheads and Announcements. A dentist may properly utilize professional cards, announcement cards, recall notices to patients of record and letterheads when the style and text are consistent with the dignity of the profession and with the custom of other dentists in the community.

Announcement cards may be sent when there is a change in location or an alteration in the character of practice, but only to other dentists, to members of other health professions and to patients of record.

Section 14. Office Door Lettering and Signs. A dentist may properly utilize office door lettering and signs provided that their style and text are consistent with the dignity of the profession and with the custom of other dentists in the community.

Section 15. Use of Professional Titles and Degrees. A dentist may use the titles or degrees, Doctor, Dentist, D.D.S., or D.M.D., in connection with his name on cards, letterheads, office door signs and announcements. A dentist who also possesses a medical degree may use this degree in connection with his name on cards, letterheads, office door signs and announcements. A dentist who has been certified by a national certifying board for one of the specialties approved by the American Dental Association may use the title "diplomate" in connection with his specialty on his cards, letterheads and announcements if such usage is consistent with the custom of dentists in the community. A dentist may not use his title or degree in connection with the promotion of any commercial endeavor.

The use of eponyms in connection with drugs, agents, instruments or appliances is generally to be discouraged.

Section 16. Health Education of the Public. A dentist may properly participate in a program of health education of the public involving such media as the press, radio, television and lecture, provided that such programs are in keeping with the dignity of the profession and the custom of the dental profession of the community.

Section 17. Contract Practice. A dentist may enter into an agreement with individuals and organizations to provide dental health care provided that the agreement does not permit or compel practices which are in violation of these *Principles of Ethics.*

Section 18. Announcement of Limitation of Practice. Only a dentist who limits his practice exclusively to the special areas approved by the American Dental Association for limited practice may include a statement of his limitation in announcements, cards, letterheads and directory listings (consistent with the custom of dentists of the community), provided at the time of the announcement, he has met in each specialty for which he announces the existing educational requirements and standards set by the American Dental Association for members wishing to announce limitation of practice.*

In accord with the established ethical rulings that dentists should not claim or imply superiority, use of the phrases "Specialist in _____" or "Specialist on _____" in announcements, cards, letterheads or directory listings should be discouraged. The use of the phrase "Practice limited to _____" is preferable.

A dentist who uses his eligibility to announce himself as a specialist to make the public believe that specialty services rendered in his dental office are being rendered by ethically qualified specialists when such is not the case is engaged in unethical conduct. The burden is on the specialist to avoid any inference that general practitioners who are associated with him are ethically qualified to announce themselves as specialists.

The following are included within the standards of the American Dental Association for determining the educational experience and other appropriate requirements for announcing a limited practice:

1. The indicated area of dentistry must be one for which there is a certifying board approved by the American Dental Association.
2. The dentist's practice must be limited exclusively to the indicated area of dentistry.
3. The dentist must have completed successfully an educational program accredited by the Council on Dental Education, two or more years in length, as specified by the Council or be a diplomate of a national certifying board.

For purposes of Section 18 those dentists who ethically limit their practices to the special area of dentistry previously identified as oral surgery may announce themselves as oral and maxillofacial surgeons and may designate their practices as oral and maxillofacial surgery.

Section 19. Directories. A dentist may permit the listing of his name in a directory provided that all dentists in similar circumstances have access to a similar listing and provided that such listing is consistent in style and text with the custom of the dentists in the community.

Section 20. Name of Practice. The name under which a dentist conducts his practice may be a factor in the selection process of the patient. The use of a trade name or an assumed name could mislead laymen concerning the identity, responsibility and status of those practicing thereunder. Accordingly, a dentist shall practice only under his own name, the name of a dentist employing him who practices in the same office, a partnership name composed only of the name of one or more of the dentists practicing in a

---

* The 1975 House of Delegates adopted the following resolution: *Resolved,* that a moratorium be imposed upon implementation of the privilege of announcing in more than one specialty under Section 18 of the *Principles of Ethics* until the report of the January 1976 Workshop Conference on Specialty Practice is received and acted upon by the 1976 House of Delegates.

The 1976 House of Delegates extended for a second year the moratorium until a Council on Dental Education report is received by the 1977 House (*ADA Leadership Bulletin,* November 22, 1976).

partnership in the same office, or a corporate name composed only of the name of one or more of the dentists practicing as employees of the corporation in the same office.

Use of the name of a dentist no longer actively associated with the practice may be continued for a period not to exceed one year.

The use of dentists' names in directories is covered entirely by Section 19.

Section 21. Corporate Designations. Corporate designations may be used.

Section 22. Judicial Procedure. Problems involving questions of ethics should be solved at the local level within the broad boundaries established in these *Principles of Ethics* and within the interpretation of the code of ethics of the component society. If a satisfactory decision cannot be reached, the question should be referred, on appeal, to the constituent society and the Council on Judicial Procedures, Constitution and Bylaws of the American Dental Association, as provided in Chapter XI of the *Bylaws* of the American Dental Association.

BIBLIOGRAPHY

Abramowitz, J.: "Expanded Function for Dental Assistants: A Preliminary Study," *J. Am. Dent. Assoc.,* **72:**386, 1966.

American Dental Assistants Association: ADAA press release, *ADA News,* May 17, 1976.

American Dental Association: "Outlook for 1976; Continued Growth in Dental Prepayment," *J. Am. Dent. Assoc.,* **92:**18, 1976a.

———: "Statement on Expanded Function Dental Auxiliary Utilization and Education," *ADA Leadership Bulletin,* November 22, 1976b.

———: Can Americans Get the Dental Care They Need? *New York Times,* Sec. 11, October 5, 1975 (special supplement).

———: "The 1973 Survey of Dental Practice," Chicago, 1973.

———: *Transactions,* Chicago, 1967a, Res. 6, p. 282.

———: "Expanded Functions for Dental Auxiliaries," *J. Am. Dent. Assoc.,* **75:**563, 1967b (editorial).

———: *Transactions,* Chicago, 1961, p. 219.

———: "Dental Auxiliaries," *Transactions,* Chicago, 1960, Res. 10 and 11, pp. 208–209.

American Dental Association, Bureau of Economic Research and Statistics: "Growth in Population and Number of Dentists to 1985," *J. Am. Dent. Assoc.,* **87:** 901–903, 1973.

American Dental Association, Commission on Accreditation: "Requirements and Guidelines for Accredited Dental Assisting Education Programs," Chicago, August 1975.

American Dental Association, Council on Dental Education: "A Compilation of Facts Related to the Teaching of Expanded Functions," Chicago, 1972.

———: *Policies and Guidelines for the Training of Dental Auxiliaries,* 3d ed., Chicago, August 1966, pp. 13—23.

American Dental Hygienists Association: "Education and Training," Chicago, 1976.

Arnold, G. T.: "The Dental Assistant, The Clinical Chairside Assistant and the Dental Hygienist as Members of the Dental Team in General Practice," *Int. Dent. J.,* **19:**12, 1969.

Baird, K. M., Purdy, E. G., and Prothero, D. H.: "Pilot Study on Advanced Training and Employment of Auxiliary Dental Personnel in the Royal Canadian Dental Corps: Final report," *J. Can. Dent. Assoc.,* **29:**778–787, 1963.

Brearley, L. J., and Rosenblum, F. N.: "Two-Year Evaluation of Auxiliaries Trained in Expanded Duties," *J. Am. Dent. Assoc.,* **84:**600–610, 1972.

Bremner, M. D. K.: *The Story of Dentistry,* 3d ed., Dental Items of Interest Publishing Co., Brooklyn, 1954.

Carnahan, C. W.: *The Dentist and the Law,* The C.V. Mosby Company, St. Louis, 1955.

Encyclopedia Britannica, Inc., Chicago, 1955.

Greene, J. C.: "Federal Programs and the Profession," *J. Am. Dent. Assoc.,* **92:**689–691, 1976.

Guerini, V. *History of Dentistry,* Lea & Febiger, Philadelphia, 1909.

Hammons, P. E., and Jamison, H. C.: "Expanded Functions for Dental Auxiliaries," *J. Am. Dent. Assoc.,* **75:**658–672, 1967.

Hammons, P. E., Jamison, H. C., and Wilson, L. L.: "Quality of Service Provided by Dental Therapists in an Experimental Program at the University of Alabama," *J. Am. Dent. Assoc.,* **82:**1060–1066, 1971.

Hollinshead, B. S., Director: *The Survey Of Dentistry; The Final Report, Commission on the Survey of*

Dentistry in the United States, American Council on Education, 1961.

Howard, W. W., and Parks, A. L.: *The Dentist and the Law,* 3d ed., The C. V. Mosby Company, St. Louis, 1973.

———: *Carnahan's The Dentist and the Law,* 2d ed., The C.V. Mosby Company, St. Louis, 1965.

Jerge, C. R., Marshall, W. E., Schoen, M. H., and Friedman, J. W.; *Group Practice and the Future of Dental Care,* Lea & Febiger, Philadelphia, 1974.

Kirk, E. C., *The Dental Cosmos,* The S. S. White Dental Mfg. Co., Philadelphia, June 1912, pp. 715–718 (editorial).

Koch, C. R. E.: *History of Dental Surgery,* vols. I, II, and III, National Art Publishing Company, Ft. Wayne, Ind., 1910.

Lotzkar, S., Johnson, D. W., and Thompson, M. B. "Experimental Program in Expanded Functions for Dental Assistants: Phase 3 Experiment with Dental Teams," *J. Am. Dent. Assoc.,* **82**:1067–1981, 1971a.

———: "Experimental Program in Expanded Functions for Dental Assistants: Phase 1 Base Line and Phase 2 Training," *J. Am. Dent. Assoc.,* **82**:101, 1971b.

Ludwick, W. E., Schnoebelen, E. O., and Knoedler, D. J.: "Greater Utilization of Dental Technicians," Report of Clinical Tests, U.S. Naval Training Center, Great Lakes, Ill., 1964, p. 11.

Morr, D. V.: Personal communication, Chapel Hill, N. C., 1976.

Myers, B. A.: "Health Maintenance Organizations," *Annual Conference of State Comprehensive Health Planning Agencies,* Washington, D.C., April 7, 1971, distributed by ADA Council on Dental Care Programs, November 10, 1971.

Myren, R. A.: "Legal Aspects of Dental Practice," Institute of Government, University of North Carolina, Chapel Hill, 1955 (unpublished).

National Center for Health Statistics: *Selected Dental Findings in Adults by Age, Race, and Sex, United States, 1960–62,* ser. 11, no. 7, Washington, D.C., February 1965.

National Association of Dental Laboratories: *J. Natl. Assoc. Dent. Lab.,* Alexandria, Va., August 1975a, p. 19.

———: "Auxiliary and Its Application to the Dental Laboratory Industry," *J. Natl. Assoc. Dent. Lab.,* Alexandria, Va., December, 1975b.

National Association of Dental Laboratories, National Board for Certification: *Who's Who in the Dental Laboratory Industry,* Alexandria, Va. 1976, p. 49.

Pelton, W. J., et al.: *The Epidemiology of Oral Health,* Harvard University Press, Cambridge, Mass., 1969.

Pelton, W. J., and Wisan, J. M.: "Dental Needs and Resources," in *Dentistry in Public Health,* W.B. Saunders Company, Philadelphia, 1955.

Prinz, H.: *Dental Chronology,* Lea & Febiger, Philadelphia, 1945.

Resnick, N.: "The Certification of Dental Assistants," *J. Am. Dent. Assoc.,* **91**:758–761, 1975.

Robinson, J. B.: "The Foundations of Professional Dentistry," in *Proceedings Dental Centenary Celebration,* Waverly Press Inc., Baltimore, 1940.

Robinson, P. A., Assistant to the Director, Office of Education, ADHA, Personal communication, Chicago, May 1976.

Rowley, M. E.: "Expansion of Education and Certification Services by the ADAA," *J. Am. Dent. Assistants Assoc.,* **36**:30–33, 1967.

Sarner, H.: *Dental Jurisprudence,* W.B. Saunders Company, Philadelphia, 1963.

Sognnaes, R. F.: "Dentistry at its Centennial Crossroads, *Science,* **130**:1681–1688, 1959.

Sullens, R. H.: Dental Assisting Education; Past, Present, and Future, *J. Am. Dent. Assistants Assoc.,* **36**:26–29, 1967.

Tawney, R. H.: *The Acquisitive Society,* Harcourt Brace and Company Inc., New York, 1920, pp. 92–95.

Taylor, J. A.: *History of Dentistry,* Lea & Febiger, Philadelphia, 1922.

U.S. Department of Health, Education, and Welfare, Public Health Service, Division of Dentistry: *Legal Provisions on Expanded Functions for Dental Hygienists and Assistants,* USDHEW pub. no. (HRA)75-21, 2d ed., rev. July 1974.

Weinberger, B. F.: *History of Dentistry,* vols. I and II, The C.V. Mosby Company, St. Louis, 1948.

World Health Organization: *Expert Committee on Auxiliary Dental Personnel Report,* Technical Report Series, no. 163, Geneva, 1959, p. 5.

2

Ethel M. Earl
Practice Administration

INTRODUCTION

The delivery of dental care to the public has become a tremendous responsibility for the dental profession. The public has become aware of the importance of dental health through education and the media. Third-party payment plans have made dentistry available to thousands of people who formerly felt good dentistry was beyond their financial means. The federal government has assumed the responsibility of providing dental care to many others who are economically unable to receive dental care. Good dental health is the right of all people; therefore, it is fitting that the dental profession assume the responsibility of delivering the best dental care in the most efficient, courteous, and economical manner possible. In order to achieve this objective, the dentist must rely upon capable and efficient personnel in the dental office.

Other chapters in this book describe the necessity of having educated, well-qualified personnel assisting in the delivery of health care in the operatory. It is of equal importance to the patient to have educated, well-qualified personnel providing efficient service in the business office. The best efforts of the dental team are soon forgotten by the patient when confronted with a disorganized, inefficient business office. Lost or misplaced records, wrong billing, or an unpleasant disposition of the business assistant discourage patients more quickly than discomfort in the operatory. Therefore, it is of extreme importance that the business office be run in an organized, efficient manner not only to maintain good public relations, but to provide the patient and the dentist with accurate records. The harmonious atmosphere of the well-run business office is immediately sensed by the patient upon entering or calling the dental office.

The career options for the assistant in the dental office are many. In the past, the dentist usually employed an assistant who was expected to handle the business office, order the supplies, answer the telephone, maintain the condition of the office, and, when needed, assist at the chair. The increase in the population and the demands of the public have made this type of practice impossible. The patient has the right not only to demand the best in dental care but to resort to the courts of law if some doubts about the delivery of the dental care exist. The right of these actions mandates that the business office keep accurate records of the patient, including thorough medical histories, diagnostic aids such as radiographs and study casts, treatment plan, charges, and agreements.

During the education and training of the dental assistant, some students may find that their talents lie in the management area of the office rather than in the technical skills required at the chair. Ideally, the assistant should be versatile in both chairside assisting and office management. However, this is not always realistic, and students should consider carefully the areas best suited for their particular abilities. Nevertheless, the entire dental health team should be familiar with the routine and management responsibilities of the dental office. Emergencies arise at times when the chairside assistant must assume the role of the business assistant and vice versa; however, definite responsibilities and roles should be firmly established to prevent confusion and misunderstanding.

THE OFFICE MANUAL

Of all the aspects of personnel management and team development, communication between the dentist and the staff and communication between the staff members is probably the most fundamental (Fig. 2-1).

Communication is not only basic to personnel relations, motivation, and job satisfaction, but serves to bridge any gap between the management philosophy of a dentist and the work attitudes of staff members. An outstanding method to start and maintain a two-way communication in the office is the composition and use of an office manual.

The manual need not be a complicated undertaking but may be constructed in the loose-leaf notebook style. The manual should clearly state the dentist's philosophy of practice. This should include the dentist's personal philosophy of his or her dental practice, treatment of patients, and method of sharing of responsibilities for the delivery of dental health care to the public. The dentist must assume the final responsibility for all patients treated in the office; however this does not absolve other personnel from assuming responsibility for the health and welfare of the patient.

The office manual should also include a section on employee policies. These policies should reflect the dentist's attitudes and intent toward the qualifications he or she feels are necessary for auxiliary personnel, the evaluation method that will be used for salary increases, policy on cost-of-living increases in salary, the number of hours that personnel are required to work each week, vacation and holiday policies, sick leave, and fringe benefits. This section may also include the method of intercommunication the dentist plans in the office. For example, staff meetings should be planned which would involve input from the entire staff to guarantee the members of the staff an opportunity to express concerns and ideas for improvement of the total operation. The staff meetings should be scheduled on a regular basis at a convenient time for all concerned. Team morale depends greatly upon the way team members perceive they are treated by the team leader(s), and productivity definitely in-

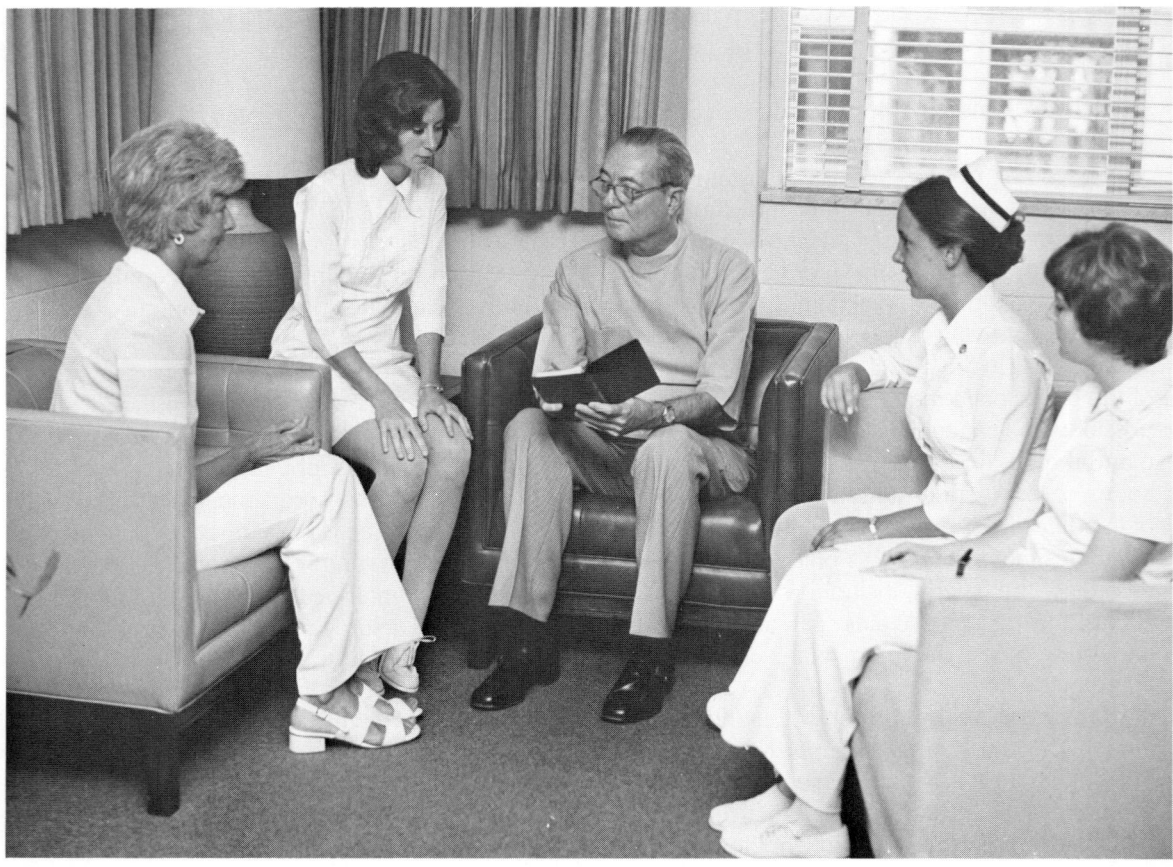

Figure 2-1 | Staff meeting scheduled at regular intervals.

creases in a harmonious atmosphere. To be completely satisfied and fulfilled, an employee must have adequate recognition and responsibility, an opportunity for achievement, and satisfaction with the work itself. Opportunities should also be made for individual staff members to consult with the dentist or office manager when problems or dissatisfactions arise.

The manual should also include sections on specific duties and responsibilities of the various staff members. An example of this could be the listing of daily duties for assistant A, assistant B, hygienist, and business assistant as follows:

Assistant A:
Turn on compressor and units
Check oxygen tank
Check and adjust temperature of office
Assist business assistant in pulling records for the day, etc.

Assistant B:
Check and restock supplies in operatories
Prepare tray setups, etc.

The dentist should continue to list weekly responsibilities and monthly responsibilities for all auxiliaries. For a change in routine, assistant A might become assistant B every other month.

Another section could include the office policies on broken appointments, telephone calls, financial arrangements, patient education, and a description of the preventive recall system. The expected equipment maintenance and inventory control could also be mentioned here.

The office manual is extremely useful when new personnel are hired; however, it should be constantly reviewed and up-dated by the existing staff at regular intervals.

THE OFFICE MANAGER

A new career option as an office manager is appearing on the horizon for qualified dental assistants. While few solo practices are large enough to employ an office manager, the group practice makes this position almost mandatory. There is a growing feeling that group practice has numerous advantages. Many dentists dislike the isolation of being the only dentist in the office and much prefer the interaction with fellow dentists provided by group practice. Such a practice would hire a person thoroughly familiar with the operation of a dental office to act as an office manager. This member of the team would assume the managerial responsibilities for personnel, relations with the laboratory, inventory control and purchase of supplies, patients' preventive program, and system of patient records and office records. Needless to say, the philosophy and policies of the participating dentists in a group practice must be compatible to ensure that all patients are treated with concern.

THE BUSINESS ASSISTANT

The business assistant's functions and responsibilities are many and may vary from office to office. The range of responsibilities may include:

Assuming the role of the receptionist in receiving telephone calls from patients
Receiving patients when arriving for appointments
Scheduling appointments for patients
Securing health histories from the patients for their records
Maintaining and filing patient records
Receiving payment of fees
Billing patients for services rendered
Processing claim forms and records for dental insurance
Controlling the inventory and ordering supplies
Managing the preventive recall system
Banking collected fees
Responding to professional correspondence

Further responsibilities which may be allocated to the business assistant are:

Maintaining the accounts receivable and accounts payable ledgers
Writing the checks for accounts payable
Maintaining and processing the staff payroll accounts
Completing financial forms such as F.I.C.A. and quarterly income tax

THE TELEPHONE

"Good morning! Dr. Smith's office, Mrs. Hale speaking. May I help you?" By this simple, courteous exchange, identification has been established, an invitation to help has been given, and precious minutes have been saved. The first impression of the dental office is established by the initial communication—be it by telephone or personal confrontation. The initial contact therefore must be professional, efficient, and, above all, courteous. Good first impressions can be changed, of course, if the rest of the communication becomes unorganized and discourteous. Therefore, it is extremely important that good telephone technique be firmly established and used routinely in the office. The telephone should be answered promptly, preferably on the first or second ring. Impatience is a common

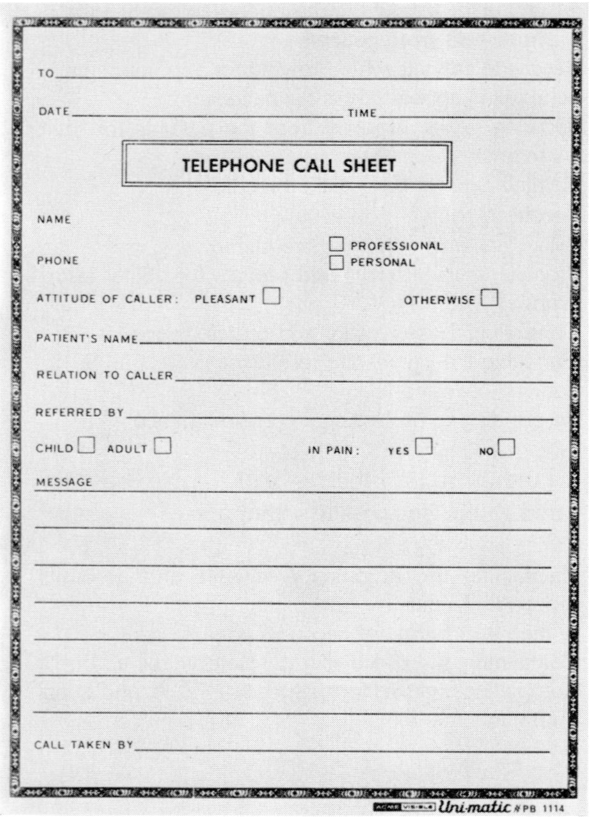

TO ____________________

DATE ____________ TIME ____________

TELEPHONE CALL SHEET

NAME

☐ PROFESSIONAL
☐ PERSONAL

PHONE

ATTITUDE OF CALLER: PLEASANT ☐ OTHERWISE ☐

PATIENT'S NAME ____________________

RELATION TO CALLER ____________________

REFERRED BY ____________________

CHILD ☐ ADULT ☐ IN PAIN: YES ☐ NO ☐

MESSAGE ____________________

CALL TAKEN BY ____________________

ACME VISIBLE Uni-matic #PB 1114

Figure 2-2 | Telephone call and message reminder. *(Courtesy of Acme Visible Records, Inc.)*

human trait and can be greatly magnified when the patient places a call to the dental office and then has to wait until it is convenient for the office to respond to the call.

Recognition

One of the basic human needs is recognition. Therefore, it is extremely important that the business assistant develop the skill of remembering people, names, and, in many instances, voices. After the initial greeting and identification of the office is made, identification of the patient is necessary. If the patient voluntarily identifies himself or herself, the assistant should immediately be able to ascertain whether the caller is a regular patient or a new patient. As previously mentioned, if the caller is a regular patient and the assistant does not recognize this, the ego of the patient is deflated, and office esteem suffers. Many patients expect the assistant to recognize their voice when calling. It may be necessary for the assistant to develop a tactful method of ascertaining the caller without harm to the caller's ego. However, once the patient's identification is established, recognition must take place. Patients' records should be within easy reach of the telephone so that during the initial conversation the assistant can easily pull the patient's record and have it handy for immediate reference. In this way the patient's problem or point of information can quickly be answered. If it is necessary for the assistant to gather additional information, the patient should be asked if he or she would mind waiting. Patient time should be valued in the same way that time in the dental office is valued. The patient is then thanked for waiting, always remembering to mention the patient's name. "Thank you very much for waiting, Mrs. Brown. I have consulted Dr. Smith and. . . ." In this manner the patient has received recognition, courtesy, and a feeling that everything possible has been done to solve the problem or that the information needed has been given. However, if the assistant is unable to give the requested information or if the dentist is unavailable for consultation, the message should be written on a telephone call memo sheet and referred to the dentist at the earliest convenience (Fig. 2-2).

The Appointment Call

Many of the telephone calls in the office will come from patients requesting an appointment. The appointment book should be within easy access to the telephone. In the case of the appointment telephone call, certain principles must be followed carefully.

1. Identify the patient.
2. Determine the need of the patient.
3. Is there pain?
4. If there is pain, secure a description of the pain for the dentist's determination of the necessity of an emergency appointment.
5. If there is no pain, ask the patient when are the most convenient times to come in.
6. Offer the patient an appointment as near his or her convenient time as possible.
7. If there is a waiting period for an appointment, inform the patient you will also put his or her name on your "call" list if an opening occurs sooner.
8. Record the patient's name, telephone number, and dental problem, in pencil, in the appointment book and on the call list. Be sure to note the patient's appointment time on the call list so that his or her name can be discarded if no opening occurs before the appointed time.
9. In closing, repeat the appointed time to the patient.
10. Thank the patient for calling.
11. Following the call, mail the patient an appointment card.

Tact, understanding, and empathy should be foremost in the assistant's attitude when making appointments for patients. It is understandable that an even flow of patients is necessary in the office and that certain times of the day must be allocated to the various types of treatment. For instance, an extraction would not be scheduled late in the day because of possible problems occurring during the night. Children should not be scheduled during an accustomed nap time, nor should complicated procedures, such as crown preparations, be set late in the day when the dentist may be tired. Nevertheless, the patient's time and convenience must also be considered. Many patients are lost to the dental office when an abrupt attitude is used. Everyone likes to feel he or she is being carefully considered.

The Fee-Shopper Call

People have been conditioned to seek the best bargain available. Some people see no difference in shopping for a TV or dental care; fortunately, not too many people have this attitude. However, the assistant should be prepared for this kind of telephone call, for example, "How much does the doctor charge for fillings?"

Fees should never be discussed over the telephone or before the dentist has determined the treatment plan. When dealing with the human body, predications cannot be made arbitrarily. Each person's dental needs are personal and require a diagnosis which is out of the realm of the assistant. The patient-shopper can be told these facts in a courteous and understanding manner. The patients will probably appreciate the personalized attention they will receive.

Telephone Control

Some people calling the dental office may ask to speak to the dentist. Upon the identification of the caller, the assistant may then determine whether the dentist should be interrupted to receive the telephone call. A predetermined listing of persons from whom calls will be taken should be made by the dentist and the staff and recorded in the office manual. Usually these calls will be from the spouse or another professional. If the caller demands to speak to the dentist after you have offered your assistance, a good approach is to take the number and name of the caller and tell the caller you will have the dentist return the call as soon as possible. Record the call on the telephone memo sheet and bring it to the dentist's attention as soon as possible. The exception may be the long-distance telephone call.

The Appointment Reminder Call

Many offices have established a policy of calling patients to remind them of their dental appointments. While this requires a lot of the assistant's time, it will promote a smooth flow of patients and is an additional courtesy to the patient. However, the assistant should be trying to be aware of the personalities and idiosyncrasies of the patients and should ask patients if they would like this service. Some patients may resent the idea that they are not capable of remembering an appointment.

Recall patients should be routinely called to remind them of their appointments unless other arrangements have been made. When the telephone call is made to remind the patient of the appointment, the assistant should not in any way infer that it is to confirm an appointment. The word confirm introduces a concept of asking if the patient intends to appear. The reminder call should be very positive in stating the date and time of an appointment which has been made. For example: "Mrs. Jones, I am calling to remind you of your dental appointment with Dr. Smith on Friday, November 6 at 2:30. We are looking forward to seeing you then."

If the office has only one telephone line, space the reminder calls so that the line will not be busy for an unreasonable length of time. Try not to have any call or series of calls exceed 10 minutes; then allow a period of time to receive incoming calls.

APPOINTMENT CONTROL

The appointment book may be seen as the heartbeat of the office. It is necessary that it be in a healthy condition to allow the smooth flow of the life blood of the office, the patients. If the appointment book becomes too crowded or too empty, the organization deteriorates. Therefore, careful control of the appointment book is extremely important.

Selection of the Appointment Book

Many different types of appointment books are available. These may be the loose-leaf, spiral, or bound book. The pages will contain a week at a glance while others may list each day on a separate page. Usually the days will be broken down into 15-minute intervals.

Appointment books can be purchased from most dental supply houses and should be purchased from 4 to 6 months prior to the new year. If a hygienist is part of the office team or if a preventive program is in use, it may be advisable to purchase two appointment books. In this way, the preventive recall patient appointments can be kept separate from the dentist's other appointments.

Preparing the Appointment Book

As far in advance as possible, the appointment book should be discussed in the office staff meeting, and, in pencil, certain days or times should be blocked out for holidays, meetings, and the regular days off each week. It is so much simpler to do this in advance rather than going ahead and making appointments during these times and then attempting to change the appointments.

The meetings mentioned may be continuing education courses which the dentist and staff plan to attend and organization meetings which are planned. These may be district, state, or national meetings, or regularly scheduled staff meetings (Fig. 2-3).

Measurement of Time

The key to a successful dental office is the prudent use of time. The organization of time must begin in the appointment book. There are several methods of allocating time for patient services, such as by the one-half hour, by the hour, or by units of time. The most satisfactory method for all concerned seems to be the division of units of time. If reference to time is in units, each 15 minutes is one unit, $1/2$ hour is two units, 1 hour is four units and so forth. Since the appointment book is usually sectioned off in 15-minute intervals, this method is easy to handle. When

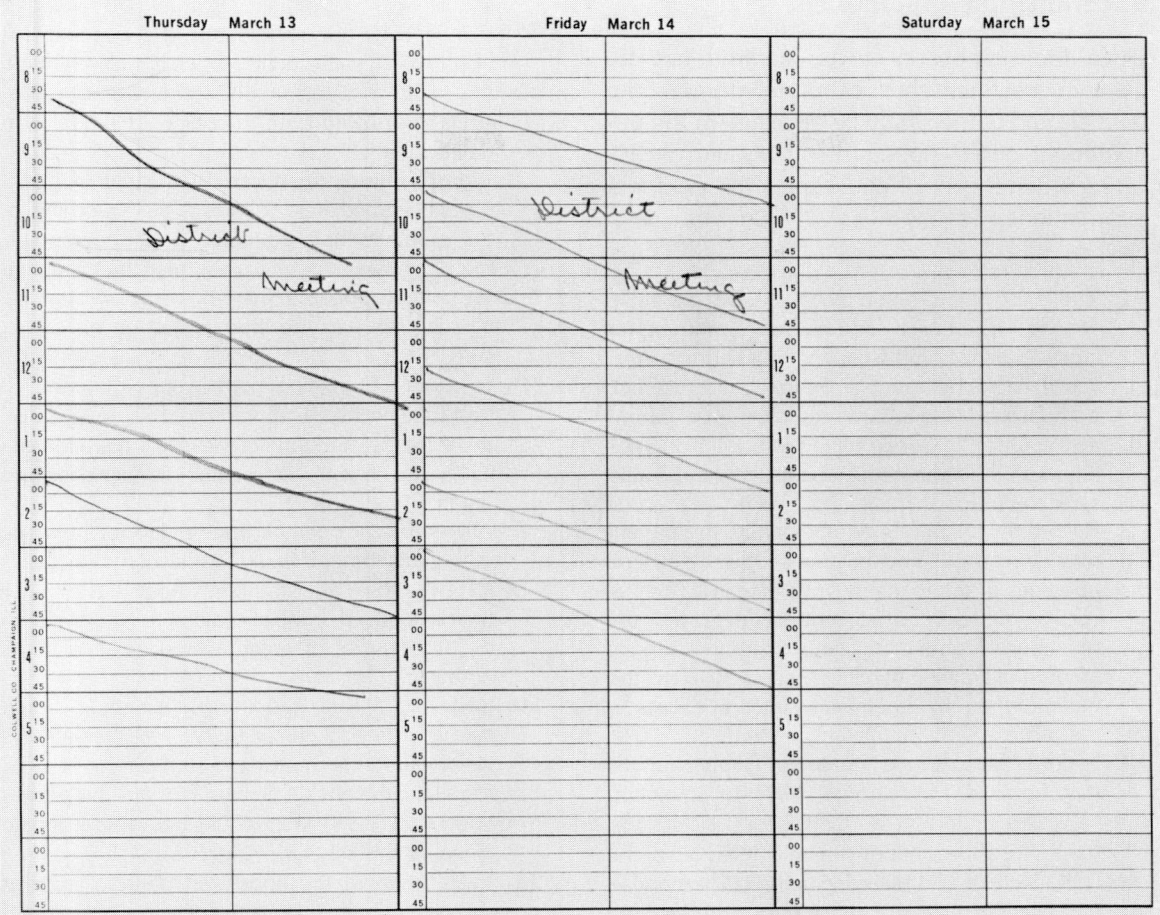

Figure 2-3 | Appointment book. Make sure all meetings and vacation times are blocked off in advance. (*Courtesy of Colwell Co.*)

the dentist is examining a patient and developing a treatment plan, he or she will indicate the number of units of time estimated for a particular restoration or treatment. After a short period of time, the assistant will easily be able to estimate the units of time necessary for a given treatment. The discussion of units of time in front of the patient indicates to the patient a professional approach rather than the work-by-the-hour approach. Patients have a tendency, when given an hour appointment, to estimate that the dentist is earning so much an hour. However, when using units of time, the thought runs to how many units are required to get the treatment accomplished. Therefore, the use of units of time not only makes the appointment schedule run more smoothly, but also has a good psychologic value for the patient.

Recording the Appointment

Once the number of units required for the planned treatment has been determined, the units should immediately be allocated in the appointment book. Appointments should always be recorded in pencil and contain all pertinent information.

1. The entire name should be written. For example: Jane Eve Thomas. If Jane Thomas is married, for cross-reference purposes Jane Eve Thomas (Mrs. John) could be used. If the patient is a child, perhaps the father's name could be put in parenthesis. Often you may have more than one patient with the same name, and this method would save confusion.
2. Record the telephone number where this patient may be reached. You may have to record several numbers if the patient is employed. The recording of these numbers not only helps with the reminder telephone call but saves an enormous amount of time if it becomes necessary to call the patient when an emergency situation occurs in the office.
3. Record the planned treatment. Abbreviations may be used, for example, "Ag" for amalgam, "RC" for endodontia, "Cons" for consultation. Codes for abbreviations can be worked out at the staff meetings and recorded in the office manual. It is necessary for the entire staff to understand the coding used in case it becomes necessary for someone else to temporarily assume the business assistant's position (Fig. 2-4).
4. Make the appointment at an appropriate time of the day for the treatment planned. Complicated treatment, such as crown and bridge, or other treatment requiring intensive concentration should be appointed to the earlier hours in the day when the operator is fresh and rested. Likewise, children should not be appointed late in the day when the child is tired or during the time the child might routinely use as nap time.
5. Do not expose the appointment book in full view of the patient. Patient appointments are private matters.
6. It is usually better to have only one person in charge of the appointment book. The dentist should be aware of this and should be reminded to not make appointments in the appointment book. Be sure the dentist does not also fall into the habit of giving verbal appointments to patients in or away from the office. This habit can create chaos.
7. Write the appointment card for the patient, in duplicate, immediately following the recording of the appointment in the book. Duplicate appointment cards are extremely helpful in the event that the patient appears in the office at the wrong time insisting this was the time written on his or her card.
8. In the case of making multiple appointments, it is best to make all the appointments, if possible, on the same day and time of the week. It is a lot easier for the patient to remember regular days and hours.
9. Allow at least one-half hour a day for buffer or emergency time. Usually the best time for this is just prior to or after the lunch hour. If the buffer time is not used, it will allow time to get caught up on other duties or enjoy a more relaxed lunch hour.
10. Each day, a daily appointment schedule should be made out and posted (away from the patient's view) where the dentist and staff can be kept informed of the day's activities. Perhaps the laboratory or sterilizing area would be an appropriate place for this schedule (Fig. 2-5).
11. Each morning the appointed patients' records should be pulled from the files, checked, and placed in an appropriate area for use during the day. Upon completion of the treatment all information is recorded and checked on the records before refiling.

Patient Appointment Problems

After working with patients a very short time, the alert business assistant will get to know the likes, dislikes, and habits of a patient. Human nature being what it is, it should not be the assistant's task to try to change people. It is far simpler for all concerned for the assistant to learn how to circumvent the problems before they happen. If a patient consistently is late for an appointment, for example, simply make the appointment card

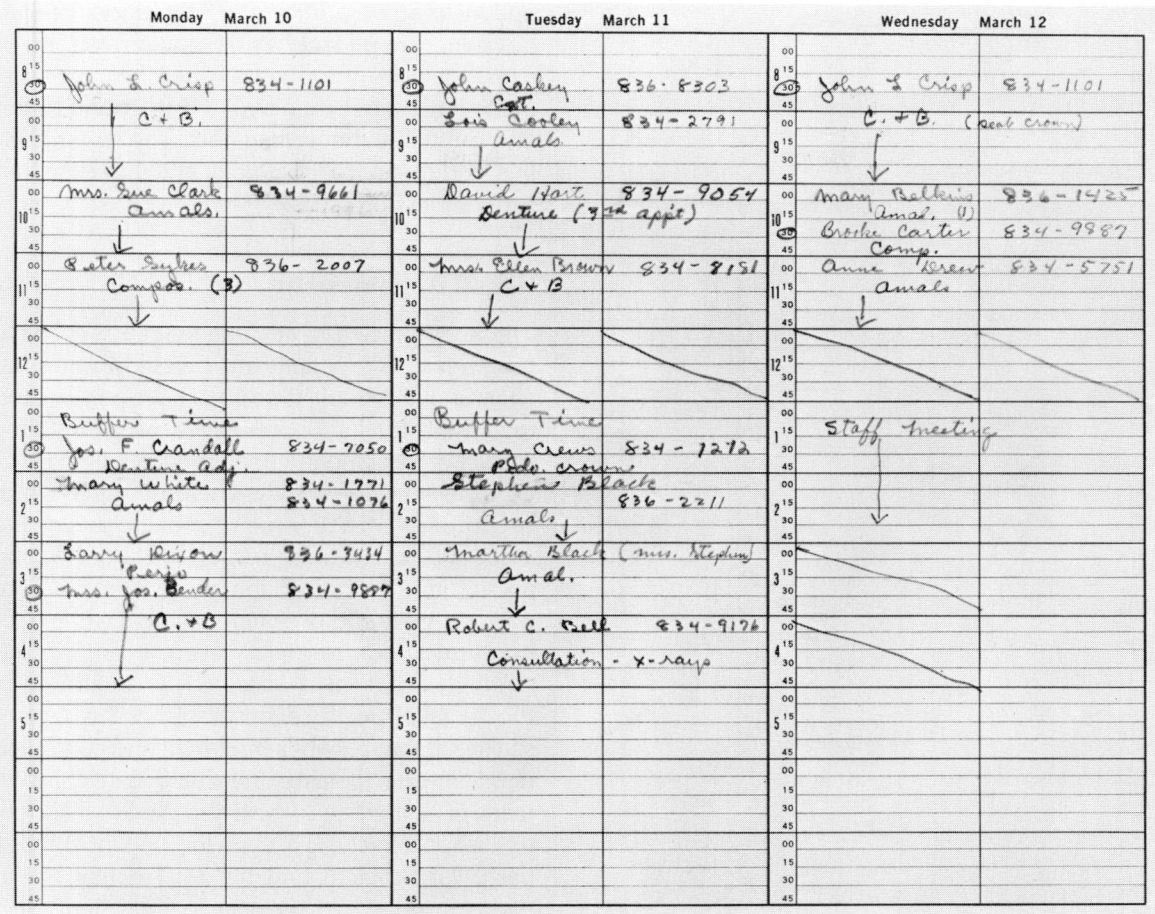

Figure 2-4 | Appointment book. Appointments are always written in pencil. Treatment to be performed is clearly indicated and the patient's telephone number is recorded for immediate contact if necessary. (*Courtesy of Colwell Co.*)

for 15 minutes earlier than the recorded time in the appointment book. On the other hand, if a patient chronically misses appointments because of forgetting, make an arrangement for you to call about an hour ahead of the appointment. Many patients have busy schedules and would appreciate this service.

The "drop-in" patient, the patient who just happened to be in the neighborhood and thought it was possible to be "worked in," should be courteously but firmly discouraged. Once this type of patient realizes the importance and the need for prior appointments, the habit will be discontinued. However, firmness is often required.

Fortunately, most people respect the value of time in the dental office and soon learn and appreciate the fact that special time has been reserved for them and will make every effort to keep their appointments. The business assistant

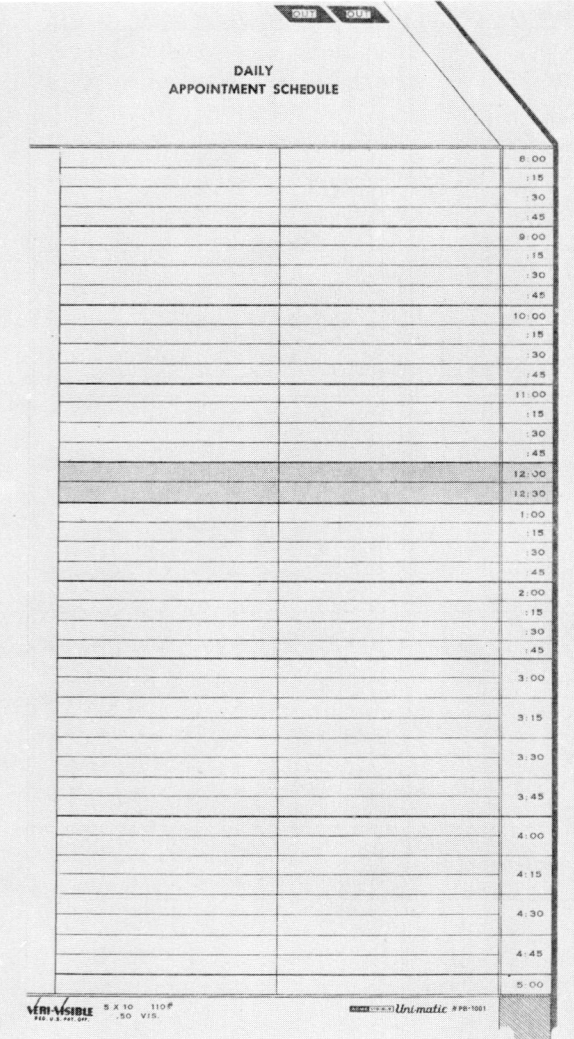

Figure 2-5 | Daily appointment schedule to be posted daily in an accessible area. (*Courtesy of Acme Visible Records, Inc.*)

stresses the fact that time has been reserved for the patient and follows through by not allowing any patient to "borrow" another's time.

If the dentist is running late with a patient's treatment, the next scheduled patient could be called and informed of this and may have the option to arrive a little later than appointed. If, however, the patient has already arrived, he or she should be informed of the circumstances. Many times a patient may have an errand to run and can utilize the waiting time. The rewards for this kind of service are untold, and the office staff is under less pressure.

Recall Appointments

The importance and advantages of a preventive program to the patient are stressed in another chapter of this book. If patients have participated in a well-structured preventive program, they readily understand the need for continuing interest in their dental health. The business assistant becomes a very active member of the preventive team and assumes the responsibility of keeping an accurate record of the preventive program patients' visits and of reminding them when a return visit is due.

When a patient is accepted for treatment in the dental office, the dentist assumes the responsibility for that patient's treatment and continued dental health. It takes the entire dental health team of that office to help the dentist carry out this responsibility. To treat the patient for one particular problem and not total dental health needs is, indeed, a disservice to the patient. Recognizing this disservice, the dental profession has assumed the responsibility of caring for and delivering total dental health treatment to the patient. In order to assure continuing treatment for and interest in the patient, a good recall system is absolutely necessary in the dental office. The business assistant would assume the major responsibility of arranging a system for patients to assure each one of continuing care.

Various types of recall systems may be used, such as (1) advance appointments, (2) monthly card coding, and (3) recall list by month. When using the advance appointment method, the 3- or 6-month recall appointment is made at the time of the last visit to the office or upon completion of the treatment. The appointment is recorded in the appointment book, and the patient is given an appointment card. The patient may then be reminded a week or two prior to the appointment by telephone or by written communication. This method works extremely well when the patient becomes accustomed to making advance appointments and assures patients of a time set aside for them in a crowded appointment book. It also has the advantage of giving the assistant an idea of the patient flow 3 to 6 months in advance.

The second method, the monthly card coding, is one in which the patient's name is placed on the appropriate monthly card for recall. An example of this might be that in March when Joseph Carter completes his dental work and the dentist decides Mr. Carter should be recalled in 6 months, the assistant will place his name on the September recall card. Prior to September 1, the assistant will pull the September recall cards and notify Mr. Carter that it is now time for his recall appointment. In order to facilitate this method, time must be left open in the appointment book for recall appointments. The appointment book, therefore, would have certain times each week blocked off for recall appointments. If this is not done in advance, time may not be readily available.

The third method, the recall system using a list, follows the same principles as the card system. The name of the patient is entered on a recall list with the date of the last appointment and the approximate date of the recall appointment. As the assistant proceeds down the list, the patients are notified that 3 or 6 months have elapsed, and it is now time for them to make another appointment. Once again, caution must be used in not filling all the time units in the appointment book on a regular basis so that time will be available for the recall patient. The office that has a hygienist on the team should appoint the patient for recall in the hygienist's appointment book, thereby assuring prompt, efficient attention for the patient.

Whatever recall system is used in the office, it is obvious that the business assistant must constantly be aware of the needs of the patient and must set aside time to look ahead in both the dentist's and hygienist's appointment books in order to advise the patient of the pending recall appointment and secure adequate time for treatment. Individual attention given to patients for recall appointments can pay off in untold dividends both to the patient's dental health and to the smooth operation of the office. Many patients can be lost to a dental practice through inefficient recall systems.

PATIENT RECORDS

An essential function of the business assistant is that of obtaining and maintaining the patient's records. The importance of accurate and complete records on all patients cannot be overemphasized. The records should be kept in an envelope-type folder and should be stored in files tightly compressed. While there are no fireproof methods available, folders tightly compressed and filed in metal file cabinets have the best chance of survival should there be a fire. The patient record folders should include

1. *Patient information form.* This form should be filled out by the patient when presenting to the office for the first visit. The information on the form should include patient's name, address, occupation, address of occupation, name of nearest kin, birth date, physician, and person responsible for the account. If the patient has dental insurance (third-party payment), this information should also be included. Be sure that each address includes a telephone number.
2. *Medical history.* A medical history should be taken on every patient treated in the dental office. In an extreme case, a complete medical history of a patient could actually save the patient's life. Printed medical history forms can be purchased, or the assistant and dentist may choose to make up their own. The information that should be included in the medical history is

a. Age, weight, and height.
b. If presently under physician's care, the name and address of the physician.
c. Whether the patient suffers from or has had heart condition, allergies, bleeding, diabetes, kidney disease, rheumatic heart disease, epilepsy, high blood pressure, anemia, or other diseases pertinent to his or her health.
d. Medication, if any, currently being taken. Many people do not know what drugs they are taking and may or may not know the reason for prescription of the medication. In such a case the patient's physician should be contacted for additional information.
e. The date and vital signs (blood pressure, pulse, and respiration) on subsequent visits, if it is necessary to record them. Open lines should be left for this on the form.
f. If there is any question at all concerning the patient's health, his or her physician should be contacted for additional information, and this new information should be entered on the record. Adequate space should be allowed on the medical forms for notation by the dentist of any change or unusual appearance or action by the patient. For example, note if the patient appeared under tension or fainted during a visit. All items of information are important for the total well-being of the patient. It is better to write something down that is not necessary than to not write something that may be quite indicative of the patient's physical or mental health.

3. *Diagnosis, charting, and treatment plan.* The chart should include complete data on the patient's existing conditions. Complete oral examination findings should be carefully recorded such as existing restorations, missing teeth, occlusion, position of teeth, tissue appearance, and other pertinent data.
4. *Record of treatment delivered.* This record should be as complete as possible with notations dated and added when necessary.
5. *Radiographs.* Current, dated radiographs should be kept in the patients' folders. Outdated radiographs, complete with the patient's name and date, can be filed for a maximum period in the outdated radiograph file. Occasionally they may be needed for comparison or history reasons. The maximum time for keeping radiographs should be referred to the dentist's legal counselor.
6. *Models and casts.* While these are part of the patient's records, obviously they cannot be kept in the folders. However, they should be filed in boxes with the patient's name clearly labeled on the boxes, and a notation card should be included in the patient's folder containing the information about the models. Make sure that each individual model is marked with the name of the patient, age, and the date the model was secured.
7. *Patient photographs and/or slides.* Many dentists prefer to use "before and after" pictures of the patient or wish to take photographs of an unusual appearance. This is a very good practice to develop and is extremely sound legally.
8. *Patient financial record.* This is the record of the charges, payments, and balance of each patient. The financial agreement or method of payment agreed upon at the case presentation would be included. Before filing the patient ledger card which shows the charges, payments, and balance, the assistant should be certain that these charges are also recorded in the daily journal. Duplicate copies of receipts for all payments made are also filed in the patient's financial records. By using a pegboard accounting system, the posting and recording of daily treatment records can be easily facilitated. The pegboard method is one in which carbon-copy interlays are used while recording the charges and payments. Various types of pegboard accounting methods can be obtained from the many office supply companies.

OFFICE RECORD KEEPING

The function of record keeping in the dental office has become both time-consuming and complex. The office record keeper or bookkeeper must be knowledgeable in completing and maintaining third-party payment plans which may include the Delta Plan, Medicaid, Medicare, and other insurance plans, maintaining tax records, sharing payroll responsibilities, maintaining the records on disbursements and expenses, and the collecting of fees by billing the patient. It is desirable for the chairside assistant to be familiar with the terminology and activity of the office record keeping. The business assistant should endeavor to pursue additional education through continuing education courses and readings to develop expertise in this area.

COLLECTION OF FEES AND BILLING

If the daily record and patient's ledger card recording all payments and charges have been accurately kept, billing can be a fairly simple and routine procedure. Patients should be encouraged to pay the fees upon completion of each treatment. However, this is not always possible for or desired by the patient, and it therefore becomes necessary to mail a statement for the treatment performed and the balance of fees due. When statements are sent to the patient, it is a good idea to have the statements completed and in the mail by the twenty-seventh day of the month. This allows ample time for the patient to receive the statement and arrange payment by the tenth day of the following month. The pegboard accounting system greatly facilitates the billing of patients. The statements must be neatly typed on letterhead-type printed statement forms. Most patients appreciate a fairly detailed account of the services rendered. If more than one member of the family has received treatment during the month, then a listing of each member's treatment can be given with a total balance due in the lower part of the statement. However, the business assistant should ascertain the wishes of the patients on this matter. A courtesy of the office may be the rendering of a total statement of fees paid to the office by a family at the end of the year for tax purposes of the patient. Once again, the patients' wishes should be referred to in this matter.

It sometimes becomes necessary to call patients to remind them of past-due accounts. While this might be a chore not particularly enjoyed by the business assistant, outstanding accounts cannot be allowed to "pyramid" or accrue in the dental office. A tactful method should be developed for the collection call and a sound step-by-step procedure used. Empathy and courtesy should be used; however, firmness and a clear explanation of office policy must be communicated. Threats and sarcasm have no place in the professional office. Many times the assistant may offer suggestions or methods of payment to the patient who is financially embarrassed. Caring about people and taking the time to help solve financial problems through suggestion builds good public relations.

INCOME, EXPENSE, AND DISBURSEMENT RECORDS

Good practice management in the office requires accurate record keeping of all payments of bills and expenses in the dental office. For tax purposes, proof of all income and expenses must be maintained and available should an audit be requested.

Income

As payments of fees are collected they should be carefully recorded on the patient's record and in the journal. Incoming checks and cash should be deposited on a daily basis. At the end of each day the deposit slip and journal entries should be checked for similarity and accuracy. Cash and checks should not be left in the dental office overnight.

Expenses

A complete record of all monies spent to maintain and operate the dental office must be maintained. This would include salaries, social security contributions for the employees, supplies, equipment, maintenance expenses such as cleaning or repair, postage, and laundry services. Proof of expenditures must be evident; therefore, receipts must be secured for those ex-

Figure 2-6 | Dental insurance form. (*Courtesy of Delta Dental Plan Association.*)

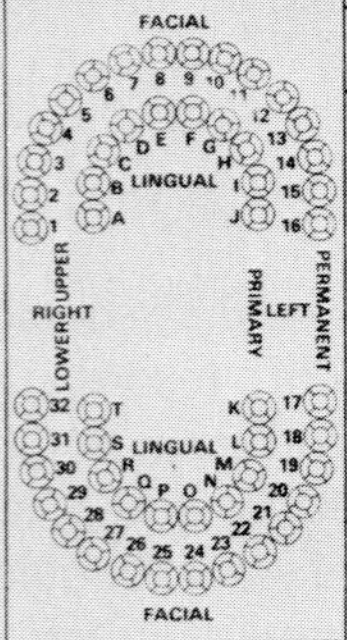

penses not paid for by check. Since canceled checks and bank statements offer excellent proof of disbursements and other payments of expenses, checks should be used whenever possible. However, there are times when a small amount of cash must be used in payment for some expenses. A small petty-cash fund can be kept in the office for this purpose; however, always be sure to place a receipt or memo in the box when removing cash to prove the expenditure. Usually the disbursements and expenses are listed under separate headings when posted in the ledger, such as maintenance, office supplies, equipment, etc. Be sure to record these headings on receipts and checks to ensure accuracy of posting in appropriate categories. Paid bills should also be kept in appropriate files, and they should be easily accessible when they are needed to check records for proof of expenses.

Convention and meeting expenses should be kept carefully for both the dentist and staff. Receipts should be secured for all meals, lodging, transportation, and registration fees. These should be carefully filed under the proper category immediately following the activity. At the end of the year all convention and meeting expenditures may be charged to expenses when filing the annual income tax form of the dentist and the practice.

THIRD-PARTY PAYMENT PLANS, PREPAID DENTAL CARE

The dental profession has rapidly become involved in the third-party or prepaid dental–health care plans. While this involves a voluminous amount of paperwork and expertise on the part of the business assistant, the end result seems to justify the cause. Many millions of Americans are eligible for dental health treatment under employee benefit programs, private policies with insurance companies, and federal and local health programs.

Delta Dental Plan

In response to the growing need for a dental profession oriented prepaid dental care insurance program, the Delta Dental Plan, with headquarters in the ADA Building in Chicago, was developed by organized dentistry. This nonprofit organization has been approved by the ADA and the various state dental societies.

Individual states organize separate plans which operate as independent corporations under the approval of state insurance commissions. Each plan contracts with individual industries to provide dental services as a fringe benefit for employees. Payment is made to the dentist for services rendered based on usual, customary, and reasonable (UCR) fees.

It becomes the function of the business assistant to help the patient complete the necessary forms and to record the treatment rendered; Fig. 2-6 is an example of the kind of treatment form required.

Insurance Company Dental Health Plans

Many insurance companies have developed dental–health plan insurance coverage. The various plans pay either directly to the dentist providing the service or to the insured patient. Although these plans are similar in many respects, thorough knowledge of the plan being utilized is necessary for the business assistant to fulfill his or her function accurately and effectively. Each plan is different regarding coverage, and most patients will not be totally familiar with their insurance coverage.

Federal and Local Health Plan Funding

Private dentists are increasingly providing treatment and services for members of the consumer public eligible to receive dental care that will be paid for by federal, state, or local agencies. This might include those patients covered under

Medicaid, Medicare, or welfare funding. The agency would contact the dentist requesting dental-care services for given patients and will guarantee payment under a restricted, preplanned, or usual, customary, and reasonable, fee. National health bills are now being considered by Congress to ensure the right of all people of the availability of dental health care. Dental offices should prepare for an increase in this type of service in the future. It will become necessary for the business assistant to participate in available continuing education courses to keep current and knowledgeable in new plans as they develop. Publications are now available containing terminology and means of completing and implementing the various plans, and the business assistant should pursue means of obtaining them through private companies and government agencies.

TAX RECORDS AND PAYROLLS

As previously mentioned in "Expenses," accurate records are extremely important for Internal Revenue Service purposes. Of equal importance is the efficient record keeping and maintenance of the payroll information. Strict requirements are legislated by federal and state governments for certain deductions to be made by the employer from the employee's salary. The employer is also required to contribute a like amount to the employee's account. The Internal Revenue Service has published information pertaining to payroll deduction which should be obtained and carefully studied by any business assistant who is required to handle the payroll.

The government requires that all employers obtain an employer's number and file quarterly returns with their respective offices. All taxable wages must be reported on in the appropriate return, along with taxes withheld. The report, to be filed quarterly (four times a year at specified dates), must be sent on time and must contain all the required information. This form is called the Employer's Quarterly Federal Tax Return and is numbered 941.

The amounts of withholding taxes are determined by the government along with the number of dependents the employee may claim. Therefore, certain withholding forms must be completed by the employee when starting employment. Also, a statement must be sent to the employee at the completion of each year stating the total amount of wages earned during the preceding year and the amount of taxes and social security which has been withheld. It is suggested that the business assistant consult carefully with the office accountant or legal council regarding these procedures.

INVENTORY CONTROL AND SUPPLIES

Every member of the dental health team in the office should be familiar with the method of inventory control and with the shelf life and ordering of supplies. However, it will probably be the function of the business assistant to organize the control and actually order the supplies. During the frequent staff meetings held by the dental team, discussion of inventory and supplies should be an item on the agenda.

In constructing the office manual, inclusion of the policy and preferences of the dentist with regard to selection of the dental supply houses to be used, responsibility for ordering, storing, and maintaining inventory and for communication with the supply sales agent should be of prime importance. To maintain efficiency and to control wasted precious minutes in the dental office, organization and planning must prevail. Personnel who have attended continuing education courses, conventions, and meetings and who have obtained information on new materials or equipment and their uses should be given every opportunity to share their knowledge with others in the office. The dentist who rigidly clings to old methods and materials taught while in dental school will not receive the advantages of the new methods and materials. The development of new methods, equipment, and materials is so extensive at the present time that it requires more than one person to seek and obtain the available information. Articles in dental journals should be read on a regular basis by the office staff and discussed at staff meetings. In this manner many minds contribute to the progress and efficiency of the dental office.

Source of Supplies

It is generally considered good practice to deal with one or two local supply companies. The reasons for this are many: ease of ordering, fast delivery, maintenance responsibilities assumed by local dealers, quality of materials provided, and information on new or faulty materials. Substantial savings on quantity and bulk purchasing are available from most dental dealers. While bulk purchasing may be financially advantageous, two very important factors must be considered: (1) adequate space for storage, and (2) the shelf life of the product.

Office supplies such as pads, pencils, staples, and folders can be purchased from the local stationary store or from office supply catalogues. Other paper materials needed, such as statements, envelopes, appointment cards, appointment books, and other bookkeeping supplies, can be ordered directly from dental office supply dealers. Usually any office supply dealer will carry a complete supply of items needed in the dental office in a variety of styles, shapes, and prices. Local printing companies can also supply reasonably fast service for the printing of letterheads, bills, and envelopes. The need for these types of items must be anticipated well in advance if actual usage is to allow adequate time for printing. Embarrassing situations, such as running out of statements, can be avoided by routinely checking the inventory of the office supplies and ordering at least 6 months in advance.

Many miscellaneous items must be purchased for the dental office. Examples of these might be tissues, soap, toilet tissue, drugs, hand lotion, coffee, and cleaning supplies. Usually these are purchased locally. The local drugstore may be a source for many of these items, and an account may be set up for the dentist to be billed once a month. The advantage of this method is that a more accurate record of purchases can be maintained, and cash would not be required. Stamps and some other miscellaneous items, however, probably would require cash. Money taken from the petty-cash account must be carefully accounted for, and a receipt should be obtained for all purchases made and paid for with cash. Remember, all tax-deductible items purchased for the running of the office must have proof of purchase in writing. This can be a receipt, a paid statement, or a canceled check.

Inventory Control

In order to know when to order supplies, whether it is office materials, dental supplies, or miscellaneous items, an efficient method of knowing what is on hand in the office at all times must be determined. This is called inventory control. There are two types of supplies in the dental office that need replacing. They are called *expendable* and *nonexpendable* supplies.

Expendable Supplies

These are the supplies that are used routinely in the office and must be replaced regularly. Examples of expendables may be amalgam pellets, mercury, composites, cotton rolls, bases, and cements. Laboratory supplies such as stone and plaster are also expendable items. A good way to remember what the expendable supplies are is to consider those supplies that are consumed or used up in a comparatively short period of time. Many of the expendable items have a definite shelf life. This means they must be used within a stated period of time due to their chemical properties. Outdated materials such as rubber-base impression material or composite material will not react after the period of time specified by the manufacturer. The material may not set up at all or may set up too fast, or perhaps the physical properties might change. Therefore, bulk or quantity buying of these supplies would not be advantageous (Fig. 2-7). Much time and energy could be consumed by the assistant if it were necessary to count the supplies on hand and decide whether to reorder. Taking an inventory is not necessary if a good method of ongoing inventory control is being utilized.

There are several methods of inventory control of expendable items presently being utilized in efficient dental offices. The business assistant may develop an individual method that is more suitable. The more popular methods used are the *red-flag tag* and the *card-index* methods.

Red-flag tag inventory control The minimum amount to be kept on hand must be determined for each item. For instance, if the minimum amount of rubber-base material is two boxes (Fig. 2-8), then a red tag should be attached to the third from the last box. This would indicate at the time of using the tagged box that it is time to reorder to maintain the minimum amount of two boxes on the shelf. The assistant should maintain a *want list* (Fig. 2-9) and, immediately upon noting the red tag, should write down "rubber-base material." With this method of inventory, stock is constantly under control, and the assistant will never face the embarrassing situation of running out of essential materials.

Card-index inventory control Indexed file cards are made up for all supplies. Each card would be headed with the name of the material, the manufacturer's name, and the supplier. When an item is purchased, the date and number purchased is recorded on the card. The price may also be recorded. When the predetermined minimum amount appears on the shelf, it is a simple matter to pull the card and reorder. The card should be kept out of the file until delivery is made. The delivery date is then recorded and the card reinserted into the card file. One of the advantages of this method is that a running check can be made of rate of materials being used up; this will indicate the use of quantity buying. A combination of red-flag tags and index-card inventory may be used in many cases.

The main point of establishing the minimum amount to be kept on hand should be the realistic time allowed for reordering and receiving sup-

TYPICAL QUANTITY RATE SAVINGS

Item	Quantity	Discount
Anesthetic	Can (50)	10 cans = 10%
		20 cans = 15%
Burs, carbide	Each	10-49 = 05%
		50-99 = 10%
		100-199 = 18%
Needles, disposable	Box (100)	10 boxes = 12%
		50 boxes = 21%
Impression material, rubber base	Box	3 boxes = 05%
		6 boxes = 08%
		12 boxes = 12%
		36 boxes = 20%

Figure 2-7 | Bulk buying advantages in saving.

Figure 2-8 | Minimum and maximum inventory list.

EXAMPLE OF MINIMUM AND MAXIMUM LIST

Item	Description	Minimum	Maximum
Anesthetic	Carpules	250	1000
Film	Periapical	3 boxes (150 each)	10 boxes
Burs, carbide F.G.	#245	10	200
Towels	Patient napkins	1 case (500)	12 cases
Impression material	Rubber base	3 boxes	36 boxes

WANT LIST

from

THOMPSON DENTAL CO.

Box 1341	Box 20067	Box 17805
Charlotte, N. C. 28201	Greensboro, N. C. 27420	Raleigh, N. C. 27609

OFFICE HOURS 8:00 A.M.–5:00 P.M. MONDAY THRU FRIDAY

ANESTHETIC
BURS, CARBIDE F.G. #½ 69L, 245, 4
COMPOSITE
DIAMONDS, F.G. #½ ¾ AF, ½ DT, 2½ J
FILM, PERIAPICAL
GINGIVAL RETRACTION CORD
NEEDLES, DISPOSABLE 27GA L
NEEDLES, DISPOSABLE 27GA. S
PASTE, BITE REGISTRATION
TRAYS, DISPOSABLE #7 & #8

Figure 2-9 | Want list. Write down supplies needed on reminder list when need is indicated. (*Courtesy of Thompson Dental Supply Co.*)

plies. The assistant should be aware that sometimes dental-supply dealers may not have on hand an item being ordered, and a back-order (Fig. 2-10) notice may be received. This means the order is being processed by the dealer but may take some time in arriving due to a present shortage of the particular item. Back orders should be followed up by the assistant within a reasonable period of time by contacting the dental-supply dealer. If the minimum supply in the office is adequate, the back order will not present a problem; however, the assistant should be prepared for unplanned delay.

ARNOLD GRAPHIC IND. INC. 17082

Dear Doctor: *Date* ______________

Goods listed below are not in stock but will be forwarded promptly, when received.

2 Diamonds Friction Grip #2 1/2J

We thank you for this order.

THOMPSON DENTAL CO., Inc.
Raleigh, N. C.

Dr. John Q. Doe
1010 Beach Drive
Shallotte, N. C. 28459

Figure 2-10 | Back order. (*Courtesy of Thompson Dental Supply Co.*)

Nonexpendable Supplies

Nonexpendable supplies are the items in the office that are not consumed but may need replacing from time to time due to wear. Usually nonexpendable supplies are thought of as equipment and instruments. The accountant should be informed of the purchase of the more expensive items of equipment such as a unit, an autoclave, or chair for longer-term tax depreciation. These larger expenses are usually grouped together as a third category called capital expenditures. The card-index inventory in this case becomes an excellent source of ascertaining the date of purchase, the manufacturer, and the life of the equipment or instruments. Any maintenance required for equipment should also be recorded on the index card.

Ordering the Supplies

As previously mentioned, a *want list* should be kept between reordering times or between the dental-supply sales agent's visit. If the office is dealing with a particular dental-supply house, regular visits are usually scheduled. The want lists can be posted in the area where supplies are kept, in the laboratory, and on the business assistant's desk. As minimal supply limits are reached or new instruments are indicated, the desired items may be listed on the want list. Prior to the scheduled or regular visit by the supply salesperson or prior to ordering supplies, the business assistant will collect the want lists, ascertain the quantities needed, and make up an order. Dental-supply sales agents are usually extremely helpful to the business assistant in providing information of maximum and minimal suggestions, new products, and sale items. Time should be allocated for discussion with the sales agent and occasionally, when time permits, to suggest to the dentist that he or she see the salesperson. The representative can usually be depended upon to give valuable information on the success or failure of new materials, instruments, and equipment. If it becomes necessary between ordering times to purchase materials, rush-order forms from supply companies are usually available. Local supply companies may also be contacted by telephone, and orders can be placed on a rush basis. An efficiently run inventory control system will probably not require this type of action; however, emergencies do occur in the best of offices.

Receiving Supplies

An invoice or packing list will usually be sent with the supplies delivered (Fig. 2-11). When the supplies arrive, they should be carefully checked with the enclosed invoice and the duplicate order form. If any discrepancy occurs, this should be immediately recorded, and the dental-supply company informed.

The supplies should immediately be placed on the indicated shelves and red-tagged or recorded on the index cards. Proper storage of supplies and materials is very important. For instance, if film is stored in the refrigerator or a very cool area, it can be used over a longer period of time.

PACKING LIST
from
THOMPSON DENTAL COMPANY

CHARLOTTE ☐ GREENSBORO ☐ RALEIGH ☐

INVOICE COVERING THIS PACKING LIST WILL FOLLOW

Your Order ______

Date ______

TO: Dr. John Q. Doe
1010 Beach Drive
Shallotte, N. C. 28459

NO.	ITEMS	
1	Case (5000) 2 x 2 Non-Sterile Sponges	
20	Lb. Carton Model Plaster	
1	Gal. Liquid Soap	
3	Each Fixer and Developer	

5M SETS—10-68—FH

Per VIA UPS

Figure 2-11 | Packing list may be delivered in lieu of invoice. (*Courtesy of Thompson Dental Supply Co.*)

Film that has been refrigerated can probably be used even after the dated expiration time indicated on the package. Darkened areas for storage of perishable materials are desirable and will extend the shelf life of many materials. Neatness, organization, and easy access to materials can save time, energy, and tempers.

Occasionally it may be necessary to return defective items or items sent by mistake. These items can usually be given to the supply salesperson on his or her next visit, and a credit will be recorded on the account. A credit form (Fig. 2-12) should be expected shortly after the return of such supplies. If the credit does not show up on the invoice or a credit form is not received, the dental-supply company should be contacted immediately.

Invoices or statements (Fig. 2-13) will be re-

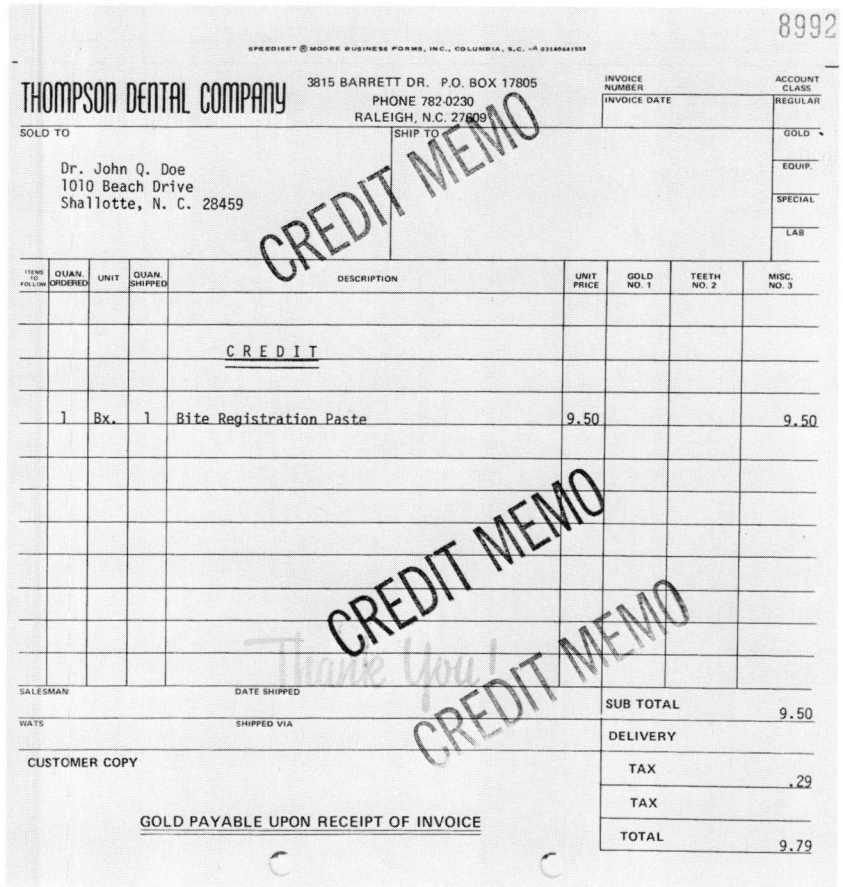

Figure 2-12 | Credit form—sent when supplies are returned. (*Courtesy of Thompson Dental Supply Co.*)

ceived on or about the first of each month. These invoices should be carefully checked for amounts, credits, and balances. It is extremely important that the dentist maintain a good credit standing; therefore, all bills should be paid promptly. A certain day each month should be set aside for the business assistant to write all the checks for accounts due that month.

As soon as the invoices and bills have been paid, they should be stamped or initialed paid, and the date paid recorded. These statements and invoices can then be immediately filed under office expenses. The canceled checks may be attached to these later. Federal or state tax authorities may wish to see these records at any time, and they should be in order at all times. The time limitations of keeping such records differ greatly; however, 5 years should be the minimum. The accountant or legal counselor should be consulted about future storage of office expense records which should never be discarded without the dentist's permission.

8993

SPEEDISET ® MOORE BUSINESS FORMS, INC., COLUMBIA, S.C.

THOMPSON DENTAL COMPANY

3815 BARRETT DR. P.O. BOX 17805
PHONE 782-0230
RALEIGH, N.C. 27609

INVOICE NUMBER | INVOICE DATE | ACCOUNT CLASS: REGULAR / GOLD / EQUIP. / SPECIAL / LAB

SOLD TO

Dr. John Q. Doe
1010 Beach Drive
Shallotte, N. C. 28459

SHIP TO

ITEMS TO FOLLOW	QUAN. ORDERED	UNIT	QUAN. SHIPPED	DESCRIPTION	UNIT PRICE	GOLD NO. 1	TEETH NO. 2	MISC. NO. 3
	20	Cans	20	Anesthetic 2%	6.45			129.00
	100	Ea.	100	Carbide Burs F.G. 50/69L, 40/245, 10/4	1.45			145.00
	1	Bx.	1	Standard Pkg. Composite	54.50			54.50
2	8	Ea.	6	Diamonds, F.G. 3/3/4AF, 3/1/2DT, 2/2 1/2J	9.00			72.00
	10	Bx.	10	Film, Periapical (150 ea.)	10.62			106.20
	3	Bx.	3	Gingival Retraction Cord	3.90			11.70
	5	Bxs.	5	Needles, Disposable, 27 Ga. Long	6.00			30.00
	5	Bxs.	5	Needles, Disposable, 27 Ga. Short	6.00			30.00
	1	Bx.	1	Bite Registration Paste	9.50			9.50
	50	Ea.	50	Trays, Disposable, 25/#7, 25/#8	.30			15.00

Thank You!

SALESMAN | DATE SHIPPED

WATS | SHIPPED VIA

CUSTOMER COPY

SUB TOTAL	602.90
DELIVERY UPS	1.89
TAX	18.09
TAX	
TOTAL	622.89

GOLD PAYABLE UPON RECEIPT OF INVOICE

Figure 2-13 | Invoice for month's purchases. (*Courtesy of Thompson Dental Supply Co.*)

Care in Storage of Supplies and Equipment

Ample storage space should be available in all dental offices to ensure safe and economical storage of equipment and supplies. However, this is ideal and not always realistic. Therefore, careful planning, knowledge of buying, and safety are important factors for consideration.

BIBLIOGRAPHY

Ehrlich, A. B., and Ehrlich, S. F.: *Dental Practice Management,* W. B. Saunders Company, Philadelphia, 1969.

Richardson, R. E., and Barton, R. E.: *The Dental Assistant,* 4th ed., McGraw-Hill Book Company, New York, 1970.

Slagon, G. J.: "Dental Receptionist Procedure Manual, Devonshire Publishing Co., Detroit, Mich.

Benjamin R. Baker
Applied Psychology

INTRODUCTION

People whose lifework is in health services need to develop a thorough working knowledge and understanding of basic psychology. It is important in dentistry because the dentist and the dentist's staff must know the variations of normal human behavior and what motivates human behavior. Applied psychology is concerned with the reactions of people to the stimulations of everyday life. With the use of applied psychology, one can program stimuli to get desired responses from people which can be predicted and controlled. Applied psychology can be used in dentistry to describe, predict, and control human activity and response so that patients' actions and decisions regarding dental services are influenced by the stimuli that are used.

The application of these researched and proven stimuli to produce a desired response is applied psychology. It implies that the knowledge of applied psychology may be enlisted for a useful purpose. This chapter is intended to introduce the student to some aspects of how people may be influenced to behave in specific ways through the use of proven methods. It serves only as an introduction to the subject. For those who desire a deeper understanding, it is suggested that the chapter references be used as a guide to learning more about human behavior.

Psychology Defined

There are as many definitions of psychology as there are authors who write about it. There is no simple explanation or definition of psychology. *Webster's New Twentieth Century Dictionary* defines psychology as "the science dealing with the mind and mental processes, feelings, desires. The sum of a person's actions, traits, attitudes, and thoughts." It might be more simply described, however, as an attempt to understand, predict, and control behavior. All definitions of psychology ultimately include two prominent words. These are *understanding* and *behavior.*

There are certain areas of study which must precede the application of psychology in dentistry. It is necessary to have some knowledge of human behavior. It is important to develop an understanding of personality and motivation. These are essential to controlling patient behavior in the dental office. Of equal importance are the art of communication with people and what goes into the development of attitudes of people. Understanding of these things is necessary for the application of appropriate stimuli in the dental office to obtain the desired patient response.

In summary, the basic emphasis of psychology is on behavior which results from adjustments to stimuli. The chief objectives of psychology are to understand, predict, and control behavior within reasonable bounds. Dentist and staff must be prepared to meet, treat, and maintain all manner of patients. They must be able to provide the proper atmosphere to keep everyone happy and satisfied. The best way to do this is through a comprehensive understanding of people. Understanding of people occurs when satisfactory adjustments to daily problems for one's self and associates is established. It is intended that the student may gain a better insight into self from this chapter.

Historical Development of Psychology

As modern sciences, psychology and dentistry developed at approximately the same time. While dentistry has been practiced for more than 4000 years, it has been developed as a modern science within the past 100 years. Psychology and dentistry as we know it today began in the final year of the nineteenth century. Psychology first gained recognition with the founding of the American Psychological Association in 1892 (Cinotti and Grieder, 1964). In the beginning, researchers in psychology would develop a theory of psychology. A school of thought would then evolve around the theory, and as each school of thought reached questions that could not be answered within the school, other schools sprang up. In order of their appearance the schools of structuralism, functionalism, behaviorism, gestaltism, and psychoanalysis succeeded each other (Cinotti and Greider, 1964). The school of transactional analysis has been the most recent to be developed. It provides the reader with a simple understanding of the behavior of people (Harper, 1975). Behaviorism appears to have excellent application in dentistry. The proponents of this area of psychology believe that behavior study is limited to overt behavior. This means that only those things which can be observed directly or manipulated are applicable in the study of human behavior. It was from this field of thought that the classic stimulus-response investigations grew and from which most true psychologic research has grown (Cinotti and Grieder, 1964). Thus, in dentistry, if the proper stimulus is known and applied to patients, it will yield the desired response in accepting treatment and maintaining optimum dental health.

Applied psychology is the outgrowth of taking the various psychologic thoughts and applying them to influence and modify behavior of people toward a desired result. Today this field has become so sophisticated that people are constantly being exposed to overt, subtle, and even subconscious stimuli to obtain predictable responses. This is best illustrated in advertising through newspapers and radio and television, where services, appliances, and commodities are sold through the use of stimuli which create a desire in the buyer. This is equally applicable in dentistry. When the dentist and his or her staff create the atmosphere of need and desirability of dental services, the patient is treated satisfactorily, and the service is rendered in an environment conducive to the well-being of all concerned.

PERSONALITY AND PERSONALITY DEVELOPMENT

The dental assistant can understand and utilize applied psychology at work and in everyday life with a better knowledge of personality. What constitutes human personality, how it is derived, and the impact of individual personalities on life and on other people are vital areas about which to learn. In the following pages some theories of the development of personality are presented. It is of the utmost importance for those who work in dental offices to have a depth of understanding of themselves in order to effectively deal with the many types of people and their personalities.

All people have a profound interest in themselves. One of their chief interests is in how they are received by others. In other words, people are interested in their own personality. Few people have the ability to describe what their personality really is. Educators in fact have some difficulty in defining personality. This is evident when more than 50 definitions of personality can be found in the *Dictionary of Psychological and Psychoanalytical Terms* (English and English, 1958). Personality deals with the whole person. It is constituted of all the factors in an individual's life which make him or her distinct from other people. The areas from which a personality is formed include the things we were born with such as intelligence, physical traits, and energy level. It includes acquired characteristics of family, culture, and the effects of motivation. Psychologists can arrive at an explanation of a personality through plotting the identifiable human traits of an individual. Since almost 18,000 human traits have been identified (Allport and Odbert, 1936), this would seem to be a colossal task. It is not the intent of this section to present such depth of insight into personality; this belongs properly in a more elaborate course of study. However, personality traits are of extreme importance since they provide tools for research in behavior. Every person has a series of traits peculiar to himself or herself which collectively are keys to his or her personality. The recognition of these traits can provide valuable knowledge in understanding why people act as they do.

The concept of personality presented here does not investigate the minutiae of psychologic research. It is a beginning to help the student see how people appear to others and to themselves. It consists of the mental and physical picture which people have of themselves (Cinotti and Grieder, 1964; Ruch, 1963). Maltz (1966) describes the personality as the total self-image a person possesses, and the self-image is the mental blueprint of all feelings, behavior, and abilities which are consistent in an individual. Cinotti and Grieder (1964) state that psychology recognizes three "selves" which make up the personality. These are the self we see, the self others see in us, and the objective self, which is our true personality since it exists independently of our own bias and of that of others. Understanding personality is important in the dental office because it is useful in channeling the approach to patients which will help satisfy their needs and interests. It is also important because the dental assistant must know about self-image before being able to function in dealing with the behavior and personalities of others.

Berne observed early in his work with transactional analysis that people literally changed before his eyes as he watched and listened to them. This occurred with vocabulary, posture, expressions, and body functions (Harris, 1973). Berne subsequently developed a theory of personality which states that all humans contain three types of ego states. An ego state is a coherent system of thought and feeling which can be directly observed and recorded in patterns of behavior in people. These ego states are the *parent ego state* (P), the *adult ego state* (A), and the *child ego state* (C). Each of the states is patterned after real people. In the child state people react to stimulus exactly the way they would do as a child prior to age 8. For those whose personality is dominated by the child ego state there is difficulty with adult responsibilities such as family and jobs. They also have frequent episodes of irrational and unrealistic behavior. In the parent ego state people think, feel, act, talk, and respond as their parents or parent substitutes did when they were small. The parent ego state is an accumulation of all the information a person perceives without making a critical analysis of it. When people are presented with problems to solve in daily living and they do not have adequate information, the parent ego state takes over, and they react in a "correct" or "suitable" manner based on their recollection of past information. The adult ego state functions as a computer. It is a data processing unit for making decisions. Adult ego state develops over the years while the parent and child states are held intact from childhood. There are no emotions in the adult state. The person appraises his or her situation objectively and makes decisions on the basis of past experience without emotion (Berne, 1964; Harris, 1973; Harper, 1975).

There are other theories of personality development which cannot be ignored. Some feel that the motivating force for behavior is a striving for superiority and power. This thesis contends that the child recognizes its inferiority early in life when parents demonstrate ability it does not have. From this point on it battles to be better. Harris illustrates this profoundly in his "I'm OK you're OK" explanation of transactional analysis. Garn (1960) has shown that personalities are controlled by four great drives of emotional appeal. These are money, romance, self-preservation, and recognition. These factors are motivating forces, one or more of which control the personality of the individual.

Bell has proposed that people have six major personality needs. These are to command, to attack, to avoid, to please, to perform, and to achieve, and that people satisfy these needs in their life-style. One of these needs will predominate in the personality with some overlap into the others. In life, people will project their personality into ambiguous situations without realizing it. For example, a person with a need to command will invariably try to control and dominate every situation she is in, while the pleaser will try to make others like him and will go to any lengths to gain acceptance. When the assistant can recognize the personality types of Garn and the personality styles of Bell, it is easier to channel them into a more receptive state in the dental office by stimulation of the specific type in evidence. Extra reading in these two books is highly recommended for personality understanding.

Culture also is a great force in the development of personality. The sociologic system in which we live dominates our life with unfulfilled needs and feelings. This leads to the development of anxiety. The personality is built and develops when we seek relief from anxiety. Gravitation is always toward anxiety relief. Those people or things which can relieve anxiety contribute to molding the personality. People have three alternatives in anxiety-relief situations, relative to other people. They may move toward them, against them, or away from them. One's adjustments in behavior and life are based upon reactions in these three directions (Horney, 1945). This theory is reinforced by the ideas of Garn and Bell above.

Human personality develops through seven stages of psychosexual development. These stages begin with the oral stage at birth and progressively include anal, genital, latency, adolescence, adulthood, and senescence stages. During each stage of psychosexual development individuals must meet and cope with all types of problems. The achievements of meeting and dealing with problems result in personality development (English, 1963). Personality maladjustments occur when the individual does not successfully meet problems which arise in psychosexual development. This creates more conflicts and reflects again in the personality of the individual. The reactions may become severe and eventually require therapy for resolution because of an inability of the individual to recognize and cope with unresolved conflicts. Psychoanalysis was developed to investigate the reasons for inner conflict and bring them out of the subconscious into conscious recognition. Hopefully it frees the individual if successful (Cinotti and Grieder, 1964). Transactional analysis also is designated to accomplish this same purpose (Harper, 1975).

In summary personality is the sum of a great complex of forces which begin at birth and contribute to behavior throughout life. There are many factors that contribute to the personality. The personality traits seen in patients in the dental office may be only one aspect of the true personality. Therefore when more is known by the assistant about personality in general and about human behavior, it will be possible for the assistant to function at a much higher level and contribute to a satisfying service for all in office contacts with people.

MOTIVATION

All human behavior is motivated by something. People employed in a health service which deals with people must know why people behave as they do. The contents of the previous pages describe the basic components involved in personality and in personality development. The factors of personality offer keys to motivations for behavior. The personality of the individual has considerable bearing upon the motivational triggers which will achieve satisfaction of needs. In the subsequent pages of this section information is presented on the factors which constitute motives and on the application of the motivational areas which may be successfully applied in dentistry. The dental assistant will learn that effectiveness in the dental office, as well as in life in general, will increase with an understanding of motivation for behavior.

Motives

A *motive* may be described as any active, driving need or force which is capable of causing action or other behavior of the individual or group. Every human act is based upon a reason. All reasons for action therefore are motives. Motivation consists of two fundamental components. The first as stated above is a drive or need. Needs may be classified as physiologic (biologic), psychologic, or social (Ruch, 1963). The second component is the object, situation, or attainment of gratification related to the need. The way in which goals are attained is also a component of motivation. Therefore behavior is determined by a need and the interaction of insight with the need. In other words, if a need exists and there is an incentive or goal which accompanies it, the activity of the individual will be directed toward meeting the need. Needs are acquired and have certain characteristics which produce behavior under given conditions. These characteristics may be called *cues* which guide persons to take action. Cues then are motives which can precipitate specific action to satisfy a need. Cues may also be directed toward escape from anxiety situations of fear, pain, or other unpleasant experiences. The latter cue has significance in dentistry, as do gratification-seeking cues. The seeking of pain relief is an example of a cue in dentistry, and the dentist is the object that provides gratification.

Currently motives may be divided into two rather broad general classifications. The first is called the *primary innate* or *internal* drives which consist of thirst, hunger, pain, and fear. Primary drives include all the basic automatic biologic functions including sexual needs. The second classification of motives is the *secondary* or *learned* drive. These are created by the nature and conditions of the surroundings in which we live (society). Learned drives are socially acquired and may vary from simple drives to those which are intricate and dynamic in structure. Learned drives are of prime importance in human behavior because they are subject to influence. This has great value in providing an approach to dental service for people. (Haney, 1962; Calhoon, 1963; Ruch, 1963).

Maslow (1943) has postulated that there is a hierarchy of needs. That is to say, needs of the individual have an order of priority. When lower needs are unsatisfied it is difficult to activate higher needs until the lower needs are met and satisfied. Some primary needs may be sidetracked so that a higher need may be met. Society has taught us to adjust and subvert some needs temporarily while seeking other satisfaction. Once a lower need is satisfied the next highest need comes to the consciousness and dominates until it is fulfilled in normal situations. This occurs because motives (drives) which have been satisfied no longer act as motivators. The order of needs begins with physiologic (primary) drives. Upon satisfaction they are replaced by safety and security needs. When these no longer motivate in a given situation, they are supplanted in turn by drives for love, regard, or affection. The higher needs of self-esteem and self-actualization are more consistent with long-range goals. They are the last to be satisfied in the order of priority of needs according to Maslow. There can be overlap of needs wherein one may be satisfying many needs at one and the same time. Age and growth and development can cause changes in needs. That is, with age some acquired needs are no longer motivators, but new ones supplant them.

Concomitant with primary and secondary needs are motives called psychologic needs. These needs may fall into both of the general classifications of primary and secondary categories. They motivate the individual to seek an environment which will satisfy all his or her social needs such as love, security, approval, and status. As such, they are basic to the maintenance of the self-image. In recent years affluence of the American community has made the satisfaction of primary needs less difficult to attain. Accordingly it is not a problem in modern living to meet the lower needs. It follows therefore that the secondary (learned) drives in modern society are the motivating forces behind most normal and abnormal behavior. Ruch (1963) has grouped these motives into what he calls a psychological social set of needs. These are the areas in which advertising and industrial psychology have formed a vast potential to influence behavior. Some of these areas are discussed below as they may be applied to dentistry.

Motivation Factors

It has been previously shown that motives (drives) are the basis for human behavior and that motives are arranged in an order of priority. When lower needs are met, higher needs dominate the consciousness for satisfaction. Higher needs (secondary drives) are acquired from society. Satisfaction of needs to relieve drives is influenced by social environment and patterns of living. One of the largest and most influential industries in the United States has developed in response to research into what influences secondary-need satisfaction. This is the advertising business. Within the past 50 years social scientists and psychologists have increasingly left academics and moved into advertising to influence buying and selling of products through application of their knowledge of motivational behavior. The extent of the influence that these people have had upon the American public is evident in the methods of selling which appeal to the individual through the media of television, radio, and newspaper. Today the science of selling is so sophisticated that people no longer pay much attention to the real value of things that they buy. Instead they buy according to the power of persuasion of advertising that appeals to their ego. Most of this is so subtle that people are not aware of it. Vance Packard has shown the American public a deep insight into the influences of advertising on behavior in two of his books, *The Status Seekers* and *The Hidden Persuaders*. In these books he explains how psychologic and social research have produced motivation analyses of the needs of the public. He also points out how the desires of the individual can be stimulated and influenced in definite directions. Motivation analysts look for reasons for behavior in people. Application of psychology toward stimulating them makes it possible to manipulate people to buy specific products. The transfer of these principles from marketing to dentistry by those in dental service would produce more and better service to more satisfied patients. This application is only beginning in dentistry. Motivation research deals not only with the conscious but also with the subconscious. In fact the subtle applications of advertising motives probably reach the subconscious more effectively than the conscious. The psychology of selling is based upon stimulation of emotional needs, compulsive acts, and unconscious actions to enhance the self-image. People are motivated for different reasons, but their actions are intricately woven around personality and personal gratification. How they react and in what direction can be significantly influenced by the proper power of suggestion. The profundity of the influence in these areas by advertising is colossal.

What are some of the motivating factors which influence behavior and which may be applied to dentistry? Garn (1960) has stated that emotional appeal is the answer to behavioral patterns. It is his thesis that there are four different emotional appeals which may influence behavior. These are the motivational factors of self-preservation, money, romance, and recognition. Every person is fundamentally influenced by all four of these areas in some way, but only one emotional appeal predominates. Garn further feels that once a pattern is established wherein one of the four emotional appeals predominates, it never changes. For instance, if money is the primary motivating factor of an individual, it will continue to influence his actions throughout life even though he becomes financially secure. Furthermore it is relatively easy to recognize what type of emotional appeal predominates in the personality of the individual. This is given away in actions, reactions, and attitudes of the person. These cues are of profound value in dentistry since recognition of the motives which cause behavior can guide the dentist's approach to the patient, resulting in good rapport as well as selling a service. Bell's theory of six personality styles (needs) of people also applies here.

There are other motives which influence behavior. They may be related to society through the culture we live in. The resultant behavior is governed by rules, custom, laws, and religious and ethnic background. The way we speak and dress and our living patterns are established by society. Conformation is the accepted thing or rejection by society can be expected. How we look and act are important drives. In certain areas of Africa missing upper teeth and alteration to the upper central incisors are symbols of manhood. All young males aspire to such symbols of recognition. In our own culture missing teeth with poor oral appearance carry entirely opposite social implications. Therefore most patients whose oral condition has deteriorated to this point have drives to seek relief in the dental office through prosthetic services and preventive dentistry. This is contingent upon the social strata in which they live.

Packard (1959) has pointed out that status seeking by the American people is one of the strongest motivational drives in many areas of living. This includes dental service. He indicates that there are many levels of social class and that there is constant effort to move up to a higher social class. Social class is a concept which tries to explain differences in behavior, thought, and feelings among people. Money, or possession of money, apparently is not the chief criterion for assignment to a social class. Rather, a style of life, values, and personality seem to be the chief factors here (American Dental Association, Bureau of Economic Research and Statistics, 1958). "Keeping up with and passing the Joneses" is the unwritten motto of status seekers. One of these areas of concern is dentistry and how it is regarded. For instance brand-name buying of commercial products is a form of status seeking. In dentistry the dentist who treats the "right" people is highly sought after for treatment, whether or not his or her talents are commensurate with this regard. Snob appeal of associating with the higher-status individual in the dental office can be a strong motivational force for some people.

Cinotti and Grieder (1964) have described other motives for behavior which have special relation to dentistry. Some of these are dependence, negative factors, recognition, and positive factors. Dependence is a learned need. Cinotti and Grieder indicate that many people who have unfulfilled dependence needs may find relief in the intimate contact of dentist and patient, because of the sustained attention which the dentist gives the patient. It is the author's experience that this is especially true in certain orthodontic and pedodontic situations. It might also be seen even more prominently in periodontics. Negative factors of pain are often the prime reason for the first contact between the patient and the dental office. Fear of loss of the teeth has been related psychologically to loss of youthful appearance and virility (American Dental Association Bureau of Economic Research and Statistics, 1958). Many patients will go to great extremes to preserve their youthful appearance. In America there is a significant negative factor of fear of bad breath. Most toothpaste advertising dwells upon this rather than the true value to be gained by tooth brushing. Fear of bad breath is a significant motivator which brings people to the dentist. Cinotti and Grieder also feel that higher needs may be reached with positive factors of good restorative dentistry and preventive dentistry in many people. The patient's appreciation of these is not basic; it must be learned. It is the responsibility of the dentist and the staff to engender these motives for two reasons. First, it provides the tools for rendering a better service while creating an atmosphere of complete understanding between patient and dentist. Second, the carry-over values to the patient for better dental health are incalculable.

ATTITUDES TOWARD DENTISTRY

Historic records reveal the practice of dentistry by professionals over 4000 years ago in Egypt. Down through the ages records, books, paintings, and pieces of sculpture have consistently emphasized the unpleasant, painful experiences related to dental service. Unpleasant association with dentistry no longer need be the case with the advent and refinement of modern anesthesia. However, early experiences which have been passed down through several generations have contributed to a strong tradition and folklore about teeth and dental service. Since self-gratification is not provided by painful experience in normal people, it is not difficult to understand how negative feelings remain prevalent even though unpleasantness and pain may be effectively removed from dental appointments. The feelings people have about teeth are deep-seated as a result of a history of pain involved encounters with the dentist in the past. It is further supported by experience, superstition, and instruction by teachers and even by the dentist. In trying to understand behavior of people so that the assistant can apply this knowledge to his or her job, some insight into attitudes toward dentistry, teeth, and the dentist should prove helpful. Feelings about teeth are strong factors which motivate people to care for or to neglect their teeth. Yet, it cannot be assumed that knowledge of teeth and of the value of good dental care will be the cues which will produce the response of seeking good care and maintaining good dental health. People just do not respond logically to comprehensive dental service even though they know that the ultimate result of neglect is catastrophic. There appear to be certain underlying factors of a subconscious nature which control the reactions that result in the care of the teeth. (See "Motivation: Satisfying a Need" in Chap. 19.)

Feelings about teeth begin to develop early in life. In the infant the mouth is the greatest source of pleasure. All the child's sources of pleasure are focused in the oral area. This involves sucking and sensations of touch and warmth. When teeth appear the pleasure aspects of the mouth may be interrupted because of the pain of teething (see "Eruption" in Chap. 26). The eruption of teeth occurs usually at the same time that other social adjustments appear. The child's intimate contact with its mother becomes more distant since nursing by the mother ceases with the appearance of teeth (Adams, 1963). Throughout the life of the child the experiences in which teeth are involved contribute to its attitude toward dentistry. What happens to its teeth is a source of social concern which has emotional overtones. Losing primary teeth, traumatic accidents, and orthodontics all bring focus upon the child from parents and other adults as well as peers. The appearance of the first cavity with the first trip to the dentist can be the initiation of negative or positive feelings toward the dentist. It also precipitates the attitude of reward and punishment with dental service. For instance all children enjoy sugar-containing foods. The appearance of decay in the teeth early in life may mean deprivation of pleasure acts of eating sweets. This is a punishment to the child which is associated with the dentist because that is where the deprivation originated. Appointments with the dentist may also come during playtime or during a favorite television cartoon program. Under these conditions it is hard for the child to associate the value of care and pleasant experiences with the dentist. The negative feelings developed carry over into adult life. As the child approaches adulthood it increasingly assumes the attitude that teeth and dental care are negative factors which have rather profound psychologic meanings (Callahan, 1964).

Adult attitudes toward dentistry are derived from a much wider range of influence. People have feelings about their teeth which vary from positive attitudes of pleasure and reward to negative attitudes of pain, trouble, and problems. This is compounded by beliefs that people are born with "hard" or "soft" teeth. This concept is one of the most difficult for the dentist to confront and dispel. Because of these predominant attitudes people seek dental care only when the condition of their teeth or related dental problems are in the late stages of breakdown. Thus the main function of the dentist for most people is to repair teeth or relieve pain. This reduces the real main function of prevention. Although people know that dental services are in their best interest, they do not act to avail themselves accordingly because of their deep-seated feelings and attitudes. Some of the predominant feelings adults have about teeth are that they inherit good or bad teeth. They feel that good dental care makes little difference because sooner or later the loss of their teeth is inevitable. People feel also that they are supposed to lose teeth as they grow older. The old wives' tale of loss of one tooth by the mother for each child born is derived from this pattern of thinking even though it is entirely false. Dental trouble is regarded as socially acceptable by the public. It is generally thought of as happening to older people or to lower-class people but it *can* happen to *anyone* sooner or later. Thus dental problems can cross social-stratum lines without loss of status to the individual. In this sense dental problems may be used as a status symbol since treatment requiring specialists has greater prestige value than treatment by the general dentist.

There is evidence that attitudes toward teeth

and dentistry may be classified according to the individual's social position. A study conducted by Social Research, Inc., for the American Dental Association revealed many attitudes about dentistry which occur in the various social classes. Social class falls into four categories. These are upper middle class, lower middle class, upper lower class, and lower lower class. The behavior of people who fall in these groups relative to dentistry can be quite distinctive. The attitudes of one group are not confined to that particular group but cross over into all positions in society to a degree. It is true, however, that certain attitudes are more prominent in one group than in another. The results of one section of the study are summarized below for each social class. (See Table 3-1.)

The upper middle class consists of people whose lifework is in the professions and also the business-executive group. Most of these people are well educated. They seek expert advice in all of their living, and it is reflected in their attitudes toward dental care. Good teeth are highly valued, and these individuals are amenable to instruction in decay prevention. Dental care begins early as they recognize the value of teeth to health as well as to personal appearance. With this attitude they are generally willing to go to great lengths to preserve their teeth and their youthful appearance.

The lower middle class is composed of people who own small businesses, lower-echelon executives, teachers, salespeople, and white-collar workers. These people make up 35 percent of the population of the United States. They are status conscious and often seek to emulate the

Table 3-1 | Class Attitudes to Dental Care*

Upper middle class	Lower middle class	Upper lower class	Lower lower class
Professional people, business executives, generally well educated	Small businessmen, junior executives, teachers, salespeople, white-collar workers	Skilled and semiskilled blue-collar workers	Unskilled laborers
1. Seek expert advice in all areas of life, especially medicine and dentistry 2. Value good teeth 3. Respond well to prevention when motivated 4. Dental care begins at early age 5. High interest in a youthful appearance	1. Status seekers 2. Compulsive attitudes toward dental care 3. Follow concepts of what is good for the child with inflexible rigidity 4. Social value of examinee in good condition is of highest concern 5. Conscious of health value of good teeth 6. Easily motivated if status value is presented	1. Modest education 2. Respectable, hard-working, law-abiding people 3. Many do not plan ahead well 4. Stoic and pessimistic demeanor 5. Feel teeth are inherited strong or soft 6. Expect dentures at an early age 7. Difficult to motivate for regular care, either restoration or prevention	1. Minimum education 2. No organized pattern of living 3. Live from hand to mouth 4. Dental care is at bottom of priorities 5. Seek only emergency care until all teeth are lost 6. Resigned to early dentures and seek early extractions 7. Consider all dental services as painful, undesirable experiences

* While the chart describes the general attitudes of people in the four groups, there are frequent exceptions in upward directions from the bad attitudes of the upper lower and lower lower classes, and there are frequently poorer attitudes in the lower middle class and the upper middle class.

upper middle class. Their attitudes toward dentistry indicate that they are the most compulsive of all social classes toward good dental care. What is good for the child is followed with inflexible rigidity for various reasons. The parents' experiences with their own teeth may motivate the compulsive behavior. The social value of sound and attractive teeth is of the highest concern. This might explain the attitude of some in seeking pedodontic and orthodontic services for the young. They are conscious of the health value as well as the social value of good teeth. Self-preservation, recognition, romance, and money motivation factors as well as status seeking affect people in this social class profoundly.

The upper lower class is composed of the skilled and semiskilled blue-collar workers. They are characterized by modest educational experience. For the most part they are respectable, hardworking, law-abiding citizens. There is very little planning ahead by this group. They are rather stoic and pessimistic in outlook. That is, they expect catastrophe to happen and are resigned to it. They assume that teeth are strong or "soft" and that dentures are the end result at an early adult age. They do not follow dental or medical advice with regularity, and they frequent the dental office only for emergency relief. It must be said that there are many exceptions to this pattern, as there are people in all classes who strive for the best in dental services. The importance of preventive dentistry is extremely hard to communicate to the majority of this group.

The lower lower class consists of the unskilled laborers. They generally have minimal education and show no organized pattern of living. They live for the present and their existence is hand-to-mouth. The care of the teeth is at the bottom of their list of health or social priorities. The resignation to the inevitable seen in the upper lower class is more prominent in the lower lower class. This group typifies the statement that people can know about good dental care and still do practically nothing about it. Pain and painful health experiences are expected by this group. For this reason they seek multiple extractions and dentures early in adult life as the escape from dental trouble. In reality they do not escape from dental trouble with this tangent.*

The dental assistant must not assume that attitudes of all people fall into the above categories according to their social class. The above only serves to illustrate the predominant attitudes of the social classes presented. There are many people in the upper middle class who have no more appreciation of the value of good dentistry than the lowest of the lower class. In turn, there are many lower-class individuals whose appreciation of good health and cleanliness is a strong motivation. These are highly motivated to seek the best dental care. Therefore judgment of what kind of dentistry a person prefers must not be hasty and should be reserved until the dentist can make a more definitive evaluation of the patient. The dentist should therefore never preassess the dentistry a patient will accept by the way the patient looks or the social stratum from which the patient comes. This is a mistake many dentists make, however, and the loss of a valuable patient is the result.

ATTITUDES TOWARD DENTISTS

The majority of dental patients have very little contact with the dentist or the dental staff outside the office. Consequently dentists frequently have little idea of the image they exhibit to patients. How people feel about dentists as health-affairs people is important to know. Information in this area may provide dentists with the key to open the doors of comprehensive patient care which otherwise might be permanently closed. It may also give them cause to improve their professional image.

* The above discussion of social classes and attitudes toward dentistry was researched for the American Dental Association by Social Research, Inc.

Generally, dentistry is regarded as a high-status profession. But the average person does not feel that it should rate with medicine since dentistry as it is commonly understood only involves the oral cavity whereas the physician is thought to treat the whole body. Most people do not realize that dental treatment affects the total health and cannot be removed from the total person. Dentists are regarded as necessary. The dentist is thought of synonymously with pain, drilling, and extractions. Very few people consider the dentist in the context of prevention. Dentists are also regarded as money conscious. That is, dental service is expensive. Many people in the lower social classes use their knowledge of the high cost of dentistry as rationale for not seeking good care. The anxieties and fears of patients relative to dental appointments are reflected in their attitudes toward the dentist. Children characteristically question the dentist about giving them a "shot." Their apprehensiveness about the administration of local anesthetic has been picked up from parents. It has been the author's experience that a logical, truthful approach reduces fear and management problems and produces trust and a good attitude in children toward the dentist. In this regard dentists are often responsible for certain attitudes by the manner in which they handle patients. Attitudes are predominantly related to anxieties created with dental appointments. The typical feelings toward dentists are that they are not sympathetic. They are rough, they are aloof, and they are concerned only with the patient's teeth instead of with the person as a whole. Some of these attitudes are produced when patients cannot be appointed at times convenient for them or when they have to wait beyond their scheduled appointment time to be treated (American Dental Association Bureau of Economic Research and Statistics, 1958; Reppert, Updegrave, and Shaffer, 1958).

Many negative attitudes toward dentists are caused by the dentists themselves. This is why it is so important to know and understand people.

Dental appointments are intimately personal experiences. Dentists who cannot take the time to explain procedures and to calm anxious people do a distinct disservice to themselves and the profession. For these reasons it is of the utmost importance for dentists and their staffs to treat all patients with respect. Society criticizes all professional people who do not accept their professional responsibility and act accordingly. The attitudes of the public toward dentistry and dentists are determined not by technical competence but by the manner in which patients are cared for in the office. Dentists who can accept people as they are morally and socially, without trying to change them, can do much for the image of their profession. They also become more popular, and there is a greater demand for their services.

DENTAL PSYCHOLOGY

The foregoing material presented in this chapter has been concerned with some of the various factors which collectively make up the personalities of people and factors which are responsible for certain behavioral patterns in people. The remaining portion of the chapter is concerned with how to use the knowledge of personality and behavior to sell dentistry and to create a satisfying atmosphere in the dental office for the patient as well as for the dentist and his or her staff.

There are certain fundamental requirements for success in dentistry. The dentist must have the technical skill to produce sound dental service. He or she must be able to manage finances with competence. The dentist must be able to influence patients toward dental goals which are beneficial and must be able to retain these patients in the practice. The dentist must have a certain amount of innate ability to do all these things. Some people are born with high manual dexterity, a pleasing disposition, and good common sense. However, the great majority of skills necessary to practice dentistry successfully are learned. There is some evidence, for instance, that the dental student who leads his or her class does not necessarily always meet with the greatest success in the business world—unless academic and manual skills are accompanied by an equally important ability to communicate with people.

In the dental office patients are not only seeking technical skill to provide solutions to their dental problems; they are also looking for complete treatment and sympathetic understanding. Consumer surveys show that people will shop where there is a warm human relationship. Dentistry offers an intangible service of knowledge, skill, experience, and advice. This makes the job of selling dentistry more difficult and is in itself a commanding reason for dentists to use all the psychologic factors available to make patients happy. Dr. Louis Marchand has often said that every patient who comes into his office must be treated as though he were a guest in his home and that he places an imaginary sign on every patient's back which reads "treat me nice"! Most unsuccessful dentists ignore the "treat me nice" concept. They ignore the application of psychologic principles to effective communication and depend upon their ability and the assumption that they are in demand. It is unfortunate that this situation occurs frequently because it lowers the image of dentistry and creates dissatisfaction and negative attitudes in patients.

Balinsky and Burger (1963) have stated that personal communication is the handle to all other executive tools and that the quality of fact-to-face contacts can determine the effectiveness of any practice or business. The gap between dental need and dental demand can be closed as a result of greater affluence in America today. Thus there is an increasing demand for services. This places dentists in an enviable position because they are needed. However, in time the dentist who uses knowledge and understanding of behavior to treat the whole person will be in even greater demand. He or she will provide a satisfying service and make people happier in their treatment, and this dentist will be a more content person. Levoy (1966) calls this serving best. He indicates that it is important to serve the entirety of the patient, including all social and psychologic needs for self-importance. The dentist who can provide dental service with a feeling of personal worth and dignity for his or her patients uses the little things to improve the patients' self-image. When people leave the dental office feeling good about their contact with the dentist, they are likely to return and bring their friends for treatment.

An increasing sensitivity toward others and the ability to understand others can be developed. It requires some study and the understanding of one's own self and goals before complete effectiveness can be achieved. Until we understand ourselves, we cannot function optimally with others. Once we do know ourselves, we are quick to recognize typical behavioral patterns in others which we can react to in order to provide the human contacts that patients need. When patients are given something of psychologic value, both parties benefit. It takes little effort to use praise or to be interested and friendly. When treatment is pleasant, the patient is reconditioned and becomes more receptive. If the patient is more receptive, more can be done in his or her behalf.

It must not be assumed that all patients can be treated alike. There are no two persons alike. Each patient must be treated individually in order to establish the most favorable communication. Calhoon (1963) has listed several factors which influence communication. These include learning, personality, motivation of the patient, and the effectiveness of the communicator. Communication involves the receptivity of the patient, the method of conveying the message, its organization, and the predisposition of the listener. In order to communicate effectively the dentist must use the approach which is most appropriate for the particular patient. Garn (1960) feels that the greatest deterrent to getting through to the patient is preoccupation with other things and the greatest asset in selling a service is in emotional appeal. If there is no emotional reaction to the seller's offer, there is no sale. Therefore being able to pick out areas of emotional appeal is essential in communication with dental patients.

Every potential patient who contacts the dental office brings a unique nature, set of motives, and personality into contact with the office personnel. In treatment the dentist must be able to identify with the patient's needs and deal with them while keeping his or her own identity. In the patient there will be various needs to be satisfied. Some of these are primitive needs such as the need for pain relief. Other needs revolve around the personality of the patient and the motivation factors which contribute to his or her drives. When needs are predominantly basic, as in threat situations to general health and the relief of pain, patients are more open to treatment suggested by the dentist. When the lower needs are not dominant, the dentist must be able to persuade patients what is best for their treatment. In this situation recognition of motivation factors and attitudes is of the utmost importance in establishing communication. Different personalities react to different persuasive appeals. For example intelligent patients may be approached with a rational and logical argument relative to their treatment needs, while people who are particularly economical tend to be influenced by the amount of money which the treatment will save them over a period of time. Individuals especially conscious of their own appearance will be influenced by the aesthetic aspects of the proposed dental treatment. All patients can be reached to a degree by the fear and guilt approaches to dental problems; this is particularly true of very young and elderly patients. This is a potentially dangerous position to take, however, because some patients may respond negatively to being made to feel guilty about neglect.

To establish good rapport with patients it is necessary for the dentist and dental staff to know and utilize the personality characteristics of people. These are factors which can be recognized through astute observation of patients. It is essential also for dentist and staff to cultivate pleasing personalities of their own. It is not always possible to get through to patients and convince them of their dental needs. Many times patients will not want to hear what is necessary to resolve their problems, and they will resist the dentist's efforts. It is in these instances that the dentist must be extremely perceptive in his or her communication. Any actions or words by the dentist in the treatment situation which are received as a threat to the self-image of the patient will also result in resistance and rejection of treatment by the patient. This is known as "tuning out" or "turning off" in more colloquial terms.

Berne felt that every communication with another person was a transaction between them. As long as transactions are complementary, they will proceed smoothly, because the lines of communication remain open. Complementary transactions occur when the ego state (P,A,C) of the receiver responds in a parallel line or positively to the ego state of the person who initiated the communication. Crossed transactions occur when the receiving ego state responds in an ego state contradictory or antagonistic to the stimulus. For example, if a patient says to the dentist, "I know I should not have waited so long to come back to you because now I am in pain, and the tooth is abscessed," and the dentist responds, "That's all right, let's get you out of pain for now, later we can get started on getting your teeth healthy," then a complementary transaction has occurred, and communication is established. If the dentist responds, "I told you so, and it serves you right for not doing what I told you," then a crossed transaction has occurred. The lines of communication cease, and the patient ego state is assaulted. The likelihood of continued treatment with the latter response is poor. The assistant must be able to assess the ego state from which the patient speaks and acts and respond at all times with complementary

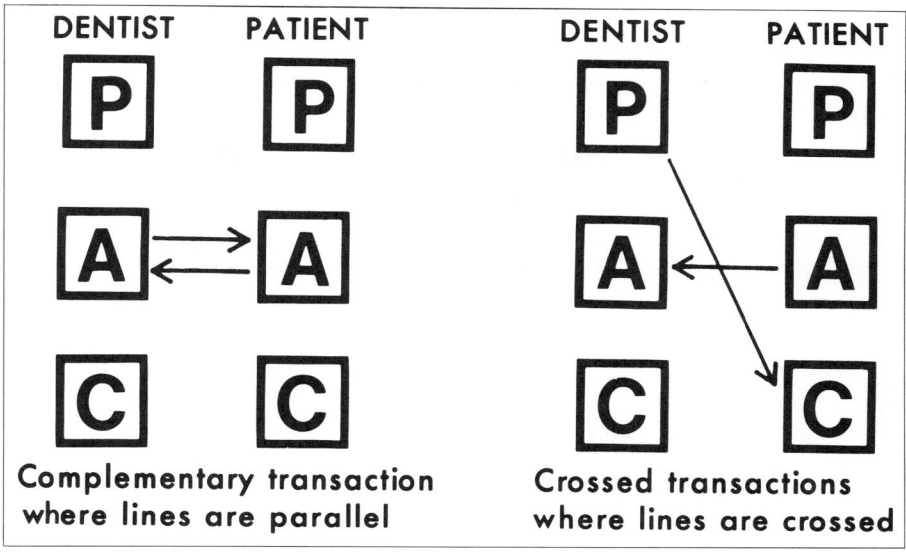

Figure 3-1 | Complementary and crossed transactions between dentist and patient.

transactions for better communication and better patient attitude about the office. (See Fig. 3-1.)

The knowledge of personality motivation and patient attitude toward dentistry are all the psychologic tools necessary to establish good patient relations. This knowledge merely needs application in the appropriate form at the appropriate time. It is advisable to know as much as possible about the patient's personal as well as dental needs. The best way to do this is to allow the patients to talk freely. When patients are allowed to talk, they will bring out many primary as well as subconscious concerns. Personality styles will always surface in these sessions and provide cues for the dentist and staff to follow for better relationships. Nothing is more pleasing to one's self-image than to have a good listener. If a patient is comfortable while talking, much more information will be made available. This will include reasons for coming in, attitudes toward dentistry and the dentist, keys to the patient's personality, and motivation factors of behavior. Every patient has an emotional weak spot which can be used to the dentist's advantage. If these areas are drawn into the open through allowing patients to talk about themselves, the dentist can use the information to establish rapport and win confidence. In turn this will lower the barriers of resistance; desirable treatment can then follow. The dental assistant who sees patients first can use the same psychology to set the stage for the dentist.

The ability to deal with people on their own level will allow one to get to know them better. Once a friendly basis has been established, patients become at ease and more open in the treatment situation. This leads to trust and confidence. When communication of this type is established, the dentist is able to do much more for patients.

A patient may often reject treatment for no apparent reason. Generally this is a result of a breakdown in communication or an error in judgment in patient handling. Most people are negative in their reactions toward expressions of disapproval, contradiction, or excessive authoritativeness from the dentist. It is not a good idea for the dentist and especially the dental assistant to show disapproval of patients' conditions and attitudes. In some situations it is necessary to be authoritative, and the dentist must always be in complete control of the patient in all treatment situations. The dentist will, however, meet all kinds of people. Therefore he or she must learn to like all kinds of people. This dentist must also learn to accept the attitudes of patients without visible opinion or disapproval. Patients may react negatively when they perceive irritability in the dentist's demeanor, either implicitly or overtly. If an awkward situation arises in the office as a result of lack of awareness of certain factors, it behooves the dentist to make every effort to remedy the situation.

The assistant and the secretary must be constantly aware of the sensitivities of patients, because their attitudes and behavior with patients may inadvertently create hostility and rejection. Patients are under stress anytime they enter a dental office. They are more vulnerable to suggestion, and they can easily misinterpret comments. Health service of any type is extremely personal, and patients expect and deserve respect and confidence concerning their health problems. Because of these things, it is of great importance for the assistant to be guarded in any comments to patients relative to their needs and treatment. When patients go to other offices for treatment, it is almost always due to a failure or breakdown in communications. Every dentist is automatically a psychologist by virtue of the nature of his or her work in dealing intimately with people. The more successful dentist is the one who is more adept at applied psychology.

PSYCHOLOGY IN TREATMENT-PLAN APPOINTMENTS

The average dental patient of today is smarter and more sophisticated than previously and comes from the middle class predominantly. However, the affluent society has made dental service more accessible to many more people. In all the patients who seek treatment there is a basic need to be informed and educated as to the benefits of good dentistry. The greatest problem among dentists in treatment-plan presentation is that they do not take time to educate their patients. Patient education as to their personal dental needs is of fundamental importance in applied psychology. Too many dentists feel that the problem of dental education is the responsibility of the patient, and they resent it when patients challenge treatment proposals and ask questions relative to the validity of treatment. In essence, however, most patients ask questions to learn what is going on and what is being planned for them and why. Recognition of this psychologic learning situation by the dentist is one of the best and lasting ways to secure patient trust and respect. Failure to recognize these factors is a travesty of the profession. More often than not the latter course of action is taken by the dentist to that dentist's detriment.

In order to present a good treatment plan the dentist must first be a good listener. Too often the dentist is more concerned with impressing the patient with his or her own knowledge and importance than with understanding the patient. In this type of office patients are not reached and either reject treatment or agree only to essential needs. The dentist must first understand the patients. When patients reveal their problems, the dentist should listen closely. The comments of the patients help the dentist tailor his or her approach to selling his or her service, because the patients have provided the dentist with clues to their personalities, fears, needs, and reasons for seeking dental treatment.

The dental assistant is of great value to the dentist when following the same protocol in contacts with patients before and after appointments. When the treatment plans are presented, the information from the patients will be used to establish a bond of trust and confidence which enhances their self-image. The self-image is further reinforced with praise, acceptance, understanding, and genuine interest in their welfare. When treatment plans are presented in an atmosphere of dignity and professional bearing with warmth and sincerity, a confidence and respect is created which results in patient acceptance. In treatment presentations patients are the same whether buying dental service or goods at the department store. People shop where there is a warm human relationship. Simply stated, if the dentist practices the rule of "treat me nice" he or she will be successful. If the assistant follows the rules of "treat me nice," his or her job security is greatly enhanced, for the dentist will appreciate these functions.

On occasion, patient misunderstanding creates unpleasant situations which must be coped with. These problems may be resolved, however, with the application of some psychologic techniques. Cinotti and Grieder (1964) recommend the following sequence. The dentist must convince the patient that he (or she) does not want to argue. He must listen until the patient is finished without interruption and try to see the patient's point of view. When possible he finds a point of agreement with the patient and settles the matter at once. This is a sound approach. In such instances the dentist and staff should do well to remember to try to establish an "I'm OK, you're OK" atmosphere quickly if possible. If not, any complimentary transaction is preferable to an intrusion or cross fire which will further antagonize. On rare occasions some patients will never be receptive to settling differences and will continue to bicker. Where this occurs, it will be better for both parties to part company; the dentist should not hesitate to dismiss a troublemaker from his or her practice. More often the objections and grievances which patients have are only misunderstandings which need to be cleared up. In these situations the dentist should listen through the complaint. The dentist should respect the feelings of such patients while attempting to win them over to his or her point of view, if it is correct. If the dentist is wrong, he or she should admit it.

It is unwise to allow personal feelings to enter into any discussion regardless of the provocation. Many personalities are strongly conditioned toward the rightness or wrongness of situations and have a drive to win at all costs in situations of grievances. If the dentist assumes an attitude of *win* in arguments, he or she may well win the argument but lose the patient in the process. This attitude must be avoided because any communication which poses a threat to the self-image of the patient will produce a breakdown of confidence between patient and dentist. From that point on satisfaction in treatment is difficult. The dental assistant *never* participates in situations of reconciling differences of treatment.

APPLIED PSYCHOLOGY AND DENTAL ASSISTANTS

The dental assistant's deportment in the office closely follows that of the dentist-employer or conforms to the image that the employer wants his or her office to convey to the public. There are certain general psychosocial concepts which can be used by the assistant to create an atmosphere of warmth and interest in the dental office. They are common-sense measures which enhance the self-image of other people, but they have proven value in patient rejection. The purpose of the dental office is to provide a health service. Service cannot be given without patients. Thus it should be recognized that patients are the most important part of the practice. They should be treated accordingly. There is nothing more disconcerting to patients than to be referred to in a treatment situation without a personal touch. The assistant should use the patient's name in all communication situations. It is much better to greet a patient with a genuine smile and say "Mr. Jones, we are ready for you now" than it is to say "You're next." Courtesy is contagious in all dealings with people. This should be a cardinal rule for the assistant in relations with patients.

The atmosphere of a dental office is reflected

in the actions of the people who work in it. Patients are sensitive to the feelings of others in dental offices. If the office is cheerful and the assistant smiles, patients will return the smile. If there is dissension among members of the staff, this also can be perceived and uneasiness can create stress situations which transfer to the patient. There is no place in the dental office for negative actions among assistants or patients or between the two. All activities of the assistants in the conduct of duties in the office should be carried out with an air of supreme confidence and pride. It is necessary for assistants to display confidence and pride sincerely. This means that they should seek employment from a dentist where they will have no difficulty in exhibiting these qualities.

Knowledge of personality types and motivational factors is of value to the assistant in the choice of appropriate words in meeting, greeting, seating, and treating patients. Patients see assistants first and last in appointments. When the assistant communicates with patients from an applied psychologic point of view, the self-image of both is cultivated and favorable impressions of the office are created with each visit. The enthusiastic patient is the only patient who means much to the practice.

The dental assistant needs and wants security in employment. This is fundamental to one's self-concept and performance. It is important that the assistant be happy in assisting. The assistant must derive a sense of importance and fulfillment in the work. Needing to be needed forms a good basis toward finding contentment. It is natural to want recognition and to seek approval for work efforts. The elements necessary for the dental assistant to be happy stem from his or her own personality as well as those of the dentist and other personnel in the office. They stem from the atmosphere in the office, which includes working conditions, compatibility of personnel, salary, and communication channels with those in authority. In health affairs the nature of the work environment can create stress in individuals. The stress may originate with duties, the dentist, personality conflicts, and many other related areas. The methods used by the dentist and the personnel in resolving staff problems will determine the success or failure of the outcome. Traditionally the methods of dealing with employees by the dentist have been centered in telling, advising, criticizing, and punishing when breaches of conduct are encountered. Today the office which clings to this approach is doomed to constant turnover of staff because mutual resolution of problems is absent. When problems cannot be adjusted, the atmosphere of the office becomes hostile and rigid. The traditional approach taken by assistants with regard to grievances is to complain to everyone but the dentist.

The most favorable approach in dealing with stress situations among employees for the dentist is to be specific in regard to responsibilities and deportment in the office. When problems arise, counsel sessions in which the employee has an opportunity to speak tend to set the stage for mutual understanding. Employer-employee problems and office management are handled best through written procedure manuals for the office. In the manual a section should be devoted to scheduled meetings of the staff in which the progress of the practice as well as any problems which have arisen are reviewed. With this arrangement the favorable outcome can be assured if all are straightforward and open in presenting their views. Essentially, satisfaction in dental assisting requires mutual trust and respect between dentist and assistant.

The individual who aspires to a career in dental assisting should establish personal suitability for this type of employment before entering the field. It is not the purpose of this section to describe the rationale of placement testing. However, there are a number of measuring instruments available from school guidance counselors and from employment services which will help determine the suitability of the individual to a career in dental assisting. These are basically personality and other types of psychologic tests designed to provide information on how a person may react in personal and social situations. Other tests are concerned with manual dexterity and visual interpretations. If favorable results from these type inventories are obtained, the individual can find a satisfying career of service and personal fulfillment in the growing field of dental assisting.

SUMMARY

Applied psychology in dentistry is derived from various areas of psychosocial discipline. In order for the dental assistant to be more conversant with applied psychology there are certain requisite areas of knowledge which should be studied. The development of psychologic theory in general is basic.

An understanding of personality and the factors of personality development is of inestimable value for the student because this area leads to self-evaluation and appraisal. The ability to know and understand oneself is essential to a comprehensive understanding of others. Personality-development factors offer the key to human behavior patterns which will help the assistant in his or her evaluation of patients and their actions.

The intricacies of motivation and the drives and needs of people which require gratification are an integral part of applied psychology in dentistry. It is important to recognize that some needs place demands upon the individual that occupy his or her mind to the exclusion of all other things. Certain lower needs must be satisfied before higher needs can be considered. Unless dental service is clearly providing for the lower needs, such as pain relief, it must have justification. The justification of dental needs or the rationale for accepting dental treatment is a major part of applied psychology.

It is important for the dental assistant to have a fundamental understanding of patient attitudes and of social classes, because the behavior of people in dental situations to some extent can be predicted upon their opinion of dentistry and the dentist. Attitudes toward dental service are rooted in some central psychologic and social concerns of people. Some of these attitudes cause people to seek dental care, and some actually prevent people from accepting dental care.

The behavior of people can be predicted with relative accuracy according to the social class to which they belong, but it should be recognized that social standing does not automatically influence people to accept or reject treatment. Individual differences in people's attitudes require the use of different motivational techniques to reach each individual.

When the dental assistant makes use of a knowledge of psychology in the dental office, he or she is functioning in the realm of applied psychology. In all contact with patients, coworkers, and the doctor, the assistant should use applied psychology to make the self-image of others and his or her own self-image comfortable. People are the same whether they are buying groceries, consulting an attorney, or seeking dental care. The same psychology which serves people in other areas of life will produce acceptance of service in dentistry. Applied psychology in dentistry is the assimilation and use of those ingredients which reach people at the proper level of their human hungers. It causes action and cooperation which result in health, happiness, and, in general, the physical and psychologic good of all of us.

BIBLIOGRAPHY

Adams, P.: "Dental Symbols and Teamwork," paper read before Florida State Dental Society, February 1963.

Allport, G. W., and Odbert, H. S.: "Trait Names: A Psycho-Lexical Study," Psychol. Monographs, **47**:1, 1936.

American Dental Association, Bureau of Economic

Research and Statistics: "A Motivational Study of Dental Care," *J. Am. Dent. Assoc.,* **56:**434–443, 566–574, 745–751, 859–860, 911–917, 1958; **57:**279, 1959.

Balinsky, B., and Burger, R.: *The Executive Interview,* Harper & Row, Publishers, Incorporated, New York, 1963, pp. 247–268, 304.

Bell, G. D.: *The Achievers,* Preston Hill Inc., Chapel Hill, N. C., 1973, pp. 3–104.

Berne, E. *What Do You Say after You Say Hello?* Grove Press Inc., New York, 1972, pp. 3–27.

Calhoon, R. P.: *Managing Personnel,* Harper & Row, Publishers, Incorporated, New York, 1963, pp. 247–267, 268–304.

Callahan, J. D.: "Emotional Problems of Childhood," paper presented to American Academy of Pedodontics, St. Louis, 1964.

Cinotti, W. R., and Grieder, A.: *Applied Psychology in Dentistry,* The C. V. Mosby Company, St. Louis, 1964, pp. 17–25, 31–44, 109–120.

English, H. B., and English, A. C.: *A Comprehensive Dictionary of Psychological and Psychoanalytical Terms,* Longmans, Green & Co., Ltd., London, 1958.

English, S. O., and Pearson, G. H. J.: *Emotional Problems of Living,* 3d ed., W. W. Norton & Company, Inc., New York, 1963, pp. 413–427.

Garn, R.: *The Magic Power of Emotional Appeal,* Ace Books, New York, 1960.

Haney, R.: "Communication in Dental Practice," paper presented before North Carolina Society of Dentistry for Children, Greensboro, N. C., Nov. 2–3, 1962.

Harper, R. A.: *The New Psychotherapies,* Prentice-Hall, Inc., Englewood Cliffs, N. J., 1975, pp. 75–90.

Harris, T. A.: *I'm OK-You're OK,* Harper & Row Publishers, Inc., New York, 1973, pp. 21–59.

Horney, K.: *Our Inner Conflicts,* W. W. Norton & Company, Inc., New York, 1945.

Levoy, R. P.: *The $100,000 Practice and How to Build It,* Prentice-Hall, Inc., Englewood Cliffs, N. J., 1966, pp. 7–23, 66, 101–104.

Maltz, M.: *Psycho-Cybernetics,* Simon & Schuster, Inc., New York, 1966.

Maslow, A. H.: "A Theory of Human Motivation," *Psychol. Rev.,* **50:**370–396, 1943.

Packard, V.: *The Hidden Persuaders,* Simon & Schuster, New York, 1960, pp. 1–19, 98–105, 38–47.

———: *The Status Seekers,* David McKay Company, Inc., New York, 1959, pp. 61–78, 253–263, 222, 246.

Reppert, H. C., Updegrave, W. J., and Shaffer, J. I.: "Public Attitude toward Dentistry," *J. Am. Coll. Dentists,* **25:**131–144, 1958.

Ruch, Floyd L.: *Psychology and Life,* Scott, Foresman and Company, Glenview, Ill., 1963.

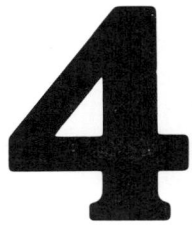

R. Jack Shankle
Dental Anatomy and Physiology

The practice of dentistry is concerned in large measure with the treatment of teeth and their surrounding structures. It is necessary, therefore, that the dental assistant become familiar with the anatomy and function of these structures.

Dental anatomy may be briefly defined as the study of the external and internal form of teeth and their surrounding structures. Dental physiology may be defined as the study of the normal function of these structures.

THE BONES OF THE ORAL CAVITY

The Maxillae

The maxillae are two in number and form the bulk of the upper jaw. They are called the right and left maxilla and join together in the roof of the mouth or palate. The union of these bones is known as the intermaxillary suture or median palatine suture (Figs. 4-1 to 4-3).

The maxillae are irregular bones from which four processes extend, namely: (1) the nasal process toward the nose, (2) the malar or zygomatic process upward above the maxillary first molar, (3) the palatal process toward the other maxilla to form the palate, and (4) the alveolar process surrounding the roots of the teeth.

The maxillae have hollow air spaces above the posterior teeth that are known as the maxillary sinuses. The air spaces communicate with the nose. The sinuses affect speech as the palate is

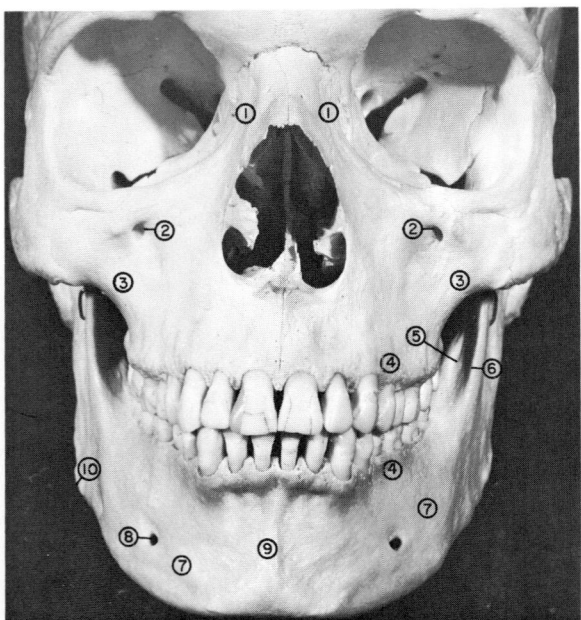

Figure 4-1 | Anterior view of skull. (1) Nasal process. (2) Infraorbital foramen. (3) Malar process. (4) Alveolar process. (5) Internal oblique ridge. (6) External oblique ridge. (7) Body of mandible. (8) Mental foramen. (9) Symphysis. (10) Angle of mandible.

made into a sounding board by their presence, giving resonance to the voice. Patients commonly suffer from infections of the maxillary sinuses. These infections produce symptoms which often cause the patient to question the health of the underlying maxillary teeth.

The maxillae function in the following manner: (1) they give shape to the face in general, (2) they form the palate, (3) they form a part of the eye socket and the nasal cavity, and (4) they support the 16 upper teeth in the permanent dentition or the 10 in the primary or deciduous (baby) dentition.

In either maxilla there are four holes, and each hole is called a foramen. Through these foramina pass nerves and blood vessels. Two of these openings are located in the palate. One of the openings is just lingual to the central incisors, and it is called the incisive foramen. Another palatine foramen is located just lingual to the last molar, and it is called the greater palatine foramen. The posterior superior alveolar foramen is located on the cheek side of the maxilla just above the last molar. The infraorbital foramen is found just below the eye socket on the anterior (front) side of the maxilla.

The Mandible

The mandible, or lower jaw, is located below the maxillae. This bone supports the 16 lower permanent teeth or the 10 lower primary or deciduous teeth, depending upon the age of the individual.

The mandible is a movable bone that is shaped like a horseshoe. It is hinged to the skull at either end, and these hinge joints are called the temporomandibular joints (Figs. 4-2 and 4-5).

The mandible is composed of a body, two rami, and five processes. The rami are the two upright portions of the mandible located at either end. Two processes are found on the superior surface of each ramus. The posterior process is called the condyloid process, and the anterior process is called the coronoid process. These processes are separated by the sigmoid notch. The alveolar process is located on the superior surface of the body of the mandible and supports the lower teeth.

The mandible functions in the following ways: (1) it gives shape to the lower part of the face, (2) it forms the framework for the floor of the mouth, and (3) it supports the lower teeth.

The mandible is the strongest bone in the head. The muscles that are attached to it bring the lower teeth into contact with the upper teeth with great force. The movements of the mandible are necessary for good speech and for the mastication of food.

There are four foramina located on the mandible, namely, the mandibular and the mental.

The mandibular foramina are two in number, one being located on the lingual side of either ramus (Fig. 4-4). The mental foramina are two in number, one being located on the left and one on the right facial surface of the body of the mandible in the premolar area (Figs. 4-1 and 4-2). Through these openings pass nerves and blood vessels supplying the lower teeth, alveolar bone, and gingivae.

THE TEMPOROMANDIBULAR JOINT

The mandible is hinged to a temporal bone on either side of the skull, hence the term temporomandibular joint.

The temporal bone presents a depression on its inferior surface just anterior to the auditory canal (ear). This depression is called the glenoid fossa and receives the condyle of the mandible, which has a knob-shaped appearance (Figs. 4-2 and 4-4).

The interarticular disc, often called the meniscus, interposes the union of bone in the glenoid fossa. This cartilaginous disc permits a smooth relationship between the bones during the various movements of the mandible (Fig. 4-5).

A dense fibrous capsule covers the temporomandibular joint. The joint is so designed that the mandible, or lower arch, may move from side to side, laterally, as well as up and down. Hence, it is termed a *diarthroidal* (freely movable) *joint,* adapting to the various movements required of the mandible as well as to many changes in occlusion resulting from tooth loss and attrition.

THE SUPPORTING STRUCTURES OF THE TEETH

The supporting structures of the teeth are (1) the alveolar bone and (2) the periodontal membrane (Fig. 4-6). The efficiency and normal func-

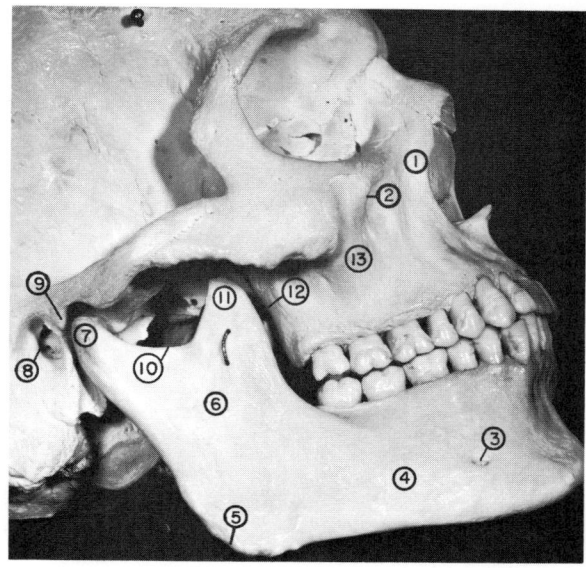

Figure 4-2 | Lateral view of skull. (1) Nasal process. (2) Infraorbital foramen. (3) Mental foramen. (4) Body of mandible. (5) Angle of mandible. (6) Ramus of mandible. (7) Condyloid process. (8) External acoustic meatus. (9) Temporomandibular joint. (10) Sigmoid notch. (11) Coronoid process. (12) Posterior superior alveolar foramen. (13) Malar process.

Figure 4-3 | The maxillae. (1) Incisive foramen. (2) Intermaxillary suture. (3) Palatal process. (4) Greater palatine foramen. (5) Malar process.

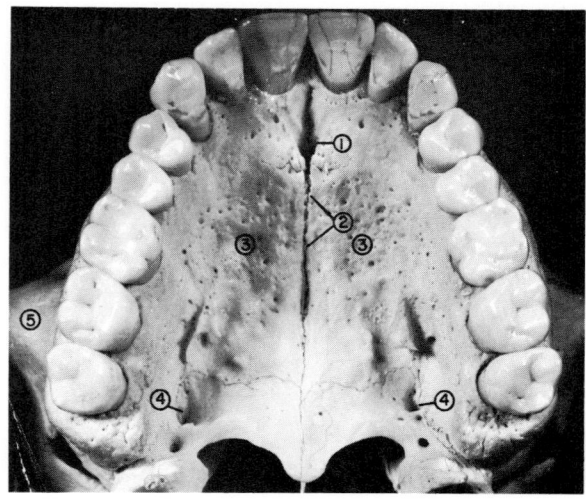

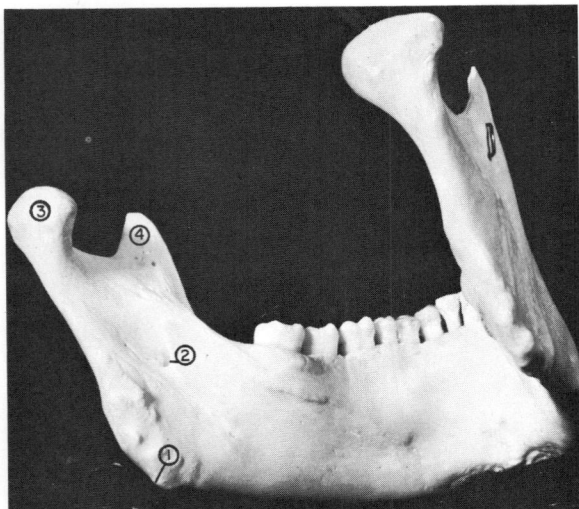

Figure 4-4 | The mandible. (1) Angle of mandible. (2) Mandibular foramen. (3) Condyloid process. (4) Coronoid process.

Figure 4-5 | Lateral view of the temporomandibular joint. A portion of the meniscus is shown interposing the body union.

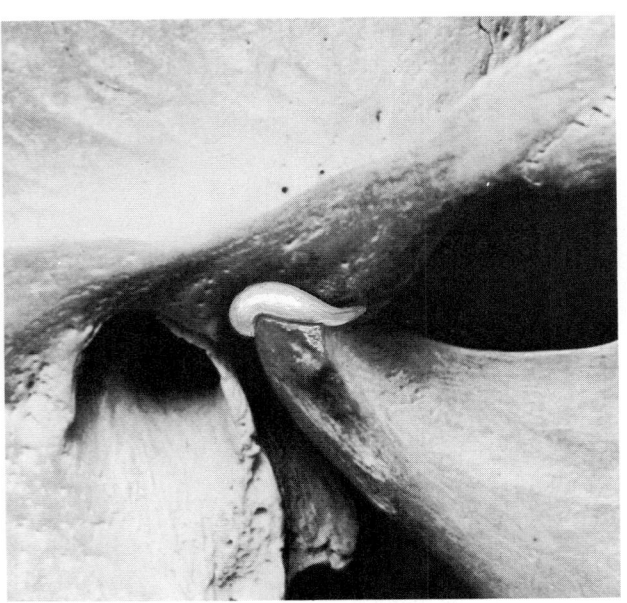

tions of the teeth, as a part of an apparatus for mastication, are dependent upon the presence and normal health of the supporting structures and the oral mucosa.

The Alveolar Bone

The alveolar bone, in the form of the alveolar process, has been mentioned previously as a supporting structure of the teeth.

The Periodontal Membrane

The periodontal membrane is a thin but very dense and tough tissue found interposing the root of the tooth and the alveolar bone. The chief functions of the periodontal membrane are to serve (1) as an attachment of the tooth to the alveolar bone and (2) as a cushion between the tooth and the alveolar bone when force is brought about during mastication.

The attachment of teeth to the alveolar bone by means of the periodontal membrane is known as *gomphosis*. The direct attachment of teeth to the bone in the absence of a periodontal membrane is known as *ankylosis*. This direct means of attachment is found in the dentition of the alligator.

The Mucosa

The mucosa is the soft tissue which covers the inside of the mouth cavity. Beneath the mucosa there is another layer of soft tissue known as the submucosa. This inner soft tissue layer contains the larger blood vessels and nerves (Fig. 4-6).

MUSCLES OF MASTICATION

The upper or maxillary arch is fixed and stable, whereas the lower or mandibular arch is movable. The movements of the mandible and the forces of mastication are carried on chiefly by the following muscles: (1) temporal, (2) masseter,

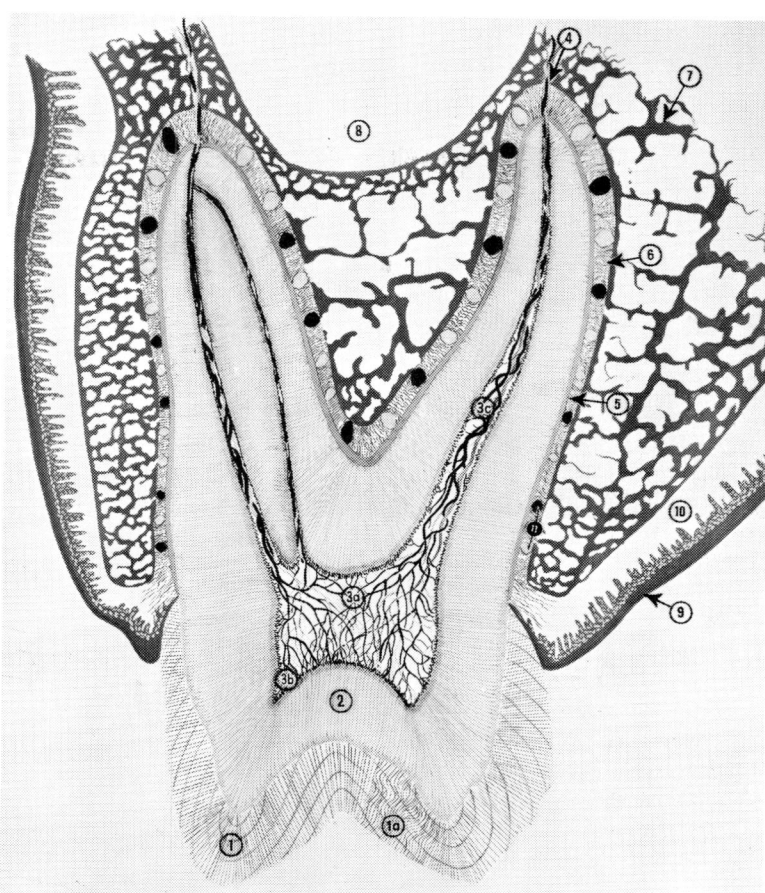

Figure 4-6 | Schematic drawing to illustrate cross section of a maxillary molar and its supporting structures. (1) Enamel. (1a) Gnarled enamel. (2) Dentin. (3a) Pulp chamber. (3b) Pulp horn. (3c) Pulp canal. (4) Apical foramen. (5) Cementum. (6) Periodontal fibers in periodontal membrane. (7) Alveolar bone. (8) Maxillary sinus. (9) Mucosa. (10) Submucosa. (11) Blood vessels. (See another version in the front endpapers of this book.)

(3) internal pterygoid, and (4) external pterygoid. These muscle pairs control the movements of the mandible from either side.

Temporal

The temporal is the largest of the muscles of mastication. It is a fan-shaped muscle, and its origin is on the broad external surface of the temporal bone, which gives the muscle its name. The muscle converges from its origin to the points of its insertion, which are the coronoid process and the anterior border of the ramus of the mandible (Fig. 4-7).

The functions of the temporal muscle are (1) closure of the jaw, (2) protrusion of the mandible, and (3) retraction of the mandible from a protruded position.

Masseter

The word is derived from the Greek word *maseter* meaning chewer. It originates from the zygomatic arch, and its main insertion is on the broad facial side of the ramus of the mandible, including the angle of the mandible. The powerful masseters function in closing the jaw (Fig. 4-8).

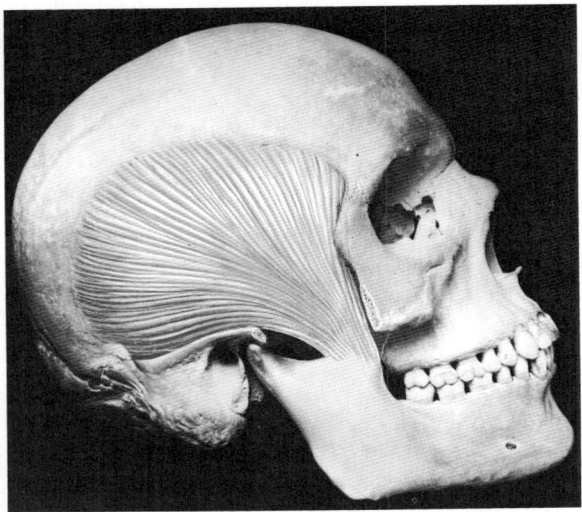

Figure 4-7 | Lateral view of the skull showing the temporal muscle. The zygomatic arch has been cut away partially.

The Internal Pterygoid

The principal origin of the internal pterygoid muscle is the pterygoid fossa of the sphenoid bone, which gives the muscle its name. The direction of the muscle is parallel to the direction

Figure 4-8 | Lateral view of the skull showing the masseter muscle.

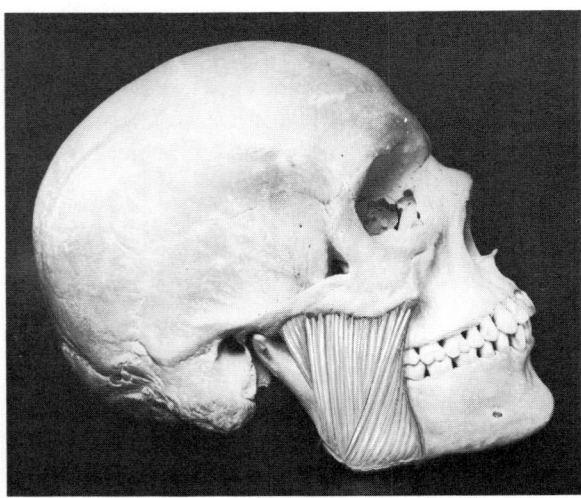

of the masseter, although it is located on the opposite side of the ramus of the mandible. The insertion of the internal pterygoid muscle is on the inner surface of the mandible near the angle (Fig. 4-9).

The functions of the internal pterygoid are (1) lateral movements of the mandible, and (2) closing the jaw.

The External Pterygoid

The origin of the external pterygoid muscle is just external to the origin of the internal pterygoid muscle, and also, just above the area, in the infratemporal fossa. Each of these sites is located on the sphenoid bone. The direction of the muscles is backward and externally to its points of insertion near the condyle of the mandible (Fig. 4-9).

The functions of the external pterygoid muscle are (1) opening the jaw, and (2) protrusion of the jaw.

THE SALIVARY GLANDS

The principle salivary glands are (1) the parotid, (2) the submaxillary, and (3) the sublingual. The combined secretions of these glands vary from 2 to 3 pt of saliva during each 24-hour period, although the exact amount differs according to the individual.

The salivary glands manufacture saliva from materials that they derive from the blood. The composition of saliva is about 99 percent water, with the remaining 1 percent composed of various salts and solids. Saliva is generally slightly acid, although the degree of acidity varies with the individual.

The smell, taste, or even thought of appropriate foods enhances the flow of saliva. This is particularly true during periods of hunger.

The saliva functions in the following ways: (1) it serves as a lubricating agent which moistens the mouth and food and facilitates swallowing, (2) it is a cleansing agent which washes away food particles that may adhere to the teeth, and (3) it is an aid in digestion, as ptyalin and erepsin are present. These enzymes act on the food, converting it into more acceptable products for use by the body.

The Parotid Gland

The parotid is the largest of the salivary glands. It lies embedded, one on each side of the face, immediately below and in front of the ear. The saliva is conveyed from the parotid gland to the mouth by Stensen's duct, which opens into the mouth from the inside of the cheek opposite the upper second molar. The saliva secreted by the parotid gland is thin and watery (Fig. 4-10).

The Submaxillary Gland

This gland, one on either side, is the second largest of the salivary glands and is about the size of a walnut. It lies beneath the posterior portion of the mandible (Fig. 4-10). Saliva from the submaxillary gland is conveyed to the mouth by Wharton's duct, which opens through the floor of the mouth just lingual to the lower incisors. The secretions of this gland are thick and mucous.

The Sublingual Gland

The sublingual gland, one on either side, is the smallest of the salivary glands. It is located beneath the tongue (Fig. 4-10).

The secretions of this gland are conveyed directly into the mouth above the gland by a number of tiny sublingual ducts and by a larger sublingual duct, which finally empties into the mouth lingual to the lower anterior teeth.

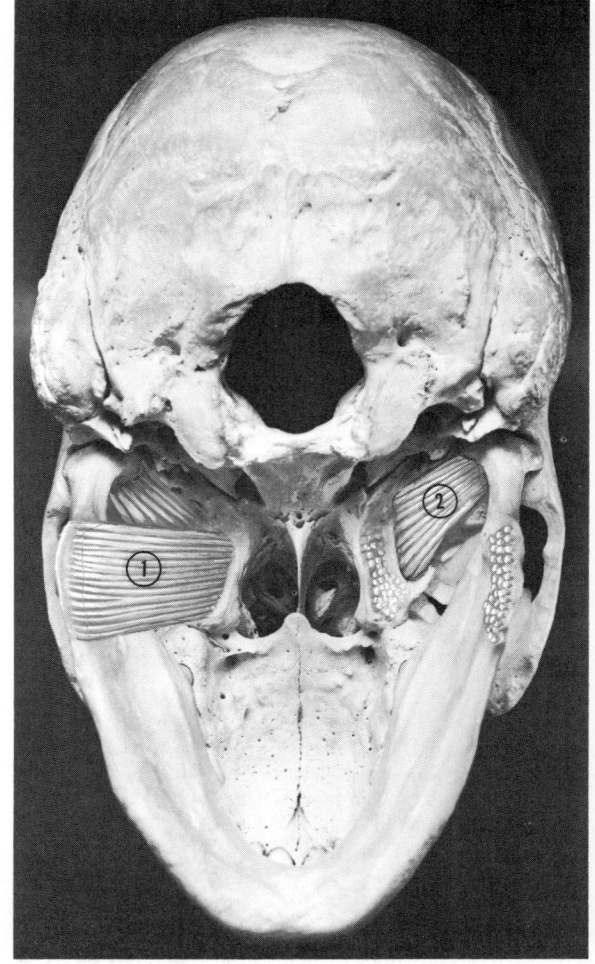

Figure 4-9 | View of the skull from beneath the mandible. (1) Internal pterygoid muscle. (2) External pterygoid muscle.

THE TEETH

Two different sets of teeth erupt during the course of a human being's life, namely, the primary dentition and the secondary or permanent dentition.

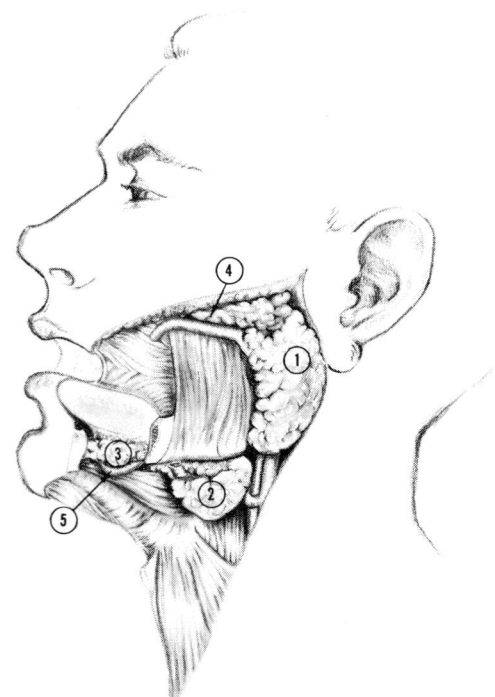

Figure 4-10 | A section of the face has been cut away in this drawing to show the salivary glands. (1) The parotid gland. (2) The submaxillary gland. (3) The sublingual gland. (4) Stensen's duct. (5) Wharton's duct.

The Primary Teeth

This is one's first set of teeth, which must function until they are replaced by secondary or permanent teeth. Primary teeth are often called deciduous teeth, because they are shed and replaced by other teeth later in life. Sometimes they are referred to as baby teeth and occasionally as milk teeth. The eruption schedule for primary teeth varies with different children but generally begins between the sixth and eighth month after birth. This eruption process continues for the various teeth during the first 2 years of life. All the primary teeth usually have been lost (exfoliated) by the twelfth year, and during this interim they have been replaced by secondary teeth. There are 20 primary teeth, designated as follows:

10 maxillary teeth (5 right, 5 left)
 2 central incisors
 2 lateral incisors
 2 cuspids
 2 first molars
 2 second molars
10 mandibular teeth (5 right, 5 left)
 2 central incisors
 2 lateral incisors
 2 cuspids
 2 first molars
 2 second molars

The Secondary Teeth

These sometimes are referred to as permanent teeth. They begin to erupt approximately at the age of 6 years, and they must function throughout the individual's life. These teeth have no successors, except those provided as substitutes, when necessary, by the dentist. There are 32 secondary teeth, as follows:

16 maxillary teeth (8 right, 8 left)
 2 central incisors
 2 lateral incisors
 2 cuspids
 2 first bicuspids or premolars
 2 second bicuspids or premolars
 2 first molars
 2 second molars
 2 third molars (commonly called wisdom teeth)
16 mandibular teeth (8 right, 8 left)
 2 central incisors
 2 lateral incisors
 2 cuspids
 2 first bicuspids or premolars
 2 second bicuspids or premolars
 2 first molars
 2 second molars
 2 third molars (commonly called wisdom teeth)

Functions of Teeth

The general functions of teeth are mastication, esthetics, and phonetics. The following functions may be listed for groups of teeth:

Incisors

The word *incisor* is derived from the Latin *incidere* which means to cut into. The incisors cut off particles of food which are forced by the tongue and muscles of the mouth between the posterior teeth where they are pulverized by these larger teeth.

Cuspids

The word *cusp* refers to the spear-shaped crown of this tooth. The incisors are rather flat from the facial to the lingual surface, but the cuspid is much thicker because of the strong ridge of enamel on the facial and on the lingual surfaces. This ridge of enamel extends from the cusp tip of the crown to the cervical line and, accordingly, makes the cuspid a much stronger tooth than the incisor. The long root also gives added stability to the cuspid, and its position at the angle of the mouth adapts it for tearing as well as for incising food.

Cuspids sometimes are referred to as canines, or incorrectly as eyeteeth or dogteeth. The cuspids are very well developed in dogs and in other animals of that family for the tearing of food and fighting.

Bicuspids or Premolars

The word *bicuspid* means two cusps. It is the term used by many American dentists to identify the fourth and fifth teeth posteriorly from the median line. The word could be misleading since not all the bicuspids possess two cusps. The lower second bicuspid usually has three cusps, and the lower first bicuspid possesses a very poorly developed lingual cusp that has little function. The word *premolar* is the choice generally, instead of bicuspid, since premolar signifies "preceding the molars in their order of arrangement from anterior to posterior."

In England and most other foreign countries, these teeth are referred to as *premolars*.

The premolars or bicuspids pulverize the food that has been cut off by the incisors and cuspids.

Molars

The word *molar* is derived from the Latin word *molaris,* pertaining to a millstone. The molars are the largest teeth in the mouth, and they also are the strongest teeth because of their crown size and root development.

The molars decrease in size, function, and strength from the first molar posterioly through the third molar. The first molars are the largest, strongest, and most functional of the molars, whereas the third molars are the least functional, smallest, and least stable.

Surfaces and Landmarks

The surfaces are named for the direction in which they face. The crowns of teeth have five surfaces:

Anterior teeth	Posterior teeth
Facial (labial)	Facial (buccal)
Lingual	Lingual
Mesial	Mesial
Distal	Distal
Incisal	Occlusal

While the crowns have five surfaces, including the incisal edge (anterior teeth) and occlusal surface (posterior teeth), the roots of teeth have four surfaces and an apex.

Angles

For purposes of classifying and identifying certain areas on teeth in operational procedures, the surfaces of the crowns of teeth are divided and designated by line angles and point angles.

A line angle divides two surfaces and derives its name from the surfaces that it divides. The mesial surface and the labial, or facial, surface of a central incisor are divided by the mesiolabial, or mesiofacial line angle. The *al* ending of the word *mesial* is dropped and replaced by *o*. For example, *mesiallabial,* or mesialfacial line angle is incorrect. However, when the *al* in mesial is dropped and the *o* is added, the correct designation of mesiolabial, or mesiofacial, is realized.

A point angle divides three surfaces and derives its name from the surfaces that it divides. For example, the point where the mesial, labial (facial), and incisal surfaces join on a central incisor is known as the mesiolabioincisal (mesiofacioincisal) point angle. The *al* endings are dropped and are replaced in each case by the letter *o* (Figs. 4-11 and 4-12).

Contact Area

The area of a tooth that touches a neighboring tooth is called the *contact area.* This frequently is called the contact point. However, as there is more than just a point of contact, it is correctly called the contact area.

Embrasure

Radiating from the contact areas between teeth are four embrasures. Because of the contour of the teeth, these embrasures are V-shaped. They are named according to the direction toward which they extend from the contact area (Fig. 4-13).

THE STRUCTURES OF TEETH

Enamel

Enamel is the hard covering that forms the outer surface of the crown. It is the hardest substance in the body and is comparable in degree of hardness to topaz, a precious gem of great hardness and durability. The thickness of enamel varies on the crown. It is thicker in areas that are subject to greatest wear (Fig. 4-6).

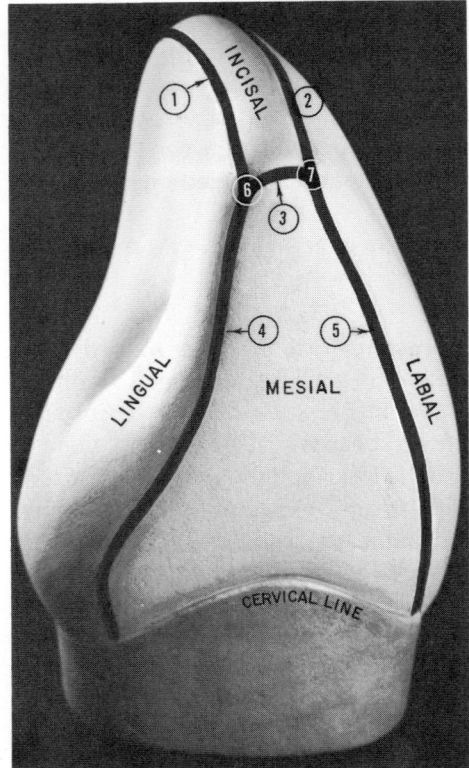

Figure 4-11 | Line angles and point angles on an anterior tooth. (1) Linguoincisal line angle. (2) Facioincisal (labionincisal) line angle. (3) Mesioincisal line angle. (4) Mesiolingual line angle. (5) Mesiofacial (mesiolabial) line angle. (6) Mesiolinguoincisal point angle. (7) Mesiofacioincisal (mesiolabioincisal) point angle. Line angles and point angles for the distal surface are not shown.

Cementum

The cementum is a bonelike substance that covers the roots of teeth. It is the softest of the hard structures of a tooth and affords attachment of a tooth to the jaw. This is accomplished by fibers from the periodontal membrane which are embedded in the cementum (Fig. 4-6).

Dentin

The dentin is the tissue that lies beneath the enamel and the cementum. It composes the

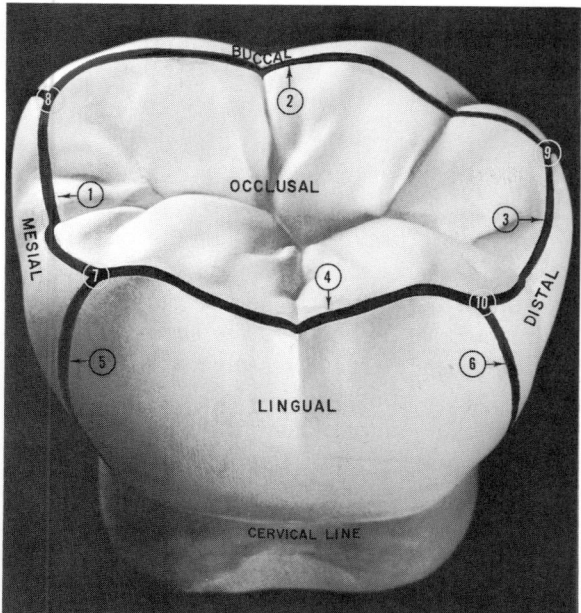

Figure 4-12 | Line angles and point angles on a posterior tooth. (1) Mesio-occlusal line angle. (2) Facio-occlusal (bucco-occlusal) line angle. (3) Disto-occlusal line angle. (4) Linguo-occlusal line angle. (5) Mesiolingual line angle. (6) Distolingual line angle. (7) Mesiolinguo-occlusal point angle. (8) Mesiofacio-occlusal (mesiobucco-occlusal) point angle. (9) Distofacio-occlusal (distobucco-occlusal) point angle. (10) Distolinguo-occlusal point angle.

greater bulk of the tooth. It is harder than cementum and softer than enamel (Fig. 4-6).

Pulp

The pulp cavity lies within the dentin. It is divided into the pulp chamber and the pulp canal (Fig. 4-6). The pulp chamber is found in the center of the crown, and the pulp canal is found in the center of the root. Some teeth (upper molars) have three roots and, accordingly, three root canals. The pulp canal opening at the apex of the root is called the apical foramen. The pulp lies within the pulp cavity and is made up of nerves, blood vessels, lymph passageways, and various tissue cells.

The tiny blood vessels and nerves that pass through the apical foramen, into and from the pulp cavity, are branches of larger blood vessels and nerves (Figs. 4-14 and 4-15). The anatomic form and relationship of the pulp cavity to the hard tooth structures are illustrated in Figs. 4-16 to 4-19.

ERUPTION OF TEETH

A table of eruption for the primary and the secondary teeth is presented which lists the average

Table of Eruption of Teeth*

Primary teeth	Age
Upper central incisor	7½ months
Upper lateral incisor	9 months
Upper cuspid	18 months
Upper first molar	14 months
Upper second molar	24 months
Lower central incisor	6 months
Lower lateral incisor	7 months
Lower cuspid	16 months
Lower first molar	12 months
Lower second molar	20 months
Secondary teeth	
Upper central incisor	7–8 years
Upper lateral incisor	8–9 years
Upper cuspid	11–12 years
Upper first premolar or bicuspid	10–11 years
Upper second premolar or bicuspid	10–12 years
Upper first molar	6–7 years
Upper second molar	12–13 years
Upper third molar	17–21 years
Lower central incisor	6–7 years
Lower lateral incisor	7–8 years
Lower cuspid	9–10 years
Lower first premolar or bicuspid	10–12 years
Lower second premolar or bicuspid	11–12 years
Lower first molar	6–7 years
Lower second molar	11–13 years
Lower third molar	17–21 years

* After Logan and Kronfeld, as slightly modified by McCall and Schour, and presently by Shankle.

age for eruption. However, this schedule may vary in individuals and still remain within a normal pattern of development (Figs. 4-20 and 4-23).

DIFFERENTIATING CHARACTERISTICS BETWEEN THE TEETH

The Maxillary Incisors

The general anatomy of the maxillary incisors is very much alike; exceptions, however, are present (Fig. 4-24).

The central incisor is a larger tooth than the lateral incisor in all dimensions. The incisal angles of the maxillary lateral incisor are more rounded than the same angles on the central, and the mesial and distal surfaces present a greater degree of curvature when viewed from the facial aspect. Marginal ridges are broader on the lateral incisor. The lateral incisor in general, is a more beautiful and gracefully contoured tooth, although its mesial neighbor is much stronger.

The Mandibular Incisors

A greater similarity exists between the mandibular central and lateral incisors than exists between the maxillary central and lateral incisors (Fig. 4-24).

The lower lateral is the larger of the two teeth, although the anatomy of the lingual surfaces is very similar. The mesial and distal surfaces of the central are almost identical; however, the distal surface of the lateral has more curvature than the mesial surface. The incisal angles are all quite sharp and similar, with the exception of the distoincisal line angle of the lateral, which is rounded in appearance. The incisal edge of the central is straight, but the incisal edge of the lateral twists lingually as it approaches its distal extremity.

The mandibular incisors are smaller than their opposing teeth and therefore they are not as strong.

The Cuspids

The maxillary cuspid is larger than the cuspid in the mandibular arch. The lingual surface anatomy of the mandibular cuspid is similar to that of the mandibular incisors, but the lingual surface of the maxillary cuspid presents more evidence of ridges and grooves (Fig. 4-25).

The mesial surface of the mandibular cuspid is straighter than the same surface of the maxillary cuspid. The cingulum of the maxillary cuspid is more prominent. The facial surface of the mandibular cuspid is whalebone-shaped when viewed from the mesial or distal aspect. The maxillary cuspid, however, is not. Maxillary cuspids that have experienced normal function show wear toward the lingual surface of the incisal edge, whereas the mandibular cuspid shows this wear to the facial surface of the incisal edge.

The Maxillary Bicuspids or Premolars

The first bicuspid possesses two roots, and the second bicuspid or premolar has only one, as a general rule. The first bicuspid is a very angular tooth, but the second bicuspid has the appearance of being rounded slightly at the angles. The occlusal pits of the second bicuspid are closer together than the pits on the first bicuspid. This gives the occlusal surface of the second bicuspid the appearance of being wrinkled. The mesial surface of the first bicuspid has a more prominent concavity beneath the contact area than the same surface of the second bicuspid. The contours of the first bicuspid lend it more grace and beauty than do the curves of the second bicuspid (Fig. 4-26).

Figure 4-13 | Embrasures of (A) anterior and (B) posterior teeth.

Figure 4-14 | Arteries. Blood supply to the teeth.

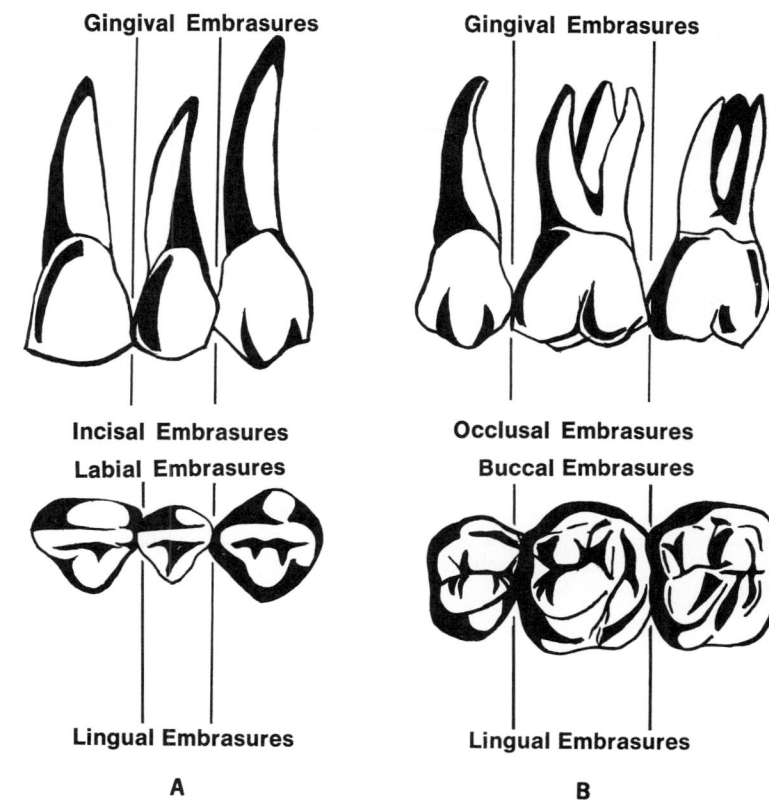

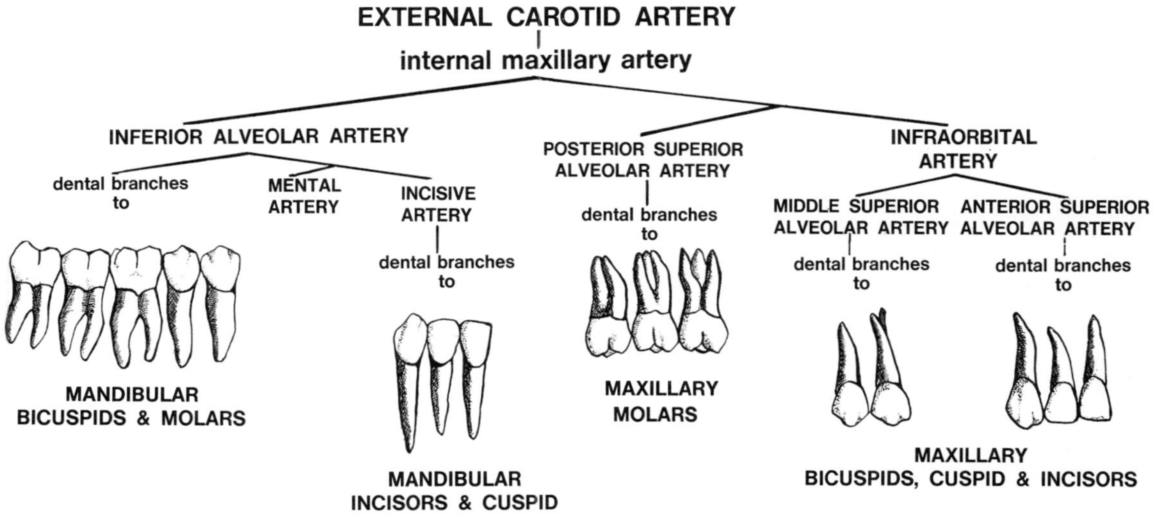

Chapter Four | Dental Anatomy and Physiology | 93

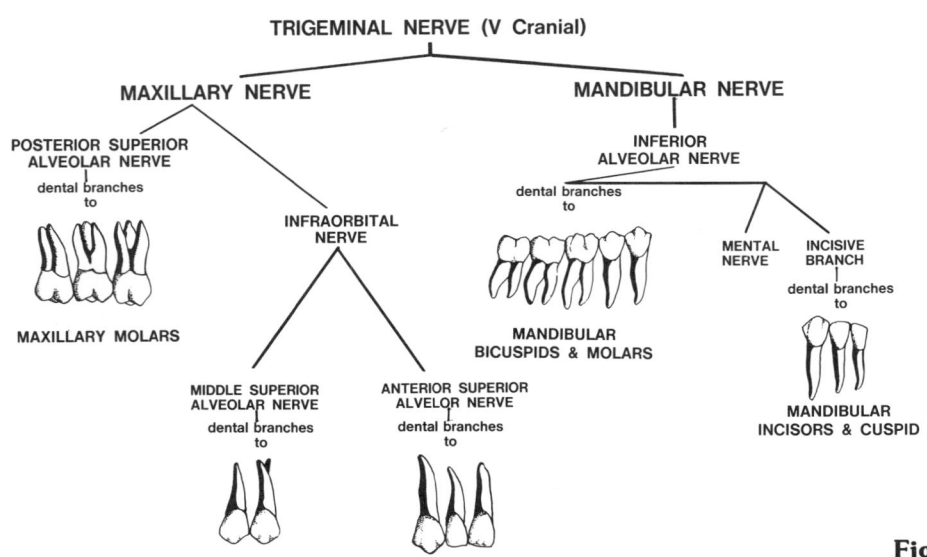

Figure 4-15 | Nerve supply to the teeth.

Figure 4-16 | Anatomic form and relationship of pulp cavity to hard tooth structure in the maxillary anterior teeth. (1) Maxillary central incisor (proximal view). (2) Maxillary central incisor (facial view). (3) Maxillary lateral incisor (proximal view). (4) Maxillary lateral incisor (facial view). (5) Maxillary canine (proximal view). (6) Maxillary canine (facial view).

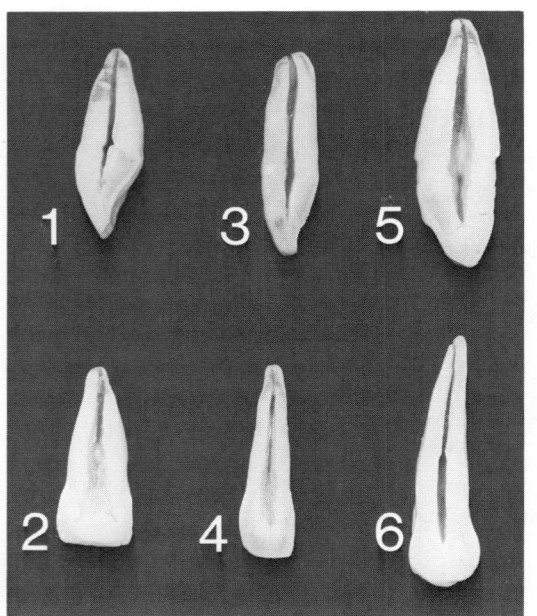

Figure 4-17 | Anatomic form and relationship of pulp cavity to hard tooth structure in the maxillary posterior teeth. (1) Maxillary first premolar (proximal view). (2) Maxillary first premolar (facial view). (3) Maxillary second premolar (proximal view). (4) Maxillary second premolar (facial view). Maxillary first molar (proximal view from mesial). (6) Maxillary first molar (facial view). (7) Maxillary second molar (proximal view from distal). (8) Maxillary second molar (facial view).

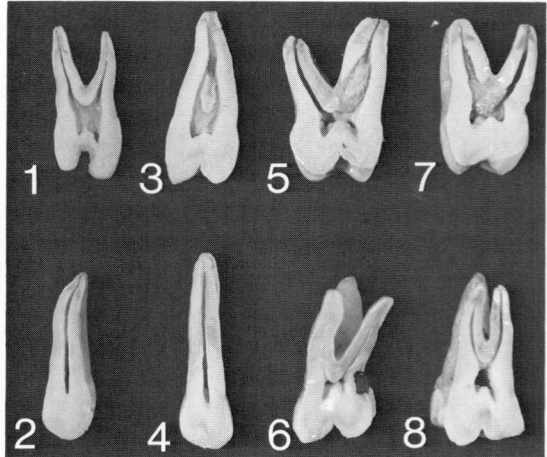

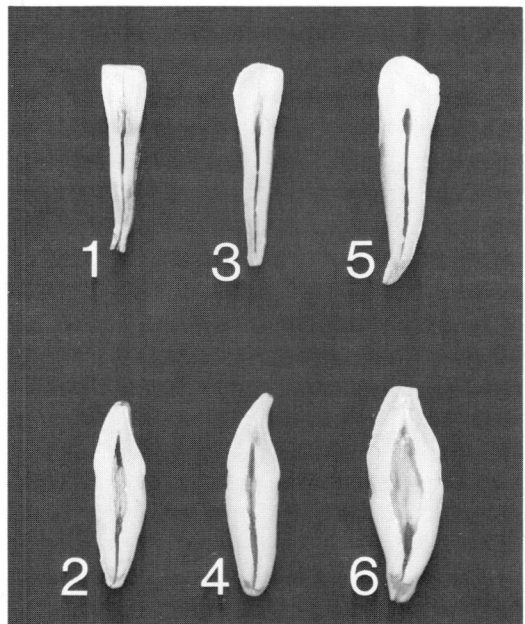

Figure 4-18 | Anatomic form and relationship of pulp cavity to hard tooth structure in the mandibular anterior teeth. (1) Mandibular central incisor (facial view). (2) Mandibular central incisor (proximal view). (3) Mandibular lateral incisor (facial view). (4) Mandibular lateral incisor (proximal view). (5) Mandibular canine (facial view). (6) Mandibular canine (proximal view).

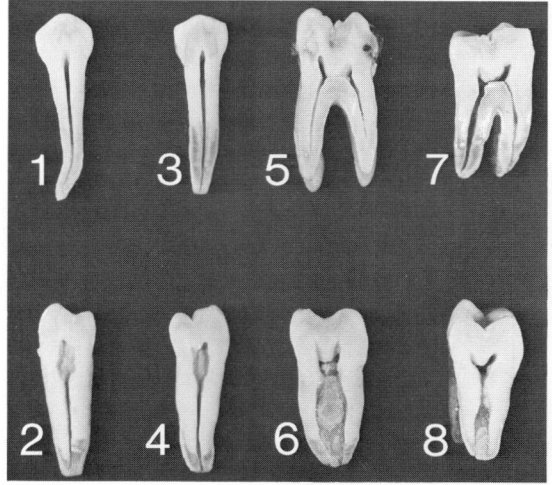

Figure 4-19 | Anatomic form and relationship of pulp cavity to hard tooth structure in the mandibular posterior teeth. (1) Mandibular first premolar (facial view). (2) Mandibular first premolar (proximal view). (3) Mandibular second premolar (facial view). (4) Mandibular second premolar (proximal view). (5) Mandibular first molar (facial view). (6) Mandibular first molar (proximal view from mesial). (7) Mandibular second molar (facial view). (8) Mandibular second molar (proximal view from distal).

Figure 4-20 | The primary teeth with approximate eruption times.

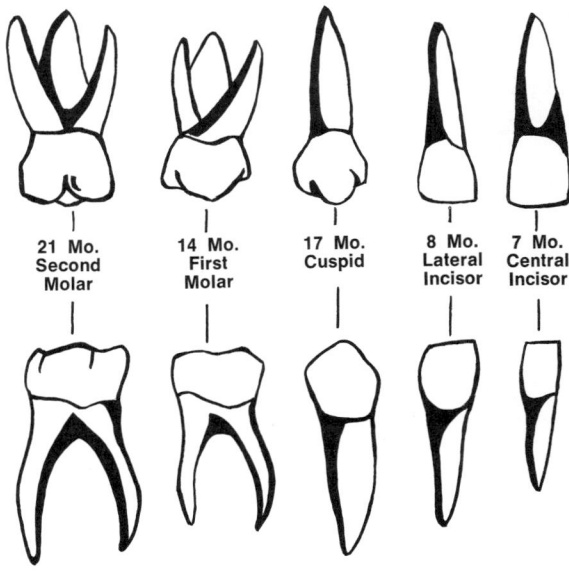

The Mandibular Bicuspids or Premolars

The first bicuspid is the smallest of all the bicuspids and possesses a small lingual cusp. The first bicuspid is quite similar to the mandibular cuspid, and the mesiolingual portion shows lack of development, since there is no occlusal function in this area.

The second bicuspid is a better developed tooth for grinding food than the first bicuspid. It is characterized by two lingual cusps and a single facial cusp. A large number of mandibular second bicuspids have only one lingual cusp (Fig. 4-26).

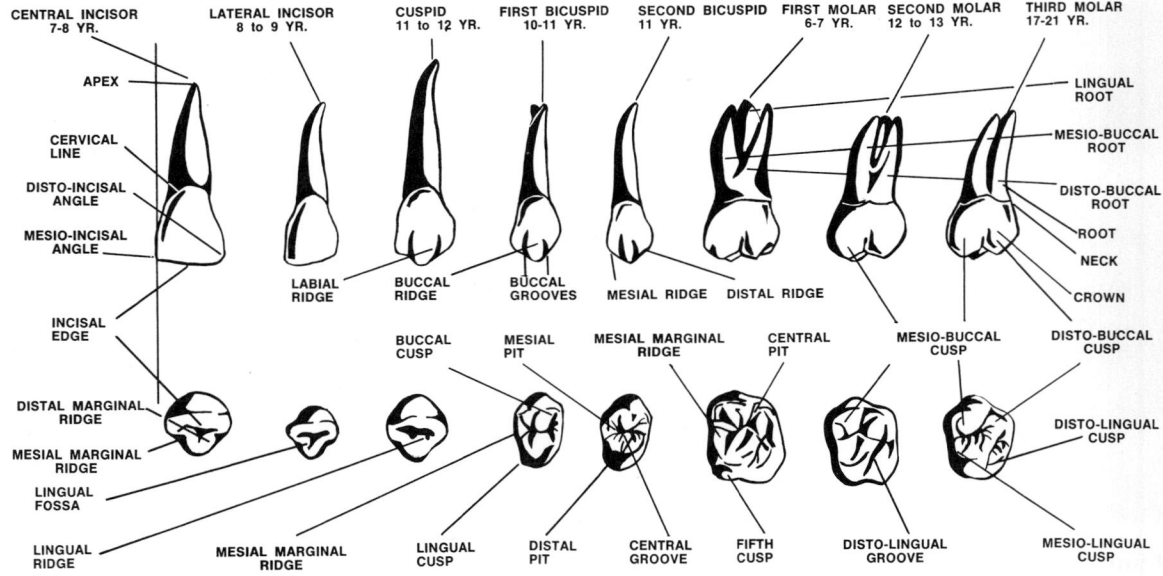

Figure 4-21 | The maxillary teeth.

The Maxillary Molars

The first molar is a larger and much stronger tooth than the second or third molars. The crown of the first molar possesses a fifth cusp, which is known as the cusp of Carabelli. This fifth cusp is found on the lingual surface of the mesiolingual cusp. The roots are more widespread in the first molar, giving it better anchorage and strength. The crowns of the maxillary

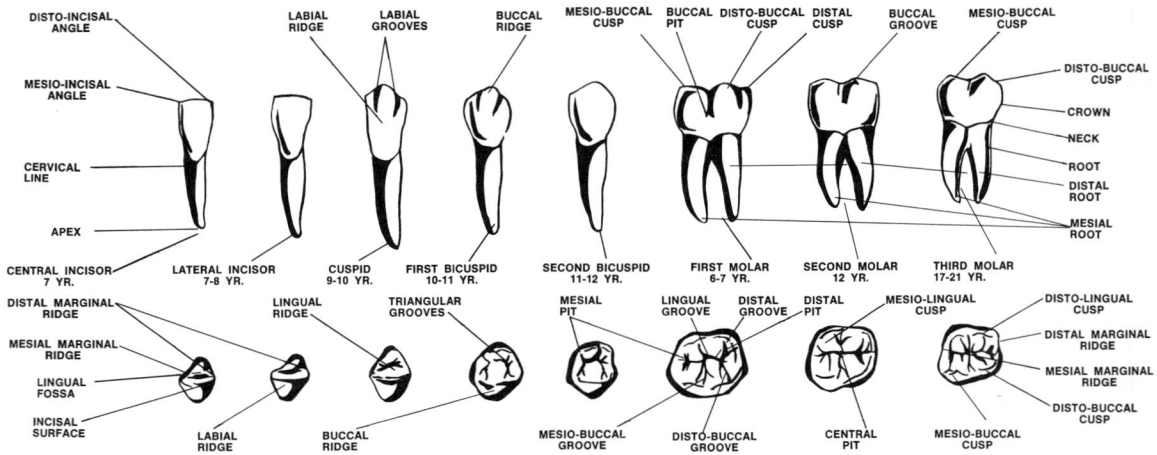

Figure 4-22 | The mandibular teeth.

molars are rhomboid in shape when observed from an occlusal aspect. The first molar, however, is less rhomboid than its distal neighbors (Fig. 4-27).

The general anatomic pattern of the third molar, commonly referred to as the wisdom tooth, is similar to that of the first and second molars, except that it presents many variations and anomalies. This tooth generally is developed very poorly and frequently has a bell crown. The occlusal surface is wrinkled in appearance as compared to the occlusal surface of the first and second molars. The cusps may vary in number from a single cusp to more than four. The roots also vary in number, some teeth having only one, whereas other third molars are multiple-rooted.

The Mandibular Molars

The crown of the first molar is larger than the crown of the second molar and possesses five cusps, whereas the crown of the second molar usually has only four cusps. The roots are more widespread on the first molar, giving it better anchorage in the mandible. The crown of the first molar is umbrella-shaped when observed from the facial or lingual aspect. The greater concavity possessed by the first molar on its mesial and distal surfaces is evident from either of those angles (Fig. 4-27).

The mandibular third molar presents as many variations and anomalies as the maxillary third molar. It is bell-crowned and usually has a wrinkled occlusal surface. The general anatomic pattern of the first and second molars is present, but the number of cusps and roots may vary somewhat.

OCCLUSION

Occlusion refers to the functional relationship of the mandibular teeth with the maxillary teeth when the jaws are closed.

Malocclusion refers to an abnormal or malfunctional relationship of the mandibular teeth with the maxillary teeth when the jaws are closed. This improper relationship may be due to malpositional eruption or missing teeth, as well as other factors which result in poor tooth alignment.

A malocclusion may pose problems in periodontics, orthodontics, prosthodontics, operative dentistry, or in temporomandibular dysfunctions. A problem in any one of these areas may be related to malocclusion, or a malocclusion may pose a problem in more than one of these areas.

The anatomy of the occlusal surfaces of teeth may vary from one individual to another; therefore, what is functional in one mouth may not be functional in another individual. Whenever there is satisfactory occlusal function, speech, esthetics, freedom from pain, and absence of damage to the supporting structures of the teeth, the occlusal pattern should not be changed. This is true although there may be excessive overbite, overjet, prognathism, and variances in occlusal curve and interproximal spaces.

The orthodontist is concerned largely with bringing teeth into a correct position by moving the individual tooth or groups of teeth or by rotating teeth.

A periodontist is concerned with occlusal function whenever treating periodontal disease. Periodontal treatment is a failure unless the general dentist or the periodontist makes occlusal selective adjustment of teeth by eliminating prematurities in occlusal contact.

A knowledge of occlusion is important in restoring teeth or groups of teeth. Failure to restore the teeth functionally may invite periodontal disease or temporomandibular dysfunction or both, with attending pain.

The prosthodontist or general practitioner is knowledgeable as to a functional occlusion for the same reasons cited above.

Mobility of a tooth or teeth during function may indicate presence of a premature occlusal

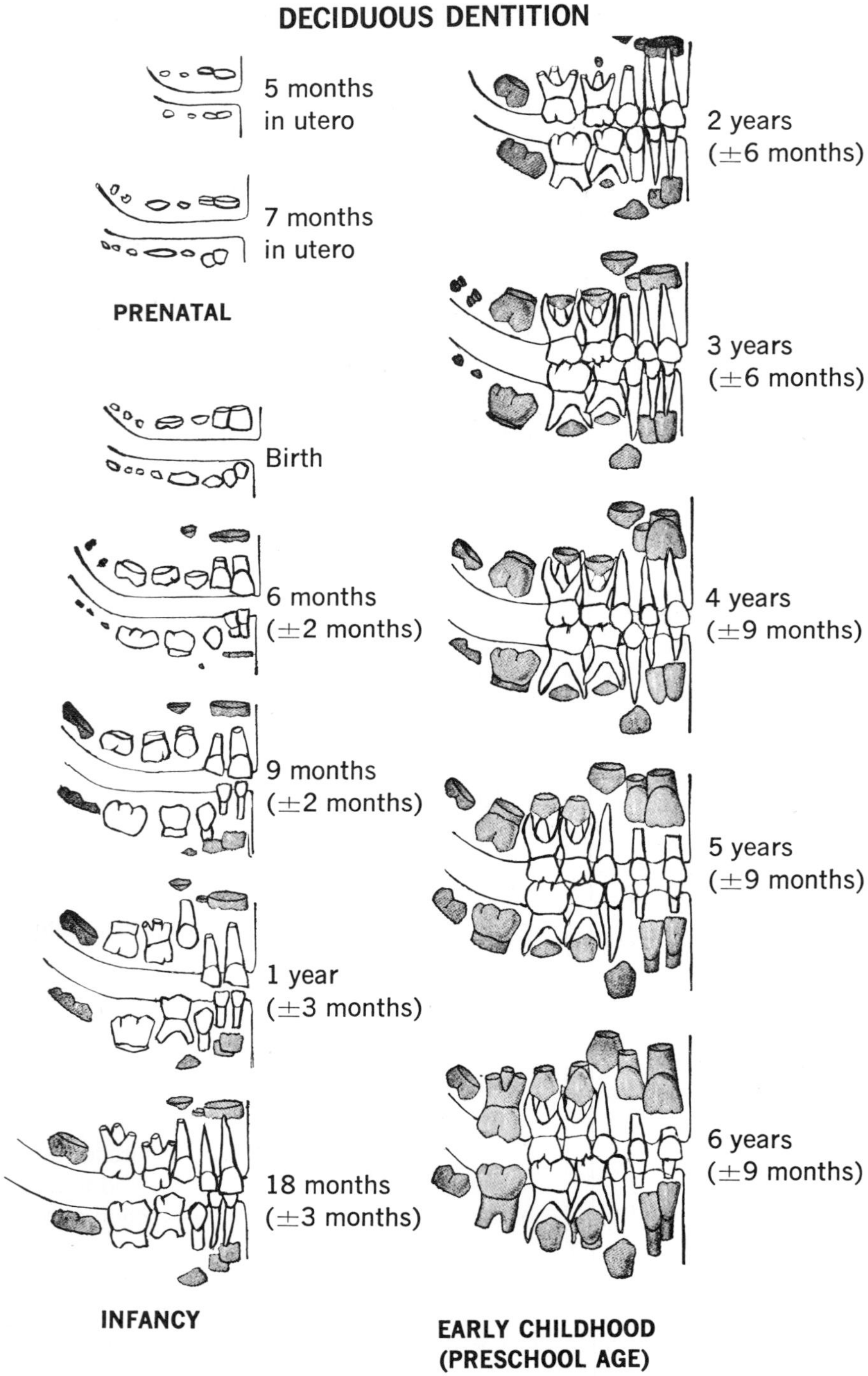

DECIDUOUS DENTITION

5 months in utero

7 months in utero

PRENATAL

Birth

6 months (±2 months)

9 months (±2 months)

1 year (±3 months)

18 months (±3 months)

INFANCY

2 years (±6 months)

3 years (±6 months)

4 years (±9 months)

5 years (±9 months)

6 years (±9 months)

EARLY CHILDHOOD (PRESCHOOL AGE)

Figure 4-23 | Chronology of the development of the dentitions. (*From M. Massler and I. Schour, Atlas of the Mouth, American Dental Association, Chicago, 1944*). See another version in the back endpapers of this book.

MIXED DENTITION

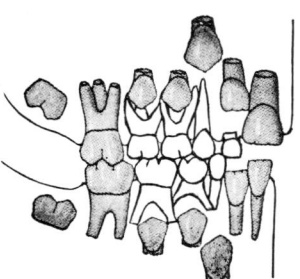

7 years
(±9 months)

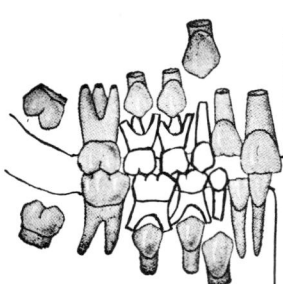

8 years
(±9 months)

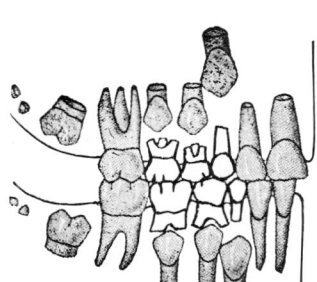

9 years
(±9 months)

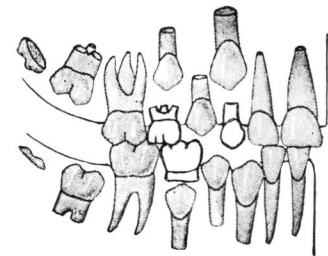

10 years
(±9 months)

**LATE CHILDHOOD
(SCHOOL AGE)**

PERMANENT DENTITION

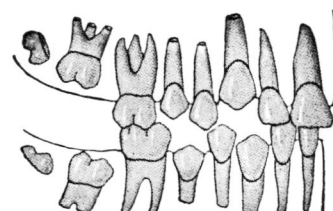

11 years
(±9 months)

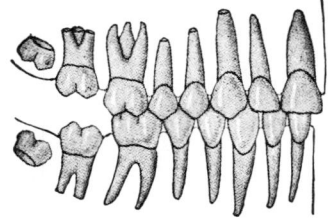

12 years
(±6 months)

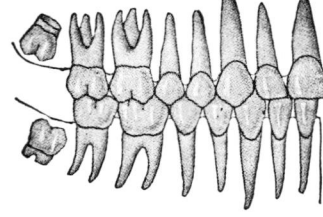

15 years
(±6 months)

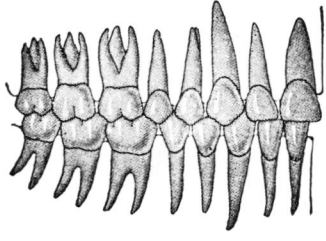

21 years

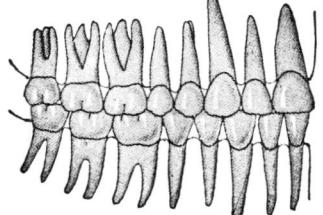

35 years

**ADOLESCENCE
and ADULTHOOD**

Chapter Four | Dental Anatomy and Physiology | 99

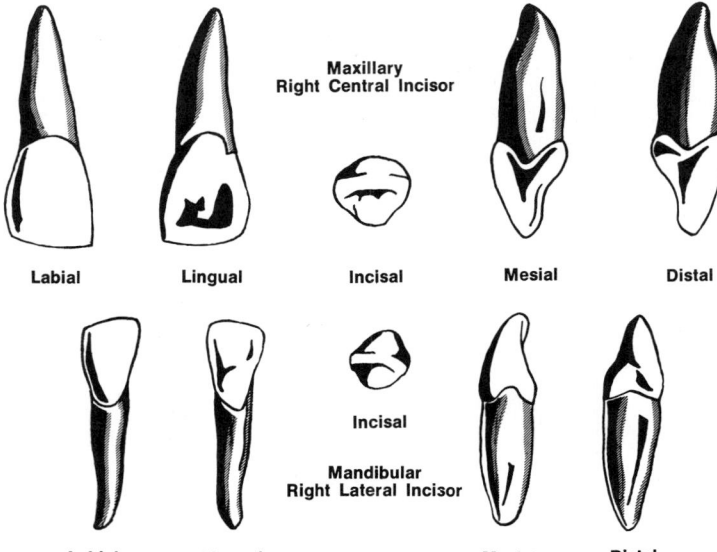

Figure 4-24 | Incisors.

relationship. By careful examination of the occlusal surfaces of natural teeth or restorations, one may observe wear facets. These wear facets may be indicative of prematurities in occlusion and undue stress on a single tooth, in groups of teeth, or individual teeth about the mouth.

More information on occlusion is found in Chap. 27.

Figure 4-25 | Cuspids.

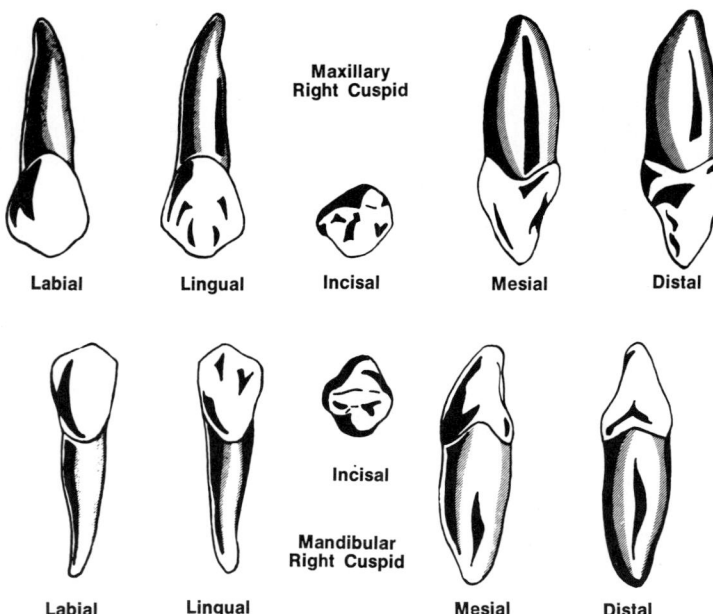

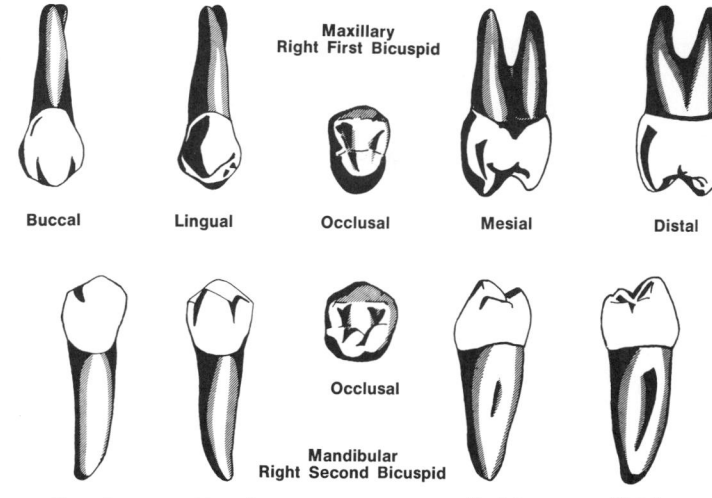

Figure 4-26 | Premolars or bicuspids.

Each tooth normally has two antagonists in the opposing arch. The exceptions are the mandibular incisors and the maxillary third molars. These teeth each have only one opposing tooth. This feature as well as the interlocking mechanism of the cusps in function ensures stability of the arches. Normal breathing, normal muscle functions of the jaws and the face, and absence of thumb sucking and other acquired habits ensure stability of the chewing mechanism.

Figure 4-27 | Molars.

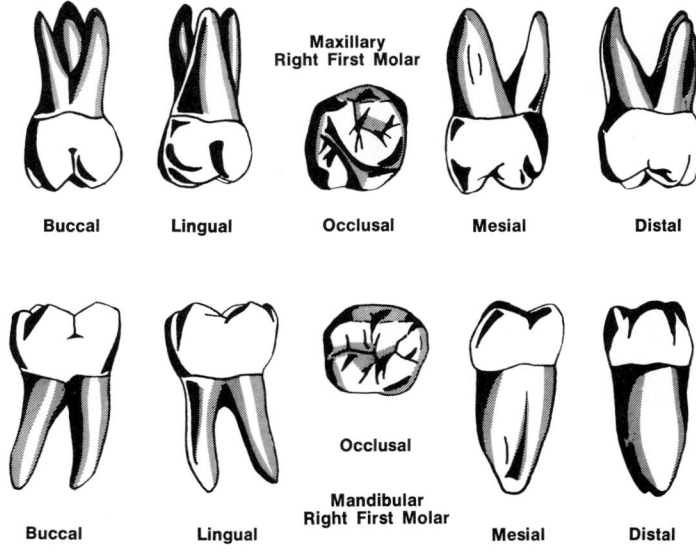

Premature loss of teeth, without replacement, may permit the drifting of teeth into these spaces resulting in inadequate occlusal relationship, loss of contact relationship between teeth in the same arch, and abnormal closing of the bite. This contributes to loss of function, possible periodontal disease, and may later require extensive treatment of the supporting structures with subsequent extensive restorative treatment. The result will be less efficient and less esthetically acceptable than the original total natural dentition.

MAINTENANCE OF TOOTH POSITION

The chief factors influencing the maintenance of teeth in position are as follows: (1) occlusal contact, (2) intercuspal relation, (3) muscles of the face and counteracting muscles of the tongue, and (4) mesial and distal contact.

Occlusal Contact

As just stated, every tooth, with the exception of the mandibular central incisor and the maxillary third molar, has two antagonists or occlusal contacts. If a tooth is lost, there is another opposing tooth remaining to aid in maintaining the arch form (Fig. 4-28).

Intercuspal Relation

The interlocking of the cusps of teeth during occlusal contact prevents facial or lingual drifting of the teeth. Obviously this intercuspal relationship aids in pulverizing foods as well (Fig. 4-29).

Muscles of the Face and Tongue

The teeth are situated between the powerful muscles of the face and tongue. The normal function of these muscles is effective in maintaining equalized pressures upon the teeth, thus ensuring proper arch form.

Mesial and Distal Contact

Mesial and distal contact between teeth prevent their movement mesially or distally. This contact also protects the gingiva and the bone structure

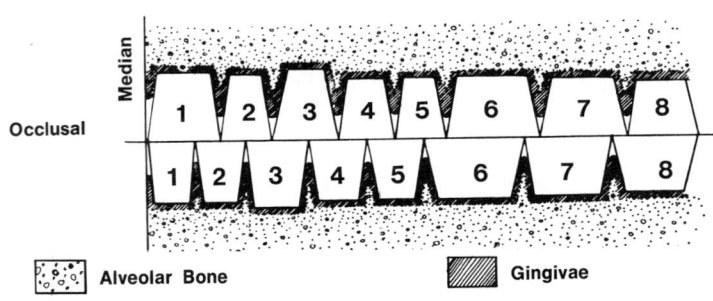

1. Central Incisor 3. Cuspid 5. Second Bicuspid 7. Second Molar
2. Lateral Incisor 4. First Bicuspid 6. First Molar 8. Third Molar

Figure 4-28 | Schematic drawing of the facial aspects of the teeth. This geometric concept illustrates the teeth as trapezoids of various dimensions. Note the relation of each tooth to its opposing tooth or teeth in the opposite arch. Each tooth has two antagonists except no. 1 below and no. 8 above. (After R. C. Wheeler, Textbook of Dental Anatomy and Physiology, 3d ed., W. B. Saunders Company, Philadelphia, 1958).

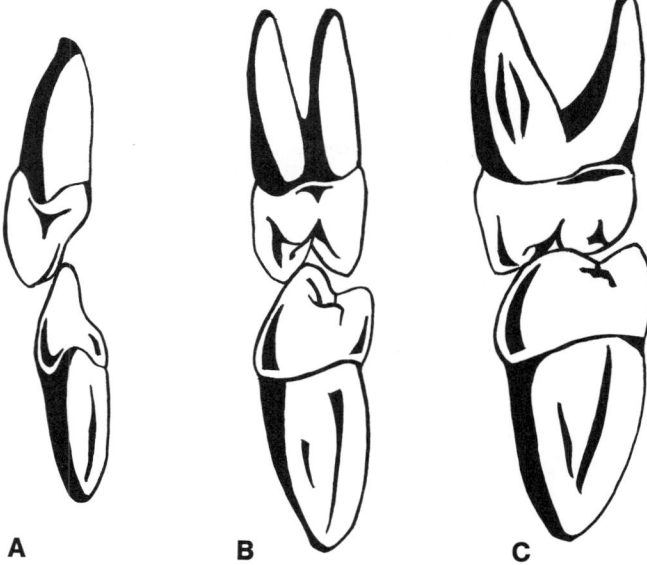

Figure 4-29 | Relative position of (A) incisors, (B) premolars or bicuspids, and (C) molars when jaws are closed in normal position.

beneath the contact area and prevents the former from being traumatized by food during mastication.

How Teeth Are Sustained by Their Own Functional Anatomy

The shape of the teeth with regard to their function in mastication has been discussed. In speaking of the teeth, Wheeler states, "They help sustain themselves in the dental arches by assisting in the development and protection of the tissues that support them." Among the various anatomic features that accomplish this are (1) contours, (2) contact and embrasure form, and (3) occlusal form.

Contours

The pronounced curvatures found on the facial and lingual surfaces act as a protection to the gingiva from the impact of foods during mastication. The gingiva will lack for adequate stimulation should the curvatures be great. However, if the curvatures are small, the gingiva may be traumatized by food (Fig. 4-30).

The contours of the mesial and distal surfaces help determine normal contact and embrasure

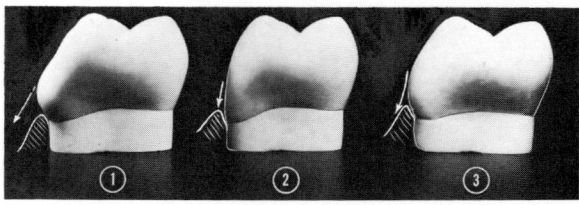

Figure 4-30 | Contours. Arrows show path of food that is propelled over the facial surface of a mandibular molar during mastication. (1) An overcontour deflects food from the gingiva and results in understimulation of the supporting tissues. (2) Undercontour of a tooth offers little protection to the tissues. The result is a traumatized supporting tissue. (3) This contour permits adequate stimulation of the supporting tissues and promotes their health.

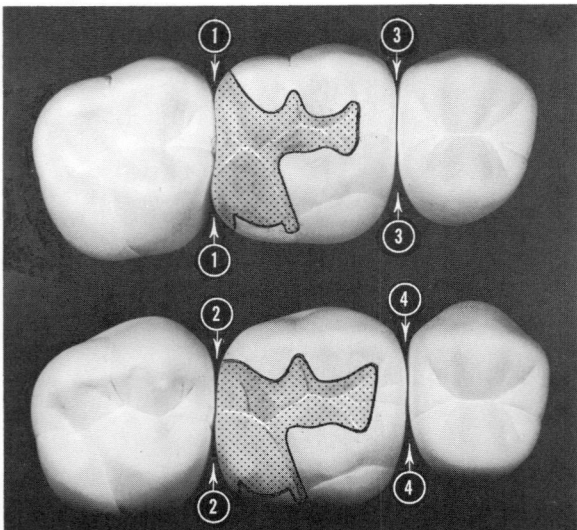

Figure 4-31 | Embrasure form. (1) Improper embrasure form as a result of the overcontouring of a restoration. Result: Gingiva unhealthy from lack of stimulation. (2) Good embrasure form. (3) Frictional wear of the contact area has resulted in a decrease of embrasure dimension. (4) Embrasure form is good. Result: Supporting tissues receive adequate stimulation from foods during mastication.

Figure 4-32 | Embrasure form. (1) Portion of tooth offering protection for the underlying tissues during mastication. (2) Contour of restoration not adequate for good embrasure form.

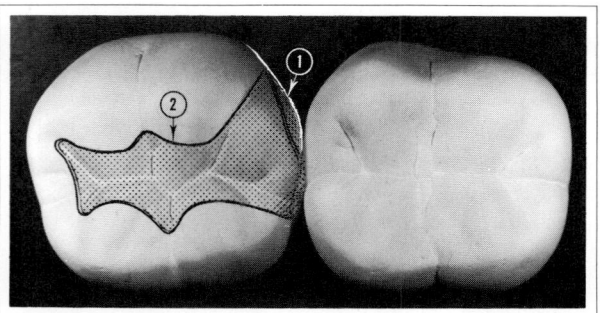

form, which lend to self-cleansing, thus further contributing to the tooth's own self-preservation.

Contacts and Embrasure Form

The lingual, occlusal or incisal, and facial embrasures provide spillways for dispersions of food during mastication. The size of these spillways determines the degree of stimulation that the supporting tissues will receive from the food during mastication. Poor anatomic form may result in a broad contact, decreasing the dimension of the spillways, thus reducing the stimulation to the underlying tissue (Fig. 4-31).

The frictional wear of the contact area by facial and lingual movements of the teeth over the years results in a broadened contact and decrease in spillway dimension (Fig. 4-31).

The correct anatomic restoration of the interproximal surfaces (mesial and distal) of teeth presents a challenge to the dentist. For example, this may involve the restoration of the distal cusp of a mandibular first permanent molar that has been lost because of caries. The failure to restore this cusp will result in an abnormally large facial embrasure. During mastication, food will be propelled downward into this embrasure by the opposing maxillary tooth, traumatizing the supporting tissue (Fig. 4-32).

The gingival embrasure is partially filled with the dental papillae. Normal contact and embrasure form are responsible for the health of this tissue.

Occlusal Form

The mesial and distal extremities of the occlusal surfaces present elevations of enamel known as marginal ridges. These ridges function to convey the food in the proper direction.

Occlusal wear gradually decreases the crown length of teeth with age. The masticatory area of the teeth increases as wear continues, accompanied by the loss of grooves, marginal ridges, and cusps. All these factors contribute to overloading of the supporting structures and cause improper direction of foods.

BIBLIOGRAPHY

Anson, B. J. (ed.): *Morris' Human Anatomy,* 12th ed., McGraw-Hill Book Company, New York, 1966.

Goldman, H. M., and Cohen, D. W.: *Periodontal Therapy,* 5th ed., The C. V. Mosby Company, St. Louis, 1973.

Kronfeld, R.: *Dental Histology and Comparative Dental Anatomy,* Lea & Febiger, Philadelphia, 1943.

McClendon, J. F., and Pettibone, C. J. V.: *Physiological Chemistry,* 6th ed., The C. V. Mosby Company, St. Louis, 1936.

Osol, A. (ed.): *Blakiston's Gould Medical Dictionary,* 3d ed., McGraw-Hill Book Company, New York, 1972.

Shapiro, H. H.: *Maxillofacial Anatomy,* J. B. Lippincott Company, Philadelphia, 1954.

Sicher, H., and Dubrul, E. L.: *Oral Anatomy,* 6th ed., The C. V. Mosby Company, St. Louis, 1975.

Wheeler, R. C.: *Dental Anatomy, Physiology, and Occlusion,* 5th ed., W. B. Saunders Company, Philadelphia, 1974.

Zeisz, R. C., and Nuckolls, J.: *Dental Anatomy,* The C. V. Mosby Company, St. Louis, 1949.

5 | Walter T. McFall, Jr.
Oral Histology

The normal dental and oral tissues presented in the previous chapter are composed of still smaller components. Invention of the light microscope and subsequent development of the electron microscope has made possible study of the minute anatomy of all bodily organs and tissues. Such study is the science of histology. Specialized investigation of oral tissues is termed oral histology. An understanding of the nature of the microscopic anatomy of oral tissues enhances comprehension of alterations resulting from disease and thus aids in return to health.

COMPOSITION AND CLASSIFICATION OF TISSUES

All body tissues contain three basic structural components—cells, intercellular substances, and tissue fluid. The basic unit of living matter (protoplasm) is the cell, and an infinite variety of designs and sizes of cells can occur. Intercellular substances can take many forms depending on the type of tissue. This material represents structures distributed among the cells, and these are usually products created by the cells themselves. Tissue fluid is a liquid, largely derived from blood, which diffuses through the tissues.

There are four major types of human tissues. These are epithelium, connective tissues, muscle, and nerve.

Epithelial tissue provides surface covering for the outer portions of the body and for those bodily cavities that open externally. Epithelium covers the lining soft tissues of the oral cavity, mucous membranes. It also gives rise to such skin appendages as hair, nails, and glands.

Connective tissues comprise much of the structure of the body. The nature of connective tissue varies widely depending upon location and functional demands. As a soft connective tissue it can be dense, fibrous, loose, or fatty. It can also assume harder forms such as cartilage, bone, and dentin and cementum of the teeth.

Nervous tissue and muscle are widely distributed throughout the body. Muscle provides for bodily movement while nerves accomplish both sensory and motor functions. With regard to the mouth, these tissues participate in the functions of jaw movement, talking, and swallowing.

TOOTH DEVELOPMENT

The first 8 weeks of intrauterine life represent the embryonic period of development. Significant stages in initiation and growth of oral and facial structures occur during this period.

Three primitive embryonic cellular layers take part in the formation of body tissue. *Ectoderm* forms the outermost layer, *mesoderm* the middle layers, and an inner layer, *endoderm*, lines the digestive tract. Structures of the oral cavity derive principally from ectoderm and mesoderm. Ectoderm subsequently gives rise to oral epithelium and enamel. Mesoderm leads to development of connective tissues of the mouth and the dentin, cementum, and pulp of the teeth.

Tooth Buds

Inception of tooth formation and subsequent tooth development is a remarkable process accomplished by ectoderm and mesoderm working in harmonious alternating control. During the sixth week of embryonic life tooth formation begins as an outsprouting of ectodermal cells in both arches. This growth initially begins near the midline and proceeds posteriorly. This early ectodermal ingrowth is the *dental lamina*. A similar process is responsible for development of the vestibule resulting in separation of cheeks and lips from alveolar ridges.

From the dental lamina at each site of a future primary tooth, 10 in each arch, further ectodermal cell multiplication occurs. This influences mesodermal cellular activity at the site resulting in the formation of a *tooth bud* or *germ*. The bud develops in three portions. The ectodermal part, termed the *enamel organ*, is the precursor of

Figure 5-1 | Cap stage of tooth development of a deciduous mandibular incisor.

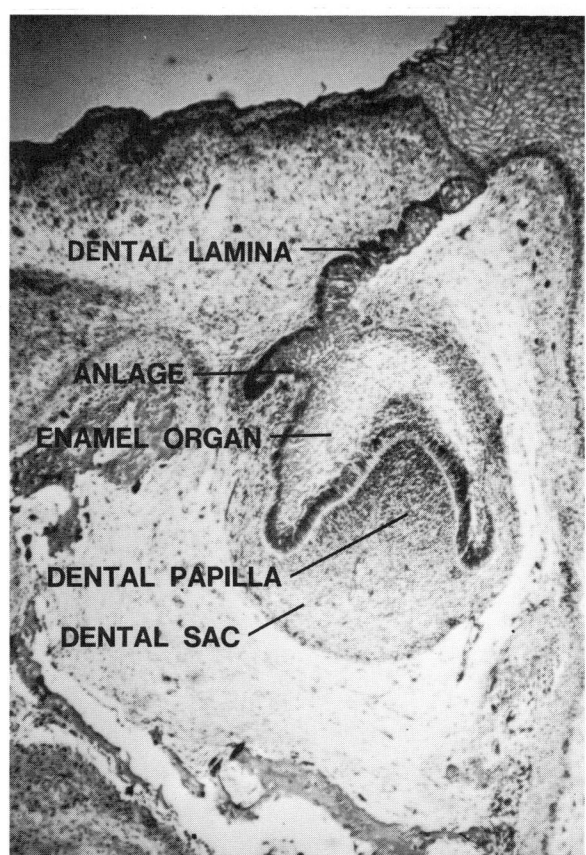

tooth enamel. Beneath the enamel organ mesodermal cells are organized as the *dental papilla,* which gives rise to the dentin and pulp. Surrounding the enamel organ and dental pulp other mesodermal cells become modified and produce intercellular substance resulting in the formation of the *dental sac.* Cementum of the tooth and supporting periodontal fibers arise from this structure.

Cap Developmental Stage

During continued growth of the developing tooth the enamel organ assumes the shape of a cap (Fig. 5-1). This occurs at about the ninth week, and further ectodermal and mesodermal modifications take place. The inner cells of the enamel organ become specialized for enamel production. These are termed *ameloblasts.* This is soon followed by alteration of mesodermal cells in the dental papillae into *odontoblasts,* which are cells capable of dentin production. Thus the dentinoenamel junction is established.

At about this same time lingual to each developing primary tooth an outgrowth from the primary bud, *anlage,* forms the start of the permanent tooth. Permanent molars arise directly by extension of the dental lamina and are not succedaneous.

Bell Developmental Stage

Further growth of the enamel organ leads to an outline of the shape of the crown and is termed the bell stage of development (Fig. 5-2). During this phase odontoblasts elaborate dentin, and then ameloblasts produce enamel. These specialized cells actually function in the production of a matrix material which subsequently becomes mineralized. The pulp aids in the support of dentin formation.

At this stage the enamel organ separates from the parent dental lamina, and crown formation proceeds, taking the shape of a primary incisor, cuspid, or molar. After crown form is completed, cells from the enamel organ shape an outline for the tooth root. These cells merely form a pattern for the odontoblasts to follow, and no enamel formation occurs in the root. Other mesodermal cells from the dental sac perform the function of cementum apposition.

Eruption of the primary teeth actually begins before the root is fully formed. The total development is completed when the tooth is in functional occlusion in the mouth. An attachment apparatus consisting of a connection between cementum and bone is established. The secondary dentition follows a similar developmental course (Fig. 5-3).

Figure 5-2 | Late bell stage of tooth development of a deciduous central incisor.

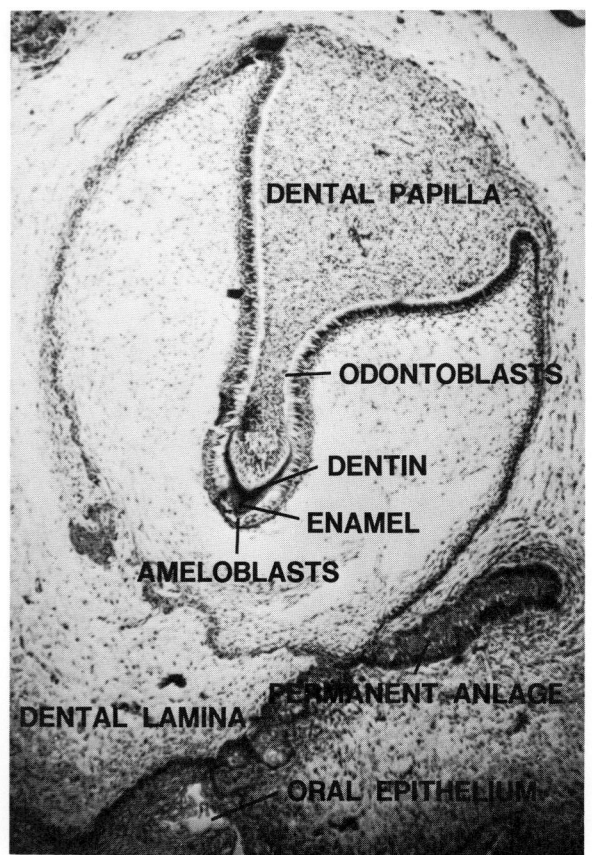

MATURE DENTAL TISSUES

The mature dental tissues consist of enamel, dentin, cementum, and dental pulp. Since enamel, dentin, and cementum are all mineralized, they are referred to as hard dental tissues. These hard structures consist of fibrous meshworks, background material, and a mineral crystalline component.

Enamel

Enamel is the hardest and most completely mineralized of all tissues of the body. Ninety-six percent of enamel by weight is composed of inorganic minerals. Organic matter and water account for the remainder. The inorganic fraction is primarily composed of calcium and phosphate salts while the organic portion is mainly a protein termed keratin.

Enamel lacks capacity for self-repair since it contains no cells. The formative ameloblasts are lost in the process of tooth eruption, and there are no living cells in enamel itself. Thus enamel resists wear only through its extreme hardness, and it does wear with age due to contact with opposing teeth during forceful occlusion.

Because of the high mineral content and relatively small amount of organic material, enamel is extremely difficult to study by conventional microscopic means. Ordinary preparation of teeth for microscopic study results in dissolution of enamel, and thus examination must be made on thin slices called ground sections (Fig. 5-4).

Enamel is composed of rods (prisms) which extend from the dentinoenamel junction to the surface of the crown. The rods are arranged perpendicular to the dentinoenamel junction and generally run a straight course. Sometimes the rods interwind as they approach the surface. Such areas are *gnarled enamel*.

Surrounding each enamel rod is a rod sheath, and between rods is a cementing material, the interrod substance. Special techniques utilizing the electron microscope reveal that the rods are

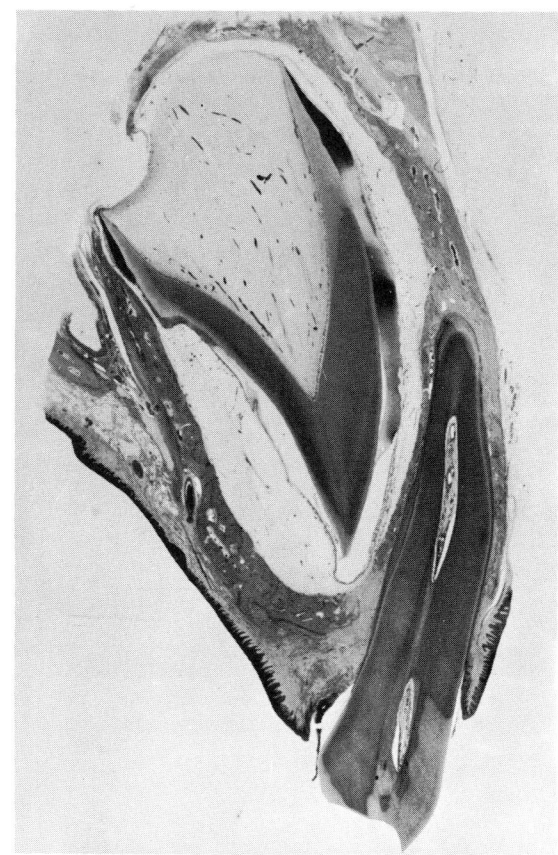

Figure 5-3 | Deciduous central incisor and developing permanent incisor.

somewhat keyhole-shaped and may share rod sheaths.

Several structural details can be found in sections of enamel. Lines termed *stripes of Retzius* are present because of the nature of enamel formations. Enamel rods are formed in a pattern of incremental growth which results in the lines and are similar to growth rings in a section of a tree. Small faults or cracks termed *lamellae* run through the enamel. Near the dentinoenamel junction occur unmineralized organic areas which appear as small brushes named *enamel*

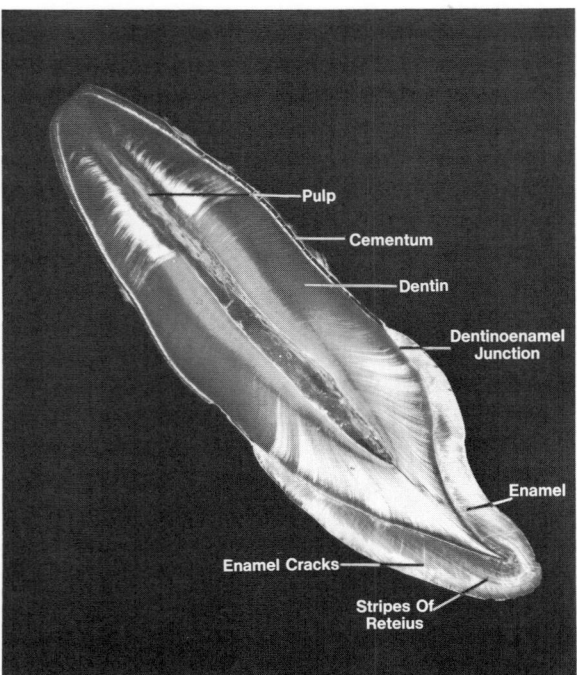

Figure 5-4 | Ground section of a permanent incisor tooth.

tufts. Occasionally in the process of formation portions of the odontoblasts, which form dentin, are caught during mineralization of enamel. These are termed *enamel spindles* (Figs. 5-5 and 5-6).

Though no new enamel is made, once the tooth erupts the mineral content and the structure of enamel may be modified. Dental caries may invade pits and fissures of the crown, and its spread may be hastened by the presence of lamellae, tufts, and spindles. Fluorides, topically applied, are taken up by the mineral portion of enamel, resulting in a stronger and more decay-resistant tooth structure.

Dentin

Unlike enamel the dentin is a living tissue containing cell processes and is capable of repair. The odontoblasts which originally formed the dentin remain viable in the pulp of the tooth. They have long protoplasmic processes coursing from dentin's junction with cementum or enamel back to the main cell body located in the pulp. These protoplasmic processes are the *dentinal fibers.* Thus odontoblasts establish a system within dentin capable of carrying nutrients, maintaining stimuli, allowing for fluid exchange, and changing structure.

Dentin is the major hard tissue of both the tooth crown and root. It contains about 70 percent mineralized material with the remainder organic portions and water. Thus dentin is considerably less hard and resistant than enamel.

Structurally, dentin is composed of mineralized tubules which enclose the odontoblastic process (dentinal fibers, Tomes's fibers). Between these tubules are intertubular matrix cementing material and collagen fibers.

Some differences occur in the composition of the dentin depending upon location. Near the dentinoenamel junction in the crown of the tooth there is much joining and overlapping of odontoblastic processes. Thus there are areas which are poorly mineralized or unmineralized. Such areas are termed *interglobular dentin.* In the root portion of the tooth just below the cementum there are usually a number of poorly calcified places (Tomes's granular layer).

Most of the dentin is composed of mature or circumpulpal dentin. Through this portion of the dentin the dentinal tubule assumes a gentle S-shaped curve. The end of the tubule near the pulp is more apical than the other end (Fig. 5-7). Nearest to the dental pulp and the cell bodies of the odontoblasts is the area of new dentin formation, the predentin. Predentin is only partially mineralized. As the minerals are deposited, predentin becomes mature dentin.

Sclerotic dentin is a modified type of structure which occurs when dentinal fibers degenerate and the tubule becomes filled with mineralized salts. This type of dentin is generally quite dense. Sometimes the dentinal fiber degenerates or is retracted and instead of filling in with mineral salts the tubule remains empty. In this instance the tubule is filled with air, and such an arrangement is a *dead tract* (Fig. 5-8).

A reparative phase of dentin formation occurs in response to some stimulus such as caries or extreme wear. In these instances *reparative dentin* is laid down by the odontoblasts to protect the pulp from danger. This type of dentin is similar to mature dentin except that it has fewer tubules.

Cementum

Lining the surface of the anatomic root of the tooth is the mineralized cementum. This thin tissue serves the important role of providing attachment for the fibers of the periodontal ligament, thus connecting the tooth securely to the alveolar bone of the tooth socket. This process must be continuous throughout the life of the tooth and is accomplished by activity of cementum-forming cells in the periodontal ligament called *cementoblasts*.

Cementum resembles bone in both composition and construction. The mineral content of cementum is about 50 percent. The coronal portion of cementum is fairly regular and is made up of alternating layers of fiber-containing zones and cementing substances. This portion of cementum lacks cells and is termed *acellular cementum*. Though there are no cells within the cementum, cementoblasts are located on the outer surface of the cementum. Where enamel and cementum meet, there may be various arrangements, but most often the cementum slightly overlaps enamel.

The portion of cementum most closely resembling bone is the apical portion of the root where *cellular cementum* is located. In this area cementoblasts are trapped in the forming cementum. Once trapped in small caves, lacunae, the cells are known as *cementocytes*. Tiny canals, canaliculi, allow protoplasmic connection of the cementocytes from lacuna to lacuna. This allows for nutrient exchange through the cellular cementum.

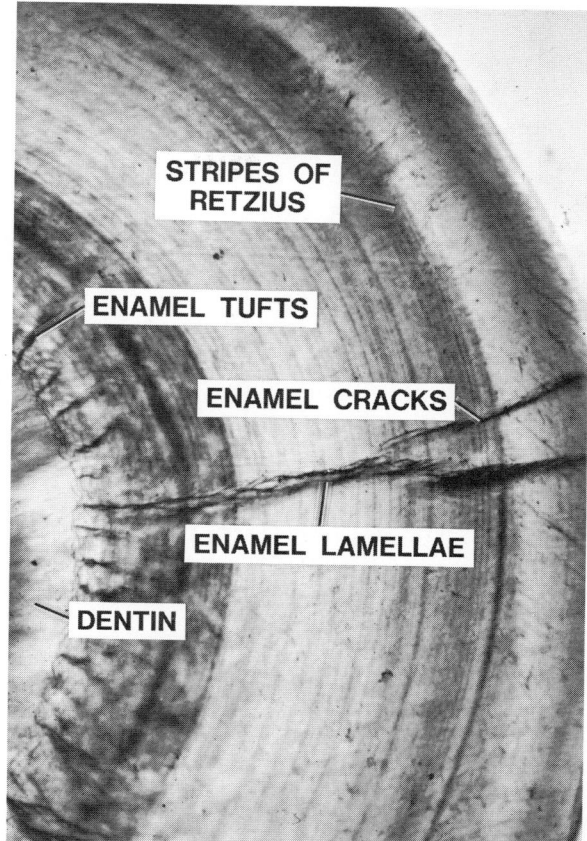

Figure 5-5 | Cross section of enamel and dentin.

Fibers from the periodontal ligament are embedded within the cementum. These Sharpey's fibers provide attachment of the tooth to bone (Fig. 5-7). Under pressure such as orthodontic tooth movement areas of cemental resorption can occur. Also, new areas of cementum may be laid down dependent upon functional demands, to repair defects or to add new Sharpey's fibers into the root.

Pulp

The soft dental tissue of the tooth is the dental pulp. Originating from the mesodermal embry-

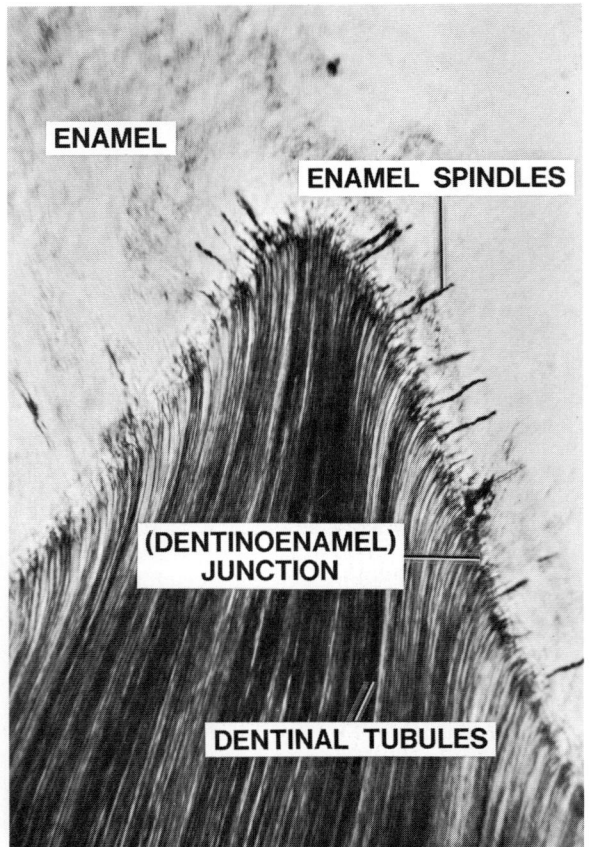

Figure 5-6 | Section of enamel and dentin at the dentinoenamel junction.

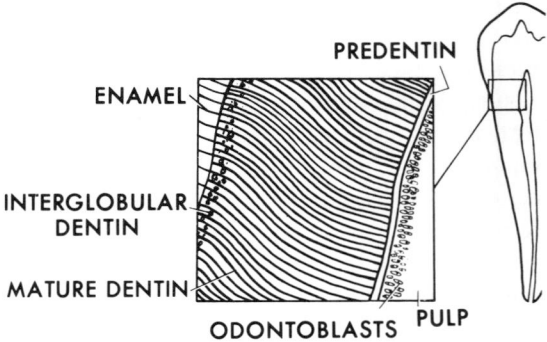

Figure 5-7 | A diagramatic drawing illustrating the S-shaped dentinal tubules and odontoblasts.

Nutritive functions for the pulp are achieved by extensive branching of tiny arteries and veins. The branching allows for rapid distribution of blood throughout the pulp chamber and canals. Usually there is one entering artery and two exiting veins, but this arrangement may vary.

Pulpal tissues play a vital role in the formation of the dentin. Odontoblastic cell bodies located in the pulp can respond to stimuli by producing new predentin matrix. Just below the odontoblasts occurs a cell-free layer (zone of Weil). Within the remainder of the pulp are cells for defense and for fiber construction, *fibroblasts* (Fig. 5-9).

onic element of the dental papillae, the pulp remains relatively primitive even in the adult tooth.

The pulp serves a variety of functions. All the sensory activities of the tooth are accomplished by nerves in the pulp. A finely developed branching network of nerve fibers occurs in the loose pulpal connective tissue. All these nerves have free endings which respond to any stimulus with the response of pain. Nerves serve also in assisting control of blood flow through the pulp and in signaling odontoblasts of the need for new dentin formation.

THE ORAL MUCOSA

Just as skin covers the external surface of the body, the oral mucosa lines the surface of the mouth. The oral mucosa, consisting of epithelium and connective tissue components, is adapted for function in the wet environment of the mouth.

Some variation in the design of the oral mucosa occurs, dependent upon location and function. Where masticatory stresses are heavy, the tissue is tough and relatively nonmobile.

Gingivae, the soft tissue surrounding the teeth and covering alveolar bone, and the mucosa of the hard palate are subject to such forces and are designated as *masticatory mucosa*.

Most of the oral soft tissues are termed *lining mucosa*. These collectively consist of the lips, cheeks, floor of the mouth, soft palate, underside of the tongue, and vestibular mucosa. These tissues are characterized by having a relatively thin, nonkeratinized epithelial surface. Connective tissue fibers are loosely woven, and there are variable amounts of fat, elastic fibers, and accessory salivary glands. These structural arrangements allow for mobility of these tissues during eating, swallowing, and speech.

The upper surface of the tongue is modified for its special function of taste. This specialized mucosa contains epithelium thrown up into little elevations with taste buds among the epithelial cells. These elevations are termed papillae and are of four major types: filiform, fungiform, foliate, and circumvallate. Most of the body of the tongue is made up of thick bands of muscle fibers.

SUPPORTING TISSUES OF TEETH

In addition to the tissues associated with the teeth themselves there are certain structures which primarily serve in support of the teeth. These comprise the *periodontium* and include gingivae, periodontal ligament, and alveolar bone. Cementum, a dental tissue, can also be properly classified as a part of the periodontium.

Gingivae

This firm oral soft tissue attaches to both teeth and bone. Facially the gingivae meet the lining mucosa at a wavy border, the mucogingival junction. On the mandible, lingually, a similar arrangement occurs where gingivae blend into lingual mucosa. On the maxilla there is smooth

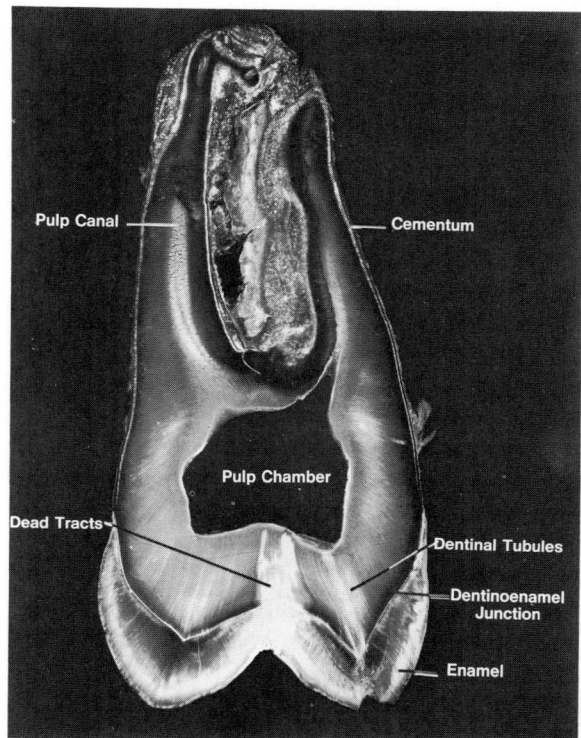

Figure 5-8 | Ground section of a molar tooth.

Figure 5-9 | A drawing illustrating the principal features of the dental pulp.

Chapter Five | Oral Histology | 113

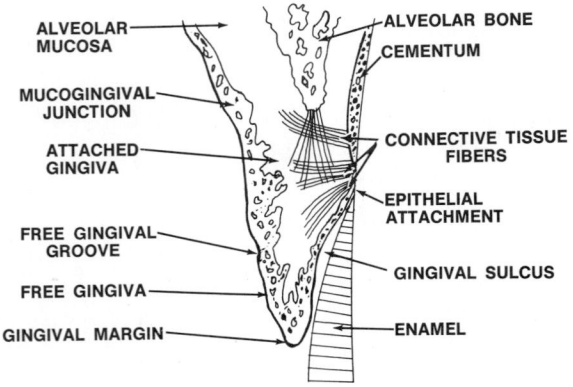

Figure 5-10 | The gingiva as viewed in a longitudinal section.

transition from the gingivae to the masticatory mucosa of the hard palate.

Most of the gingivae is securely fastened to tooth and bone and is attached gingivae. The color of this tissue in health is usually pale pink; but may be darker in individuals with more pigmentation. Attached gingivae are pebbled in texture, resembling the surface of an orange peel. This phenomenon is referred to as stippling. The gingival embrasures between the teeth are filled by the gingivae which form cone-shaped interdental papillae.

Figure 5-11 | A drawing showing the principal fiber groups of the periodontal ligament.

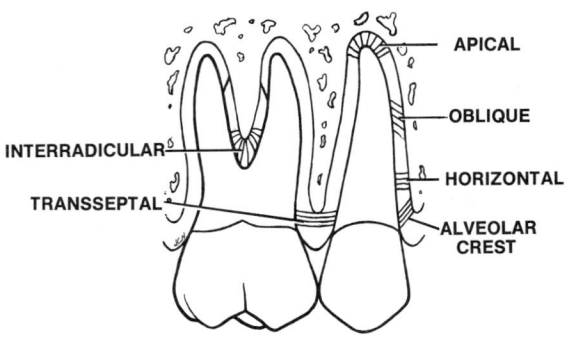

A portion of the gingival tissue encircles the neck of the teeth like a cuff. This portion of the gingivae, the *free gingivae,* fits snugly to the tooth, but may be blown free with a blast of air. Thus a space exists between the free gingivae and the tooth. This space is the *gingival sulcus.* The boundaries of the gingival sulcus are the tooth on the inner surface and nonkeratinized sulcular epithelium on the outer surface. Where the sulcular epithelium joins the tooth, the bottom of the sulcus occurs. This junction is the *epithelial attachment.*

Most of the attached gingivae is composed of dense connective tissue fibers which firmly bind gingivae to either bone or teeth. These collagen fibers are arranged into thick bundles or fiber groups. Also present in this connective tissue, *laminia propria,* are fibroblasts. A rich blood supply and an intricate nerve pattern are also located in this lamina propria (Fig. 5-10).

Overlying the lamina propria is a surface of epithelial cells. These are arranged in several layers. Nearest to the connective tissue are basal epithelial cells which multiply to provide new cells which are constantly being lost from the outer surface. The cells mature through several layers until they reach the outermost layer. The cells here are so arranged as to form a tough, keratinized surface which protects the underlying connective tissue. As the cells die, they are shed from the surface.

Periodontal Ligament

An attachment apparatus exists for support of the teeth consisting of cementum, alveolar bone, and an intervening soft tissue, the periodontal ligament. This ligament connects the tooth to the surrounding bone, allowing the tooth to yield to forces applied upon it.

The periodontal ligament consists of collagen fibers arranged into specific fiber groups (Fig. 5-11). The principal fiber groups are the alveolar crest group, horizontal group, oblique fiber group, apical fibers, and, in multirooted teeth, interradicular fibers. Perhaps the most important of these is the oblique group, which resists vertical forces applied to the tooth. Another important group of fibers runs from tooth to tooth interproximally and helps support the interdental gingiva. This is the transseptal fiber group.

Between the fiber groups is a loose connective tissue which contains blood vessels and a variety of cellular elements. The vascularity provides a cushioning effect which helps protect the principal fibers and tooth socket from sudden shocks. Important functions are served by cells present in the interstitial connective tissue. Fibroblasts are abundantly present for making new fibers for insertion in bone or cementum. The cells which form cementum, *cementoblasts,* are located here, as are bone-forming cells, *osteoblasts.* A number of cells for defense against disease are also located in this loose connective tissue.

Alveolar bone

A portion of the attachment apparatus is made up of alveolar bone. This is the part of the mandible and maxilla which functions in support of the tooth and consists of bone forming the tooth socket and supporting osseous tissues (Fig. 5-12).

Supporting bone is made up of two types of bone, compact and cancellous. The dense compact bone is arranged in layers and forms the outer surfaces of the mandible and maxilla. These dense osseous plates are separated from one another by the cancellous spongy bone. In this type of bone there is a scaffolding arrangement with marrow intervening between bone spicules. In the young this is red blood–forming marrow, while in the adult the marrow is yellow because of the fat content.

On a dental radiograph the bone which forms the tooth socket appears as a white, compact, radiopaque line surrounding the root or roots of the teeth and is called the *lamina dura*. Actually this is the *alveolar bone proper.* Fibers from the

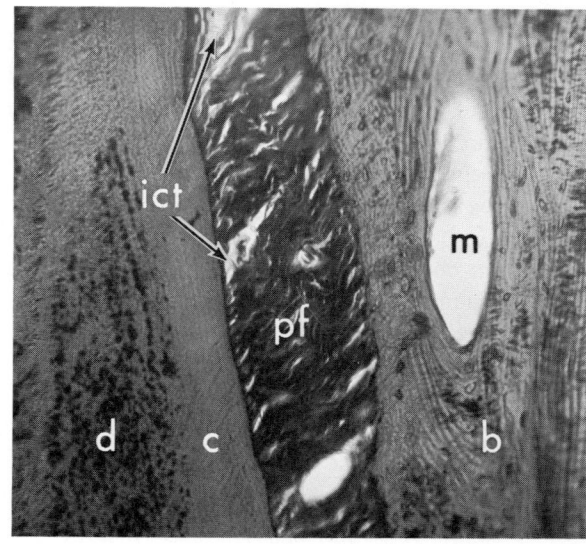

Figure 5-12 | The attachment of tooth to bone: (d) dentin, (c) cementum, (pf) principal fibers, (ict) interstitial connective tissue, (m) marrow, (b) bone. (From D. L. Allen, W. T. McFall, Jr., and G. C. Hunter, Jr., Periodontics for the Dental Hygienist, Lea & Febiger, 2d ed., Philadelphia, 1974.)

periodontal ligament insert into this alveolar bone proper for tooth support. The surface of the tooth socket is penetrated by channels which communicate with bone marrow and allow nutritional transfer to the periodontal ligament and aid in cushioning the stresses on the teeth.

Bone is manufactured by osteoblasts. These elaborate a bone precursor material, osteoid, which is subsequently mineralized. Osteoblasts may be trapped in the material they produce and remain viable in small lacunae. Once trapped the cells become *osteocytes* and are connected by canaliculi.

Many arrangements of bone are possible. It can be formed in flat layers or arranged in circular form around a central nutritional vessel. This circular arrangement is a *Haversian system.*

Alveolar bone functions for tooth support, and, if the tooth is extracted, it no longer has a function and is resorbed. This resorptive or removal process is accomplished by cells named *osteoclasts*. Actually both bone construction and removal are accomplished almost continuously depending upon demands placed upon it.

On the outer surfaces of bone is a dense connective tissue called *periosteum*. The inner surfaces of bone and marrow cavities are lined by a thinner connective tissue, the *endosteum*. Both periosteum and endosteum function in the deposition and removal of alveolar bone.

BIBLIOGRAPHY

Allen, D. L., McFall, W. T., Jr., and Hunter, G. C., Jr.: *Periodontics for the Dental Hygienist,* 2d ed., Lea & Febiger, Philadelphia, 1974.

Bhaskar, S. N.: *Synopsis of Oral Histology,* The C. V. Mosby Company, St. Louis, 1962.

Bhaskar, S. N. (ed.): *Orban's Oral Histology and Embryology,* 8th ed., The C. V. Mosby Company, St. Louis, 1976.

Goldman, H. M.: "The Topography and Role of the Gingival Fibers," *J. Dent. Res.,* **30:**331, 1951.

Gottlieb, B.: "Biology of the Cementum," *J. Periodontol.,* **13:**13–17, 1942.

McFall, W. T., Jr., and Kraus, B.: "Histological Studies of Human Prenatal Oral Mucous Membranes," *Periodontics,* **1:**20–27, 1963.

Meckel, A. H., Griebstein, W. J., and Neal, R. J.: "Structure of Mature Human Dental Enamel as Observed by Electron Microscopy," *Arch. Oral Biol.,* **10:**775–783, 1965.

Orban, B.: Clinical and Histological Study of the Surface Characteristics of the Gingiva, *Oral Surg.,* **1:**827–841, 1948.

Permar, D.: *Oral Embryology and Microscopic Anatomy,* 5th ed., Lea & Febiger, Philadelphia, 1972.

Provenza, D. V.: *Fundamentals of Oral Histology and Embryology,* J. B. Lippincott Company, Philadelphia, 1972.

6

James J. Crawford
Microbiology

INTRODUCTION

In the last 100 years the study of microbes, termed microbiology, has grown from the discoveries of a few pioneers into a vast, vital science. Microbiology now contributes greatly to the survival, health, and comfort of all people. It has become a vast basic and applied science, indispensibly woven throughout all of the health sciences as well as major areas of agriculture, industry, and even space exploration.

The major concerns of persons involved in oral-health care are mainly the bacteria and viruses. These do not include all microbes that interact with human beings or even all that relate to oral health. Only a few examples of greatest relevance to oral health can be described here without devoting an entire textbook to this important and fascinating subject of microscopic life forms and their interactions and contributions to human life.

Because of the emphasis we must place upon disease, it will be difficult to accept the accurate realization that a *very few microbes cause human illness*. There is nothing mysterious, sinister, or terribly difficult to understand about these few. They obey laws of physics and biology, and can be controlled. Information will be provided here to help the assistant to understand and perform the role of an oral-health educator of dental patients, as well as to perform technical duties in the protection of self, other personnel, and patients from infection in the dental operatory.

THE SCOPE OF MICROBIOLOGY

Many fundamentals of microbiology can only be touched upon here and should be supplemented by outside readings and/or course work to provide a more thorough understanding of microorganisms and the many ways in which we interact with them in our everyday lives as well as in the clinic, and the ways in which they grow and can be detected and observed. Basic fundamentals include study of the various microbes found on our bodies and in our environment in health and illness; their anatomy and composition; how they reproduce and change genetically in relation to their ability to harm us and to resist our efforts to control them; what their requirements are for growth and survival with regard to environmental factors of temperature, light, moisture, acidity, and nutrition; how they change food into energy and growth materials; how these facts can be used in their control; how some bacteria can live fairly peacefully on our bodies while others cause disease; what kinds of diseases they can cause; how the body responds to infection to become more resistant, or at times to become more susceptible; how infections can be treated with antimicrobial drugs; how infections can be prevented by immunization; how the spread of harmful bacteria and their activities can be controlled by purification and preservation of water, food, utensils, and all the materials used in health-care clinics. Still other fundamentals deal with how we critically depend upon microbes as part of the biologic ecology, within our bodies as well as in nature, for our survival and for the balance of nature; and how we make use of microbes in many ways to produce numerous chemicals such as alcohol, antibiotics, and foods such as cheese and bread.

FUNDAMENTALS AND HISTORY OF MICROBIOLOGY

A few of the fundamentals of microbiology can be seen from its history. Little was known about microbes until Antony van Leeuwenhoek first took the minute bacteria from between his own teeth and examined them with hand-ground lenses in the early 1700s. Most bacteria, just as those he first observed, are about 0.5 μm in diameter. About 2000 of them can be laid side by side across a thick line drawn with a pencil. They vary in shape from spheres called *cocci*, to rod or sticklike forms called *rods* or *bacilli*, to long threads or *filaments*. Some cocci form chains that resemble a string of pearls and are called *streptococci*. Other cocci that form clusters of spheres are called *staphylococci* (Fig. 6-1).

Genera or family names of bacteria have been derived from their appearance, from the names of persons who discovered them, from diseases they cause, or from products they form.

Several hundred years ago, microbes that

Figure 6-1 | Microscopic shapes of bacteria. (1) Sphere-shaped cocci. (2) Streptococci. (3) Staphylococci. (4) Rod forms of bacilli. (5) Branching and nonbranching filaments. (6) Rod forms containing round, heat-resistant spores. (7) Spirochetes.

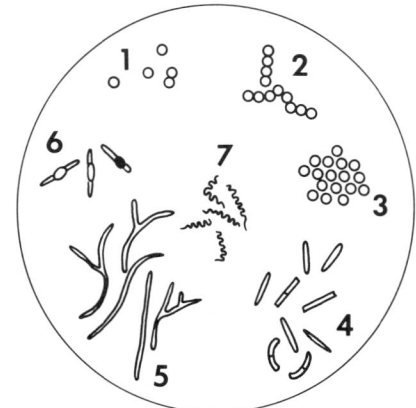

spoiled food, and even the rodents that infested homes, were believed to originate spontaneously as an act of creation. While soups generated bacteria, old rags and corn would generate mice. Diseases and plagues were believed to be a vindictive curse or punishment from the heavens. A number of researchers in the mid-nineteenth century changed those beliefs. They didn't disprove the concept of creation, but showed that it didn't happen the way other's ignorance and superstition believed it to happen. They also showed that human beings are endowed with reason that can learn to bring infectious disease under control.

Pasteur showed that fresh beef broth was spoiled by microbes that settle with dust from the air. He showed that fresh beef broth could be made sterile and free from bacteria by heating with steam under pressure. (We use his principle of cooking with steam under pressure in the home pressure cooker for canning, and in office steam sterilizers called autoclaves.) Then as long as Pasteur kept dust out of the sterilized containers, the broth in them remained pure and did not spoil (Fig. 6-2). When dust was deliberately admitted, the broth became cloudy with bacteria and spoiled. The bacteria in the air of closed rooms was found to be associated with the movement of people, their clothing, and hair which shook germ-laden lint and dust into the air. Moving feet stirred dust up from the floors. From his studies Pasteur also learned that bacteria could be enclosed and safely grown in closed test tubes of broth and that cultures of pure bacteria could be studied and identified in that way. The bacteria in the tubes didn't magically fly out to infect the researchers but remained there where they were placed, unless they were carelessly spilled, splashed, or sprayed around, the way cold germs are spread by sneezing. From investigations of bacteria grown in broth in test tubes it was found that bacteria reproduce by dividing in two. They do this by forming a new wall across the parent cell. When most bacteria found on or in the human body are placed in a suitable broth, each can divide about every 20 minutes. By repeated divisions they can actually reproduce millions of new bacteria that make a broth cloudy in about 24 hours. Infectious bacteria can also grow like this in a wound. When a few bacteria are placed on the surface of broth that has been jelled with seaweed extract called agar, they can reproduce enough times in 24 hours to form a small oval pile of bacteria that can be seen by the naked eye and resembles a tiny droplet of butter or soft wax. This is called a colony and comprises millions of individual bacteria (Fig. 6-3). Bacteria in the mouth actually form tiny colonies on teeth, where they can cause decay or injure the gums.

All bacteria were found to have a firm cell wall, like their plant relatives, which enables them for a few hours to a few days to withstand immersion in plain water or drying without bursting.

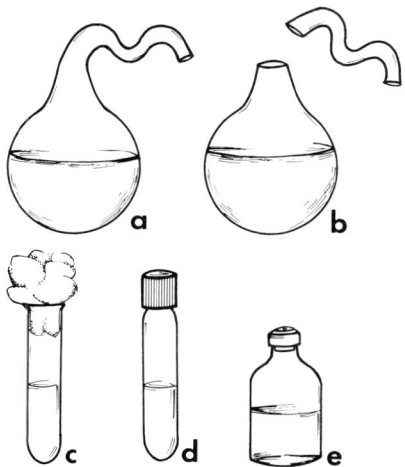

Figure 6-2 | Kinds of culture vessels and tubes used to exclude or safely confine bacteria. (A) Pasteur flask with a bent neck to exclude dust-borne bacteria. Broth sterilized in the flask remained sterile until (B) the neck was broken off to admit dust. (C) A cotton-plugged culture tube. (D) A tube of broth with a screw cap. (E) A sealed sterile serum vial used for sterile injectable solutions.

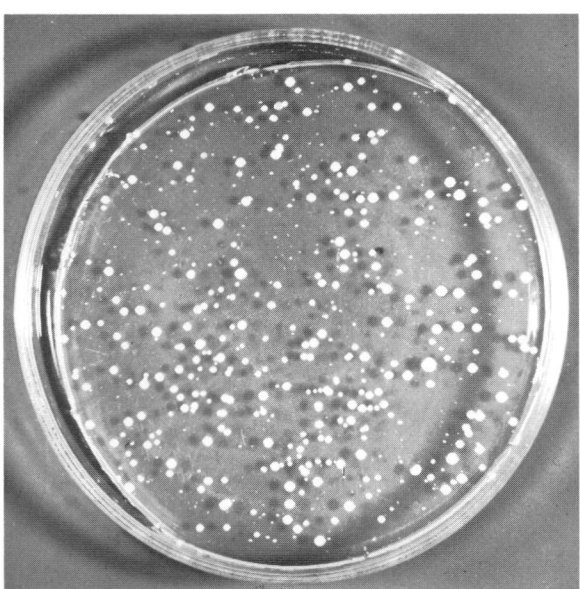

Figure 6-3 | Colonies of oral *Lactobacillus acidophilus* growing on selective culture medium.

Certain bacilli (rod forms) also produce a hard, dense particle called a spore (Fig. 6-1). The spore retains its ability to grow, but it is enclosed in a dense cell wall that can withstand drying for months and years. It can also withstand boiling. Bacteria that cause tetanus (lockjaw) and gas gangrene, as well as many harmless bacteria, form spores that can survive in the soil and dust for years. The infectious varieties can enter puncture wounds and cuts to cause severe infections. Special sterilization processes had to be designed to kill all life forms including spores in medicines for injection and surgical instruments because spores can even withstand boiling water for hours. Wrapping of surgical instruments is designed to keep dust and spores off instruments so that they will remain sterile. Now most materials used for health care and canned foods are sterilized.

In studying certain diseases Koch found that he could culture the same type of bacteria from each person with a certain kind of disease. These bacteria were of a different type from the bacteria normally found in the human body. He then found that he could inject experimental animals with the bacteria and produce a similar infection from which he could recover the same bacteria in pure culture. He postulated that whenever this series of events could be carried out, it would prove that type of bacteria to be the cause of the disease, called the *etiologic agent* of the disease. Tuberculosis was one of the diseases for which he successfully cultivated and identified the etiologic agent.

Pasteur and others further showed that when a vaccine prepared from killed or weakened microbes was injected into an animal, the animal became immune or resistant to further infection. Pasteur produced a vaccine against rabies that saved countless lives (including the life of this author). These discoveries led to the fascinating, almost miraculous discoveries of disease agents and vaccines for them that helped stop many epidemics. Diphtheria was one. It was a severe throat infection that terrorized Europe and killed hundreds of thousands of people throughout the world. Insects that helped spread microbial plagues were also recognized and controlled, such as mosquitoes that spread malaria. Bubonic plague was spread by rat fleas and lice. Vaccines have not been made against all microbes that can cause disease, such as those that cause colds, but vaccines have been found to keep the major plagues under control.

Unfortunately, at the beginning of the twentieth century surgeons did not immediately take heed of Pasteur's and Koch's findings. Hospitals remained filthy, and the death rates of mothers and infants were much higher when births occurred in hospitals than when infants were born at home. This was especially because physicians at that time didn't wash their hands before they delivered babies after dissecting cadavers. Mothers often died of "blood poisoning," a fatal infection caused by streptococci. Pasteur ranted at the surgeons and gynecologists, saying that it was they who killed these mothers by carrying the microbes on their hands from the infected corpses they studied. Today illegal abortions performed outside of hospitals in filthy surroundings still unnecessarily claim the lives of women because of poor sanitation and sterilization. Oral infections can also be caused by lack of proper sanitation and instrument sterilization in dentistry.

Lister, an English surgeon, applied Pasteur's discoveries to surgery and instituted the sanitary procedures now in use which include handwashing, gloving, draping of patients, cleaning the surgical site with antiseptic, and using sterilized instruments. These are termed *aseptic surgical procedures*, i.e., procedures free of sepsis or infection. Principles of asepsis have become an ethical and legal tradition in medicine and have a direct carry-over into surgical and general treatments of the oral tissues in dentistry. Surprisingly, all dentists who perform oral surgery do not yet wear gloves, although handwashing in dentistry is usually conscientiously used before examining patients. This is still not adequate to prevent surgeons and patients from contracting serious infections such as viral hepatitis.

Figure 6-4 | Aseptic surgical treatment.

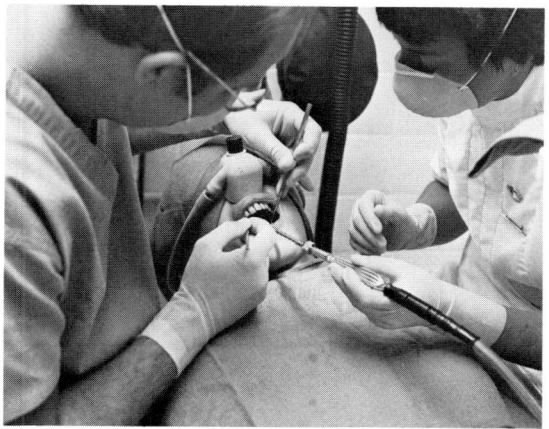

Oral surgeons now recognize their vulnerability to infection with viral hepatitis, and now most wear masks and gloves to protect themselves (Fig. 6-4). Avoidance of postoperative staphylococcal infections caused by the surgeon's skin bacteria and improved healing with less pain are some of the advantages for surgical patients when surgeons wear gloves. Because of the complexity and delicacy of dental instruments, and the amazing resistance of the oral tissues to infections, dentistry had lagged about 20 years behind medicine in instituting thorough aseptic controls. Also, because of the complexity of oral diseases, dental caries, gingivitis, and periodontal disease, we are still working to better understand these diseases and in order to bring them under better control in the population.

The discovery that chemicals called antibiotics produced by molds can kill infectious microbes provided an almost miraculous treatment for bacterial infections. This discovery and the development of the polio vaccine near the middle of the twentieth century were the climax of an age of major discoveries in microbiology in medicine.

A new age of discovery in oral microbiology probably really began in the 1940s when Orland and his associates at Notre Dame used germ-free animals to study dental caries. His work heralded an explosion of research in dentistry into the microbiology of dental caries, gingivitis, and periodontitis that has made great progress toward an understanding of the therapy and prevention of these bacterial diseases.

BACTERIAL GROUPS OF CLINICAL IMPORTANCE

In recent years we have also learned that not all bacteria found on and in our bodies and in our environment are harmful. Many are beneficial. Out of thousands of species of bacteria that exist in nature, less than 100 happen to be able to survive on or in the human body. A few microbes happen to produce substances that can injure human tissues. These are called *pathogens*. Their tendency to cause disease is called their *virulence*. The more virulent bacteria are, the fewer are required to cause illness. The bacillus of tuberculosis is highly virulent because a single bacillus can infect a susceptible person if it enters his or her body by the proper route. Thousands of bacteria of low virulence normally live in our mouths. We would not want to totally get rid of our oral bacteria, because their growth prevents the growth of foreign virulent pathogens that would begin to grow on and infect our oral tissues. Normal oral bacteria also combine with food and aid our digestion. Bacteria in our intestines synthesize vitamin K without which our blood would not clot. Thus, microbes have several different relationships with human beings. Microbes can be classified into four general groups according to our relationship with them.

Group I

The first group comprises those microbes that live separate from human beings in nature. For example, this group includes the yeasts found on fruits that ferment sugar into wines and other alcoholic beverages. Certain soil bacteria convert nitrogen in the air into compounds that are utilized by plants for growth. Most soil bacteria have no ability to cause disease if eaten or on contact. There are some exceptions to the concept that microbes that live in the soil are harmless, but most harmful ones come only from soil polluted by human and animal waste. *Private water supplies for home or office use must be tested by the county health service to ensure that no intestinal diseases are spread by waste-polluted water.*

An example of harmful soil microbes that are important in dentistry are the *Clostridium* species. Three main species can cause infections. One, *Clostridium tetani,* causes tetanus. Tetanus bacteria enter the soil through animal waste and form spores that can survive for years. *These spores can enter tissues through cuts and punctures* and cause minor infections. But their powerful toxins diffuse into the body and can cause rigid paralysis of the body and death. The disease is often called lockjaw. Everyone should be immunized against tetanus as a child. Patients treated for traumatic facial injuries usually require an injection to provide or to stimulate their immunity against the potent toxins. Other species, such as *Clostridium welchii,* can cause gas gangrene of severely traumatized limbs, such as an injured leg. *Clostridium botulinum* is a species that does not infect people but can grow in inadequately sterilized canned foods, especially in beans of all kinds. It produces a toxin that can be fatal if the food is even tasted before being thoroughly boiled for 10 minutes. Spoiled or questionable foods are the biggest hazard and should be discarded without hesitation. However, boiling will make such foods safe.

Group II

A second group of bacteria comprise the *indigenous* or *normal* flora of human beings. These consist of bacteria that commonly live on our skin and in the mouth and other body cavities. Despite the popular belief that our own bacteria can't hurt us, these can act as pathogens when introduced into injured tissues in sufficient numbers. Severe swelling and infections can result when these organisms are introduced into oral-facial tissues (Fig. 6-5). These involve many anaerobic species of bacteria that grow without air in the gingival crevices, such as the *Bacteroides* species. These can produce massive abscesses of the facial tissues. Oral bacteria as well as similar bacteria from the intestines cause severe infections in other parts of the body, particularly following abdominal injuries. Severe oral-tissue infections can extend to cause swelling of the eyelids and fever. Such infections can spread to the brain and cause death. Infections with oral bacteria can result from abscessed teeth and gingival abscesses. Infections some-

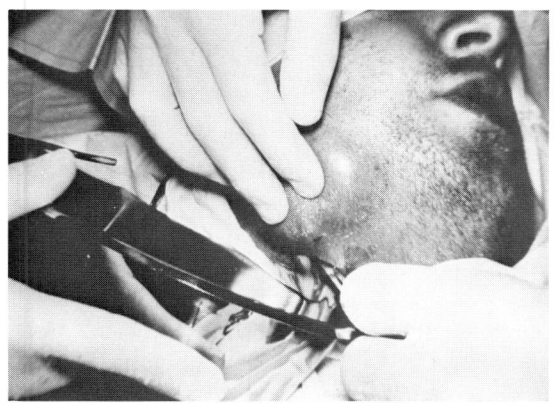

Figure 6-5 | A severe oral-facial infection. (From Lawrence and Block, Disinfection, Sterilization and Preservation, Lea & Febiger, Philadelphia, 1976, p. 694.)

times occur after extractions and are rarely caused by anesthetic injections. Posttreatment infections can be avoided by use of topical antiseptics and mouth washes to reduce the numbers of living bacteria introduced into the tissues by dental treatments. Patients with a history of heart disease or rheumatic fever are susceptible to heart valve infections and must be protected before dental treatments with antibiotics.

The same bacteria that live normally in the mouth form deposits on patient's teeth called *plaque*. This in turn, if not properly controlled with good oral hygiene, can cause gingivitis and periodontal disease. Certain species of bacteria in plaque also cause dental caries. These will be described in more detail.

Group III

A third group comprises pathogens common to most human populations. These are important to consider because they cause severe infections, some of which are quite common. They can be easily transmitted in a dental office. *Staphylococcus aureus* is a pathogen often carried in the vestibule of the nose and sometimes on the skin. It can cause painful boils and abscesses. It is sometimes found on oral surgeons' and assistants' hands and can infect injured oral tissues if gloves are not worn by all personnel during surgery. Patients who have artificial heart valves are highly susceptible to heart infections by either *S. aureus* or *S. albus,* which are normally present on the skin and in the pores. Skin staphylococci cannot be removed by washing.

In health our nasal passages are fairly free of bacteria, and the sinuses, middle ear, and lungs are sterile. During infections of the sinuses, middle ears, and lungs, a number of pathogens may be found. Viruses initiate colds and influenzas which are often followed by bacterial infections of the sinuses, middle ears, or lungs. Rarely, if not properly treated, these can spread to the spinal chord or to the brain. Bacteria that can cause such infections include *Streptococcus pneumoniae, Hemophilus influenzae, Staphylococcus aureus,* and *Neisseria meningitidis. Unless proper precautions are used, cold germs are easily and commonly spread in the dental office.*

Antibiotics can be used to treat severe bacterial infections but have no effect on viral infections. Any patient or clinical person with a fever or a sore throat or who feels very ill with a respiratory infection should be seen by a physician so proper medication can be prescribed.

Mycobacterium tuberculosis is an uncommon pathogen of the lungs causing tuberculosis, or TB. Signs of tuberculosis take several months to appear. These include tiredness, loss of weight, low-grade fever, night sweats, and finally a chronic cough. Tubercle bacilli are coughed into the mouth from cheesey lesions that break open in the lungs. Infection is spread by saliva contamination and by coughing. Tuberculosis used to be a severe, often fatal disease requiring that patients be isolated in a hospital. Now, most patients can be treated at home with antibiotics and other drugs. Infected persons can be detected by a simple skin test and by chest x-rays. Dental personnel can be exposed by infected patients who are not aware of their illness. *Personnel should have a skin test every 6 months.*

The throat normally contains the same bacteria found in the mouth. A sore throat, tonsillitis, or pharyngitis indicates an infection by either a virus or by *Streptococcus pyogenes* bacteria. Viral sore throats are accompanied by redness or painful spots or ulcers on the throat and usually fever. Antibiotics have no effect on viruses, and only symptomatic relief and rest can be prescribed. *S. pyogenes* or "strep" sore throat is less painful. There is usually a low fever, weakness, redness, and swelling of the tonsils, with distinct yellow pus to be seen, and possibly small white or yellow abscesses. Persons who also have a rash are said to have *scarlet fever*. Penicillin is highly effective against *S. pyogenes* infections. A serious concern is that streptococcal sore throats that go untreated can result in *rheumatic fever* (rheumatic heart disease) which damages the heart valves, in kidney disease (acute glomerulonephritis), or in joint disease (rheumatoid arthritis). These occur in a small percentage of instances several weeks after the throat infection has subsided. They do not respond to antibiotics. However, antibiotics are often prescribed for long periods to help affected patients avoid other infections. Patients with rheumatic fever remain very susceptible to heart valve infections caused by normal oral streptococci (*Streptococcus viridans*). Subsequent heart valve infections are termed *bacterial endocarditis*. These can most easily occur when patients who have a history of rheumatic fever receive any kind of dental treatment. These patients usually must receive antibiotics just prior to all dental treatments and when they are being trained to floss their teeth. The dentist determines whether antibiotics are needed and what kinds by consulting the patient's physician. Use of oral antiseptics before treating a patient with a history of rheumatic fever also helps to protect the patient.

Some of the questions asked patients in taking a history elicit whether the patient has a present or a past history of some of these serious diseases, and also if the patient is allergic to antibiotics and other drugs used for medications.

Group IV

A fourth group of microbes is comprised of the virulent plague and epidemic infection agents. Epidemic infections that we have under good control by vaccines are polio, diphtheria, tetanus, whooping cough, and smallpox. Through public health control of food, water, and pests, we control infectious hepatitis, typhoid fever, dysentery, typhus, bubonic plague, cholera, and malaria. Tuberculosis was also a serious plague at one time. When a person leaves the United States, a series of injections and medications are needed to protect them from contracting these infections. Patients who newly arrive in this country by air, especially from tropical countries, Asia, or the Orient, may have infections such as these. The assistant should be alert to unusual symptoms in such dental patients or in clinic personnel after a world traveler has been treated.

Although measles, chicken pox, influenza, mumps, and other children's diseases usually do not threaten lives, their spread in dentistry must be avoided. A vaccine for German measles is now available and should be used by any woman who was not infected as a child. It protects her from being infected with this disease during early pregnancy, which can cause deformities of the fetus. A vaccine against mumps is also available which can prevent a severe infection of adult males.

Prior to an influenza epidemic, all dental personnel should receive the influenza vaccine, because they will surely be exposed by their patients.

BACTERIOLOGY OF GINGIVITIS AND PERIODONTITIS

Since the first microscopic observation of bacteria in the oral cavity about 200 years ago, researchers have become aware that the mouth teems with millions of bacteria. In the early 1900s, W. D. Miller suggested the relationship of bacteria to dental decay, but absolute proof was not available.

Public health surveys in recent years have shown gingivitis to be present in most adults, but the role of bacteria was only theorized until 1965. At that time Harold Loe and his associates in Denmark carried out the first conclusive investigations into this disease. They taught a group of young adults how to remove all bacterial deposits from their teeth. Tissue samples examined from the volunteers showed an absence of inflammatory cells which indicate infection. Once they had established good oral health, the subjects were asked to stop all oral hygiene and brushing for a month. Samples were scraped from their teeth at the gingival margins and examined daily. Bacterial changes observed are shown in Fig. 6-6.

The day before oral hygiene was stopped, only a few spherical cocci could be observed together with epithelial cells.

At 24 to 48 hours a film composed of masses of cocci with short rods was beginning to cover the teeth. This was the initial stage of plaque formation. The cocci were mainly *Streptococcus sanguis* and some *Neisseria* species.

Approaching the end of a week, elongated, slender, pointed bacteria, *Fusobacterium* species, appeared in increasing numbers together with much longer, thicker filaments, *Leptotrichia buccalis,* and branching forms, *Bacterionema* species. These were seen in addition to the coccal masses present.

After 1 week, tiny, rapidly moving, tumbling, comma-shaped forms and twirling, serpentlike, or springlike spirochetes, *Borrelia* and *Treponema* species, appeared.

Shortly after the last two forms became very abundant in the plaque, gingival redness and bleeding and other signs of acute gingivitis were observed.

Many more bacterial species may be present, but those named were the easiest to see at the end of the first week. Many white blood cells, also known as pus cells, appeared then, indicating a tissue reaction to bacterial injury.

After having developed gingivitis, the patients were asked to restore brushing and other hygiene procedures. After 3 to 5 days of removing the plaque bacteria, gingivitis disappeared, and good gingival health was restored.

Thus the uncontrolled masses of normal oral bacteria commonly found in plaque on the teeth are not "normal" in the sense of contributing to health. Plaque produces gingival disease. Plaque bacteria are "normal" only in the sense of being found in almost all adults, and most adults have gingival disease.

Periodontitis (pyorrhea) results when gingivitis is allowed to continue for months or years without adequate hygiene. After long periods the gingiva lose their attachment to the teeth exposing more and more of root surface and allowing deep pockets to form around the teeth. These fill with plaque which continues the inflammation. Bone that surrounds and supports the teeth gradually resorbs, leaving the teeth loose. The pockets often become infected and abscess, and the teeth may be extracted. When plaque is left in place, calcium deposits form in it which harden it into calculus that can no longer be removed by a brush. Calculus prevents effective brushing, and teeth must be scaled in a dental office. Gingivitis can be stopped or prevented simply by daily flossing and brushing. Dental treatments and careful education of the patient are necessary to prepare the patient to practice good oral hygiene.

Most patients do not know how to properly clean their teeth. Dentists did not define how to teach their patients effective hygiene until recently. Before, they scolded patients who did a poor job and blamed them for poor oral health which created poor dentist-patient relationships. It is now recognized that patients can and must be carefully taught how to clean their teeth effectively, and that it is the job of the dental staff to carefully guide the patient's learning process through motivation, careful instruction, careful

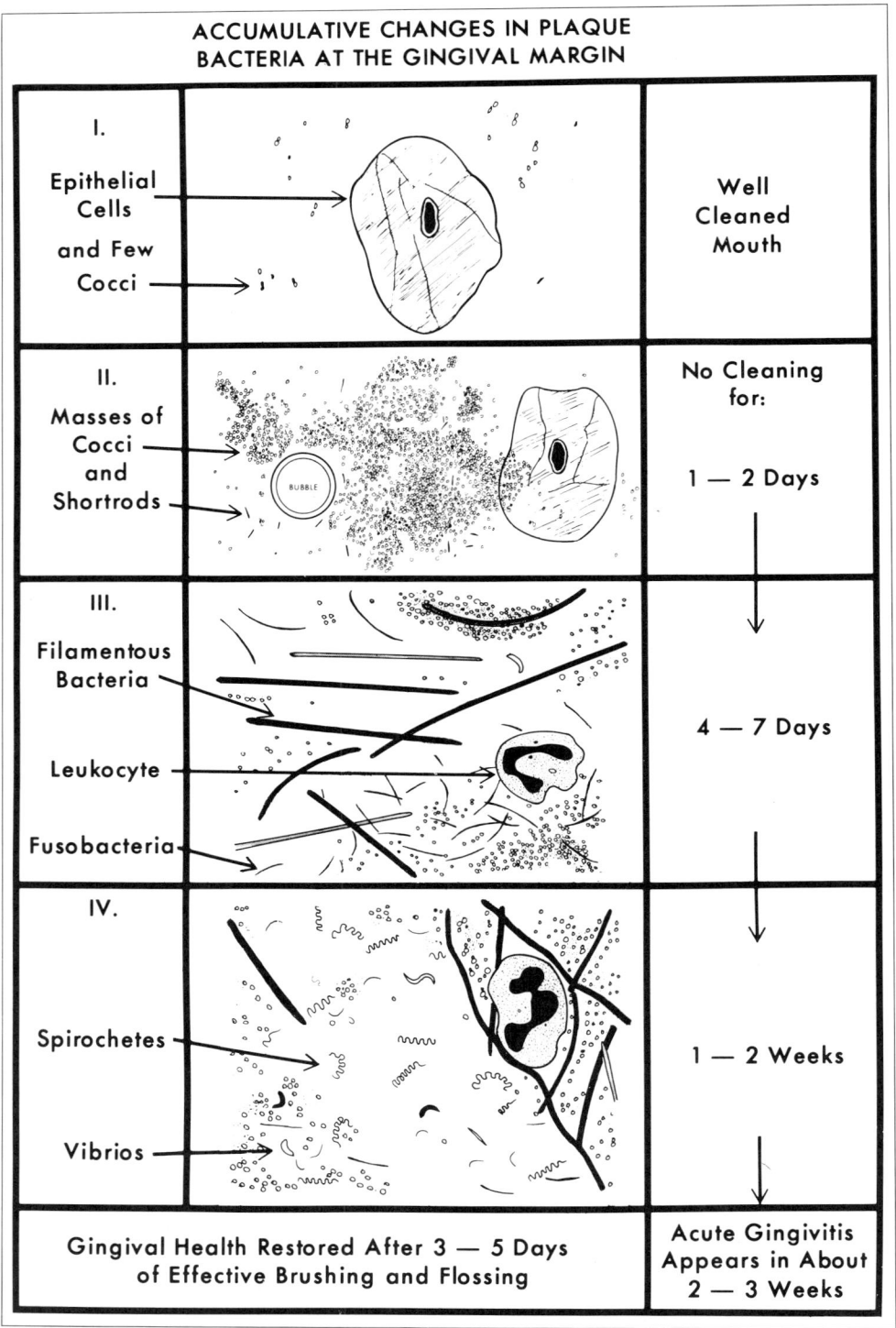

observation, repeated evaluation, and reinforcement of the patient's efforts for several days, until mastery of the skills and comfort are achieved. This may even take a week or more, and it must be followed by periodic checking and reinforcing. The patient now is approached as an equal and an ally against a microbial disease that results when oral bacteria are allowed to get out of control.

PHASE CONTRAST MICROSCOPY OF PLAQUE BACTERIA

In recent years Sumpter Arnim realized that looking at microbes in one's own plaque with a microscope could be as impressive for patients as it is for students of dental sciences. So he made movies of plaque bacteria and showed these to patients and then let them look at their own living bacteria in plaque from their own mouths with the aid of a phase contrast microscope. Using this demonstration together with disclosing dye to show the patient just where plaque occurred on his or her own teeth, Arnim found that he had a highly effective means of reaching the patient's own level of understanding of the disease problem firsthand. This proved to be a strong motivating factor in training patients in the use of flossing and brushing to remove the plaque from their teeth. Today many preventive dentists, hygienists, and assistants use these methods to educate and motivate patients. Patients are charged a fee to learn how to prevent diseases rather than just to receive treatment for it after it happens. This can include letting the patients meet the bacteria that cause their disease firsthand.

Materials needed for a phase microscopic demonstration of plaque bacteria are simple. They include a box of clean glass slides 1 mm thick, a box of cover glasses, #1 thickness, and a phase contrast microscope. These are all obtainable from dental-supply companies. Fluid is needed to disperse the specimen on a slide. The ordinary kitchen type of beef boullion broth can be prepared for this purpose from a boullion cube; it is boiled and can be stored in a covered pan in the refrigerator for several days. It should be discarded if it becomes the least bit cloudy. A small amount can be kept in a clean dropper bottle for half a day at a time without being spoiled by heavy growth of contaminating bacteria.

Microscopes of Japanese manufacture sold for patient education are of good quality at a reasonable cost. A small closed-circuit TV camera and monitor can also be obtained at low cost (Fig. 6-7). These televise the microscopic image of the bacteria on a TV screen so plaque bacteria can easily be pointed out to the patient. This proves to be highly effective in practice.

The procedure for examining a sample is not complex, but each detail is important. Using a curette, remove a tiny speck of plaque from the molars at the gingival margin, preferably near an interproximal space. Tease the sample apart in a drop of the broth on a slide and place a cover glass upon it. Press on the glass with a rubber pencil eraser in a circular motion briefly to disperse the plaque. Place a paper towel over the cover glass and press firmly to seal and blot the slide. Place the slide on the microscopic stage.

Now the slide can be examined. Adjust the transformer to the brightest light setting, or nearly so. Turn the $40\times$ objective into position for use pointing straight down. Consult the manufacturer's directions on how to adjust the condenser beneath the stage of the microscope. This is usually done by turning a dial to the proper setting, or by adjusting the condenser to a setting that corresponds to the objective in use. Focus on the edge of the sample. At the edge of the sample individual single bacteria or epithelial cells can be seen.

From the bacteria observed, the stage of

Figure 6-6 | Changes in plaque deposits at the gingival margins that lead to gingival disease.

plaque development and the least amount of time which has passed since the patient cleaned that area can be roughly estimated. In a well-cleansed mouth only a few nonmotile cocci and epithelial cells will be seen. Most plaque samples from the mouth of a patient who brushes ineffectively every day will consist of masses of cocci and a tangled network of filamentous bacteria. Most of these will not be motile (swimming) because they lack the fine, hairlike projections (flagellae) that make these microbes move. But, like weeds in a lawn, they are very much alive. Flowing and streaming of water under the cover glass and molecular movement may give a bouncing motion to single forms. Despite patients' efforts at hygiene, the finding of filamentous plaque indicates that the bristles of the brush have not reached this area for about 4 days. If one finds numerous spinning, vibrio, and spirochete forms in addition to the filamentous and coccal masses, it suggests that plaque in the area has not been reached with the brush for more than a week, or possibly for several weeks. Bleeding and redness of the area suggests gingivitis. The dentist will have to determine what degree of gingivitis and periodontitis may be present. Usually samples taken around the incisors show a less advanced plaque, indicating that the patient brushes better anteriorly.

The smaller microbes are easier seen at higher magnifications. Turn the 100× objective into place. Place a drop of immersion oil on the slide and, using the course adjustment, lower the objective into the oil until it just barely touches the slide. Adjust the substage condensor to the correct setting. Looking at the field, focus using the fine adjustment knob. Show the patient the types of bacteria. Explain how they injure the mouth.

Bacteria injure tissues because of the irritating chemicals they release that cause inflammation. They call forth many pus cells, up to several million every 30 seconds in irritated gingiva to combat the bacteria. In doing so they also appear to injure the gingival tissues. All of the destructive factors at work are not well under-

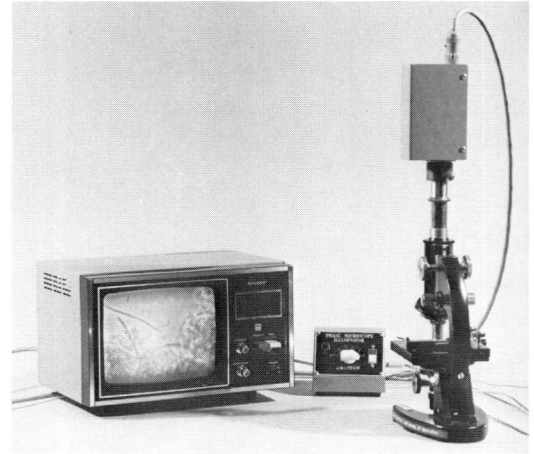

Figure 6-7 | A closed-circuit television camera and monitor (Sharp) attached to a phase contrast microscope (Unitron) effective for plaque demonstrations in patient education. Acceptable models and makes are available from dental-supply companies.

stood. What is important is that removing the bacteria daily stops the disease process.

The microscopic demonstration is usually performed only at the first visit. It may be repeated later, but plaque scoring after the use of a disclosing dye is done each time. Observing their own teeming plaque bacteria has a fair amount of shock value for most patients. A few may have no reaction to what they see. It is not advisable either to try to shame the patient, to scold, or to exaggerate the grotesque quality of what you are showing in a sadistic manner. Your goal rather is to provide realistic information to teach the patient, to help the patient understand the disease problem in order to help him or her learn adequate hygiene skills and habits. This has not occurred if the patient fails to reduce subsequent plaque scores.

DENTAL CARIES

What we have recently learned about how plaque bacteria cause dental decay is as interesting as it is complex. Both patients and dental personnel need to understand the role of bacteria in decay in order to understand how to control the disease.

The first plaque bacteria that adhere to the teeth have been found to be *Streptococcus* species. As soon as the mouth is closed after polishing, a microscopic film of salivary mucin covers the mouth. *Streptococcus sanguis* rapidly begin to attach and grow in the mucinous deposit to form the early stages of bacterial plaque. These apparently do not cause decay but form a plaque in which grow other bacteria that can cause decay. Bacteria that produce caries are believed to be *S. mutans* and *Lactobacillus* species. Lactic acid is produced by such bacteria from sucrose, i.e., table sugar found in the patients' diet. When lactic acid is produced by bacteria on the teeth, it reacts with and dissolves calcium from enamel, leaving a cavity. This takes months, so it is related to long-term habits of frequent sugar consumption. Flossing and brushing remove plaque from smooth surfaces of teeth. Eating sugar frequently during the day causes the plaque to be rapidly replaced, possibly even faster than it can be removed by one or even two daily brushings. Moreover, flossing and brushing cannot effectively clean occlusal pits and fissures in which decay most frequently occurs.

Fluoride treatments improve the resistance of smooth surfaces of the teeth to decay, and occlusal sealants help to protect pits and fissures, but the protection dentists can provide by these measures is far from complete for masses of people who are susceptible to decay.

Without sugar, bacteria cannot produce lactic acid. It is possible to prevent some patients from eating sugar, but it is not possible to restrict the sugar intake of everyone in the population at the present time. Therefore, it is important to study the bacteria that produce decay in order to learn how they can be controlled. Also, if tests can be used to detect bacteria that produce decay, patients can be tested to learn when they are infected and are most likely to develop decay. Patients can also be tested to determine whether preventive measures are working to control decay-producing bacteria. Research in caries bacteriology has made much progress, but there is still much to learn. Early findings are still useful.

In the 1930s *Lactobacillus* species, which are small, chain-forming rods, were found to be abundant in the mouths of people with decaying teeth. These ferment sugar and form more lactic acid than any other species of oral bacteria. Lactobacilli can also grow in the presence of more acid than can most other bacteria. Thus, they are called *acidogenic* and *aciduric*. Lactobacilli could be more easily detected by culturing saliva on an acid medium (Fig. 6-3). This seemed to clearly identify the agent of dental caries, since *Lactobacilli* are also found in virtually every carious lesion. Sugar was strongly suspected of causing caries when fermented to lactic acid by *Lactobacilli*. This was borne out by European research that showed feeding sticky sweets to children between meals accelerated dental caries and generally increased the counts of *Lactobacillus* colonies that grew from their saliva. Restricting children's sweets reduced *Lactobacillus* counts. A sugar-free diet plan devised by Philip Jay is still used for caries control. Tests for *Lactobacilli* were performed to keep a check on the patient. Tests related fairly well to dietary sugar restriction, and counts would decrease in about 2 weeks if the patient followed the diet.

In the 1940s Orland and his associates developed ways of keeping animals in germ-free chambers so they could study effects of various foods and single strains of bacteria upon the animals. They fed germ-free rats large quantities of sucrose and obtained no decay. When various bacteria that could break down protein were introduced, no decay resulted. This disproved an old theory that proteolytic bacteria may be important in decay. When rats were fed sugar together with *Streptococcus fecalis*, which formed lactic acid from sugar, the rats' teeth did decay. Surprisingly, their studies did not show that lactobacilli could produce decay. Further studies by other scientists showed that *Streptococcus mutans* is the most effective bacterial species for producing decay in rats and hamsters kept in regular cages and fed a sucrose diet. Now, *S. mutans* has been found in all human dental-decay lesions examined. More recently some strains of *lactobacilli* have been found to produce decay in otherwise germ-free rats fed sucrose. An interesting point is that human beings seem to be most vulnerable to occlusal surface pit and fissure caries, and *S. mutans* is found in these susceptible areas before decay occurs. Occlusal fissures without *S. mutans* do not tend to decay. Unfortunately, practical tests for *S. mutans* that would help identify conditions leading to decay are not available for office use.

Thus, the decay process has three requirements: (1) a constant supply of sugar for acid production, (2) specific bacteria such as *S. mutans* and possibly *Lactobacillus* species, and (3) susceptible teeth with vulnerable enamel and decay sites.

Decay prevention in individual patients is not easy to achieve. Susceptible decay sites in children's teeth can be reduced by providing 1 ppm of fluoride in the water supply, and by use of topical fluorides and occlusal sealants. Unfortunately, fluorides reduce decay only about 30 to 60 percent rather than 100 percent. Occlusal sealants can protect pits and fissures but wear away. Flossing and brushing apparently help to reduce decay, especially on smooth surfaces, to some degree. However, as long as excessive amounts of sucrose exist in the diet, especially in the form of between-meal and bedtime snacks, decay will still occur. Pits and fissures remain the hardest to clean and protect. An anticaries vaccine may be available some day, but it still seems years away. Therefore, diet evaluation and sucrose restriction are still an essential critical factor that cannot be overstressed to prevent or arrest decay in caries-prone children and young adults. Instituting a period of total sucrose restriction for children who have extensive or rampant caries together with indicated dental hygiene and restorations is imperative for decay control.

The patient's teeth remain at the mercy of the patient's dietary whims unless the dentist has some method of checking up on how well the patient adheres to a sucrose restriction diet. Regardless of the role of *Lactobacilli* in caries etiology, once carious lesions are treated, tests for *Lactobacilli* and other such acid-producing bacteria serve as a good index of oral hygiene and as a monitor for the frequency of sucrose intake in patient education and motivation.

Tests for Acid-forming Bacteria

Most tests for *Lactobacilli* such as *Lactobacillus* counts are complex, but Alban's modification of a test developed by Snyder is fairly simple to use. A small tube, 3 by $1/2$ in, of Snyder's test medium is used. This is available from dental-supply companies. The patient drools saliva into the culture tube; or a swab can be wiped over the buccal surfaces of the teeth and inserted just under the surface of the agar, and the stick is broken off so the cap can be replaced. The tube is incubated at 37°C and read every day for 4 days. The medium contains sugar and an acid indicator, which is green to begin with at pH 5.0. As acidity increases to pH 3.5 or below, the indicator turns yellow. A yellow color at the top of the medium is scored as +1; half-yellow is +2; all yellow except for the bottom quarter inch is +3; and all yellow is +4 (Fig. 6-8). A score is given the test every day, and the scores are totaled on the last day. Any distinct yellow-color change in 4 days indicates *Lactobacillus* activity; more rapid change or more rapid movement of the color change indicates more activity; distinct yellow color evident at 1 day at the top half of the tube moving rapidly throughout the tube would indicate a very high *Lactobacillus* count. Grainger described a similar test that can be evaluated more accurately using a pH meter.

Bacterial tests for *Lactobacilli* are not tests for dental caries, nor are they meant to be. Caries

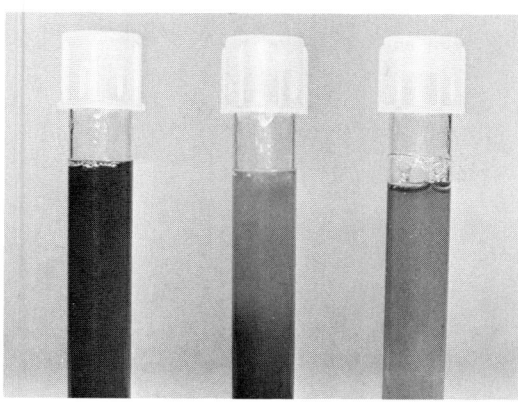

Figure 6-8 | Tubes of Snyder's test medium used according to Alban's method, incubated for 3 days. From left to right, the tubes show no activity, moderate activity, and high *Lactobacillus* activity.

can be actually measured only by radiographs and visual oral examinations for carious lesions. *Lactobacillus* tests are only tests for acidogenic bacteria which indicate conditions conducive to carious activity. Numerous preventive dentists have demonstrated the usefulness of such tests in patient education and for monitoring oral hygiene and sucrose restriction in diet control.

All measures that reduce caries risk, fluorides, restoration of lesions, good oral hygiene, and sugar restriction will lower *Lactobacillus* counts. Test results approach zero in a few weeks if adequate treatment and dietary sucrose restriction are provided. These also reduce and control *S. mutans*. Duplicate or triplicate tests performed on alternate days are more reliable than a single test. When used with preventive patient training and with an explanation of how the bacteria decay teeth, they are an aid to patient education. Tests are also of value at follow-up examinations. *Of greatest significance and concern are times when tests suddenly become positive when they have been negative previously.* If teeth have any susceptible sites under these renewed acidogenic conditions, the teeth appear to be highly vulnerable to rapid decay.

OTHER ORAL AND RELATED INFECTIONS

A severe form of gingivitis that is common to young adults is known as *necrotic ulcerative gingivitis,* or NUG. The common name is trench mouth because of its occurrence among young soldiers in the first world war when they were under conditions of poor oral hygiene, poor nutrition, loss of sleep, and stress. These factors seem to be universally associated with the disease. NUG is characterized by bleeding gingivae covered with a grey-white film of pus, resembling a false membrane (pseudomembrane) over the gingivae with ulceration of the dental papilla. A metallic taste and putrid mouth odor are also typical. Fever and lethargy may be present. The disease is sometimes precipitated by a viral infection of the gingivae, herpes simplex, which usually causes the fever. Herpes virus may make the condition more painful, and, as an infectious predisposing factor, accounts for the apparent transmissibility of NUG. NUG alone is not contagious or transmissible. NUG consists of a massive penetration and infection of the gingivae by fusobacteria and spirochetes commonly seen in advanced stages of plaque development. NUG is the only common condition in which these bacteria become so invasive and infective. They are easily seen with a phase contrast microscope and resemble the last stage of plaque development (Fig. 6-9). Saltwater rinses and careful cleaning and scaling of the teeth are therapeutic. Antibiotic therapy is mainly used in extensive cases associated with a fever.

Herpes simplex can take the form of a painful gingival inflammation, especially initial infections of children, or it can take the form of fever blisters on and around the lips. There is no effective treatment other than symptomatic, but the infection subsides after a few days. It may reoccur in the form of cold sores whenever the person has a cold.

Aphthous stomatitis is a similar kind of recurrent canker sore or ulcer that occurs on the tongue or the oral mucosa. The cause is not known, but it may be associated with oral streptococci.

Candidiasis or *moniliasis* is an irritating infection of the tongue and mucosa caused by the yeast *Candida albicans,* which causes white patches to appear on the tissue surfaces.

A number of other infections can occur on or in the mouth, such as syphilis. Since these can be infectious to anyone on contact, clinical personnel should not directly handle a patient's mouth without gloves if an infection appears to be present until it has been diagnosed and determined to be safe.

Syphilis may be seen as gray mucous patches inside the mouth, or a button-hard sore on a patient's lip (a chancre). Syphilis is transmitted only by direct contact. Syphilis, like gonorrhea, is a microbial genital infection transmitted mainly by sexual intercourse. Syphilis is caused by a spiral microbe or spirochete called *Treponema pallidum.* Lesions of syphilis can occur on or in the mouth as well. Patient's blood can be tested by any hospital laboratory using the VDRL, Kahn, Wassermann, or other *serum test for syphilis (STS).* The patient's test report will record the name of the test and the result, positive or negative. Tests become positive about 2 weeks after an initial ulcer appears. Gray mucous patches may occur later. Treatment is simple. A physician must be consulted. He or she will prescribe penicillin and be sure that a complete cure results as well as locate contacts who must also be treated. If left untreated, the chancre will disappear, but the infection will not be cured. Years later vital organs are very likely to be affected, causing brain damage, crippling, or death.

VIRUSES

Viruses are unique in being 10 to almost 1000 times smaller than bacteria, and they can reproduce only in suitable body cells. An influenza virus must contact mucous membranes of the respiratory tract. Only mucous cells are infected by it. Following infection, the virus is reproduced by the cell. The cell ruptures and dies, releasing many new virus particles. Most viruses die rapidly outside of the body. A few do not. Some, like herpes simplex and possibly cancer viruses, can lie dormant inside a cell until something triggers their growth. Tumor and cancer viruses appear able to lie dormant until they are triggered by certain chemicals or by irradiation. Then they stimulate very rapid cell growth in the form of a cancer or tumor. Cancer cells can invade blood vessels and be carried to the other vital organs, where they begin to grow, eventually causing death.

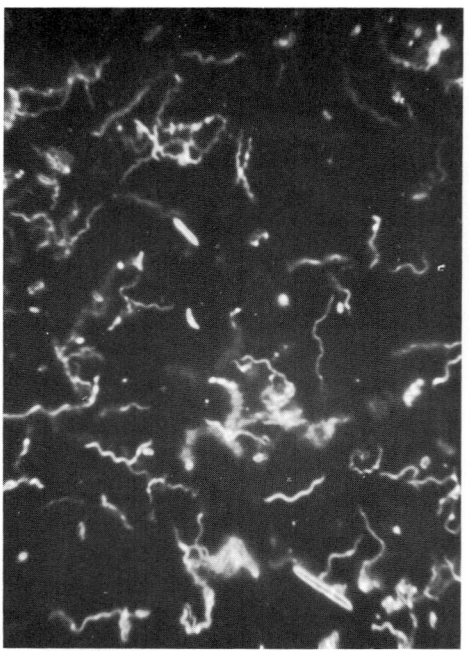

Figure 6-9 | Microorganisms associated with Vincent's infection, NUG (dark field).

Viral Hepatitis

Hepatitis is a term used for any disease of the liver. Certain viruses can cause severe liver diseases termed viral hepatitis. Two viral diseases, *hepatitis A* (infectious hepatitis) and *hepatitis B* (serum hepatitis) are of great concern to dentistry because they can be easily spread by dental treatments if the proper precautions are not taken. Dentists, dental auxiliaries, and patients are all highly vulnerable. Methods used in the past to disinfect instruments are no longer adequate to cope with the increase of viral hepatitis in the population. Hepatitis viruses appear to survive for weeks on dry surfaces of a dental unit, and they are resistant to most disinfectants that can be safely and feasibly used on surfaces in a dental office. They both cause serious illnesses that can hospitalize a person for weeks or months. Hepatitis A causes death in 0.2 to 1 percent, and hepatitis B in 1 to 30 percent of patients infected. About 5 percent of persons who contract hepatitis B can become carriers and spread the disease to others. This has happened to some dentists who have had to stop their practice. Infected dentists have unintentionally infected 12 to 50 dental patients in different outbreaks. Most people do not remain carriers longer than the time of illness. Then blood tests for the viral antigen will show when they are free of the virus. Rarely a person can remain a carrier for years.

Hepatitis A is mainly spread by feces and sewage-contaminated foods and drinking water. This is well controlled now. It can also be spread by blood and saliva. Hepatitis B was believed to be spread only by blood transfusions, by needles, and by surgical instruments. Recently we have learned that it is spread about one-half as frequently by saliva as by blood and that the virus does not have to be injected. *Just taking the virus into one's mouth in saliva or blood from an infected person or a carrier can transmit the disease.* This has serious implications for dentistry. Adequate sterilization of all instruments that enter the mouth is required. Wearing gloves for routine treatments is also desirable, especially when a patient is suspected of hepatitis.

Public concern is also needed about other sources. Many teenagers have been infected by passing cigarettes and drinks around among large groups of friends at parties. Serious questions are being raised about restaurants that do not wash and steam reusable dishes and utensils.

An increase of hepatitis B in the population of 6 to 100 times in recent years (depending on the group surveyed) now places the dental office in a much more difficult situation than before. Measures that were barely adequate to deal with viral hepatitis in 1965 are not adequate now. About 14 of 100 dentists have been exposed and 25 to 30 out of 100 oral surgeons have been exposed; almost 1 in 100 dentists may be a carrier, and 2 in 100 oral surgeons may be carriers. About 6 percent of persons who are infected remain carriers for up to a year or more. Dentists who were found to be infectious carriers have had to close their practice.

No statistics are available for dental-auxiliary personnel, but cases are continuously being reported. There is no treatment for infection with hepatitis B, although hepatitis A can usually be prevented by an injection of gamma globulin. Blood tests are available for hepatitis B, so a person can at least know if he or she is a carrier or has stopped being a carrier.

One problem is that *there is no way to recognize at least one-half of the patients who may carry the virus into a dental office,* because they give no history of the infection and because the incubation periods range from about 1 to 5 months, during which a person can be infectious. The best one can do is to upgrade the standards of office disinfection and sterilization to try to protect everyone all of the time and to take a careful medical history prior to treatment.

CONCLUSION

Of necessity, microorganisms that cause disease must be studied so we can learn how to best protect ourselves and our patients. Yet relatively few of the millions of microbes that occur in nature are harmful. Many are beneficial. Without those that live in the soil, leaves would not decay, and many plants would not grow. Without certain

Lactobacilli we would not have cheeses, bread would not rise without yeasts, nor would grapes ferment to make wine. Without bacteria in our intestines that make vitamin K, our blood would not clot.

Microbes that cause severe diseases concern us but are often forgotten because most are not visible. The patient with heavy plaque may have bad breath and an obnoxious appearance. The plaque bacteria threaten that patient's own tissues and teeth much more than they threaten the dentist or assistant. On the other hand, the patient with perfect oral hygiene and sweet breath may carry sore throat streptococci or hepatitis B virus which could seriously threaten your health. No matter whether an instrument has been used to treat the first patient or the second, no matter how clean and shiny it may look, unless it has been thoroughly sterilized, it can transmit disease.

Although microbes can't be seen directly, they are neither magic or more powerful than our understanding and ability to control them. With rational understanding and a responsible attitude in place of the irrational thoughts and imaginings that people use to charge their emotions and fears, effective measures can be carefully planned, and skills can be mastered so we can live at peace with the microbial world. As part of the assistant's responsibility for patient management and patient education, the assistant has a job of helping patients achieve a measure of responsibility and control over their oral microflora, avoiding its harmful effects as well. This is a task well worth mastering.

BIBLIOGRAPHY

Alban, A.: "An Improved Snyder Test," *J. Dent. Res.*, **49:**641, 1970.

Alban, A.: "Caries Prevention in Pedodontic Practice," *J. Dent. Res.*, IADR Abstracts no. 639, 1971.

American Association of Dental Schools: "Report of Actions of the 1974 House of Delegates; Res. No. 9-74-H," *J. Dent. Educ.*, **38:**316, 1974.

Crawford, J. J.: "New Light on the Transmissibility of Viral Hepatitis in Dental Practice and Its Control," *J. Am. Dent. Assoc.*, **91:**829–836, 1975.

Grainger, R. M.: "Swab Test for Caries Activity," *J. Can. Dent. Assoc.*, **31:**515–526, 1965.

Sims, W.: "The Interpretation and Use of Snyder Tests and *Lactobacillus* Counts," *J. Am. Dent. Assoc.*, **80:**1315–1319, 1970.

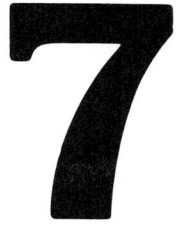

James J. Crawford
Sterilization and Disinfection

INTRODUCTION

A major responsibility of all members of the health-care profession is to protect patients and fellow staff persons from the risk of infection while patients are undergoing treatment. The risk of transmitting or causing infections is especially great in treating the oral cavities of many patients in a busy private dental practice and in large dental clinics.

The greatest risk is that of *cross-infections,* that is, transmitting serious infections from one patient to another, from clinic personnel to patients, or from patients to clinic personnel. Transmissible infections include all minor and serious respiratory infections ranging from colds to tuberculosis, childhood infections such as chickenpox, measles, and mumps, which can also be dangerous to adults, and herpes simplex, which can cause serious primary infections in children.

Presently the dental assistant faces the critical responsibility of helping dentists to implement new improved standards to prevent cross-infections among patients and clinic personnel. A serious need to update clinic standards has resulted from an increase of viral hepatitis in the population and an alarming increase in exposure and infection among dentists. A few dentists have even become carriers, and unknowingly caused infections among many of their patients. Cross-infections between patients are harder to document, but the risk of their occurrence is implied by the incidence of exposure of dentists to viral hepatitis. About 14 percent of general dentists have been exposed, 25 to 30 percent of oral surgeons have been exposed, and 6 to 14 percent of all dentists have been seriously ill. The characteristics of viral hepatitis infections and how they are spread have been described in the chapter on microbiology. It is important to recall that hepatitis viruses A and B are found in the saliva of infected persons, that they are resistant to many disinfectants, and that they can survive on operatory surfaces for 2 weeks. For these reasons the American Association of Dental Schools has supported a resolution stating that *cold disinfectant solutions are not acceptable for sterilization of instruments between patient treatments and that only accepted methods of heat and gaseous sterilization should be used.* This information has caused instrument sterilization practices to be changed in dental schools and many dental offices, but many dentists may still not be totally aware of the need for the changes or how to carry them out completely. This, then, becomes a major challenge of the dental assistant—to understand the reasons why the improved methods must be used, what methods are most effective, and which are less effective or not at all effective for clinic use.

The assistant must also master the effective methods and ways in which they can best be implemented. This is not a simple task, because different situations require different methods, and as yet we do not have all of the methods we need to provide perfect protection against each type of cross-infection problem. So the assistant must be willing to seek improved methods as well.

The risk of becoming infected can be worrisome. There appears to be less of a risk among assistants than among dentists. Only about 5 percent of persons who become infected with hepatitis become carriers for prolonged periods. This still remains a major concern to the practicing dentist, because the dentist may be prevented from practicing as long as he or she remains a carrier. Certainly, if clinic personnel were not willing to take risks, we would no longer have a health-care profession. Most important, many risks can be avoided by judicious and conscientious use of acceptable protective methods to protect both clinic personnel and the patient. This is a major responsibility of the dental assistant.

Another risk is that of causing *posttreatment infections* of patients by introducing excessive numbers of their own salivary and plaque bacteria into their tissues. Normally, people all have heavy populations of bacteria in their mouths, but local infections of the oral and facial tissues can result whenever excessive numbers of oral bacteria enter these tissues from diseased gingivae or infected dental pulps or as a result of traumatic treatments or injections.

Infections following treatments are not common, despite the fact that the mouth cannot be entirely freed of bacteria. However, it is now recognized that simple measures used by the assistant can greatly reduce the numbers of bacteria that can enter tissues during injections and treatments, and thus reduce the risks of infection that patients face. This becomes of greatest importance to patients who have a high risk of heart valve infections because of a prior illness or heart condition.

TERMINOLOGY

When considering adequate methods of protecting patients and personnel against infections, it is important to understand the terms often applied to materials and methods involved.

Sterilization

Clinical sterilization methods are those designed to destroy all microbes, including the most chemical- and heat-resistant hepatitis viruses and bacterial spores such as those that cause tetanus. The accepted test for sterilization is the total destruction of a dried preparation of nonpathogenic (non-disease-producing) heat-resistant bacterial spores that withstand boiling in water at 100°C (212°F).

Disinfection

In dentistry, disinfection commonly means the destruction of most infectious microorganisms. Disinfection is usually achieved by the use of boiling water or chemicals that commonly do not kill bacterial spores. Many disinfectants also do not kill tuberculosis bacteria. Even some that do, do not destroy hepatitis viruses. Presently no chemicals are available that are practical for routine office use that can destroy hepatitis viruses. Therefore, in routine use, thorough cleaning of all surfaces touched during patient treatment becomes a vital part of disinfection. Chemicals used for disinfection are called *germicides,* meaning that they kill germs. Since some kill certain microbes and not others, different prefixes are often used. The terms viricidal, bacteriocidal, tuberculocidal, sporicidal, and fungicidal indicate specifically what the chemical can destroy. Many chemicals are said to be *bacteriostatic,* meaning that they only stop the growth of bacteria but do not kill them. That is true of most antibacterial substances added to hand cleansers. Only those that contain *iodine* tend to be germicidal.

Asepsis; Aseptic Technique

Since *sepsis* means infection and *asepsis* means without infection, *aseptic technique* would be that which avoids contamination of patients and objects used in treating infected patients. Asepsis also involves careful use of items that have been sterilized or disinfected to avoid contaminating them with infectious microbes.

Antiseptic means against infection and is applied to chemicals tolerated by skin and mucous membranes that can kill or inhibit infectious bacteria.

These terms were first applied early in this century to surgery performed by surgeons who first began to wash their hands and who put on sterile gloves and sterile outer clothing before operating. They also covered the patient, except for the disinfected area to be treated, with sterile drapes and used only sterilized instruments. Before that time many surgeons wiped their hands with a dirty towel and pulled their instruments from their pockets.

Almost all dental treatments result in injury to the oral tissues with some bleeding. We are now confronted with a serious infection, hepatitis, that can be spread by blood and saliva. We are now making use of terms relating to aseptic technique to mark a change in dentistry, because they were used to mark a change in medicine nearly 100 years ago.

CROSS-INFECTIONS

The most serious infections transmissible as cross-infections in dentistry and the most difficult to control can be considered "target infections" against which control measures are aimed. These are (1) tuberculosis, which can be transmitted by saliva, and (2) infectious (A) and serum (B) varieties of viral hepatitis, which can be transmitted by saliva and by invisible amounts of blood left on any instruments or needles that routinely penetrate tissues. Blood is about twice as effective as saliva in transmitting hepatitis B. (From a growing knowledge of dental assisting, the reader may think about how many kinds of dental instruments might transmit these diseases.)

Infectious hepatitis is also excreted in feces of infected persons during active stages of the infection. Other persons become infected when the virus enters the mouth on soiled hands not adequately washed after handling contaminated objects such as paper holders and faucets in a rest room.

Serum and infectious hepatitis and tuberculosis are still common in the United States. Incubation periods last several months. During that time the patient is infectious, but symptoms are not detectable. Some cases of hepatitis are never diagnosed, and the patient will be unaware of having the infection. Some patients who have recovered from hepatitis can remain infectious for years. For every patient who is suspected of hepatitis, probably at least one more patient is an unrecognized carrier.

Tuberculosis organisms can be destroyed by boiling, by dry heat, and by some varieties of alcoholic, diphenolic, and iodine disinfectants under ideal conditions. Detergent disinfectants such as Zephiran chloride or benzalkonium chloride do not kill tuberculosis organisms. Hepatitis viruses are only known to be destroyed by heat or gas sterilization. Iodine detergents, sodium hypochlorite, and glutaraldehyde may be effective against hepatitis viruses, but their use has many limitations.

CONTROL OF CROSS-INFECTIONS

Cross-infection control would be very simple if all personnel wore disposable gloves and if the entire operatory and instruments could be sterilized before each patient treatment, or if the operatory materials and instruments could be made disposable and all surfaces could be covered with disposable materials. Research efforts are actually working in some of these directions. Disposable needles are one great advance. But right now the composition of operatory surfaces and instruments as well as the kinds of microbes transmitted complicate the selection of methods we can use to try to provide the safest oral-health treatments possible.

Therefore, methods of cross-infection control are divided into (1) methods of personal hygiene, (2) methods for disinfecting surfaces, (3) aseptic procedures used to avoid cross-contamination in the handling of instruments and dispensing of materials during patient treatments, and (4) methods for the sterilization of instruments.

Clothing and Personal Hygiene

It is important to wear clean, fresh clothing into the operatory each day for appearances and for infection control, to protect both yourself and your patient. Saliva mists and splatters cover your clothing and hair. Long hair must be carefully tied back away from your face so it never touches the patient or instruments or the surfaces you touch. For your own protection against these aerosols your hair should be covered, since it goes home to your pillow with you without always being washed before you retire. Eyes and nasal passages should actually always be protected whenever you are near aerosols and splatters produced by ultrasonic scaling devices used to clean teeth, or produced by a handpiece when teeth are cut or polished. Exposure to the heavy mists and aerosols causes dental personnel to have about 50 percent higher incidence of respiratory infections than individuals in other health-care professions. Glasses and a mask will not completely protect you from this exposure, but they can greatly reduce the *dose* of infectious bacteria to which you are exposed. Many dentists now wear masks just while mists are being created by treatment procedures. This rarely raises questions from patients. They accept a simple explanation that they have some resistance to their own bacteria but that you are exposed to those of every patient treated in your office unless precautions are taken. Germicidal lamps and disinfectant mists do little to protect you, because you are so near the exposure. An operatory should be well ventilated with fresh air. Special air filtration devices can be placed in an operatory to bathe the treatment field in a comfortable, rapidly moving, moist laminar flow of air that can completely protect personnel from aerosols and mists.

When you leave work, replace your uniform

with uncontaminated clothing to wear around home.

Hand Washing

Hands should be washed with a liquid soap dispensed from a foot-operated dispenser (Fig. 7-1). Bar soap and squeeze or hand-operated dispensers can hold bacteria and viruses for long periods. Sink faucets should turn on with foot pedals or have handles operated by your wrist. If they do not, use a paper towel to turn off the faucet.

Lather hands vigorously and rinse with cool water, 3 times between patients. This can take less than a minute. Use a brush or plastic nail cleaner to clean under nails during the first lathering. This brush should not be used to clean instruments. Paper towels are safe for use, since manufacturing processes kill all bacteria on them.

The kind of soap used is not critical unless a germicidal soap is needed, like an iodine surgical scrub. Mild soaps can be obtained from druggists for persons with sensitive skin. Low pH or nonalkaline detergents used for hair or dishes appear to be the least irritating to hands. Soaps containing 0.25 percent hexachlorophene are not harmful and are preferred to suppress staphylococci that grow on the skin, but hexachlorophene is not germicidal and will not kill infectious bacteria.

Gloves made of plastic or latex must be worn for your protection and that of the patient during oral surgery. These must be removed and discarded or cleaned and sterilized for reuse after the patient treatment, since the risk of viral hepatitis is so high in the presence of much blood. Since saliva can also transmit hepatitis, gloves also can and probably should be worn routinely. These can be changed and sterilized. If there are no breaks in them, they can be washed cleaner than hands. Wearing gloves is gradually becoming more common among general dentists.

Surface Disinfection

In preparing for a patient treatment, operatory surfaces that will be repeatedly touched are best covered with disposable paper covers whenever possible. The head rest is the most common example. The lamp handle can easily be covered with a small piece of paper fastened with a bit of plastic tape or with a disinfectant-moistened gauze sponge. Routinely, a clean paper cover is placed on the instrument tray after the tray has been carefully disinfected or sterilized. During surgery, operatory surfaces and the patient are draped with sterilized towels.

For disinfecting surfaces 70 percent isopropyl alcohol or a 2 percent solution of a phenolic detergent disinfectant are commonly used. Skin irritation can be avoided by wearing a household glove. These chemicals are *not* known to destroy

Figure 7-1 | Effective hand washing involves repeated lathering and rinsing using liquid soap.

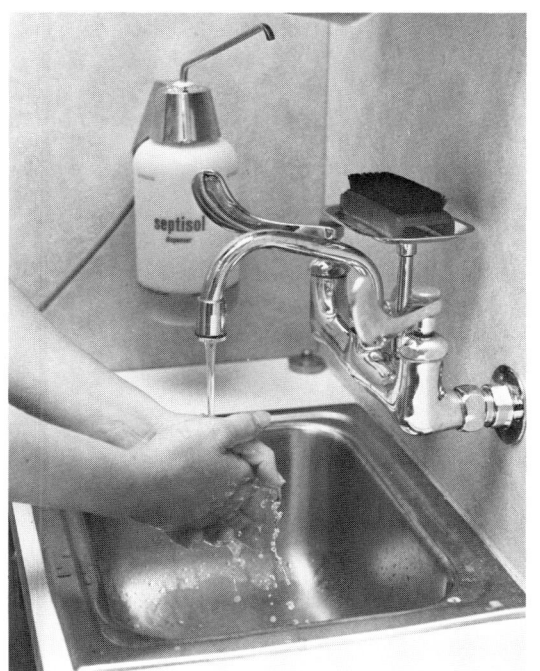

hepatitis viruses, but they are good cleansers and are effective against tuberculosis bacteria and most other disease agents. Therefore, thorough scrubbing of all surfaces disinfected is essential. Since gauze sponges or small paper towels used for this purpose quickly become saturated with saliva, do not wipe more than two or three surfaces with a single sponge or towel. Turn the material as you wipe. Large 4 by 4 in sponges work best.

Because the size of the dose of infectious microbes determines whether a susceptible person becomes infected, this is probably the only reason that surface disinfection protects so many patients. Thorough cleaning was shown to reduce the spread of viral hepatitis in one hospital.

Whenever a patient suspected of viral hepatitis is treated, wipe all contaminated surfaces with an iodophor iodine detergent or surgical scrub diluted with an equal part of alcohol. Allow it to remain on the surface for 20 minutes, or as long as possible. Then remove the yellow iodine film with an alcohol sponge. Iodophors do not generally harm surfaces, but they tend to leave a sticky film, especially around crevices. They do stain the starch in clinic uniforms, but stains wash out. Dentists tend to reserve iodophor for special situations.

Spray disinfectants are ineffective and wasteful. The unit still has to be scrubbed to remove films of saliva that protect even susceptible bacteria from the disinfectant.

All surfaces that are often handled during patient treatments by the dentist or assistant and may become directly or indirectly contaminated by saliva must be scrubbed before the next patient is seated (Fig. 7-2). This suggests the need to cut down the number of surfaces that are touched by saliva-coated hands. If the assistant's right hand is used to handle instruments, he or she may be able to reserve the left for adjusting the chair, holding the water spray, opening drawers, etc., if that is practical. This has to be determined by what works in a given operatory. Using a disposable sponge or clean paper towel

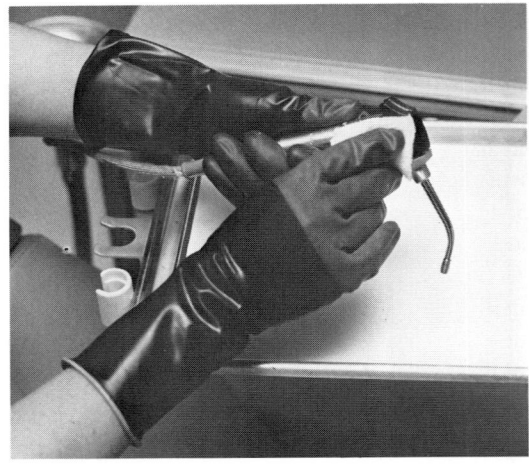

Figure 7-2 | All surfaces touched during treatment must be scrubbed with a disinfectant before each patient treatment.

to grasp contaminated switches, etc., can prevent contamination of hands.

Caution should be used to avoid repeatedly grasping air and water hoses where they are covered with cloth which can't be disinfected. If this isn't possible, a suitable area of the hose can be neatly wrapped with waterproof plastic tape which can be disinfected. A strip of plastic tape can be used to cover the entire row of recessed switches and discarded later.

These are some surfaces frequently contaminated that should be disinfected: lamp handle, lamp switch, instrument tray, tray pull handle, holders for handpiece and air-water syringe, chair-control switches, chair-arm release lever, knobs and places touched on the x-ray unit, and the cuspidor. The air-water syringe and handpieces present problems that will be described later.

Splatter and dust should be wiped from the entire unit each day or whenever surfaces appear soiled. Alcohol or a 1:200 dilution of phenolic disinfectant can be used.

If your dental unit has a removable hand-held

cuspidor, this should be the last item you disinfect. Use a paper towel saturated with disinfectant to first thoroughly scrub the outside and lip of the cuspidor. Patients frequently place this part to their mouth. Next scrub the inside of the cuspidor and discard the paper towel. Be careful not to contaminate the outside with the towel used to clean the inside. Wash your hands before handling other items or the unit. To eliminate this cross-infection hazard some dentists replace this type of cuspidor with an evacuator tip that the patient can hold. The suction is sufficient that the patient can rinse and evacuate easily. A replaceable tip is used that is disposable or can be sterilized.

Dispensing Clean and Sterile Items

A number of items are dispensed in the operatory before and sometimes during patient treatment. This must be managed to avoid contaminating all of the items by hands or by aerosolized microbes that settle on all exposed objects in the operatory during many patient treatments. Except for disinfectant sponges all materials should be stored dry. The practice of storing anesthetic cartridges in alcohol is not desirable because, as the solution collects debris and dust containing resistant microbes, all of the cartridges become contaminated. Cartridges are best dispensed from their dry, covered shipping canisters. Before use they are wiped with an alcohol sponge. For surgery they can be steam sterilized.

Other objects include cotton rolls, disposable needles, sponges, x-ray film tabs, and holders, swabs, and evacuator tips. All items should be stored in covered containers such as covered metal or glass hospital jars; or they can be stored in the shipping container if it is suitable. Some items such as wire, rubber dam, etc., can be stored in clean drawers. All items whether clean or actually sterile should be dispensed in a way that does not bring fingers into contact with other items in the container. Items are removed from covered jars with a set of forceps or pickups reserved for that purpose, kept in a separate container (Fig. 7-3). These and their container are replaced with a sterilized set or disinfected every day. Used materials, such as bands, clamps, or orthodontic wire, are never returned to a container, even if they were just tried and didn't fit. They must be sterilized or otherwise suitably treated first.

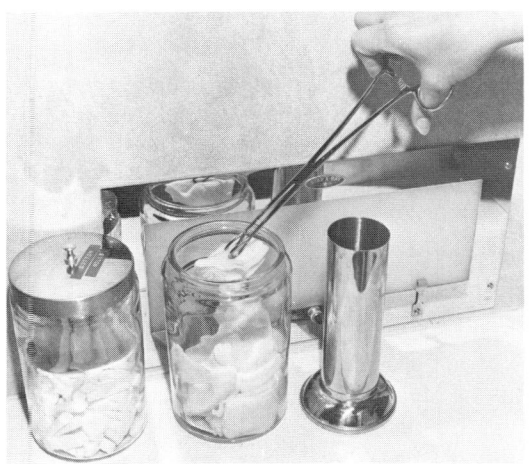

Figure 7-3 | Sterile and clean disposable items must be protected from dust and dispensed with sterilized transfer forceps.

Instrument Sterilization versus Disinfection

According to a resolution passed by the American Association of Dental Schools (AADS) in 1974 and given support by the ADA Council on Dental Therapeutics

Disinfection of dental instruments with chemical agents is *unacceptable* in preventing the transmissions of infectious disease. Therefore, the Association strongly recommends the use of auto-claving, dry heat, and gaseous sterilization, which are *acceptable* and effective methods of preventing the transmission of disease-causing agents.

The term *cold sterilization* coined by disinfectant manufacturers has been in common office use for many years. Its basis was that many common germicides *appeared* to destroy all bacteria of common importance. They were neat and inexpensive. The dentist believed that he or she was sterilizing until dentistry began to focus on resistant organisms such as agents of tuberculosis and viral hepatitis. In fact, most of these chemicals probably never sterilized in the 15- to 20-minute exposure periods used. They could at best only disinfect. Moreover benzalkonium chloride, possibly still used in some offices, did not even disinfect instruments after several uses and never had the ability to kill tubercle bacilli.

Cold disinfection or disinfection at room temperature is an accurate term, and, as the AADS resolution indicates, it has no acceptable application to instruments reused in oral treatments. This is because few chemicals are viricidal for hepatitis viruses in a reasonable period of time for clinic use and because penetration of even effective chemicals through organic debris on instruments in a reasonable period of time cannot be guaranteed. Therefore, chemical germicides such as glutaraldehydes only fill the purpose of surface disinfection and can provide some stopgap measures with an uncertain degree of safety until acceptable means of sterilization can be instituted.

Acceptable Methods of Instrument Sterilization

Autoclaving

The autoclave is a chamber that sterilizes by use of steam under pressure (Fig. 7-4). Steam under pressure can reach much higher temperatures than free-flowing steam. The high temperatures together with the steam under pressure are critical in bringing about effective rapid sterilization.

Autoclaving is one of the most effective methods of killing all microorganisms, and can provide total sterilization in a short time. All pathogens and spore forms will be destroyed. The autoclave is essentially an elaborate pressure cooker such as those used for home cooking and canning. In fact an ordinary pressure cooker can be used for instrument sterilization if used at the same temperature and pressure. Autoclaves are manufactured so the temperature can be selected electronically. Then the cycle is carried out automatically.

In using an autoclave, reliance should be placed on the internal temperature of the autoclave, as indicated by a thermometer placed in the discharge line. Autoclaving requires at least 121°C (250°F) with a steam pressure of at least 15 lb. Bacterial spores are more resistant to heat than hepatitis viruses and are destroyed in 15 minutes. An additional 5 to 15 minutes is needed to achieve penetration of large loads of materials. So, cycles require 20 to 30 minutes. Autoclaves that sterilize more rapidly at higher temperatures are also available commercially.

For the autoclave to be effective, the steam must be able to penetrate to all parts of the instruments. Therefore packaging and arrangements of articles to be sterilized must serve this

Figure 7-4 | A combination steam autoclave and dry-heat sterilizer. (*Omniclave, courtesy of The Pelton and Crane Company.*)

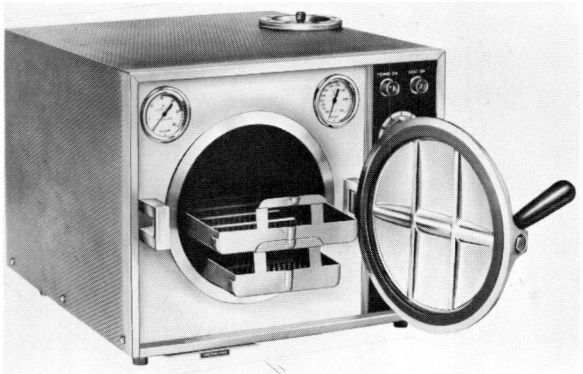

purpose. Instruments can be wrapped with paper or cloth or steam-permeable plastic. Closed metal or glass containers will not allow steam to penetrate. Containers are left uncovered or laid on their sides with lids partly removed if contents will not spill out.

Cotton and fabric materials will contain moisture after sterilization but will dry rapidly if left in the hot inner chamber with the control knob set on "vent."

The main disadvantage encountered in the use of an autoclave is rusting of instruments, unless preventive chemicals are used. To prevent rusting and corrosion of instruments, cleaned instruments can be dipped before sterilization in a milky emulsion of oil in water or in a fresh solution of 1 percent sodium nitrite. In some portable electric autoclaves, rusting can be prevented only by the additional use of a volatile alkaline solution. For this purpose an open beaker containing 15 ml of fresh household ammonia solution may be placed in the autoclave with each load of the oil emulsion–treated instruments. The milky emulsion leaves no noticeable residue on the instruments.

Dry-Heat Sterilization

Dry heat is a valuable method of sterilization, especially for materials which cannot be autoclaved safely. These include non-stainless-steel dental instruments, zinc oxide and other powders, wax, petrolatum, and other oils free of water.

Dry heat at a carefully regulated temperature is very effective for sharp or delicate instruments such as curettes and orthodontic pliers, since dry heat will not cause corrosion or rust. This method is also used for glassware, syringes and syringe needles, towels, sponges, and particularly for root canal instruments, where rusting is frequently a problem.

Dry-heat sterilization possesses some disadvantages; a greater length of time is necessary to achieve sterilization than with moist heat. Also rubber and plastic materials cannot be treated in this manner.

For the dental office small sterilizing ovens are available which are capable of reaching sterilization temperatures in a few minutes (Fig. 7-5). At temperatures of between 160 and 168°C (320 to 335°F) *sterilization is achieved in about 30 minutes in a preheated oven once the instruments reach that temperature.* Time is added to permit the instruments to come to the sterilization temperature, plus a safety factor. For efficient preheated ovens this requires a total of about 1 hour for sterilization of light loads. Needles and syringes should be given $1^{1}/_{2}$ hours.

Careful attention must be paid to the temperature range. The resistance of spores undergoes a change at about 160°C (320°F); consequently sterilization might not be accomplished below that temperature. However, soldered tips may loosen and impression trays come unsoldered if they are exposed to a temperature much above 168°C (335°F). Adjusting the oven to 165°C (335°F) provides a safe, adequate sterilization temperature.

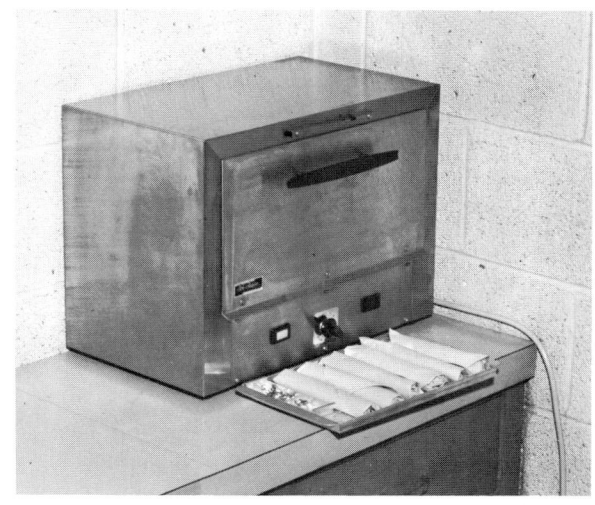

Figure 7-5 | A small, efficient dry-heat sterilizing oven equipped with an automatic timer. (*Dri-Clave, Courtesy of Dri-Clave Corporation.*)

Instruments to be sterilized must first be well cleaned and dried to prevent rusting. They may be placed loose in perforated trays or wrapped in small packages with paper or aluminum foil. The sterilizing oven must be loaded in such a manner that air is able to circulate adequately between the packages or individual instruments. Many dentists have installed built-in home wall ovens in their offices for dry-heat sterilization of instruments. This is particularly applicable for sterilizing trays of instruments.

Hot Bead and Salt Sterilizers

These are basically small dry-heat sterilizers used in endodontics. They operate at a temperature of 218 to 246°C (425 to 475°F). They consist of an electrically heated cup containing beads about 2 mm in diameter or table salt. Salt is the best conductor of heat. These must be turned on about 20 minutes before use to preheat.

Burs and endodontic instruments and surfaces of absorbent points that are not heavily contaminated can be sterilized by being submerged in such a sterilizer. Root canal instruments and burs require 15 to 20 seconds. Larger instruments require about 30 seconds. Surfaces of absorbent points require about 5 to 10 seconds. Sterile points exhibit a slight color change to yellow when they become sterile. Brown points will fragment in the canal and should not be used. Absorbent points are the most awkward objects to sterilize in this manner. These can be purchased already sterile.

Formaldehyde-Alcohol Vapor Pressure Sterilization

One means of sterilization combines heat with a gaseous vapor of formaldehyde and alcohol under pressure (Fig. 7-6). This method of sterilization operates a little above 121°C (250°F) and will sterilize all metal instruments including burs, mirrors, and curettes in 30 minutes without rust.

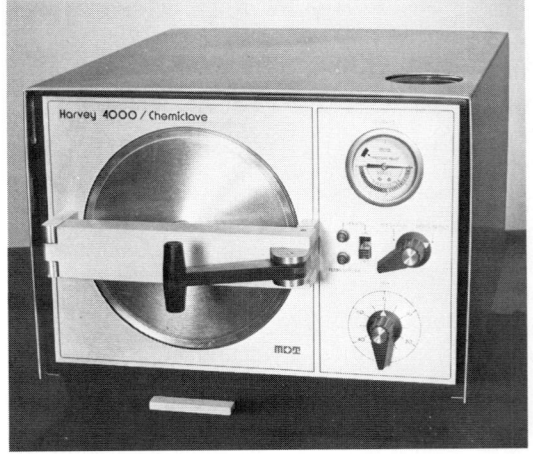

Figure 7-6 | Formaldehyde-alcohol vapor pressure sterilizer. (*Harvey 4000 Chemiclave, Courtesy of MDT Corporation.*)

It is especially valuable for sterilizing orthodontic pliers.

It is not recommended for sterilization of used needles since debris in a needle may obstruct penetration of the gas. Only a steam autoclave or dry heat should be used for that purpose. It is now almost imperative that disposable needles be used and discarded after one use, since they are so difficult to clean, sharpen, and resterilize, and the risk is so great.

New models of the vapor sterilizer are automatic, efficient, and reliable, having been tested and approved by the U.S. Environmental Protection Agency. Cost is about the same as an autoclave. The chamber measures 6 by 11 in. Larger models are under development.

Operation requires filling the reservoir with a sterilization solution which must be obtained from the manufacturer. Water or other solutions will not work. Older manual models are still in use in some offices. If these are loaded, just turned on, and left to operate for 30 minutes, they will not sterilize. They must be preheated with the reservoir chamber lever left in the closed position. Once preheating is completed, instruments are loaded into the tray, and the door is closed. The preheated vaporized solution is admitted into the chamber until the proper pressure is obtained, and the reservoir chamber is closed off again. Then timing is commenced for sterilization. The older machines released a vapor of formaldehyde into the room which made extra ventilation desirable. In the new model formaldehyde is condensed into a closed compartment beneath the sterilizer, and ordinary good room ventilation is adequate. The odor is slight and does not seem to be offensive or hazardous.

Testing Sterilizers

Spore strips can be obtained commercially for testing sterilizers. These consist of paper impregnated with dried living spore forms of noninfectious bacteria. Spores of certain infectious bacteria such as tetanus can cause serious illness. Spores of infectious and noninfectious bacteria are more resistant to heat than any other form of life, including heat-resistant viruses that cause hepatitis. Spores of a harmless species are therefore ideal for testing sterilizers. Tests should be made every week or two or whenever packaging is changed or loads are increased, or whenever temperature- or pressure-gauge indications suggest altered operation of the sterilizer.

Spore strips are provided with directions for use in a divided paper envelope. Two spore strips are removed from the open half of the envelope. Each spore strip is left in its small tissue-paper envelope; one is placed in the center of a standard test load, another is placed near the surface, and the load is sterilized. The small envelopes containing the strips are labeled and returned to the large envelope. These can be tested by most hospital or medical laboratories. If culture tubes used by most dentists for endodontic cultures are available, these can be inoculated according to the directions on the envelope.

Beginning with the test strips, each strip is re-

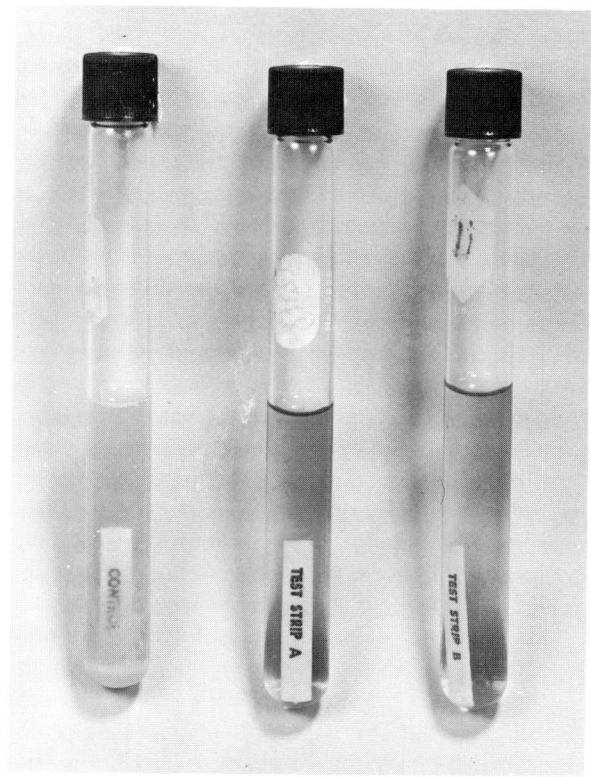

Figure 7-7 | Culture tubes showing cloudy growth of unheated control strip (A) and no growth from test strips (A) and (B). (Fluid thioglycollate medium, Baltimore Biological Laboratories.)

moved from its tissue envelope with sterile scissors and forceps and placed directly into a separate tube of culture medium. The closed side of the large envelope contains an unheated control strip that should produce growth. It is cultured in the same manner. Growth produces cloudiness in the broth, indicating that the spores placed into the tube were alive. If sterilization was effective, broth containing test strips should remain clear and therefore sterile (Fig. 7-7). *Bacillus subtilis* strips are best suited for testing sterilizers in offices and clinics, because they will grow at room or body temperature; 37°C (99°F) is preferable.

Ethylene Oxide Sterilization

Ethylene oxide is a germicidal gas that will destroy all microbes, including spores and hepatitis viruses, at room temperature in about 10 hours. It has amazing penetrating abilities for rubber, plastic, and debris. Its activity can be accelerated by using heat and by increasing its speed of diffusion by placing the materials under a vacuum before admitting the gas to the chamber. Inexpensive devices such as a simple 1-gal canister can be used for room-temperature sterilization (Fig. 7-8). A cartridge wrapped in plastic is broken and dropped into a plastic bag with instruments. The bag is placed into the canister which is locked and is simply allowed to stand overnight. Gloves, plastic evacuator tips, endodontic instruments, and surgical and high-speed handpieces all can be sterilized this way.

Cloth, plastic, and rubber goods must be aerated for 24 hours or more after sterilization to allow the toxic gas to escape. Metal instruments can be used immediately. More expensive automatic elevated-temperature ethylene oxide sterilizers can be purchased at about 2 to 3 times the cost of an autoclave. These can sterilize at temperatures below those used in an autoclave in 1 to 3 hours per total cycle. These are especially valuable for large clinics. Many disposable items from gloves to evacuator tips can be cleaned and recycled by use of ethylene oxide sterilization. However, it is still advisable to discard disposable needles.

Other Methods

The dentist or assistant may be confronted with situations where acceptable sterilization procedures are temporarily not available for all items, or for nondisposal plastic items, because the procedures have never been instituted, or because of equipment failure, shortages, etc. What can be done? Following are comments on some less acceptable stopgap methods and how they are best used until acceptable methods can be instituted.

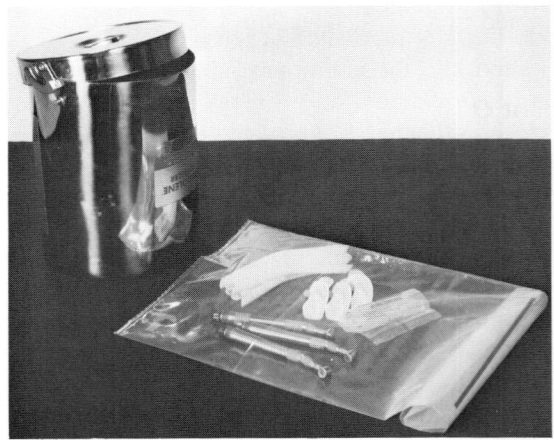

Figure 7-8 | An ethylene oxide sterilizer that uses overnight cycle; must be used in a well-ventilated area. (*Courtesy of H. W. Anderson Products, Inc.*)

Boiling Water

Boiling will kill bacteria and hepatitis viruses in 30 minutes, but not spores. While boiling in water can be an effective means of disinfecting instruments, it has proven hazardous for routine use because it has so often been abused. Instruments are often placed in and taken out of the water chamber without a set time period of heating; instruments that have just been placed in the sterilizer are not distinguished from those that have been boiled for 30 minutes; instruments develop scale and rust that can retard sterilization; the water gradually boils away and instruments are no longer exposed to the temperature of boiling water. In years past because of these abuses many patients were infected in physicians' offices when boiling was used for sterilization.

However, boiling under carefully controlled conditions may be the safest stopgap for disinfection of routine instruments, especially for plastic evacuator tips and other items that can be boiled without damage. Boiling is the only rapid procedure accepted by the World Health Organization for field use.

Instruments boiled must be covered with

one-half in of water. Antirust tablets can be obtained from dental suppliers.

Hot Oil

A heated bath of silicone oil is sometimes used to disinfect or sterilize hinged instruments, contra-angles, and prophylaxis angles, although most of these can now either be dry-heat sterilized or autoclaved with less mess. Where hot oil is used, instruments should be washed and dried thoroughly before sterilization. The oil reaches a temperature much higher than the boiling point of water, and so instruments should never be wet when immersed in the oil. Only disinfection is achieved when the instruments are heated at 150°C (302°F) for 20 to 30 minutes. Actual sterilization will not be achieved until the instruments have been heated for at least one-half hour at 160°C (320°F). Hepatitis viruses are probably destroyed by the disinfection temperature.

Following sterilization in oil, contra-angles with oil holes need to be run for about a minute with the opening kept downward in a paper towel so excess oil can run out. After instruments have been drained and cooled, they need to be wiped with clean towels or sterilized towels. Any oily film can be removed with an oil solvent.

For handpieces and contra-angles, only those silicones providing good lubrication should be used. Silicone fluid becomes dark after use, but this has no effect on its value. It may be filtered with paper towels or filter paper. Silicone fluid remains stable for 2 or 3 years, and it does not vaporize. If instruments are properly drained following its use, little will be lost.

Disinfection of Instruments

Acceptable disinfection of metal instruments with chemicals in 30 minutes is not possible to ensure destruction of hepatitis viruses. Chemicals that might be effective in that period of time are too corrosive for this. If this is the only procedure available, a glutaraldehyde solution should be used as the best choice. The action of this chemical in 30 minutes against hepatitis viruses has not satisfactorily been tested. This chemical is known to destroy bacterial spores only after 10 hours. There is a critical time limit of 2 weeks on the effectiveness of the solution. In heavy use it should be changed once a week. This solution can seriously *sensitize and irritate hands,* so direct contact must be avoided. Glutaraldehyde disinfectant is available from dental-supply companies.

Phenolic solutions and alcohol are not satisfactory for disinfection of instruments. Benzalkonium chloride, Zephiran chloride, and other quaternary ammonium chlorides are hazardous for instrument disinfection. In heavy use aqueous solutions not only become inactive but support the growth of gram-negative infectious bacteria.

Cleaning and Preparing Instruments for Sterilization

Instruments must be cleaned thoroughly by scrubbing with a brush or by use of an ultrasonic cleaner. The latter method is preferred to avoid puncturing the hand with contaminated instruments. If hand scrubbing is used, a heavy duty household glove to hold the pointed instruments should be worn (Fig. 7-9).

Some instruments are made of stainless steel and will not rust easily. Some instruments marked "stainless," like orthodontic pliers, are not truly rustproof. Instruments that can rust must be completely dry before sterilizing by a method that will not cause rust, such as by formaldehyde vapor or dry heat.

Orthodontic pliers require special care. These must be wiped clean with alcohol only, without letting the alcohol enter the hinge, before they are sterilized.

Instruments for nonsurgical use need not be kept wrapped during or after sterilization. They must be handled with clean hands and placed in drawers disinfected once each week or placed on covered trays in cabinets. If you wish to keep them packaged, color-coded bags or small, heavy brown grocery bags can be used. Paper and aluminum foil wrappings lend themselves well to dry-heat sterilization. Cloth is preferred for autoclaving.

Treatment of Specific Instruments

Routine Instruments: Mirrors, Rubber, and Plastic Items

Additional instruments that must be sterilized if reused include mouth mirrors, burs, clamps, amalgam pluggers, plastic and metal impression trays, stones, prophylaxis cups and brushes, prophylaxis and contra-angles, as well as all explorers, curettes, and other instruments used in oral treatments. Most can be sterilized by autoclaving, dry heat, or gas. Prophylaxis cups and brushes cannot withstand dry heat. Mirrors tend to withstand dry-heat sterilization better than steam.

Disposable items need not be sterilized if they can be discarded after one use. These include burs, prophylaxis cups, needles, and plastic impression trays.

Plastic evacuator tips can be purchased that withstand the heat of autoclaving, or disposable ones can be purchased. If only those are available that would be harmed by heat, they are best sterilized in ethylene oxide overnight at room temperature. If sterilization is not possible, they can be cleaned thoroughly and soaked for a minimum of 30 minutes in fresh household sodium hypochlorite bleach. This is diluted 1:4 for use and must be replaced daily. Another alternative is to soak the items overnight in glutaraldehyde disinfectant. For either treatment, all items must be covered by one-half in of solution. All items must be thoroughly rinsed with clean water before use.

Removable and fixed prosthetic appliances, including custom trays, occlusal rims, and dentures, that have been prepared or altered using

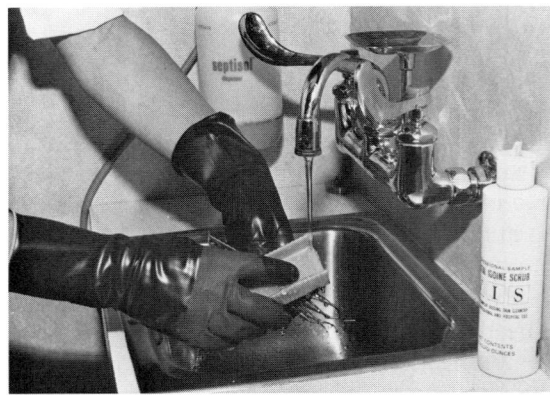

Figure 7-9 | For instrument cleaning before sterilization, hands must be protected by heavy household gloves.

nonsterilized instruments and materials, should be disinfected before returning them to the patient. These are soaked in a 1:10 dilution of household bleach (containing 5.25 percent sodium hypochlorite) for 20 minutes, but never longer than 60 minutes. Rinse well with water before returning them to the patient.

Rubber bowls, wooden handled instruments, and all other prosthetic instruments that cannot be sterilized should be scrubbed with a brush using surgical iodine scrub under running water after use.

Handpieces, Prophylaxis Angles, and Contra-Angles

A special problem is presented by handpieces because many are damaged by heat and ethylene oxide sterilization takes too long for practical routine use. The handle of some straight, air-driven handpieces is covered by a sleeve that can be removed and sterilized by any method. The remaining surfaces can only be scrubbed with a disinfectant and touched as little as possible during use. *Prophylaxis angles* and *contra-angles* used with the straight handpiece can be sterilized by dry heat or by autoclaving.

Consult the manufacturer or try one experimentally to determine which is suitable. Angles are usually cleaned with grease solvent, sterilized, and relubricated with fresh, clean oil or grease before use. Consult the manufacturer's directions. Careful cleaning will usually prolong the life of the angle, but despite what some manufacturers state, *cleaning alone does not sterilize an angle.*

Presently only a few manufacturers make an air-driven handpiece that can be steam sterilized in an autoclave without damage. For surgery, handpieces must be sterilized with ethylene oxide before use unless they can be autoclaved. *For routine operative use,* most dentists may have not yet obtained enough sterilizable high-speed handpieces to permit their routine sterilization between patients. If that is the case, the handpiece can only be disinfected between patient treatments.

Handpiece disinfection requires thorough scrubbing in order to remove resistant infectious microbes. Most angled handpieces can be scrubbed with a brush, soap or iodine surgical scrub, and water under a faucet before you disinfect them. Then wipe the surface and any removable parts thoroughly with two separate gauze sponges saturated with 70 percent alcohol (isopropyl or ethyl).

The air-water syringe must be treated the same way. The removable tip should be sterilized. Instead of scrubbing the syringe, you can cover it with a fresh finger cot with a hole for the tip, or you can wrap it with disposable plastic wrap. This must be replaced after each treatment.

After use for treatment of any infected patients, heat or gas sterilization of handpieces and other items is imperative. Use an iodine surgical scrub to clean surfaces and items that cannot be sterilized. The iodine should not be removed for 20 minutes. It then can be wiped away with alcohol.

Many units also aspirate saliva and aerosols into the handpiece and hose when the water coolant spray is turned off. To help prevent transfer of infection from one patient to another, hold the handpiece over the sink or cuspidor and operate the water spray for at least 30 seconds before and after each treatment. Consult the handpiece manufacturer for further information on problems of handpiece disinfection and sterilization.

Treating Patients Suspected of Viral Hepatitis

Patients suspected of hepatitis are best treated in a hospital dentistry clinic. If that is not possible, all reasonable precautions should be used to protect all personnel. Use a rubber dam. Place an air evacuation tip near teeth being cut with a bur to evacuate aerosols.

All individuals should wear a mask while aerosols are being generated or while they are in close proximity to the patient. Gloves should be worn by all personnel involved in treating the patient. These should be sterilized afterwards. Aluminum foil covers should be placed on all surfaces to be touched and on instrument trays that can't be heat-sterilized. All instruments and all covers should be heat-sterilized after use. Any uncovered surfaces touched should be wiped with an iodine surgical scrub solution. The iodine should be removed after 20 minutes with an alcohol sponge. Gowns and smocks should be autoclaved after the treatment. Face, hands, and arms should be thoroughly washed to remove aerosol deposits. Disinfect glasses with iodine.

AVOIDING POSTTREATMENT INFECTIONS IN PATIENTS

Posttreatment infections result when excessive numbers of oral bacteria enter oral wounds or injection sites in the mouth. For patients with an unusual susceptibility to infection, a small number of bacteria may constitute an infectious dose. Patients who have had rheumatic fever or who have an artificial heart valve implant have such a high risk of cardiac infection that they must be protected with antibiotics before any dental treatment. Oral antiseptics used before an oral treatment usually cannot sterilize the mucosa, but they *can greatly reduce the numbers of oral bacteria that are carried into the tissues by treatments.*

Oral antisepsis is imperative for high-risk patients because antibiotics alone do not necessarily give them complete protection. Before a patient treatment, have the patient rinse his or her mouth with one of the so-called stronger commercial mouth washes containing essential oils or phenolic compounds. Before surgery and injections, block saliva from the site with cotton rolls. Apply an iodine or iodophor compound or one of the more effective mouthwash solutions with a cotton swab to the site, twice. For injections apply the topical anesthetic to the site with a cotton swab and leave it in place until the injection is made.

These are simple precautions that are not absolute, but they clearly favor the patient rather than the bacteria. Should an infection occur despite your efforts, you have at least made a responsible, ethical effort to provide as much protection as possible.

CONCLUSION

All the above described methods of disinfection and sterilization are virtually useless in controlling cross-infections if any aspects of dental-operatory asepsis are neglected, from adequate cleansing of hands, to disinfection of objects touched or handled on or around the unit during patient care, to adequate sterilization of instruments. The ultimate responsibility for clinical sanitation rests with the dental clinician, but his or her reliance for proper use of sanitary aseptic clinical procedures, as well as for helpful recommendations in this regard, rests with the dental assistant. Health care is an important responsibility. Knowledge is now available for it to be administered safely. It is a prideful job, well worth the conscientious effort of those involved in order to preserve their own health and the health of their patients.

BIBLIOGRAPHY

American Association of Dental Schools: "Report of Actions of the 1974 House of Delegates; Res. No. 9-74-H," *J. Dent. Educ.,* **38**:316, 1974.

Crawford, J. J.: "New Light on the Transmissibility of Viral Hepatitis in Dental Practice and Its Control," *J. Am. Dent. Assoc.,* **91**: 829–836, 1975.

———: *Clinical Asepsis in Dentistry: Advanced Programmed Instruction for Dental Students, Practicing Dentists, Dental Hygienists and Certified Dental Assistants,* R. A. Kolstad Publisher, Baylor College of Dentistry, Dallas, Tex., 1976.

Kolstad, R. A., and Crawford, J. J.: *Sterilization, Disinfection and Asepsis in Dental Practice: Programmed Instruction for Students in Dentistry, Dental Hygiene and Dental Assisting,* R. A. Kolstad Publisher, Baylor College of Dentistry, Dallas, Tex., 1976.

8 Grover C. Hunter, Jr.
Oral Pathology

INTRODUCTION

Pathology is the study of disease processes, of the causes, manifestations, and effects of disease upon the living organism and the alterations in structure resulting from disease. It is the *what, why,* and *how* of disease. Dental pathology is a division of general pathology and is concerned primarily with disease processes of the oral cavity.

Since the cell is the individual unit of the living organism, one might justifiably conclude that all pathology goes back ultimately to the behavior of cells and their structural changes resulting from unfavorable stimulation, irritation, or injury. Cold, heat, x-ray, pressure, trauma, bacteria, and chemicals are some of the injurious agents or irritants which may cause pathologic changes in tissue cells.

Recent studies have been directed at exploring the alterations in molecular and biochemical processes of cells and tissues. This knowledge helps explain the dysfunctional behavior of cells and tissues before clinical and microscopic changes can be seen as alterations in structure under the microscope.

REACTION OF TISSUES TO INJURY

Inflammation and Repair

Inflammation is one of the most common reactions of tissues and cells to injury. It is a nonspecific response of the body and, while it may serve a useful purpose at times, there are instances in which the end result is detrimental to the host. Biochemical products of injured cells are now known to mediate the vascular and cellular reaction in the injured tissues and to influence the general reaction of the body in terms of fever and leukocytosis (increase in the total white blood cell count). Almost everyone has had a boil or toothache. This is an inflammatory condition. The cardinal symptoms of inflammation are pain, swelling, heat, redness, and often an interference in function of the part involved. In terms of cells and tissues, the redness is accounted for by an increase in blood flow to the part; the small blood vessels become enlarged, and fluid escapes from them, causing swelling. White blood cells (leukocytes) from the blood also find their way out into the tissue spaces. Some of them have the ability to engulf bacteria and to destroy them by a process called *phagocytosis*. In so doing the leukocytes die, and collections of these dead cells along with dead tissue cells cause the formation of *pus,* which is the fluid product of inflammation. The pain produced is caused by pressure of the fluids upon the sensory nerve supplying the part. The pain in toothache (pulpitis) is caused by pressure of excess fluids on sensory nerves enclosed in the dental pulp.

The usual outcome of inflammation is healing or repair. After the defense cells (principally leukocytes) have destroyed the irritant (in this case bacteria), new connective tissue fills in the area. This tissue is called *granulation tissue* and consists of new blood vessels, young connective tissue cells (fibroblasts), and varying numbers of leukocytes (principally lymphocytes). The end result of this process may be the formation of dense connective tissue with a gradual elimination of blood vessels, leaving *scar tissue.*

Degeneration and Hypoplasia

Another pattern of response by cells and tissues to injury is referred to as *degeneration*. Degeneration is a normal process physiologically, when considered as part of the process of aging, but it may take place in younger tissues and cells as a result of injury to the cells during development or when highly specialized structures, such as bones or tooth tissue, are being formed. Injury to cells during their formative period may bring about serious consequences. An example of this type of injury is *enamel hypoplasia* of the tooth, a condition in which an insufficient amount of enamel forms; the enamel-forming cells (ameloblasts) are injured during the time they are producing and forming enamel. If the injury takes place in cells that are no longer actively growing, such as mature skeletal muscle cells, then *atrophy* or diminution in size of the muscle may be the result.

Degenerative changes in tissues and cells may be caused by many injurious agents, such as chemicals and drugs, or by a lessened oxygen supply to them. The end result of degenerative changes often is cell or tissue death, but in some cases the cells may recover if the process has not gone too far and if the injurious agent has been withdrawn in time.

Senile degenerative changes take place in the pulps of teeth, in the supporting periodontal tissues, and in the oral mucosa and its underlying connective tissue. In the case of the dental pulp, the dentin-forming cells called *odontoblasts* show changes in size and cellular detail, and there are fewer of them present than in the young pulp. Also there are fewer blood vessels and connective tissue cells (fibroblasts) present. Calcifications in old pulps become more frequent, and these may become large enough to be seen as *pulp stones* in the radiograph (x-ray picture).

Hyperplasia and Hypertrophy

There is still another way in which cells may react to unfavorable environmental conditions or to irritation. They may multiply and increase in number (*hyperplasia*) or actually increase in size themselves (*hypertrophy*). In either case (hyperplasia or hypertrophy), there is a visible increase in size of the tissue. Thus, it is possible to have hyperplasia of the gingivae as a result of irritation or ingestion of certain drugs such as diphenylhydantoin, which is given to control seizures in patients with epilepsy. Hyperplasia of the soft tissues may also occur under an ill-fitting denture which is irritating the maxillary or mandibular ridge. An example of hypertrophy is seen in compensatory heart disease, in which individual muscle cells or fibers actually enlarge and produce a visible increase in size of the organ.

Neoplasia

Normally when cells multiply, there is a restraint mechanism to keep them within reasonable bounds. They sometimes, however, start multiplying wildly without regard to serving a useful purpose for the organism, and then there is a resultant condition known as *neoplasia* (new growth). A *neoplasm* is a new growth started by cells which serves no useful purpose and which sometimes is the result of chronic irritation or injury. It is frequently difficult to say where hyperplasia leaves off and where neoplasia begins.

Neoplasms (tumors) may be classified as benign or malignant. Malignant tumors if untreated always kill the patient, usually by spreading from the original site of occurrence to distant organs and tissues of the body. This type of spread is called *metastasis*. Benign neoplasms (tumors) do not usually kill the patient but may do so indirectly if they occur in certain locations. For instance, a fibroma (a benign connective tissue tumor) may obstruct the trachea and eventually cut off the air supply to the lungs.

Neoplasms may be distinguished according to their origin from different tissues. They may be derived from epithelium, from connective tissue, and sometimes from both. Malignant epithelial tumors are called *carcinomas*. Malignant connective tissue tumors are called *sarcomas*. Laypersons usually use the term *cancer* to cover all malignant tumors.

DEVELOPMENTAL ANOMALIES

The life history of tooth development is a complicated one. Since cells are involved in this life history, any injury to them during the time of development may result in a change in pattern. Most organs of the body, such as the liver, are mature when the functioning cells are fully mature (differentiated). A tooth, like a bone, however, must become calcified and, unlike a bone, must also *erupt* in order to perform its normal function. The developing tooth, according to Schour and Massler (1958), passes through the following stages:

1. *Initiation.* Primitive cells from the oral mucous membrane begin to bud and grow.
2. *Proliferation.* These original cells multiply.
3. *Differentiation.* Certain of these original cells take on the duty of forming each type of tooth tissue. Thus, ameloblasts prepare to form enamel; odontoblasts, dentin; and cementoblasts, cementum.
4. *Apposition.* The specialized cells mentioned immediately above form an organic framework to receive inorganic salts of calcium and phosphorus.
5. *Calcification.* The organic framework becomes hard (calcified) from calcium and phosphorus salts brought in by small blood vessels.
6. *Eruption.* When the crown of a forming tooth becomes calcified, it begins to force its way through the gums. After eruption 2 or 3 years are required for the entire tooth root to form and calcify.
7. *Attrition.* The chewing surface becomes worn.

Enamel Hypoplasia

From the previous account of tooth formation, it is apparent that any disturbance during the time when the cells are actively engaged in laying down enamel will cause defects in the finished product (*enamel hypoplasia*) (Fig. 8-1). The amount of the defect depends upon the severity

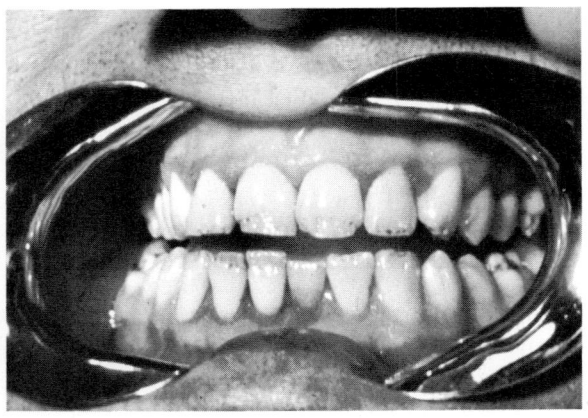

Figure 8-1 | Enamel hypoplasia. Note pits and groove defects in central incisors.

and length of the disturbance. Disturbances of adjustment during the first 2 weeks of life, including birth trauma, probably account for a great many of the tooth defects known as enamel hypoplasia. Also, in deficiency states such as rickets (vitamin D deficiency), calcium and phosphorus absorption from the intestinal wall is interfered with, and so the tooth-forming cells cannot get the necessary building blocks to form high-quality tooth substance.

Figure 8-2 | Hutchinsonian incisors. Note screwdriver shape of maxillary and mandibular central incisors.

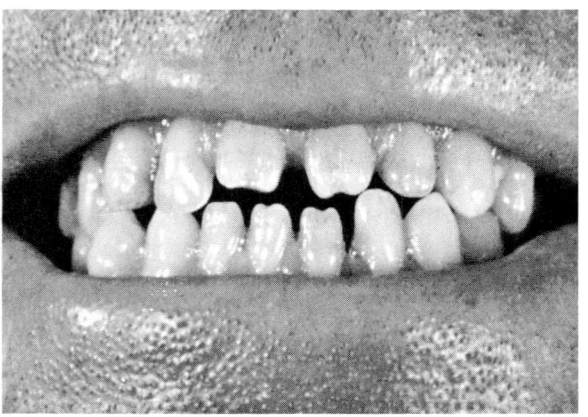

Depending upon the severity of the disturbance, the clinical picture of enamel hypoplasia may vary from small pits and grooves to large crown defects as seen in what has been called *mulberry molars*. It is significant that the defects will appear only in those areas of tooth substance that were growing and calcifying at the time of the disturbance. Thus, we can actually date the approximate time of disturbance by a study of the location and distribution of the enamel defects.

It is interesting to note that one does not see enamel hypoplasia as frequently in the primary teeth as in the secondary teeth. The reason for this lies in the fact that the crowns of primary teeth are at least partially formed and calcified before birth. Nature gives protection to the developing embryo, sometimes even at the expense of the mother. The mother would have to undergo a very critical illness in order to affect the ameloblasts of the embryo that are forming the prenatal enamel of the primary teeth. Postnatal enamel of primary teeth is, however, subject to hypoplastic defects just as readily as is the enamel of secondary teeth.

Hutchinson's Teeth

This is a developmental defect sometimes seen in the teeth of patients who have a history of a congenital syphilis (Fig. 8-2). There is injury to the tooth-forming organ during development, causing an absence of a part of the tooth crown. The effect on the central incisor results in a narrow crown at the biting edge and often a notching in the center. Thus, it is referred to by many authors as being screwdriver-shaped.

Mottled Enamel

This is a disturbance in calcification of the enamel as a result of toxic amounts of fluorides in the drinking water in areas where large amounts of fluorides are found (Fig. 8-3). In most instances the amount of fluorides must exceed 1.5 or 2.0 ppm before visible effects on the enamel are produced. Only developing teeth are affected by excessive fluorides; fully developed teeth are unaffected. Thus, an adult could move into such an area, and none of his or her teeth would be affected.

Mottled enamel is usually brownish in appearance, the color resulting from stains picked up by the incompletely calcified enamel. The tooth surface is smooth when tested by a dental explorer.

While large amounts of fluorides in drinking water are known to be harmful, scientific investigation in recent years has shown that small amounts can be helpful as a caries-control measure, especially for the younger population groups. In the past few years small amounts of fluorides have been added to the drinking water of various cities and communities on the strength of these investigations. These fluoridation projects have the approval of a large number of health organizations such as the American Dental Association and the U.S. Public Health Service.

Hereditary Opalescent Dentin

As the term implies, this is a hereditary trait carried by a gene and has its effect primarily upon the quality and amount of dentin produced by the odontoblasts (dentin-forming cells). These cells produce too much dentin of poor quality and eventually obliterate the dental pulp. Since the tooth substance is of poor quality, these teeth wear down excessively under the stresses of mastication.

The clinical appearance of these teeth is a dull opal color without the normal translucency. Radiographs show complete absence of the dental pulp.

Anodontia

This term implies absence of teeth either because of lack of formation or because of lack of eruption. In true anodontia there is a complete absence of tooth formation. This absence seems to be a dominant hereditary character and most

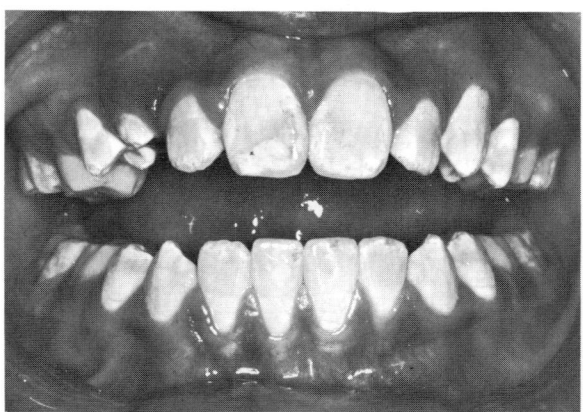

Figure 8-3 | Mottled enamel resulting from excessive amounts of fluorides in drinking water.

often affects lateral incisors, bicuspids (premolars), and third molars of the secondary dentition. True anodontia affecting all the secondary teeth is very rare indeed. For some reason the primary dentition is very seldom affected, either partially or completely.

Delayed Eruption

The process of eruption is not yet fully understood, but it is known that the ductless glands have a role in this particular phase of tooth physiology, the pituitary and the thyroid glands probably being the principal ones involved. Of course, there are sometimes local conditions which prevent eruption of teeth. For instance, the premature loss of a primary tooth may permit shifting of teeth and close up the space necessary for the eruption of the secondary tooth. Also the scar tissue left after the extraction of a primary tooth may prevent eruption of the underlying secondary tooth.

Harelip and Cleft Palate

While thus far the discussion has mainly concerned tooth formation and development, a little thought will suggest facial and body changes in development occurring also during intrauterine life. The bones of the face and jaws as well as overlying soft tissues are derived from primitive cells and structures called *branchial arches*. A disturbance in the formative stages of these primitive cells and tissues may result in the following defects:

Harelip is a defect in the upper lip caused by failure of the two halves or sides to join properly.

Cleft palate is a defect resulting from the failure of the right and left halves of the palate to join properly.

These defects occur during the first 3 months of intrauterine life and are now thought to be a connective tissue failure rather than a lack of epithelial union.

DENTAL CARIES

The whole story of caries is yet to be told. How decay begins and its causes are still disputed. There is considerable agreement, however, that caries is a demineralization process brought about by certain mouth bacteria with a supply of fermentable carbohydrates (sucrose) in susceptible persons. These bacteria are able to penetrate both enamel rods and the interprismatic substance. The end process results in cavitation and dissolution of tooth substance (Fig. 8-4). For more detail, consult Chap. 6, Microbiology.

Acidity is expressed in terms of hydrogen-ion concentration (pH), with 7 as the neutral point. Any pH with a number higher that 7 is on the alkaline side, while any pH with a number less than 7 is on the acid side. If the pH on any tooth surface drops sufficiently on the acid side (below 5.5), decalcification begins. Aciduric bacteria thrive on sugars and carbohydrates, and so the consumption of excessive sweets and carbohydrates may be dangerous in spite of the neutralizing effects of saliva. In addition, carbohydrates furnish the material necessary for the sticky plaques which form on uncleansed tooth surfaces and harbor within them the acid-producing organisms. The presence of these plaques allows the pH to drop sharply on the tooth surfaces, and in most instances saliva cannot neutralize these acid products. Any defects in a tooth, such as pits and fissures, furnish an ideal breeding ground for these bacteria and also trap their food requirements.

Decay starting in these defects of tooth formation results in what are called *pit* and *fissure cavities*. Decay starting on smooth surfaces usually begins between the teeth near the contact point and results in *smooth-surface cavities*. Buccal and lingual smooth-surface cavities beginning near the gum line sometimes become chalky white in appearance and thus have been given the name *white decay* by some clinicians.

If decay progresses far enough into the tooth, the soft tissue of the pulp is finally reached by the bacteria. Then inflammation of this soft enclosed tissue results, and the patient has a toothache. This progression of decay, according to Massler (1958), goes through certain stages (Fig. 8-5):

1. The enamel alone is involved.
2. In addition to the enamel, the dentin is becoming involved.
3. Enamel and dentin are involved; the pulp is approached but not yet involved.
4. In addition to enamel and dentin, the pulp (nerve) is also involved.

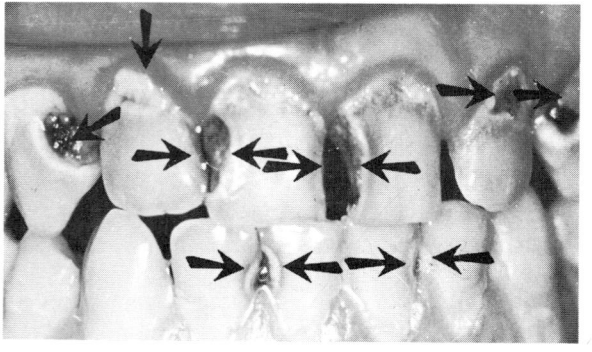

Figure 8-4 | Rampant dental caries. Arrows indicate multiple surface involvement in anterior teeth.

Clinical observations have shown that age influences caries susceptibility and activity. This has been confirmed by clinical laboratory tests which rely on the count of the numbers of colonies of aciduric bacteria (mainly streptococci and *Lactobacilli*) grown from the saliva of the patient. High counts of lactobacilli from a patient's mouth may indicate a high rate of caries activity. Apparently caries activity reaches a peak in children 10 to 15 years of age and then gradually tapers off until the sixth decade when increased activity may be observed.

Sometimes the progress of caries may come to a halt, and this period is called *arrested caries*. This is seen more often in older people when the conditions which helped bring about the original caries have changed. An example of this is seen on occlusal surfaces of molars where attrition and occlusal wear have made the area self-cleansing and where the points of origin (pits and fissures) have been erased by the continuous wear from mastication. Arrested decay appears dark yellowish in color, and the underlying dentin is firm and hard when tested with an explorer.

EROSION

Erosion is a loss of tooth substance by a chemical process not clearly understood. It may start in the enamel near the gum line on the facial surfaces of the teeth and progress toward the pulp (Fig. 8-6). The destruction of tooth substance is even and gradual, leaving a highly polished surface which is smooth to an explorer. This condition should not be confused with decay or with enamel hypoplasia.

PULPITIS

When bacteria in a carious lesion of a tooth pass through the dentinal tubules and enter the pulp, inflammation sets in, and the end result is a toothache. The pulp, like other soft tissues of the

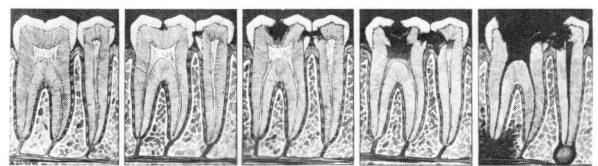

Figure 8-5 | Progress of dental caries from enamel involvement alone to pulpal and periapical involvement with formation of abscess. (*Courtesy of M. Massler and I. Schour, Atlas of the Mouth, American Dental Association, Chicago, 1944.*)

body such as the skin, can become inflamed. No such reaction, however, is possible in the hard tissues of the tooth, because enamel and dentin contain no blood vessels. But as soon as the pulp is reached, pain, swelling, redness, and abscess formation begin, just as in any other soft tissue. The pulp is housed in rigid calcified walls of dentin; hence, pressure is built up quickly, resulting as a rule in pulpal death. This condition is called acute pulpitis (toothache).

Some forms of pulpal inflammation in which bacteria have not yet gained a foothold may be cured by proper dental treatment. Heat shock from a deep filling may cause pulpal inflammation which may be stopped by removal of the filling and the placement of a soothing material in its stead.

Figure 8-6 | Dental erosion.

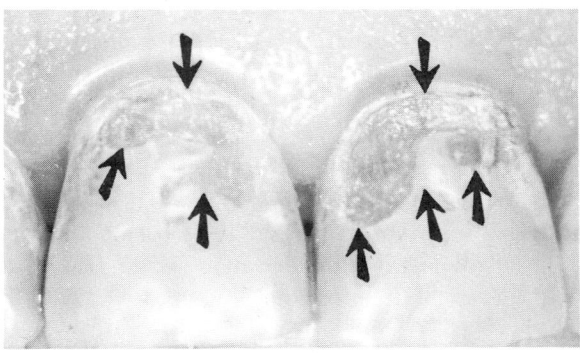

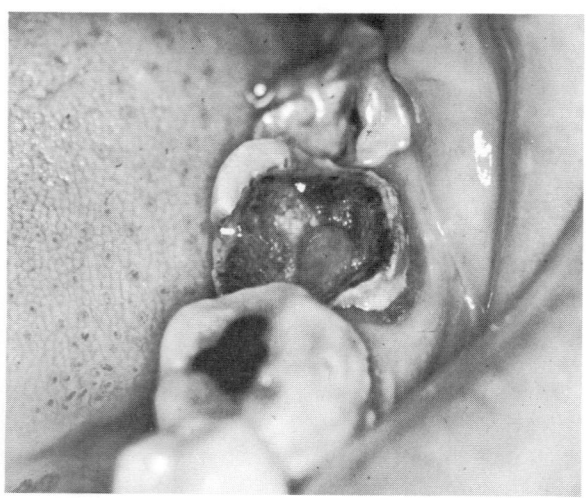

Figure 8-7 | Pulp polyp.

In young teeth where there is a large open cavity and the pulp chamber is large, the pulp may grow out and fill the cavity, forming a bulbous mass called a *pulp polyp* (Fig. 8-7).

It must be remembered that the pulp can and does put up a fight against invading bacteria. The dentin-forming cells (odontoblasts) which lie next to the dentin on the surface of the pulp continue to function through the life of the tooth by building *secondary dentin*. As the tooth ages and wears, this process goes on evenly and slowly, but when these cells are irritated by filling materials, bacteria, heat, or cold, they work faster in building more dentin to protect the pulp. Sometimes irritants finally overcome the pulp defenses, causing its death. The chemical irritation from silicate fillings may sometimes cause pulp death. Friction from the rotating stones or burs of the dental engine may generate enough heat to cause pulp damage. Gold foil when pounded too close to the pulp also may set up pressure and thermal (heat or cold) irritation.

PERIAPICAL ABSCESS, FISTULA, PARULIS, AND OSTEOMYELITIS

After the pulp becomes inflamed and minute abscesses form in it, the inflammation spreads down the pulp canal and out through the root end of the tooth into the soft and hard tissues of the jawbone. The result is a condition known as a *periapical* (root-end) *abscess*. As the abscess forms, pressure from inflammatory swelling and pus at the root end causes the tooth to be pushed up in its socket, making it feel high and sore to touch. This acute stage is marked by local bone and soft-tissue destruction, and the involved area appears dark on the radiograph. The cells responsible for bone destruction are known as *osteoclasts*.

If the accumulated pus at the end of the tooth finds no pathway of immediate drainage, the jaw may swell, and the patient will have much pain and discomfort. Sometimes spontaneous drainage may occur through the bone and gums adjacent to the root end of the abscessed tooth. The pathway through which the pus has burrowed in order to drain into the mouth is called a *fistula*. The gum tissue where the pus finally drains may swell, causing an abscess of the gum (*parulis*). These abscesses are more frequently seen in children than in adults.

If drainage of an abscess is not successfully established by the dentist or if the patient's health is poor, the inflammation may spread deeper into the jawbone, causing a widespread infection (*osteomyelitis*) which is hard to manage and which may have serious consequences. Large areas of bone may die as a result of this infection and may separate from the healthy bone. Patients in the acute stage usually require hospitalization.

In some instances teeth may abscess without the patient's knowledge until the dentist discovers the condition on a radiograph. These blind abscesses may be injuring the general health of the patient. Bacteria may be constantly migrating from the root end of such teeth throughout the entire body by way of the bloodstream. This spread of bacteria from a focal point (in this instance the root end of an abscessed tooth) is called *focal infection*. Root canal treatment or extraction should be performed to clear up this condition in order to prevent further damage to the patient's health.

GRANULOMAS AND CYSTS

The body may have strong enough resistance to wall off an acute abscess, and thus the abscess may enter a chronic stage. This chronic state of inflammation is productive of new connective tissue at the root end of the tooth and is called a *periapical granuloma*. It can be seen after the extraction of the tooth as a small bulbous sac attached to the root.

The production of this replacement and healing tissue (granulation tissue) also stimulates the old abandoned cell remnants of the tooth germ to multiply. These epithelial remains (rests of Malassez) may grow and form a lining inside the sac or granuloma. A cavity thus formed and lined by epithelium is called a *cyst*. Such a cyst would be classified as a *periapical cyst*. The contents of the cystic cavity break down into a thick yellowish fluid which is usually sterile. Cysts may be classified as either of tooth origin (odontogenic) or developmental (fissural). Developmental cysts are derived from enclaved epithelial cells at the site of union of embryologic processes which unite during the time of embryologic development and closure. An example of a developmental cyst is a *median palatine cyst*, which occurs in the midline of the palate.

ORAL LESIONS

Canker Sores (Aphthous Ulcers)

Canker sores are circumscribed, usually small ulcers which have necrotic yellow centers and

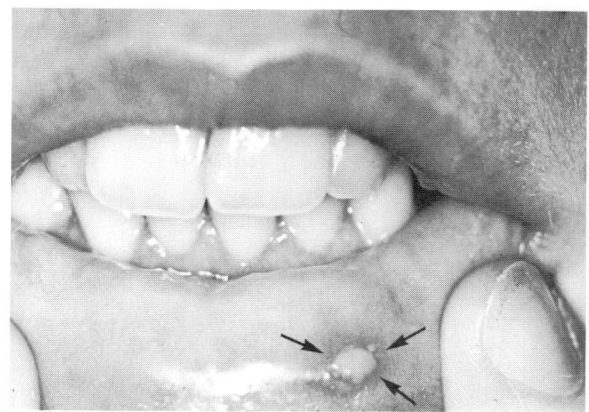

Figure 8-8 | Aphthous ulcer on mucous membrane. Note necrotic center.

bright-red inflammatory halos around them. The origin is believed by some to be viral in nature (Fig. 8-8). This virus resides within tissue cells of the oral mucosa and usually remains dormant unless some trigger mechanism sets off the inflammatory reaction. Others believe these aphthae to be associated with a special form of streptococcal infection. The predisposing factor may be irritation from dental instrumentation or cheek or lip biting. Systemic conditions sometimes influence the condition, especially when the patient has recurrent multiple aphthae (ulcers). Among these conditions are temporary metabolic upsets during menstruation, excessive fatigue, lack of sleep, and anxiety states.

Herpes Labialis (Herpes Simplex)

Cold sores appear as crusted single or multiple lesions most commonly found at the vermilion border of the lips (Fig. 8-9). They leave a dry crusted exudate. They are believed to be of viral origin, and similar trigger mechanisms as with canker sores probably are operative in producing the lesions.

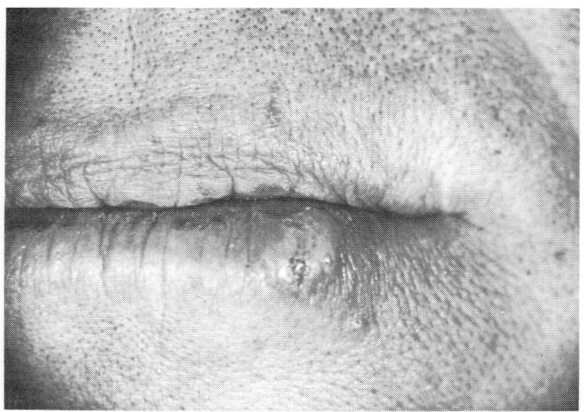

Figure 8-9 | Herpes labialis. Note vesicle formation characteristic of this viral lesion.

Geographic Tongue

This condition (wandering rash) is a wandering inflammation of the top surface (dorsum) of the tongue (Fig. 8-10). The affected areas, which migrate from time to time, give the surface of the tongue a pattern somewhat resembling a geographic map. The centers of the affected areas appear slick and smooth, while the edges are red and inflamed. This condition is poorly understood but is harmless.

Hyperkeratosis ("Leukoplakia")

This condition is characterized by white raised patches found on any of the mucous membranes of the oral cavity. Since it has so often been associated with smoking, it has been called by some writers *smoker's patches*. It is probably a protective reaction of the mucosa to irritation just as calluses on the palm of the hand are a reaction from working in the garden or using golf clubs without gloves. Clinically it varies from rather smooth irregular patches to rough, raised, highly hornified areas (Fig. 8-11). It may also be localized in small areas or may cover large sections of the oral mucosa. Some types of white patches are precancerous in nature and are prone to break down into carcinoma (squamous cell cancer). *Hyperkeratosis* occurs more often in the male than in the female. Chronic irritation from tobacco, spices, and broken-down teeth seems to be the most important causative factor, but certain systematic diseases and conditions such as syphilis may be predisposing factors.

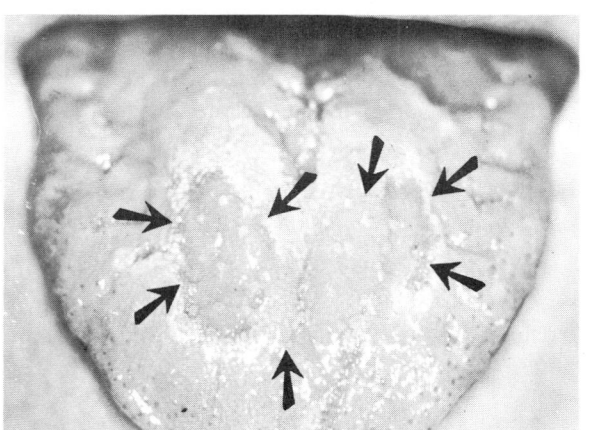

Figure 8-10 | Geographic tongue. Arrows indicate large areas of papillary desquamation on the dorsum.

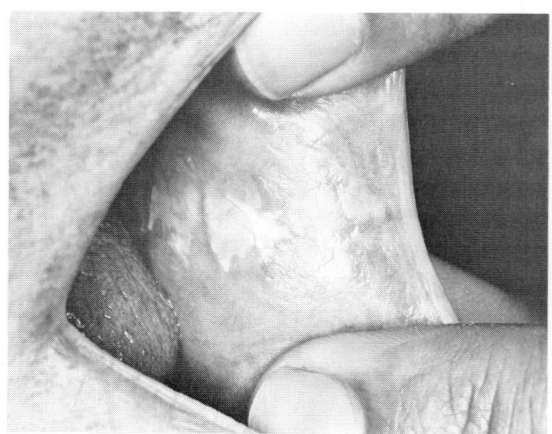

Figure 8-11 | Hyperkeratosis of the buccal mucosa. (*Courtesy of R. Richardson.*)

Lichen Planus

Lichen planus is a skin disease that may have associated mouth lesions resembling, in some ways, leukoplakia. It is generally characterized by raised, smooth, pearly white lines or patches and may be found on the inner surface of the cheek and lips and on the tongue. Lichen planus is harmless and, therefore, must be distinguished from the potentially more dangerous lesion of *leukoplakia*. Microscopic examination of excised tissue will help in making a correct diagnosis. This type of examination is called *biopsy*.

Syphilis

This is a generalized infectious disease caused by *Treponema pallidum* and transmitted by contact with infected individuals. Sexual contact, kissing, and objects such as unclean dental instruments which are conveyed from one mouth to another are the main methods of transmission.

The first lesion of syphilis is called the *chancre*, a papule or erosion which appears about 3 weeks after the initial infectious contact. Often it may be located on the lips and may be confused clinically with a fever blister or cold sore. It will disappear with or without treatment, and the second stage may appear 6 to 8 weeks later. The organisms at this time have invaded the body and multiplied, and a generalized body rash may be observed. Analogous lesions may appear in the mouth as mucous membrane eruptions known as *mucous patches*. This second stage is highly infectious, and care should be exercised in not placing the unprotected fingers or hands in such a patient's mouth. There are case histories of dentists who have contracted the disease by lack of precaution in this respect.

The tertiary (third) stage may set in after varying intervals of time have elapsed. The large blood vessels (especially the aorta) and central nervous system are affected in this stage. The only oral lesion at this stage may be a large indolent perforating lesion known as a *gumma*. This lesion most frequently involves the nose and palate.

Pyogenic Granuloma

This lesion represents an exuberant vascular and connective tissue response to irritation or injury, usually by bacteria. The degree of vascularity determines the color of this sessile or pedunculated lesion, which may vary from red to bluish red. In the oral cavity it is frequently associated with a deep periodontal pocket (Fig. 8-12). Since white blood cells can be seen microscopically in sections from the excised lesion, the term *pyogenic* (pus-producing) is applicable. It is clinically and microscopically indistinguishable from the so-called pregnancy tumor. Pyogenic granuloma is an inflammatory lesion and is not neoplastic.

Benign Neoplasms (Tumors)

Exostoses, or *tori,* are hard, bony enlargements of the outer plate of the jawbone (Fig. 8-13). They are not neoplasms in the true sense but are simply localized areas of overgrowth of normal bone. They are seen in the midline of the hard palate (*torus palatinus*) and on the lingual side of the lower jaw near the floor of the mouth,

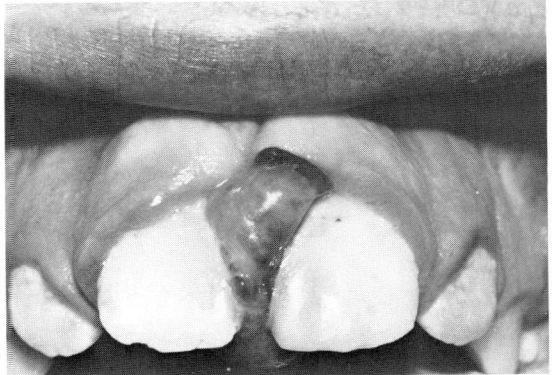

Figure 8-12 | Pyogenic granuloma. (*Courtesy of J. Burkes.*)

usually in the bicuspid region (*torus mandibularis*). Pressure from a dental plate on an exostosis may cause discomfort to the patient; for this reason exostoses should be removed surgically if they interfere with the mechanical requirements of a good restoration.

Papilloma is a soft-tissue tumor having a warty or mushroom-like appearance. It may occur in almost any place in the mouth and should be surgically removed if constantly irritated.

Fibroma is a soft-tissue tumor having a pink, smooth appearance. It is the most frequently occurring benign tumor of the oral cavity. It should be removed if it interferes with chewing or if it is uncomfortable.

Epulis is the name given to any benign tumor of the gingivae. It has been classically associated with giant-cell tumors of the gums in the lower bicuspid region. Most of these tumors, however, are simple fibromas (Fig. 8-14).

Squamous Cell Carcinoma (Epidermoid Carcinoma)

This condition is by far the most frequently occurring malignancy of epithelial origin in the oral cavity. In its more advanced stage it appears clinically as a raised indurated (hard and gristle-like to touch) lesion with rolled borders and a necrotic center (Fig. 8-15). The early clinical lesion is often difficult to diagnose; therefore, tissue from suspicious lesions should be excised and sent to a pathologist for diagnosis. A patient's life may depend upon keen observation by the dentist, who may be the first to see the condition. These tumors spread (metastasize) to distant parts of the body through the lymph channels.

Sarcomas

Sarcomas are malignant tumors of connective tissue origin that are much rarer than carcinomas and usually occur in young individuals, often in children. They grow very rapidly as a rule and

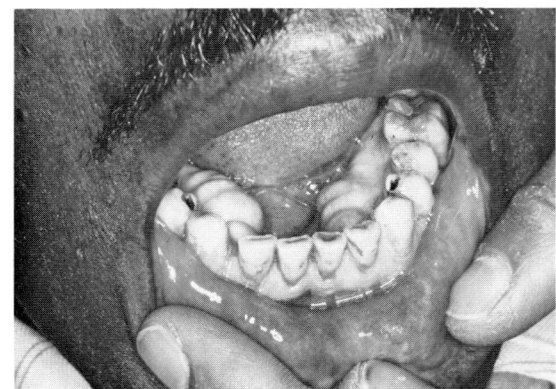

Figure 8-13 | Mandibular tori (excessive localized normal bone enlargements). These are slow, harmless growths but sometimes complicate dental-treatment planning. (*Courtesy of J. Burkes.*)

are almost always fatal. There are many varieties of this type of tumor.

Odontogenic Neoplasms (Ameloblastoma and Odontoma)

Ameloblastoma is a tumor derived principally from the epithelial portion of the enamel organ

Figure 8-14 | Epulis between mandibular cuspid and lateral incisor. (*Courtesy of J. Burkes.*)

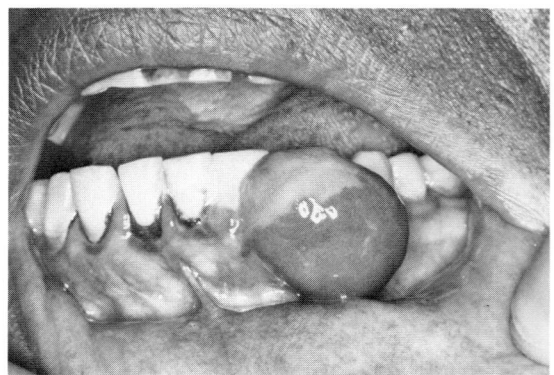

or its remains in the jaw; it occurs more frequently in the mandible than in the maxilla. It is usually a very slow-growing tumor, destroying the body of the bone by extension, and is usually detected in the age range 25 to 40. Radiographically it produces large, dark cystic areas (multilocular cysts). Surgery is necessary in its treatment.

Odontomas are benign tumors derived from tooth-germ components in the jaw just as are ameloblastomas, but, unlike ameloblastomas, they consist of more specialized tissue and produce hard structures such as enamel, dentin, and cementum. In a radiograph they appear white and dense (radiopaque) and are irregular in outline. Some of them contain poorly formed and odd-shaped teeth. Many of them have been discovered because they blocked the normal eruption of a tooth.

BIOPSY AND CYTOLOGY

Biopsy and oral exfoliative cytology are important aids in the diagnosis of oral lesions. *Excisional biopsy* refers to the removal of the entire growth or lesion along with a small amount of normal tissue surrounding the lesion for submission to the pathologist for microscopic examination. *Incisional biopsy* refers to removal of part of the growth or lesion along with some contiguous normal tissue for surgical pathology examination. Excisional is used more for small growths or lesions, and incisional for larger growths or lesions. Proper fixation of the excised tissue plus filling out the information form required by the pathologist for an examination may be a duty assigned to the assistant.

Oral exfoliative cytology refers to examination of surface cells of a lesion obtained by vigorous scraping with a tongue blade or small metal spatula. The cells are spread on a slide, properly prepared to keep from losing the smeared specimen, and fixed. The prepared slide specimen

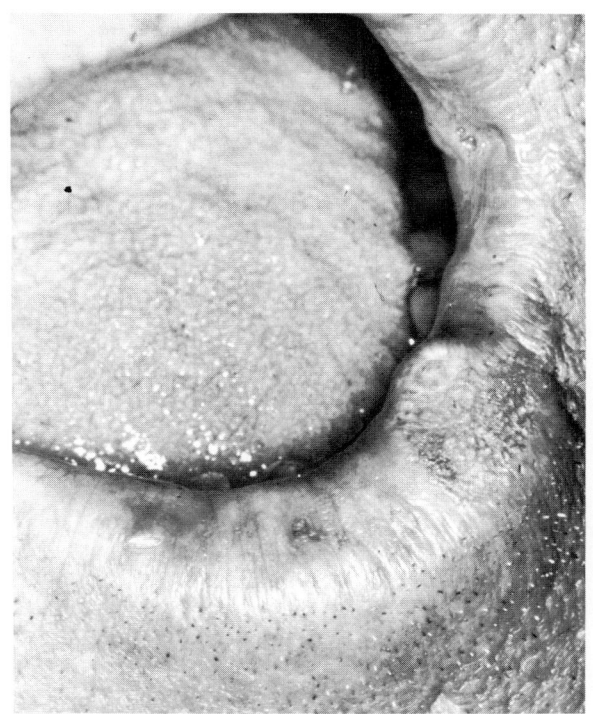

Figure 8-15 | Squamous cell carcinoma of lower lip.

plus a completed information sheet are then sent to the pathologist for an examination and diagnosis. Oral exfoliative cytology is used more frequently for erythematous and ulcerative-type lesions and is an important screening type of examination. If the report from the pathologist indicates abnormal cells, then a biopsy, which is a more definitive diagnostic tool, is mandatory (Fig. 8-16).

ORAL PIGMENTATION

Melanin, a normal dark-brown pigment produced by the basal epithelial cells lining the oral cavity, is seen easily in dark-skinned individuals (Fig. 8-17). In certain pathologic conditions, this

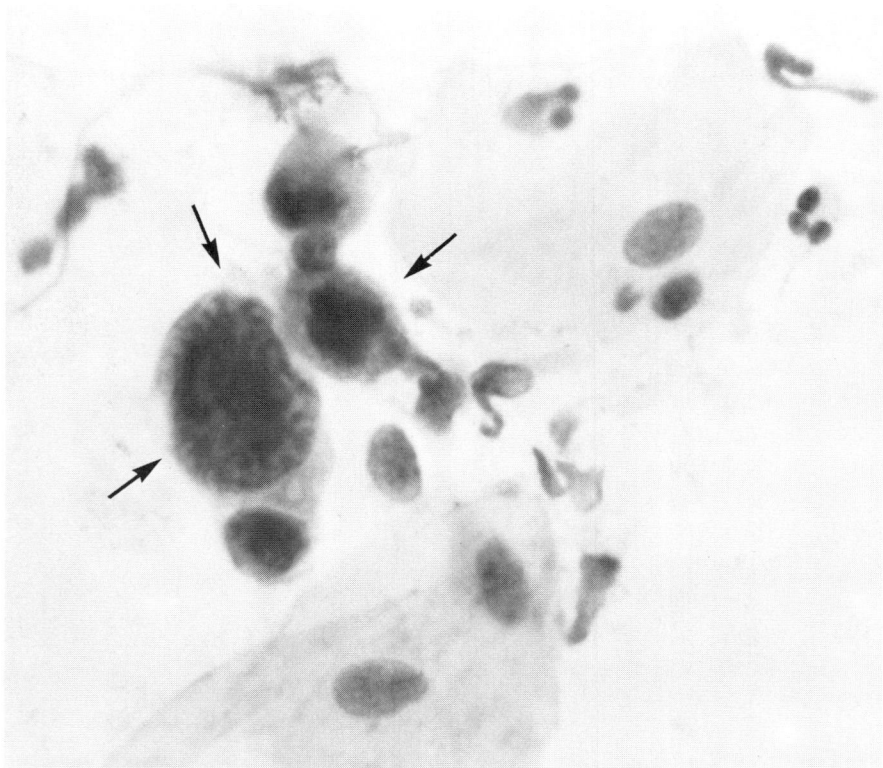

Figure 8-16 | Abnormal oral squamous epithelial cells from a stained smear. (*Courtesy of J. Burkes.*)

Figure 8-17 | Normal melanin pigmentation in the gingivae of a dark-skinned individual.

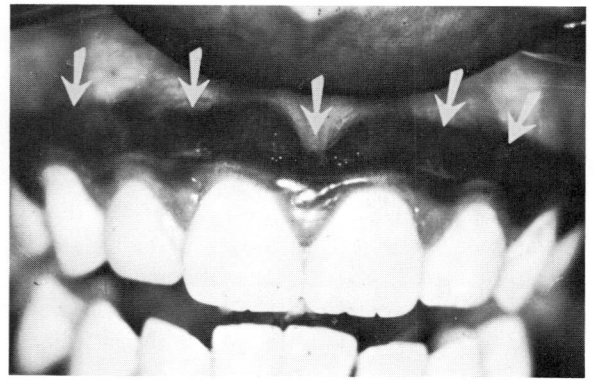

pigmentation may be accentuated and can thus be helpful in diagnosis.

Pathologic pigmentation may be seen in the gums and oral mucous membranes after exposure to heavy metals such as silver, lead, bismuth, and mercury. In lead poisoning, there is a characteristic bluish line in the gingivae. Amalgam fragments sometimes become accidentally embedded in soft tissue during dental procedures and produce a characteristic discoloration ("amalgam tattoo"). Silver nitrate is also capable of causing discoloration of the teeth and surrounding tissues.

Pathologic pigmentation by the various frac-tions of disintegrated red blood cells is usually the result of trauma, accident, or rupture of small vessels in the lip, buccal mucosa, tongue, or pulp of a tooth.

INJURIES TO THE TEETH AND RELATED ORAL STRUCTURES

The principal injuries to teeth and related oral structures are usually traumatic, thermal, or chemical in nature.

Traumatic injuries result from rough and broken-down teeth, from improper toothbrush techniques, from impaction of foreign bodies such as fish bones, and from loss of control by the dentist of burs, stones, or discs during dental operations. Traumatic ulcers of the alveolar ridge from improperly fitted dentures resemble cancer in clinical appearance, but heal and disappear when the irritating factor is removed. Acute traumatic injury in accidents accounts for a large number of fractured anterior teeth and soft-tissue mutilations.

Thermal injuries of the soft tissue result from ingestion of hot foods such as coffee. Heat produced by inadequate use of coolants on burs and stones during cavity preparations may cause severe pulpal damage in the tooth operated on. Large metallic fillings without bases or insulation also may result in pulpal injury.

The more common chemical burns occur either from imprudent self-medication of drugs such as aspirin (Fig. 8-18) or from loss of control by the dentist in the use of such drugs as phenol, alcohol, zinc chloride, and trichloroacetic acid during dental procedures.

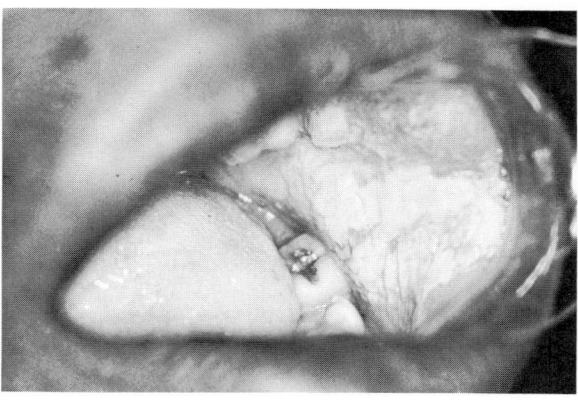

Figure 8-18 | Severe aspirin burn of buccal mucosa resulting from self-medication (holding aspirin tablets in buccal fold against a painful tooth).

Irradiation burns from therapeutic doses of x-ray for treatment of oral cancer may result in severe soft-tissue and bone injury.

BIBLIOGRAPHY

Bhaskar, S. N.: *Synopsis of Oral Pathology,* 4th ed., The C. V. Mosby Company, St. Louis, 1973.

Giunta, J.: *Oral Pathology,* in M. J. Dunn, series ed., *Module 3 for Dental Auxiliary Practice,* The Williams and Wilkins Company, Baltimore, 1975.

Kerr, D. A., and Ash, M. M., Jr.: *Oral Pathology,* 3d ed., Lea & Febiger, Philadelphia, 1971.

Massler, M., and Schour I.: *Atlas of the Mouth,* rev. ed., American Dental Association, Bureau of Public Relations, Chicago, 1958.

Shafer, W. G., Hine, M. K., and Levy, B. M.: *A Textbook of Oral Pathology,* 3d ed., W. B. Saunders Company, Philadelphia, 1974.

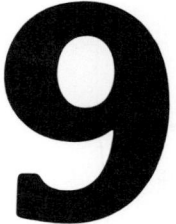

Cecil R. Lupton
Pharmacology

INTRODUCTION

Pharmacology, the science which deals with the study of drugs in all its aspects, is an important element of the practice of dentistry. The use of drugs in dentistry to treat disease processes in many instances also involves conditions and areas of the human body that are not associated directly with the teeth and their surrounding tissues. One of the dental problems which confront every dentist is that of infections, and modern drugs have indeed revolutionized the treatment of infections associated with the structures of the oral cavity.

Historically, it was about 3500 B.C. that the Egyptians began to use drugs and other remedies in competition with witchcraft and magic for the relief of dental pain. The Chinese, much later, some 3000 years ago, cited a number of dental ailments and also listed a number of prescriptions. The ancient biblical city of Nineveh is referred to by archaeologists who excavated some tablets there which were written about 700 B.C. and which contained a story of a king who became critical of his physician for not curing him of his dental problems. Later, however, the fall of Rome brought forth the Dark Ages, and for several centuries witchcraft and magic again became the most widely used remedies for dental pain.

It was not until the eighteenth century that dentistry began to emerge as a member of the healing arts when a Frenchman, Pierre Fauchard, published his famous book *Le Chirurgien Dentiste.* He has been designated as the Father of Modern Dentistry. Oil of cloves and cinnamon were employed commonly for the relief of toothache.

Books on the history of dentistry indicate that no one group or nation can claim all the credit for the advancement of the profession. Dr. Crawford W. Long was the discoverer of ether as a general anesthetic, and the site of the first surgical operation in the history of the world under a general anesthetic was in Georgia in 1842. Following Dr. Long in 1844, Dr. Horace Wells, a practicing dentist in Hartford, Connecticut, was the first to use nitrous oxide as a general anesthetic (Bremner, 1954; Prinz, 1945; Robinson, 1940; Weinberger, 1948).

The histories of dentistry, medicine, public health, and other health sciences present many dramatic and valuable discoveries related to drugs, which have saved countless numbers of lives as well as contributed greatly to the productivity of individuals and nations. For example, there is insulin, which commonly is used therapeutically in the deficiency condition known as diabetes to assist in the regulation of carbohydrate (sugar) metabolism, and penicillin, a powerful drug used in the control of infections, and then there are various vaccines administered for the prevention or treatment of infectious diseases. The number of such drugs is large and the list is increased annually.

The research within universities, drug companies, and federal agencies continues to discover and produce new drugs and methods of utilizing drugs for the prevention, control, and cure of diseases and other conditions of humans and animals. Thus, the subject area of pharmacology is too vast in its scope and dynamics for any one individual to comprehend or evaluate.

The objective in this chapter is to provide an introduction to the subject for the dental assistant. Some of the legal aspects pertaining to the diagnosis and treatment of patients have been discussed in Chap. 1, and, accordingly, the responsibility for the prescribing of drugs and the writing of prescriptions in the dental office rests with the dentist. However, it is important that the dental assistant be familiar with the various sources of information on drugs, as well as with certain procedures and other factors that relate to drug administration and action.

RESPONSIBILITY AND STANDARDS RELATED TO DRUGS

The Food and Drug Administration of the Department of Health, Education, and Welfare has the responsibility for the enforcement of the Federal Food, Drug, and Cosmetic Act. Such enforcement relates to the labeling of drugs, food, cosmetics, and related items. The manufacturer of a new drug, for example, must provide evidence to the Food and Drug Administration that the product is *effective* for the conditions indicated before it is released for marketing. There also must be assurance of the safety, identity, strength, quality, and purity of the product.

The Federal Trade Commission, as cited by the Wheeler-Lea Act, has jurisdiction over the advertising of drugs. This act, coupled with the Federal Food, Drug, and Cosmetic Act, provides substantial protection to the public and the health professions, as well as to the drug manufacturers.

Current (1977) regulation of the manufacture, distribution, and dispensation of controlled substances is the responsibility of the Drug Enforcement Administration. Dentists may purchase and prescribe controlled substances following registration with the above agency. The Drug Enforcement Administration outlines definitive procedures for the handling of controlled substances, and information regarding such may be obtained by requesting DEA registration information from the U.S. Department of Justice,

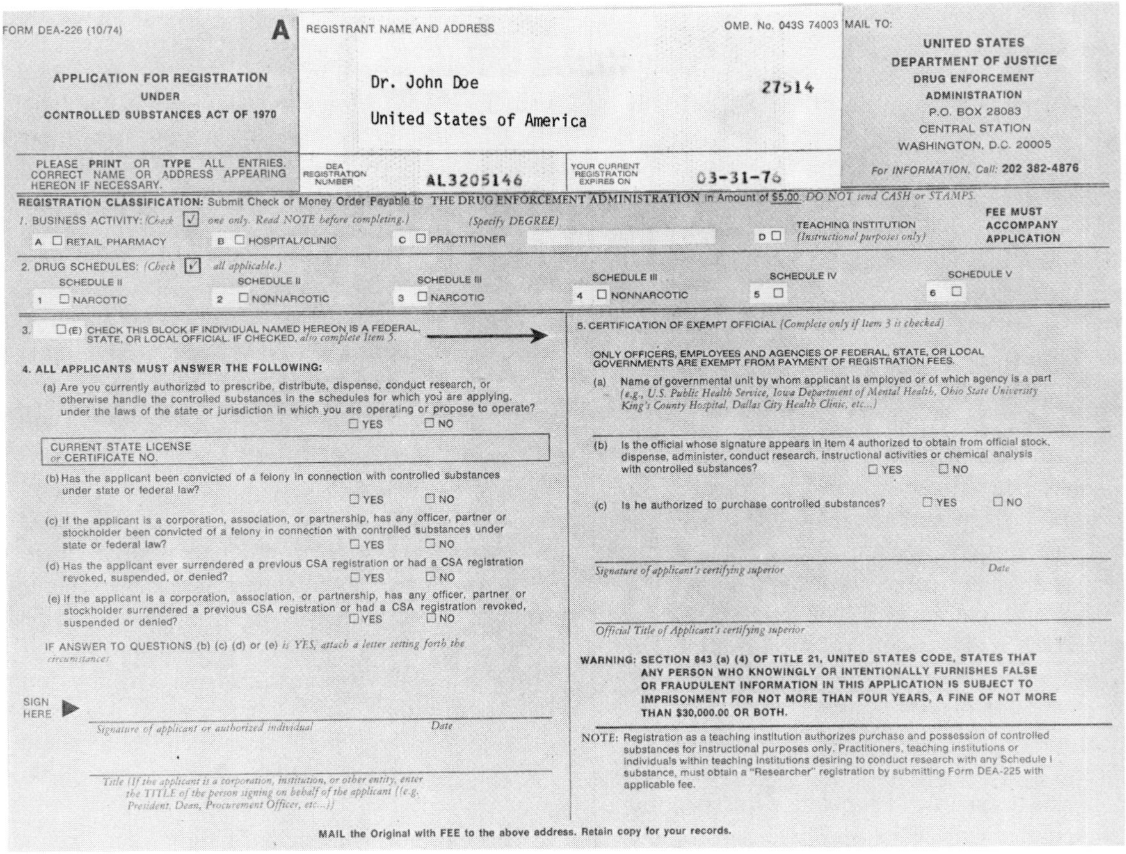
FORM DEA-226 (10/74)

A

APPLICATION FOR REGISTRATION UNDER CONTROLLED SUBSTANCES ACT OF 1970

REGISTRANT NAME AND ADDRESS

Dr. John Doe

United States of America

27514

OMB. No. 043S 74003

MAIL TO:

UNITED STATES DEPARTMENT OF JUSTICE
DRUG ENFORCEMENT ADMINISTRATION
P.O. BOX 28083
CENTRAL STATION
WASHINGTON, D.C. 20005

For INFORMATION, Call: 202 382-4876

PLEASE PRINT OR TYPE ALL ENTRIES. CORRECT NAME OR ADDRESS APPEARING HEREON IF NECESSARY.

DEA REGISTRATION NUMBER AL3205146

YOUR CURRENT REGISTRATION EXPIRES ON 03-31-76

REGISTRATION CLASSIFICATION: Submit Check or Money Order Payable to THE DRUG ENFORCEMENT ADMINISTRATION in Amount of $5.00. DO NOT send CASH or STAMPS.

FEE MUST ACCOMPANY APPLICATION

1. BUSINESS ACTIVITY: (Check ☑ one only. Read NOTE before completing.)

A ☐ RETAIL PHARMACY B ☐ HOSPITAL/CLINIC C ☐ PRACTITIONER (Specify DEGREE) D ☐ TEACHING INSTITUTION (Instructional purposes only)

2. DRUG SCHEDULES: (Check ☑ all applicable.)

SCHEDULE II 1 ☐ NARCOTIC SCHEDULE II 2 ☐ NONNARCOTIC SCHEDULE III 3 ☐ NARCOTIC SCHEDULE III 4 ☐ NONNARCOTIC SCHEDULE IV 5 ☐ SCHEDULE V 6 ☐

3. ☐ (E) CHECK THIS BLOCK IF INDIVIDUAL NAMED HEREON IS A FEDERAL, STATE, OR LOCAL OFFICIAL. IF CHECKED, also complete Item 5.

4. ALL APPLICANTS MUST ANSWER THE FOLLOWING:

(a) Are you currently authorized to prescribe, distribute, dispense, conduct research, or otherwise handle the controlled substances in the schedules for which you are applying, under the laws of the state or jurisdiction in which you are operating or propose to operate? ☐ YES ☐ NO

CURRENT STATE LICENSE or CERTIFICATE NO.

(b) Has the applicant been convicted of a felony in connection with controlled substances under state or federal law? ☐ YES ☐ NO

(c) If the applicant is a corporation, association, or partnership, has any officer, partner or stockholder been convicted of a felony in connection with controlled substances under state or federal law? ☐ YES ☐ NO

(d) Has the applicant ever surrendered a previous CSA registration or had a CSA registration revoked, suspended, or denied? ☐ YES ☐ NO

(e) If the applicant is a corporation, association, or partnership, has any officer, partner or stockholder surrendered a previous CSA registration or had a CSA registration revoked, suspended or denied? ☐ YES ☐ NO

IF ANSWER TO QUESTIONS (b) (c) (d) or (e) is YES, attach a letter setting forth the circumstances.

SIGN HERE ▶

Signature of applicant or authorized individual Date

Title (If the applicant is a corporation, institution, or other entity, enter the TITLE of the person signing on behalf of the applicant (e.g. President, Dean, Procurement Officer, etc...))

5. CERTIFICATION OF EXEMPT OFFICIAL (Complete only if Item 3 is checked)

ONLY OFFICERS, EMPLOYEES AND AGENCIES OF FEDERAL, STATE, OR LOCAL GOVERNMENTS ARE EXEMPT FROM PAYMENT OF REGISTRATION FEES.

(a) Name of governmental unit by whom applicant is employed or of which agency is a part (e.g., U.S. Public Health Service, Iowa Department of Mental Health, Ohio State University King's County Hospital, Dallas City Health Clinic, etc...)

(b) Is the official whose signature appears in Item 4 authorized to obtain from official stock, dispense, administer, conduct research, instructional activities or chemical analysis with controlled substances? ☐ YES ☐ NO

(c) Is he authorized to purchase controlled substances? ☐ YES ☐ NO

Signature of applicant's certifying superior Date

Official Title of Applicant's certifying superior

WARNING: SECTION 843 (a) (4) OF TITLE 21, UNITED STATES CODE, STATES THAT ANY PERSON WHO KNOWINGLY OR INTENTIONALLY FURNISHES FALSE OR FRAUDULENT INFORMATION IN THIS APPLICATION IS SUBJECT TO IMPRISONMENT FOR NOT MORE THAN FOUR YEARS, A FINE OF NOT MORE THAN $30,000.00 OR BOTH.

NOTE: Registration as a teaching institution authorizes purchase and possession of controlled substances for instructional purposes only. Practitioners, teaching institutions or individuals within teaching institutions desiring to conduct research with any Schedule I substance, must obtain a "Researcher" registration by submitting Form DEA-225 with applicable fee.

MAIL the Original with FEE to the above address. Retain copy for your records.

Figure 9-1 | Sample renewal application form received from the Drug Enforcement Administration.

Drug Enforcement Administration, Registration Section, P. O. Box 28083, Central Station, Washington, D.C., 20005. An application for registration may be obtained from the same address. When requirements for registration have been met, a certificate will be issued, and an annual renewal application will be forwarded (Fig. 9-1). Dispensing or prescribing any controlled substance prior to receipt of the certificate of registration is a violation of federal law. Also, some states have registration requirements for dispensing and prescribing particular classes of pharmaceuticals. The appropriate agency in a particular state should be contacted in regard to such activity.

A publication issued every 5 years which is recognized as an official standard by the Federal Food, Drug, and Cosmetic Act is the *United States Pharmacopeia.* It gives the source, appearance, properties, standards of purity, and other specifications of drugs that are commonly used by the health professions. The drugs which meet these specifications may bear the label U.S.P.

The *National Formulary* is a publication issued by the Committee on the National Formulary that is elected by the Council of the American Pharmaceutical Association. It is recognized as an official standard under the Food, Drug, and Cosmetic Act, and contains a history of drugs not included in the *United States Pharmacopeia* and also a description of important standard mixtures of drugs frequently employed in prescriptions.

All drugs listed in the *United States Pharmacopeia* and in the *National Formulary* are referred to as *Official Drugs,* and they are so designated in the Federal Food, Drug, and Cosmetic Act. These books also are recognized by the courts.

The most useful publication for the day-to-day practice of dentistry is probably the *Physician's Desk Reference* published by Medical Economics. It contains a therapeutic index, brand name index, generic name index, other useful information, and, most importantly, a drug identification section. This identification section is most helpful in identifying medications that potential patients may have in their possession. This publication is revised annually and, in addition, supplementary drug information is provided during the year.

Another valuable publication, one that should be present in every dental office, is *Accepted Dental Therapeutics,* which is published biennially under the immediate supervision of the Council on Dental Therapeutics of the American Dental Association. It is considered a handbook on therapeutics and not a textbook of pharmacology, and includes information concerning

(1) drugs of recognized value in dentistry, (2) drugs of uncertain status more recently proposed for use by the dentist, and (3) some drugs once employed extensively but now generally regarded as obsolete. Only brands of drugs of recognized value in dentistry which are labeled and advertised to dentists in accordance with the Council's Provisions for Acceptance of Products are included in the listing of accepted dosage forms. Description of other drugs are provided for information only. (American Dental Association Council on Dental Therapeutics, 1966)

SOURCES OF DRUGS

All the drugs and medicaments used in modern medicine are obtained from four main sources. Many of the products are used in their pure form, while others are combined chemically to form entirely different compounds. Some are combined physically to permit the combined action of two or more drugs that are synergistic in their therapeutic action. The four main sources of drugs are (1) plants, (2) minerals, (3) animals, and (4) synthetics.

Plants

Many plants have medicinal value in a portion called the active principle. This active principle is extracted from the part of the plant in which it exists. For example, cascara sagrada is obtained from the bark of a tree, while strychnine is obtained from the seeds of a tree. The active principle of other plants may be in the leaves, the roots, or even the flowers.

Minerals

Naturally occurring mineral substances are commonly used in medicine, usually in a highly purified state or in chemical union with other elements. Some examples are magnesium sulfate (Epsom salt), zinc oxide, and sodium chloride (common salt).

Animals

Researchers continually are finding more extracts of animal tissue which are useful. One of the more common is insulin, which is obtained from the pancreas of cattle, sheep, and hogs; this drug is used in the treatment of diabetes.

Synthetic Drugs

As previously stated, the research programs in the field of organic chemistry have added materially to our supply of drugs and medicaments. These have been produced at a volume and price to permit their broad use in medicine. Many drugs, scarce in nature but essential to treatment of human ills, now are being produced synthetically in the chemical laboratory. These synthetic products may equal or even surpass in quality those obtained from natural sources.

THE ADMINISTRATION OF DRUGS

When a therapeutic agent is being selected, it is important for the dentist to know if the patient is receiving any other medication, such as for diabetes or a cardiovascular disease. The dental treatment to be provided, as well as the drugs to be selected, may be modified by the dentist depending upon the medication received by the patient, who also is under the care of a physician. Further, the dentist's plan of treatment and medication may be changed as a result of a physician's diagnosis of the patient's condition or disease. Thus, the dental and medical histories of every patient are a vital consideration in the examination and plan of treatment. Reference is made in Chaps. 2 and 17 to the records pertaining to histories.

General Considerations

In the administration of drugs, the following items are deemed important:

1. The drug should be administered at the time specified, accurately, and in the best way to bring results.
2. The intelligent administration of drugs requires some knowledge of the following:
   a. Nature of the drug, including potential side reactions.
   b. Maximum and minimum dosage.
   c. Factors that modify the dose.
   d. Disease or condition being treated.
   e. The effect desired.
   f. Symptoms of overdosing.
   g. Effect of habit-forming drugs.
3. The medicine cupboard should be kept locked.
4. Labels must be clear and legible. They should be changed as often as necessary as a precaution against administering the wrong drug.
5. Bottles should have well-fitted stoppers, since some drugs undergo a change on exposure to air.
6. All drugs should be discarded that show change in color or consistency, unless the manufacturers state such changes do not affect their action.
7. Certain preparations must be kept under refrigeration.
8. Security and records for controlled substances should be handled in accordance with DEA and state regulations.

Suggestions for Drug Administration

The following general rules are recommended office routine:

1. Know the various modes of measuring drugs, and do not use them interchangeably. For example, minims and drops are not the same.
2. Obtain calibrated measures, and use them for all drugs. Do not guess.
3. Read the label at least three times. First, when taken from the cabinet, then before administering the drug, and again when returning it to the cabinet.
4. Do not handle pills, tablets, etc., with the fingers.
5. Remain with the patient until after the medication has been taken.
6. Do not pour excess back into the bottle or container. Be careful to pour out only that amount required, since drugs are expensive.
7. If in doubt, do not administer the drug until checking to be sure that both the drug and dose are correct.

Recording of Medication and Patient Reaction

Accurate records may mean the difference between successful and unsuccessful treatment of a patient. All drugs administered should be recorded on the patient's chart, and the record should include:

1. The drug or medicament given.
2. Date and time.
3. Dose and route (oral, I.V., etc.) of administration.
4. If the patient is ambulatory and a prescription is given, all prescription information should be recorded.

It is also of importance to record any reactions of the patient following administration of a drug. In many cases these records determine the future course of therapy by the attending dentist or physician.

Methods of Administering Drugs

Although there are numerous channels by which drugs may be given, the desired effects of the drug will determine in most cases the routine of administration. If local action is desired, the drug may be administered by one method, while systemic results may be obtained much faster or better by another route. These channels of administration are as follows:

Mouth (p.o.)

This usually is the easiest route by which one may obtain local or systemic results as desired. When drugs are administered by mouth (or per os, meaning "by mouth" and abbreviated p.o.), flavoring agents should be used when necessary to avoid unpleasant tastes.

Rectum

Drugs may be administered by this route for various reasons:

1. Unpleasant taste of the drugs.
2. Mentally ill or unconscious patient.
3. For slow absorption through the walls of the colon.
4. As a medicament applied directly to the colon wall.
5. For anesthesia.

Inhalation

The lungs offer one of the fastest routes of absorption of drugs. Inhalation therapy can, therefore, be used in the following cases:

1. In the treatment of infections of the respiratory tract, usually by means of a steam inhalator or a vaporizer.
2. For relief of angina pectoris, drugs such as amyl nitrite being absorbed rapidly through the lungs and producing systemic results.
3. For relief of anxiety and analgesic effect, nitrous oxide (N_2O).

Inunction

The drug, usually in ointment form, is rubbed into the skin thoroughly and absorbed slowly through the sweat glands and hair follicles. The nurse should use rubber gloves in applying these medicaments, because prolonged exposure to some of the chemicals may be dangerous.

Sublingual

The mucous membrane in the floor of the mouth absorbs some drugs readily and rapidly. Nitroglycerin, given for the relief of angina pectoris, is one of the more common drugs applied sublingually, although many others may be administered in this manner.

Injection

There are a number of methods used to inject drugs for therapeutic purposes, depending upon the drug given or results desired. Two types of injections that are of importance to the dentist will be discussed briefly

1. *Intramuscular injection.* The medicine is injected into a muscle by hypodermic syringe and needle. The needle is thrust into the muscle at a right angle to the skin surface and to the desired depth. Injection is made rather slowly, and the area should be

gently massaged after the needle is withdrawn. Before injecting, the syringe plunger should be pulled back to aspirate. This is to ensure that the needle tip is not in a blood vessel.

Drugs administered by this method are absorbed into the bloodstream rapidly, and a therapeutic blood concentration is reached much faster than by administration by mouth. This method is also used to administer drugs that cannot be tolerated in the stomach.

2. *Intravenous injection.* The needle is inserted in a vein, and the drug is injected into the bloodstream directly. This method gives the most rapid response to medication. The intravenous route of administering medication in the dental office is becoming more prevalent, and dental assistants are a part of the team when using this modality of administration.

In any technique of administering drugs by injection, several things must be kept in mind:

1. Equipment must be absolutely sterile.
2. Medicine or drug must be absolutely sterile.
3. The area of injection must be prepared to render it as nearly sterile as possible. An alcohol sponge or other appropriate antiseptic agent should be used to prepare the skin prior to injection. In an acute life-threatening emergency, such a procedure is a secondary consideration.

Conditions Modifying Action of Drugs

In the past, practitioners of medicine and dentistry have gone through periods of prescribing fixed drugs and fixed dosages for certain illnesses. In more recent times, however, it has been learned that not all drugs have the same effect on all persons. It has been learned also that there are a number of factors that may contribute to the reaction or response of a patient to any and all medication. A few of these more important factors will be discussed here.

Tolerance

Prolonged use of a drug causes the body to build up a tolerance to that drug, and increasingly larger doses are necessary to produce the desired results. This is easily demonstrated in the use of narcotics or alcohol.

Age and Weight

The modern concept of drug therapy is that weight has more to do with the dosage required than does age. It is reasonable to assume that the greater the bulk present, the larger will be the dose required to produce comparable results. Hence, a child of 50 lb does not require as large a dose as an adult of 150 lb. However, the dosage of the child in the above case does not equal one-third that of the adult; accordingly, some rules have been established to determine children's dosages. The manufacturer will usually provide the accepted dosages if you request them, and these figures are a good guide.

Allergy

In the antibiotic therapy used so widely today, it has been found that some patients are allergic to penicillin or other antibiotics and must be given substitute drugs. Many patients will be found to display idiosyncrasies to specific medicaments, and it will be necessary to discontinue their use. For example, one occasionally finds patients who are sensitive to certain local anesthetics. In all instances of allergic manifestation, the medication should be stopped at once and appropriate measures instituted to counteract any life-threatening sequelae.

Cumulative Effect

Some drugs are destroyed or eliminated from the body very slowly. When this is true, continued intake of the drug at a rate faster than it is eliminated will result in excessive amounts being present in the body, and harmful effects will result.

Channel of Administration

Six major routes of administering drugs have been listed. It is known that drugs given by mouth, for example, will not produce results so fast as those given by intramuscular injection. It is true also that larger doses must be given if the drug is to be absorbed through a living membrane of the body, i.e., skin, mucous membrane of the mouth, or stomach.

Pathologic Condition

The infecting agent determines the drug to be used in most cases. Too, the number of organisms present, whether localized or systematic, chronic or acute, will determine the amount of the dose as well as the route of administration.

Important Pharmacologic Actions

Although a multitude of drugs are in use today, their action on the body may be reduced to six basic pharmacologic actions. These actions are (1) stimulation; (2) depression; (3) irritation; (4) demulcent (soothing or bland); (5) salt (or osmotic) effect; and (6) replacement of deficient biologic functions. Any of the above may be systemic or local, and the extent of their action may depend on the amount of the drug administered.

WEIGHTS AND MEASURES IN DRUG PREPARATIONS

The science of weights and measures is known as metrology. In the United States there are two accepted systems of recording weights and measures in prescription writing, i.e., the apothecaries' and the metric or decimal. The apothecaries' is the oldest, but the metric system was legalized by an act of Congress in 1866 which made its use mandatory in Army, Navy, and Marine hospitals. It is the method of choice and should be used in preference to the apothecaries' system. The metric system was adopted by the *United States Pharmacopeia* and is, therefore, considered legal in the United States.

In the metric system there are three basic units of measure. The *meter* is the linear measure, the *gram* is the unit of weight, and the *liter* is the unit of capacity. In expressing subdivisions of these units, the Latin prefixes are used as follows: deci- = 10, centi- = 100, and milli- = 1000. Therefore, a centimeter equals $1/100$ of a meter. If one wishes to express the multiples of the three basic measures, it is done by prefixes from the Greek numerals as follows: deca- = 10, hecto- = 100, kilo- = 1000, and myria- = 10,000. Thus, a kilogram is equal to 1000 grams.

Knowing the above methods and simple arithmetic, it is easy to express units of measure by the use of a decimal point and the arabic numerals 1, 2, 3, etc. If the dosage of a drug is $1/10$ of a gram, it is expressed by 0.1 gram. Another unit of measure which must be understood in mixing or giving drugs is the *milliliter*. This unit of capacity measure is equal to $1/1000$ of a liter. Thus, 1000 milliliters equals 1 liter. The milliliter is used in the measurement of liquids. The *cubic centimeter* is equal to $1/1000$ of a liter, and is also used in the measurement of liquids.

Abbreviations are often used in expressing these units of measure. Care must be taken in writing the abbreviation for gram. The accepted abbreviation for *grain* is gr and it must not be confused with g for *gram*. The following abbreviations are important to know:

$$\begin{aligned}
\text{Gram} &= \text{g} \\
\text{Cubic centimeter} &= \text{cc} \\
\text{Milliliter} &= \text{ml} \\
\text{Liter} &= \text{l} \\
\text{Kilogram} &= \text{kg}
\end{aligned}$$

It becomes necessary on occasion to use some units of home measure. The following table gives a comparison of common home measures and the metric equivalent:

1 drop = 0.06 ml
1 teaspoonful = 4.0 ml
1 tablespoonful = 15.0 ml
1 cupful = 120.0 ml
1 glassful = 240.0 ml

The solution commonly prepared in the dental office is a percentage solution. In preparing this, one should start with ingredients of known strength. If, for example, a 10 percent solution of sodium chloride is desired, start with the solid (table salt), and add enough distilled water to make 100 ml. In this case it is 10 g sodium chloride with sufficient distilled water to make 100 ml of the solution.

Percentage solutions simply mean the number of grams or milliliters of the concentrated material in 100 ml of the completed solution. By starting with 10 ml of a liquid concentrate and adding 90 ml of distilled water, the desired 100 ml of a 10 percent solution is obtained. Any larger quantities are made by simple multiples. Thus, 1000 ml of a 10 percent saline solution would be 100 g salt with enough distilled water added to make 1000 ml or 1 liter.

PRESCRIPTIONS

A prescription may be defined as a written order authorizing a pharmacist to dispense a certain drug or a combination of drugs for a patient. Drugs which are habit-forming or too hazardous for use without professional supervision may not be dispensed by a pharmacist except upon prescription by a dentist, physician, or veterinarian. A prescription for a controlled substance must include the DEA number of the individual signing the prescription.

The Prescription

Simplicity is desired and thus Latin rarely is used in the modern prescription. However, a few abbreviations derived from the Latin phrases generally are used by the prescriber.

A prescribed drug may be designated by its brand (proprietary) name or by its generic name. If the generic name is used, it permits the pharmacist a choice in using a brand that is in stock.

Prescription blanks, which are printed especially for the dentist, are not essential. However, such blanks are desirable, and they conserve time. They should contain the name, address, and telephone number of the dentist, and the DEA registry number. The blank also should have a notation directing the dentist to indicate the number of times the prescription may be refilled. A notation for age, too, may be included on the form. The other items on the prescription form include areas for the name and address of the patient, for the date, and for the signature of the dentist.

The form and content of a prescription are divided into the following parts: (1) heading, (2) superscription, (3) inscription, (4) subscription, (5) signature, (6) prescriber's (dentist) signature, and (7) refill information.

1. *Heading.* The heading contains the name, address, and telephone number of the individual or institution (hospital, dental school, clinic, etc.) prescribing the medication. Also, the name, address, and age (optional) of the patient plus the date.
2. *Superscription.* This portion of the prescription is the symbol Rx. It is an abbreviation of the Latin word for recipe and literally means "take thou." It is an order for the pharmacist or other appropriate individual to take the medication(s) listed below and dispense them to the patient.
3. *Inscription.* This is the body of the prescription and lists the name and strength of the drug to be dispensed. The generic or brand name may be used to convey this information.
4. *Subscription.* This is the amount of the drug to be dispensed. For pills, capsules, inhalents, or suppositories this would be a number. For a liquid, volume designation would be written.
5. *Signature.* This is usually a confusing term as it does not denote the usual meaning of the word. It comes from the Latin word *signa* meaning "mark a label." This portion is the directions or instructions

to be placed on the container label for the patient to follow in using or taking the medication.
6. *Signature of the prescriber.* This is the written signature of the doctor and, when indicated, should include his or her DEA registry number.
7. *Refill information.* This is information regarding the refilling of the prescription or specific orders not to refill. In accordance with the Durham-Humphrey Act, all medications which require a prescription in order to be filled cannot be refilled unless specified on the prescription. All prescriptions should be typed or written in ink. For future reference, the prescription information should be recorded in the patient's record.

PHARMACEUTIC PREPARATIONS: ACTION AND DOSAGE

Central Nervous System Depressants

Hypnotics and sedatives are drugs that produce sleep or decrease excitability by depression of the central nervous system. In normal doses they do not appreciably affect the medullary centers of circulation or respiration; their action is primarily on the cerebral cortex and midbrain. It should be remembered that natural sleep is better than that induced artificially, so that hypnotics should not be used promiscuously.

There are many hypnotics available today, but those most commonly used are the barbiturates, the salts of barbituric acid, which are odorless and bitter to taste. Mild doses will usually have a sedative effect and will allay nervousness, while stronger doses will produce drowsiness and sleep. Ordinarily one-half the hypnotic dose will produce sedative effects. The barbiturates produce only slight analgesic effect, and so one should prescribe a pain-relieving drug with them if necessary.

Patients with an allergy to the barbiturates may develop a skin rash and experience a prolonged mental depression.

Some of the more commonly used barbiturates, with the adult hypnotic and sedative dosage, are presented as follows:

Name	Oral hypnotic dose	Oral sedative dose
Barbital	0.3 g	0.15 g
Barbital sodium	0.3 g	0.15 g
Phenobarbital	0.1 g	0.05 g
Secobarbital	0.1 g	0.05 g

The above preparations usually are given in capsule or tablet form. However, liquid preparations are available as elixirs and are preferable in many cases because:

1. Patients may have difficulty in swallowing a capsule or tablet.
2. The taste is camouflaged by the addition of syrups, and children do not mind "taking their medicine."
3. They are absorbed into the bloodstream more rapidly, thereby giving much faster results.

These preparations can be purchased from a drug company, and the label will state the quantity of the medicament contained per volume. If one prefers to have the elixir prepared by the local druggist, it can be made in the concentration desired.

Narcotics

Narcotics are obtained primarily from opium, although Demerol (meperidine) is produced synthetically. All are governed by the Controlled Substances Act, and it is necessary to keep accurate records of their dispensation.

There are a number of narcotic drugs obtained from opium, including morphine and codeine. Morphine, codeine, and Demerol are the three most commonly used in dentistry. Morphine in average doses inhibits the entire function of the cerebrum, abolishes sensibility to pain, and produces sleep, thus acting as an analgesic and a hypnotic. Prolonged use will produce addiction; it should be used only when other analgesics will not relieve the condition.

For dental use codeine is better than morphine as an analgesic. It does not produce a depressing feeling and will, in half-grain doses, allay most dental pain. The patient should be cautioned, however, that his or her reflex actions are inhibited by any narcotic drug and that for 6 hours following administration, he or she should not engage in any work or activity that might therefore be dangerous.

Demerol is comparable to morphine in its analgesic qualities but does not produce constipation. It is replacing morphine as the most ideal analgesic, and is being used extensively in preoperative and postoperative medication. It is very effective when given orally, while morphine should be given by hypodermic injection for best results.

Name	Oral dose
Codeine sulfate	0.03 g–every 4 to 6 h as needed
Codeine phosphate	0.03 g–every 4 to 6 h as needed
Demerol	0.08 g–every 4 to 6 h as needed
Morphine	0.01 g–hypodermic injection only

Tranquilizers

These drugs are being widely used for preoperative and operative relief of anxiety for dental patients. Chlordiazepoxide hydrochloride, diazepam, and hydroxyzine hydrochloride, or pamoate, are the most frequently used of these drugs. These drugs secondarily produce varying degrees of muscle relaxation that is desirable during dental procedures. Administration as therapy for some dental problems is a frequent prescription where muscle relaxation is desired. The brand names of some of these drugs are Librium, Valium, and Vistaril. Each has its own specific and secondary action. The routes of administration are variable for each and may be either oral, intramuscular, or intravenous, depending on the specific preparation and desired effects.

Patients administered or given these drugs should be cautioned that their reflex actions will be inhibited and, as with narcotic drugs, they should not engage in any work or activity that might be dangerous while under the influence of such drugs.

Analgesics

Analgesics are a group of drugs that relieve pain without loss of consciousness. Strong, narcotic analgesics have been described in previous paragraphs, and this section will deal primarily with the mild and moderate analgesics.

Acetaminophen is the most widely prescribed drug in the United States at the present time. Aspirin, a salicylate, is also in this group of drugs and has the properties of being analgesic, antipyretic (causes fever reduction), and anti-inflammatory.

Occasionally, as with all drugs, a few patients are hypersensitive to aspirin and will develop allergic symptoms such as upset stomach, skin rash, and edema. Most of the other salicylates have one or more side reactions that make them less desirable as analgesics.

There are on the market numerous prepared mixtures of analgesic drugs that give better and faster analgesic action than the individual drug alone. Trade names of some of these analgesic drugs alone and in combinations with other drugs are: Tylenol, Bufferin, Anacin, and Darvon. Reference should be made to *Accepted Dental Therapeutics* for amounts and other names of analgesic drugs. Possible allergy to such drugs should always be checked prior to prescribing.

Ordinary dental pain can be relieved by one of the milder analgesic drugs and, if a stronger drug is necessary, it is wise to prescribe one of the narcotics.

Central Nervous System Stimulants

The use of this class of drugs in dentistry is limited almost exclusively to emergency measures.

These stimulants are discussed under the classification of emergency drugs and their uses. In that context, they should be used only when a specific diagnosis of the problem has been made.

Anesthetics, General and Local

These drugs are discussed in Chap. 22.

Antibiotics

The medicinal value of the antibiotic is derived from the antagonistic effect of one organism upon another in its vicinity. It has been known for many years among biologists that this inhibitory effect existed among certain organisms, and this knowledge led to the discovery that certain molds and bacteria excreted substances that inhibited or destroyed bacteria. An antibiotic may be defined as an agent obtained from molds and bacteria that tends to destroy other organisms.

Treatment by chemotherapy has been difficult because there is no direct access to an infection. The bloodstream, therefore, becomes the medium of transmission for the medicinal agent to the source of infection. Chemotherapy was made difficult, because it required a concentration of the medicament at the site of infection without the concentration's injuring tissue or endangering the life of the patient. The discovery of the antibiotics has been a boon to humankind, since they have been very effective in treating bacterial infections.

The first antibiotic discovered was penicillin, and since that time a number of others have been found which are of therapeutic value.

There are many available antibiotics for patient treatment, and each case should be treated with sound clinical judgment as regards the type of infection present. Patient records should show the name of the drug used, and, most importantly, the record should contain a drug allergy reminder that is placed in an eye-catching position on the record. *Any allergy is a life-threatening condition.*

Astringents, Styptics, Hemostatics, and Vasoconstrictors

There is considerable overlapping in thought and usage of astringents, styptics, and hemostatics. All are applied topically, and in many cases the same drug is used to fit all three groups. A brief discussion of each is presented here.

Astringents are intended to reduce or condense the mucous membrane or skin surface of inflamed, engorged, or edematous tissue. By doing this, bacterial invasion is prevented at the site, and further serum and leukocyte effusion is prevented.

Styptics, usually concentrated astringents, are used where capillaries have been broken and where oozing of blood and serum has occurred. The effect is superficial, and local coagulation is promoted.

A *hemostatic* may be a styptic or another drug that is used to stop a more profuse flow of blood by aiding the normal coagulation mechanism. It is not effective against a profuse flow from large vessels, for which mechanical aid is usually necessary.

Vasoconstrictors act by constricting or closing blood vessels, but they do not coagulate blood. They may be applied topically or injected into the immediate area of bleeding.

The following chemicals or agents are used commonly in a dental office, and they will be discussed briefly.

Alum is an astringent, styptic, and hemostatic when applied locally. It is obtained in stick or powder form and is freely soluble in water.

Copper sulfate is an astringent and is slightly caustic in strong solutions. This chemical is obtained as blue crystals and is soluble in water.

Ferric subsulfate (Monsel's salt) is a styptic that is effective when applied topically. It should not be used internally.

Tannic acid is an astringent used for local application in solutions of 0.5 to 2.0 percent concentration. Stronger solutions may be purchased, and they may be diluted for office use as required. Tannic acid also is available in powder form that may be mixed into a paste with thrombin solution and then applied directly to the area of bleeding.

Gelatin sponge is a gelatin substance which is absorbed by the body. The dentist can apply the sponge to bleeding areas, after moistening it thoroughly with sterile saline or thrombin solution. It also may be placed in a tooth socket without necessity of removal later.

Oxidized cellulose is a specially treated surgical gauze or cotton that exerts an unusual hemostatic effect and that possesses the property of absorbability when buried in tissue. Oxidized cellulose should not be used as a surface dressing, because it inhibits epithelial growth.

Thrombin accelerates the blood-clotting mechanism. It may be applied topically as a solution or in powder form. Thrombin must not be injected, since it will cause clotting in the vein. It is stable in the dry state but may lose its potency after 8 hours in solution at room temperature.

Epinephrine is the most widely used vasoconstrictor in dentistry. It is used in varying concentrations in local anesthetics and also is available in solutions of $1:1000$ or $1:100$ for noninjectable topical application. Injectable solutions of epinephrine are available, but care must be taken that the dosage is not too great. Its use may result in a general rise in blood pressure due to the constricting of the blood vessels.

Antiseptics

An antiseptic is considered to be an agent which stops or inhibits the growth of microorganisms, while a bactericide or germicide is any substance or agent which destroys bacteria. A fungicide is an agent which kills fungi (molds are one class of fungi). A disinfectant kills pathogenic microorganisms.

Many drugs are available for use as antiseptics in the dental office, and a few of the more commonly used ones will be given here.

Benzalkonium chloride (Zephiran Chloride) is one of the ammonia derivatives and has been used widely as a skin and mucosal antiseptic (see Chap. 7). Solutions in concentration of $1:1000$ and higher are effective for general oral antisepsis and can be used prior to injections and surgical procedures.

Dyes such as acriflavine and gentian violet have decreased in usage in dentistry. They exhibit antiseptic action when applied locally in concentrations of 1 percent. Saliva and serum seem to inhibit the action of the dyes; accordingly, care should be taken to apply them to dry areas. They are used in gingival and pericoronal infections.

Iodine is used in dentistry as a local antiseptic and as a disclosing solution. It is more irritating to the mucous membrane than to the skin and is, therefore, used in dilute solution.

Betadine is an iodine preparation that is used as a topical solution on oral mucosa. It is not irritating to mucous membranes, as the release of iodine from the compound is slow as opposed to the iodine tincture. It is used as a preinjection germicide, to prepare tissue prior to surgery, and in hand washing prior to surgery. There are different kinds of solutions for each use.

Metaphen is a mercurial antiseptic compound. It is obtainable in the tincture for topical antiseptic action.

Miscellaneous Drugs and Preparations for Office Use

Calcium hydroxide is a powder which may be obtained from the pharmacist. It is commonly used in pulp capping or pulpotomy operations.

Laxatives are prescribed by the dentist in some cases of infection. Usually a mild laxative such as milk of magnesia, or a saline laxative, is sufficient. An adult dosage of 15 ml aromatic cascara sagrada fluid extract also is considered a mild laxative; it is most effective in chronic constipation. The oral dosage of cascara for the adult is 30 drops.

Oil of cloves is one of the essential oils that serves as an anodyne or counterirritant. Eugenol is the active principle of oil of cloves and is used as an anodyne cement when mixed with zinc oxide powder.

Fixed oils commonly used are mineral oil and liquid petrolatum. Their primary use in the dental office is as lubricants for dies, models, etc.

Fluoride solutions are applied to the teeth topically as a caries-control measure (see Chap. 19).

Phenol compound is a caustic liquid mixture consisting of 2 parts phenol, 2 parts thymol, and 1 part camphor.

Hydrogen peroxide is a 3 percent U.S.P. solution which may be diluted with 1 part water to 1 part hydrogen peroxide as a mouthwash or irrigating solution.

Ethyl alcohol may be purchased on prescription from the druggist. It has multiple uses in the dental office such as antiseptic and solvent.

Emergency Drugs

The following drugs may be found in many dental offices. The assistant should be familiar with their names and possible uses in dentistry.

Adrenalin may be referred to by the scientific name *epinephrine.* It is an extract of the suprarenal glands of animals. It is a powerful vasoconstrictor, acting on the heart to increase its rate and on the blood vessels to cause constriction. It is useful in cases of shock and collapse when blood pressure drops. Caution must be exercised in administering this drug to those who have a heart problem.

Epinephrine is prepared in ampule form for intramuscular injection in 1:1000 strength.

Caffeine and sodium benzoate is one of the most important and most frequently used respiratory stimulants. The drug may be given by intramuscular injection in doses of 0.5 g, or if the patient is conscious, strong black coffee may be given orally.

Amyl nitrite, one of the volatile nitrites, is absorbed readily through the lungs, the action being to dilate the small blood vessels and thus decrease the blood pressure. The nitrites are used for several purposes besides lowering blood pressure, such as in attacks of angina pectoris and to relax contracted muscles in attacks of asthma. Amyl nitrite is prepared in glass pearls of 0.2 ml which are broken in a handkerchief and inhaled. The effect of amyl nitrite lasts 10 to 15 minutes.

Glyceryl trinitrate is also one of the nitrites, it has a longer acting time, usually about $1/2$ hour. It is prepared in tablet form of $1/200$, $1/150$, $1/100$, and $1/50$ gr and is held under the tongue and allowed to dissolve.

Barbiturates, discussed previously, are used as central nervous system depressants and should be used preoperatively and postoperatively as necessary to combat excitability.

Oxygen is one of the most important adjuncts for general all-around emergency use in the dental office. Many of the so-called emergency drugs are dangerous to use unless one is sure of the cause of the trouble. One always is safe, however, in administering oxygen. A mixture of 5 percent carbon dioxide and 95 percent oxygen is a good respiratory stimulant in all cases.

Aromatic spirits of ammonia (U.S.P.) is a standard preparation used extensively in the dental office to prevent fainting or psychic shock. It may be used as an inhalant, or, instead, about 30 drops may be placed in a few swallows of water for the patient to drink.

The bottle containing aromatic spirits of ammonia should be kept tightly sealed at all times. Ammonia is a volatile substance, and the solution will soon lose its potency if it is left in an open container.

BIBLIOGRAPHY

American Dental Association Council on Dental Therapeutics: *Accepted Dental Therapeutics,* 36th ed., 1975.

Bremner, M. D. K.: *The Story of Dentistry,* 3d ed., Dental Items of Interest Publishing Co., Brooklyn, 1954.

DEA Registration Information: "Drug Enforcement Administration."

Dunn, M. J., Booth, D. F., and Clancy, M.: *Dental Auxiliary Practice,* The C. V. Mosby Company, St. Louis, 1974.

Holroyd, S. V.: *Clinical Pharmacology in Dental Practice,* The C. V. Mosby Company, St. Louis, 1974.

Prinz, H.: *Dental Chronology,* Lea & Febiger, Philadelphia, 1945.

Robinson, J. B.: "The Foundations of Professional Dentistry," in *Proceedings, Dental Centenary Celebration,* Waverly Press Inc., Baltimore, 1940.

Weinberger, B. F.: *History of Dentistry,* vols. I and II, The C. V. Mosby Company, St. Louis, 1948.

10

James E. Overberger

Dental Materials: Gypsum Products

DENTAL MATERIALS

Introduction

A wide variety of materials are used in dentistry, and the assistant should be familiar with the general structure, composition, properties, and uses of these materials. A basic conceptual knowledge of these aspects is necessary to understand the reaction of materials to biting forces and other destructive conditions in the mouth, and to scientifically select, evaluate, and successfully manipulate these materials as well as to understand standards which exist for these materials. Some of these materials are used only for restoring teeth at the chairside, and others are used only in the laboratory as a part of the restorative fabrication procedure. The effect of manipulation on the properties should be particularly understood so that the proper handling of the materials by the assistant both in the laboratory and at the chairside can be reflected in clinical success.

The assistant should be aware of the limitations and rigid conditions imposed upon restorative materials by the oral environment. The varying temperature changes, changes in acidity and alkalinity, varying biting stresses, and corrosive conditions contribute to their destruction. The limitation of design and access by the dentist as well as the fact that only a certain amount of tooth structure can be safely removed must be considered. The material must be biologically compatible with the hard and soft tissues, simple to use, pleasing in taste and color, able to reproduce natural contour, and relatively inexpensive. These rigid conditions therefore dictate unique compositions and precise manipulative techniques for clinical success.

Structure

Dental materials display the basic characteristics of matter by occupying space, possessing mass, and being composed of atoms and molecules. Most dental materials are solids and a brief, simple explanation of the solid state will facilitate an understanding of the reactions and properties of the various materials.

Solids can be classified generally as being crystalline or noncrystalline. Crystalline solids are characterized by a definite long-range repetitive atomic arrangement called a space lattice (Fig. 10-1). Other characteristics of crystalline solids are rigidity and definite melting temperatures. Gold alloys are examples of crystalline solids.

The noncrystalline solids or amorphous solids are characterized by a nonuniform arrangement of the atoms or molecules; however, a limited amount of grouping of the molecules may occur. These substances are not as rigid as crystalline materials, soften under heat rather than melt at a definite temperature, and when placed under load exhibit a slow, continuous change in shape. Sometimes amorphous solids are called supercooled liquids. Waxes are examples of amorphous solids.

Properties

A wide variety of physical and mechanical properties are used to characterize dental materials and can be used to compare different materials. These properties also indicate how a certain material will behave under laboratory and clinical conditions. Those properties that are unique to each material will be discussed in relation to each material that will be presented in the suc-

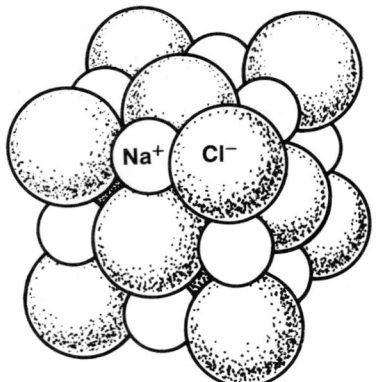

Figure 10-1 | Crystal structure. The sodium and chlorine atoms are arranged in a repeating, three-dimensional pattern called a space lattice.

ceeding chapters, although several properties common to most materials will be discussed here.

As a result of biting and chewing forces acting on restorations and appliances, stresses and strains are induced in the materials. Stress is the internal force in the restoration or appliance that resists the external applied biting force. Stress is classified by the direction of the force, and tensile (pulling), compressive (crushing), and shear (sliding) stresses can be identified. Stress is expressed in terms of force acting across a unit area as pounds per square inch (psi). The maximum stress that can be induced in a restoration such that it will return to its original shape when the biting forces are removed is known as the elastic limit and should be high in magnitude so that restorations and appliances will return to their original shape when biting forces are released. The proportional limit and yield strength are other terms that indicate the stress at which a material no longer behaves as an elastic structure. For dental purposes, the terms elastic limit, proportional limit, and yield strength are used synonymously.

Table 10-1 | Mechanical Properties

Material	Yield strength, psi	Compressive strength, psi	Knoop hardness number
Enamel	50,000*	58,000*	300
Dentin	24,000†	43,000†	65
Amalgam	30,000‡	57,000‡	90

* Craig, 1961.
† Craig, 1958.
‡ Stanford, 1960.

The maximum stress that occurs when a structure fractures or ruptures defines the strength of a material, and tensile and compressive strengths are used generally to compare the fracture characteristics of materials.

As a result of the force of application, a change in shape or deformation of the restoration or appliance will occur. The deformation is known as strain and is expressed in terms of change in length per unit of length, as inch per inch or as a percentage. The amount of elastic strain or deformation that occurs under biting forces in a restoration as an inlay should be minimal to preclude undesired major dimensional change. The permanent or plastic strain or deformation that occurs when the structure fractures under tensile load expressed as percent elongation is a measure of the ductility of a material. A high value for elongation would indicate a high ductility. One of the reasons gold alloys are used for restorations is their relativity high ductility.

Surface hardness is another property to be considered in relation to general wear resistance of different materials. However, it should be used to compare the wear resistance of the same class of materials, as resistance to wear is best determined by carefully designed laboratory tests using experimental conditions similar to that in the mouth. There are two surface penetration hardness tests usually used to indicate hardness for dental materials, mainly the Brinell and Knoop hardness tests. In both of these tests, the higher the numerical value associated with the test, the greater the surface hardness. Table 10-1 lists several of these mechanical properties for tooth structure and dental amalgam.

The time-dependent deformation of a material under a specified load expressed as percentage change in shape is called flow or creep. Flow or creep are often used to evaluate the deformation changes occurring in dental amalgam. Flow is used to evaluate the changes occurring before the amalgam is fully hardened and is an indirect measure of the strength of amalgam; creep is used to evaluate the changes occurring in a hardened amalgam and may indicate resistance to marginal deformation and resultant fracture.

Two physical thermal properties are also of common interest: the coefficient of thermal expansion and contraction and thermal conductivity. Upon differential thermal changes in the mouth as a result of the ingestion of hot or cold foods and beverages, the restoration should expand and contract similar to tooth structure. If the material differs from that of tooth structure, then leakage of saliva and fluids can occur at the interface between the restoration and tooth structure upon differential thermal change, leading to the recurrent caries and tooth sensitivity. This leakage occurs to a greater or lesser extent with all restorative material, depending on the relationship of the thermal coefficient of expansion and contraction and tooth structure.

Restorations should be low in thermal conductivity, as are dentin and enamel, to protect the vital pulpal tissues from thermal shock. Unfortunately, metal restorations are good thermal conductors so that cements that are poor thermal conductors have to be used to provide insulating bases or layers in the deeper areas of the prepared cavity. Table 10-2 lists the properties for tooth structure and certain restorative materials.

The assistant should have a conceptual knowledge of these and other properties and behavioral characteristics of those materials which are used in the dental office.

Standards

The American Dental Association (ADA) through its Council on Dental Materials and Devices has maintained through the years a specification program for establishing properties and other requirements for particular materials and/or devices so that their quality and usefulness can be determined by the standardized tests as described in the specification. Through this council, the ADA is represented in national and international organizations and federal agencies concerned with standards, evaluation, safety, and effectiveness, and other requirements of dental materials and devices. The council administers an extensive evaluation program for improving and maintaining the quality, safety, and effectiveness of certain materials and devices and for promoting truthful advertising in the labeling of materials and devices. This evaluation is accomplished by means of the certification and acceptance programs.

Under the certification program, the manufacturer of a dental material certifies that the product complies with the specifications which have been approved as official specifications of the ADA so that he is in compliance with the ADA advertising and exhibit standards. If the product is found to comply with the specifications, its name is placed on the list of certified dental materials which is maintained and published periodically by the Council on Dental Materials and Devices in the *Journal of the American Dental Association* and *Guide to Dental Materials and Devices* (ADA, 1974).

The council also conducts an acceptance program for determining the qualities, safety, and effectiveness of those materials, and devices are considered for which evidence of safety and effectiveness has been established by biologic, laboratory, and/or clinical evaluations where

Table 10-2 | Thermal Properties

	Linear coefficient of expansion, $\times 10^{-6}/°C$	Thermal conductivity, $cal/s \cdot cm^2 \cdot °C/cm$
Tooth (across crown)	11.4	Enamel 0.0022
		Dentin 0.0015
Amalgam	25.0	0.055
Zinc oxide–eugenol cement	—	0.0011
Dental resin (polymethyl methacrylate)	81.0	0.0005

Source: Phillips, 1973; Craig, 1975.

appropriate. Under this program, the manufacturer supplies appropriate data and information relative to specific guidelines developed by the council and agrees to abide by the advertisement and exhibit standards. After consideration of a product under the provisions of this program, the council classifies the product as acceptable, as provisionally acceptable, or unacceptable, and the material as classified is placed on the list of classified materials and devices which is also published in the *Journal of the American Dental Association* and *Guide to Dental Materials and Devices* (ADA, 1974). The assistant should know that the list of certified and classified dental materials and devices is a reliable and impartial guide for the purchase of those materials and devices for which a specification and/or acceptance program exists.

GYPSUM PRODUCTS

Gypsum products are supplied as fine powders that are mixed with water to form a fluid mass which can be poured and shaped, and which subsequently hardens into a rigid, stable mass (Fig. 10-2). Gypsum products are used mainly for making positive reproductions of oral structures, called casts, from negative impressions, as well as other related uses where shaping followed by rigidity is necessary. Since most dental restorations are fabricated on these casts, it is essential that the particular gypsum product be carefully manipulated to ensure an accurate restoration.

Types of Gypsum Products

Gypsum products are made from gypsum rock, which is a mineral found in various parts of the world. Chemically, gypsum is calcium sulfate dihydrate, $CaSO_4 \cdot 2H_2O$. Pure gypsum is white; however, in most deposits it is discolored by impurities. The pure natural form of gypsum is called alabaster, which in ancient times was used for making urns and lining the walls of tombs.

In this chapter three types of gypsum products will be discussed: plaster, stone, and improved stone. Chemically, they are all calcium sulfate hemihydrate, and are produced as a result of heating gypsum and driving off part of the water of crystallization by a process called calcination. This process is shown in the following diagram:

$$CaSO_4 \cdot 2H_2O \xrightarrow[\text{and other modifications}]{\text{heat}} CaSO_4 \cdot \tfrac{1}{2}H_2O$$
$$+ 1\tfrac{1}{2}H_2O$$

Gypsum products differ in the physical characteristics of their powder particles as a result of differing calcination methods; this is responsible for their differing uses and properties.

Plaster was the first gypsum product available to dentistry. It is manufactured by grinding the gypsum rock to a fine powder followed by heating the powder in an open container. This direct and rapid heating in open air drives part of the water of crystallization from the crystal in a shattering manner so that the resulting powder consists of porous, irregular particles. Plaster is the weakest and least expensive of the three gypsum products. It is used mainly where strength is not a critical requirement, as for making preliminary casts for complete dentures

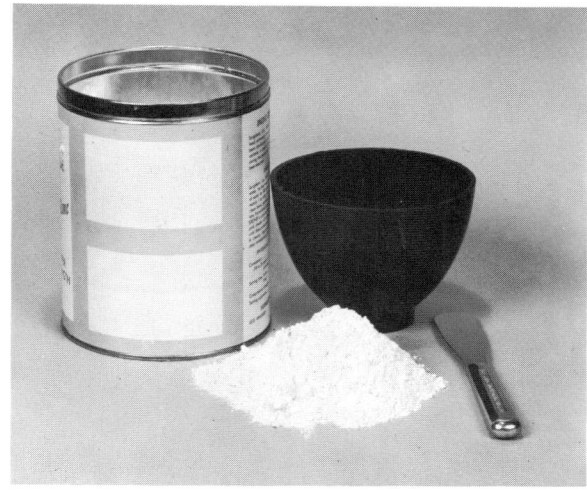

Figure 10-2 | A can of improved stone is shown along with the powder, mixing bowl, and spatula.

and for attaching casts to a mechanical device called an articulator which simulates the masticating apparatus (Fig. 10-3). Plaster is usually white in color and sometimes is referred to as beta-hemihydrate.

Stone is made from gypsum by carefully controlled calcination under steam pressure in a closed container. This method of calcination releases the water of crystallization from the crystal

Figure 10-3 | Preliminary plaster casts for complete dentures.

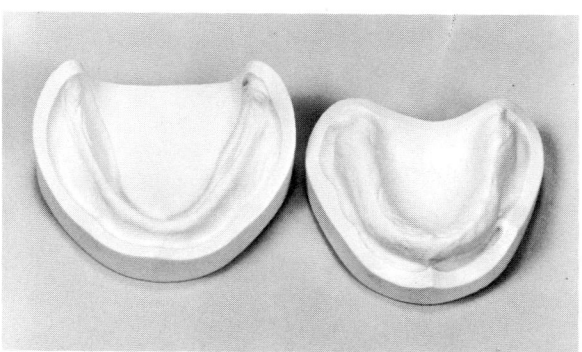

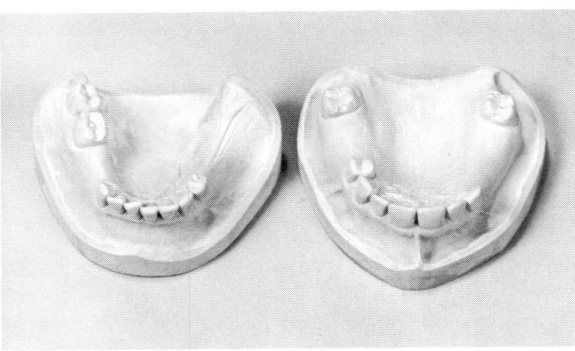

Figure 10-4 | Stone casts for partial denture construction.

slowly so that the resultant powder particle is more regular, more uniform in shape, and less porous when compared with the powder particle of plaster. Stone is stronger and more expensive than plaster and is used mainly for making diagnostic casts and casts for complete and partial denture construction where greater strength and surface hardness are desired (Fig. 10-4). The stone is usually yellow in color; however, it can be obtained in other colors. It is often referred to as alpha-hemihydrate, Class I stone, and Hydrocal.

Figure 10-5 | Improved stone casts for crown and inlay fabrication.

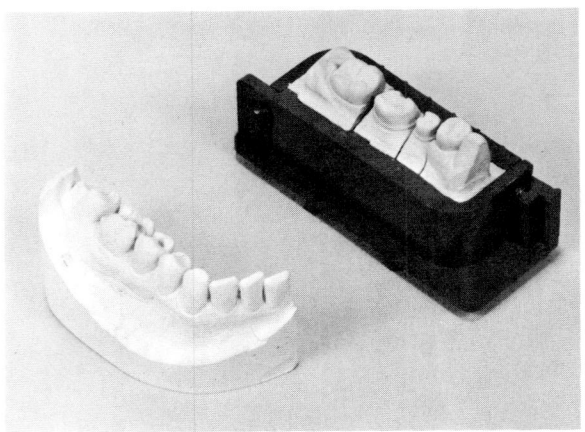

Improved stone also is made from gypsum by calcining the gypsum in a calcium chloride solution. This method of calcination results in a powder particle that is very dense, cubical, and spherelike in shape. Improved stone is the strongest and most expensive of the three gypsum products and is used mainly for making casts or dies for inlay and crown fabrication where high strength and surface hardness are required (Fig. 10-5). Improved stone is often referred to as Class II stone, die stone, densite, and modified alpha-hemihydrate.

Setting Reaction

When any of the three types of calcium sulfate hemihydrate is mixed with water, the hemihydrate is changed back to the dihydrate by the process of hydration and heat is liberated, as shown by the following diagram:

$$CaSO_4 \cdot 1/2 H_2O + 1 1/2 H_2O \longrightarrow CaSO_4 \cdot 2H_2O + heat$$

The calcium sulfate hemihydrate dissolves in the mixing water and the dihydrate is formed which is less soluble than the hemihydrate. The calcium sulfate dihydrate precipitates out of solution as nuclei of crystallization and forms interlocking crystals which cause the formation of a hard mass.

Water/Powder Ratio

The relative amounts of water and powder used to make a workable mix of a particular gypsum product are called the water/powder ratio. For dental use, an excess amount of gauging water is always necessary above the theoretically correct amount required for hydration to make a workable mix that can be utilized for pouring and shaping. This excess water is distributed as free water in the set mass without taking part in the chemical reaction and contributes to subsequent porosity in the set product. The proper water/powder ratio for each product is dependent upon the physical characteristics of the powder particles. Therefore, plaster will require more gauging water to wet and fill the pores and float the irregular porous particles. The dense particles of stone will require less gauging water to float them and the regular shape will allow them to roll over one another more easily. The improved stone, because of its very dense and spherical type of particle, will require even less gauging water than stone. For dental use, the proper water/powder ratio for the average mix of plaster is 50 ml/100 g; for stone, 30 ml/100 g; and for improved stone, 24 ml/100 g.

This difference in the amount of gauging water required to make a workable mix results in different consistencies for the products when first mixed at the proper water/powder ratio. Plaster generally is thin in consistency, while improved stone is putty-like; stone possesses an intermediate consistency. The water/powder ratio has a direct effect on the properties of each gypsum product and must be controlled for optimum properties.

Setting Time

A knowledge of the setting characteristics of a gypsum product is important for proper manipulation. The length of time from the start of mix until the setting mass reaches a semihard stage represents the available time for manipulating the product. This time interval is called the working or initial setting time and represents some point in the progress of the setting reaction. The length of time from the start of the mix until the setting mass becomes rigid represents the time interval necessary before such further procedures as separation of the impression can be performed. This time interval is called the final setting time and indicates the major completion of the hydration reaction.

The setting times are usually measured by the use of a surface penetration test. The Gillmore needles are commonly used as shown in Fig.

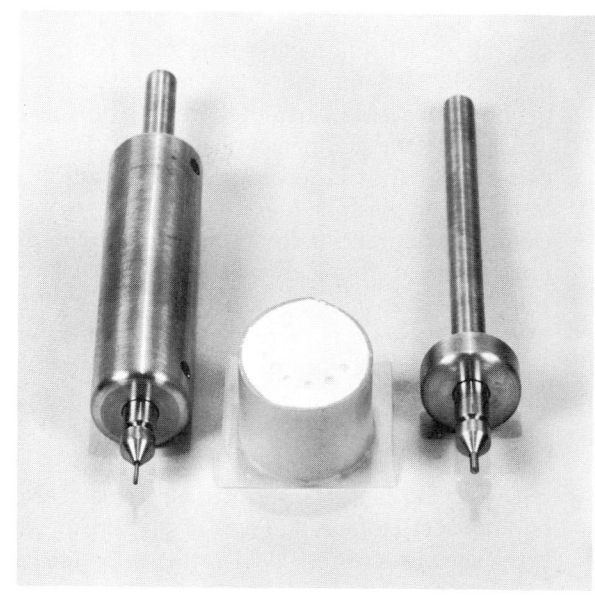

Figure 10-6 | The 1-lb (*left*) and ¼-lb (*right*) Gillmore needles are shown with a test sample of a gypsum product.

10-6. When the surface of the setting product has developed sufficient strength to support the weight of the ¼-lb needle and the 1-lb needle, the initial and final setting times as determined by this method have occurred. This method is somewhat arbitrary and difficult to correlate directly with the setting reaction, and the values are used mainly for valid comparisons of different manufacturers' products. Practically, loss of surface gloss can be used as a determination of the working time, and the time when a fingernail or knife indicates relative rigidity or no indentation can be used as an indication of final set.

The setting time of a gypsum product is controlled by the manufacturer by his particular formulation so that there are gypsum products of varying setting characteristics on the market. Thus, either a fast-setting or slow-setting product can be purchased. It may occasionally be necessary to modify the setting time of a particular product in the dental office, and there are several methods available. Increased mixing, a lower water/powder ratio (thicker mix), and addition of certain chemicals called accelerators result in a faster-setting product. Decreased mixing, higher water/powder ratio (thinner mix), and the addition of certain chemicals called retarders will result in a slower-setting product. Chemicals often used as accelerators or retarders are potassium sulfate and borax, respectively. Other chemicals can be used but their effect on the setting time is dependent upon concentration and other factors.

The setting characteristics can be changed also by improper storage and use of gypsum products. Since water is essential for the setting reaction, any moisture inadvertently coming in contact with the product can change the setting time. Thus, gypsum products should be stored in airtight containers to prevent pickup of water due to high relative humidity. In routine laboratory use, water should not be introduced to the product in the container. The first indication of moisture contamination is faster setting of the product. If the contamination continues, then a slower setting occurs.

Setting Expansion

All gypsum products expand externally upon setting, plaster exhibiting the most expansion: 0.3 percent; stone: 0.10 percent; and improved stone, the least: 0.06 percent. Theoretically, a contraction on setting can be calculated; however, the growing crystals of the gypsum cause an outward crystal thrust that results in an external expansion with resulting internal porosity in the set mass. A minimal setting expansion is desirable for accurate dimensional reproduction for casts and dies. Most gypsum products that are used for casts and dies have been modified by the manufacturer to provide for minimal expansion by addition of chemicals which also control the setting characteristics. Thus a particular gypsum product has both the setting and expansion characteristics controlled by the manufacturer. The expansion characteristics can be controlled by manipulative variables in that a thicker mix and increased spatulation will cause an increase in the amount of setting expansion and conversely; however, in most dental offices there is little need to change the expansion characteristics of gypsum products used for cast construction by varying the manipulative variables.

If gypsum materials are immersed or come in contact with water during the setting process, the setting expansion increases. This is called hygroscopic expansion and will be discussed later in relation to casting investment. Hygroscopic expansion, while small, is approximately twice as great as the normal setting expansion; therefore, to prevent an inadvertent increase in size, casts should not be immersed in water during setting.

Strength and Surface Hardness

The strength of the gypsum product is usually measured in terms of crushing or compressive strength. As expected from the setting reaction, strength develops rapidly during the first 30 to 45 minutes as the hydration is completed. The strength is dependent upon the porosity of the set material, which is related to the water/powder ratio necessary to make a workable mix. Plaster (which requires the most gauging water to make a fluid mix) is the weakest, with improved stone the strongest and stone intermediate in strength.

The presence or absence of the excess or free water affects strength, and two strengths are recognized—wet and dry strengths. The wet strength is the strength measured when the sample contains some or all of the water in excess of the theoretical amount required for hydration. The dry strength is the strength measured when the excess water is not present. The dry strength may be two or more times the wet strength. The strength of a particular product is dependent upon the water/powder ratio in that thicker mixes will increase the strength within limits and conversely. However, extremely thick mixes, particularly of stone and improved stone, are heavy in consistency and can cause distortion of the impression as well as entrapment of air voids; thin mixes cause a detrimental decrease in strength. Therefore, it is good office procedure to follow the manufacturer's recommended water/powder ratio for optimum strength and consistency properties.

The surface hardness is related to the compressive strength but reaches its maximum more rapidly because the surface is the first to dry out. The greatest surface hardness occurs when the product reaches its dry strength, which often cannot be realized under practical conditions. Therefore, casts and dies should be allowed to set for 1 to 2 hours or preferably overnight or longer before beginning subsequent operations. The surface hardness of set gypsum is not very desirable, and many methods have been advocated to improve it. To date there are no practical methods that will significantly increase the surface hardness.

Dimensional Stability

The dimensions of a hardened or set gypsum cast are relatively constant under ordinary conditions of room temperature and humidity. However, gypsum is slightly soluble in water so that if the cast is soaked in water for prolonged periods of time, the surface may be dissolved away. If the cast must be soaked in water, the water should be saturated with gypsum to prevent erosion of the surface. The safest way to soak a cast is to place it in a water bath that has particles of gypsum in the water so as to provide a saturated solution of calcium sulfate at all times.

Technique of Use

The technical use of gypsum products is relatively simple, requiring only a mixing bowl, mixing spatula, room-temperature water, and the respective gypsum product. As pointed out previously, the water and powder must be proportioned accurately for optimum properties. The water can be conveniently dispensed by volume in a graduated cylinder, as 1 g of water has a volume of approximately 1 ml. The powder can be weighed in grams by a simple balance. A dietetic balance is a convenient method of weighing the powder since the water can be added to the mixing bowl, the dial rotated to 0, and the powder sifted into the water with a suitable scoop until the desired weight of powder is obtained (Fig. 10-7). Volume dispensers may be used, but volume dispensing of the powder is not as accurate due to the varying packing effect of the powder. Weighing with the dietetic scale is a simple and convenient method to ensure accurate proportions.

Figure 10-7 | Equipment used for measuring and mixing gypsum products.

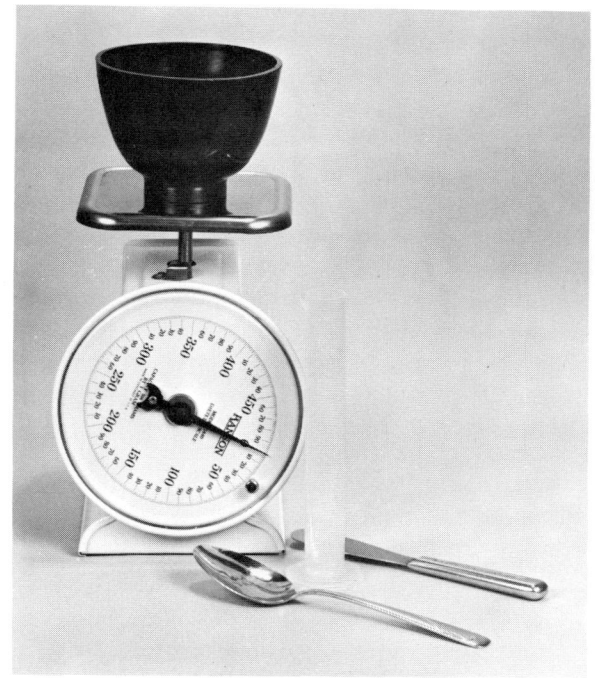

Mixing is usually done in a flexible plastic or rubber bowl with a stiff-bladed spatula. The objective of mixing is to rapidly combine the powder and water into a smooth, homogeneous, workable mix free of air bubbles. A minimum of air inclusion in the mixed product is desirable to prevent surface and internal defects due to air voids. Mixing generally is accomplished with a wiping motion against the sides of a bowl, to eliminate lumps and air bubbles, and is continued until a smooth, homogeneous mix is obtained in approximately one minute. A whipping motion should be avoided. Often mixing is done mechanically, which provides for a more homogeneous mix, freer from air bubbles. Vacuum can also be utilized to minimize the formation of air bubbles and provide for a dense mix. There are many devices available that will mix gypsum products mechanically with or without vacuum and are used where the application of the product is critical (Fig. 10-8). Often the fluid mixture needs to be flowed into an impression and the flow of the material ahead of itself may be aided by the use of a vibrator (Fig. 10-9). Vibrating the mix after mixing can also be used to bring air bubbles to the surface. Manipulation of gypsum products, while relatively simple, requires careful attention to detail for accurate results.

STUDY MODELS

In many dental practices, a complete dental examination, diagnosis, and treatment plan includes the use of diagnostic aids such as study models. The dentist is better able to study and evaluate the patient's complete dental situation by having a positive reproduction of the dental arches. Study models provide this positive reproduction of the maxillary and mandibular arches in either plaster of paris or dental stone. They are prepared from a negative reproduction of the dental arches known as a dental impression (Fig. 10-10). The material used in obtaining the impression for study models is usually an irreversible hydrocolloid (alginate) impression material. One distinction between study models and other models or casts used in dentistry is that they provide a permanent record of the patient's dental arches and are not used for the fabrication of appliances or restorations.

The role of the dental assistant in preparing study models varies from assuming responsibility for the complete procedure, including tray selection and impression taking, to performing the laboratory procedures only, depending on the respective state dental practice acts. The primary purpose of this section is to provide information on the trimming of plaster models to present a usable, uniform, and esthetic-appearing set of study models.

Impressions

Regardless of who actually takes the impression, the dentist or assistant, the procedure should be

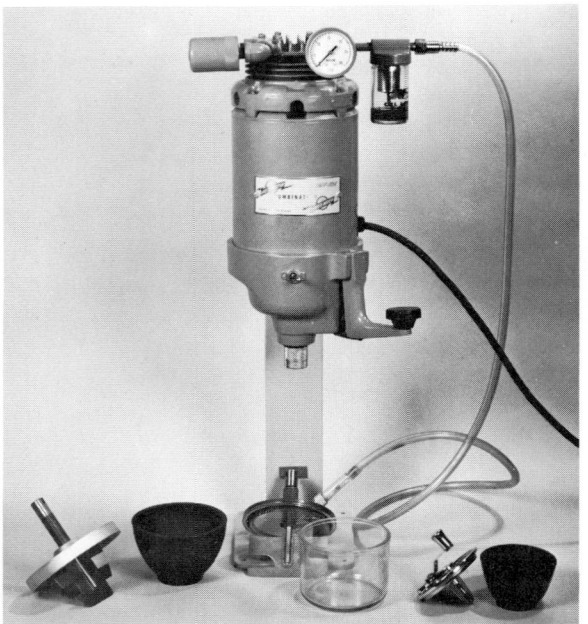

Figure 10-8 | Mechanical devices for mixing gypsum products with or without vacuum.

thoroughly explained to the patient since some patients are apprehensive about having a large bulk of material placed in their mouth. Taut muscles and stimulation of the gag reflex are not conducive to obtaining good impressions. The patient should be seated upright with the head tipped slightly down to help prevent saliva and the impression material from flowing toward the throat. Every attempt should be made to keep the patient's attention diverted from the procedure. The lower impression should be taken first since there is less chance of gagging than with the maxillary impression.

The mixing of alginate impression material, loading the impression tray, seating and removing the impression are discussed elsewhere in this book (see Chap. 30). In addition to the impressions, a wax bite must be obtained as an aid in positioning the models together for certain trimming procedures and for articulation, if this is to be accomplished. To obtain a wax bite, a single thickness of beeswax, cut in the shape of a horseshoe, is placed on the occlusal surfaces of the mandibular teeth and the patient guided into centric occlusion. The wax bite must be handled with care since it is easily distorted. It is also important that the alginate impressions are poured immediately to prevent distortion. If pouring cannot be accomplished immediately, the impressions should be washed with running water to remove any saliva and debris and carefully wrapped in a damp paper towel or placed in a humidor. If accuracy is expected, the impressions should not be allowed to remain in this atmosphere for more than 20 minutes.

Pouring Procedures

There are three methods of pouring models or casts: the *boxing* method, the *inverted* method, and the *double pour* method. The use for which the model or cast is intended may have some bearing on the preferred method. As an example, where a more dense model with a uniform land area and complete mucobuccal fold is

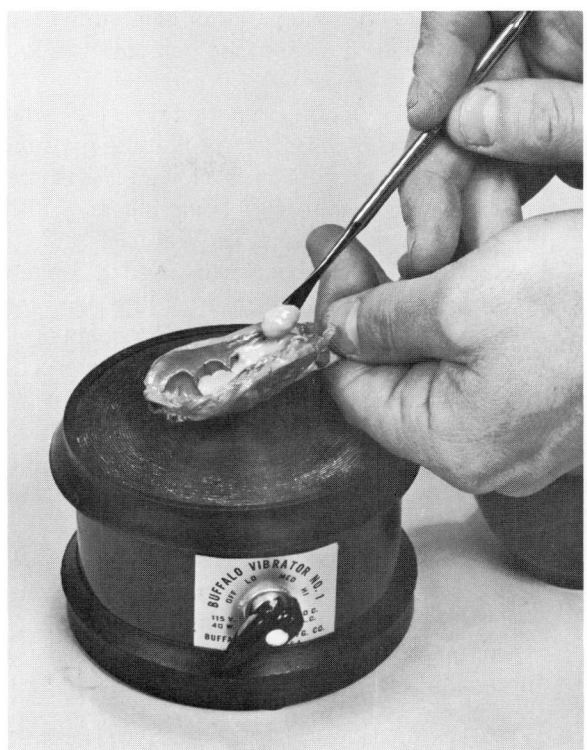

Figure 10-9 | Use of vibrator to aid flow of gypsum products into a rubber impression.

required, the boxing method is the pouring method of choice. The boxing method is reviewed in Chap. 30. The inverted method or double pour method is used in study model construction. In the inverted method the entire impression is poured and immediately inverted onto a mass of gypsum on a glass slab. While holding the impression tray handle, a plaster spatula is used to form and smooth the base portion of the model (Fig. 10-11). Unless extreme care is used with this method, the gypsum may pull away from the impression or the impression may be distorted by too much pressure being exerted while the base is being formed. The double pour method has the advantages of being accurate and not consuming a lot of time during the initial pour since the base may be poured at any time.

Basically, the double pour method is the same as the inverted method except that the gypsum material in the impression is allowed to assume an initial or final set before being inverted onto the second gypsum mass on the glass slab. A base-former (Fig. 10-12) may be used to contain the base gypsum, thus eliminating the need for shaping this material with the plaster spatula.

Pouring a model is a relatively simple procedure, but it must be accomplished in a precise manner to produce an acceptable model. Study models are usually poured in plaster, and the first step is to properly measure and mix the plaster as detailed earlier in this chapter. The impression is placed on a vibrator and small amounts of the mixed plaster are added until the teeth imprints are filled. The small increments of plaster are added to the palate on the maxillary impression (Fig. 10-13) and to the lingual flange area on the mandibular impression. Larger portions are then added until the impression is filled up to and covering the mucobuccal fold. Wax or damp paper placed between the flanges on the mandibular impression will prevent plaster from filling the tongue area. The surface of the plaster is left rough and undercut (Fig. 10-14) to assist in forming a mechanical lock with the base portion of the model to be poured later.

The plaster mix for the base portion should be slightly thicker than that used to fill the impression. This mix is placed either in a base-former or on a glass slab and the poured impression rough surface placed on it. If the poured impression has assumed its final set, it should be allowed to soak in water for at least 5 minutes before being placed on the base-pour plaster.

A poured impression should be allowed to set for approximately 1 hour prior to separating the impression from the model. Separation of the two must be done carefully to prevent breaking of the teeth on the model. The margins of the impression tray must be free of all plaster and fully exposed. This is accomplished with a plaster knife. The impression tray is removed with a straight pull from the model. Rocking or twisting the tray during removal will tend to fracture teeth on the model. Any blebs or excess plaster that would interfere with occluding the models is then removed, and they are ready for trimming.

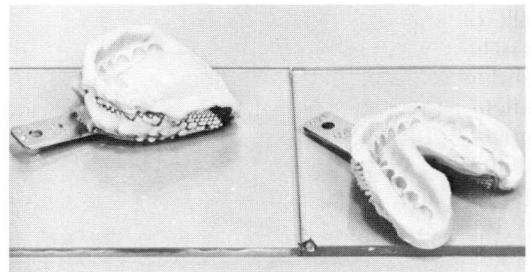

Figure 10-10 | Alginate impressions taken in perforated trays of maxillary (*left*) and mandibular (*right*) arches. Note impressions include the mucobuccal fold and lingual flange areas.

Figure 10-11 | Smoothing the sides of the base in the inverted method of pouring a model. If tray is not held, the weight of the impression may cause the base portion to be too thin.

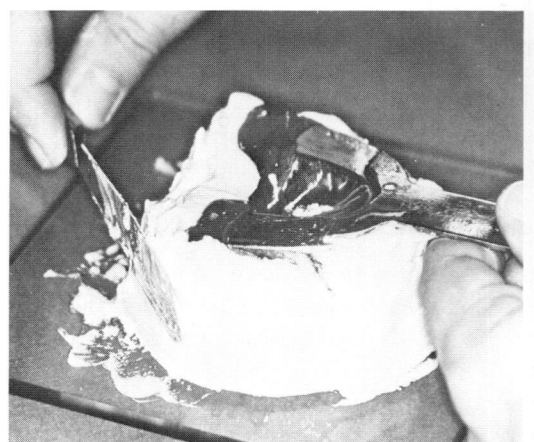

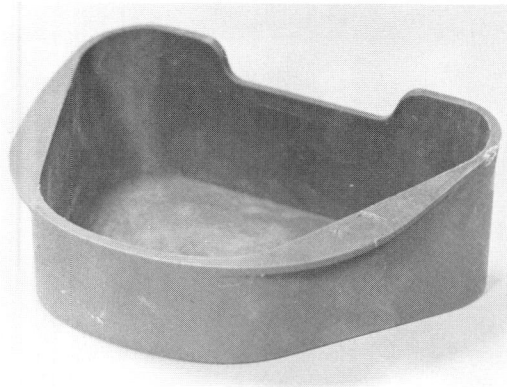

Figure 10-12 | Use of a base-former conserves time and material, and provides some uniformity for starting the trimming procedures.

Figure 10-13 | Tilting the impression on the vibrator table enables the plaster to flow into the teeth imprints in a thin film.

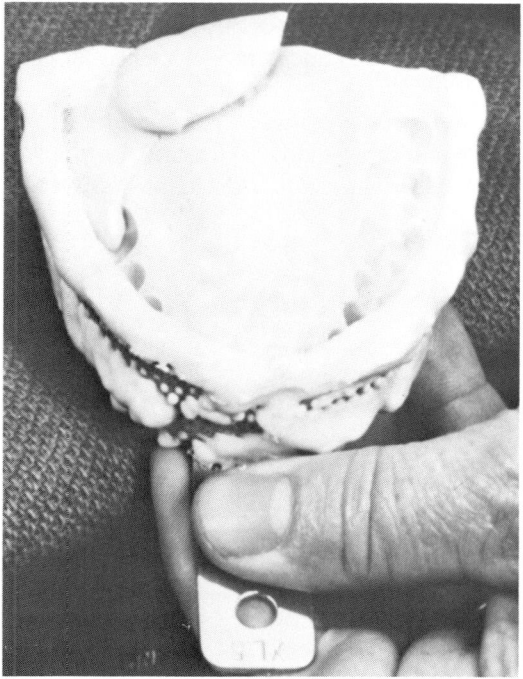

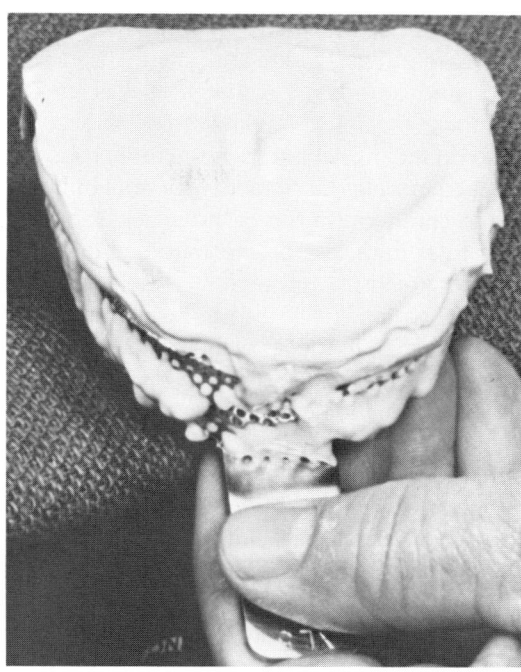

Figure 10-14 | Completed first pour. Note mucobuccal fold is covered with plaster.

Trimming Procedures

Dental models are considered to consist of two portions, the *anatomic* portion and the *art* portion. The anatomic portion is that which was formed by the impression and consists of teeth and tissue reproduction. The art portion is the remainder of the model or the base portion. Model trimming is confined to the art portion to form an esthetic appearance. The teeth and tissue portion should not be cut or altered. Every attempt should be made to produce a symmetrical art portion, but the various arch shapes and sizes plus missing and malpositioned teeth do not make this a routine procedure. The assistant must exercise an esthetic viewpoint while following the fundamental procedures in model trimming.

The larger of the maxillary and mandibular anatomic portions (width and length) is determined, and trimming on that model is begun first. However, before any trimming is accomplished on the model trimmer, the model should be soaked in water for 5 minutes or until bubbles cease to come to the top of the water.

The total thickness of the model should be one-third greater than the greatest height of the anatomic portion (height from the depth of the mucobuccal fold to the tip of the canine or incisal edge of the anterior teeth). With dividers set to the total height, the model is placed on a flat surface, tooth surface down and the incisal edges of the anterior teeth touching the surface, and a line is inscribed around the base of the model (Fig. 10-15). If the model is held firmly as indicated, this line will be parallel to the plane of occlusion. The base is then trimmed to this line. (Refer to the use of the model trimmer in Chap. 16.)

The posterior plane is next cut on the larger model (usually the maxillary) perpendicular to the midline or midpalate suture and at least one-fourth in posterior to the most posterior tooth or the last anatomic registration, whichever is greater (Fig. 10-16).

The total height of the smaller model is determined by the same method used on the larger model, and a mark is made on the base. With the models occluded properly with the wax bite and the larger model base resting on a flat surface, the marking around the base of the smaller model is continued with the use of dividers. The smaller model base is then reduced to that line.

With the models again occluded and the wax bite in place, the posterior plane trim is made on the smaller model by placing it base down on the model trimmer table and moving it against the revolving wheel until it is in the same plane as the previously trimmed model (Fig. 10-17).

The side cuts are made on the larger model by making a mark one-fourth in facially (buccally) to the bony ridge just below the gingival margin of the second premolar on both sides and then trimming a plane back to the mark, as parallel as possible to the mesiodistal centers of the posterior teeth.

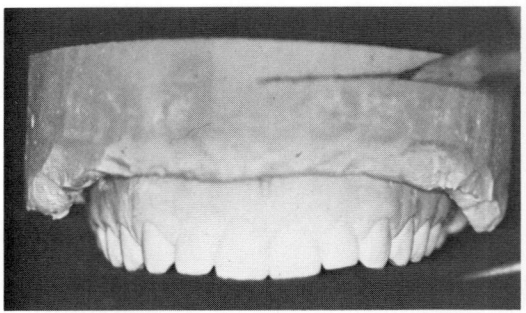

Figure 10-15 | Depending on the teeth complement in the arch, the model may have to be held to keep the anterior teeth in contact with the flat surface while inscribing the line.

The two heel cuts are made on the same model about $1/2$ in long and parallel with the mesiodistal plane of the canine on the opposite side of the arch (Fig. 10-18).

The models are again occluded with the aid of the wax bite, the uncut model placed on the model trimmer table, and the side and heel cuts made to the same planes.

Three marks are made on the anterior portion of the maxillary model to assist in making the an-

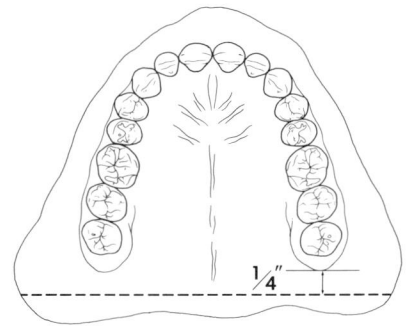

Figure 10-16 | The posterior cut must be posterior to the third molars if they are present in either arch.

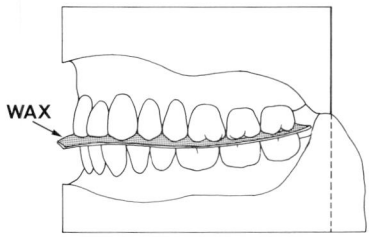

Figure 10-17 | Articulated or occluded models should never be trimmed on a model trimmer without the wax bite in place. The broken line indicates the plane to which the smaller model posterior cut is made.

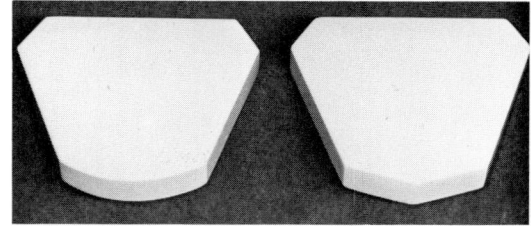

Figure 10-19 | Trimmed maxillary base at right and mandibular at left. Note similarity of all cuts except the anterior.

terior cuts. These marks should be ¼ in facially to the bony ridge just below the gingival margins of the canines and between the central incisors and opposite the mesiodistal centers of the canines and the median line. The canine markings are repeated on the mandibular model. The maxillary model is trimmed back to the described marks, making a V-shaped appearance. The two canine marks on the mandibular model are joined in the form of an arc maintaining the ¼ in clearance of the bony ridge (Fig. 10-19).

Finishing the trimming of models includes smoothing the land area and the tongue area of the mandibular model with a sharp plaster knife, filling in all voids and discrepancies with plaster, smoothing all trimmed areas with fine-grit sandpaper, and placing a small bevel on the edges of all trimmed sides (Fig. 10-20). Beveling is accomplished by placing a piece of fine-grit sandpaper on a flat surface, holding the art portion of the model at a 45-degree angle to the

Figure 10-18 | Malpositioned posterior teeth may alter the location of the side cuts. Care must be exercised in these cases that teeth and tissue reproduction is not cut during trimming.

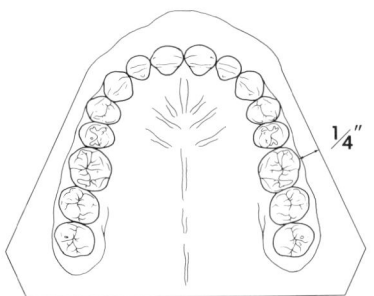

Figure 10-20 | Final smoothing is important for esthetic appearance. Teeth and tissue reproduction should not be sanded.

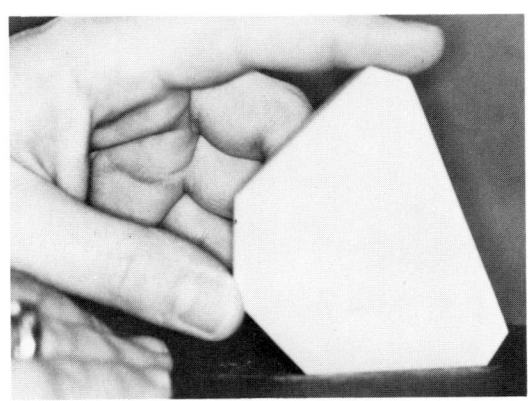

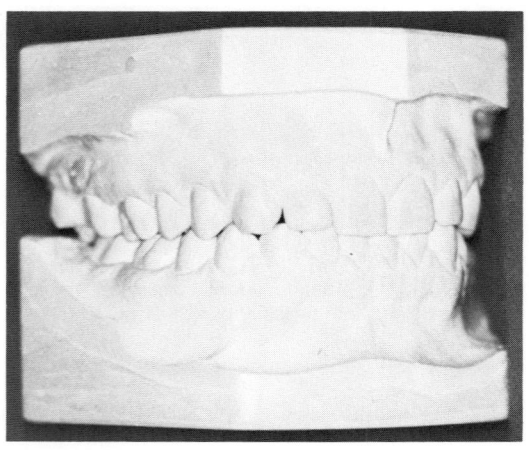

Figure 10-21 | Completed study models.

sandpaper, and drawing the model across the sandpaper for 4 in.

Polishing and Identifying

After the models have thoroughly dried, they may be polished by being soaked in a concentrated soap solution for 1 hour, removing and rinsing, and rubbing with a soft cloth to produce a glossy finish. Another method of producing a glossy finish is to apply several coats of plastic model spray. It should be applied in thin layers since a heavy application will run and produce an uneven surface.

Both the maxillary and mandibular models should be identified with the patient's name, age, and the date the impression was taken. This identification is placed with an indelible pencil on the posterior portions of the models.

Models prepared following the described method will present an esthetic appearance for case presentations and will provide a permanent record for the dental office.

BIBLIOGRAPHY

American Dental Association: *Guide to Dental Materials and Devices,* 7th ed., Chicago, 1974, pp. 13–18.

Craig, R. G., and Peyton, F. A.: *Restorative Dental Materials,* 5th ed., The C. V. Mosby Company, St. Louis, 1975, p. 47.

———: "Elastic and Mechanical Properties of Human Dentin," *J. Dent. Res.,* **37:**710–718, 1958.

Craig, R. G., Peyton, F. A., and Johnson, D. W.: "Compressive Properties of Enamel, Dental Cements and Gold," *J. Dent. Res.,* **40:**936–940, 1961.

Phillips, R. W.: *Skinner's Science of Dental Materials,* 7th ed., W. B. Saunders Company, Philadelphia, 1973, p. 49.

Stanford, J. W., Weigel, K. V., Paffenbarger, G. C., and Sweeney, W. T.: "Compressive Properties of Hard Tooth Tissue and Some Restorative Materials," *J. Am. Dent. Assoc.,* **60:**746–756, 1960.

11

Roger E. Barton

Impression Materials, Dental Waxes, and Synthetic Resin Materials

IMPRESSION MATERIALS

It is more convenient for the dentist and the patient to have certain types of restorations processed outside of the mouth. In order to accomplish this, certain areas of the oral cavity must be reproduced in exact detail in the form of a model, cast, or die on which the restoration or appliance can be fabricated. The term *die* refers to the reproduction of a single or multiple tooth preparation, while *model* or *cast* denotes more extensive reproduction of oral tissue. The first step in obtaining this exact reproduction of an area of the mouth, after the dentist has made the necessary preparations, is to secure an impression of the area. An *impression* is an accurate and detailed negative or reverse reproduction of either the hard or soft tissue or both. From this impression a positive reproduction or exact duplicate of the oral tissues can be produced (Fig. 11-1).

To produce a dental impression a material in a plastic or moldable state is placed in a special tray, placed in the mouth, and held in position until the material is set or firm. The tray together with the material is removed from the mouth and into this negative reproduction or *mold* is placed a suitable material which will harden and form the duplication of the oral tissues.

Desirable Properties

There are certain desirable properties that impression materials should possess. Although

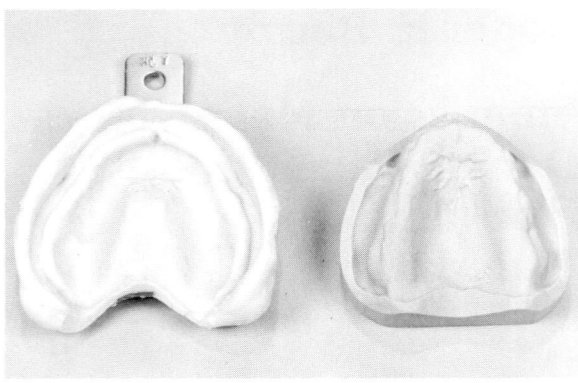

Figure 11-1 | *Left:* An impression or reverse reproduction of the edentulous maxillary arch. *Right:* A stone model or positive reproduction made from the impression.

there are many different impression materials available, no one material fulfills all the desirable qualities. The dentist, therefore, must select the material best suited to the technique to be performed.

The desirable qualities are essentially based on patient acceptance, ease of manipulation, and requirements of the procedure being used. The impression material should have a pleasant odor and taste and an appropriate color, and it should be free from toxic or irritating ingredients for patient acceptance. For ease of manipulation the material should not require extensive preparation, should have adequate flow properties, should be prepared with a minimum of equipment, and should have convenient working and setting times. Since accuracy is an important requirement in producing a dental model, the material should exhibit elastic properties to permit its withdrawal from undercuts without permanent change in shape; it should have adequate strength when set so that it will not break or tear during manipulation; it should possess dimensional stability under normal clinical and laboratory procedures when set; it should be compatible with the model, cast, or die material; and it should have satisfactory texture and accurate detail potential.

Classification

Through continuing research, the dental profession now has at its disposal three basic types of impression materials, namely, (1) rigid, (2) plastic, and (3) elastic. Quick-setting plaster of paris and metallic oxide paste are rigid impression materials. The plastic impression materials consist of waxes, impression compound, and other materials that are softened by heating and hardened by cooling. Materials that react accordingly with little or no chemical change are known as *thermoplastic* materials. Rubber-base impression materials and reversible and irreversible hydrocolloids are examples of the elastic-type impression materials.

Rigid Impression Materials

Plaster of Paris

Plaster of paris has been used in dentistry to take impressions, by various methods, for over 100 years. Before the advent of the more versatile impression materials, plaster was used in bulk to accomplish the entire impression procedure. The plaster becomes rigid upon setting and, therefore, has limited application in bulk where undercuts or similar irregularities are present in the mouth. When using plaster for an impression where undercuts are present, it is necessary to break the impression to remove it from the mouth. The pieces must later be reassembled and secured before a cast can be poured. It is obvious that the advent of newer materials brought welcome relief to both patient and dentist.

Quick-setting (impression) plaster is still used in impression taking in the making of various prosthetic appliances. This, however, is usually in the form of a *plaster wash* or as a *corrective wash* and is capable of recording fine detail. This procedure requires that an initial or preliminary impression be made with a suitable impression material. The plaster is then used as a thin lining of material to produce fine detail when reseating the initial impression, or as a lining in a custom acrylic tray made on a cast from the initial impression. The custom tray and lining are reseated in the mouth to obtain an accurate final impression. It is important to remember that when an impression is made in plaster, the surface of the impression must be coated with a separating medium before another gypsum product is poured over it in constructing the model or cast. Plaster is also used in making *transfer registrations* of crown positions in crown and bridge and jaw relations in full denture techniques.

Some impression plasters contain coloring agents, flavoring agents, natural gums, starches, and other materials to enhance desirable properties. These plasters should have a suitable setting time of between 3 and 5 minutes, have little or no dimensional change upon setting, and exhibit a fine grain for satisfactory surface detail. The manufacturer will note on the container that the plaster is of the impression type. The water-powder ratio for impression plaster will usually be 60 parts water by weight to 100 parts powder by weight. It is very important that the assistant follow the rules governing the proper manipulation of gypsum products, as discussed in Chap. 10, when dealing with impression plaster. A mix that is lumpy, incompletely mixed, contains trapped air, or does not set within the prescribed time cannot be utilized by the dentist in obtaining an impression. The assistant must master the proper spatulation and manipulation of impression plaster.

Metallic Oxide Impression Paste

During the 1930s zinc oxide–eugenol pastes were introduced as corrective-wash impression materials for use in completely edentulous mouths. These materials set by chemical action as does plaster but are not quite so rigid. This type of material is commonly called *metallic oxide impression paste* and is used to register final impressions, stabilize baseplates in bite registration, and in bite registration procedures in crown and bridge techniques. The material is primarily utilized as a thin corrective-wash lining in initial impressions or custom trays. It is capable of producing fine and accurate detail, is quite strong, and is dimensionally stable. However, the tray material used to contain the paste may be subject to dimensional change. Therefore, to prevent distorted models, the impression should be poured within a reasonable length of time before the tray material warps and distorts the lining material.

Zinc oxide–eugenol impression pastes are classified as hard and soft types with the set soft type not so brittle as the hard type. The essential ingredients of this material, as indicated by the name, are zinc oxide and eugenol. Certain fillers, additives, and accelerators such as gum rosin and inert oils are included by the manufacturer to produce a material of dimensional stability, smooth and homogeneous consistency, and proper setting time. The material is dispensed in two tubes, one tube containing the active ingredients (base material) and the second tube containing the eugenol in paste form (accelerator). The material from the two tubes is placed in equal lengths, but not necessarily equal volume, on a mixing pad (Fig. 11-2). Mixing on a glass slab results in a considerable problem in cleaning the slab. The two pastes are mixed together for approximately 40 seconds to 1 minute, in which time a smooth, homogeneous mass results. The mix is then placed in the impression tray. The material will remain plastic for an additional 2 to 3 minutes during which time it should be positioned in the mouth. Depending on the brand of material, the final set may occur in as little as 5 minutes or as long as 10 minutes. The set material consists of unreacted zinc oxide contained in a matrix of zinc eugenolate.

The setting time of this material is important and is controlled by the manufacturer. However, the assistant may alter the setting time by several means. (1) With many pastes, the longer the mixing time (within limits), the shorter the setting time. (2) A change in the ratio of one paste to the other will alter the setting time. When the paste containing the accelerator is increased in

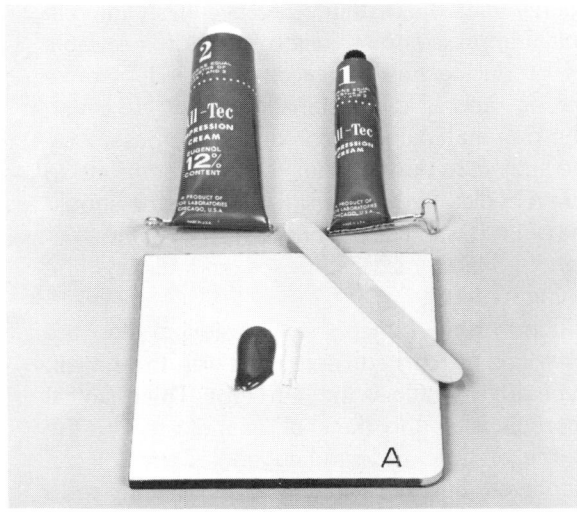

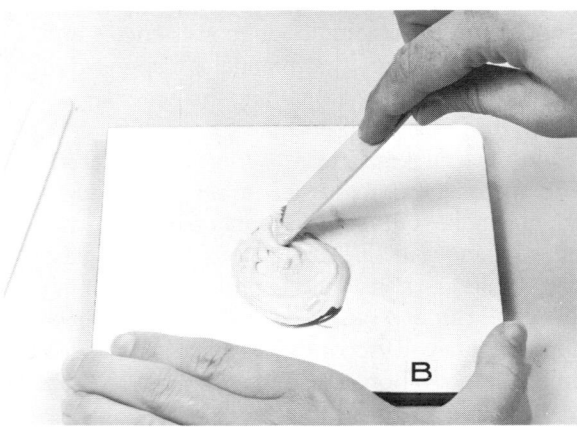

Figure 11-2 | A. Metallic oxide impression paste dispensed for mixing. Note equal lengths but not equal amounts of material on the pad. The tube orifices are designed to provide the correct paste proportions. A wooden tongue blade is a satisfactory spatula and eliminates the need for spatula cleaning. B. Mixing is begun with a rotary motion to incorporate the two materials, followed by a back-and-forth spatulation to produce a homogeneous mass.

amount, the setting time will be shortened. Conversely, a decrease in the amount of paste containing the accelerator will lengthen the setting time. (3) Cooling the tubes of material and the mixing equipment will lengthen the setting time.

(4) Adding a drop or two of mineral oil will retard the setting time. (5) A drop or two of water will act as an accelerator with most pastes. Primary alcohol will also act as an accelerator to shorten the setting time.

Noting that water may be used to reduce the setting time, it must be realized that inadvertent contact with moisture will produce the same result. This applies to storage as well as manipulation. The assistant must be aware that mixing during periods of high humidity may very likely shorten the setting time and precautions must be taken to prevent too rapid setting.

It must be realized that any method employed to alter the setting time may also affect other properties of the material, possibly to the detriment of the technique. Since various manufacturers produce metallic oxide impression pastes with different setting times, it would be advantageous for the dentist to select a material to suit particular needs rather than attempt to alter an existing material.

Since this material is used primarily in removable prosthodontic procedures, additional information is included in Chap. 30.

Plastic Impression Materials

Plastic impression compounds are amorphous, resinous, waxlike materials and are often referred to as modeling compounds. They are thermoplastic materials which may be used for impressions where no undercuts are present. Although it is still used in some practices in specific procedures, the use of this type of material is declining due to the development of other impression materials.

Impression Compound

This plastic-type material is available from manufacturers with varying softening temperatures and plastic ranges (Fig. 11-3). The harder and higher-fusing compounds are used as tray compounds to support other impression materials and to ensure an even distribution of pressure when the impression is taken. Slightly softer and lower-fusing compounds may be used to make any needed corrections or repairs on the impression proper.

The low-fusing stick or cone materials may also be used for impressions of teeth prepared for inlays or crowns. In this procedure, a copper tube is properly adapted to the tooth, the compound is heated over a flame until uniformly plastic, and then the compound is placed in the tube which in turn is carried to the tooth. An impression of fine detail is obtained provided there are no undercuts on the tooth.

Some desirable properties of impression compound may be listed as follows: (1) It should soften at a temperature just above mouth temperature and exhibit flow in this state; (2) it should harden at mouth temperature; (3) it should remain homogeneous during manipulation; (4) it should exhibit a smooth surface after flaming; and (5) the margins should be firm and smooth after trimming with a sharp knife.

The composition of the modern dental impression compounds is a trade secret. However, certain basic types of materials enter into their composition, such as (1) thermoplastic resins (shellac, copal resin, kauri gum, etc.); (2) plasticizers (fatty acids, glycerin, etc.); (3) fillers (talc or chalk); (4) coloring pigments; and (5) flavoring agents.

The low thermal conductivity of impression compound necessitates special considerations during the softening process, whether it be by hot water or over a flame. When the material is softened by either method, the outside surface will soften quite rapidly while the internal material remains stiff. On the other hand, overheating by a flame or by extended immersion in hot water will result in adverse alterations of the physical properties due to the loss of some of the ingredients or incorporation of water.

The temperature of the water bath should be approximately 130°F for softening impression compound. When using a water bath, the material may be kneaded to bring the unsoftened material to the surface and to improve the han-

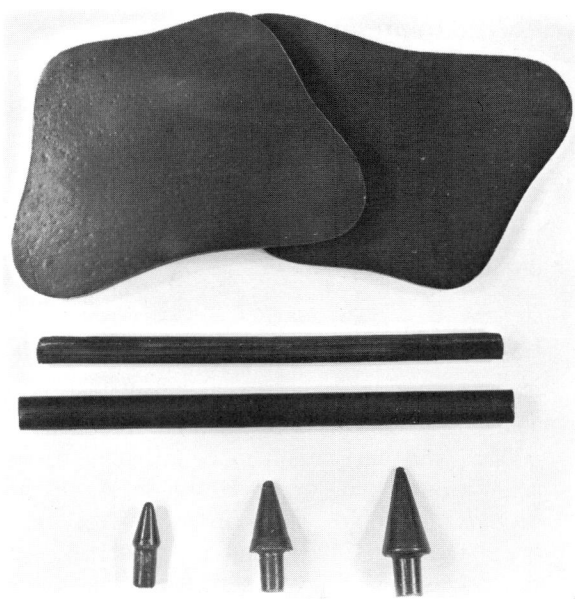

Figure 11-3 | Various types of impression compound. *Top:* Cake compound used in full impression techniques. *Center:* Stick compound for corrective procedures on compound impressions. *Bottom:* Cone compound used in copper tubes to secure impressions of individual teeth.

dling qualities. This kneading with the fingers can be overdone, resulting in an increase in the flow property of the material. However, to facilitate complete softening of the material throughout, in a reasonable length of time, kneading is advisable in moderation.

If an open flame is used to soften compound, the material should be rotated in the flame to distribute the heat over the surface of the material and not concentrate it on one spot.

The amorphous materials are notable for the fact that they are sluggish in the release of strains. A stone or plaster cast made 1 day after the impression is taken is not so accurate as the cast made soon after the impression is obtained. The compound tends to change shape slowly in an attempt to reach physical equilibrium; therefore, most accurate results are obtained by pouring the cast within 2 hours.

Elastic Impression Materials

This type of impression material will permit the taking of accurate impressions of the mouth, or parts thereof, where undercuts are present. This presents a considerable advantage over the rigid and plastic materials. Consequently, the elastic materials are used almost exclusively when teeth are involved in the impression.

Hydrocolloids

Colloidal solutions are called colloidal sols. Those colloidal sols which change to gels upon cooling and back again to liquid solutions (or sols) upon heating are called *reversible hydrocolloids*. Examples of reversible hydrocolloids are agar and gelatin. If the colloidal sol changes to a gel, as by chemical reaction, and the change cannot be reversed to the liquid condition (or sol), it is classified as an *irreversible hydrocolloid*. An example is calcium alginate.

It was not until the 1930s that the hydrocolloid impression materials were adopted in the practice of dentistry. Before that time, obtaining an accurate impression of some areas of the mouth proved to be an arduous task with the available materials.

Figure 11-4 | Full maxillary arch water-cooled tray used with reversible hydrocolloid impression material. Note the tube handle for water hose attachment.

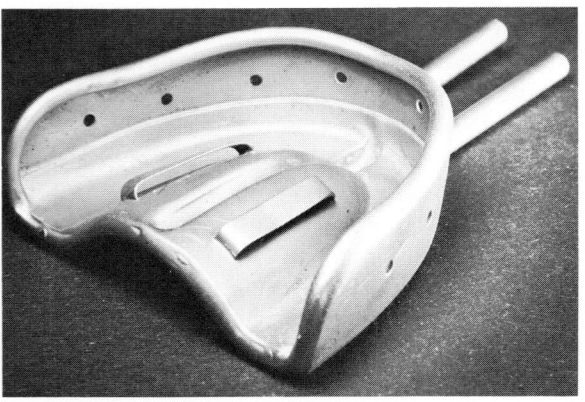

The reversible hydrocolloids were the first elastic impression materials to become available to the dental practitioner. The basic ingredient is agar, a product made from a type of seaweed. Minor ingredients such as fillers, preservatives, and flavoring are included in the formulas. A typical formula may contain as much as 85 percent water by weight, 12 percent agar by weight, and the remainder additives.

The reversible hydrocolloids are used for tray impressions of arches where teeth are present, for impressions of teeth prepared for inlays or crowns, and for duplicating models or casts. Application of this type of impression material in the mouth is gradually being replaced by other impression materials and techniques.

When the material is used in the mouth, the method of preparation should be followed with accuracy to prevent poor results and accidents. The hydrocolloid should be carried through three steps in preparation for use.

Since the material is purchased in the gel form, the first step is to change it to the liquid (sol) form. This is accomplished by placing the container of material in boiling water for a period of 8 to 10 minutes. The container must be completely submerged in the water. This is followed by placing the material in a storage bath of water at 155°F. It may remain in this bath for several hours without damage, and it will remain workable. Before it can be placed in the mouth, the hydrocolloid must be tempered. This is accomplished by placing the material in a water bath at 115°F for 10 minutes. To avoid burning the mouth tissues and yet to assure enough working time the 10-minute time period should be strictly adhered to.

When the material is placed in the impression tray, which, in turn, is placed in the tempering bath, possible surface contamination of the material may result. Therefore, just before the tray is carried to the mouth, the assistant should scrape away the surface material to a depth of about $1/8$ in.

The material being reversible, unused material

may be reboiled for use at a later time. Where material is reliquefied, an additional 2 minutes should be added to the original boiling time for each reboiling procedure. Due to changes in physical properties from repeated heating and cooling, the material should be reboiled no more than 4 times.

The material is applied to the tooth or teeth with a specially designed syringe, and the bulk of material is carried to the mouth in a special water-cooled tray (Fig. 11-4). The assistant should never allow the water to pass through this tray until the tray and material are properly positioned. The water should be turned on gradually so there is no sudden surge of cold water through the tray.

There are several types of automatically controlled devices available for heating and controlling the temperature of the hydrocolloids. Some of these "conditioners" have separate water baths with separate temperature controls for the three steps in preparing the material (Fig. 11-5).

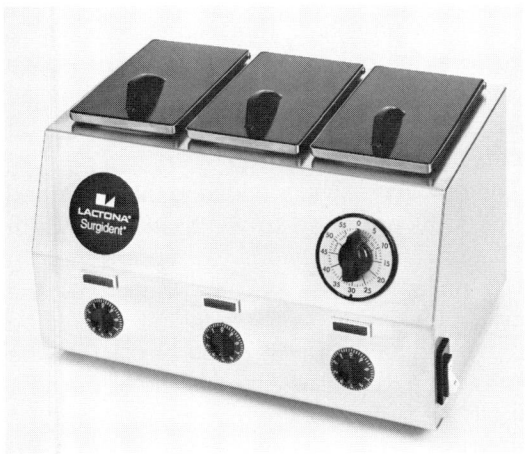

Figure 11-5 | Hydrocolloid conditioner with separate water temperature controlled baths for the three steps in preparing the impression material. The tank on the left is for liquefying, center for storage, and right for tempering. The large dial is a time switch. (*Courtesy of Lactona Corporation, subsidiary of Warner Lambert Company.*)

If this material is used routinely in the office, this piece of equipment is helpful and time-saving.

By virtue of their composition, the reversible hydrocolloids are very susceptible to atmospheric conditions. Some show shrinkage of as much as 1.0 percent over a period of 1 hour in air. Then when immersed in water at room temperature, the same materials not only swell to their original volume but may exceed the original dimensions by 0.6 to 0.8 percent. These phenomena may be attributed in whole or in part to the loss of water from the material (*syneresis*) or the gain of water by the material (*imbibition*). The casts made from impressions subjected to atmospheric conditions for a period of time, therefore, are inaccurate. It is advisable for this reason to pour the casts immediately after the impression is completed. When it is found necessary to delay the pouring for a few minutes (this delay should never exceed 30 minutes), the impression should be stored in a humidor in order to minimize dimensional change. In all instances, the surface of the impression should be cleared of all saliva, drops of water, and exudates before the plaster or stone cast is poured. The surface of the cast can be injured by this surplus water or salt solution.

Alginate

The irreversible hydrocolloids are referred to as alginate-base impression materials. These materials were developing during World War II because of the inability to acquire the seaweed from the Japanese coast for the agar used in the reversible hydrocolloids.

The alginate impression materials have several advantages, such as their pleasant odor and taste, that they are nonirritating to the oral tissues, their good reproduction of detail, their ease of mixing and manipulation, their low cost, that they require minimum equipment, their variable setting times, and that they are easily cleaned from tissue and instruments.

The alginate-base materials are used primarily

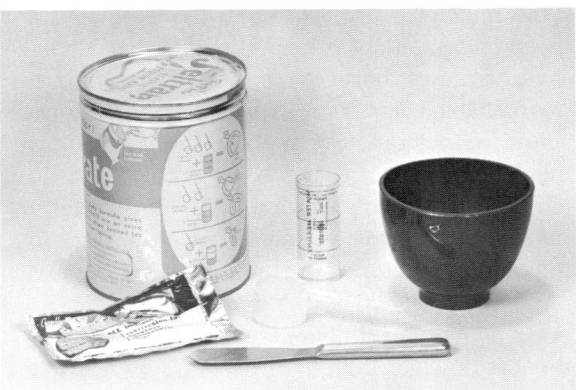

Figure 11-6 | Irreversible hydrocolloid may be supplied in bulk form or full impression individual packages. Equipment necessary for mixing are flexible bowl, semistiff spatula, water-measuring device, and powder proportioner when bulk material is used.

for impressions of arches where teeth are present, such as in partial denture procedures, in the preparation of study models for diagnostic aids, and to construct models for the preparation of athletic mouth guards. They are not used for impressions of cavity preparations.

The irreversible hydrocolloid (alginate-base) material is supplied as a powder (Fig. 11-6). It

Figure 11-7 | A type of perforated metal tray used with irreversible hydrocolloid impression material.

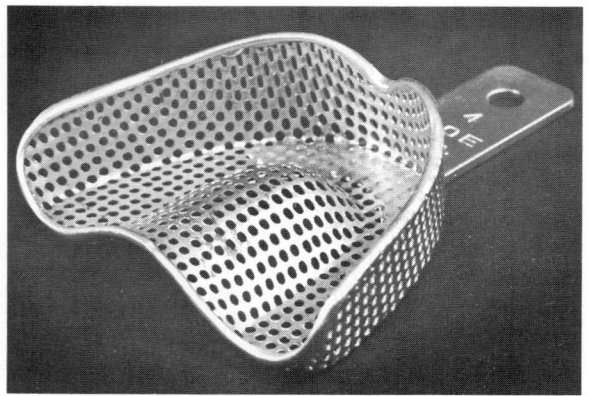

contains, as a basic ingredient, a by-product of marine plant life. This product is a salt of alginic acid which is extracted from marine kelp. Other ingredients include calcium sulfate, sodium phosphate, an inert filler, and coloring and flavoring agents. The powder is mixed with a specified amount of water within 1 minute to produce a paste. The paste is then placed in a properly prepared perforated tray (Fig. 11-7) and seated over the area of which an impression is desired. Manipulation time is critical since a mix that is not homogeneous or has begun to set cannot be used by the dentist in securing a satisfactory impression. The paste sets chemically (changing from the soluble salt to an insoluble salt) within 3 to 5 minutes, forming a strong, elastic gel which may then be removed from the teeth and mouth.

Proper mixing technique is important with alginate materials as it is with other dental materials. Both the powder and room temperature water should be measured accurately and mixed in a flexible bowl with a spatula having a wide and somewhat stiff blade. The powder is available in bulk or preweighed packages. A special scoop is provided with bulk material to dispense the alginate. The water measuring cup is usually marked with two or three lines indicating the proper amount of water to be used with a similar number of scoops of powder. Before measuring the powder, it should be fluffed up by gently shaking the container. The measuring scoop is filled level full but not compressed. The scoop should be tapped several times to fill any air voids and the mixing spatula used to scrape off excess powder from the top of the scoop.

The powder is always added to the water and a stirring motion used to wet the powder with the water. This is followed by a strong stropping action pressing the mix against the side of the bowl. At the end of 1 minute the mix should be creamy and smooth and ready to place in the impression tray. The assistant should fill the tray, smooth the surface of the mixed material with a wet finger, and pass the tray to the dentist—handle first. These procedures must be accomplished quickly so that the material does not begin to set before being placed in the mouth.

The dental assistant, in mixing alginate material, can exercise some control over the setting time by altering the temperature of the mixing water from normal room temperature. Cooler water will increase the setting time. Changing the water/powder ratio will also alter the setting time, but this is not advisable because the consistency of the mix and the strength and quality of the impression are also altered.

Impressions made from alginate-base material must be poured immediately (within several minutes after removal from the mouth), because the material changes in dimensions as time elapses, just as with the previously mentioned agar-base hydrocolloid. If a delay is necessary in pouring, the impression should be stored in a humidor or wrapped in a wet towel.

It should be noted that the strength of hydrocolloid impression materials is quite low. The set material will tear or break easily and, therefore, added precaution is necessary in handling hydrocolloid impressions during the pouring procedure.

Rubber Impression Materials

Continued research with impression materials has produced another elastic material for impression procedures. This rubber-like material possesses many of the ideal properties desired and is the only material that can be classified as a universal impression material for any dental procedure. The materials may be classified as mercaptan-base, silicone-base, or polyether, according to their composition.

Most manufacturers of the rubber impression materials produce the material in two types according to the viscosity of paste formed. These are generally known as a "light" or "syringe" type of low viscosity and a "heavy" or "tray" type of high viscosity. These two types of material add to the versatility of the product in allowing it to be adapted to many different impression procedures.

The mercaptan-base materials (frequently referred to as polysulfide materials) are distributed in two tubes. One tube contains the base material in paste form. The other tube contains the chemical accelerators in paste form. The accelerators, such as lead peroxide and sulfur, when mixed with the base material, cause a chemical reaction resulting in the formation of a rubber-like mass. The accelerator paste may also contain a rubber plasticizer and odor-masking agent.

The silicone-base materials, likewise, are dispensed as a base material and an accelerator, or catalyst. The base material (methyl polysiloxane) is in a paste form; the catalyst (tin octoate) is usually supplied as a liquid but may also be in a paste form.

There are two time periods associated with the rubber impression materials. The first time period is known as the *working time* and is that period from the start of mixing until the material is placed in the mouth. The second period is known as the *setting time,* or that period necessary for sufficient curing (vulcanization) before the impression can be removed from the mouth. For clarification, the setting time may be defined as the time elapsing from the beginning of mixing until the cure has proceeded to the extent that the impression can be removed from the mouth, and includes the working time.

The dental assistant should be aware of the fact that temperature will affect the length of these times. The warmer the temperature, the shorter the time element. The working times are decreased in both materials by an increase in temperature and humidity, but to a lesser extent in the silicone materials than in the mercaptan materials.

The control of the time elements can be accomplished to a certain extent by changing the ratio of the accelerator to the base material. A reduction in the amount of accelerator will produce additional working and setting times, but appreciable alterations should not be practiced

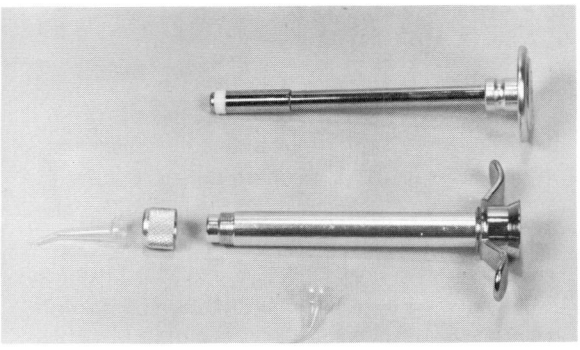

Figure 11-8 | Syringe for injecting rubber-base impression material into a cavity preparation. The syringe consists of a plunger with adjustable Teflon washer, barrel with finger grips, plastic tip, and hub for securing disposable tip to barrel.

because of the adverse effect on the elastic properties of the cured material.

The mixing of either the mercaptan-base or silicone-base material should be accomplished in a specified time, with the end result a homogeneous mass.

For cleaning purposes, the mercaptan material is best prepared on a paper mixing pad. This paper should be of the oil-impervious type and should be secured on at least three sides. The

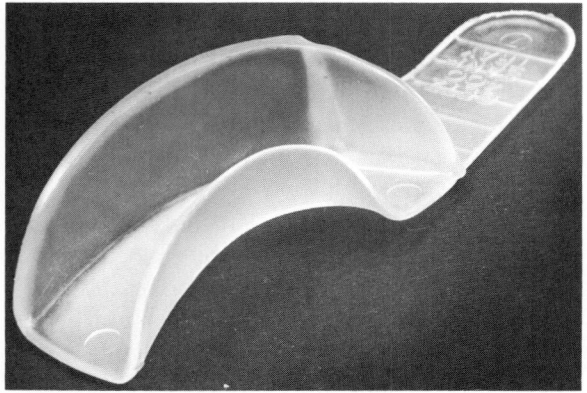

Figure 11-9 | Stock plastic tray used with rubber impression materials for a quadrant impression.

spatula should have a stainless steel blade that is flexible, wide, and at least 4 in long with a tapered flat side to assist in gathering up the material. If the mixed material is to be injected onto a prepared tooth, the syringe (Fig. 11-8) should be prepared prior to mixing the material. Likewise, if a tray (Fig. 11-9) is to be used, it should be selected and coated with an adhesive before the impression material is mixed. A band used for a single tooth impression should also be coated with an adhesive so that the impression material will be held firmly in the band when the impression is withdrawn from the tooth.

The mixing of mercaptan rubber impression materials of different viscosities is essentially the same. Depending on the amount of material needed, a strip of base material 2 to 4 in in length is placed on the mixing pad. An equal length (not amount) of the accelerator material is then placed on the pad. The accelerator material is picked up on the spatula blade and incorporated in the base material with a wiping, pressing motion. Considerable force must be used in this back-and-forth mixing motion. The spatula blade is held parallel to the pad and as much of the blade surface as possible is used. During the mixing the material is gathered up with the straight edge of the blade and redeposited on the pad and the wiping, pressing motion is continued until a homogeneous mix results. This must be within the time limits as expressed in the manufacturer's instructions. Failure to produce a uniform mix within the specified time will result in an inaccurate impression. The technique for taking an impression of prepared teeth is discussed in Chap. 28.

In the case of hydrocolloid materials, bulk of material is necessary in the tray to provide ample strength and body to the impression. When using the rubber impression materials the amount of material between the impression and the tooth should be only 2 mm thick. This minimum amount will minimize shrinkage. However, it also dictates that the container (tray or tube) must be rigid and of the proper size.

Table 11-1 | **Classification and Uses of Waxes**

Classification	Types	Basic uses
Pattern	Inlay	Inlay, crown, bridge patterns
	Baseplate	Denture base patterns
	Casting	Removable partial denture metallic frameworks
	Sheet Shape	
Processing	Sticky	Temporarily holding materials in position during procedure
	Utility	Customizing stock impression trays plus multiple applications
	Boxing	Forming a collar or matrix around an impression before pouring
	Undercut	Filling in undercuts on working dies or casts
Impression	Beeswax	Initial impression of edentulous arch, bite rim, bite registration
	Corrective	Final corrected impression of edentulous arch
	Bite	Bite registration

The mixing technique for the silicone materials is basically the same as that for the mercaptan materials. When the catalyst is in liquid form, the manufacturer's instructions should be carefully followed regarding proportions and mixing time. In such cases, the proportions are indicated as a prescribed number of drops of liquid per unit length of paste.

At times the dentist may ask the assistant to hold the tray once it has been placed in the mouth and the initial set has occurred. It is important that the tray is held steady with firm pressure. The impression is removed with a quick pull away from the occlusal surfaces after setting has occurred. The setting time varies between 6 and 10 minutes depending on the material.

Rubber impression materials are as elastic and reproduce detail as fine as hydrocolloid materials. They are also stronger than hydrocolloid materials and are not subject to the critical dimensional change when set. However, dies and casts should be poured in 1 to 2 hours. These materials may be electroplated successfully with silver where plated dies are desired.

The silicone-type impression materials have had several deficiencies overcome as result of continued research. They are, therefore, increasing in use over the mercaptan type because they are easier to manipulate and have a more pleasant odor and taste, they do not stain cloth materials, they are more esthetic regarding color, and the equipment used with them is easier to clean.

The polyether rubber impression materials were developed after the mercaptan and silicone types. Polyether materials are provided as a base and accelerator in paste form which must be mixed in equal lengths. The working time is less and the mixed material is more stiff with these than with the other rubber impression materials. Although some properties of the polyether materials are similar to the mercaptan or silicone types, electroplating is not recommended. Impression storage conditions are more critical, requiring dies and models to be poured promptly, and the accelerator may be irritating to the skin and oral tissues.

DENTAL WAXES

The dentist employs several kinds of waxes in the practice of dentistry. Waxes are generally classified in three categories, according to use: (1) pattern, (2) processing, and (3) impression (Table 11-1). The special physical properties desired of dental waxes dictate that they are not composed of any one wax but are blends of natural and synthetic waxes, fatty acids, oils, gums, resins, and pigments of various types. The types and amounts of the various ingredients are dictated by the desirable properties required for the various uses of the waxes. Although synthetic materials are used, most dental waxes are basically of natural origin. These products are derived from plants, animals, or mineral sources.

Examples are carnauba from leaves of a tree, beeswax from insects, and paraffin from petroleum.

Properties that are common in all waxes include melting or softening range, strength, flow, thermal conductivity, and residual stress. These properties are directly related to the use of the particular waxes and their manipulation for proper results.

Pattern Waxes

The pattern waxes are used to form the exact size and shape of a restoration or appliance. They are prepared on the teeth or a replica of the teeth or oral tissues. Through the processes of investing, eliminating the wax (thus forming a mold), forcing metal or plastic material into the mold, recovering the metal or plastic, and finishing and polishing, the final restoration or appliance is produced.

It is extremely important that individuals working with waxes, particularly waxes employed in gold or any alloy castings, be considerate of the properties and limitations in use. A thorough working knowledge of the inlay waxes is most important from a professional as well as from an economic point of view. Factors relating to warpage, shrinkage, and expansion must be controlled if an acceptable wax pattern is to be realized. It has been stated properly that "the casting can be no better than the wax pattern."

The American Dental Association establishes specifications for various materials. Materials meeting these specifications are certified, indicating to the profession their acceptance as qualified materials. Because of the critical role played by inlay wax in the production of precision castings, it is advisable to use only certified inlay waxes.

Composition

Inlay wax is a semicrystalline amorphous material. The composition and, consequently, the working characteristics of inlay waxes vary considerably. The formulas of some inlay waxes are complicated, but the essential ingredients of a successful inlay wax are paraffin wax, ceresin wax, candelilla wax, beeswax, and carnauba wax along with some coloring matter.

The paraffin wax constitutes 40 to 60 percent of the formula and controls the softening and melting range, thus producing the desired degree of plasticity at different temperatures.

The other ingredients of inlay wax provide resistance to cracking and flaking, add hardness and toughness, and enhance the smooth and lustrous surface. The coloring matter is added to give a desired contrast to the dental and oral tissues.

Inlay waxes generally are cast or rolled into sticks about 3 in long and $1/4$ in in diameter (Fig. 11-10), are blue in color, and are available as type I, regular (for direct technique), and type II, hard (for indirect technique).

Physical Properties

A desirable property of type I inlay wax is that it exhibits a plasticity or flow at a temperature slightly above that of the mouth. This property is essential where the wax is used in the direct-pattern technique. If the flow were not attained until a higher temperature, the patient would suf-

Figure 11-10 | *Top:* No. 7 wax spatula used in preparing a wax pattern. *Center:* Completed inlay wax pattern on a model tooth. *Bottom:* Inlay wax stick.

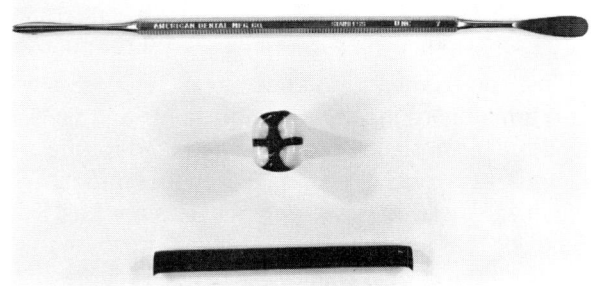

fer discomfort or injury to the pulp of the tooth when the wax was placed in the prepared cavity.

The thermal coefficient of expansion of waxes is quite high. This fact must be kept in mind when manipulating waxes in order to keep dimensional changes and warpage to a minimum. After a wax pattern is completed, distortion is increased as storage temperature and time increase. If a pattern must be stored for a considerable length of time, it should be kept in a refrigerator to minimize distortion. When so stored, the pattern should be allowed to return to room temperature before investing.

The thermal conductivity of wax is very low; therefore, adequate time at a constant temperature is essential for uniform softening or hardening. The surface condition does not always indicate the condition of the wax throughout.

Manipulatory Procedures

Wax should be softened for use by being heated in air (over a flame) to the highest temperature tolerable to the comfort of the tooth and compatible with the proper working plasticity. In heating, care must be exercised not to volatilize any of the ingredients. The wax should be so heated that it will be homogeneous in temperature and plasticity.

Commercially available wax annealers (using dry heat) are excellent for the heating of wax. Wax annealers not only ensure a homogeneous material of a definite uniform plasticity but also save time, since at this point the wax can be ready for use. The wax should not be softened in a water bath, inasmuch as the liquid portion of the softened wax may be washed out into the water, thereby changing the physical properties of the wax.

Inlay wax that has been softened and pressed into a cavity in a tooth should be cooled slowly by compressed air or water in decreasing temperatures to aid in minimizing warpage of the carved wax pattern while it is stored prior to investing. This gradual cooling should be done while the wax is under pressure. The wax pattern, whether made directly or indirectly, should be accomplished with as little repairing and recarving as possible. Additional heat or "pooling" of a portion of the pattern is contraindicated. The pattern should be withdrawn from the tooth or die with extreme care, never touched with the hands, not subjected to unnecessary temperature changes, and invested without extensive delay. Such precautions are necessary in order to minimize dimensional change and warpage. Manipulation of the wax pattern in the fabrication of an inlay is discussed in Chap. 15.

Baseplate Waxes

Baseplate wax is usually supplied in sheets approximately 3 by 6 in and is slightly brittle as compared with other sheet waxes. It may be purchased with various compositions and working qualities and is designated as type I, soft, type II, medium, and type III, hard. This wax is used principally to produce the pattern for a full or partial denture base to be molded of acrylic. It is that material in which the artificial teeth are placed for the "setup." Residual stress is built up in baseplate wax as a result of manipulation of the material in placing the teeth in the setup and, therefore, to reduce distortion of the denture base and minimize movement of the teeth, the case should be flasked as soon as possible. Baseplate wax is also used in the construction of bite rims (Fig. 11-11).

Casting Waxes

Casting waxes are frequently called sheet or shape waxes and are used to produce patterns for full or partial denture frameworks to be cast in gold alloy or chrome-cobalt alloy. The sheets are usually available in 28- and 30-gauge thickness. The shape waxes are available in round, half-round, and half-pear-shaped strips in various guages. Using these waxes helps to establish minimum thickness and smooth contour

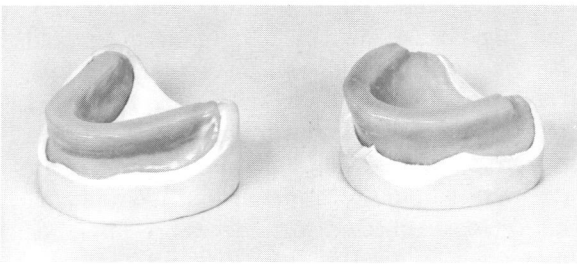

Figure 11-11 | Bite rims (wax occlusion rims) prepared on casts. The built-up rim portion is baseplate wax.

on frameworks in minimum time. This reduces the time required in grinding and finishing the cast framework. The casting sheet wax is also used for checking occlusion for premature contact points.

The composition of casting wax is similar to that of inlay wax with various combinations of the ingredients. In addition, some of the shape waxes possess a slight degree of tackiness to help hold them in position on the cast during construction of the pattern. When final positions are established, the wax must be sealed to the cast with a hot spatula.

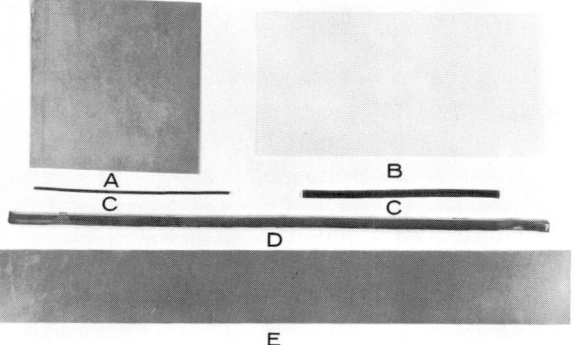

Figure 11-12 | Various types of processing waxes. A. Sheet or gauge wax. B. Baseplate wax. C. Shape waxes. D. Rope or bead wax. E. Boxing wax strip.

Processing Waxes

These waxes are very useful to the dentist, laboratory technician, and dental assistant as aids in various steps of processing dental restorations fabricated outside of the mouth (Fig. 11-12).

Sticky Waxes

This type of wax contains rosins in addition to other ingredients. Such a material is sticky when melted and will adhere to plaster, metal, acrylic, or other waxes. At room temperature the wax is hard and not sticky, but it is brittle. It is used primarily to hold materials together in a temporary position such as pieces of a plaster impression or a broken denture prior to repair.

Utility Waxes

Utility wax is a soft adhesive wax that is tacky and pliable at room temperature. It is usually dark red or orange. It is supplied in sheets or rope form. This type of wax finds many uses in the operatory as well as in the laboratory. It is often used to alter impression trays by providing postdams, lengthening flanges, or providing stops. It is composed largely of beeswax, petrolatum, and other soft waxes.

Boxing Waxes

Boxing wax may be used in boxing impressions or in making a collar around an impression (Fig. 11-13) to hold the cast material (gypsum product) in place until it sets. Boxing wax is provided in strips and is similar in consistency to utility wax. This type wax must be pliable at room temperature so that it is easily adapted to the impression without causing distortion of the impression.

Undercut Waxes

Undercut or blockout wax is used as a filler to correct or eliminate undercuts on working casts or dies before the preparation of wax patterns.

Impression Waxes

Impression waxes are usually used in nonundercut areas of the mouth and are used in registration procedures rather than for impressions in the strict sense of the word. An example of an impression wax used in prosthetic techniques for many years is *beeswax*. Other waxes have metallic fibers such as bronze and aluminum powders which alter their characteristics regarding hardness and rigidity at room temperature, making them useful in a variety of registration procedures.

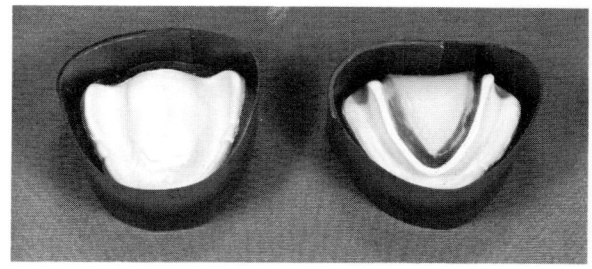

Figure 11-13 | Edentulous arch impressions boxed with wax strips in preparation for pouring of final casts. Baseplate wax was used to build support for tongue area on mandibular case. (*Courtesy of Dental Assisting, Course VI, Laboratory and Technical Application, University of North Carolina, Chapel Hill, 1965.*)

SYNTHETIC RESIN MATERIALS

Synthetic resins or plastics were perfected for the dental profession in the form of acrylic polymers in the 1930s. The material was originally used in the construction of denture bases. Gradually, through research, the synthetic resins have been refined, changed, and improved until they are presently used in many areas of dentistry. In addition to denture bases, plastics are used for repairing, rebasing, and relining dentures, for making custom impression trays, in manufacturing artificial teeth, in facings for crowns and bridges, in orthodontic splints, as luting cements, as restorative materials, and in numerous other applications.

The resin materials used in dentistry may be classified into two main categories—thermoplastic and thermosetting. Thermoplastic materials are softened under heat, molded into the desired shape, and harden upon cooling while exhibiting no chemical reaction. Thermosetting plastics solidify during fabrication as a result of a chemical change. Thermosetting plastics may further be classified as heat-curing resins, which require the application of external heat to cause polymerization, and self-curing resins, which cure as a result of chemical reaction between the ingredients without the application of external heat.

In 1938 a synthetic resin called acrylic was introduced to the dental profession. Acrylic is the methyl ester of methacrylic acid and is known as methyl methacrylate. This type acrylic resin is presently the most common resin or plastic material used in dentistry. Modifications permit a variety of uses.

A single molecule of acrylic is called a *monomer,* and when many molecules are linked together, a *polymer* is formed. Simply diagrammed (where M symbolizes a molecule):

$$M$$
monomer

$$-M-M-M-M-M-$$
polymer

When acrylic is supplied as a powder and a liquid, the powder is referred to as the *polymer* (Fig. 11-14) and the liquid as the *monomer*. The polymer is formed from monomer by a process known as *polymerization*. To polymerize means to change (by union of two or more molecules of the same kind) into another compound having the same elements in the same proportions but with a higher molecular weight and different physical properties. The more polymerization that occurs (converting monomer into polymer), the longer the polymer linkage (chain) becomes, resulting in a higher molecular weight, thus increasing the strength and hardness of the final product.

Polymerization may be characterized as either *addition* or *condensation*. In addition polymerization the monomers are linked together and no by-product results as with condensation polymerization. Due to the formation of by-products, condensation polymerization is not common in dental products.

The chemistry of polymerization can become quite involved in forming various bonds and chains in the polymer. One method of increasing the desirable properties of a resin is through *copolymerization*. This is a process whereby two or more monomers are polymerized at the same time, and the molecules are blended in the same chain.

Basically, the mixing of acrylic resins consists of adding the liquid to the powder in a sufficient amount to wet all the powder particles. Excessive stirring or mixing is not necessary. As the resin polymerizes or cures, it progresses through four stages. These stages are identified by the physical condition of the material as (1) sandy; (2) sticky or tacky; (3) doughlike; and (4) stiff or solid. To prevent polymerization of the monomer during storage an *inhibitor* such as hydroquinone is incorporated. The polymer contains a chemical known as an *initiator* (benzoyl peroxide) which when activated will begin the polymerization process. In heat-curing resins, the application of heat will activate the initiator. In self-curing resins, a second chemical is added to the monomer known as an *activator* (dimethyl-*p*-toluidene). When the powder and liquid are mixed together, the activator reacts with the initiator, and polymerization occurs at room temperature.

Denture Base Materials

A denture base is that portion of an artificial denture in which the artificial teeth are fixed and

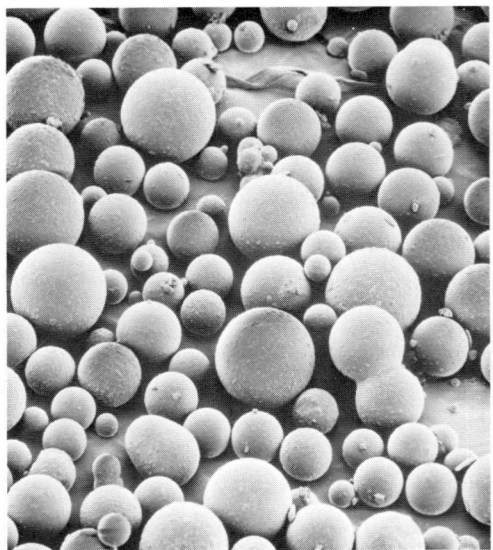

Figure 11-14 | Photomicrograph of a denture base polymer (original magnification ×160). Note large spherical particles. (*Courtesy of Dr. Karl Leinfelder, University of North Carolina at Chapel Hill, School of Dentistry.*)

which is in contact with the soft tissues of the alveolar arches and the palate.

Ideal Properties

For the complete satisfaction of the dentist as well as of the patient, denture base materials should possess certain properties. The dental assistant should have an understanding of some of the physical properties that are necessary for a satisfactory denture base material. These materials should possess good color-matching qualities that will not change over a period of time. They should also be dimensionally stable and should not expand, contract, or warp during use of the denture. The material should possess strength, but in case of breakage, it should be capable of being repaired easily and efficiently. It should be compatible with the mouth tissues, insoluble, and capable of resisting stain and odor accumulation. It should be impermeable to mouth fluids and resistant to normal abrasion. Additional requisites that pertain to the material as it is processed are of more interest to the technician than to the assistant.

Different materials such as cast metal, porcelain, rubber, and synthetic resins have been used as denture bases. The synthetic resins have all but replaced all other denture base materials.

Manipulation

There are a variety of processing techniques utilized in processing acrylic denture bases, and these are routinely used in commercial laboratories rather than in the dental office. Most dental assistants, therefore, do not become involved in denture base processing. However, a brief summary of the process adds to the general understanding of dentures.

After the dentist obtains a final impression, a dental stone cast of the arch is poured and trimmed. A pattern of the denture base (that portion contacting the soft tissue) is made of baseplate wax on the cast. The artificial teeth are positioned in the baseplate wax and the wax contoured and shaped.

The waxed denture and cast are then placed in the lower portion of a denture flask and the cast surrounded by plaster, leaving all wax and teeth exposed. When the plaster sets, a separating medium is applied to the plaster, the upper portion of the flask positioned, filled with plaster, and the flask top applied.

After the plaster has set, the flask is separated and the wax removed, thus making a mold for the acrylic base material. The teeth are held in place in the plaster. This area is filled with acrylic in the doughlike stage, closed tightly several times, and then placed under pressure for heat curing. After processing, the flask is again separated and the plaster chipped away, leaving the molded denture base with the artificial teeth embedded. Suitable textbooks on prosthetic dentistry describe this procedure in more detail.

Even though acrylic denture base resin has a high softening temperature, patients should be cautioned never to subject an acrylic denture to water hotter than 160°F. Higher temperatures will cause a denture to warp badly due to stress release in the base material. Also, a denture removed from the mouth for a length of time should be stored in water to prevent loss of absorbed water and accompanying contraction.

Denture Liners

The tissue side of denture bases may be lined with a hard or soft resin material to improve the comfort or fit of the denture. If this becomes necessary, the patient should have it accomplished by the dentist. If confronted with the question of denture liners, the dental assistant should discourage patients from using over-the-counter materials and procedures since some of the products contain ingredients that may be harmful to the oral tissues as well as the denture base. Such procedures may also result in an improper fit, thus causing tissue trauma and improper occlusion which may create additional problems for the patient.

Denture Repair Material

The material of choice for denture repairs is the self-curing or autopolymer acrylic resins. These resins cure by chemical reaction and, therefore, excessive heat need not be applied to the denture. The assistant may be requested to process a denture repair using a self-curing resin material. The procedure for replacing a tooth is described in Chap. 30.

If the assistant does use self-curing resin material in the laboratory there are several precautionary measures that should be observed. (1) The liquid is highly flammable and very volatile and must not be used around an open flame. (2) The liquid is a skin irritant and contacted skin should be immediately washed with water. (3) The liquid may be subject to premature polymerization by heat and/or light and should be stored in a cool dark place in an amber bottle. (4) Large bulks of curing material should not be confined in the hands because of the heat given off during the curing reaction. (5) Contamination of the liquid and powder should be avoided.

The usual method of mixing the self-curing resins is simply wetting of the polymer with the monomer until excess liquid appears. No mixing or stirring is usually required.

Other Resin Uses

The self-curing resins have many applications in addition to repair materials in both the dental laboratory and operatory. The assistant will be using these materials, and they will differ in composition and manipulative procedures. Therefore, it is essential that the proper instructions be followed in all instances.

In addition to denture-related usage, resins are used as temporary restorations, as cements, to fabricate custom trays, as pit and fissure sealants, and as esthetic restorative materials. They are also used as maxillofacial tissue replacement materials. With the exception of the latter, these materials and their application are discussed elsewhere in this textbook. Although the materials are all classified as resins, the physical properties differ, the actual composition differs, and each is manipulated differently. Likewise, they are all constantly being improved, and this requires constant attention and evaluation of the various products.

The most striking example of improvement may be noted in the resin restorative materials introduced about 1945 in the same formulation as the denture resin materials but with a reduction in the size of the spherical particles. These materials have been perfected and changed in many respects and now provide the most satisfactory esthetic material to date for use in non-load-bearing restorations.

BIBLIOGRAPHY

American Dental Association: *Guide to Dental Materials and Devices,* 7th ed., Chicago, 1974.

Craig, R. G., O'Brien, W. J., and Powers, J. M.: *Dental Materials Properties and Manipulation,* The C. V. Mosby Company, St. Louis, 1975.

Leinfelder, K. F.: Personal communication, University of North Carolina at Chapel Hill, School of Dentistry.

Peyton, F. A., and Craig, R. G.: *Restorative Dental Materials,* 4th ed., The C. V. Mosby Company, St. Louis, 1971.

Phillips, R. W.: *Elements of Dental Materials for Dental Hygienists and Assistants,* 2d ed., W. B. Saunders Company, Philadelphia, 1971.

12

Roger E. Barton

Dental Cements and Resin Restorative Materials

INTRODUCTION

The dental assistant's ability to mix the various cements and restorative materials properly is expected and appreciated by the dentist. To excel in this work, the assistant must have a fundamental knowledge of the nature, properties, and behavior of the cements and restorative materials and must know the manipulative variables and their effects.

Dental cements are utilized by the dentist in a variety of circumstances and are employed in one form or another in one-half of all restorations. They may be used as a luting medium under cast restorations, as a pulp capping material, as a base under metallic restorations, as a palliative cement in prepared teeth, as temporary restorations, and as restorative materials.

ZINC OXIDE–EUGENOL CEMENT

Zinc oxide–eugenol cement may be used in the form of pure zinc oxide powder and eugenol liquid. However, this mixture is extremely slow-setting and has very low strength. The material is also available with additives in the powder and liquid and in the form of two pastes similar to metallic oxide impression pastes.

Composition

A typical formula with percentages of powder and liquid by weight is as follows:

Powder		Liquid	
Zinc oxide	70.0%	Eugenol	85%
Rosin	28.5%	Cottonseed oil	15%
Zinc stearate	1.0%		
Zinc acetate	0.5%		

Source: From American Dental Association. *Accepted Dental Remedies.* Chicago, 1965.

When spatulated together, the zinc oxide and eugenol react to form zinc eugenolate which in the hardened form is a meshlike matrix binding together the remaining particles of unreacted zinc oxide. This hardened mass is formed in 2 to 3 minutes, depending on the composition of the material plus other factors. The addition of *zinc acetate* in the powder reduces the setting time to a few minutes. *Rosin* is added to the formula to increase the strength of the cement to approximately 5500 psi.

Table 12-1 | **Classification of Dental Cements**

Cement	Uses
Zinc phosphate	Luting fabricated restorations
	Luting orthodontic bands
	Insulating base
	Temporary restoration
Copper phosphate (red and black)	Insulating base
	Temporary restoration
	Luting orthodontic bands
Zinc oxide–eugenol and Zinc oxide–eugenol–EBA	Insulating base
	Obtundent base
	Temporary restoration
	Luting fabricated restorations
	Surgical dressing
	Root canal sealer
Zinc-silicophosphate	Luting fabricated restorations
	Luting orthodontic bands
	Temporary restoration
Polycarboxylate	Luting fabricated restorations
	Luting orthodontic bands
	Insulating base
Resin	Luting fabricated restorations
Silicate	Anterior restorations
Resin restorative materials	Esthetic restorations

Eugenol is a colorless, aromatic liquid found especially in oil of cloves. Either eugenol or oil of cloves may be used in the practice of dentistry as a sedative to allay pain in a tooth. Similarly, the set zinc oxide–eugenol cement is palliative to the tooth.

The primary disadvantages of this cement are that the compressive strength is low and the solubility is high. In an effort to overcome these deficiencies, ingredients have been added to the powder and the liquid. The most effective additives to date are polymers and alumina in the powder and orthoethoxybenzoic acid (EBA) in the liquid. The resulting cement has a compressive strength of over 10,000 psi and solubility comparable to zinc phosphate cement. The *Guide to Dental Materials and Devices* (1974–1975) lists a formula for zinc oxide–eugenol–EBA as zinc oxide 64 percent, alumina 30 percent, and hydrogenated resin 6 percent for the powder, and EBA 62.5 percent, eugenol 37.5 percent for the liquid.

Mixing

Since very little heat is generated by the reaction between the powder and liquid, mixing (spatulating) the zinc oxide–eugenol cement is usually accomplished on a paper pad to facilitate cleaning. The pad is comprised of sheets of treated paper which are glued together at their edges in a manner which permits removal of one sheet at a time. Before mixing, the powder is placed on the pad in slight excess, along with the eugenol. Then enough powder is spatulated into the liquid to produce a mix of the desired consistency (sometimes the dentist may desire a thin mix and at other times a thick mix, depending upon the intended use). The powder is incorporated by increments, a large amount at first, then smaller amounts to produce a mix of the desired consistency. If the cement is of the fast-setting variety, the assistant must learn to incorporate the powder rapidly; otherwise, the mix may set before it can be applied. The rate of addition of the powder does not affect the setting time of this type of cement.

"Brand" preparations of zinc oxide–eugenol are also mixed on a paper pad (Fig. 12-1). This material is fast-setting and is primarily used as a base material. Since only a small amount is usually necessary, ¼ to ⅜ in of the paste from each of the tubes (equal lengths) is dispensed on the pad. Using a small-blade metal spatula, the pastes are mixed together with a firm, steady, stirring motion until a homogeneous mass results. The mix is immediately ready to place in the cavity.

Water will accelerate the setting of zinc oxide–eugenol cement. For example, on days of high humidity, some of these cements may set so rapidly as to almost preclude their use. The thicker the mix, the faster the set; and the higher the temperature, the faster the set.

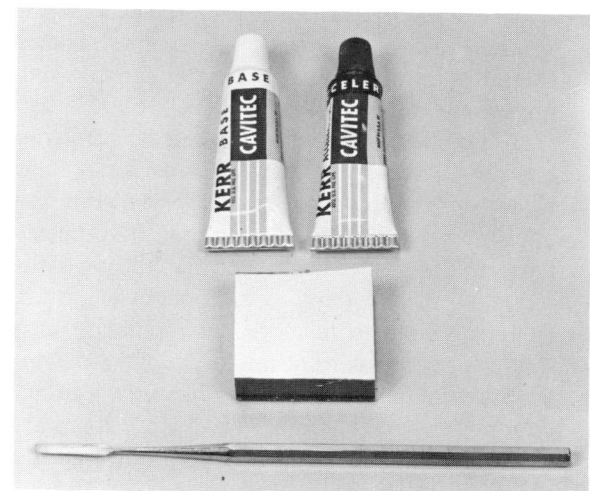

Figure 12-1 | Paste preparation of zinc oxide–eugenol cement. Note small-size mixing pad and small-blade spatula.

ZINC PHOSPHATE CEMENT

Zinc phosphate cements are used principally for the luting (cementing) of inlays, crowns, and bridges, as cement bases under metallic restorations, and for temporary restorations.

Composition

The powder of these cements is chiefly zinc oxide with a small proportion of magnesium oxide. The actual formulas of many cements are trade secrets. The liquid is composed of phosphoric acid, phosphates, and water. The average water content of the liquid is approximately 33 percent. Since the water in the liquid is balanced to match the powder, liquids and powders of different brands cannot be interchanged. When the powder and liquid are mixed, the surface of the powder is dissolved by the acid liquid, and considerable heat is generated. Although mixing is continued, not all of the powder dissolves, and the set cement is a crystalline network surrounding the undissolved zinc oxide particles.

General Characteristics

The zinc phosphate cements are not strong enough for the restoring of lost tooth structure subjected to occlusal stress. As a comparison, the crushing strength of silver amalgam is 60,000 to 80,000 psi, while that of zinc phosphate cement is approximately 12,000 psi. Another disadvantage of zinc phosphate cement, which is true of all cements except the resin type, is its solubility. Other serious disadvantages are its acidity and lack of hydraulicity. The acidity of the cement mix is very high at first and, therefore, may seriously irritate the pulp. This acidity is neutralized in about 1 hour. Hydraulicity refers to the ability of a cement to harden under water. A mix of zinc phosphate cement does not possess this property inasmuch as water (or saliva), if allowed to come in contact with the mix while it is hardening, will leach out the phosphoric acid, rendering the affected surface cement chalky and permeable.

Zinc phosphate cement is a good thermal insulator, which makes it a good lining (or base) under metallic restorations in deep cavity preparations. However, due to acidity, an intermediary should be placed between the dentine and zinc phosphate cement.

The chemical reaction between the powder and liquid is exothermic (evolves heat), and while considerable heat can be generated in the improper, rapid mixing of cement, the ordinary temperature realized with a correct mixing technique is not disturbing to the patient when the cement is applied to a cavity preparation in a tooth. A special word of caution is given to warn the assistant *never to mix zinc phosphate cement on a paper pad.* The mix must always be made on a glass slab. The paper pad will not keep the cement mix as cool as the glass slab. The increased temperature (of the cement mix on the paper pad) will cause the cement to set too rapidly for practical use and may cause permanent injury when applied to the tooth.

Control of Setting

The setting time of zinc phosphate cement can be controlled by the manufacturer and the operator by

1. The composition of the powder
2. The composition of the liquid, which includes buffering salts and water
3. The particle size of the powder, which will affect the surface contact of the powder with the liquid
4. Reducing the temperature of the mixing slab
5. Reducing the rate of addition of the powder to the liquid
6. Reducing the amount of powder used in ratio to the liquid
7. Prolonging (within limits) the mixing

The first three methods are under the control of the manufacturer. However, with reference to item 2, it is most important that the manufacturer's concentration be retained by keeping the liquid bottle stoppered tightly at all times (when not in use) to maintain the water content. Also, liquid dispensed on the slab must not be left in contact with the air for any length of time. If the water content is increased, as might happen on a humid day, the setting time will be shorter; if the water content is reduced, as might happen on a dry day, the setting time will be longer. The manufacturer provides 20 percent more liquid in the bottle than required for the amount of powder supplied. This excess liquid should be discarded when the powder is used up, inasmuch as the liquid has been exposed to the air for the maximum safe length of time during the periods of dispensation. Also, the liquid should be discarded if a cloudiness is detected, which is an indication of chemical imbalance. Some cement liquids are dispensed in squeeze-type bottles, thus reducing the possibility of acid/water ratio change since the bottles must not be opened.

The last four items, namely, items 4 to 7, are controlled in the dental office. The dental assistant, therefore, has an opportunity to control the setting time and also to present a cement mix that is most favorable for use by the dentist. For luting purposes the cement mix should remain sufficiently fluid long enough for careful application to the tooth or inlay (or both); yet the final set must not be unduly prolonged.

1. Cooling the glass slab retards the setting while mixing and allows the incorporation of more powder for a given consistency (workability). The increased powder/liquid ratio increases strength and decreases solubility, shrinkage, and acidity. Never, however, cool the slab to the point that dew forms on it, because the effect is the same as that mentioned previously when the water content is increased.
2. Reducing the rate at which the powder is added will increase the setting time; the faster the powder is added, the quicker is the set. This is within certain limits.
3. The thick mix sets faster than the thin one.
4. Within limits, prolonged mixing lengthens the setting time.

The American Dental Association specification for an acceptable dental zinc phosphate cement states that the time of setting shall not be less than 5 nor more than 9 minutes.

Technique of Mixing

It is recommended that the assistant follow the manufacturer's instructions for proportioning and mixing the powder and liquid. However, the procedures described herein are generally accepted in principle and serve to emphasize important manipulative fundamentals.

1. Use a glass slab that is thick enough (about 1 in), provides a generous working area, is perfectly level, and is highly polished. If the slab is deeply scratched or chipped in the spatulation area, it is well to replace it with a new one. The spatula should be of noncorrodible metal. Keep the slab and spatula absolutely clean, free of any hardened cement particles (Fig. 12-2).
2. Cool the slab to approximately 65°F. (Caution: Do not cool the slab below the dew point, which would produce a cloudy, moist slab surface.)
3. Place the powder on the slab near one end, the amount being determined by the powder/liquid ratio (included in the manufacturer's instructions) and also by the amount of cement mix desired. Some manufacturers provide a device for dispensing the powder (Fig. 12-2D); such volume proportioning of the powder is satisfactory if done in a consistent and careful manner. Instructions for use of the device illustrated call for packing the powder tight in the well of the dispenser by pushing it through the powder, and then firmly pressing it against the bottom surface of the bottle. The well on one end of the device is half the volume of the well on the other end. One dispensing of powder from the large well supplies powder necessary to produce a cementing consistency with four drops of liquid. One dispensing of powder from the large well, together with one dispensing from the small well and four drops of liquid, will make a mix that will be of correct consistency for a temporary restoration, liner, or base.
4. With the spatula, pat the powder level, about 1 mm thick. Next, divide it into halves, and then di-

Figure 12-2 | Dispensing the zinc phosphate cement powder. A. Glass slab. B. Noncorrodible spatula. C. Powder bottle. D. Powder-measuring device, each end having a well, one large and one small, for full-portion and half-portion dispensations of powder.

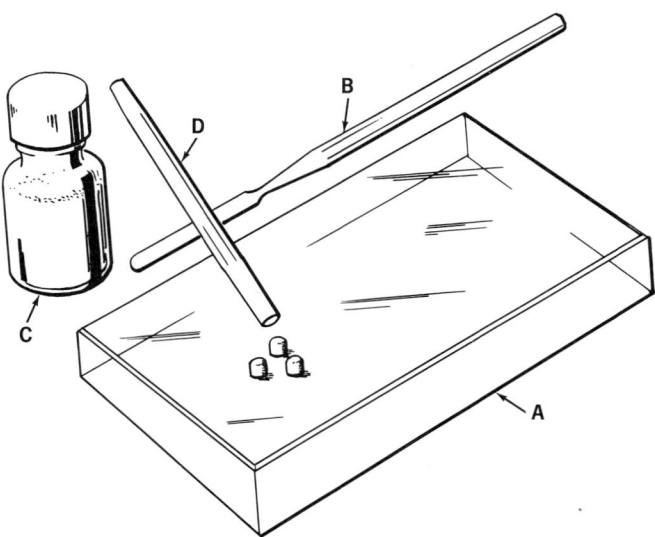

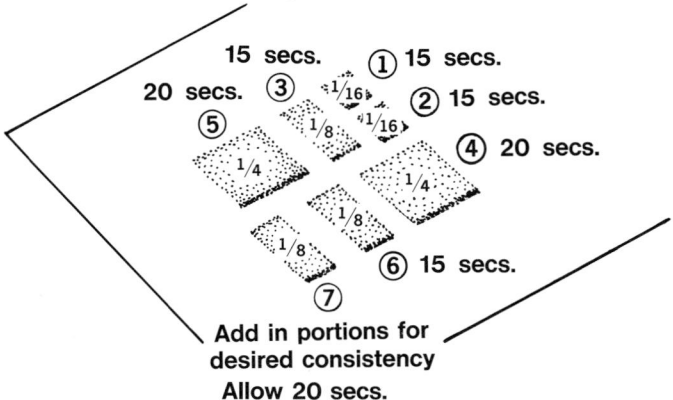

Figure 12-3 | The division of zinc phosphate powder into portions, the sequence of incorporation of the portions (circled numbers), and the mixing time for each portion.

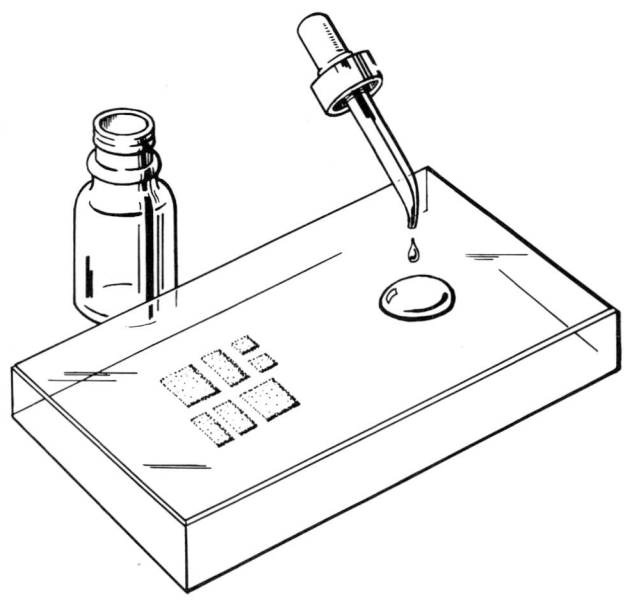

Figure 12-4 | Dispensing the zinc phosphate cement liquid. Note dropper end is parallel to surface of glass slab and about $1/2$ in away from slab.

vide each half, thus making four quarter portions of powder. Finally, divide two of the quarter portions into eighths, and then one of the eighth portions into sixteenths, as illustrated in Figs. 12-3 and 12-4. *Caution:* Move the portions far enough apart so that later, during the mixing, each portion can be moved into the mix by the "wet" spatula (wet with the mix) without contaminating the remaining portions of powder.

5. Before unscrewing the medicine dropper type cap from the liquid bottle, shake the liquid a few times and also pump the liquid out of the dropper several times by alternately pressing and releasing the rubber bulb. Then dispense the recommended number of drops, as shown in Fig. 12-4. (For uniform drops, the dropper end should always be held parallel to the slab surface.)

6. Keep the liquid bottle tightly stoppered except when withdrawing liquid.

7. Spatulate one of the sixteenth portions into the liquid in 15 seconds. In mixing, use one-half or more of the surface of the slab (i.e., spread the mix widely) to aid in the dissipation of the exo-

thermic heat (Fig. 12-5A). Hold the spatula blade flat against the slab (Fig. 12-5B), and use rotary motions in combination with a linear motion, with firm pressure. Interrupt spatulation several times to gather up the edges of the mix into the central mixing area, using a scraping motion of one edge of the spatula against the glass slab. After the incorporation of this or any subsequent powder portion, the mix should be homogeneous, with no free liquid or unmixed particles (in the form of liquid streaks or particle lumps) at the side of the mix or in the mix itself. This homogeneity always must be attained before the incorporation of any additional powder. A firm pressure is necessary to smooth out (break down) any visible granules of powder, often noticeable when the mix is spread in a thin film over the slab. It is helpful to learn the movements of the of the spatula illustrated in Fig. 12-6, by which the spatula blade can be wiped "clean" of the mix, before reaching for the next portion of powder.

Spatulate the remaining powder portions into the mix, following the time schedule shown in Fig. 12-3.

8. Incorporation of powder is complete when the desired consistency is obtained, and this should be accomplished in approximately 2 minutes. Cementing consistency is correct when the mix is creamy and will follow the spatulate about 1 in before breaking in a thin thread (Fig. 12-7A). The mix will fall from the spatula in a gummy drop, hold its form for a moment, and then spread slightly on the mixing slab (Fig. 12-7B).

Filling consistency is correct when the cement hangs but does not drop from the spatula (Fig. 12-8A). This mix will be tacky and have putty-like consistency. It will not follow the spatula when it is raised from the mix on the slab, but will appear as in Fig. 12-8B.

9. Use the maximum amount of powder possible for the operation at hand. This reduces the solubility and acidity of the cement and increases its strength.
10. Never add liquid to a mix. Make a new one.
11. Never reach in the powder bottle for more powder with a "wet" spatula.
12. Discard any unused powder on the slab, as it may be contaminated from the mix.
13. For some cements, additional working time,

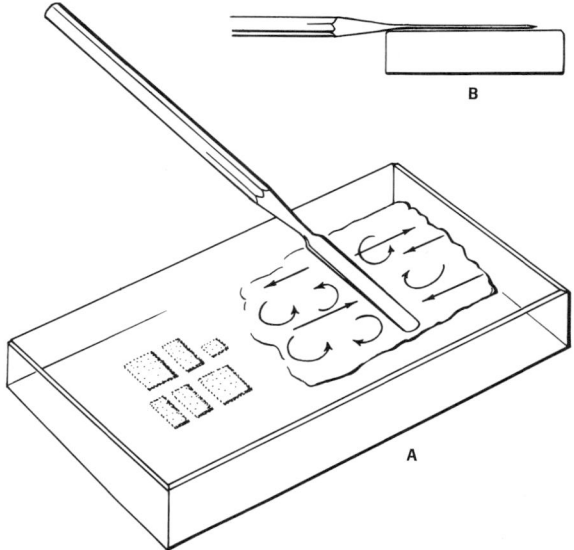

Figure 12-5 | Depicting the mixing technique of zinc phosphate cement. A. The mix is spread over a large area of the slab using a rotary-linear spatulation motion. B. The spatula is held flat against the slab and firm pressure applied.

when desired, can be obtained by spatulating a very small amount of powder (a one-sixty-fourth portion of powder) into the liquid to initiate the mixing and allowing this clouded liquid to rest approximately 1 minute before continuing incorporation of the powder as previously described.

The services of an assistant are desirable when cementing inlays, crowns, and bridges, not only in preparing the cement mix, but in applying the cement to the cavity side of these restorations while the dentist is applying the cement to the teeth. Both the assistant and the dentist must exercise care not to incorporate or trap air in this phase of the cementing operation. The assistant must learn to apply the cement slowly enough (consistent with the working time of the cement mix) to prevent bridging over remote corners (Fig. 12-9). During the seating of the restoration, trapped air as depicted in Figure 12-9A may be

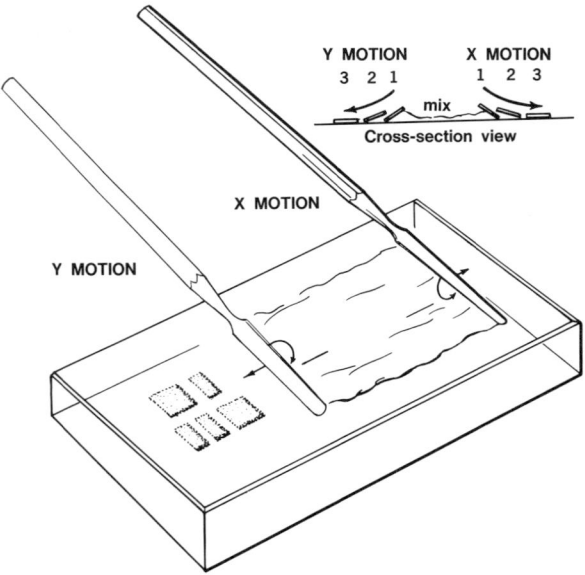

Figure 12-6 | The two rotary sliding movements of the spatula blade used to clean the sides of the spatula before reaching for the next portion of powder (X motion for cleaning one side of the blade and Y motion for the other side).

Figure 12-7 | Cementing consistency is correct when the mix is creamy and will follow the spatula before breaking in a thin thread (A). The mix will fall from the spatula, hold its form for a moment, and then spread slightly on the glass slab (B).

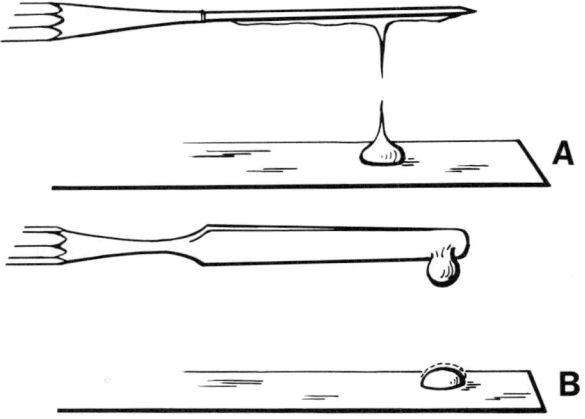

displaced to a region near a margin, thereby resulting in leakage and early failure of the restoration. The cemented restoration and surrounding region must be kept dry while the cement is setting.

It is important to realize that most cements used as luting agents have no adhesive qualities, and retention is obtained by mechanical locking of the cement in the irregularities of the surfaces being cemented.

COPPER PHOSPHATE CEMENT

Generally, these are zinc phosphate cements to which copper oxide has been added to the powder. If the red copper oxide (cuprous oxide) is added, the powder and the cement are a characteristic red. If the black oxide of copper (cupric oxide) is added, the powder and the cement are black.

The main object in the addition of these oxides of copper is to render the cements germicidal. However, their germicidal value is questionable, and they are seldom used in present-day dentistry.

SILICATE CEMENT

Silicate cement is used mainly as a restorative material in anterior teeth. These restorations are commonly referred to as porcelain restorations because the set material resembles porcelain. However, this is an incorrect application of the term.

The present silicate cements possess an esthetic advantage in resembling tooth structure and are easy to manipulate and insert in the prepared cavity. On the other hand, they possess such disadvantages as solubility, staining, shrinkage, acidity, and lack of strength. With these inherent shortcomings, it is of the utmost importance that the handling and manipulation of silicate cements by the assistant be as exacting as

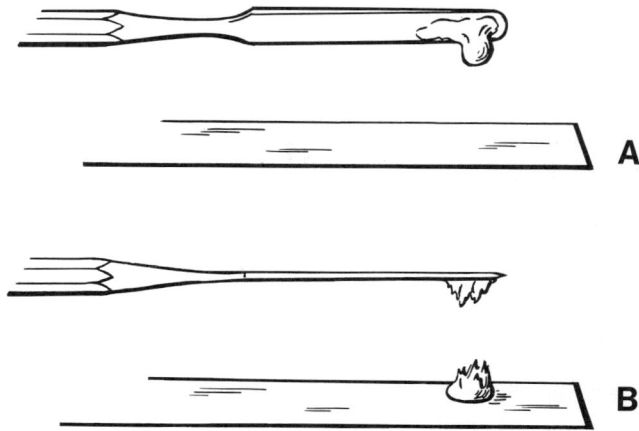

Figure 12-8 | Filling consistency is correct when the mix hangs but does not drop from the spatula (A). This mix should be tacky and have a putty-like consistency. It will not follow the spatula when it is raised from the mix on the slab, but will appear as in (B).

possible in order to produce a restoration of maximum quality.

The development of another esthetic restorative material, namely composite resin, has reduced the routine use of silicate cement in anterior teeth. However, it is still used by many dentists and, therefore, is discussed in detail.

Composition

From the time of the introduction of a translucent cement by Fletcher in England in 1871 constant improvements have been made in silicate materials. Presently the silicate powders are supplied in a variety of shades to provide a close color match with the tooth.

The powder consists primarily of silica (SiO_2), alumina (Al_2O_3), and a flux of either sodium fluoride (NaF) or calcium fluoride (CaF). These materials are proportioned and fused. The glasslike mass is crazed and then ground into fine particles.

The liquid, which contains phosphoric acid, phosphates, and water, is very similar to zinc phosphate cement liquid. However, the liquids should not be interchanged since the silicate liquid contains more water (approximately 40 percent) and less acid than the phosphate cement liquid.

The set silicate cement is composed of particles of undissolved powder surrounded by a silicic acid gel matrix.

General Characteristics

The crushing strength of silicate cement averages about 24,000 psi, which is twice that of zinc phosphate cement and about one-third that of amalgam. Silicate cements are brittle and, therefore, cannot absorb shock.

The solubility of the silicate cements is the major handicap of this restorative material. A large percentage of practicing dentists agree that the average life expectancy of a silicate restoration is not more than 5 years and that it probably is less. The poor physical properties of a silicate cement restoration (lack of strength, shrinkage, staining, solubility, and acidity) must be attributed to the matrix material which is formed around the powder particles in the setting reaction, inasmuch as the powder particles in themselves are strong, relatively insoluble, nonstaining, and dimensionally stable. Therefore, good technique is based on the principle of incorporating in the mix as much powder as possible to reduce the amount of matrix material in the mass.

The shade for a silicate cement restoration should be selected from a shade guide (Fig. 12-10) which is generally provided by the manufacturer. Both the tooth and shade guide must be wet when the shade selection is made. Always take the shade of a tooth before the application of a rubber dam, because the tooth when isolated by the dam for a period of time becomes lighter because of a partial loss of water content. Also, the dam creates an abnormal background and shading.

In the selection of silicate cements, only those certified to meet the specifications of the American Dental Association should be used.

Setting Time

The importance of maintaining the composition of the liquid needs to be understood by the dental assistant. Just as with the liquid used in zinc phosphate cement so, also, the water content of the silicate cement liquid is critical and must be maintained by keeping the bottle tightly stoppered except when dispensing the liquid. The liquid solution always tends to come to equilibrium with the water vapor of the air. Loss of water increases the setting time, and an increase in water content decreases the setting time, just as with the zinc phosphate cements. If either change occurs (loss or gain of water in the liquid), a silicate mix made using such liquid will be less strong, more soluble, and more subject to staining, and will shrink more.

If the slightest cloudiness or sediment appears in the liquid, the bottle should be discarded, since such a condition indicates a chemical imbal-

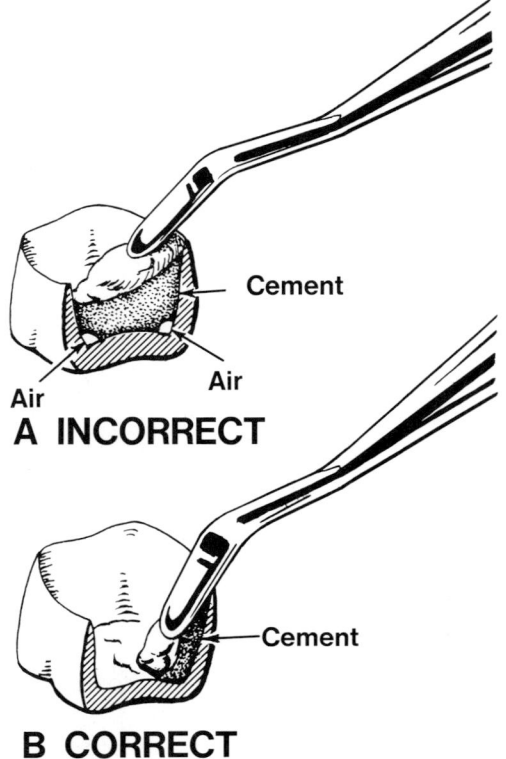

Figure 12-9 | Placing large increments of cement in a restoration may trap air (A) in line and point angles.

ance. As with the zinc phosphate cement liquid, the silicate cement liquid should be discarded when four-fifths of it has been used, inasmuch as the remainder is likely to be affected unfavorably by the repeated exposures during the many withdrawals of liquid.

The mixing time should *never be prolonged beyond 1 minute,* because if more time is consumed, the cement will be weaker, more soluble, and more subject to staining.

The powder/liquid ratio should never be reduced less than that recommended by the manufacturer, which provides the standard consistency. Increasing the liquid proportion decreases the strength and increases the solubility, staining, shrinkage, acidity, and setting time.

The setting time is decreased (shortened) by increasing the temperature of the slab, and vice versa.

Adding the powder to the liquid all at one time, rather than in increments during the prescribed 1-minute mixing period (i.e., the rate of adding the powder), has only a slight tendency to decrease the setting time. The reaction between the silicate powder and liquid is not exothermic. This explains why the rate of addition of the silicate powder (within the mixing period by the manufacturer) has only a small effect on the setting time, in contrast to the marked effect this variable has on the setting behavior of the zinc phosphate cement which is exothermic in its reaction.

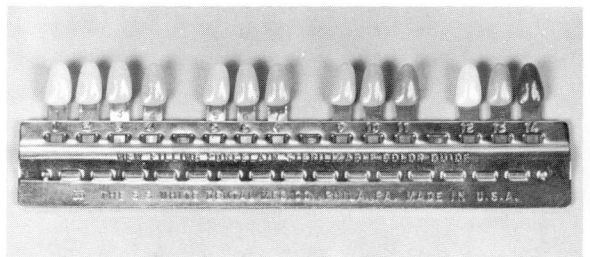

Figure 12-10 | Silicate cement shade guide as provided by one manufacturer. Shade matching should not be accomplished under bright operating light alone.

Technique of Mixing and Placement of Silicate Cement

The manufacturer's directions should be carefully followed; however, a technique is described herein which is generally accepted in principle and which will serve to emphasize important fundamentals in the manipulation of silicate cement.

1. Use a thick, smooth, transparent glass mixing slab of generous size, a spatula made of agate or stellite type (to avoid discoloring the silicate material), and a powder-measuring device supplied by the manufacturer of the silicate material (Fig. 12-11). The slab should be clean and dry.
2. Chill the slab to approximately 65°F (not below the dew point). The cooled slab decreases the rate of reaction between the powder and liquid, thus aiding the wetting of each powder particle during mixing, the incorporation of a maximum amount of powder, and the formation of a minimum of matrix material prior to insertion of the mix into the cavity.
3. Carefully dispense the powder according to the manufacturer's directions. First vibrate the powder bottle to settle its contents, then press the powder measurer deep into the powder several times to make certain that the dispensing well of the measurer is packed tight with powder. Two dispensings of powder from the deeper well to two drops of liquid are the recommended quantities of powder and liquid. It is recommended that a small amount of extra powder be placed on the slab [note (E) in Fig. 12-11], available for use to develop the proper consistency at times when the cool slab permits the incorporation of more powder than indicated in the manufacturer's directions. (There is not sufficient time during mixing to open the bottle and obtain more powder.)
4. Divide the powder into half portions. Then divide one of the half portions, making two quarters. Finally, divide one of the quarter portions, making two eighths (Fig. 12-12).
5. Note that the powder was dispensed and divided before dispensing the liquid; recall that this is also true when preparing to make a mix of zinc phosphate cement. Shake the liquid in the bottle, and agitate it by squeezing the bulb of the pipette, drawing the liquid in and out several times. Draw the liquid from the bottom of the bottle and dispense two drops. (Fig. 12-13). Replace the pipette in the bottle and screw the bottle cap tight.
6. Start mixing immediately after the liquid has been placed on the glass slab, thereby never exposing the liquid to air longer than necessary.
7. Incorporate the large (half) portion of powder into the liquid (in 10 seconds or less), mixing over a small area. Spatulation is accomplished either by a circular stirring motion (Fig. 12-13) with the end of the spatula or a folding motion with the spatula blade. No heavy stropping motion is used

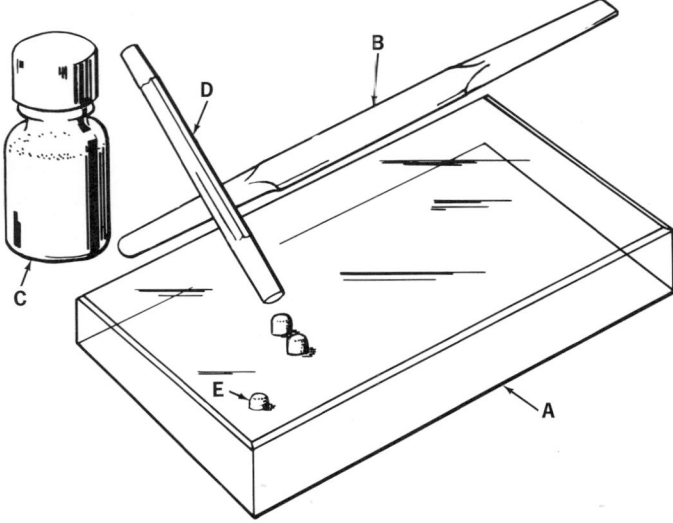

Figure 12-11 | Dispensing the silicate cement powder. A. Glass slab. B. Agate spatula. C. Powder bottle. D. Powder-measuring device. E. Extra powder from small end of dispenser.

Figure 12-12 | The division of the powder, the sequence of incorporation of the portions (circled numbers), and the mixing time for each portion. Note that the small amount of additional powder is not included in the portions.

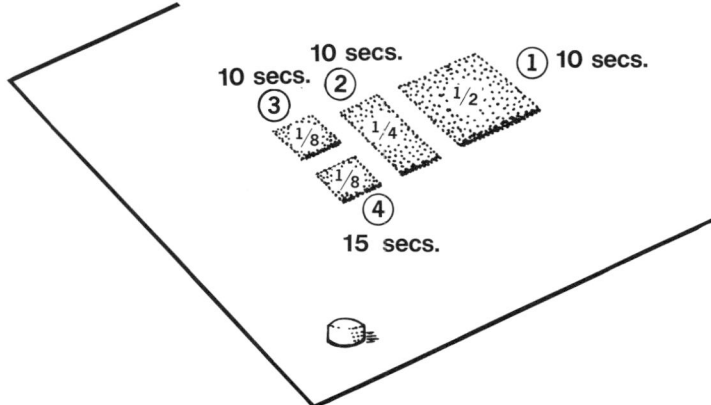

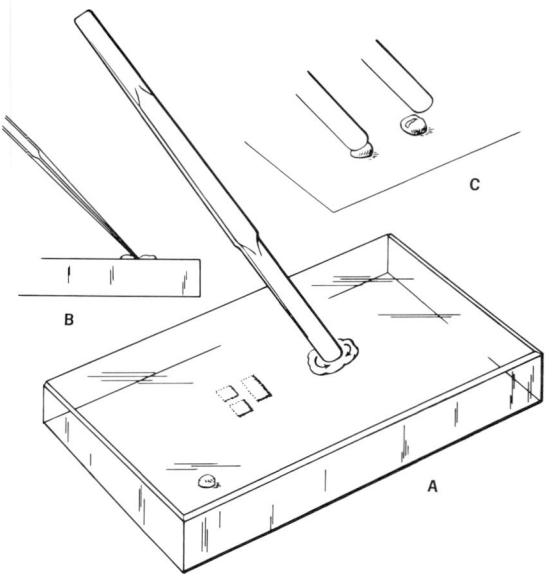

Figure 12-13 | A. The mixing is commenced by drawing the large (one-half) portion of powder into the liquid. B. The spatula is held at an angle with the slab, and a stirring motion is used over a small area of the slab. C. The completed mix should have a consistency which does not follow the spatula. Two light taps from the spatula should bring a liquid sheen to the surface of the mix.

as with zinc phosphate cement. Continue this manner of mixing with all subsequent additions of powder, endeavoring to wet every powder particle and to develop the thickest usable homogeneous mix in as short a time as possible.

8. Draw in the one-quarter portion of powder and mix thoroughly during the next 10 seconds.
9. Bring in one of the eighth portions of powder and mix thoroughly during the next 10 seconds.
10. From the remaining eighth portion, bring in and mix the required amount to develop the correct consistency. The consistency of the mix is correct when it does not follow the spatula and when two light taps of the spatula bring a liquid sheen to the surface of the mix (Fig. 12-13C). If no moisture appears when the mix is tapped, it is too dry. Such a mix should never be used. Never add liquid to a dry mix. Make a new mix.
11. The mixing operation can be completed easily in 45 seconds. The maximum mixing time is 1 minute.

Silicate cement may also be mixed mechanically similarly to amalgam. This requires purchase of preportioned powder and liquid capsules. Mechanical mixing usually is accomplished in 10 seconds.

The dentist generally places a cavity varnish or a lining of calcium hydroxide or zinc oxide–eugenol cement in the prepared cavity prior to placing the cement. The dental assistant should time his or her activities to permit the placement of the silicate cement by the dentist immediately after mixing. Following placement, the cement should remain undisturbed until set, being held in place by a plastic strip or other desired matrix. This matrix generally is kept in place for 5 to 12 minutes, depending on the type of cement used. Holding in the fingers a portion of extra cement which has been rolled into a ball is an excellent guide to indicate the setting time.

Immediately after the matrix is removed, the restoration is covered by a varnish (or wax, a cocoa butter preparation, or a silicone grease) as a protective covering, thereby preventing exposure to the air or to the saliva for the first few hours. The alert assistant will always see that the covering material desired by the dentist is ready for application. Exposure to air or saliva in the early "life" of this restoration causes serious damage to the surface material, making it soft, opaque, more soluble, and more subject to staining.

The final finish of the restoration generally is deferred for at least 24 hours. Because the setting reaction is only partially completed during the first few hours after the insertion, the silicate cement is too soft to finish properly by discing at the time of the insertion appointment.

The two most common causes of failure of silicate restorations are use of liquid changed through exposure to the atmosphere or by contamination and improper mixing technique. The previous statement emphasizes the role of the dental assistant in silicate cement restorations.

ZINC SILICOPHOSPHATE CEMENT

The zinc silicophosphate cements are basically combinations of zinc phosphate and silicate cement powders and are sometimes called zinc silicate or silicate zinc cements. They are classified as type I, a luting or cementing agent, type II, a temporary posterior restorative material, and type III, a dual purpose cement (luting and temporary restoration).

The primary use as a luting agent is in placing porcelain restorations, because the cement is more translucent than zinc phosphate cement and stronger than silicate cement. These cements are also used for cementing orthodontic appliances because of strength, low solubility, and anticariogenic properties due to the fluoride content.

The manipulation of these cements generally follows that of silicate cement.

RESIN CEMENT

Resin cement may be used for the cementation of inlays, crowns, fixed bridges, and facings.

Composition and Setting Reaction

The cement is the result of mixing a powder with a liquid. The powder is comprised of small particles of polymethyl methacrylate, plus a small amount of benzoyl peroxide, together with a filler and plasticizer. The filler and plasticizer aid in increasing the smoothness of the mix. The liquid is methyl methacrylate, with a minute amount of hydroquinone and some tertiary amine added. When the powder is mixed with the liquid, the resulting mix is fluid for a brief period of time, and then it sets to a hard resin because the liquid (which surrounds the powder particles) is converted by a polymerization reaction to solid polymethyl methacrylate.

The benzoyl peroxide in the powder and the tertiary amine in the liquid are termed initiator and activator, respectively, and are necessary for the polymerization to occur at room or mouth temperature. The hydroquinone aids in the inhibition of polymerization of the liquid during storage.

General Characteristics

The resin cement has the advantage of not being so soluble in the mouth fluids as the zinc phosphate, silicate, and zinc oxide–eugenol cements. The resin cement and the zinc phosphate cement have approximately the same strength and the same degree of adhesion to the cavity walls. These two cements also rate equally with regard to the amount of irritation to the pulp of the tooth. The disadvantages of the resin cement, when compared to the zinc phosphate cement, are the difficulties often encountered in cleaning away the hardened cement from between the teeth and the difficulties associated with a shorter working time. These two disadvantages have limited the acceptance of these cements since they do not provide other distinct advantages as luting agents.

POLYCARBOXYLATE CEMENT

One of the most recently developed dental cements is polycarboxylate cement. The cement is supplied as a powder which is modified zinc oxide and a liquid which is an aqueous solution of polyacrylic acid. The cement is somewhat weaker than zinc phosphate cement but is less irritating to the pulp and exhibits an adhesion to tooth structure. However, the cements do not adhere to gold alloys, resins, or porcelain. Thus, there is little advantage over zinc phosphate cement from a bonding action. The adhesive quality does present the possibility of attaching orthodontic brackets directly to the tooth surface, thus eliminating the need for bands.

The setting reaction between the zinc oxide powder and the polyacrylic acid produces zinc polyacrylate which acts as a binder for the unreacted zinc oxide particles.

Manipulation

The polycarboxylate cements may be mixed on a cool glass slab to slow down the setting time or on a disposable treated pad. The powder is dispensed by a powder-measuring device, and the liquid dispensed by a squeeze bottle. The proportions are approximately 1 $^1/_2$ parts powder to 1 part liquid by weight (1 scoop of powder to 3 drops of liquid). As with other cements, the bottles should be capped as soon as possible to prevent the evaporation or absorption of water.

A flexible stainless steel spatula is used to incorporate the powder rapidly into the liquid. Spatulation should be complete in 30 seconds to a smooth, creamy consistency for luting. When the cement is to be used as a base, the mix should be 1 scoop of powder to 2 drops of liquid; the resulting mix should be putty-like. Both consistencies are slightly thicker than zinc phosphate mixes for similar uses. The cement can be manipulated while shiny, but it should not be applied when it becomes stringy. The working time, including mixing, is about 3 minutes, and therefore a coordinated effort between dentist and assistant is essential.

Since polycarboxylate cements do adhere strongly to some materials, instruments used with the cement should be cleaned immediately after use. If the cement is set, it can be removed with a 10 percent sodium hydroxide solution.

In order to take advantage of any adhesive qualities, all surfaces to which the cement is to be applied must be absolutely clean and free of any oily materials, saliva, or medicaments. If surfaces are cleaned with water, they must be dried thoroughly.

RESIN RESTORATIVE MATERIALS

The continuing search for an ideal esthetic restorative material resulted in the introduction of resin material for restorative purposes in the mid 1940s. This material had the same basic formulation as the acrylic denture base materials with reduced spherical particle sizes plus the addition of certain chemicals necessary for self-polymerization of the material. One or two types of chemical combinations (catalyst/accelerator) are employed to produce the self-polymerization, namely, the benzoyl peroxide–tertiary amine combination or the sulfinic acid–thionyl chloride combination.

These materials at first were accepted as having great promise as esthetic restorative materials since they exhibited excellent initial properties. However, it soon became apparent that the anticipated results were not available due to the high coefficient of thermal expansion, poor abrasion and wear resistance, low strength and surface hardness, shrinkage during polymerization, discoloration, and recurrent decay around the restoration. Improved manipulative techniques such as the *brush* or *bead* technique helped to some extent in controlling polymerization shrinkage. Color stability was also improved by the manufacturer by changing the added chemical combinations.

Further refinements followed by the addition of fillers in the form of ceramic powders as fibers or glass beads. The intended improvement in mechanical properties did not materialize since the fillers did not bond to the resin, and the percentage of ceramic powder was too low.

The next change was the development of "composite" resins. In this group of materials the inorganic filler content of fine particles of glass or quartz was increased to approximately 75 percent, and these particles were coated with an agent (vinyl silicone) that bonds with resin (Fig. 12-14). The resin composition is also different. These materials are now available in a variety of forms, i.e., paste-paste, paste-liquid, and powder-liquid (Fig. 28-43). The use of composite resins together with the *acid-etch* technique of application to the tooth provide the most satisfactory esthetic restoration to date, since the combination of the newer material and technique exhibit greater compression and tensile strength, superior hardness and resistance to abrasion, lower polymerization shrinkage, good color stability, and a reduced coefficient of thermal expansion.

Neither the improved unfilled resin material or the composite resin material have universal application as an esthetic restorative material, nor do they replace the metallic restorative materials in stress-bearing restorations. Since both types of resin materials (unfilled and filled) are used by the profession, a discussion of both is included in this chapter. The acid-etch technique of application is discussed in Chap. 28. The application of pit and fissure sealants is included in Chap. 26.

Application Techniques

A number of manufacturers produce resin restorative materials, and each has its own characteristic and proper manipulative procedures to follow. It is important that the assistant follow the manufacturer's instructions for each material used and not attempt to apply a common technique to all resin materials.

Unfilled Materials

The unfilled resin restorative materials are supplied as a powder and a liquid. The powders are available in a variety of shades. A shade selector should be available to assist in the proper powder to use in a given situation. Two different techniques are used in applying the material to the prepared tooth. Each requires a different preparation of the material by the assistant. The *bulk* or *flow* technique requires the mixing of the powder and liquid, while the *brush* or *bead* technique simply necessitates placing the powder and liquid in separate small vessels such as dappen dishes.

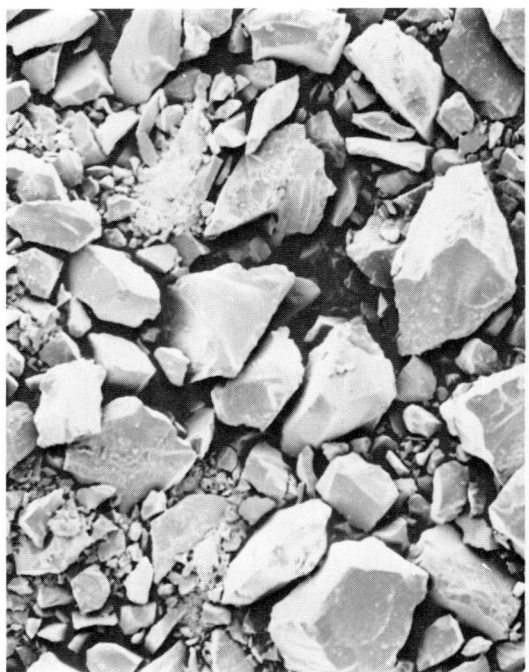

Figure 12-14 | Scanning electron micrograph of inorganic filler content of a composite restorative material. Note irregularity of particles. The matrix material is not present in this illustration. ×600. (*Courtesy of K. F. Leinfelder, University of North Carolina at Chapel Hill, School of Dentistry.*)

The glass-filled acrylic resins are manipulated similar to the unfilled materials.

The bulk or flow technique requires the mixed material to be of the proper consistency for successful application to the prepared tooth. Essentially there are five steps in mixing this type material (Fig. 12-15):

1. Place eight drops of monomer in the mixing vessel.
2. Add the correct shade of polymer to the monomer until an excess of polymer is noted.
3. Tap the vessel twice and then invert and discard the excess dry polymer with one tap.
4. Add three additional drops of monomer (four drops when room temperature is high).
5. Stir in one direction with a glass rod for 10 seconds.

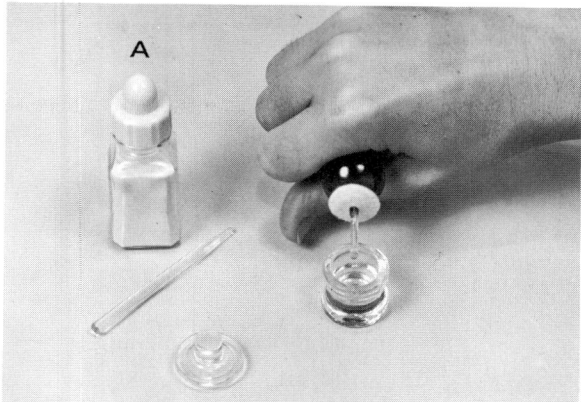
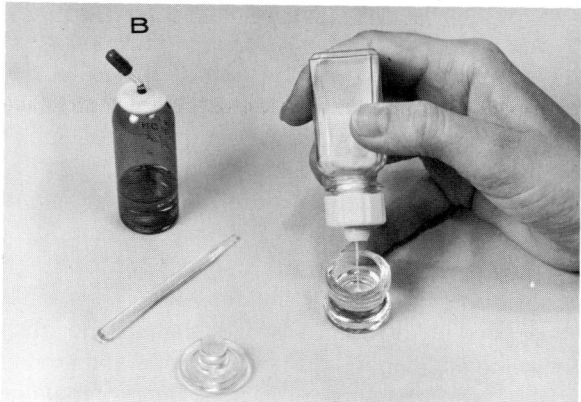
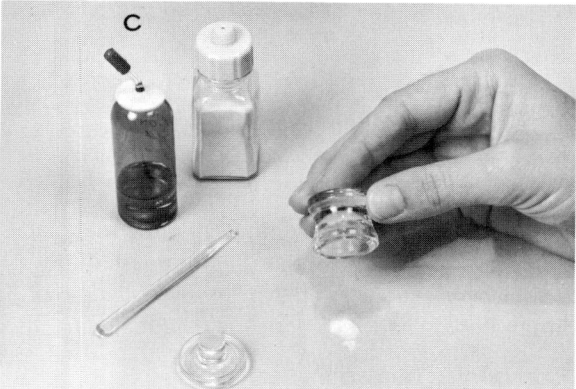
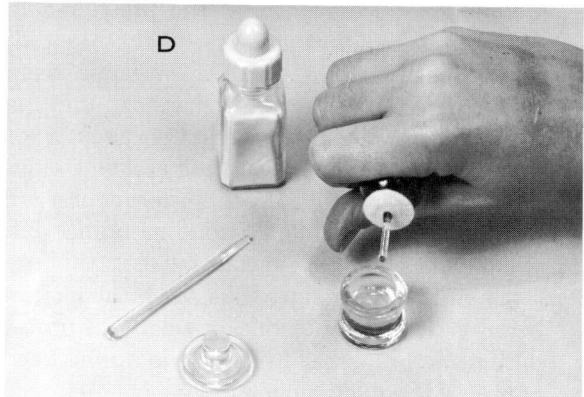
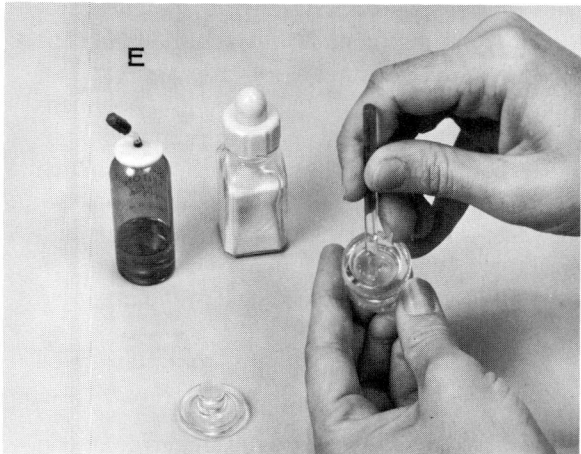

Figure 12-15 | Mixing resin for flow technique. A. Grasp liquid bottle in palm of hand to assist flow of liquid in dispensing eight drops. B. Add polymer (powder) to excess. C. Invert mixing vessel and discard excess polymer. D. Add an additional three drops of monomer (liquid). E. Stir with glass rod for 10 seconds.

The material is then ready for immediate use. It is carried in increments by an instrument (Fig. 12-16) to the cavity which has been treated with a primer or sealer, or it is placed in a small plastic tube and carried to the treated cavity. When the cavity is slightly overfilled, the material is covered either by a matrix strip or a special protective film, supplied by the manufacturer, to prevent the escape of monomer. The resin is usually hard in 5 to 10 minutes and, after the removal of the matrix or protective covering, it may be finished and polished. The dappen dish and metal instruments are easily cleaned by soaking in water, which separates the glass or metal from the set resin.

When the brush or bead technique is used, the assistant does not have to mix the resin material. Essentially, the resin is mixed as it is placed in the cavity. The assistant should place the following items in the setup: a small sable-hair brush (No. 00) either straight or angled depending on access, a gauze 2 × 2 sponge, and three dappen dishes. The selected shade of powder is placed in the one dappen dish and monomer is placed in the other two. The resin is applied by the dentist as he or she dips the brush in the first dappen dish of monomer and then in the polymer to pick up a small bead of material to be carried to the cavity. The brush should never be placed in the first monomer dish without being cleaned. An efficient dental team will operate in the following manner. After the dentist places a bead of resin in the cavity, he or she will hold the brush while the assistant wipes the end with the gauze sponge; the dentist will then dip the brush in the second monomer dish several times and hold it while the assistant dries it with the gauze sponge. Thus, the brush is clean before picking up additional powder. The procedure is then repeated from picking up the bead of resin through drying the brush until the cavity is slightly overfilled. If additional monomer need be applied to the material in the cavity because it is too dry, the same procedure is followed except the brush wet with monomer is not dipped in the powder. The chief concern is to prevent contamination of the monomer during the application process.

When the cavity is overfilled, a protective strip or coating is applied to prevent the escape of monomer or early exposure to moisture during polymerization. Finishing and polishing are the same as for the bulk technique.

In using either of the above techniques, unused monomer and polymer should never be returned to the containers.

Although the restoring of a tooth with resin material is less complicated than with some other restorative materials, the assistant must prepare the proper setup (including the surface conditioner and protective covering), mix the material properly when appropriate, and assist in the actual application. Therefore, a knowledge of the materials and techniques is essential.

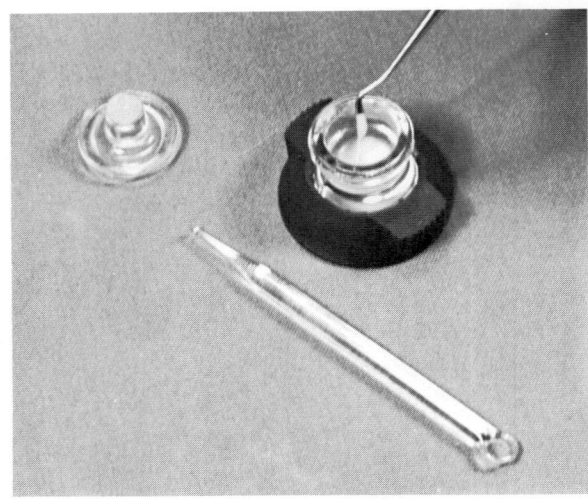

Figure 12-16 | A plastic instrument may be used to convey creamy mix to the prepared cavity. The small glass lid is used on the mixing vessel to prevent dust contamination of mix during insertion.

Composite Materials

The composite resin restorative materials not only vary in the manner in which they are supplied in the combinations of base and catalyst, but also in methods of color variation, polymerization activation (such as by concentrated ultraviolet light), and dispensing mechanisms (such as predispensed capsules). These variations necessitate different manipulation procedures and the manufacturer's instructions must be followed. The materials are placed in the prepared tooth by the bulk method.

Several considerations are common to all composites:

1. The filler particles are abrasive and irregular, and therefore a metal spatula should never be used in mixing since the filler particles will abrade the metal, causing pieces of the metal to be incorporated in the mix and resulting in discoloration of the restoration.

2. The materials should be worked at room temperature (75°F) since polymerization is affected by temperature. Increased temperature will shorten the working time, and cool temperature will increase the working time. Working time (from start of mix to insertion) averages from $1\frac{1}{2}$ to 2 minutes. When the material begins to set, it should not be disturbed.
3. Water may interfere with the reaction of the material. Thus all working surfaces, instruments, and the prepared tooth should be free of moisture.
4. Eugenol and other oils inhibit the setting reaction. Any oil that may accumulate during cavity preparation must be thoroughly removed from the prepared tooth. The composites should not be placed over a zinc oxide–eugenol base.
5. Since the filler particles are stronger than the resin matrix, finishing and polishing does not produce as smooth a finish as is obtained with unfilled resins. The best finish is that acquired as a result of contact with the matrix strip and as little mechanical finishing as possible.
6. Prolonged or repeated contact of the components or mixed material with the skin can cause a burn or allergic reaction. The skin so contacted should be washed thoroughly.

When the *paste-paste* system is used, one end of the disposable mixing spatula is used to place a small amount (about one-half the size of the restoration) of the base paste on the mixing pad, and the other end of the spatula is used to place an equal amount of the catalyst paste on the pad. The two pastes are mixed together thoroughly for 20 seconds, producing a stiff and homogeneous mass. The mixed material is then inserted in the prepared cavity with a nonmetallic instrument or a special syringe and covered with a matrix. The matrix should be held firm for at least 2 minutes. Upon removal of the matrix a sharp knife or a finishing bur is used for initial contouring. If additional finishing is necessary, it should not be initiated sooner than 6 minutes after the start of mixing.

The manipulation of the *paste-liquid* system and the *powder-liquid* system are essentially the same as the paste-paste system except for component ratios or specific mixing time instructions by the manufacturer.

There are several types of predispensed powder and liquid capsules available for use in a mechanical mixer (amalgamator). After the powder and liquid are united in the capsule the material is mixed 10 seconds if a high-speed mixer is used and 30 seconds if a low-speed mixer is used. Two considerations must be kept in mind prior to mixing. The capsule containing the proper shade must be selected, and the medium separating the powder and liquid must be broken to permit powder and liquid contact.

The wide variety of manipulation procedures of all composites cannot be discussed in detail in this text, only the typical techniques. Dramatic advancements have been made in resin restorative materials thus far, and continued improvements and new techniques are certain to follow. The competent dental assistant as well as the dentist will be expected to evaluate and utilize future refinements.

BIBLIOGRAPHY

American Dental Association: *Guide to Dental Materials and Devices,* 7th ed., Chicago, 1974.

Craig, R. G., O'Brien, W. J., and Powers, J. M.: *Dental Materials Properties and Manipulation,* The C. V. Mosby Company, St. Louis, 1975.

Leinfelder, K. F.: Personal communication, University of North Carolina at Chapel Hill, School of Dentistry.

Peyton, F. A., and Craig, R. G.: *Restorative Dental Materials,* 4th ed., The C. V. Mosby Company, St. Louis, 1971.

Phillips, R. W.: *Elements of Dental Materials for Dental Hygienists and Assistants,* 2d ed., W. B. Saunders Company, Philadelphia, 1971.

Sturdevant, C. M., Barton, R. E., and Brauer, J. C.: *The Art and Science of Operative Dentistry,* McGraw-Hill Book Company, New York, 1968.

13

James E. Overberger

Amalgam

INTRODUCTION

Dental amalgam is the material most often used for restoring carious posterior teeth. Its popularity is based on the simplicity of its preparation and ease of chairside insertion into the prepared tooth with a resulting restoration that is adequate in strength, hardness, and sealing qualities, and that provides good clinical service. Its major clinical deficiency is its tendency for marginal fracture. If amalgam is manipulated properly, a very serviceable restoration results (Fig. 13-1). Therefore, a dual responsibility between the dentist and the assistant is necessary in the placement of an amalgam restoration. The dentist must properly prepare the tooth and insert and carve the amalgam; the assistant must properly prepare the amalgam.

An amalgam is an alloy of which one of the constituents is mercury. Dental amalgam is an

Figure 13-1 | Polished amalgam restorations.

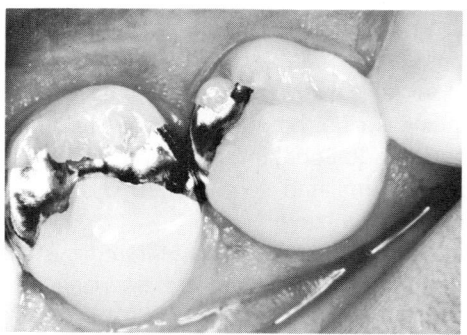

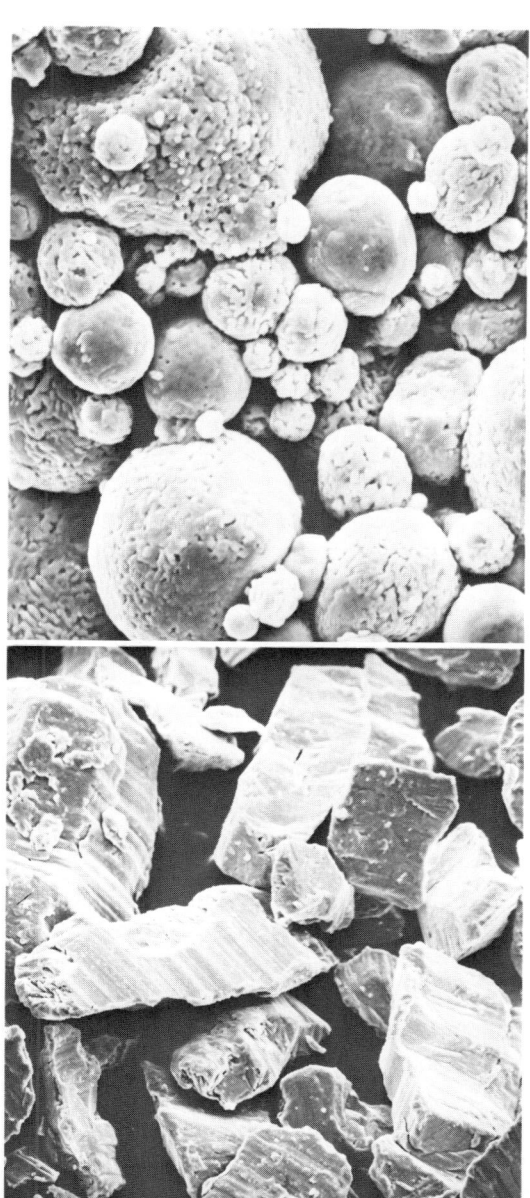

Figure 13-2 | A. Amalgam alloy spheres. B. Amalgam alloy filings. *(Courtesy of K. L. Leinfelder, University of North Carolina at Chapel Hill, School of Dentistry.)*

alloy of mercury with silver, tin, and copper, and sometimes zinc.

Mercury is a metal that is liquid at room temperature; it will combine or amalgamate with certain other solid metals and alloys at room temperature to form new alloys. If mercury is improperly handled, intoxication may occur. However, if simple precautions are taken, mercury can be used safely. Mercury is volatile at room temperature, and every precaution should be exercised to prevent inhalation of mercury vapor. The volatility of mercury increases with temperature, and it should never be heated. Offices should be well ventilated, and procedures should be designed to minimize spillage of mercury. If spilled, mercury should be cleaned up as soon as possible with a vacuum bottle with a water trap. Mercury as well as waste amalgam removed during condensation should be stored in well-sealed, unbreakable containers. Mercury should not be touched by the fingers, and finger cots should be used with techniques that would require contact of mercury with the fingers. The possibility of toxic reactions to patients from traces of mercury penetrating the tooth or from vapor during insertion of restoration is quite remote. The Council on Dental Materials and Devices has published in the *Journal of the American Dental Association* a series of recommendations for mercury hygiene that should be followed in all offices (1976).

Amalgam alloy is the complex, powder-like alloy supplied in the form of filings or spheres or a combination of these particles (Fig. 13-2). These filings or spheres can be supplied in bulk form in small bottles, preweighed and placed in small plastic packets, or compressed into pellets (Fig. 13-3). When the amalgam alloy is mixed with mercury, a plastic mass is formed (similar to a melt of other metals that takes place at elevated temperatures) that can be placed into the prepared tooth surfaces or cavity with special instruments under pressure, and the anatomic form of the tooth then reconstructed. The proper anatomic form and occlusion are developed by

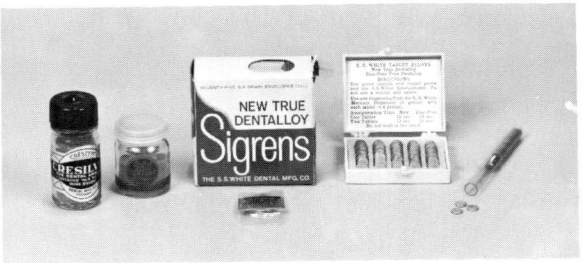

Figure 13-3 | Amalgam alloy in bulk form in bottles and in preweighed packets and pellets.

carving as the plastic mass hardens. Further hardening occurs, and the restoration is finished and polished at a later time.

One of the reasons amalgam restorations provide good clinical service is their tendency to diminish in marginal leakage. No restorative material chemically bonds to tooth structure, so that penetration of fluids and debris around the margins may be one of the causes for recurrent caries and failure. Under the best manipulative conditions, amalgam is only reasonably close in adaptation to the tooth structure. However, the amount of leakage which occurs initially diminishes in time due to the deposition of corrosion products or other debris at the tooth-amalgam interface (Phillips, 1973).

PROPERTIES

The main properties which characterize amalgam and relate to its clinical behavior are strength, flow, and dimensional change on hardening. A detailed discussion of these properties and their clinical application is somewhat complex, and only a brief explanation of interest to the assistant will be given.

Due to the complex nature of the amalgamation and setting process, minor dimensional changes take place with proper manipulation, and most amalgams exhibit a very slight expansion or contraction during hardening that has no adverse clinical effect. The specification for amalgam permits a limit of ± 20 μ/cm or ± 0.2 percent. Extreme changes as a result of faulty manipulation should be avoided to prevent either excessive expansion leading to protrusion of the restoration from the prepared cavity or excessive contraction leading to leakage occurring around the restoration. Most modern amalgams exhibit a slight contraction at the end of 24 hours.

The strength of amalgam indicates its resistance to fracture under biting forces and is usually expressed as compressive strength. Amalgam exhibits relatively high values for compressive strength but is low in tensile strength, and clinical failure often occurs when high tensile forces are exerted, as on the isthmus of proximal-occlusal restorations or at thin marginal areas. Amalgam does not develop adequate strength to resist the biting forces without proper enamel support, and therefore the cavity prepared by the dentist should be designed to provide a certain bulk of amalgam where stress will be applied and to prevent thin ledges at the marginal areas. Amalgam is low initially in strength but develops its strength fairly rapidly after placement in the tooth cavity, and the major portion of its maximum strength is reached in 3 to 6 hours. Newer alloys of very fine filings or of spherical shape develop their strength more rapidly than older alloys, and recently developed high-copper-containing alloys develop rapidly in strength and also are higher in final strength.

Flow may indicate the resistance of the amalgam to change in shape under biting forces and also gives an indication of the strength since the flow test as used in the specification applies the load before the amalgam is fully hardened. Time-dependent deformation of a fully hardened amalgam is called *creep*, and clinical studies have shown a relationship between creep and resistance to marginal fracture. Therefore, those alloys that exhibit low values for creep may exhibit improved marginal integrity. Typical properties of an amalgam made from filings,

Table 13-1 | Properties of Amalgam

	Compressive strength, psi at 24 h	Compressive strength, psi at 1 h	Static creep, %	Dimensional change, μ/cm
Filing alloy	54,000	25,000	3.72	−5
Spherical alloy	53,000	26,000	0.32	−4
High-copper spherical alloy	63,000	46,000	0.02	−6

Source: Adapted from Eames, 1976.

spheres, and high-copper-containing spheres are shown in Table 13-1.

These properties are controlled by the manufacturer in the formulation of the product so that optimum properties can be obtained. However, manipulative variables affect these properties, and thus all manipulation by the dentist and assistant also must be done properly for the attainment of optimum properties in the finished amalgam restoration.

COMPOSITION

The compositions of the various alloys on the market are similar. The average composition of a modern amalgam alloy and the composition limits as stated in the specification are as follows:

	Specification limits, % maximum	Average, %
Silver	65*	69
Tin	20	26
Copper	6	4
Zinc	2	1
Mercury	3	0

* Minimum
Source: American Dental Association, 1974.

To produce the amalgam alloy, these constituent metals are melted together and are either cast into cylindrical ingots which are made into small filings or atomized to produce spheres. Heat-treatment procedures are performed on the ingot, filings, or spheres by the manufacturer, as are other carefully controlled procedures relative to particle shape, size, and distribution to improve manipulation characteristics and to impart more desirable and stable properties to the amalgam.

Recently developed new alloys are the combination of conventional filings to which are added spheres of silver-copper alloy. Other new alloys are spherical alloys of high copper content. Both these alloys have copper contents above the specification limits. However, the specification permits deviation from the composition, provided the manufacturer supplies clinical and laboratory data to support the deviation along with the information about the composition.

An understanding of what each constituent metal imparts to the amalgam is also an important consideration. Silver is the main component and imparts high strength, low flow, high expansion, rapid hardening, high luster, and the silver-colored appearance to the finished amalgam.

Tin constitutes approximately one-quarter of the composition, and it aids amalgamation by its affinity for mercury. It reduces the expansion and strength and slows the setting of amalgam.

Copper is added in small amounts to conventional alloys to replace the silver and imparts high strengths, low flow, and high expansion to the amalgam.

Zinc is added to remove oxides and impurities during manufacturing and amalgamation. Since it is added in very small quantities, it has little effect on the properties of amalgam. Unfortunately, zinc will react with moisture in any form to form hydrogen gas which becomes incorporated in the amalgam and makes the restoration unsatisfactory. Clinical aspects of the effect of moisture contamination of a zinc-containing alloy are excessively delayed expansion leading to possible postoperative pain and growth out of the cavity; reduced strength; pitting; and blister formation on the surface of the amalgam. Therefore, any type of moisture contamination, such as contact with saliva, must be avoided to prevent these adverse effects. Alloys are available that do not contain zinc and do not exhibit the adverse effects of moisture contamination. Their use is justified where it is impossible to keep the operating field dry, such as in the mouth of the unmanageable patient. Nevertheless, all efforts should be directed toward the maintenance of a dry, clean field of operation regardless of which alloy is used.

AMALGAMATION

The amalgamation or setting reaction is complex and only a simplified explanation will be given. When amalgam alloy is mixed with mercury, the mercury diffuses into the surface of the alloy particles, and new, complex silver-mercury and tin-mercury alloys are formed, as shown in the following diagram:

Amalgam alloy + mercury $\longrightarrow$
    new alloys + surface-reacted particles

This reaction progresses rapidly during mixing and placement of the amalgam into the prepared tooth and continues for several hours. The alloy particles are composed mainly of the complex silver-tin alloy called the gamma (γ) phase; the silver-mercury alloy is called the gamma$_1$ (γ_1) phase; and the tin-mercury alloy is called the gamma$_2$ (γ_2) phase. The γ phase is the strongest of the phases, and the more of this phase in the hardened amalgam, the stronger the restoration. The γ_2 phase is the lowest in strength, and it is less resistant to corrosion. These new alloys or phases crystallize and bind the surface-reacted alloy particles, together causing the amalgam to harden and develop its characteristic properties. The amount of new alloys formed can be determined by performing an analysis of the mercury content of the hardened amalgam. Optimum properties of strength, flow, and dimensional change are achieved when the mercury content is below 50 percent. As will be mentioned in subsequent sections, all manipulative efforts are directed toward controlling the progress of the reaction so that the mercury content of the hardened amalgam is kept below 50 percent. If the reaction progresses too far and the residual mercury content goes above 55 percent (indicating the formation of the weaker phases), a drastic reduction of strength occurs, along with an increase in flow and creep. Also a greater amount of expansion will occur, since the amount of expansion is related to the amount of new alloys formed. It should be understood that once amalgamation has occurred, for all practical purposes no free mercury remains in the restoration.

With the newer alloys in which spheres higher in copper content are dispersed in filings as well as with spherical alloys higher in copper content, the silver-copper phase that is present reacts in time with the tin-mercury phase to form an additional silver-mercury phase and a tin-copper phase that exhibits less corrosion. This later reaction eliminates the undesired weak and corrodible γ_2 phase. Present data indicate that these alloys are higher in strength characteristics, improved in corrosion resistance, and lower in creep that may lead to improved marginal integrity (Craig, 1975).

MANIPULATION

The success or failure of an amalgam restoration greatly depends upon the techniques of manipulation, as manipulation controls the setting reaction and the resultant properties. Every detail of manipulation must be controlled and performed with precision for clinical success of the amalgam restoration. The following discussion covers the general aspects of manipulation of importance to the assistant.

Selection of Alloy and Mercury

There are many alloys available of varying particle sizes, shapes, and working qualities, and the selection of an amalgam alloy is a matter of personal preference by the dentist. The dentist should select an alloy that meets the requirements of the American Dental Association (ADA) specification. The mercury used must be pure and free from contaminating elements and must meet the requirements of the respective ADA specification.

Alloy/Mercury Ratio

The amounts of alloy and mercury used to make a suitable plastic mix of amalgam is referred to as the alloy/mercury ratio and indicates the parts by weight depending upon the alloy and technique to be used. The manufacturer's directions should be followed as to the correct ratio to be used with any particular alloy or technique, as this ratio is a distinct characteristic of a particular alloy, depending upon alloy composition, surface condition, and particle size and shape.

There are two techniques commonly used: the excess- and the minimal-mercury techniques. The excess-mercury technique employs an excess of mercury to alloy to allow the particles to pass over one another easily during mixing, particularly if hand mixing is utilized. After mixing, the excess mercury is removed before and during placement of the plastic mass in the prepared cavity. The usual ratio used for the technique is five parts alloy to eight parts mercury (1.6 times as much mercury as alloy), although newer alloys can be used at lower ratios such as 5:6. This technique can be used with all alloys and mixing devices.

The minimal- or controlled-mercury technique does not add the excess mercury before mixing; uses approximately equal parts of alloy and mercury, depending upon the particular one used; and eliminates the necessity for removing excess mercury after mixing. The usual ratio used for this technique is 1:1 (equal amounts of mercury and alloy), although the mercury content can vary 2 to 4 percent above or below this amount with different alloys. The least amount of mercury should be used which still permits formation of a coherent mix. Exact proportioning is required. This technique can be used only with a mechanical mixing device when alloys made of filings are used. The technique is usually used with newer filing alloys and with spherical alloys. This technique is the most popular technique, as it eliminates the necessity for removal of excess mercury from the mix, thus reducing the possibility of spillage and potential finger contact with mercury. It also establishes the precondensation percentage of mercury around 50 percent so that the desired mercury content of 50 percent or less for optimum properties can be more easily achieved in the hardened amalgam.

Regardless of which technique is used, the alloy/mercury ratio must be controlled for consistent mixes in the dental office and for the development of optimum properties. If too little or too much mercury is used for a particular alloy, the resulting amalgam will have poor properties.

There are devices available for dispensing amalgam alloy by volume or by weight; however, most dental offices use the preweighed alloy pellets or envelopes since this method of dispensing is more accurate and convenient. Mercury, being a liquid, can be dispensed accurately by volume, and there are many mercury

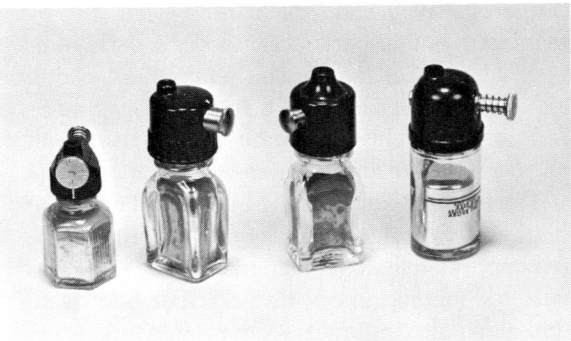

Figure 13-4 | Different types of mercury dispensers.

dispensers on the market that are quite accurate (Fig. 13-4). They should be held vertically and kept at least one-half full for accurate, uniform spills. Usually the manufacturer will provide settings or adjustments that will allow the proper amount of mercury to be dispensed for either the excess- or the minimal-mercury technique; otherwise calibration against a standard weight and adjustment of the dispenser may be necessary.

The desired alloy/mercury ratio must be established before mixing. The addition of mercury or alloy after mixing has started results in an amalgam with poor properties. The pelleted-type alloy and mercury should be kept separate until immediately before mixing to prevent inadvertent amalgamation.

Mixing

Traditionally, the alloy and mercury have been mixed in a mortar and pestle, but some form of mechanical mixing is presently more commonly used. Regardless of which method is used, the objective of mixing is to initiate the reaction between the alloy and mercury and to produce a plastic mix that subsequently can be inserted into the prepared tooth. The alloy particles are covered with a film of oxide and the mixing process (sometimes called trituration) is designed to disrupt the film of oxide so that the mercury can come in contact with the alloy particles.

Mortar and Pestle

There are several varieties of shapes of mortars and pestles available that are acceptable. Pestle pressure and speed are usually established by the convenient pen grasp which will result in a pressure of approximately 2 lb and a speed of around 200 rpm. If greater pressure is desired, a palm grasp can be used. The mortar should be placed on the bench top and the pestle rotated through the properly proportioned alloy and mercury with the objective of bringing the alloy and mercury into contact so that the mercury wets and coats the alloy particles and a smooth, homogeneous plastic mix results. The size of the mix will determine the time of mixing. For average restorations the mix will be completed in approximately 1 minute. The proper amount of mixing can be judged by the appearance and consistency of the mix and can serve as a guide for establishing the mixing time for the particular alloy and technique. When the mix develops a sheen, rides upward on the sides of the mortar, and tends to adhere to the walls of the mortar, the mix is complete. Hand mixing requires careful control to achieve a satisfactory and consistent mix.

Figure 13-5 | Different types of capsules and pestles.

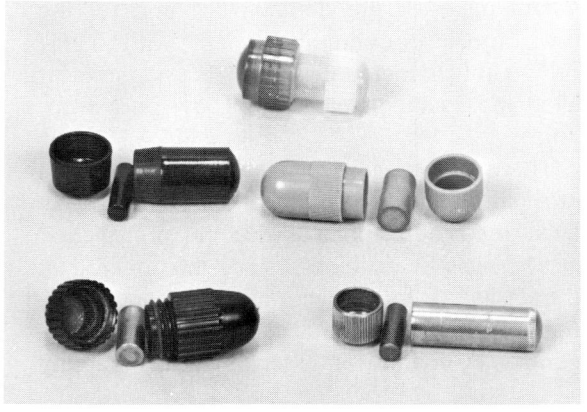

Mechanical

There are several mechanical devices available for mixing the alloy and mercury (Fig. 16-46). These devices rapidly mix the alloy and mercury together with a reciprocating or eccentric rotary motion. A plastic or metal capsule serves as the mortar, and a plastic or metal piston which is placed in a capsule serves as the pestle (Fig. 13-5). Screw-type capsules are preferred as they eliminate the possibility of mercury leaking from the capsule during mixing. There are available disposable plastic capsules and pestles containing preweighed quantities of alloy and mercury separated by a membrane; these are discarded at the end of mixing (Fig. 13-5, *top*). These are more expensive and do not permit a change in the alloy/mercury ratio. The proper quantities of alloy and mercury are placed in the capsule with the pestle, and the capsule is placed into the mechanical device. The timer on the device is set for the proper amount of time as specified by the manufacturer, the device is started, and the mixing is accomplished automatically. The operating speed of different mechanical amalgamators varies, and low- and high-speed as well as variable-speed units are available so that the correct mixing time as well as the proper capsule and pestle must be used as recommended by the manufacturer. The proper mixing can be determined by the consistency of mix. Using the controlled mercury technique, the mix should be shiny, coherent, and smooth in texture with sufficient plasticity to permit ease of condensation (Fig. 13-6). These devices greatly simplify the mixing procedure and provide for rapid, consistent mixes. The time of mixing is reduced to a few seconds, which expedites the use of multiple mixes for large restorations.

The capsule must be kept free of amalgamated particles. Removal of the pestle at the end of mixing, followed by several seconds of mixing in the amalgamator, will gather the amalgam into a ball and facilitate cleanliness of the capsule. Mechanical mixing standardizes the mixing procedure but requires careful control to achieve a satisfactory and consistent mix.

Regardless of which method is used, thorough mixing in which all particles are incorporated and uniformly coated by the mercury is essential. Undermixing should be avoided as it produces an amalgam with poor properties.

Condensation

After the mix is made it must be used immediately, and condensation of the plastic mass into the prepared cavity must proceed as rapidly as possible; thus close cooperation between the assistant and dentist is necessary. If the time interval from the end of mixing to the completion of condensation exceeds 3 minutes, the reaction will have proceeded too long with accompanying decrease in the desirable properties of the amalgam. Therefore, if the condensation procedure exceeds 3 minutes, the amalgam should be discarded and a new mix made. Several mixes may be required for a large restoration.

The purpose of condensation is to force the surface-reacted alloy particles as close together as possible so that the greatest possible density free of voids is obtained and with sufficient bind-

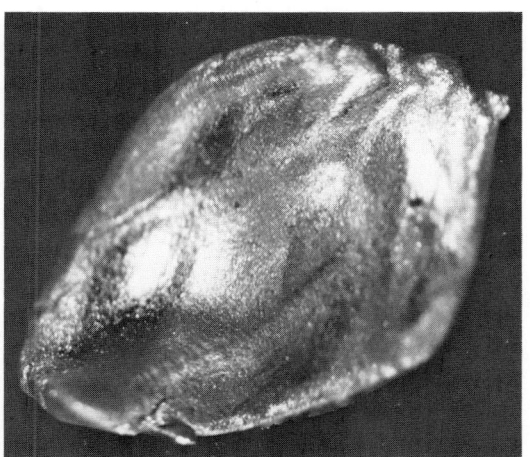

Figure 13-6 | Appearance of a properly mixed amalgam using the controlled-mercury technique.

ing alloys present to ensure a continuous structure. A second objective is to force the plastic mass into intimate contact with the tooth structure as the missing tooth contour is reconstructed. This compacting process is done with special instruments called condensers (Fig. 16-44). Condensation can be done with either hand or mechanical condensers of varying design characteristics (Fig. 13-7). Acceptable clinical results can be achieved by either method; the selection of the method depends on the preference of the dentist.

There are several acceptable condensation techniques that can be used with the excess-mercury technique. The techniques differ in the amount of mercury present in the mix before condensation and in the amount in each increment. Regardless of which technique is used, every effort should be made to remove as much mercury as possible during condensation by the use of as great a force on the condenser as possible with a use of a condenser that will be most effective in mercury removal. Generally, the more mercury left during condensation, the more the restoration will expand during setting and will flow or creep under biting forces. An increase in the mercury content also reduces the strength of amalgam. In the increasing-dryness technique, the freshly mixed amalgam is rolled into a rope in a linen cloth called a squeeze cloth and cut into several pieces. Each piece is squeezed in the squeeze cloth with finger pressure, using finger cots, to remove some of the excess mercury before insertion into the prepared tooth. The amount removed from each piece will depend on the preference and consistency requirements of the dentist; generally enough mercury is left so that slightly more can be removed or expressed under the condensing instrument; thus close cooperation between the assistant and dentist is essential. This squeezed amalgam is picked up with a special instrument called an amalgam carrier which is used to carry a small increment of amalgam to the prepared cavity (Fig. 16-45). The condensation of the increment is done with heavy pressure to accomplish the previously stated objectives, and excess, or "plashy," amalgam brought to the surface is removed and discarded. After the first piece is condensed, the mercury is removed from the second piece with heavier pressure so that each piece has less mercury. The compaction process is repeated until the tooth is reconstructed and filled to a slight excess. Often the remaining amalgam is squeezed with pliers to remove more mercury, and this extremely dry amalgam is used to "blot" the excess mercury at the surface.

When the minimum-mercury technique is used, there is no need to squeeze out the excess mercury before condensation. The freshly mixed amalgam can be picked up immediately with the amalgam carrier, carried to the prepared cavity, and condensed. During condensation less effort needs to be directed toward removing excess mercury since an optimum amount of mercury is already present. However, depending upon the particular alloy and the alloy/mercury ratio used, some excess mercury may need to be removed during condensation. Otherwise, the condensation technique or objectives do not differ from other methods.

The spherical alloys are generally used with the minimal-mercury technique and because of

Figure 13-7 | Mechanical condenser with condenser points.

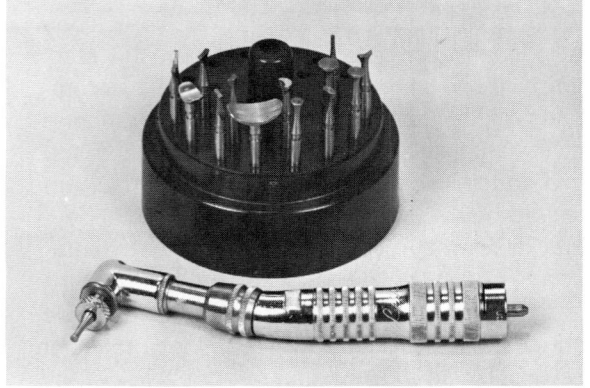

their round shape require less condensation pressure for proper compaction. However, spherical alloys have to be carefully condensed for good density and adaption to tooth structure. The spherical alloys are more plashy when mixed and generally condensers with larger working surfaces are used.

Carving

After the amalgam has been condensed and the missing tooth structure reconstructed, the amalgam is carved with carving instruments to proper occlusion and contour (Fig. 13-8). The amalgam must be sufficiently hard to offer resistance to the carver; otherwise, the amalgam may be so plastic that it may be pulled away from the margins and is difficult to contour. Most modern alloys set sufficiently fast that carving can begin shortly after condensation is completed. The carving should remove all excess amalgam from the tooth surfaces and leave the surface of the amalgam as smooth as possible. Burnishing or rubbing of the surface with an instrument with a smooth surface or with a wet pledget of cotton can be used to further smooth the surface and adapt the amalgam to the enamel margins. Care should be taken to remove thin fins of amalgam that extend beyond the enamel margins. Alloys of fine filings or spherical shape usually produce a smoother carved surface. The patient is cautioned not to place biting forces on the restoration for at least 3 to 6 hours to prevent fracture.

Finishing and Polishing

Final finishing and polishing should be delayed for at least 24 hours to allow the amalgam to harden thoroughly. The restoration is not completed until it is polished. Polishing makes the restoration more hygienic, more resistant to corrosion, more compatible to soft tissues, and makes the interface between the amalgam and tooth structure smooth and continuous and less susceptible to decay.

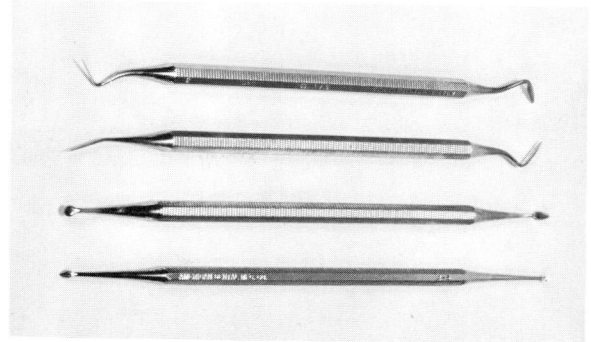

Figure 13-8 | Amalgam carvers.

The surfaces are smoothed and recontoured if necessary with finishing burs, abrasive discs, and other instruments, depending on the dentist's preference. Any excess amalgam not removed during carving must be removed; otherwise thin fins may be fractured during clinical service, resulting in a "ditched" margin. Final polishing is done with a mild abrasive followed by a polishing agent in a rubber cup or a soft brush. Frictional heat must be avoided during the polishing, as high temperatures can cause an alteration in the desired surface properties of the restoration.

BIBLIOGRAPHY

American Dental Association: *Guide to Dental Materials and Devices,* 7th ed., Chicago, 1974, p. 32.

Council on Dental Materials and Devices: "Recommendations on Mercury Hygiene," *J. Am. Dent. Assoc.,* **92:**1217, 1976.

Craig, R. G., and Peyton, F. A.: *Restorative Dental Materials,* 5th ed., The C. V. Mosby Company, St. Louis, 1975, pp. 178–179.

Eames, W. B., and MacNamara, J. F.: "Eight High-Copper Amalgam Alloys and Six Conventional Alloys Compared," *J. Op. Dent.,* **1:**98–107, 1976.

Phillips, R. W.: *Skinner's Science of Dental Materials,* 7th ed., W. B. Saunders Company, Philadelphia, 1973, pp. 302–303.

14

Roger E. Barton
Gold and Gold Alloys

GENERAL CHARACTERISTICS OF METALS AND ALLOYS

Metals

A metal may be defined as any chemical element which ionizes positively in solution. Atoms composing metals are arranged in regular formations with definite periodic spacing. This uniform arrangement in all directions results in a single crystal known as a *space lattice*. Metals in the solid state possess a certain characteristic metallic luster which is seldom duplicated in other types of solid matter. Metals also exhibit a definite fusion temperature. They are crystalline in character and generally are good electrical and thermal conductors. They possess high density, strength, ductility, and malleability in comparison to the nonmetals.

Many different metals and types of metals are used in dentistry. These metals are used as restorative materials or as processing materials in the construction of dental appliances. Some of the metals are used in their pure form, but the majority are used in the form of alloys.

Evidence has been found which indicates that gold was used for dental purposes before the birth of Christ. From that early beginning, gold has seen favor in dentistry even though new metals and alloys have been introduced for use in dental procedures. Gold and gold alloys still constitute a high percentage of all dental restorations.

Metalloids

Three chemical elements do not ionize positively in solution, but they do possess many characteristics of metals under certain circumstances. They are fairly good electrical and thermal conductors, but they are neither ductile nor malleable. These elements are carbon, silicon, and boron and are known as *metalloids*.

Alloys

The use of a pure metal in dentistry is quite limited; therefore, most common "metals" used are a combination of two or more metals. This combination of metals is termed an *alloy*, and may be defined as a metallic substance composed of two or more metals that are mutually soluble in a molten or liquid state.

When solidification of two metals takes place and the metals remain completely mixed, i.e., the atoms of the metals are scattered randomly through the crystalline structure (Fig. 14-1), the alloy formed is called a *solid solution*. However, in some alloy combinations similar atoms precipitate out at lower temperatures. In such a situation the atoms of one metal occupy a definite space in the crystalline structure of the other metal. These are *heat-hardened* alloys. Casting gold alloys fall in the above two categories. In the case of *eutectic mixtures,* where two metals are only partially soluble in each other, the metals precipitate as very fine layers of crystalline structure of differing composition.

The properties of solid solutions basically resemble the properties of the metals making up the alloy. Heat-hardened alloys are less malleable than many other alloys. Eutectic alloys are usually harder than the individual component metals, are relatively brittle, and the properties do not resemble those of the metals making up the alloy. These alloys usually have poor corrosion resistance. The eutectic alloys also possess a melting *point* rather than the melting *range* of most other alloys. They are used in some dental solders to take advantage of the decreased melting temperature.

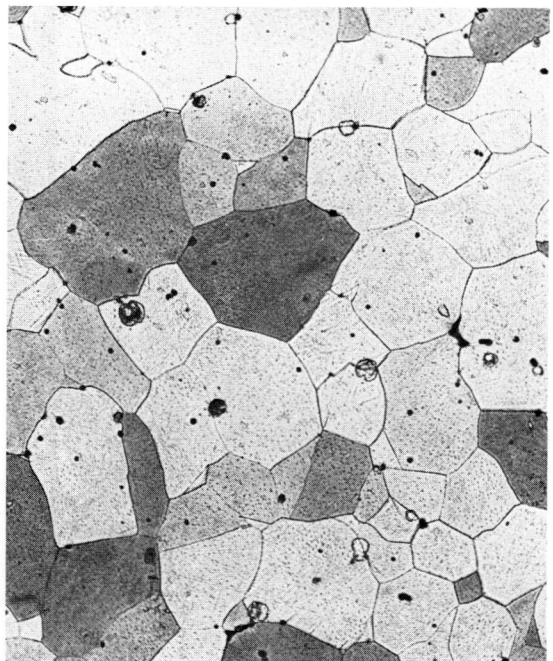

Figure 14-1 | Photomicrograph of casting gold alloy. This type of grain structure is typical of a cast metal. ×400. (*Courtesy of K. F. Leinfelder, University of North Carolina at Chapel Hill, School of Dentistry.*)

Properties

Pure metals as well as alloys used in dentistry possess many physical and mechanical properties that, to some extent, dictate their use. A complete study of these properties is in the realm of metallurgy and is not appropriate for this textbook. However, two terms repeatedly used in referring to metals are malleability and ductility. *Malleability* refers to the ability of a metal or alloy to be hammered or rolled into thin sheets. *Ductility* refers to the ability of a metal or alloy to be drawn into wire form.

PURE GOLD AND ITS MANIPULATION

Gold is an exceptional metal in that it is used in dentistry in its pure form; however, because of its extreme softness, it is not indicated for use in the mouth other than in the form of cold welded gold. Gold is the most malleable of all metals; accordingly, it can be rolled into thin sheets and beaten until it is so thin that it will transmit light.

Properties

Pure gold is a noble metal and will not tarnish or corrode in the mouth; therefore, it can receive and maintain a high polish. Other advantages of this material are (1) it is completely insoluble in mouth fluids, (2) it is capable of being adapted closely to the cavity walls, and (3) proper condensing produces great density. Properly constructed condensed gold restorations are considered ideal as permanent restorations. They do, however, have the disadvantages of high thermal conductivity, color, and difficulty of manipulation.

Pure gold exhibits the peculiar property of welding at oral temperature, provided that the surface of the gold is free from adsorbed gases and other impurities. This property is utilized in the construction of condensed gold restorations by forcing pieces of gold together in a prepared cavity, thus building up a gold mass by cold welding. The forcing of the pieces of gold together (condensing) is accomplished by gold condensers. The majority of condenser points have a small, flat serrated surface at one end. The assistant must keep these serrations clean and free of material to prevent burnishing of the gold while it is being condensed.

Types of Pure Gold

Pure gold may be referred to as a direct filling material in deference to gold alloys which are cast to form restorations in the dental laboratory.

Pure gold, as a direct filling material, is available in three basic forms: foil, crystalline or mat, and powdered. In addition, these basic forms may be classified as cohesive or noncohesive, and are available in ropes, sheets, strips, or pellets.

As previously stated, pure gold will cohere or weld to itself at oral temperature when placed under pressure and when the surface is clean and free of all impurities. The manufacturer will usually supply the gold free of surface impurities and classified as cohesive gold. However, since gold does attract gases, its surface may be rendered noncohesive during storage. On the other hand, the manufacturer may treat the surface of the gold with ammonia gas to protect the surface and produce a noncohesive material. Since ammonia gas is adsorbed on the surface of the gold and does not form a compound, it actually acts as a protective film against other elements. Some gases are capable of adhering directly to the gold and are extremely difficult to remove, thus preventing the gold from becoming cohesive. The conversion of noncohesive gold to cohesive gold will be discussed later.

Gold Foil

One form of pure gold used as a direct filling material is gold foil. Because of the great malleability of pure gold, it may be rolled or beaten into extremely thin sheets. The foil is manufactured in 4-in^2 sheets which are extremely thin and packaged in books of 12 or 24 sheets totaling 48 grains. Gold foil is also available in cylinders. These are produced by rolling the sheets to form a compact mass. In some instances these cylinders may be cut into small pellets before dispensing. The gold foil may be used to make up the entire restoration, or it may be used as a veneer over other forms of pure gold to complete a restoration.

In some instances, dentists prefer to use noncohesive gold foil for the bulk of the restoration and then use cohesive foil as a veneer.

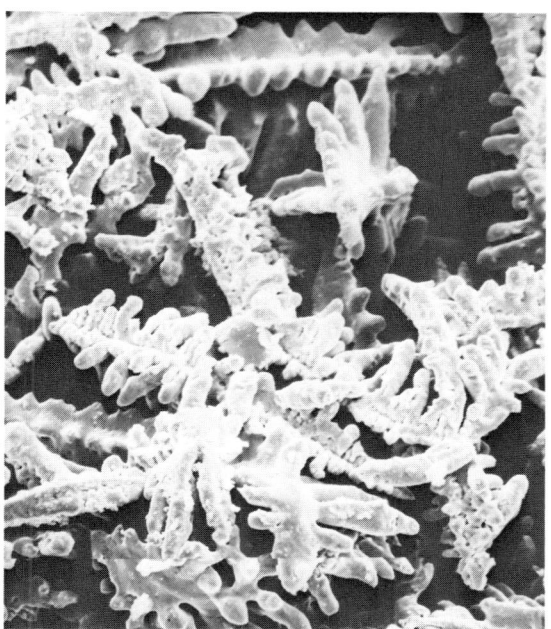

Figure 14-2 | Scanning electronmicrograph of mat gold. ×800. (*Courtesy of K. F. Leinfelder, University of North Carolina at Chapel Hill, School of Dentistry.*)

Mat Gold

Another form of pure gold is a finely divided crystalline gold (Fig. 14-2) prepared by electrolytic precipitation. This type of gold is available in narrow or medium strips about 2 in long. It may also be obtained in the form of cylinders. Due to the size of the crystalline structure and the amount of gold in a given volume, it is advantageous to use mat gold to form the bulk of the restoration to save time in condensation. However, it cannot be cold welded into as homogeneous a mass as gold foil and, therefore, it is usually veneered with foil to present a more suitable surface for strength and finishing.

Powdered Gold

The most recent form of pure gold to be used in dentistry is powdered gold. This material consists of very fine gold spheres pressed together to form pieces large enough to handle. However, in this form the pieces tend to fall apart upon manipulation. To correct this situation, some manufacturers wrap the pressed spheres in gold foil to hold them together. This type of gold possesses all the qualities of gold foil when condensed into a preparation, is easier to manipulate and condense than foil, and will cold weld as does gold foil; the pellets of it have a heavier mass than foil pellets requiring fewer additions of the material to the restoration, and it does not require a veneer as does mat gold.

Removing Impurities

As previously stated, in order for pure gold to cold weld the surface must be free from impurities. These impurities may have accumulated during storage or may have been placed by the manufacturer to render the gold noncohesive. When gold is purchased in the cohesive form, it is essential that it be stored in a closed container and exposed to the atmosphere for as short a time as possible. Exposure to the atmosphere will permit a number of surface gases to accumulate. However, regardless of the condition of the gold, all pure gold should be heated immediately before being placed in the preparation. This procedure is commonly known as *annealing*. Although the heating may remove some strain hardening, the primary purpose is to remove the surface gases and promote a clean surface. Therefore, the process of heating gold before condensation in a cavity preparation is more aptly termed *degassing*.

Degassing may be accomplished in an open gas flame, on a mica or enamel tray placed over a gas or alcohol flame, or by an electric annealer.

When one is utilizing the open gas flame, the gold should be held with a foil carrier, not with tweezers, because that portion of the gold touching the tweezers will not be cleaned. Care must also be taken that the gold is not melted by this method. Even with these precautions, this method is the least desirable because of the

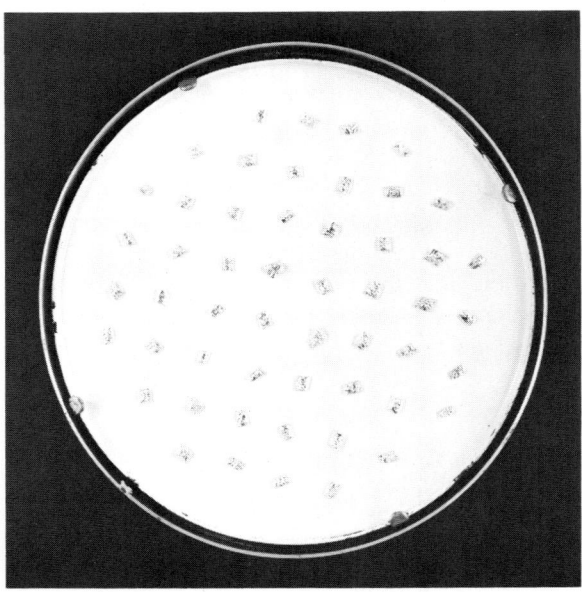

Figure 14-3 | Spacing of gold foil pellets on an enamel tray prior to heating.

It, naturally, eliminates the hazards of an open flame in the operating room.

Since the dental assistant will be primarily responsible for preparing the gold for delivery to the cavity preparation, it must be understood that a poor restoration will result from under- or overheating. Underheating (underannealing) will permit the retention of surface impurities and, therefore, will result in incomplete welding of one piece to another. This may not be realized until the restoration is completed and layers of gold begin to flake off. On the other hand, if the temperature is too high or the gold is heated too long the metal will become brittle, making it impossible to condense properly.

Condensation

Pure gold is condensed by a force applied to a condensing point by a condensing instrument; thus, each piece of gold is welded by driving it against the mass already placed in the prepared cavity of a tooth. This process strain hardens the gold foil, making it harder than pure cast gold. The degree of condensation depends, in part, on the size of the condensing point and the impact force applied. The condensation must be complete to ensure sufficient density and the hardness required for a permanent restoration. Properly condensed gold will have a density approaching that of cast 24-carat gold, and a higher Brinell hardness number than cast pure gold.

The condensing force may be applied by one of several means, depending on the preference of the operator. One method is known as the hand method and includes the use of a hand condenser and a mallet. When this method is used, the assistant will very often use the mallet to tap the condensing instrument lightly as the dentist moves it across the gold. Another instrument used for condensing gold is the automatic plugger. It is mechanically operated by spring action activated by pressure on the instrument.

The pneumatic condenser is the third type of

danger of the adsorption of gas due to the incomplete combustion of the flame and the possibility of uneven heating. If an open flame is to be used, the alcohol flame is preferred over the gas flame because it reduces the possibility of contamination of the gold.

In the degassing method using the tray, the gold is placed on the tray, which is supported by a hood over the flame. The pieces of gold should not touch one another while on the tray (Fig. 14-3), and the flame should be kept low to ensure a low degassing temperature. From 5 to 10 minutes of heating time should be allowed to ensure complete elimination of impurities before the gold is carried to the cavity.

The most desirable method of degassing is the electric "annealing" system. The electric bulk "annealer" eliminates all possibilities of gas adsorption and can be regulated so that the proper temperature (650 to 700°F) is easily maintained.

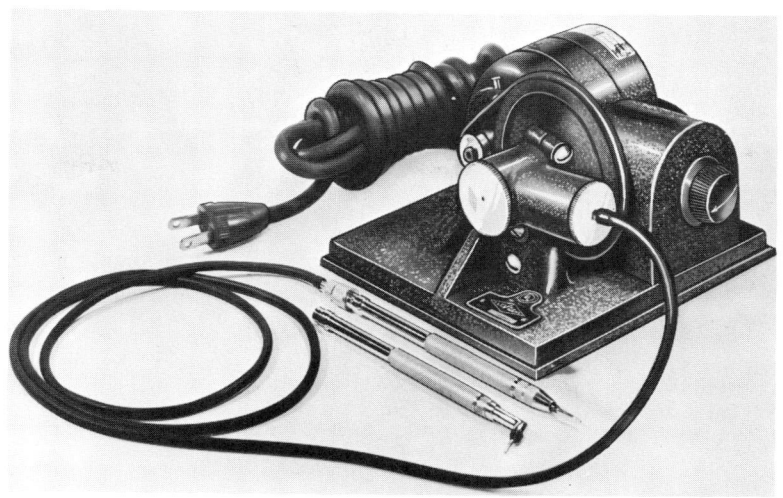

Figure 14-4 | Portable pneumatic condenser with electric motor, and straight and angle handpieces. (*Courtesy of Clevdent, Division of Cavitron Corp.*)

condensing instrument (Fig. 14-4). It is operated by means of compressed air which activates the plunger in the handpiece. The unit has an electric motor to run the small compressor. Another condensing unit is an electronically operated mallet with electronic control over the frequency and intensity of the blows (Fig. 14-5).

Both the pneumatic condenser and the electronic condenser may be used in condensing amalgam as well as pure gold.

The assistant, in addition to preparing the gold, should assume other responsibilities during the condensing procedure. First, the magnitude of the force of the condenser should be tested so that it is at a level that will be tolerated by the tooth and supporting structures and at the same time provide the necessary force for complete welding. Then as the gold is required by the operator, the assistant may carry it via a gold carrier directly to the cavity preparation. The gold should not be released by the assistant until the operator has begun condensing the particular piece. This team operation will save considerable time in building a gold restoration. The systematic placing and condensing of pure gold in a cavity preparation and the finishing of the restoration are discussed in detail in books on operative dentistry.

Figure 14-5 | Electronically operated mallet. Straight or angle adapter is placed on handpiece in foreground. (*Courtesy of McShirley Products.*)

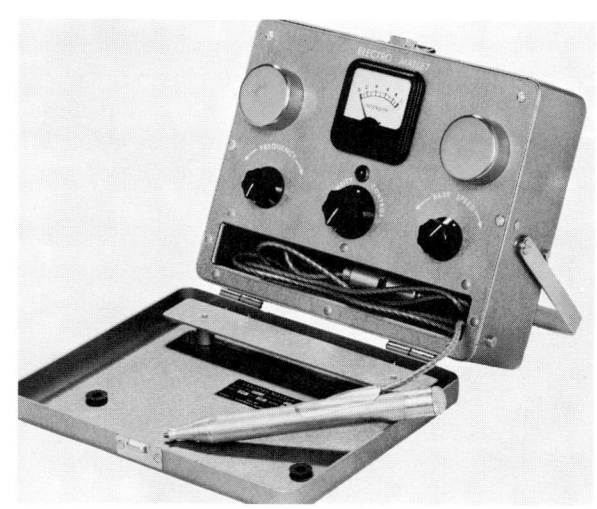

Chapter Fourteen | Gold and Gold Alloys | 249

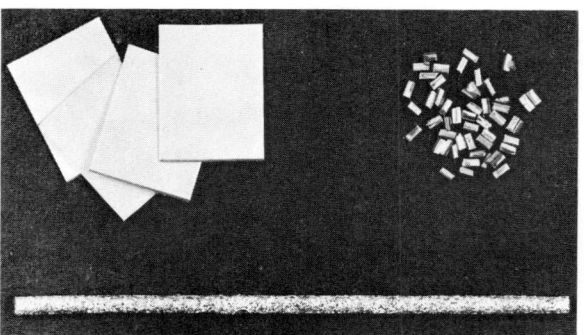

Figure 14-6 | Three types of gold used in dentistry. *Top left:* Casting gold alloy ingots. *Top right:* Gold alloy solder pellets. *Bottom:* Gold foil rope.

GOLD ALLOYS AND THEIR USES

In addition to pure gold, gold alloys are used extensively in dentistry (Fig. 14-6). These gold alloys may be divided into three categories according to their use as follows: (1) casting gold alloy, (2) wrought gold alloy, and (3) soldering gold alloy. In these gold-colored alloys, the principal ingredient is gold, along with such metals as copper, silver, platinum, palladium, and zinc.

Carat and Fineness

The gold content of a dental alloy is designated as either the carat or the fineness of the alloy. The *carat* of an alloy is based on the number of parts of pure gold, with 24 parts as the maximum. Pure gold would then be designated as 24-carat gold. A 20-carat gold indicates that there are 20 parts of pure gold with the remaining 4 parts composed of other metals. Gold foil is 24-carat; casting gold ranges from 14 to 22 carat. The carat is designated by the small letter k as indicated in 22k.

The *fineness* of a gold alloy is the number of parts of pure gold per thousand. Pure gold is designated as 1000 fine. An alloy of 850 fine indicates that there are 850 parts of pure gold plus 150 parts of other metals in the alloy.

The carat and fineness assist the dentist in determining the properties of the alloy and the tarnish resistance.

Troy Weight

Dental golds are dispensed on the basis of the troy weight system. The most frequent means of receiving gold is by the pennyweight (dwt). The assistant should become familiar with this table of weights in order to facilitate the ordering of gold supplies from the dental supply house. The troy weights are as follows:

24 grains = 1 pennyweight
20 pennyweights = 1 ounce
12 ounces = 1 pound (troy)

General Effects of Constituents

Gold

Gold is the principal metal in gold-colored alloys. The chief contribution of gold to the alloy is to increase its resistance to tarnish and corrosion. It also contributes ductility and malleability to the alloy.

Copper

The most important contribution of copper in a gold alloy is that it increases the strength and hardness of the alloy. Copper is also important in combination with gold in heat treatment of the alloy. It generally reduces the melting point of the alloy, adds ductility, and tends to impart its own reddish color to the alloy. Copper lowers the tarnish and corrosion resistance of the alloy.

Silver

Silver helps to reduce the deep yellow color of the gold by the addition of a whitish hue.

Platinum

The principal benefit derived from platinum is that it adds strength and hardness to the alloy. It also increases the resistance of the alloy to tarnish and corrosion and helps to whiten it. Platinum is used in moderation because it increases the melting range of the alloy.

Palladium

In general, palladium imparts the same properties to an alloy as platinum and is often used as a substitute for the latter since its cost is less. It will also increase the melting range.

Zinc

Zinc reduces the melting range of the alloy and also acts as a scavenger by combining with any oxides present.

Fusion Temperature

In simple terms, the temperature at which the alloy changes from the solid state to the liquid state is the *fusion temperature*. Alloys generally do not possess a melting point as do pure metals, but rather exhibit a melting range. The temperature range of fusion is supplied by the manufacturer of the alloy in most instances. In the process of making a dental gold casting, the alloy must be completely liquid so that it can be forced into the mold. The fusion (melting) temperature, therefore, must be within the realm of dental office equipment. The fusion temperature for most casting gold alloys averages about 1725°F.

Heat Treatment

The physical properties of some gold alloys, such as hardness and ductility, can be altered in the dental office by heat treating the metal. In dental terminology, there is softening heat treatment and hardening heat treatment.

Softening heat treatment is accomplished by heating the alloy for 10 to 15 minutes at 1292°F (700°C) and then quenching it in water. Note that this temperature is below the melting range. This treatment increases the ductility but decreases the tensile strength, elastic limit, and hardness. (Refer to the Glossary for definitions of these physical properties.)

Hardening heat treatment may be accomplished by cooling the alloy slowly (bench cooling) from the 1292°F temperature. In this instance, the tensile strength, elastic limit, and hardness are increased while the ductility is decreased.

The assistant should not attempt heat treating of a gold alloy unless specifically instructed to do so by the dentist, because the resulting changes in physical properties may not be indicated for the purpose for which the specific casting is intended.

Dental Casting Gold Alloys

Casting gold alloys are used to fabricate dental inlays, crowns, bridges, partial denture frameworks, etc., the combination of which compose the largest percentage of all dental castings. The base-metal alloys of the chrome-cobalt type are used in constructing denture frameworks but do not lend themselves to the smaller dental castings.

In general, the composition of casting gold alloys is as follows: gold, 70 percent; silver, 15 percent; copper, 10 percent; palladium, 3 percent; platinum, 1 percent; and zinc, 1 percent. In the white gold alloy, the composition is altered to increase the palladium and reduce the gold; the percentages of other metals remain relatively the same. The general mechanical properties of the two types of gold are similar, and they are used for the same purpose. The white gold alloy is not to be confused with the silver alloys or chrome-cobalt alloys used in prosthetic dentistry.

Dental casting alloys can be classified according to their hardness as well as their use.

They are classed as type I, type II, type III, and type IV. The various types differ in percentages of the metals in the alloy, thus changing the mechanical properties to best suit the specific need. When casting alloys are purchased, special attention should be paid to the type of gold desired and a check made by the assistant to verify the delivery of the proper type. The manufacturer will indicate, on the package, the type classification of the alloy.

Type I

These alloys are known as the soft alloys and are used to cast restorations that will not be subject to great stress during mastication. They seldom contain any platinum or palladium, and the fusion temperature range is 1800 to 1900°F. This type of alloy is quite ductile and can be burnished easily. These alloys cannot be hardened by heat treatment.

Type II

The alloys belonging to this group are used to cast most types of inlays and some crowns and bridges. This type of casting gold is the most popular for operative procedures. These alloys are known as medium hard alloys and have a fusion temperature range from 1650 to 1750°F. They contain a very small amount of platinum and palladium.

Type III

These alloys are termed hard alloys and contain the greatest amounts of platinum and palladium. Therefore, these alloys are stronger and harder than the first two types, are lighter yellow in color, and have decreased ductility. They are used primarily in inlays, crowns, and bridges that will be subject to great stress during mastication. They can be hardened by heat treatment. The fusion temperature range is slightly higher than that of type II alloys—1700 to 1800°F.

Type IV

This is a special type of alloy used for casting denture frameworks and is known as extra hard. Ductility is low in this type of alloy but strength and hardness are high. Because a large bulk of this alloy must be melted at one time in the casting procedure for a denture framework, the fusion temperature range is the lowest of all alloy types—1600 to 1700°F. The lowering of the fusion temperature is accomplished by replacing some of the gold content of the alloy with additional copper. These alloys are effectively hardened by heat treatment and may easily fracture if adjustments are attempted in this condition.

White Gold Alloys

The casting alloys previously discussed all have the characteristic gold color. The white golds have a silver appearance due to the fact that most of the gold in the alloy composition has been replaced with palladium and silver. The fusion temperature maximum may be as high as 1950°F. The high temperature creates difficulties in melting large quantities of the alloy with a gas-air torch. These alloys have low ductility compared with the gold-colored alloys and are, therefore, extremely difficult to burnish. Their tarnish resistance is also lower than that of gold-colored alloys. Although white gold restorations are as satisfactory as other cast restorations and more esthetic to some, the manipulation procedures are more critical in the casting operation; and they are more difficult to finish and polish. Therefore, the majority of white gold castings are made in commercial dental laboratories rather than in a dental office laboratory.

High-Temperature Casting Alloys

The most recent development in casting alloys are the types capable of having porcelain fused to the cast restorations. These alloys are not processed in the dental office due to the high fusion temperatures required to resist melting during the porcelain firing procedure and the special skills needed for processing. New alloys (some gold-colored) have been developed that have a high degree of rigidity and a coefficient of thermal expansion that approaches that of porcelain and is lower than the value for standard gold alloys.

In addition to gold, the gold-base alloys contain platinum, palladium, silver, and small quantities of iron, indium, and tin as hardening agents. A satisfactory degree of bonding occurs between the special porcelain and the alloy. As a result, esthetic restorations capable of withstanding the stresses of mastication can be fabricated. The porcelain fused to alloy restoration combines the strength and rigidity of metal with the esthetic appearance and abrasion resistance of porcelain. This type of restoration is being used, in many instances, in place of those where a porcelain facing or pontic is luted to a casting.

Remelting of Casting Alloys

A good casting gold alloy may be remelted several times without adversely affecting the proportions of the constituent metals. When this practice is followed, the proper melting procedure must be used and only alloys of the same type should be remelted together. It is a fairly common practice in many dental offices to remelt gold for casting with the addition of one or two pennyweights of new gold of the same type. In addition to adding bulk, the new gold adds zinc which is lost during fusion in the form of zinc oxide. Some dentists prefer the use of new gold for all castings, and the assistant who assumes the responsibility of the casting procedure should not remelt an alloy without the consent of the dentist. When remelting an alloy, special care must be taken to include only alloys of the same type and to have the metal free of debris and oxides. The same melting technique is used as for new gold.

Casting Shrinkage

Most metals and alloys shrink when they change from the liquid state to the solid state. Casting gold alloys follow this phenomenon in that they shrink within a range of 1.2 to 1.4 percent upon solidifying. Since the alloy replaces the wax pattern, which is an accurate duplication of the missing tooth structure, the resulting casting will be too small due to shrinkage. This fact requires special consideration during the investing and casting procedure in order to produce suitable castings. The compensation for the gold shrinkage is discussed in Chap. 15.

Porosity

Porosity in castings is not inherent to the procedure as is shrinkage, although it is frequently experienced as a result of faulty technique. Porosity should be minimized, since it reduces the strength and hardness of the casting; when on the surface it prevents acceptable finishing, thus leading to tarnishing; it is unesthetic; and if it extends through the casting, it provides a source of leakage.

The most common causes of porosity are the lack of sufficient molten gold bulk during casting; the trapping of gases and air in the molten metal as it is forced into the mold; mold not sufficiently heated; and the premature freezing of the molten metal before solidification of the metal in the mold. Porosity is not the same as incomplete casting although some of the causes are common to each.

Porosity can be minimized by following in detail the casting procedures discussed in Chap. 15.

Dental Wrought Gold Alloys

The appliances made from wrought gold alloys are not cast in that configuration. They are worked into the desired shape. Any metallic structure that has been mechanically worked into shape is called *wrought metal.* Wrought metal is used in dentistry to construct denture clasps, lingual bars, etc. Some orthodontic appliances contain wrought gold wire. The most common form of wrought metal used in dentistry is wrought gold wire.

The composition of wrought gold alloys differs slightly from that of casting gold alloys. The general composition is as follows: gold, 60 percent; platinum, 15 percent; copper, 12 percent; silver, 8 percent; palladium, 4 percent; and zinc, 1 percent. Nickel is sometimes included in wrought alloys in a small amount. In comparing wrought and cast alloys of the same composition, the wrought metals will have better mechanical properties due to the fibrous structure (Fig. 14-7) rather than the metallic grain structure found in cast metals.

The general effects of the constituents are the same as those in the casting gold alloys. The nickel is a strengthener of the alloy, but in excessive amounts it reduces ductility and the resistance of the alloy to tarnish. Heat treatment, both softening and hardening, is used frequently when fabricating appliances with wrought metal.

The fusion temperature of wrought gold wire should not be less than 1750°F to ensure that the alloy will not melt under normal soldering conditions. Just as important is the maintaining of low heat during any soldering operation where wrought metal is concerned. If excessive heat is used, recrystallization of the internal structure will result in the loss of the fibrous structure and a reduction of the desired mechanical properties.

Dental Soldering Gold Alloys

Soldering is the process of joining two metals by fusion, usually by the fusion of an intermediary alloy of a lower melting temperature called *solder*. This union of the solder and metal is metallic bonding and does not involve fusion of the metal parts to be joined. Gold alloy solders are used in dentistry for building up or forming parts of restorations, for building contour to gold restorations, for joining wrought metal parts such as clasps or wires, and for joining cast parts as in the construction of a bridge.

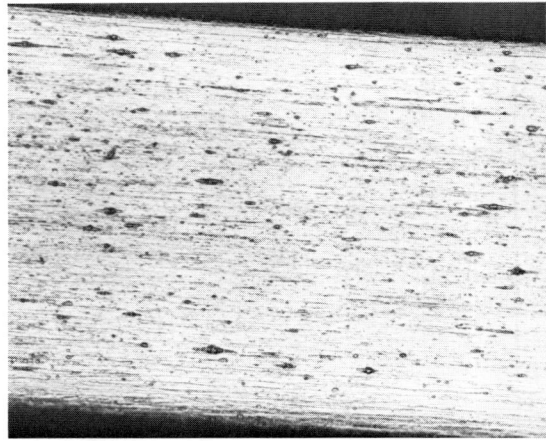

Figure 14-7 | Photomicrograph of a typical grain structure of a wrought metal wire. Note grains are elongated and fibrous in nature in deference to the grain structure of a casting metal (Fig. 14–1). ×100. (*Courtesy of K. F. Leinfelder, University of North Carolina at Chapel Hill, School of Dentistry.*)

The basic composition of gold solders is essentially the same as that of casting gold alloy. Tin is added to reduce the fusion temperature, and platinum and palladium are usually eliminated. In general, the composition of a gold solder is as follows: gold, 65 percent; silver, 16 percent; copper, 13 percent; zinc, 4 percent; and tin, 2 percent.

Solders are usually designated by their fineness. If, however, the manufacturer indicates gold solder by carat, the designation does not refer to the gold content of the alloy as previously discussed. When the term *carat* is applied to solder, it indicates the carat of the gold casting on which the solder is to be used. An 18-carat solder does not mean there are 18 parts of gold out of 24 parts in the solder, but rather that the particular solder should be used on a gold alloy that is 18 carat.

The selection of a solder for a particular application is somewhat critical because of the changes in properties of the solder with changes in fineness. The properties of most concern are resistance to tarnish, hardness, and the fusion temperature. In general, as the fineness number decreases, the fusion temperature and the resistance to tarnish decrease while the hardness increases. It should be apparent then that when selecting a solder, consideration must be given to the fusion temperature of the metals being soldered, the carat of the parts to be soldered, the stresses to which the soldered join will be exposed, and the ability to remove the appliance from the mouth for frequent polishing. As an example, when resistance to tarnish and discoloration is important, a solder of no less than 650 fineness should be used.

Dental gold solders are usually dispensed by the grain. For the convenience of the operator in the soldering procedure, they may be purchased in wire form, as cubes, or as squares.

Dental solders are known as *hard* solders, in contrast to the soft solders used by plumbers and metalworkers. Although they are termed hard, the fusion temperature is below that of the casting gold alloys and ranges from 1350 to 1550°F. The higher-fusing solders are preferred in most dental procedures for several reasons: (1) when a second or third successive soldering procedure is necessary, a lower-fusing solder may be employed without fear of remelting the solder previously used; (2) with the variety of fusion temperatures of the various casting gold alloys, the range of the fusion temperatures of the solders allows the use of one with a fusion temperature at least 180°F (100°C) less than that of the parts to be soldered; (3) the color and strength of the higher-fusing solders compare favorably with those of the casting gold alloys.

Requisites for a Dental Solder

An ideal dental solder should have certain general properties.

1. The melting point must be lower than that of the metals upon which it is employed so that these metals will not be melted during the soldering procedure. The fusion temperature of the solder should be 180°F below that of the parts to be soldered.
2. The composition of the solder should be such that it will flow freely, spread easily and quickly over clean metal surfaces, and penetrate small voids. This property depends upon the surface tension, viscosity, and adhesive properties of the molten solder.
3. It should not cause pitting of the soldered joint when the proper soldering technique is employed. The proper technique pertains to the distance between the parts to be soldered as well as to the cleaning and heating of these parts.
4. The strength of the solder should be at least as great as that of the metal to be soldered in order that the solder joint will not be a source of weakness.
5. The color of the solder should match that of the metal on which it is applied.
6. It must not corrode or tarnish in the mouth fluids, and its resistance to them should approximate that of the parts on which it is used.

The fineness of the solder dictates the degree to which the above requisites are exemplified in a particular solder. Since some of the properties change with fineness, the dentist must decide which solder is best suited for each particular type of procedure.

Considerations in Soldering Procedure

Dental soldering may be accomplished by either the freehand method, as employed primarily in orthodontics, or by the investment method, as used when joining heavier pieces than wire.

Briefly, the freehand technique utilizes a small pinpoint flame directed toward the parts to be soldered. These parts are held in the hands, flux is applied, a small piece of solder is fused to one piece, and then the pieces to be joined are brought in apposition over the flame until the solder fuses and joins the parts.

The investment method requires a longer procedure and is used when the parts are too large or too complicated to be held in the hands.

The first consideration in any soldering procedure is to have the surfaces of the parts to be soldered absolutely clean. Once this is accomplished, the surfaces may be kept free from oxidation by the use of a *flux* during the soldering operation. The flux may be applied in the form of a paste or powder. The most common flux used in dentistry is borax or a combination of borax glass, boric acid, and silica compounded into a powder.

As a precaution in the control of the flow of the solder, an *antiflux* may be placed on the parts where solder is not desired. A common method of applying antiflux is to mark the parts with a lead pencil.

Before investing, the pieces are temporarily held in position with wax and a gap between the parts of approximately 0.005 in is maintained to prevent warpage. A controlled soldering investment is placed around the parts, with only those portions to be soldered exposed. This step is often overdone, with the result that the joint is buried in investment, thus preventing proper heat from being applied to the area. As with other gold alloys, solder will shrink upon solidifying. This is compensated for by the use of the controlled soldering investment. An investment of high expansion is undesirable because it will alter the space between the parts to be soldered.

When the investment has set, the flux is applied and the entire unit (investment and metal parts) is heated until the metal parts become visibly red and the flux flows. At this stage the solder is added in the smallest amount possible to ensure a complete union, and the gas-air flame is changed from a brush flame to a thin needle-like flame which is directed at the joint area. As is always the case in melting metals, only the reducing zone of the flame as described in Chap. 15 should come in contact with the metal. This will allow rapid melting, protection from oxidation, and better control of the flow of the solder. If the solder "balls," it indicates that the surfaces to be soldered are contaminated, and the use of additional flux may be necessary. The actual soldering process should be accomplished in as short a time as possible. Overheating will cause pitting of the solder and will also reduce the strength and ductility of the parts.

Once the solder is observed to flow, the flame is immediately removed; the piece is allowed to cool for 5 minutes and is then quenched in water. This leaves the parts annealed and will allow the piece to respond to heat treating if desired. The piece is then cleaned and polished.

Successful soldering is an art that requires attention to details, patience, and practice. The preceeding information is basic, and if the assistant desires to become proficient at soldering, additional information should be obtained from dental-materials textbooks.

Welding

Welding is another means of joining metals. Gold foil is welded by *pressure welding,* in which the parts are not melted but rather are united by a recrystallization across the surface between the parts. Most other welding requires heat along with pressure and is known as *fusion welding.* In this method, the parts to be joined are melted and fused under heat and pressure. The fusion welding unites the parts by fusion, but does not employ an intermediary solder. Electricity now is commonly used to weld metals, and the spot welder is an instrument frequently used to join stainless steel orthodontic wires and bands (Fig. 14-8).

Tarnish and Corrosion

Metals used in the oral cavity will tarnish and corrode when not properly manipulated and finished in the dental office and when the patient neglects oral maintenance. Not only is tarnish and corrosion of metallic restorations unsightly, but the process may lead to the alteration of physical properties of the material resulting in the failure of the restoration or appliance. The conditions of the oral environment are conducive to tarnish and corrosion, and the best efforts of the dental team and the patient are necessary to maximize resistance to these situations.

Tarnish is basically a discoloration on the surface of the metal and is caused by the formation of hard and soft deposits on the surface of the metal. Plaque is an example of a soft deposit, while calculus is the chief hard deposit. Tarnish may be the forerunner of corrosion if not removed.

Corrosion is an actual chemical reaction between a nonmetal and a metal, resulting in a deterioration of the metal. Rusting of a metal is *chemical* corrosion. Elements contained in food or drink such as sulfur, oxygen, or chlorine plus various acids remaining in contact with metal restorations will result in corrosion. Good oral hygiene will minimize this chemical corrosion.

The oral cavity is also favorable for another type corrosion known as *electrolytic* or *electrochemical corrosion*. When two metals are placed in a solution that is capable of carrying electricity (an electrolyte), an electric cell (battery) is created. Since saliva, containing salts, is an electrolyte, and the metals used in restorations are bathed in saliva, batteries can be formed with accompanying current. When this situation exists, one of the metals goes into solution with a resulting surface roughness and pitting of the restoration. Thus, corrosion occurs.

When two different metal restorations come in contact, a *galvanic current* is produced causing corrosion and also causing discomfort to the patient. This is not common, but when it does occur it is very annoying to the patient. If the restoration is painted with a varnish, it will not be contacted with saliva, and thus the battery cannot be formed.

FINISHING AND POLISHING AGENTS

When dental restorations or appliances are constructed, they are usually rough and irregular. To

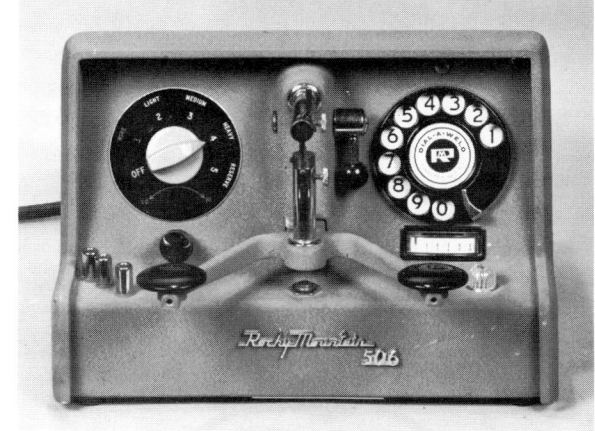

Figure 14-8 | Electric welding machine used to join orthodontic wires and bands.

be comfortable to the patient, to improve the appearance, to resist staining, and to resist tarnish and corrosion, the exposed surfaces must be smoothed to a shiny finish. To accomplish this, agents known as *abrasives* are used. An abrasive is a substance or material capable of cutting or scratching. Polishing is basically the utilization of finer and finer abrasives causing smaller and smaller scratches until they are undetected by the unaided eye. The surface will then appear smooth and shiny. A coarse abrasive is first used to remove all irregularities and produce the required contour and shape. This is followed by a series of less coarse and finer abrasives to create the desired results. In any finishing and polishing technique, the surface being worked on must be cleaned between the use of each agent to remove all remnants of the previous agent.

The degree or rate of finishing and polishing will depend on the particle size of the abrasive, the amount of pressure of the abrasive against the surface being finished, and the speed with which the abrasive is carried across the surface. However, this process (pressure and speed) also generates heat, and this is not desirable, especially in the mouth. Not only is it uncomfortable for the patient, but it may also damage vital tissue.

The dental assistant may be called upon to finish and polish in the mouth as well as in the laboratory. Recognizing the proper abrasive agents to use under various circumstances is very important. Some basic points to remember include: (1) Do not generate excessive heat by using heavy pressure and high rotating speeds; (2) use progressively finer grits, do not jump from coarse to fine; (3) clean the surface between agents; (4) do not use the same wheel (cloth or felt) for different agents; (5) use care in using coarse agents so as not to remove too much material; (6) do not use agents that stain such as rouge on nonmetallic substances; (7) hold objects to be polished firmly as they may easily be caught by the revolving wheel or disc and thrown to the workbench top or floor; and (8) do not polish the tissue surface of dentures or the internal surface of crowns or inlays.

Specific finishing and polishing procedures for restorations and appliances are at the discretion of the employer dentist. These instructions should be followed explicitly. Detailed information on finishing and polishing may also be found in operative and prosthodontic textbooks.

Abrasive Agents

Dentistry uses many abrasive agents of various coarsenesses or grits. They may be used as a powder, as a paste, placed on discs, impregnated in stones or wheels, or placed on cloth strips. They are used in the mouth as well as in the laboratory. Some abrasive stones and discs are illustrated in Chap. 16.

Diamond is the hardest known substance. Diamond chips are impregnated in a binder in the form of stones, wheels, or discs. These instruments may be used for finishing as well as for cutting tooth structure, but the chips are not fine enough for actual polishing.

Sand as a form of quartz is bonded to paper discs in coarse, medium, and fine grits.

Carborundum is actually a trademark for a compound of carbon and silicon produced in various grits as a powder or placed on discs or impregnated in wheels.

Pumice (Fig. 14-9) is ground volcanic ash and is produced in various particle sizes from coarse to fine. It is usually used in the powder form.

Garnet (Fig. 14-10) is a composition of several mined minerals and is used on discs and strips ranging from coarse to extra fine.

Cuttle is presently a fine grade of quartz, but its original name applied to an abrasive prepared from bones of fish. It is applied to discs and strips and is available in coarse, medium, and fine grits.

Emery is aluminum oxide and is placed on discs in coarse, medium, and fine grits.

Tripoli is produced from certain porous rocks

Figure 14-9 | Scanning electron micrograph of pumice. Note irregular size and shape of particles. ×400. (*Courtesy of K. F. Leinfelder, University of North Carolina at Chapel Hill, School of Dentistry.*)

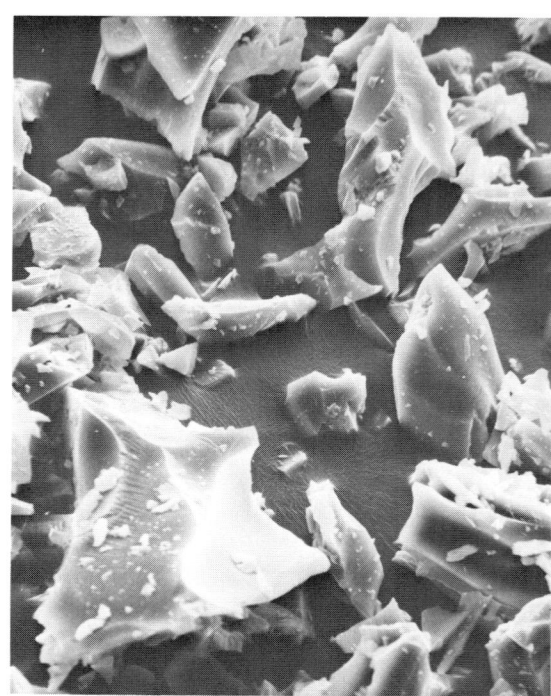

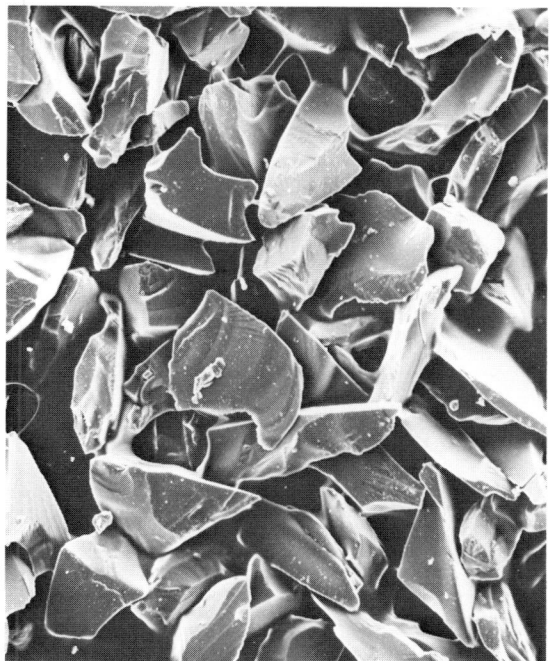

Figure 14-10 | Scanning electron micrograph of garnet particles. (*Courtesy of K. F. Leinfelder, University of North Carolina at Chapel Hill, School of Dentistry.*)

found in Africa and is a fine or mild abrasive agent. It is sold as a bar (as soap) and is used with a rag, felt, or chamois wheel. The wheel is rotated against the bar to pick up the agent and then moved against the surface to be polished. It is routinely used in the laboratory.

Rouge is a fine red powder of iron oxide produced in cake or bar form. It is used in the same manner as tripoli but is a finer agent. It is not used in the mouth because it may stain teeth and nonmetallic restorations. It is a fine agent for polishing gold outside of the mouth.

Tin oxide is a pure white powder commonly used as a final polishing agent in the mouth. It is used as a paste mixed with either water, alcohol, or glycerin.

Chalk is a form of calcium carbonate used much the same as tin oxide. It is also used in dentrifices. Both tin oxide and chalk when used in the mouth are applied to the area with a rubber cup attached to a prophylactic handpiece angle.

Dental Assistant's Role

Although the majority of metals used in dentistry take the form of restorations or appliances, the dental assistant may become involved in many ways before the restoration or appliance is placed in the mouth. A basic knowledge of golds, casting alloys, wires, solders, abrasives, etc., is necessary to order these materials correctly. The assistant may be required to cast an inlay, polish a casting, or solder in the office laboratory. When pure gold is used as a restorative material the assistant will prepare the material for insertion into the cavity. The assistant who is knowledgeable of dental metals will be of greater value in the dental office.

BIBLIOGRAPHY

American Dental Association: *Guide to Dental Materials and Devices,* 7th ed., Chicago, 1974.

Craig, R. G., O'Brien, W. J., and Powers, J. M.: *Dental Materials Properties and Manipulation,* The C. V. Mosby Company, St. Louis, 1975.

Leinfelder, K. F.: Personal communication, University of North Carolina at Chapel Hill School of Dentistry.

Peyton, F. A., and Craig, R. G.: *Restorative Dental Materials,* 4th ed., The C. V. Mosby Company, St. Louis, 1971.

Phillips, R. W.: *Elements of Dental Materials for Dental Hygienists and Assistants,* 2d ed., W. B. Saunders Company, Philadelphia, 1971.

15

Karl F. Leinfelder
Investments and Casting Procedures

DENTAL CASTING INVESTMENTS

Introduction

Cast restorations such as crowns, inlays, and partial dentures require a technique which is not only complex but exacting in every detail. In general, most dental casting procedures involve the *lost wax* process. Essentially, this method consists of developing a wax pattern of the object to be reproduced. The pattern in turn is surrounded with a molding material referred to as an investment. The entire ensemble is subsequently heated to temperatures sufficiently high to eliminate the wax pattern from the mold. At this point a gold alloy or other appropriate metal is heated to the molten state and cast into the evacuated mold. After cooling, the casting is surfaced and polished and finally cemented to the tooth previously prepared by the dentist.

Although the concept of casting metals by the lost wax process has been known for many centuries, it was only after the turn of the century that the technique was first used by the dental profession. Since that time however, technologic advancements have made it possible to produce castings so accurate that tolerances of 0.05 percent can be routinely attained.

Composition

There are a number of different types of dental casting investments depending upon the casting temperature of the alloys with which they are used. Regardless of the type of investment, however, they all contain three specific ingredients:

1. *Refractory material.* The refractory is added for a number of purposes. Primarily, however, it serves to not only protect against elevated temperatures but also to help regulate thermal expansion. The refractory material generally consists of some form of silica (SiO_2) such as quartz, cristobolite, tridymite, or some combination thereof. Refractory content of most investments for casting gold alloys ranges from 60 to 65 percent.
2. *Binder.* The purpose of the binder is to hold the refractory particles together as well as to control setting and hygroscopic expansion. Most commonly the hemihydrate form of calcium sulfate is used. The binder content generally ranges from 30 to 35 percent.
3. *Chemical modifiers.* Since the binder and refractories alone are not sufficient to provide the desirable properties of a casting investment, it is necessary to add other chemicals. Such additives generally include boric acid, graphite or copper powder, sodium chloride, and coloring agents. The graphite or fine copper particles provide a reducing atmosphere in the mold during casting. Without the reducing agent the surface of the casting would become oxidized and blackened at elevated temperatures. Sodium chloride in small amounts helps to eliminate the contraction caused by the binder and increases the expansion without an excessive amount of silica. Not only does the boric acid help to control the dimensional change of the investment but it also contributes to its hardness. Coloring agents are commonly used to help identify one type of investment from another. The modifiers usually constitute about 5 percent of the total composition.

In order to produce castings with any type of precision it is necessary to use an investment that can compensate for the dimensional changes which occur during the casting process. For example, when the gold alloy is cooled from a liquid state to a solid state, it undergoes a certain amount of shrinkage. Although the amount of shrinkage varies from alloy to alloy, the amount generally ranges between 1.2 and 1.3 percent. However, some precious metal alloys depending upon their fusion temperature may contract as much as 1.7 percent or more (Peyton and Craig, 1975).

To compensate for this shrinkage the investment must correspondingly expand to the same amount. Inadequate compensation for shrinkage of the gold alloy will result in an undersized casting. By the same token, too much expansion will result in a casting which will be larger than the original wax pattern.

In order to compensate for the shrinkage of gold alloys, the casting investment undergoes three types of expansion: setting, hygroscopic, and thermal.

1. *Setting expansion.* The setting expansion of an investment is the linear expansion which takes place due to the normal setting of the gypsum ingredient. It is produced by the outward thrust of growing dihydrate crystals. The proper combination of refractory particles and gypsum ingredient allows even greater setting expansion. The additional expansion probably results from the silica particles interfering with normal entanglement of the developing dihydrate crystals. Although the normal setting expansion of most inlay casting investment may somewhat vary, a value of 0.3 to 0.4 percent can be expected.
2. *Hygroscopic expansion.* If water is added to the mixed investment at about the time of initial set, the overall expansion will increase by as much as 5 to 6 times that produced by normal setting expansion. This is normally accomplished by adding known quantities of water to the end of the invested casting ring or merely by submerging the invested pattern in a water bath at a controlled water temperature. For all practical purposes hygroscopic expansion is actually a continuation of normal setting expansion. The addition of water at the proper time will allow further expansion of the growing dihydrate crystals by providing a greater space for crystal thrust. Although the amount of hygroscopic expansion depends upon the particular technique employed, it normally amounts to approximately 1.0 percent.

3. *Thermal expansion.* The third type of expansion used to increase the mold size is thermal expansion. This form of expansion is directly related to the amount and type of refractory added. As the investment is heated, the refractory ingredients undergo a change in crystal structure with a resulting increase in crystal volume. As a result an overall expansion will occur. At high enough temperatures expansion values of as much as 1.0 percent can be attained.

None of the three types of expansion is employed to its maximum. They are, instead, regulated in such a way that the maximum amount of expansion equals the total amount of contraction of the gold alloy.

Effect of Water/Powder Ratio

One of the most important considerations in handling casting investments is the use of a proper water/powder ratio. Increasing the water/powder ratio by only a slight amount, for example, will cause a decrease in setting and thermal expansion as well as a decrease in crushing strength. It is necessary, therefore, to carefully weigh or measure the investment powder and the water. Some investment materials, however, are available in premeasured packages.

Manipulation

All investments should be kept in airtight containers to prevent moisture contamination. Exposure to water will result in premature formation of dihydrate crystals which in turn may cause considerable and unpredictable changes in setting time, expansion, and strength of the investment.

Although the investment may be successfully mixed by hand, it is generally better to use a mechanical spatulator which is so designed that the mixing is carried out under vacuum. Such a technique will minimize the amount of air bubbles in the investment. Directions regarding water/powder ratio, time of spatulation, and heating technique should be closely followed.

DENTAL CASTING PROCEDURES

The objective in making or processing an inlay or crown is to cast an exact duplicate of the missing tooth structure. Since both the tooth structure and the gold alloy of which the casting is made are hard substances, accuracy cannot be overstressed, because neither substance can be manipulated to fit the other accurately in case a considerable discrepancy exists.

In general there are two methods that may be used in preparing for the casting procedure. They include the thermal expansion method or *high-heat* technique and the hygroscopic expansion method or *low-heat* technique. In the high-heat technique an investment of high thermal expansion is used, together with a furnace temperature of 1250 to 1300°F (677 to 704°C), to provide the principal means of acquiring the compensating expansion. In the second method, a hygroscopic investment is used, together with a furnace temperature of 900 to 950°F (482 to 510°C). Since the manufacturer designates, in some form, the type of investment in the container, a compatible technique of investing and furnace treatment must be followed.

The Wax Pattern

There are two general methods for obtaining the wax pattern, namely direct and indirect methods. The first consists of forming the pattern directly in the cavity preparation by the dentist. The pattern is then removed from the tooth, placed on a sprue pin, and invested in preparation for casting. The use of such a technique has declined in popularity, and presently the technique is used relatively little.

The indirect method, on the other hand, con-

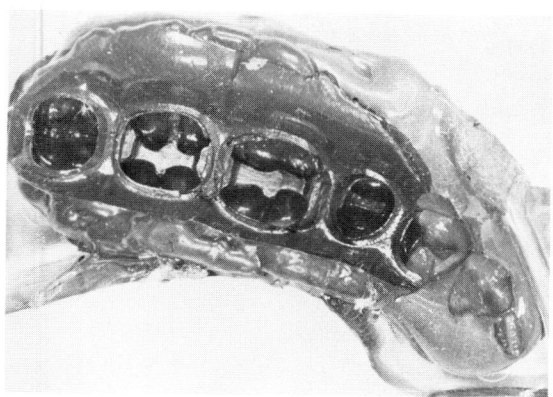

Figure 15-1 | A quadrant impression taken with a rubber-base impression in a stock plastic tray in which the die and model are poured.

sists of developing the wax pattern outside of the mouth, usually by a technician. The pattern in this case is constructed on a model or a die of the prepared tooth obtained from an impression.

The procedure for obtaining the die for purposes of waxing the pattern consists first of taking an impression of the prepared tooth or teeth. Although a number of impression materials may be used, the most common generally consists of either polysulfide or silicone rubber base. The type of material used is up to the discretion of the dentist. After the impression is removed from the mouth (Fig. 15-1), the coronal portions of the teeth in the impression are filled with a high-strength dental stone (die or improved stone). At this point dowel pins are placed into the poured stone so that they extend from the impression in a vertical and parallel manner (Fig. 15-2). Two unused dowel pins can be seen in the foreground. When the die stone has hardened a separating agent is placed on the surface and then cast stone is poured on top. Once the stone has hardened the individual teeth containing the dowel pins can be removed from the casts (Fig. 15-3). Instead of pouring the impression with die stone, the impression can be electroplated with silver or copper and thereby provide the dentist or technician with a die that is substantially harder and more abrasion resistant than the conventional stone die.

It should be remembered that the die is a reproduction of the prepared tooth and any fault on the die will cause a discrepancy in the fit of the restoration. It must, therefore, be constructed and handled with care to help ensure a satisfactory result.

Once the die has been properly constructed and the margin of the preparation clearly defined, it is coated with a lubricant of a fine film thickness. The purpose of the thin film (die separator) is to prevent the molten wax from adhering to the surface by sealing off any microporosity on the surface of the die. Excess application of the lubricant should be avoided so as not to impair close adaptation of the wax to the walls of the cavity preparation. To be effective the lubricant needs to be dry before wax is applied.

The inlay wax may be applied to the stone die in a number of acceptable ways. The best method, however, consists of flowing the wax onto the die to ensure uniform adaptation and then to cool it under pressure. Such a technique

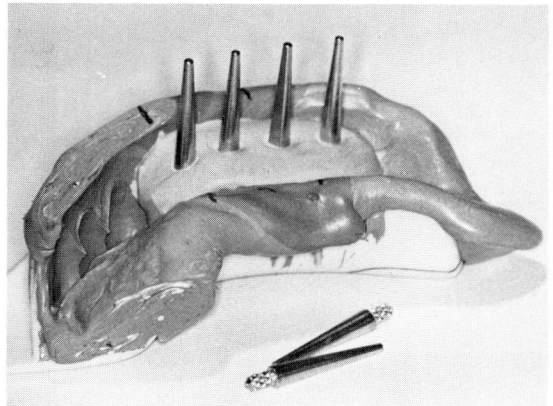

Figure 15-2 | Coronal portion of impression filled with die stone after which dowel pins are inserted in a vertical and parallel manner.

prevents the wax from pulling away from the margins as it shrinks. It also aids in minimizing distortion or warpage of the pattern. Furthermore, the wax should not be overheated, worked excessively, reheated more than absolutely necessary, or subjected to wide temperature changes once it is formed.

After the wax is properly cooled under pressure, it is carved to shape with one or more of a variety of wax instruments. Another technique for fabricating a wax pattern consists of adding wax in small increments until normal shape and functional relationships are attained. The wax pattern is frequently contoured to shape using a warmed carving instrument. Such a technique facilitates easy removal of wax with little pressure and thereby helps to preserve the margins of the die when carving in such areas.

Once the pattern has been completed, the surface is polished with a smooth, soft cloth or flame-polished while still on the die. The smoother the surface of the pattern, the easier it will be to finish and polish the casting. Just prior to removal of the pattern from the die all margins are carefully examined for discrepancies. If the margins have pulled away from the die, they must be readapted with a heated instrument.

In most practices there is little time for the dentist to fabricate the wax pattern. Instead the dentist normally relegates this duty to a laboratory technician who in part has been trained for this purpose. In some instances, however, the dentist may prefer to "wax-up" the patterns personally. Under normal circumstances the dental assistant will not carve the wax patterns. However, with a sufficient background and under the guidance of the dentist it is possible that the dental assistant may assume this responsibility.

Spruing

Once the pattern has been completed, the next step in the casting process is to place a sprue pin on the wax pattern (Fig. 15-4). The purpose of the sprue pin or ingate is to form a channel

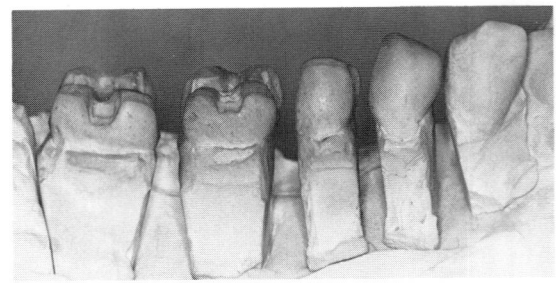

Figure 15-3 | Cast containing removable dies.

through which the molten metal can flow into the evacuated mold. The diameter and length of this channel is of utmost importance in its influence on the soundness of the casting. When the evacuated mold fills with the molten metal and the temperature decreases, solidification will begin. As the alloy solidifies, it is accompanied by shrinkage. Simultaneously, additional molten alloy flows through the channel to compensate for this shrinkage. It is imperative, then, that the channel remain open or unsolidified at least until the entire mold chamber has solidified. If the

Figure 15-4 | Attachment of sprue pin to wax pattern. A collar or fillet is formed at the area of attachment of sprue pin to wax pattern. Such an arrangement prevents the onrushing molten alloy from breaking off investment particles into the mold chamber.

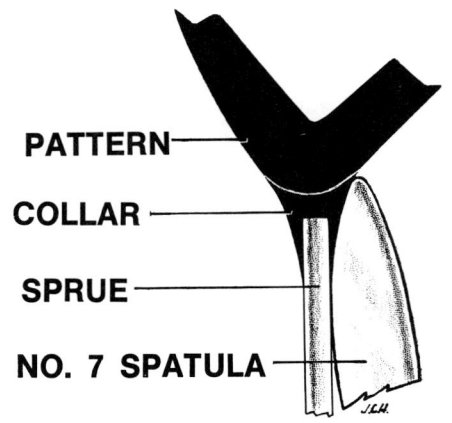

sprue pin is too narrow, for example, the channelway will solidify prematurely, and as a result the supply of molten alloy necessary to compensate for casting shrinkage will be unavailable. Such a casting will be clinically unacceptable because of large voids at the junction of the sprue pin and the casting surface. The size of the sprue pin, therefore, depends upon the size and thickness of the wax pattern. The diameter of the sprue pin should not be smaller than the thickest portion of the wax pattern. A sprue pin with an excessively large diameter, on the other hand, may also cause problems serious enough to prevent the casting from being usable. If the diameter of the sprue pin is great enough, the molten alloy will enter the mold so rapidly that a higher than desired cooling rate will occur. As a result gases within the mold become entrapped in the alloy. Such castings may have rounded and incomplete margins.

The thickest portion of the pattern is generally designated as the location for the sprue pin. A small bead of inlay or sticky wax is added to this portion, and the warmed end of the sprue pin is inserted into this soft, added wax. If the warm end of the sprue pin is inserted into the pattern proper, a distortion of the pattern may occur. The direction of the sprue should be such as to cause the least change in direction of the molten gold while it is flowing into the mold.

A small collar or fillet of inlay or sticky wax (Fig. 15-4) is added to this area of attachment in a uniform manner to aid in securing the pattern firmly to the sprue.

The sprued pattern is then mounted on a sprue base by carrying the sprue pin with pointed-tip serrated pliers and inserting the free end of the sprue into the base. The length of the sprue pin (distance from junction of the pattern to top of the sprue base) should be approximately ⅜ in (8 to 9 mm). After the sprued wax pattern is placed on the sprue base, additional wax should be added to the union of the two to provide stabilization during the investing procedure. When placed inside the casting ring (Fig.

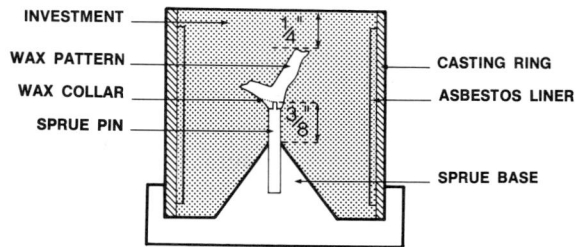

Figure 15-5 | Cross section of sprued and invested wax pattern.

15-5), the top of the wax pattern should be approximately ¼ in (6 to 7 mm) from the open end of the casting ring.

If the pattern is closer than ¼ in (6 to 7 mm) to the end of the ring, the force of the molten metal hitting the investment during casting may cause the investment to break, with the result that the gold will pass through the mold. On the other hand, if it is more than ¼ in (6 to 7 mm) from the end, the air in the mold may not be forced out through the porous investment as the molten gold enters. If this air is not eliminated, incomplete castings result.

Before the mounted wax pattern is placed inside the casting ring, the inside surface of the ring is lined with a layer of asbestos. The purpose of the asbestos liner is to provide a cushion for the expanding investment mold. Note that as seen in Fig. 15-5 this liner is short of both ends of the ring. This arrangement is necessary so as to lock the liner inside the ring. The casting ring could otherwise separate from the investment before the casting has been made. The purpose of the casting ring is to give support to the invested mold during the casting procedure.

Investing

Essentially there are two methods for investing wax patterns. The first is a vacuum investing technique whereas the other is a hand investing procedure. The mechanical investing method (Fig. 15-6) consists of mixing the investment powder and water under vacuum and subsequently filling the casting ring containing the wax pattern which is also under vacuum. The amount of air in the investment material as well as the casting ring is reduced to such a degree that the investment will adapt smoothly to the wax pattern. If the vacuum is insufficient, bubbles or nodules will occur on the surface of the casting. These defects which range in size can be removed without too much trouble if they occur on the outside surface of the casting. If, however, they occur on the margins or on the internal surface, the crown or inlay may not be salvageable.

Care must be taken not to overmix the investment when using the mechanical investor. Overspatulation will affect the setting time of the investment as well as the setting expansion. The recommended water/powder ratio as well as time of mixing is given by the manufacturer of each investment material.

The hand investing method is used less frequently than the mechanical mixing procedure, because results are more subject to variation. The technique consists of first dispensing the appropriate amount of water into a rubber bowl. The powder (usually 50 g) is added to the water in the bowl and briefly mixed with a plaster spatula. At this point a mechanical hand-turned spatula (Fig. 15-7) is placed over the bowl and rotated for a number of turns recommended by the respective manufacturer. Typical mixing time ranges from 30 to 45 seconds using 60 turns of the handle.

Since no vacuum is used in this procedure, the wax pattern should be painted with a wetting agent to permit the investment to cover the wax pattern uniformly. Failure to do so may cause surface nodules on the casting.

After the investment has been mixed, it is applied to the wax pattern with a soft camel's hair brush. When the pattern has been completely coated, it is inserted into a casting ring. At this

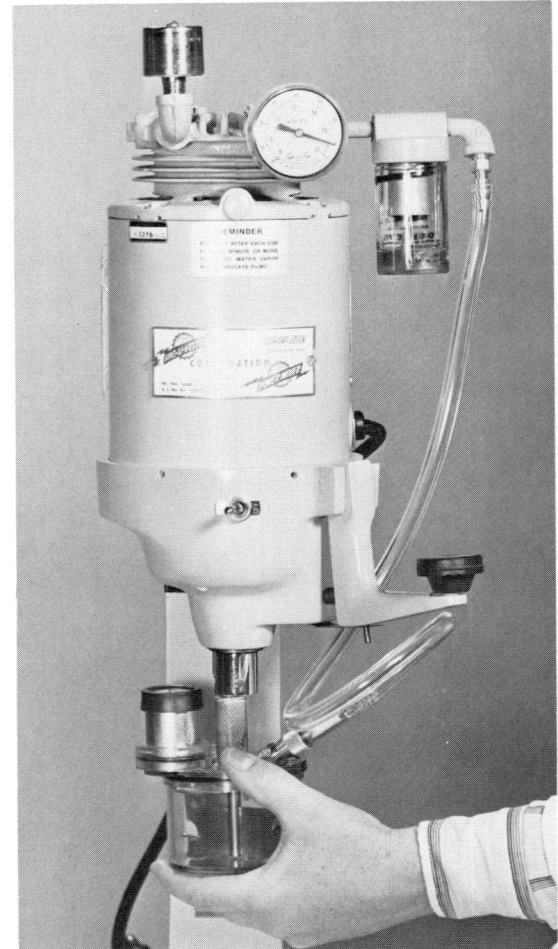

Figure 15-6 | Mechanical unit for mixing investment under vacuum. After mixing, the bowl is inverted and the investment is vibrated into the ring under vacuum.

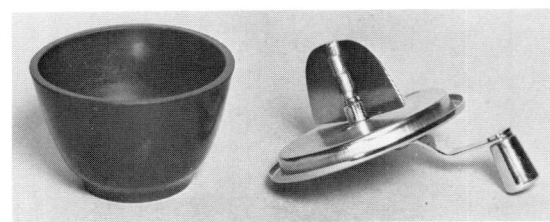

Figure 15.7 | Mixing bowl and mechanical hand-turned spatula.

point the rest of the investment is gently vibrated into the opened end of the casting ring. Excess investment extruding from the ring is removed with a spatula in such a way as to make the surface even with the ends of the ring.

Special Considerations

When the hygroscopic technique is used, the additional water necessary to produce the desired expansion must be applied immediately after the investing procedure. This can be accomplished in one of two ways. The first consists of submerging the invested wax pattern into a water bath at 100°F (37°C) for at least 30 minutes (Fig. 15-8). The second method consists of adding a controlled amount of water to the investment filled ring (Asgar, Mahler, and Peyton, 1955). When this technique is used, special equipment is necessary. Basically it consists of a flexible sprue base, a metal collar or water reservoir, a flexible rubber ring, a metal sleeve for handling the flexible ring, and a syringe for adding water in an accurate manner.

When the thermal or high-heat technique is employed, the invested ring is allowed to "bench" set for 45 to 60 minutes before the next step is initiated.

Wax Elimination

After the investment has fully set, it is trimmed flush with the upper end of the ring. In addition, all excess investment is removed from the sides of the ring. Next the rubber sprue base and sprue pin are removed. If plastic rather than metal sprue has been used, it may be left in place since it will be eliminated by the heat of the furnace. When the sprue is removed from the investment, care must be taken to keep the open end down so that loose particles of investments will not fall into the sprue channel.

Next the casting ring is placed into a furnace (Fig. 15-9) which is then heated to a temperature or range of temperatures depending upon the particular expansion technique employed. If the hygroscopic expansion technique is used, the

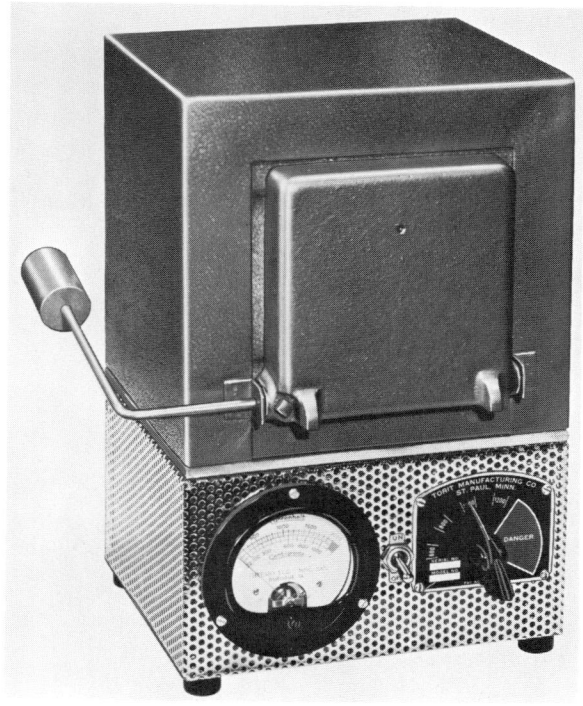

Figure 15-9 | Electric burnout furnace designed for wax elimination and controlled heating of the investment. (*Courtesy of Torit Manufacturing Company.*)

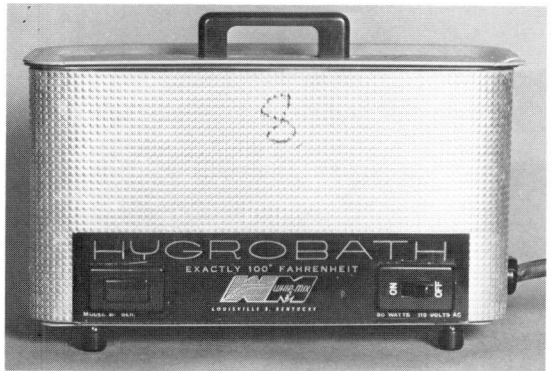

Figure 15-8 | Hygroscopic water bath. When using the hygroscopic technique the invested pattern is submerged in water heated to 100°F (37°C) for 30 minutes.

casting ring is placed into a furnace preheated to 850 to 900°F (454 to 482°C) for at least 60 minutes. If a thermal expansion technique is used, then the casting ring is inserted into a room temperature furnace or one that is preheated to 250°F (121°C). The temperature of the furnace is then elevated to 1200 to 1300°F (649 to 704°C) over a prescribed period of time. The ring is allowed to "heat soak" for about an hour at that temperature, after which it is ready to cast. Under no condition must the temperature of the investment be raised above 1300°F (704°C) due to a breakdown of the investment and subsequent sulfur contamination of the gold casting (O'Brien and Nielsen, 1959).

Regardless of the technique the casting ring should be inserted into the furnace with the sprue end down for the purpose of allowing the molten wax to flow from the mold. Although the inlay wax melts at relatively low temperatures, complete elimination is possible only at higher temperatures. If the wax is insufficiently removed during the burnout procedure, the casting will be incomplete, particularly in the areas of thin margins.

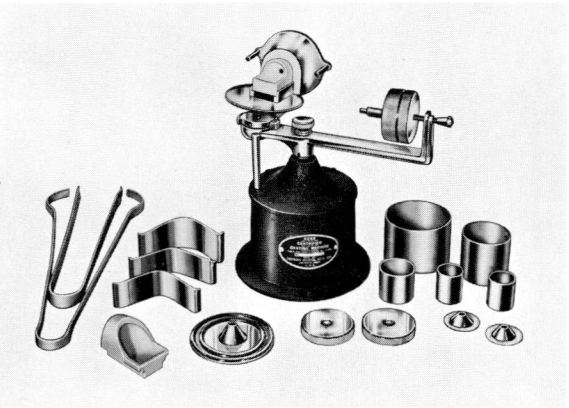

Figure 15-10 | Centrifugal casting machine with tongs, cribs, clay crucible, sprue bases, and rings. (*Courtesy of Kerr Manufacturing Company.*)

Casting Procedure

Although a wide variety of casting machines currently exist for the purpose of forcing the molten alloy into the evacuated mold, there are only two general types. The first and most common is a centrifugal force type, whereas the other uses air pressure to fill the chamber.

The centrifugal casting machine is available in a wide variety of sizes, designs, and modifications. An example of the most basic type is illustrated in Fig. 15-10. Essentially this machine consists of a casting arm with a crucible (in which the alloy is liquified) at one end and a counter or balancing weight at the other. The base, which generally holds the casting arm in a horizontal position, contains a spring for the purpose of spinning or rotating the crucible. When a sufficient centrifugal force is attained, the molten alloy is forced through an opening in the back of the alumina or clay crucible and into the mold chamber of the casting ring which lies just behind it.

Before the gold alloy is placed into the crucible, the floor must be covered with an asbestos liner. Failure to do so may result in adherence of the alloy to the surface of the crucible.

Melting of the gold alloy in this type of casting machine is generally accomplished with a gas-air blowpipe flame. The proper adjustment and use of this flame are very important. A properly adjusted flame has a dark-blue inner cone near the tip of the blowpipe, followed by a lighter blue center cone and a dark purplish-blue outer cone (Fig. 15-11). The light-blue center cone is the hottest part of the flame and is slightly reducing. This portion of the flame should cover the gold completely for rapid melting and protection from oxidation.

When using gold alloy that has been previously melted, it is generally advisable to use a casting flux to absorb oxides formed on the metal surface. The fluxing agent is applied to the alloy as it starts to turn red and again just before casting. When the metal becomes liquid and mobile with a bright shiny surface, the casting ring is removed from the furnace and placed into the casting machine just behind the crucible. At this point the molten alloy is forced into the casting ring by means of centrifugal force.

After casting the ring is quenched in water as soon as the sprue button loses its dark-red color. Quenching facilitates the removal of the casting from the investment.

A more automatic type of centrifugal casting machine is illustrated in Fig. 15-12. No flame is needed to melt the alloy with this type of casting machine since gold is heated in a small electric furnace located at the end of the casting arm. Such an apparatus offers greater consistency from casting to casting since the procedure is comparatively automatic. The main disadvantage to this method, however, is that melting of the gold takes somewhat more time than the blowtorch.

An example of the air pressure type of casting machine is illustrated in Fig. 15-13. In this type of apparatus the gold alloy is melted in the impression or crucible formed by the sprue base.

Cleaning and Pickling the Casting

After the investment has been removed from the casting with a medium-hard bristle brush, it is ready for pickling. Normally the casting will appear dark with oxides and tarnish when removed from the investment. This superficial surface can be removed by submerging in a hot acid solution. Although there are a number of proprietary solutions for this purpose, a 50 percent solution of sulfuric acid can be effectively employed.

For a safe and reliable way of cleaning the surface, the casting should be pickled in a glass beaker or porcelain dish. For best results the solution is gently warmed until the surface of the casting takes on a bright appearance. Since the pickling solution is an acid, the casting should be carefully rinsed in running water before it is handled with the fingers. When removing the casting from the pickling solution, plastic-coated

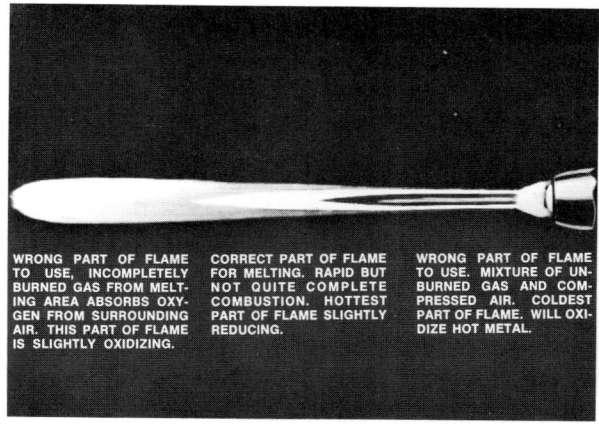

Figure 15-11 | Gas-air blowpipe flame, illustrating the three cones of the flame. (*Courtesy of The J. M. Ney Company.*)

Figure 15-12 | Centrifugal casting machine with electrically controlled heating elements incorporated in it for controlled melting of the casting alloy. (*Courtesy of J. F. Jelenko and Company, Inc.*)

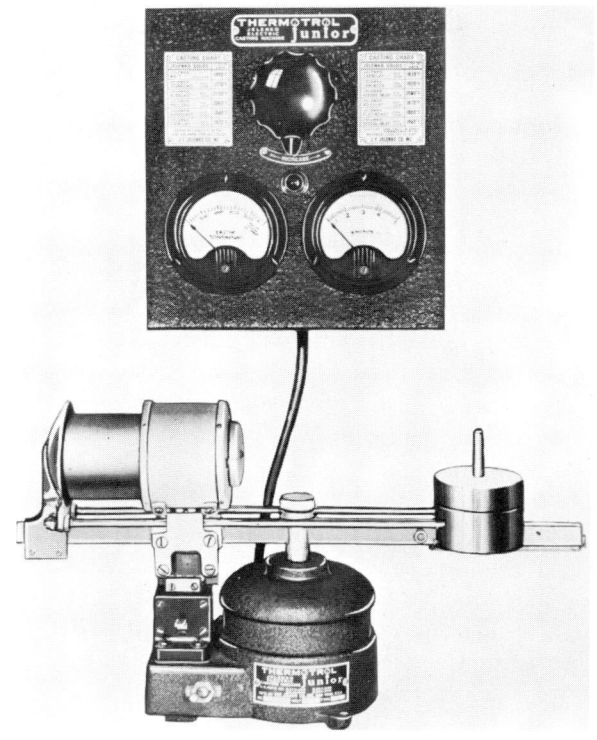

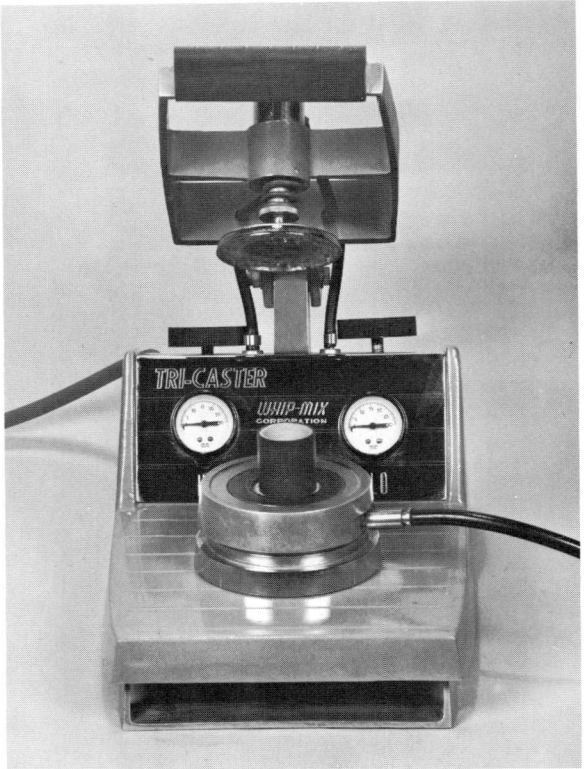

Figure 15-13 | Air pressure casting machine.

tweezers should be used. Using steel or other metal tweezers will result in an attack of the acid on metal surface which in turn may cause plating of some of the base metals from the tweezers on the surface of the gold casting. When the pickling solution has been contaminated or discolored, it should not be used.

CASTING DEFECTS

Although there are many types of casting defects, they may all be grouped into the following categories: incomplete castings, improper fit, surface defects, and internal defects.

Incomplete Castings

This type of defect is characterized by short, rounded margins as well as missing sections. The most common causes for this type of defect include inadequate casting pressure, insufficiently heated casting mold or gold alloy. Smooth, shiny margins may also result from incompletely burning out the investment mold or by trapping air in the chamber by using a nonporous investment or by positioning the pattern too far from the open end of the casting ring.

Improper Fit

When the casting does not fit or it "rocks" in the preparation and there is no apparent visible reason for the misfit, generally the wax pattern has been distorted. Although the distortion may have occurred during the hardening of the investment, usually the wax distortion has taken place prior to the investment procedure. The distortion may result from insufficient pressure as the wax cools, heating the pattern during spruing, or delayed investing. One of the most frequent causes for distorting the wax pattern is the improper removal of the pattern from the die. However, if the casting is undistorted but is either too large or too small, one or more of the following variables was inadequately controlled: burnout temperature, water/powder ratio, or time of immersion into the water bath (hygroscopic technique).

Surface Defects

The most common type of surface defects include bubbles or nodules, roughness, and fins. Large bubbles generally are the result of an insufficient vacuum during mixing or using an investment which is too thick. Small bubbles result from air being mixed into the investment or by overvibrating the casting ring during the investment procedure. Generalized surface roughness, on the other hand, may result from using a thin mix in addition to overvibrating the casting ring. It may also result from using too much surface tension–reducing agent.

Small projections called fins may also appear on the surface of the casting. These thin, sheet-like extensions which generally occur on the outside of the casting result from heating the investment too fast (Phillips, 1973), inserting a dry, cold ring into a hot oven, heating too long, or using too much casting pressure or excess water in the investment.

Internal Defects

The two most common defects inside dental castings include porosities as well as various types of inclusions. The first type of porosity is called *localized shrinkage porosity*. It results when the molten alloy freezes in the areas of the sprue attachment before the mold is filled. This type of porosity may result from insufficient sprue diameter, reduced casting pressure, or failure to attach the sprue pin in the thickest section. The second type of porosity is called *subsurface porosity* and occurs just below the surface of the casting. It normally results from sprue pins which are too short and too thick.

The last type of porosity is termed *microporosity* and consists of small irregular voids throughout the casting. This type of porosity results from either the investment or alloy being insufficiently heated (Ryge, Kozak, and Fairhurst, 1957).

Inclusions result from foreign particles being carried into the mold chamber during the casting process. Most common inclusions include fluxing agents and particles of casting investment.

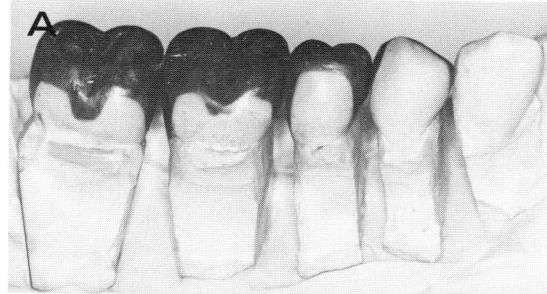
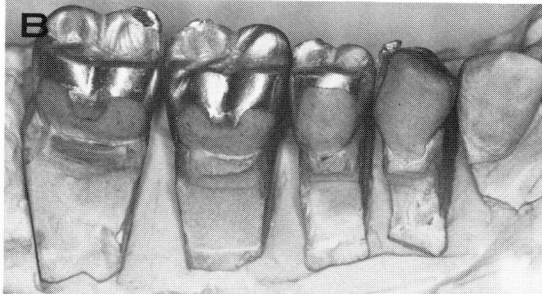
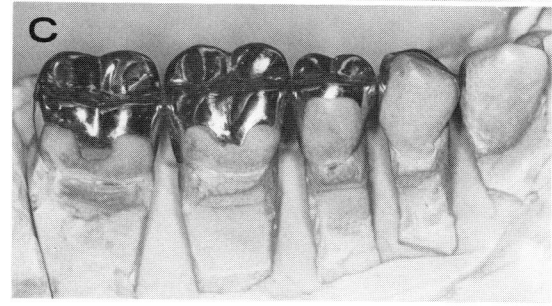

Figure 15-14 | A. Completed wax patterns on removable dies in stone model. B. Castings cleaned, pickled, and seated on dies. C. Polish inlays on stone dies.

FINISHING AND POLISHING

In some dental offices the dentist may prefer to finish and polish the casting personally. If so, he or she may delegate a portion of this responsibility to the dental assistant. There are numerous ways and many agents that can be used to finish small castings such as crowns or inlays. Nonetheless there are certain general steps that have to be followed in sequence:

1. After cleaning and pickling, the casting should be inspected for the various types of defects such as nodules, porosity, or incompleteness. Particular care should be directed to inspecting the inner surface of the casting for small artifacts before seating it on the die since such defects will seriously damage the die. Small protruberances can often be removed with a small, sharp bur.
2. Next the casting should be checked on the die for marginal fit. At this point the sprue pin is removed.
3. The casting is then surfaced and polished with a series of abrasive and polishing agents. A polished surface is attained by rubbing the metal surface with a series of abrasive particles of progressively smaller sizes. The surface attains a highly reflected appearance when the scratches produced by the polishing agents become so small that they cannot be detected by the naked eye.
4. Before the casting is permanently cemented, it is first seated on the tooth and tested for fit, and marginal adaptation is accomplished on the tooth by burnishing, usually with hand instruments. When polishing the casting in the mouth, care must be taken to polish toward the margins so that they cannot be caught or nicked.

The dental assistant who not only has a basic understanding of the process for fabricating inlays but can assist in any portion of the process will be a considerable asset to the dental office.

BIBLIOGRAPHY

Asgar, K., Mahler, D. B., and Peyton, F. A.: "Hygroscopic Techniques for Inlay Casting Using Controlled Water Addition," *J. Prosthet. Dent.,* **5:**711–724, 1955.

O'Brien, W. J., and Nielson, J. P.: "Decomposition of Gypsum Investment in the Presence of Carbon," *J. Dent. Res.,* **38:**541, 1959.

Peyton, F. A., and Craig, R. A.: *Restorative Dental Materials,* 5th ed., The C. V. Mosby Company, St. Louis, 1975, p. 345.

Phillips, R. W.: *Science of Dental Materials,* 7th ed., W. B. Saunders Company, Philadelphia, 1973, p. 448.

Ryge, G., Kozak, S. F., and Fairhurst, C. W.: "Porosities in Dental Gold Castings," *J. Am. Dent. Assoc.,* **54:**746–754, 1957.

16

Roger E. Barton

Instruments, Equipment, and Their Care

INTRODUCTION

It is immediately apparent to individuals being introduced to dental assisting that they must become acquainted with a large assortment of dental equipment, instruments, and materials before they can be completely successful at their work. It is essential not only to easily recognize hundreds of items, but also to learn the care and maintenance of equipment and instruments, plus the behavior of dental materials. The study of dental materials is presented in other chapters. This chapter concentrates on the recognition and care of equipment and instruments found in the dental operatory, plus several items located in the laboratory. Since all items in the operating room and laboratory cannot be included in this chapter, a representative selection of equipment and instruments is discussed.

The assistant will find that the dentist will have "pet" instruments for some operations. These may be of standard design or specially made. It is advisable to learn the use and care of these instruments, as well as of the standard equipment and instruments, as soon as possible.

Every year new equipment and new materials are developed for dentistry. The conscientious dental assistant will keep abreast of these developments and will be able to discuss them with the dentist if and when the occasion arises. Much time, money, and effort are wasted by dentist and assistant if inferior equipment or materials are purchased. The assistant, as well as the dentist, must be able to screen all new products with an open but critical mind.

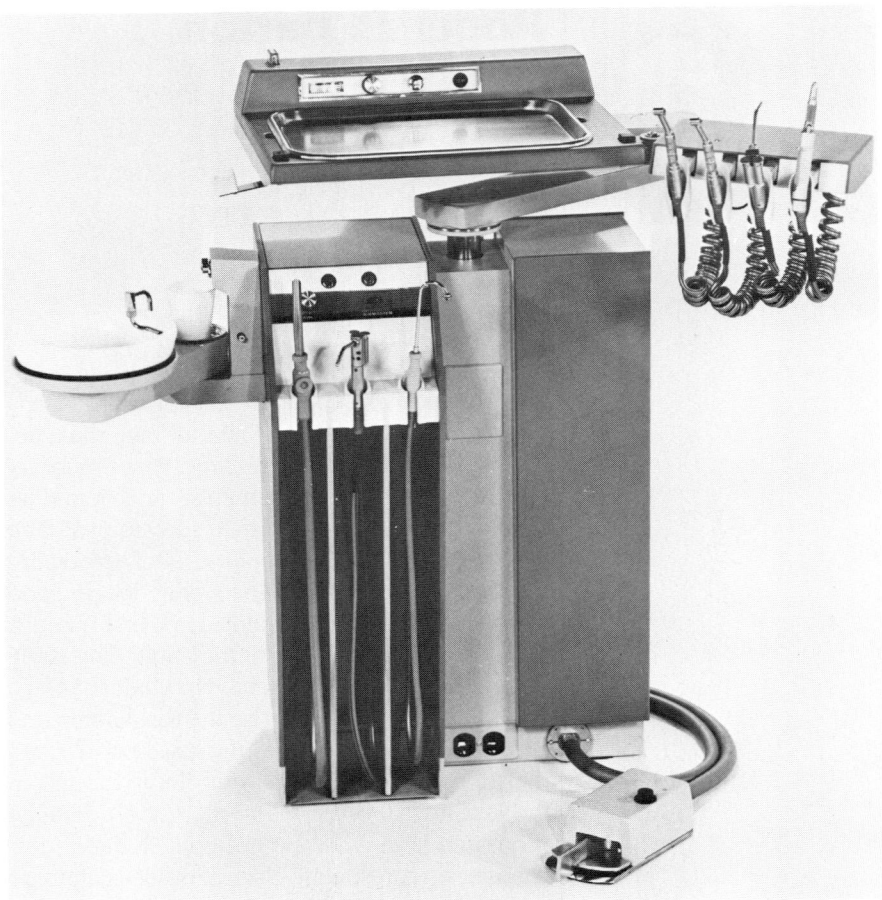

Figure 16-1 | Pedestal-type basic unit providing instrument table and handpiece module movement both vertically and horizontally for the operator, and an assistant component containing evacuation, syringe, and cuspidor systems. Accessories such as operating light and ultrasonic unit may be added. (*Courtesy of S. S. White Dental Products International.*)

In the past, the basic dental-office equipment was quite standardized, with minor variations by different manufacturers. The modern dental equipment varies widely to accommodate the various concepts of dental practice and, in some respects, the specialty areas of dentistry. However, since such items as the dental unit, chair, and cabinets are expensive as well as sturdy, not all dentists are able to purchase new equipment with every improvement or concept change. As a result, some assistants will be working with the older "conventional" equipment, others with the newest and most modern equipment, and still others will be working with both types of equipment. Regardless of the vintage, all equipment requires specific and routine care and maintenance. The dental assistant must, therefore, assume the responsibility of obtaining the proper

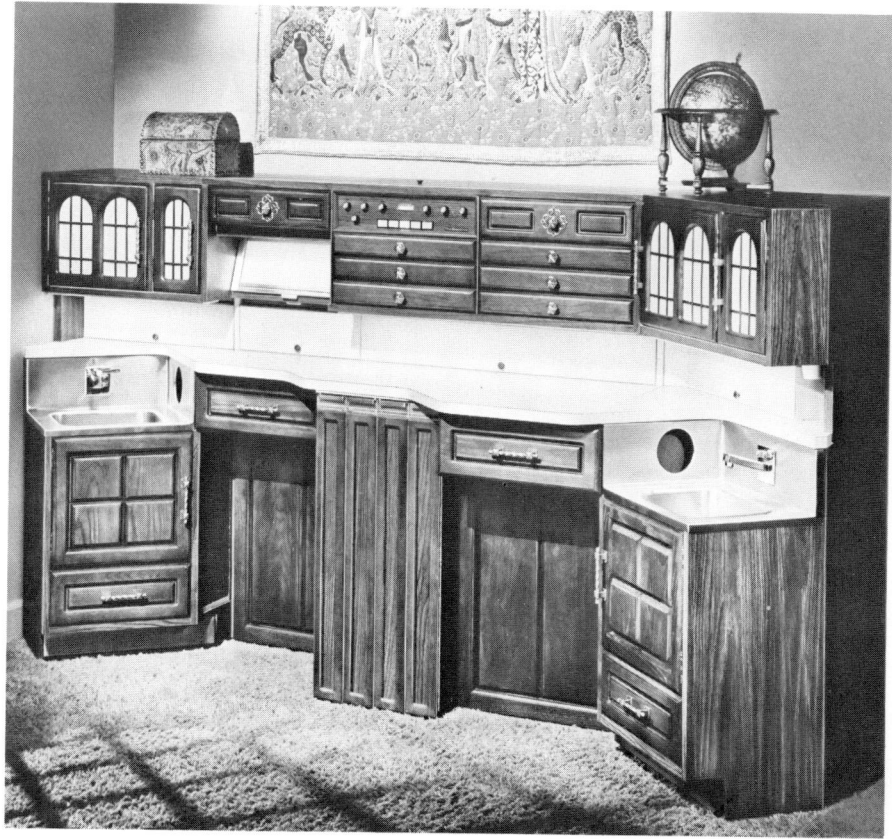

Figure 16-2 | Console unit combining all support elements of an operatory for the operator and assistant. The instrument delivery system (for handpieces, evacuation, etc.) is provided in the base module in the center of the console. (*Courtesy of The Pelton and Crane Company.*)

maintenance information for specific equipment. Since there is such a great variety of equipment design, make, age, and function, the information presented in this chapter must be considered general in nature.

The dental assistant is not expected to assume the role of a maintenance or repair technician, but proper care and some preventive maintenance functions should be performed by the assistant. There is nothing more annoying to the dentist than malfunctioning equipment, particularly if it results from improper routine care.

Proper cleaning, adjusting, and use of equipment by the assistant can prolong the functioning and useful life of such items.

THE DENTAL UNIT

The dental unit is that piece of equipment that provides the basic utilities for dental operations. These include electricity, water, compressed air, and vacuum. The unit not only provides the utilities in a convenient, centralized area, but it may also furnish the support for, or include, such

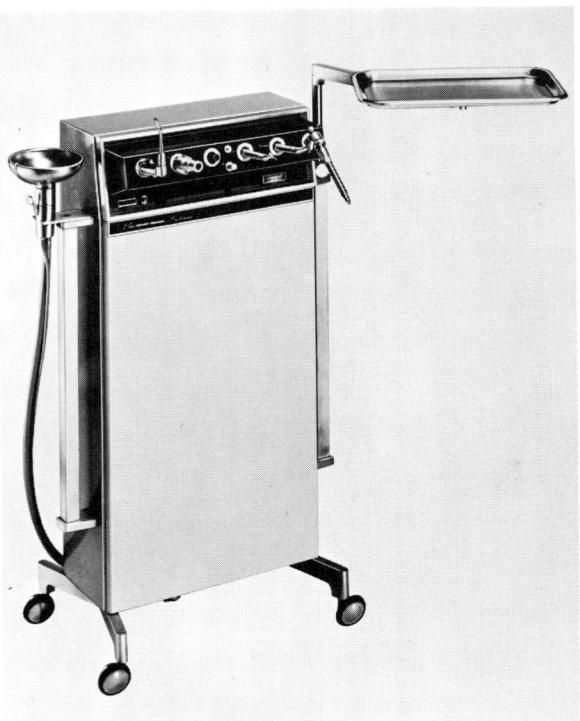

Figure 16-3 | Mobile dental unit containing small, hand-operated flush cuspidor, multipurpose syringe, oral evacuator connection, saliva ejector hose, air-driven handpieces, and tray arm. (*Courtesy of Midwest American Division of American Hospital Supply Corporation.*)

items as the cuspidor, view box, bracket table or tray arm, operating light, syringes, handpieces, suction instruments, and other auxiliary appliances as required by the mode of operation and techniques employed by the dentist.

Experimentation in dental procedures has resulted in the general adoption of seating of the dentist and assistant during most dental operations, and the more effective use of a chairside assistant. This change, from the traditional standing position of the operator and assistant, has resulted in the development of dental units other than the fixed-pedestal type (Fig. 16-1). In addition to the variety of pedestal types, units are available that attach to the dental chair, that can be custom-assembled from modular parts, that are built into console cabinetry (Fig. 16-2), that are mobile with a flexible tubing containing the utility lines which run from the unit to a central utility outlet (Fig. 16-3), or that split into two units or carts (Fig. 16-4), one conveniently placed for the dentist and the companion placed for use by the dental assistant.

Although there is a wide variety of unit designs, there are certain basic components that are provided in one configuration or another and warrant consideration by the dental assistant. Once these basic components are understood, there should be little difficulty in accommodating to the various unit designs.

The Master On-Off Switch

Every dental unit is provided with a master *on-off* switch. When it is turned off, none of the appliances on the unit can function. The reliable dental assistant can be depended upon to turn this master switch to the *off* position at the close of work each day. She thereby relieves the dentist of any worry concerning the possibility that electricity is running some appliance on the unit throughout the night, causing the appliance to be ruined or its length of service to be materially shortened. Some of the small heating elements on the unit are particularly vulnerable to an excessive flow of electricity. The assistant should also realize that leaving electricity turned on overnight will increase the hazard of fire.

One of the first duties of the assistant on arriving at the office in the morning is to turn the master switch of the dental unit to the *on* position. This will allow time for the heating elements to become effective. The unit provides separate controls for the degree of heating of some of these elements, and when these controls are once set by the dentist, they should not be changed by the assistant without instruction.

Depending on the mechanical construction of the unit, a master water cutoff valve may be

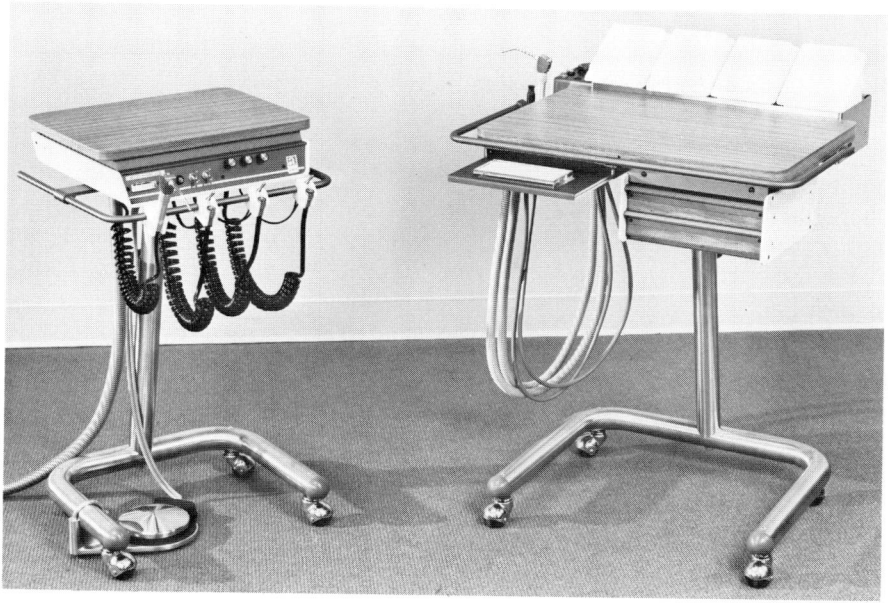

Figure 16-4 | Split mobile units. *Left,* operator unit with work surface, syringe, handpieces, and controls. *Right,* assistant unit with tray surface, instrument drawers, storage compartments, mixing slab module, syringe, and evacuating system. (*Courtesy of A-dec.*)

present, or the master switch may control the flow of all utility services. If a separate master water valve is located on the unit, it should be cut on and off at the beginning and close of each day. If a flooded operatory is ever experienced, the value of this valve is more appreciated.

The Cuspidor

The cuspidor on the dental unit is a round bowl either of white glass or stainless steel provided for expectoration by the patient. The cuspidor may be fixed to the unit and have continuous running water provided by water tubes which extend into the bowl and along its outer perimeter, or it may be detachable from the unit and hand held by the patient (Fig. 16-3). In the former design, the unit is provided with a water valve usually located near the cuspidor. In the latter situation, the cuspidor is usually attached to the central evacuation system and may have a finger lever on the bowl to provide a water flush when actually in use by the patient. When the detachable cuspidor is used, the assistant should instruct the patient in its proper use.

The dental assistant is expected to keep this cuspidor clean. It is most important that the bowl be wiped with towels between patient visits. Both the inside and the outside surfaces must be clean. In the bottom of the bowl is a trap, which should be removed and cleaned daily.

The Saliva Ejector

On the dental unit is a flexible suction tube called the saliva ejector hose. This hose is long enough to reach from the unit to the patient's mouth. Into its end is inserted a curved tube, usually of metal, called the saliva ejector mouthpiece, the function of which is to aspirate (suck) saliva from the mouth as it accumulates. This piece is placed in the mouth, with the curved end running over the lower teeth and ending near the floor of the mouth. In addition to the ordinary saliva ejector mouthpiece (just described), several different shapes and sizes are available that perform more than the fundamental function of the ejector mouthpiece (Fig. 16-5).

For the operation of the saliva ejector, the unit is provided with a two-way valve which when turned to the *on* position causes running water to create suction in the tube. Before the saliva ejector works, it is also necessary to turn on the master and the cuspidor flush valves. Some units do not utilize the running water to create suction. Rather, the saliva ejector is placed on the hose of the evacuating system and is operated through that mechanism.

After each use, the saliva ejector and tubing should be rinsed by inserting the open end of the mouthpiece into a cup of warm water and activating the mechanism thereby removing saliva and debris from the mouthpiece and tubing. Also, the holes (slots) in the end of the mouthpiece may become clogged with debris, and it is the duty of the assistant to thoroughly clean the mouthpieces. This should be accomplished when cleaning up at the close of each patient's appointment. The saliva ejector mouthpiece is then sterilized if it is not of the disposable type.

The receptacle at the end of the suction tube, which receives the saliva ejector, contains a screen, or trap, to collect debris and prevent it from clogging the tube. This screen should be removed and cleaned weekly to assure efficient suction.

The Air and Water Syringes

The majority of units have a combination syringe that is capable of accomplishing from three to six operations (Fig. 16-6), providing a warm or cool spray, warm or cool stream of water, and warm or cool air blast. The control for these syringes may be on the unit panel or on the syringe itself. If automatic syringes are not available on the unit, or if they are temporarily not functioning properly, the dentist is forced to use bulb-type, hand-operated syringes.

If the syringes are of the automatic type provided on the dental unit, the assistant is required to wipe them between visits of patients with a gauze sponge saturated with a germicidal solution. The automatic syringes that are provided with removable tips should have the tips removed and sterilized after each patient. This will necessitate an additional supply of syringe tips.

The Operating Light

The operating light provides illumination upon the mouth (Fig. 16-7). It usually is supported by an arm attached to the dental unit, but it may be suspended from wall or ceiling brackets. Through suitable joints, this arm provides the necessary mobility to the light fixture to facilitate directing the light beam.

Figure 16-5 | Saliva ejectors. *Left,* saliva ejector–tongue retractor type available in right and left design. *Center,* ordinary saliva ejector with replaceable rubber tip. *Right,* disposable plastic saliva ejector with wire inside tube to allow for custom shaping of ejector.

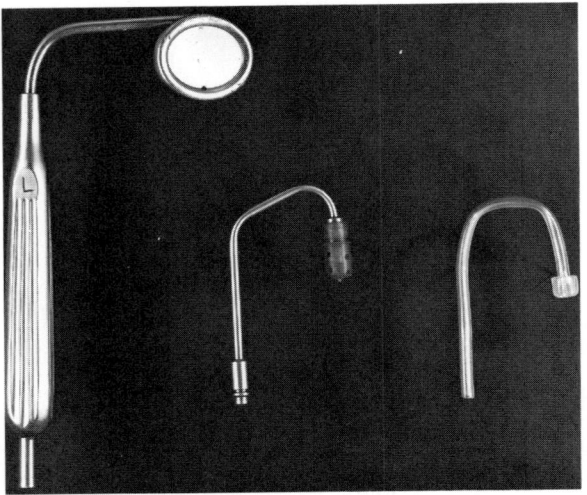

The assistant should take care to see that this fixture, particularly the glass cover over the bulb and the reflector, if exposed, is free of fingerprints and debris from the hands. Cleaning is best accomplished with a lint-free cloth dampened with a glass-cleaner solution.

The assistant should also be able to replace the operating bulb if it burns out. Keeping these bulbs in stock for replacement is one of the assistant's responsibilities. The dentist usually must stop operating in a patient's mouth if he is without this illumination.

The Dental Engine and Foot Controller

For a number of reasons, the dental profession has generally converted from the electric engine to compressed air as the power source for dental handpieces. However, the dental engine may still be utilized by some practitioners. When present in the dental office, certain maintenance practices must be performed on the dental engine and the three-piece cord arm. The engine should be wiped clean of dust daily and oiled according to the manufacturer's directions. Usually only a few drops of high-grade engine oil, provided by the manufacturer of the engine, are required about twice a year. The motor will run if the pedal on the foot controller is pushed and the master electric switch is on. The foot controller rests on the floor, usually just behind the chair, and is connected to the dental unit by an electric cord.

The three-piece cord arm is the jointed arm that extends from the dental engine. The dental handpiece is connected to the free end of this arm. Through a series of pulleys and an engine belt extended over these pulleys, this three-piece cord arm transfers the rotating action of the dental engine to the handpiece, thereby causing the moving parts of the handpiece to rotate.

The assistant should take special care to wipe the cord arm and keep the pulleys clean and bright. Every month or two the pulleys should be lubricated with a few drops of good-quality light

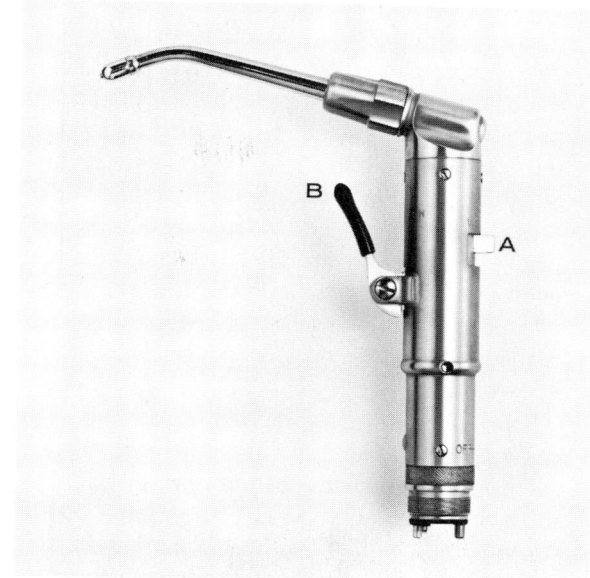

Figure 16-6 | Multipurpose syringe which by manipulation of the selector (A) and on-off control (B) can produce a stream of warm water, air, or air-water spray. This syringe may be easily removed from the unit hose by a special coupling if necessary for repair. (Courtesy of Midwest American Division of American Hospital Supply Corporation.)

Figure 16-7 | Dental operating light produces proper light intensity in operating area. (Courtesy of The Pelton and Crane Company.)

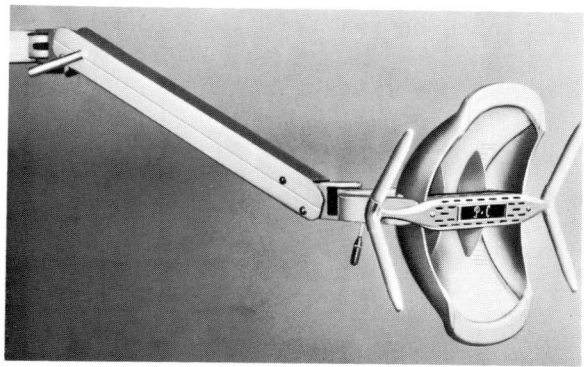

Chapter Sixteen | Instruments, Equipment, and Their Care | 279

oil. Care should be exercised to apply this oil directly to the oilholes provided in the equipment piece, without getting oil "all over." Letting the oil run down a toothpick, the end of which is positioned into the oilhole, is one method of guiding the oil into the hole. Too often oil is carelessly spread over the equipment surface adjacent to the oilhole and on the pulleys, which when in operation are likely to sling oil upon everyone and everything in the room. Careless oiling of the arm plus a lack of careful wiping will readily cause it to take on an unclean, grimy appearance.

The capable assistant will know how to change the engine belt whenever replacement seems indicated. The assistant will watch for the first evidence of wear, which is indicated by the fraying of the belt, and will replace the worn belt with a new one. Excessive fraying of the belt may lead to a complete break during an operation, creating an annoying and expensive loss of operating time while a new belt is being placed. Furthermore, a frayed belt is not desirable because it increases vibration in the handpiece, and this is discomforting to the patient.

Learning to change the belt should not prove difficult, if the assistant practices immediately following a demonstration by the dentist. It is extremely important that the assistant be aware of the correct degree of tautness, or tension, of the belt and of the mechanical feature on the arm which provides for adjustment in this degree of tautness. If the belt is too tight, excessive wear of the pulleys and the belt will ensue. If the belt is too loose, there will be slippage, that is, loss of traction of the belt over the pulley on the handpiece or over the pulley on the motor. When the belt is at rest, that is, when the motor is not running, it should sag just a little from pulley to pulley.

The dental engine and cord arm are also located in many dental office laboratories. The same maintenance procedures should be followed as previously outlined.

The air-driven handpiece does not require an electric motor mounted on the unit nor a three-piece cord arm, but it does require a foot controller to activate the handpiece. The foot controllers are usually a disk depressor type rather than a lever type. If there are several handpieces on the unit, the same foot controller is used for various handpieces, and a selector switch is located on the unit to direct the air flow to the desired handpiece.

The alert assistant will help to keep the foot controller in close proximity to the operating foot of the dentist when he or she is using the rotary instruments.

The air supply to drive the handpiece is conveyed through a flexible tubing which may also provide for an oil line, a water line, and an air exhaust line. The proper couplings between the handpiece and the tubing are very important because all tubings and handpieces are not interchangeable. The various types of handpieces will be discussed later in this chapter.

The Bracket Table

The bracket table is a round glass tray supported on an extension arm from the unit. The arm moves in a horizontal plane. The glass tray holds the hand instruments and should be covered with a paper cover or towel. After dismissing the patient, the assistant should wipe the glass tray with a gauze sponge saturated with a germicidal solution.

Many bracket tables also hold a fixed gas burner. The assistant should keep the shield and burner clean of melted wax and debris.

Most of the advanced types of dental units have replaced the conventional bracket table with a tray arm (Fig. 16-1). This arm is capable of moving vertically as well as horizontally and usually holds a stainless steel tray. With the expanded arm movements and the interchangeable tray, this feature of the unit becomes more versatile.

THE AIR COMPRESSOR

An air compressor, although not located in the operating room, is an essential piece of equipment in the modern dental office. It supplies the air to such instruments as the air syringe, spray attachments, and air-turbine handpiece. In addition, the air is used with various pieces of equipment in the laboratory. Quite frequently this piece of equipment is located in the laboratory.

It is the duty of the dental assistant to see that the air compressor is running before the dentist begins work for the day. Then he or she will not have to wait for air pressure to build up before using certain pieces of equipment. If the compressor supplies air to only one dentist's office, the assistant should turn off the machine before leaving the office for the day.

All manufacturers have their own specific suggestions for maintenance. The machines are usually sealed units and require no lubrication. The instructions should be reviewed, however, and the specific suggestions followed to prevent excessive wear and breakdown of the equipment.

THE DENTAL CHAIR

The dental assistant, responsible for seating the patient in comfort as well as for the operator's convenience, should know the purpose of the various manipulative features of the dental chair. There are a variety of dental chairs, including the manually operated chair, motor chair, contour chair, vibrating chair, and those chairs combining several features. The manually operated chair must be raised and lowered by the foot pedal. The backrest, headrest, foot platform, etc., are adjusted by means of levers.

When the patient is seated properly and comfortably in a conventional chair the backrest is so placed that it provides support to the lumbar region and the headrest contacts the lower posterior portion of the head with the head in the same relation to the spine as when the patient is standing. The backrest and headrest adjustments should not be made while the patient is contacting the parts. The patient should lean slightly forward as the adjustments are made. After these adjustments are made, the chair is then reclined.

The contour chair is designed to add to the patient's comfort and is usually electrically operated (Fig. 16-8). Because of the design of the seat, back, and legrest, few adjustments are necessary to accommodate the patient. Some contour chairs are constructed to utilize a variety of headrests, including a doughnut or U-shaped rest, contoured neck cushions of various sizes, or the conventional adjustable headrest.

Regardless of the type of chair in the office,

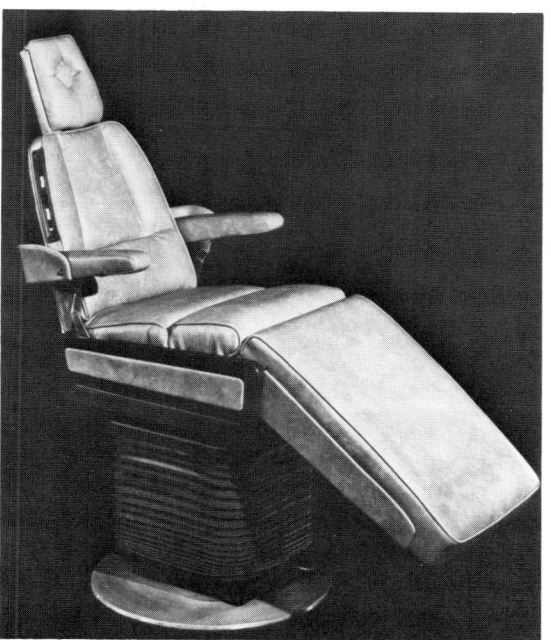

Figure 16-8 | Modern electromechanically operated dental chair. Back and leg supports are independently controlled. The headrest is adjustable. The thin back permits the operator to have unobstructed leg room. (*Courtesy of Chayes Virginia, Inc.*)

the assistant must learn to make chair adjustments for the patient smoothly. It is very annoying to the patient to be "bumped" into a comfortable position or left in an awkward or unrelaxed position. During an operation it is not uncommon for the dentist to desire the chair position to be altered. If the dental assistant can accomplish this smoothly, it will save the operator time, because once the operator touches the levers, hand scrubbing is in order.

The dental assistant is also charged with the responsibility of keeping the dental chair clean. This includes the maintenance of a clean headrest cover and clean armrests, free of hand prints and fingerprints.

When the office is closed, it is advisable to lower the chair to the lowest position to increase the length of trouble-free service of the lifting mechanism.

OPERATING STOOLS

To increase ease of operation, make patient, dentist, and assistant more comfortable, and lessen physical fatigue, operating stools may be used. They are designed to give the dentist and assistant complete freedom in approaching the patient as well as access to the necessary equipment and instruments.

The stool may be completely mobile, being mounted on casters (Fig. 16-9), fixed in a certain position in relation to the dental chair, or it may be stationary. The fixed stool allows movement of the seat through a combination of arms, posts, and joints; the stationary stool allows the seat to be moved by means of a ball-and-socket joint between the base and the seat post.

When a contour chair (which has no adjusting levers on the back) is used, it can be tilted back, and the dentist can work comfortably from a seated position. At the same time, the assistant can carry out the chairside duties from a seated position. The suggested seated position is that the assistant's eye level be 4 to 6 in higher than

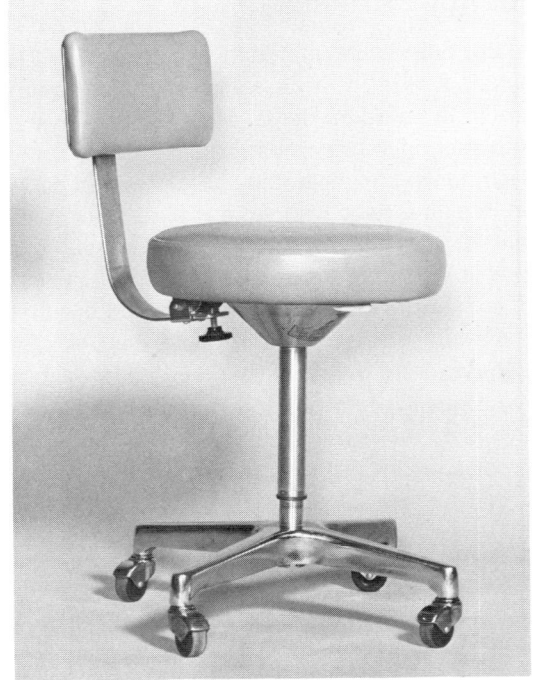

Figure 16-9 | Operator's stools range from a simple style (as illustrated) with adjustable seat and backrest to sophisticated styles with multiple adjustments, seat, and backrest designs.

the operator. Therefore, quite often the assistant's feet cannot touch the floor. The stool for the assistant should, therefore, have a footrest ring (Fig. 16-10) to allow sitting with the thighs parallel to the floor and feet resting on the ring.

DENTAL OPERATORY CABINETS

Cabinets used in the dental operatory vary in size, design, and function to meet the needs of the dentist and his or her methods of operating. The cabinets may be mobile, stationary, wall hung, or modular components (Fig. 16-11). They may be designed with instrument drawers; compartments for supplies of various types; sec-

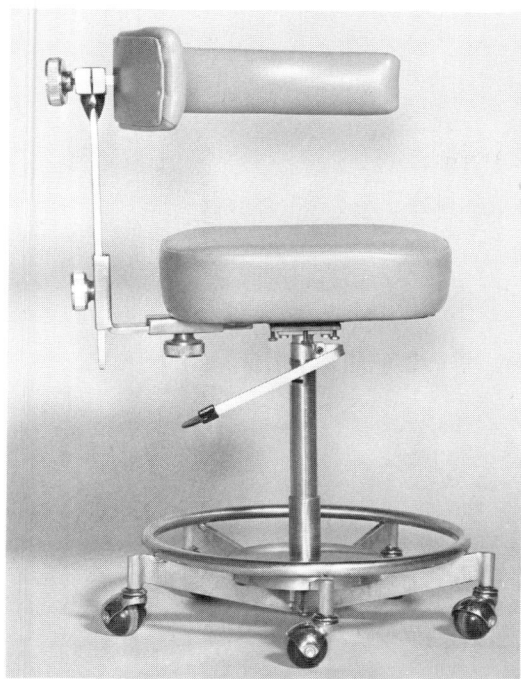

Figure 16-10 | Assistant's stool should have a footrest ring in addition to other features. The extended trunk rest may be moved to support the back, side, or chest. The five casters help prevent tipping.

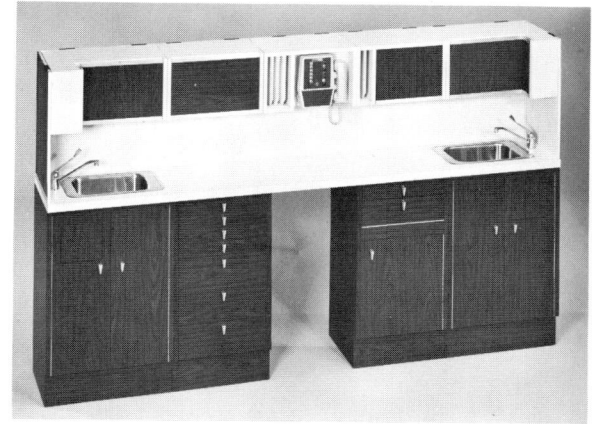

Figure 16-11 | Modular cabinet arrangement. A variety of stock cabinets may be arranged with a continuous work surface to fit the desires of the dentist and the available office space. (*Courtesy of The Valtronic Corporation.*)

tions for equipment such as mechanical amalgamator, electric welder, instrument sharpener, hydrocolloid conditioner, oral evacuating unit, etc.; or they may even house the air-turbine control unit and handpieces.

Cabinets are also available that are placed next to the dental chair and are used by the assistant for placement of the operating instrument setup and as a work surface (Fig. 16-12). These cabinets are mobile and are moved out of the operating area when not in use.

No matter what design or type of instrument cabinet is utilized, it should be easily accessible to the operator as well as to the assistant, and it should contain a neat, systematic arrangement of instruments and materials. Each instrument in the cabinet must have a definite position so that both the dentist and the assistant can easily select any instrument from the cabinet without causing an annoying delay while searching. Whenever possible, the small glass trays which are grooved for instruments or partitioned for small items should be used in the cabinet drawers (Fig. 16-13).

In addition to keeping the instruments in a regular or systematic arrangement, the assistant is also expected to maintain the drawers in a condition of the utmost cleanliness. The interior of these drawers often is observed by patients, and certainly an untidy drawer will not reflect favorably upon the dentist's competence. The exterior of the cabinet should be kept spotless.

After the assistant has been associated with the dentist for a while, suggestions from the former regarding improvements in instrument arrangement will be welcomed. Fortunate is the dentist who finds an assistant sincerely interested in keeping the contents of the dental cabinet neat and clean and who also displays initiative regarding improvements in the instrument arrangement.

ORAL EVACUATING MACHINES

The oral evacuating machines produce a powerful, yet gentle, vacuum air flow. These machines are capable of eliminating saliva, water, blood, and debris from the oral cavity at a much greater speed than the ordinary aspirators or unit-operated saliva ejectors. The high air velocity allows the machine to pick up liquid without being immersed in it, and the size of the suction tips prevents clogging to a greater extent than do the saliva ejector tips.

The machines are designed for various office needs. The central system construction is a means of servicing several operating rooms with a centrally located power apparatus with outlets in each operatory where simple brackets hold the suction hoses, tips, and debris containers. The individual room units may be mobile (Fig. 16-14), or they may be incorporated in modular cabinets or advanced unit designs. This type of equipment, therefore, is versatile and can be adapted to almost any office arrangement.

Fundamentally, the oral evacuating machine is used to remove the water that serves as a coolant during cutting operations on teeth, although it has been adapted in special fields such as periodontia, oral surgery, and orthodontia. In some dental units, this apparatus often replaces the cuspidor completely.

The dental assistant has a twofold duty in connection with this type of equipment. The first has to do with its application in the office. While the dentist is concentrating on cutting tooth structure, the assistant must manipulate the suction tip in such a manner as to effectively remove liquid and debris at the site of the operation without interfering with the dentist's movements or sight (Fig. 16-15). This operation requires perfect concentration and attention at all times. The proper method will be learned through practice and study. There are also attachments, other than the regular tips, that can be used which are held in place in the mouth thus freeing the operator or assistant from holding the apparatus in place.

The second duty of the assistant in regard to

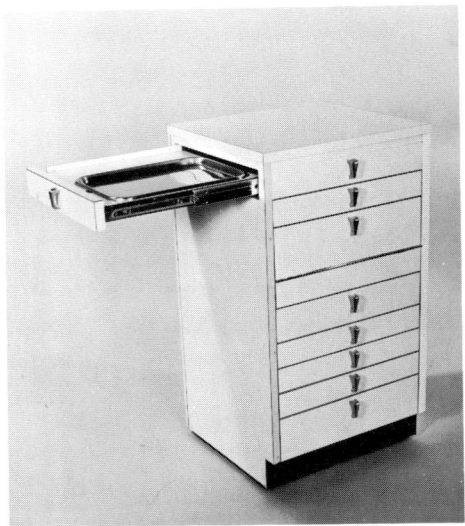

Figure 16-12 | Mobile cabinet with side pullout surface for setup tray. Cabinet may be moved next to dental chair and provide assistant with double working surface and easy access to items stored in the cabinet.

an oral evacuating machine is in operation and cleanliness. The assistant should learn the full operating procedure, not only starting and stopping the machine. If the equipment should cease to work during an operation, the assistant should

Figure 16-13 | Glass trays for instrument drawer. Tray in foreground is grooved for instrument storage. Second tray is partitioned for separation of small supply items.

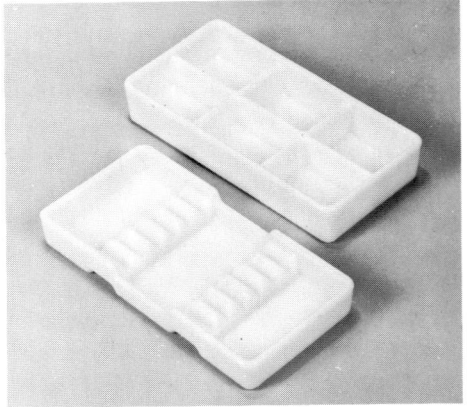

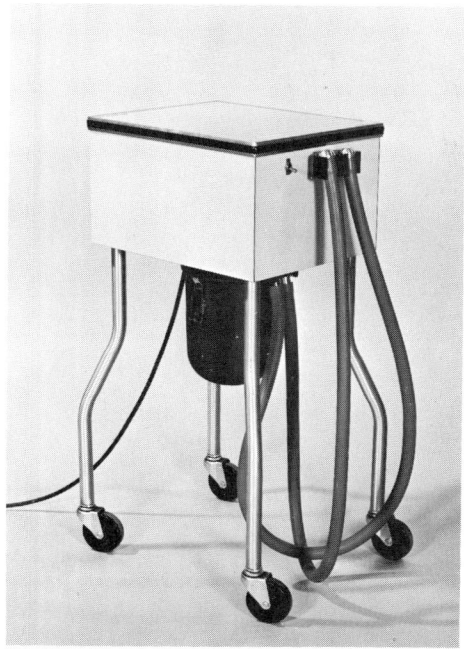

Figure 16-14 | Mobile oral evacuating machine that may be moved from office to office. The unit is self-contained and requires only an electrical connection.

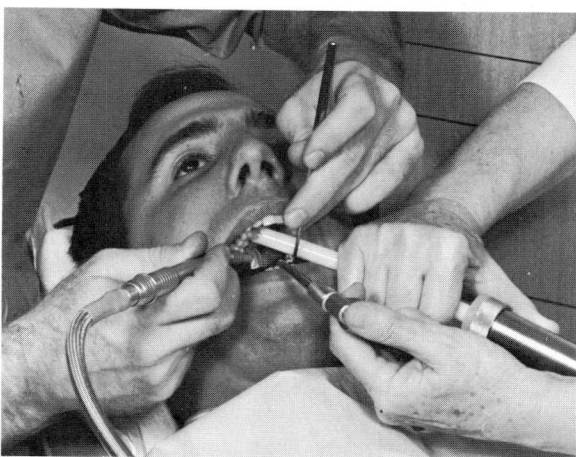

Figure 16-15 | The suction tip is so placed that it does not interfere with the operator. Note the use of the syringe to keep the mouth mirror clean during the cutting operation.

know the possible reasons for this and how to overcome them so that the operation may continue with the least amount of interruption.

Keeping this piece of equipment clean cannot be stressed too much. Each manufacturer has specific instructions for maintenance. The tips must be cleaned with a brush and sterilized, the hoses flushed, and a germicide sprayed into them after each patient. If the machines have collection tanks, these should be emptied at least twice a day and thoroughly cleaned. The accumulation of debris, blood, etc., in this equipment will very shortly produce a most unpleasant odor.

ULTRAVIOLET ACTIVATOR LIGHT

Resin-type pit and fissure sealants and restorative materials have received wide acceptance by the dental profession. There are several resin systems available. One system utilizes ultraviolet light to produce polymerization of the resin materials. The light should be used only when the material instructions indicate its use.

Ultraviolet rays can be a health hazard and, therefore, proper maintenance and use of ultraviolet light equipment is extremely important. This equipment (Fig. 16-16) has protective components that must be properly maintained and properly used. Basically, such components may include a filter to prevent the emission of harmful rays, a second filter to reduce the light brightness, a shutter switch which when closed prevents the transmitting of light, a thermostatic control which shuts off the lamp if it begins to get too warm, and a plastic sleeve which covers the quartz rod. The assistant should follow the manufacturer's instructions for checking, maintaining, and using these components.

The ultraviolet light is stored in a special console where it remains during the warm-up period prior to use. When not to be used, the console should remain covered to prevent an accumulation of dust and debris. The quartz rod and plastic sleeve are sterilizable, and both items must be thoroughly dry after cleaning before being reassembled. Any resin material must be removed from the tip of the quartz rod, since an accumulation of such material will reduce the light transmission.

The output of an ultraviolet light decreases with repeated use. If improper polymerization of the resin material appears, the light should be tested according to the manufacturer's instructions. In fact, it is a good policy to test the effectiveness of the light on a periodic basis.

ANALGESIC APPARATUS

The dental assistant should not assist in the administration of gases for analgesic purposes unless fully trained in the procedure. The dentist should not expect an assistant to acquire this knowledge from technical literature alone. The assistant is not prepared to handle this equipment just because of acquired knowledge of the operation of all the mechanical features of the apparatus. This type of equipment, when used properly, is not dangerous to the health and welfare of the patient, but it must be kept in mind that the patient is conscious at all times. This fact is important in that any undue commotion or indecision on the part of the dentist or the assistant may tend to produce an adverse psychologic effect on the patient and thus render this phase of treatment unsuccessful.

When the assistant has become thoroughly familiar with all aspects of this procedure, he or she may assume a large part of the responsibility for it. This particular piece of equipment should be located where it is least conspicuous to the patient. Like any other dental equipment, it must be kept spotless and in perfect working order. Before the nosepiece is used, it should be sprayed with alcohol to which a small amount of volatile oil has been added. It is then dried off with a gauze square or compressed air and is ready for use.

In storing the apparatus, care must be taken

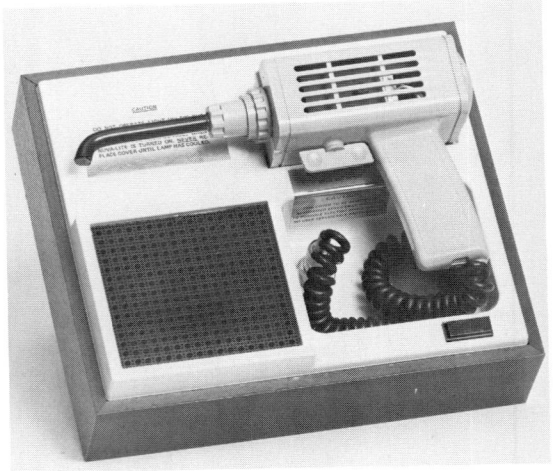

Figure 16-16 | Ultraviolet light equipment used to activate polymerization of certain resin systems. The light must remain in the console as illustrated during the warm-up period. When curing the resin material, the light shutter is opened, and the flat tip of the quartz rod is held parallel to and approximately 2 mm away from the tooth surface. (*Courtesy of The L. D. Caulk Company, Division of Dentsply International Inc.*)

that the necessary valves controlling the gases are closed tightly (Fig. 16-17). The assistant should also check the connections and hoses for leaks and the pressure in the tanks to assure a continuous supply of gases during the operation.

ULTRASONIC UNIT

The ultrasonic instrument is not a rotary instrument and is not used to cut tooth structure. This type of instrument converts electrical energy into mechanical energy in the form of tiny mechanical vibrations. This energy activates a metal tip to move back and forth within a distance of one thousandth of an inch at speeds up to 25,000 times per second. The tips which are mounted in a handpiece are available in various sizes and shapes.

The instrument is a self-contained unit, light in weight, and portable (Fig. 16-18). The primary

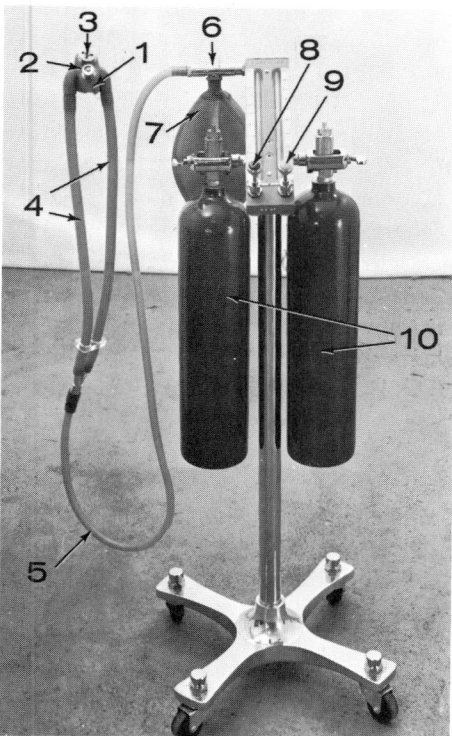

Figure 16-17 | Analgesic apparatus. (1) Latex nosepiece. (2) Air vent. (3) Exhaling valve. (4) Breathing tubes. (5) Delivery tube. (6) Outlet T piece and bag holder. (7) Breathing bag. (8) O_2 control valve. (9) N_2O control valve. (10) Gas cylinders. (*Courtesy of The Foregger Company, Inc.*)

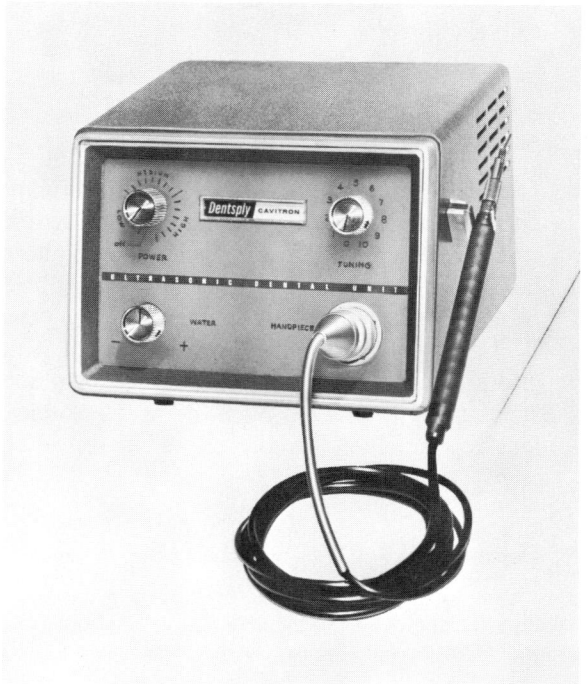

Figure 16-18 | Ultrasonic portable unit with handpiece is used primarily in oral prophylactic procedures. (*Courtesy of Dentsply International, Inc.*)

function of the instrument is in the oral prophylactic procedure and in minor periodontal procedures. During these procedures water is passed over the activated tip. It is beneficial in removing calculus and stain but does not preclude the use of hand scalers. Proper sterilization of the tips is the responsibility of the assistant.

HYDROCOLLOID CONDITIONER

Reversible hydrocolloid impression material (discussed in Chap. 11) is best prepared for use in special equipment known as a hydrocolloid conditioner. These units contain three separate water baths, one for liquifying, a second for storing of the material, and the third for tempering the hydrocolloid immediately before use. Each bath has a separate temperature control (Fig. 11-5). The manufacturer's instructions in adjusting the temperatures should be followed. A timer is also built into the conditioner. Most conditioners are designed to be left on day and night, thus assuring constant temperatures in the various baths.

Outside of cleaning the water bath inserts, the conditioner requires little if any maintenance. For best results in cleaning the inserts, remove them from the conditioner, pour out the water, refill with a special hydrocolloid cleaner, return the filled inserts to the conditioner for 1 hour with the conditioner on, remove the solution, dry

Chapter Sixteen | Instruments, Equipment, and Their Care | **287**

the inserts with a soft cloth, and refill the inserts with clean water.

SURGICAL EQUIPMENT

Cleaning, sterilizing, and storing of instruments and equipment used in conjunction with oral surgery procedures must be given special attention. These instruments should be stored in a cabinet other than the operating cabinet.

The actual care of surgical equipment over and above the exacting routine of cleaning and sterilizing is minimal. Such items as surgical knives (scalpel) and needles should be discarded when dull; no attempt should be made to sharpen them. Surgical burs and chisels are treated as operative burs and hand cutting instruments, except for sterilization methods. Chisels may be sharpened on an oilstone when necessary.

In a fully equipped office with a general anesthesia machine and/or an oxygen machine, the assistant should assume the minor maintenance operations as dictated by the manufacturer's instructions. In offices utilizing aspirators and electric cautery machines, the assistant has an additional responsibility of sterilizing the tips and keeping these machines clean and in proper working condition. It must be remembered that in many instances these pieces of equipment are used unexpectedly or even as an emergency measure. This equipment, therefore, must not be neglected and must be ready for immediate use at all times.

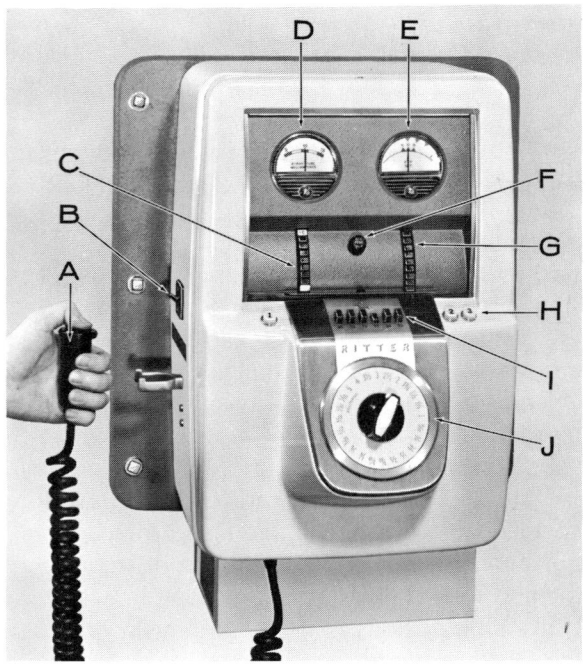

Figure 16-19 | X-ray unit control panel. A. Timer switch. B. Main switch. C. Milliampere control. D. Milliampere meter. E. kVp set meter. F. Fuse holder. G. kVp set control. H. Head selector indicator lights (this control panel will operate several different x-ray heads, and the lights indicate which x-ray head is in use). I. Kilovoltage selector buttons. J. Electronic timer. (*Courtesy of Ritter Company, Division of Sybron Corp.*)

X-RAY UNITS

The parts of an x-ray unit and the principles of operating it are discussed in Chap. 18. However, a few remarks concerning the various types of units and their maintenance are in order.

The units may be permanent (i.e., mounted on the floor or wall in a convenient location) or mobile, or the less powerful x-ray head may be mounted on the unit. They may also have a centrally located control panel with the unit heads located in two or more separate operatories.

The dental assistant should assume the duties of checking the maintenance of the x-ray unit but should not attempt any repairs on defective parts. The voltage compensator (Fig. 16-19), the pilot light, the reset timer, and the movement of the extension arm should be checked, and any faults observed should be reported to the dental dealer.

Several radiographic units have been developed that expose panoramic films (radiograph of the entire oral region on a single film). A panoramic film includes the mandible and maxilla with their associated teeth, the temporomandibular joint structures, and the maxillary sinuses all in their correct relationship. Films are not placed in the mouth for exposure. The film holder and x-ray tube are automatically rotated around the patient's head, which is stationary. This type of machine is a special unit and is not used for routine intraoral films.

HANDPIECES AND HANDPIECE EQUIPMENT

The handpiece and handpiece equipment, including coolant apparatus for high-speed handpieces, and the rotary instruments used in handpieces, such as burs, stones, and discs, are probably the most important pieces of equipment in the dentist's armamentarium. When these items are inoperable, a large percentage of the operations in many dental practices must be eliminated. This can substantially reduce income if the condition exists over a prolonged period of time.

Conventional Handpieces

Essentially, handpieces are of three basic designs: straight, contra-angle, and right angle, including the prophylaxis angle (Fig. 16-20). The power source is an electric engine connected to the handpiece by a belt which runs over a series of pulleys on a three-piece cord arm. The straight handpiece is the basic instrument and is attached to the cord arm and belt. The angle handpieces are attached to the front end of the straight handpiece and are utilized by the dentist to afford better access in various portions of the mouth.

When cutting on posterior teeth, the dentist needs the angle (direction) afforded by the angle handpiece. The contra-angle is used more frequently; it has two angles which bring the point of the working instrument almost into line with the straight handpiece, thereby making the instrument easier to handle and better balanced. The "angle" burs and stones are inserted in the end of the angle handpiece, and the rotary power is obtained from the straight handpiece by a shaft and gears inside the angle section (Fig. 16-21).

The prophylaxis handpiece is attached to the straight handpiece in the same manner. The right angle operates on the same principle as any other angle handpiece and is used with removable rubber cups and/or bristle brushes in polishing the teeth and restorations.

The conventional handpieces are designed to operate at speeds of from 4000 to 9000 rpm.

The care, sterilization, and lubrication of these

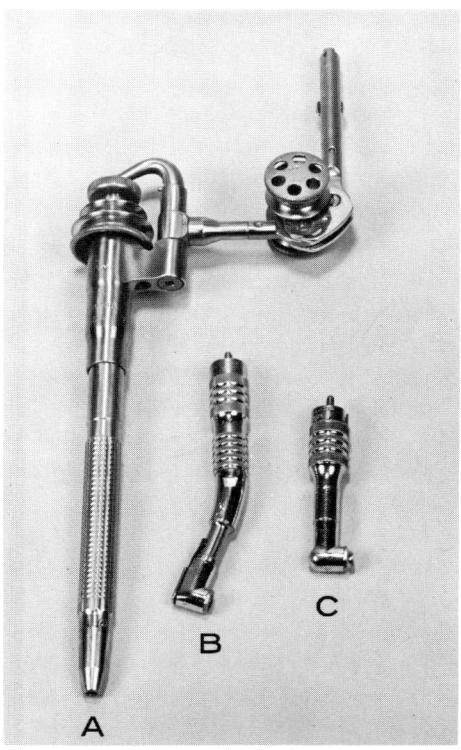

Figure 16-20 | Conventional handpieces. A. Straight. B. Contra-angle. C. Prophylaxis angle. The two angle handpieces attach to the straight handpiece.

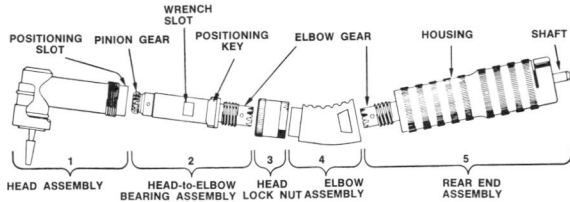

Figure 16-21 | Parts assembly for conventional contra-angle handpiece. (*Courtesy of Teledyne Dental, Densco Division.*)

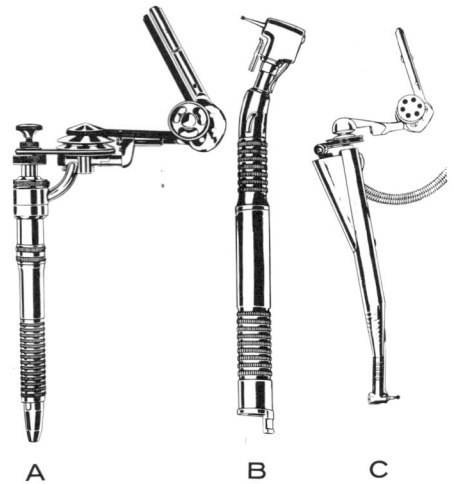

Figure 16-22 | Belt-driven high-speed handpieces. A. Needle ball bearing straight handpiece. B. Long-sheath ball bearing contra-angle used with needle ball bearing straight handpiece. C. Gearless one-piece contra-angle handpiece capable of speeds up to 150,000 rpm.

dental handpieces are the responsibility of the dental assistant. No other piece of equipment in the operating room is more deserving of proper attention. It would be impractical to list the maintenance instructions for all the types of straight and angle handpieces. It must be noted, however, that daily handpiece care is essential and that the recommendations of the handpiece manufacturer should be followed. The daily care of the handpiece must be followed by a weekly concentrated and more detailed effort in cleaning and lubricating these pieces of equipment. The manufacturer provides adequate instructions on care, adjustment, sterilization, and lubrication, and the assistant should refer to these instructions. The local dental supply dealer will gladly provide them if they have been lost or destroyed. The dentist will appreciate the interest shown by the assistant in mastering the proper care of the handpieces.

High-Speed Handpieces

High-speed handpieces are "belt-driven" handpieces and can attain speeds of 150,000 rpm. Although high-speed handpieces are attached to the source of power as are conventional handpieces, they must be precision-built instruments to accommodate the increased speed potential. These handpieces may be designed with gears and ball bearings for speeds up to 50,000 rpm, or they may be the single-unit gearless type of contra-angle handpiece which operates on a special internal belt and is capable of speeds in excess of 150,000 rpm (Fig. 16-22).

The high-speed, belt-driven type of handpiece is relatively free of maintenance problems because the bearings are factory sealed.

The maintenance of the high-speed type of handpiece is considerably less of a problem than that of the conventional type, but it is more critical if the life of the handpiece is to be preserved. Angle handpieces operating at higher speeds (usually sleeve-type, Fig. 16-22) must be cleaned and lubricated after a specific number of minutes of running time. This is usually accomplished simply by running the head of the contra-angle in a cleaning solution for a few seconds, shaking off the excess, and running it in the lubricant for a few seconds. Other types of handpieces have self-lubricating equipment and, therefore, require only cleaning and sterilization. Finally, there are those handpieces that require no lubrication because no gears are involved.

Many of the high-speed angle handpieces will not receive the latch-type burs, stones, or mandrels. The friction-grip shank is often required. Since these types of shanks vary in design, the dental assistant must be certain to specify the exact design desired when reordering instruments for the angle handpiece.

Handpieces of the high-speed type are available in many speed ranges and are of several different types of mechanical construction. It is of the utmost importance that the dental assistant become thoroughly familiar with the proper care and maintenance of the instruments used in the office.

Some manufacturers request that high-speed straight handpieces and contra-angles be returned to the factory for specific maintenance. In offices where this routine is followed, the assistant should keep an accurate record of each instrument so that proper procedures are followed and costly repair bills kept to a minimum.

Figure 16-23 | Air-driven handpieces. A. Standard contra-angle. B. Miniature head contra-angle. C. Straight handpiece. The straight handpiece provides lower speeds and higher torque than contra-angles, and has a removable sleeve that permits attachment of long-sleeve angles. (*Courtesy of Midwest American Dental Division of American Hospital Supply Corporation*).

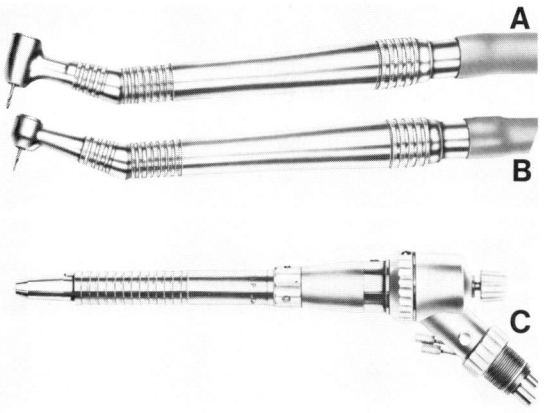

Ultraspeed Handpieces

The air-driven handpieces (Fig. 16-23) are the classic example of the ultraspeed handpieces capable of speeds of approximately 300,000 rpm. The air-driven angle handpieces can attain the ultraspeeds but have low torque and will stall with moderate lateral pressure. The air-driven straight handpiece will attain speeds of only 25,000 rpm but has high torque and will not stall easily. Conventional gear-driven angle handpieces may be attached over the front end of the air-driven straight handpiece. However, this is not advisable, and angles designed for the air-driven straight handpieces should be used.

The air-driven (air-turbine) handpiece is propelled by compressed air carried by a flexible tube to the back of the handpiece. The air is forced against the blades of the small turbine in the head of the handpiece and produces the rotation of the bur. Some handpieces utilize ball bearings to support the turbine shaft while others use air bearings. The latter type is capable of higher speeds and is very quiet in operation. In addition to the built-in spray, handpieces are also available with built-in lights that focus on the cutting site.

The majority of dental offices utilize air-driven handpieces in the operatories. They may either be incorporated in the unit or may be attached to a conventional unit in the form of a control box with attached handpieces.

The burs and stones used with these angle handpieces are $1/16$-in shank instruments and are not the type used in conventional angle handpieces. The burs and stones are held in the handpiece by friction grip in a plastic or metal chuck or by a wrench-tightened metal chuck. In some cases special bur-changing tools are necessary to change burs where plastic or metal chucks are used in the angle handpiece.

The handpieces are cleaned by wiping with a gauze sponge soaked in a disinfectant, and they should not be placed in cold disinfectant solutions. Some types may be autoclaved, but the manufacturer's instructions should be checked for proper sterilization methods.

Instructions for maintenance of these instruments vary with the manufacturer but are usually simple. Maintenance is not the same on all air-turbine units; therefore, only the accompanying specific instructions should be followed. Some minor repairs can be made in the dental office, but for major repair, the handpiece should be returned to the manufacturer.

Electric Handpiece

Handpieces have also been developed that attach directly to a miniature electric motor (Fig. 16-24). This type of handpiece is light in weight, has variable speeds up to 20,000 rpm, and has high torque. Since all that is necessary to run the unit is a source of electricity, it is portable and may easily be used outside of the dental operatory. This type of handpiece has found considerable favor with dental hygienists, periodontists, and orthodontists.

Coolant Equipment

Frictional heat generated in tooth preparation, regardless of operating speeds, induces pain and may seriously traumatize tooth structure. To overcome this hazard in cavity preparation, a coolant should be directed to the tip of the bur, diamond, or other abrasive point. The coolant may be air, water, or an air-water spray.

There are several ways in which this coolant may be supplied. Most of the high-speed handpieces (air-turbine) supply the coolant, and no other equipment is necessary. For those handpieces not supplying a coolant, permanent or temporary attachments are available. The more complete cooling systems are provided with a selector for air, air-water, or water and are operated in conjunction with the foot rheostat for the dental engine.

The assistant may also provide the coolant by means of the unit air or water syringe. When using either of these syringes, strict attention must be paid to the operation. The assistant must learn to position the tip of the syringe so that the stream of air or water is directed at the point of operation and at the same time does not impair the field of operation.

Whether the coolant is supplied automatically or by the assistant, the excess water is best removed by an oral evacuating unit. When the assistant is supplying the coolant by means of a syringe, the placing of both the syringe tip and the evacuating tip is critical; the vision of the dentist must not be obstructed. This is a procedure that must be worked out with the dentist and practiced to ensure complete efficiency in the operation.

Rotary Cutting Instruments

The instruments placed in the various types of handpieces and caused to rotate by the handpiece for the purpose of cutting tooth structure or restorative material are manufactured in many sizes, types, and shapes (Fig. 16-25). Burs are the most common rotary cutting instruments. Other classifications include stones, diamond instruments, and discs.

Generally, these instruments consist of a

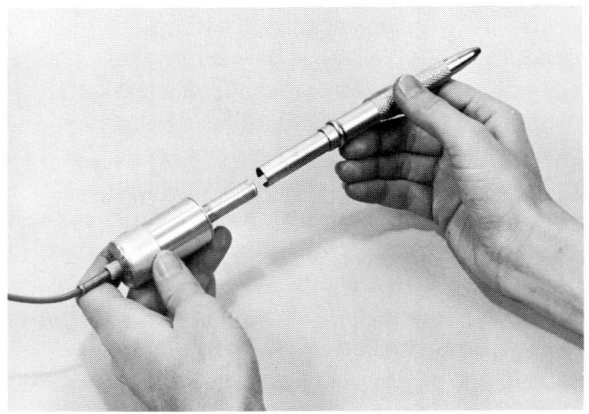

Figure 16-24 | Electric handpiece. Special handpiece sleeves are attached to small electric motor.

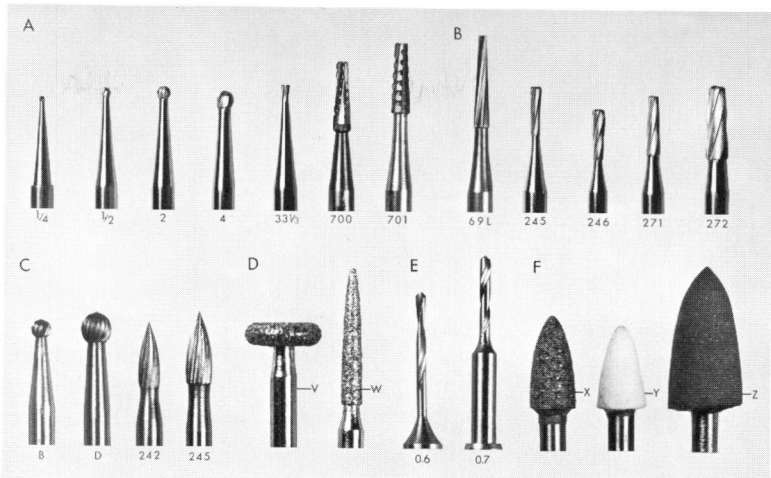

Figure 16-25 | Rotary cutting instruments. A. Carbide excavating burs, ADA standard sizes. B. Carbide excavating burs, modified designs (Densco, no. 69L; Premier, nos. 245, 246, 271, and 272). C. Steel finishing burs. D. Diamond instruments: (v) wheel (Star, no. 110); (w) flame (Star, no. 265-8F). E. Twist drills. F. Molded abrasive points: (x) silicon carbide, (y) aluminum oxide, (z) rubber-bonded. (*From Sturdevant, Barton, and Brauer (eds.),* The Art and Science of Operative Dentistry, *copyright 1968 by McGraw-Hill, Inc. Used with permission of McGraw-Hill Book Company.*)

shank, neck, and head. The shank portion fits into the handpiece and may be one of three designs: straight handpiece, latch type, or friction grip (Fig. 16-26). When the assistant orders these instruments the type of shank must be specified in addition to the type of cutting head.

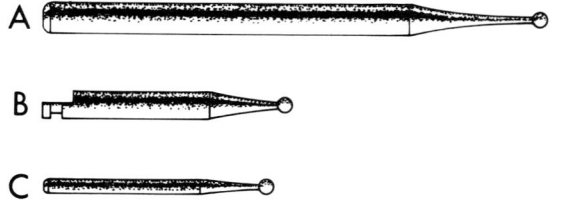

Figure 16-26 | Typical bur shank designs for (A) straight handpiece, (B) latch-type angle handpiece, and (C) friction-grip angle handpiece.

Burs

Burs are used to cut tooth structure in the process of shaping cavities and for removing old restorations from teeth. These instruments come in many sizes and shapes (Fig. 16-27). The five most common shapes are referred to as (1) round, (2) straight-fissure crosscut, (3) tapered-fissure crosscut, (4) plain fissure, and (5) inverted cone. Each of these shapes comes in several sizes which are referred to by numbers, the smaller numbers always indicating the smaller sizes. The inverted-cone burs are designated as nos. 33½, 34, 35, 37, 39, etc. The round burs are nos. ¼, ½, 1, 2, 4, 6, 8, etc.; the straight-fissure crosscut burs are nos. 556, 557, 558, 559, 560, etc.; the tapered-fissure crosscut burs are nos. 700, 701, 702, etc.; and the plain straight-fissure burs are nos. 56, 57, 58, 59, etc. There are other types of burs such as plain

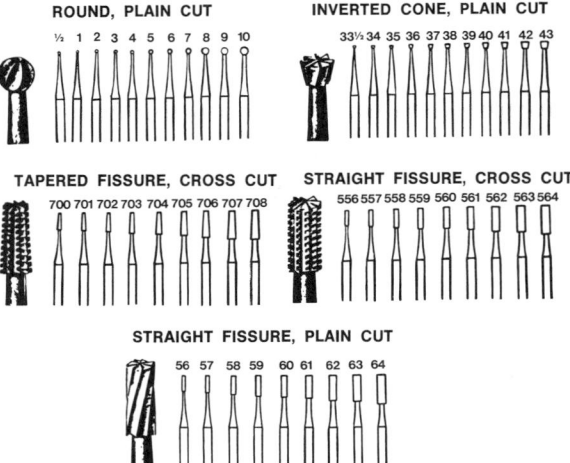

Figure 16-27 | Common bur designs and sizes. *(Courtesy of Star Dental Manufacturing Company, Inc.)*

tapered-fissure burs, round-end fissure burs, end-cutting burs, wheel burs, finishing burs, etc., all designated by their series of special numbers.

With the advent of ultraspeed and the air-turbine handpieces, the basic shapes have had small variations added such as domed ends and increased head lengths. Likewise, the majority of the burs used with ultraspeed are the small sizes. With these changes have naturally come additional numbered series and name designations (Fig. 16-25).

Burs made of exceptionally hard steel (called tungsten carbide burs) are used extensively by the dentist, and the assistant must keep them separate from the burs made of ordinary steel, realizing that the former are expensive in comparison. All burs used with ultraspeed angle handpieces are carbide burs. The carbide bur, because of its hardness, may be used many times in cutting the hard enamel tooth structure without becoming dull. The ordinary steel bur, on the other hand, will become dull after it is used only once in cutting the hard enamel of the teeth and should be discarded. If it is used only on dentin, the dulling action is much less.

The assistant should see that all the various sizes and shapes of burs are convenient for use by the dentist at all times.

The burs are cleaned free of ground tooth structure and other debris by brushing with a special steel bur brush. They are then sterilized by any prescribed method that will not harm the cutting edges or the temper of the steel.

Stones

Stones are the small grinding wheels and points that are held and caused to rotate by the handpiece. They are used for many grinding operations in and out of the mouth.

Stones are available in many sizes and shapes, various grits, and mounted or unmounted designs. Unmounted stones are placed on a suitable mandrel (a metal rod that is gripped and rotated by the handpieces) for use (Fig. 16-28). Mounted stones and mandrels are designed for use in the straight handpiece or the angle handpiece. Stones are generally divided into two groups: (1) those made of an abrasive, such as Carborundum, held in a binding matrix material, and (2) those having diamond particles as the abrasive. The latter are called "diamond instruments" and are fairly expensive.

Some of the Carborundum stones are called heatless, because the binder disintegrates at a low temperature. If placed in boiling water, they are ruined; therefore, cold disinfection is recommended. The dental assistant should also keep

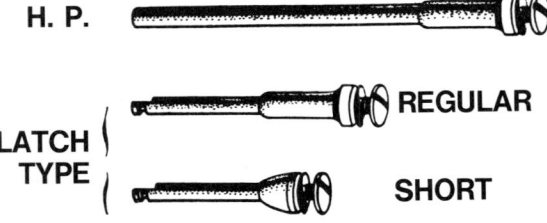

Figure 16-28 | No. 303 mandrels for straight handpiece and latch-type angle handpiece to which unmounted stones or discs may be attached.

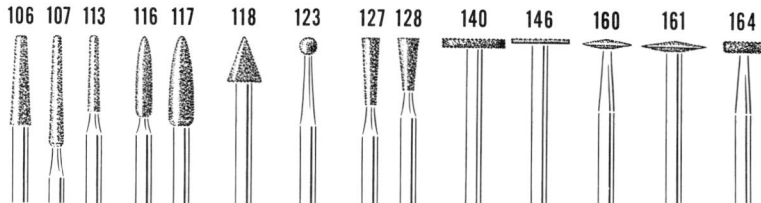

Figure 16-29 | Mounted diamond stone assortment. Some conventional uses are as follows: 106, 107, 113, taper cylinder for tapering walls in inlay and crown preparations; 116, 117, flame for enlarging pulp-canal chambers, subgingival grinding and beveling, and rounding corners; 118, cone for occlusal beveling; 123, ball for opening and gross extension of cavities; 127, 128, inverted cone for undercutting walls in establishing retention; 140, square-edge wheel for opening fissures, reducing occlusal and incisal surfaces; 146, top-cutting thin wheel for jacket crown and slice preparations; 160, 161, knife-edge wheel for opening occlusal fissures and making grooves; 164, round-edge wheel for gross enamel reduction. (*Courtesy of The S. S. White Dental Products International.*)

the Carborundum stones separated into two groups—those to be used on metal only and those used on tooth structure, porcelain, and synthetic filling materials. Stones are available in different colors to aid in maintaining this distinction.

Diamond Instruments

Diamond instruments were introduced to dentistry in the United States in 1942 and became popular because of their long life and great effectiveness in cutting enamel and dentin. Diamond instruments are commonly used in bulk reduction of tooth structure in addition to other preparation procedures. The designs vary from shapes similar to bur designs to large stones and even discs (Fig. 16-29). The grit will also vary from very fine to coarse; this degree of fineness, together with the shape of the stone and the rotational speeds at which it is used, determines its use. A diamond stone loses its cutting efficiency because of either loss of the abrasive particles or clogging with debris. If clogging is the cause, the stone may be run over a rubber and Carborundum wheel to restore the cutting efficiency.

Discs

For various polishing operations in and out of the mouth, the dentist uses paper discs which have an abrasive glued to one side (Fig. 16-30). These discs are available in various sizes with coarse, medium, or fine grits in garnet or cuttlefish abrasive. The discs can be quickly mounted on a suitable mandrel for use. The heads of mandrels are of various designs, some intended especially for paper discs and others for wheels. The dental assistant must become familiar with

Figure 16-30 | A disc rack provides a convenient storage and arrangement for various grits and sizes of discs and wheels.

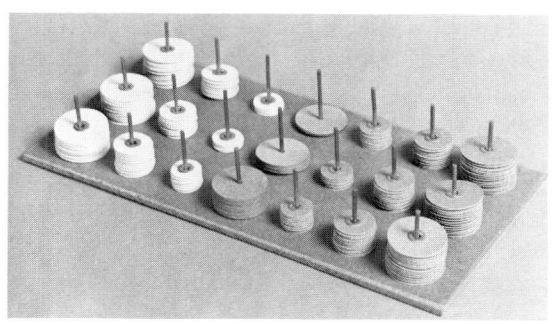

the different designs of mandrels and their applications.

Another familiar disc in the dental office is the Carborundum or diamond "separating" disc. When abrasive is on one side only, the disc is often termed "safe-sided." In addition to having an abrasive on both sides, these discs may be flat as well as cup-shaped. The Carborundum disc is quite brittle and must be handled with caution.

INSTRUMENTS AND ITEMS IN THE DENTAL OPERATING CABINET

The chairside assitant is of little help if he or she does not know the instruments in the operating cabinet. In order to assist efficiently and effectively, the assistant must make setups before operations and must pass instruments during an operation. In both these procedures, to avoid disaster, the assistant must have a thorough knowledge of the instruments and their use. In addition to studying instruments as they are in the operating cabinet, the assistant may obtain a dental supply house catalog which will provide valuable information for identifying instruments.

Hand Cutting Instruments

These instruments are commonly found in the top drawer of the cabinet (Fig. 16-31). They are rodlike pieces of steel and consist essentially of three parts—handle or shaft, shank, and blade or nib. The handle, or shaft, may be small or large in diameter, depending on the work to be accomplished with the particular type of instrument. The shank connects the handle and the blade. The blade contains the cutting edge and may be on one end (single-ended) or both ends (double-ended) of the handle. When the instrument is a condensing instrument, the working end is termed the *nib*. The cutting edge of the blade is produced by placing a bevel on the blade. The location of the bevel and the shape

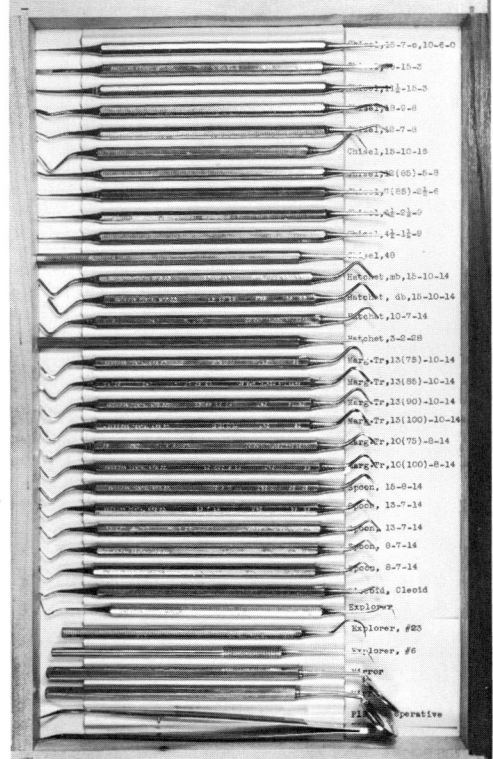

Figure 16-31 | Instrument drawer. Each hand instrument has an appropriate place which should be clearly indicated.

of the shank determine, in part, the area of the mouth and the surface of the tooth on which the instrument is used.

In order for the dentist to have adequate access to various surfaces of various teeth, the shanks of some instruments must be angled. One classification of instruments is by the number of angles in the shank: monangle (one), binangle (two), triple-angle (three), and quadrangle (four). When the instrument shanks are angled and the cutting edge is removed from the long axis of the handle, the instrument loses working balance. To overcome this, the instruments are contra-angled, which places the cut-

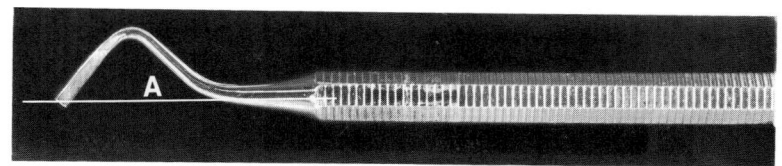

Figure 16-32 | Enamel hatchet with cutting edge brought to within 2 mm of long axis of handle by contra-angle A.

ting edge within 2 mm of the long axis of the handle (Fig. 16-32). Instruments that are contra-angled may be termed binangle contra-angle, triple-angle contra-angle, and quadrangle contra-angle.

In order to standardize instruments, the manufacturers produce hand cutting instruments in accord with an instrument formula. This formula appears on the instrument handle as a number or series of numbers. These numbers actually indicate the measurements of the blade in the metric system (Fig. 16-33). When more than one number appears, the first figure represents the width of the blade in tenths of a millimeter, the second figure indicates the length of the blade in millimeters, and the third figure designates the angle the blade forms with the long axis of the handle as expressed in centigrades. On instruments such as gingival margin trimmers, a fourth figure is included in the formula and is placed in the second position. This figure indicates the angle made by the cutting edge with the long axis of the handle. These numbers are not to be confused with the manufacturer's stock number appearing near the end of the handle. The formula numbers are essential in obtaining the correct instrument when ordering new instruments.

A suggested aid to the assistant in keeping the hand cutting instruments in proper order is to cut a piece of white paper to place under the blades of the instruments when they are in correct position in the drawer (Fig. 16-31). Then the name of the instrument together with the formula numbers can be typed in a position directly adjacent to the respective instruments. Later the paper can be covered with transparent tape or any coating that will preserve its clean appearance.

In relation to operating on tooth structure, hand instruments are usually placed in two groups—excavators and chisels. The excavators are used for removal of caries and the refinement of the internal parts of the cavity. The chisels are used for cutting of enamel.

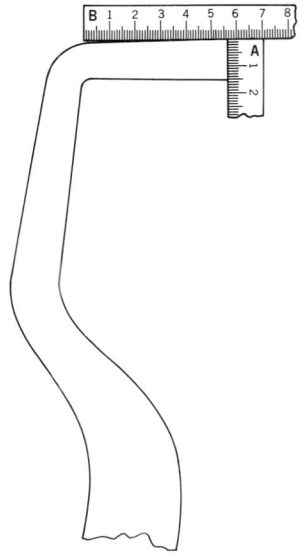

Figure 16-33 | Measurements for instrument formula. A. First figure of formula, width of the blade in tenths of a millimeter. B. Second figure of formula, length of the blade in millimeters.

Chapter Sixteen | Instruments, Equipment, and Their Care

Excavators

Instruments such as the spoon, the hoe, and the ordinary hatchet are forms of excavators (Fig. 16-34).

The *spoon* excavators are used for removal of soft decay from the cavity and are shaped like a margin trimmer (curved blade) with the cutting edge either rounded (*discoid*) or clawlike (*cleoid*). The shanks may be binangled or triple-angled, and they are available in pairs (rights and lefts).

The *hoe* excavators are used primarily on anterior teeth for removal of caries and forming line angles. The cutting edge of the blade is in a plane perpendicular to the long axis of the handle. Instruments of similar design but with longer and heavier blades are used for cutting enamel on posterior teeth.

The *ordinary hatchet* excavators are used on anterior teeth in refining internal line angles and removing the hard-type caries. The cutting edge of the blade is in the same plane as the long axis of the handle, and it is bibeveled (beveled on both sides of the blade).

The *angle formers* may also be classified as excavators. They are used for sharpening line angles and obtaining retention form in dentin. They are monangled and have the cutting edge at an angle to the blade (requiring a fourth number in the instrument formula as with gingival margin trimmers).

Chisels

Instruments such as straight or binangle chisels, enamel hatchets, and gingival margin trimmers are forms of chisels (Fig. 16-35). They are used in cutting enamel.

The *chisel* resembles a miniature wood chisel with a straight or curved blade or a binangled shank. The binangle and Wedelstaedt (curved blade) chisels may have the bevel on the mesial or distal side of the blade.

The *enamel hatchet* is similar to the ordinary

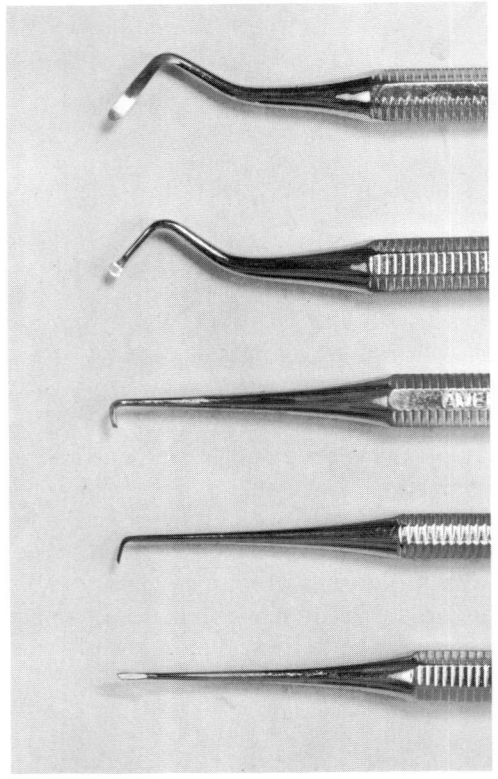

Figure 16-34 | Excavators. Beginning with instrument at top of illustration: spoon, 15–8–14; binangle spoon, 13–7–14; ordinary hatchet, 3–2–28; hoe, 8–3–22; and angle former, 12–85–8.

hatchet except that the blade is larger and heavier and beveled on only one side. All enamel hatchets are contra-angled to bring the working edge of the blade to within 2 mm of the long axis of the handle. They are also made in pairs for working on the right or left side.

The *gingival margin trimmer* is a special chisel designed for placing bevels on gingival enamel margins of proximoocclusal cavity preparations. The blade is similar to that of an enamel hatchet but is slightly curved, and the cutting edge is at an angle with the blade. These instruments are made in pairs for either the mesial or distal surface of the tooth, as well as being paired for right

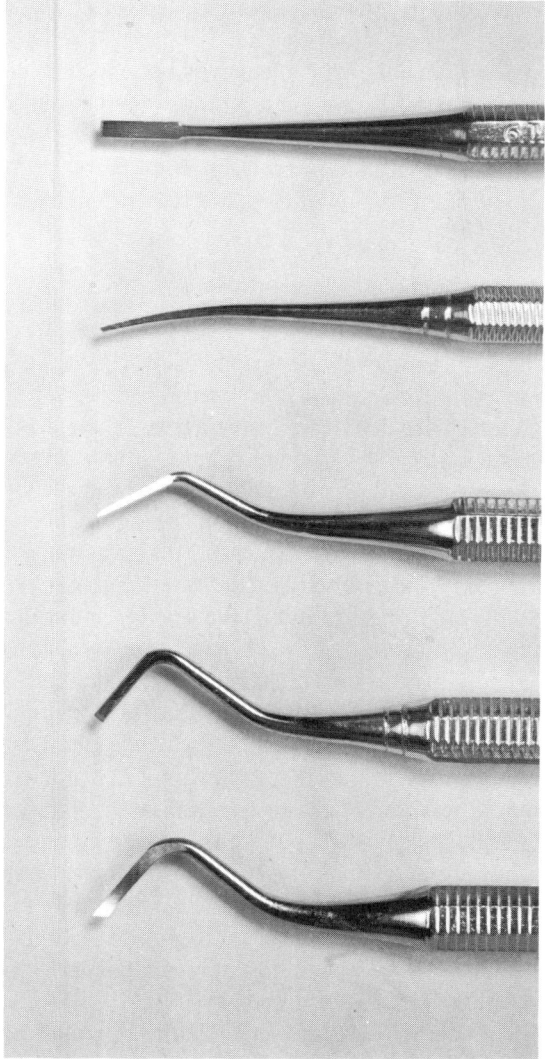

Figure 16-35 | Chisels. Beginning with instrument at top of illustration: straight, 15–7–0; Wedelstaedt, 11½–15–3; binangle, 12–7–8; enamel hatchet, 10–7–14; and gingival margin trimmer, 10–100–8–14.

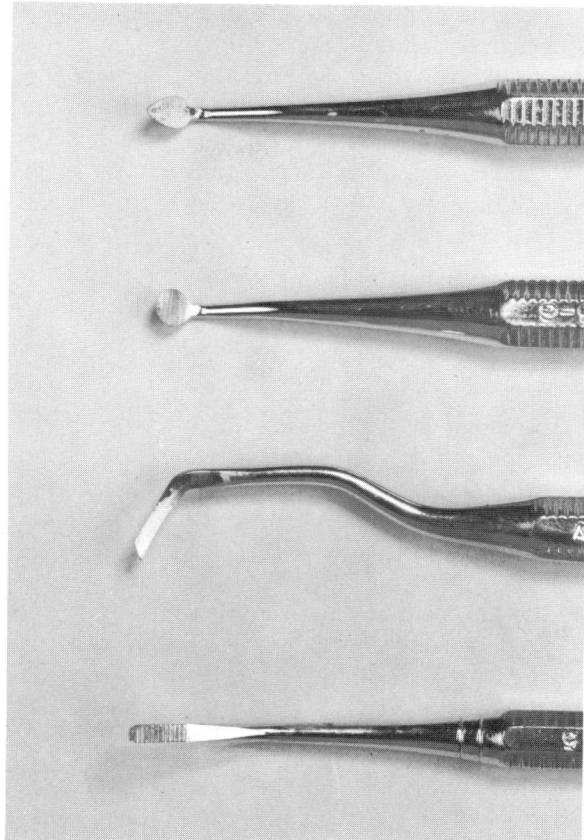

Figure 16-36 | Miscellaneous hand cutting instruments. Beginning at top of illustration: cleoid, discoid, finishing knife, and dental file. These instruments do not have instrument formulas in the same context as the excavators and chisels.

and left. When the second number in the instrument formula is 90 or above, the margin trimmer is used on the distal surface, and when it is 85 or below, the instrument is used on the mesial surface.

Miscellaneous Hand Cutting Instruments

Instruments such as the knife, file, and discoid-cleoid are classified as hand cutting instruments (Fig. 16-36). However, these instruments are used in trimming restorative material rather than in cutting tooth structure.

The *knife* may be known as a finishing knife, an amalgam knife, or a gold knife and has a very small, thin, knifelike blade.

The *file* is designed in various shapes and sizes with a thin blade. The teeth on the blade are very short and are so designed to make the file either a push or a pull instrument.

The *discoid-cleoid* instrument has working ends similar in shape but larger than the ends of excavators. In addition, the plane of the working ends is perpendicular to the long axis of the handle.

Sterilization of Hand Cutting Instruments

Hand instruments are made of one of three metal alloys—stainless steel, high-carbon steel, or cobalt-chromium alloy. Hand cutting instruments made of high-carbon steel retain the cutting edge better than those made of stainless steel alloys. However, they are subject to rust and corrosion if they are sterilized in boiling water. Rust inhibitors help prevent this reaction, but the hand cutting instruments are best sterilized by other methods. Various methods of sterilizing instruments and materials are discussed in Chap. 7, and the assistant should follow the dentist's suggestions regarding this matter.

When an ultrasonic cleaner is used in the office (Fig. 16-37), the assistant must keep in mind that this piece of equipment does not take the place of sterilization procedures even though it is an excellent means of cleaning instruments.

Prophylaxis and Periodontia Instruments

These instruments are usually kept in one section of the cabinet not immediately associated with the hand cutting instruments. Their construction is similar to that of hand cutting instruments in that they are rodlike pieces of steel and consist of a handle, shank, and blade. In many instances, the handles of these instruments are somewhat larger and heavier than those of hand cutting instruments, and a cutting edge is usually not on both ends of the handle (Fig. 16-38).

These instruments are used for the mechanical removal of concretions (calculus and debris) from around the teeth and subgingival pockets. The areas in which these instruments are used are not always easily accessible; therefore, various designs and configurations of the cutting edges are available. The selection of the proper instruments for specific purposes is a matter of personal choice of the dentist. For ease in identification, these instruments may be classified as *scalers, curettes,* and *files.*

The dental assistant must learn the names, uses, and identification of these instruments, as for the hand cutting instruments. Their sterilization and care are very similar to those of the hand cutting instruments.

Mirrors

The assistant must be constantly alert to the condition of the dental mirrors. Usually they are detachable from their handles by simply unscrewing them. This feature saves the expense of the handle when it becomes necessary to discard

Figure 16-37 | Ultrasonic cleaner. Instruments are placed in the tank, which contains the proper cleaning solution. Instruments are cleaned in a few minutes; because of the gentleness of the process, even the most fragile instruments are not damaged. This apparatus, however, is not to take the place of sterilization procedures. (*Courtesy of L & R Manufacturing Company.*)

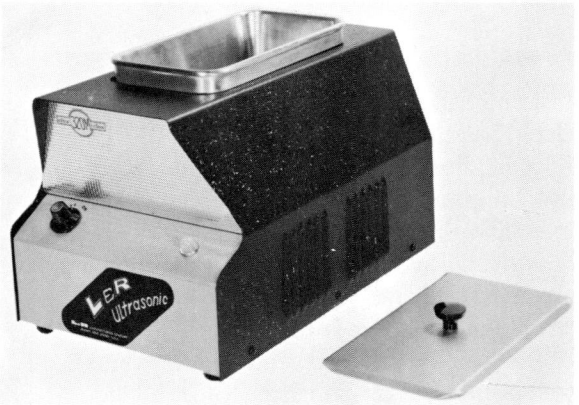

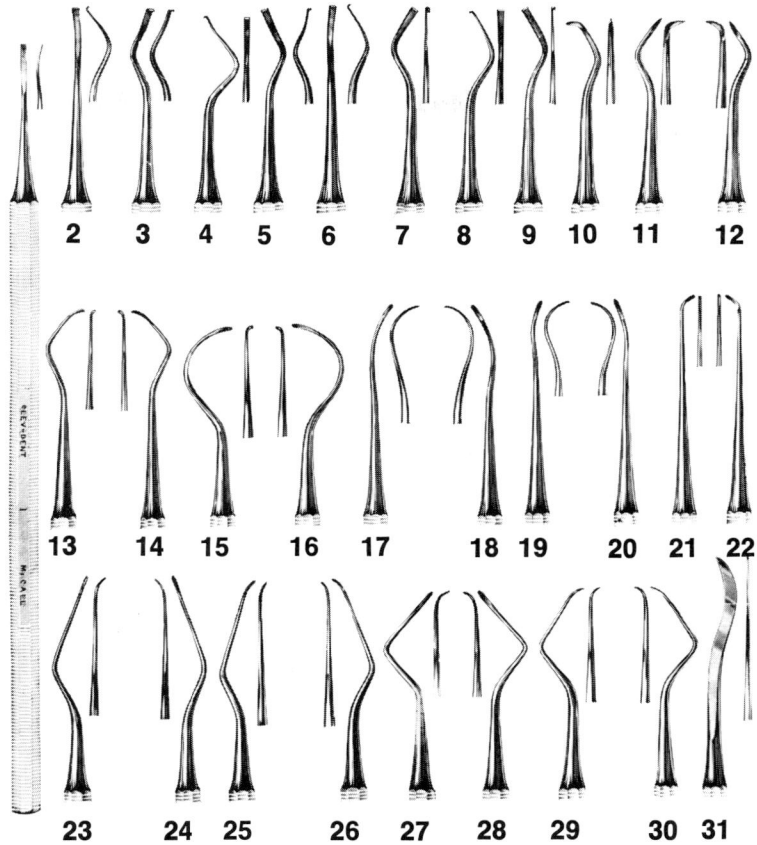

Figure 16-38 | Scalers and prophylactic curettes designed by Dr. John Oppie McCall. Nos. 1 to 12, scalers; nos. 13 to 30, curettes; no. 31, interproximal scaler. (*Courtesy of Clev-dent, Division of Cavitron Corp.*)

the mirror. The handles used are termed *cone-socket handles,* and the mirrors are mounted on a cone-socket stem (Fig. 16-39).

The dental mirror is used not only for viewing areas of the oral cavity, but also for reflecting light on dark areas and for retracting the lips, cheeks, or tongue for better visibility and for protecting this tissue from injury in case an instrument slips off the working surface. Replacing old mirrors with new ones, when they become badly scratched or permanently fogged, is the responsibility of the assistant. Therefore, the assistant must watch to see that additional mirrors are always stocked in the supply closet.

Some dentists use dental mirrors that are magnifying; others use plain mirrors or front-surface mirrors. Dental mirrors also come in various sizes. The assistant must become acquainted with the dentist's wishes in these respects.

In most dental operating rooms a hand mirror is kept for occasional use by a patient. The assistant must see that this mirror is clean at all times and free of fingerprints or other signs of use by previous patients.

Explorers

The dentist uses explorers to examine teeth through the sense of touch. These instruments are used not only in the initial examination of the teeth, but also during the entire cavity preparation and restoring procedures to locate decay and check the walls and angles of the preparation as well as the margins of the restoration. These instruments are made of steel, have sharp tines, and come in many different shapes (Fig. 16-40A). The assistant is expected to maintain a few of each of the dentist's favorite explorers in the supply closet as replacements for those which are broken.

Operating Pliers

Operating pliers are commonly referred to as the cotton pliers or tweezers (Fig. 16-40B). They are used to convey objects such as cotton pellets, cotton rolls, small lengths of wire, etc., to and from the mouth.

Since these pliers are used in the mouth, they should never be placed over an open flame. This will destroy the temper of the metal and discolor the tips, making them unsightly. There are other types of pliers of similar design that should be used in conjunction with open flames.

The setup for each patient always includes (1) operating pliers, (2) explorer, and (3) dental mirror. The dentist expects the assistant to have these items out of the cabinet and ready for his use.

Plastic Instruments and Mixing Spatulas

Plastic instruments are steel instruments with handles similar to those of the cutting instruments but with paddles and/or nibs (or condensers) instead of blades with cutting edges (Fig. 16-41). These instruments are used to insert plastic materials into cavities in the teeth. These plastic materials include the thermoplastic (i.e.,

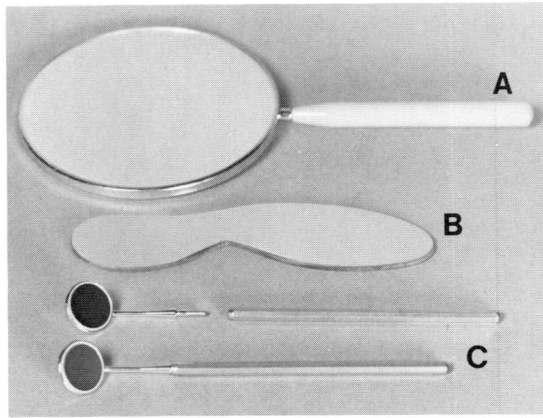

Figure 16-39 | A variety of mirrors are used in dentistry. A. Patient hand mirror. B. Photography mirror utilized in producing intraoral pictures. C. Cone-socket dental mirror and handle.

softened by heating and hardened by cooling) temporary materials (such as temporary stopping and gutta-percha) and the cements (silicate cement, zinc phosphate cement, resin cement, and zinc oxide–eugenol cement).

An alert assistant will soon observe which instruments the dentist prefers when inserting the various plastic materials and will, accordingly, anticipate the need for a certain instrument.

The assistant should take special note of those instruments used for inserting the silicate cements. These are the cements used in filling cavities in the anterior teeth. Generally, these instruments should never be used for any other purpose. Care must be taken not to heat them in an open flame, since heating will cause them to turn black and thus render them unsuitable for use in handling the silicate cements. The special plastic instruments used with silicate cements are made of stainless steel to prevent the forming of rust on the instrument surface.

Often, after use, other plastic instruments have wax, compound, temporary stopping, or gutta-percha on them. As previously mentioned, these materials are thermoplastic. Therefore, any resi-

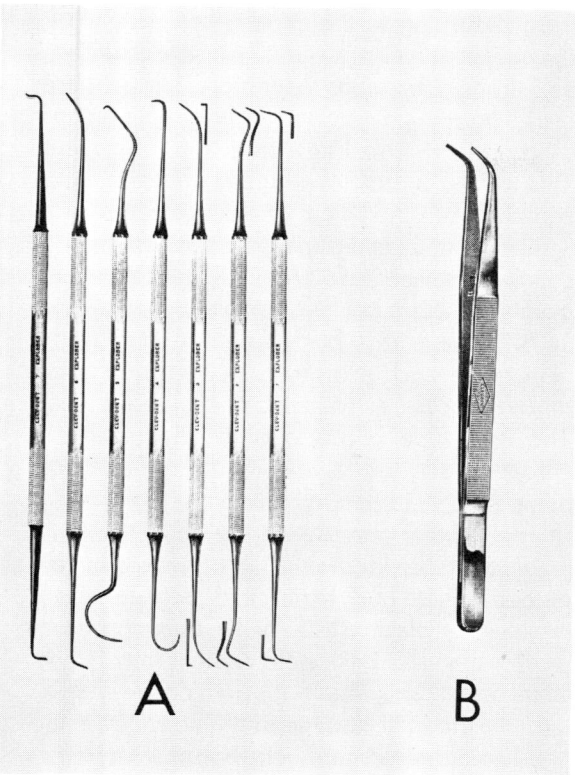
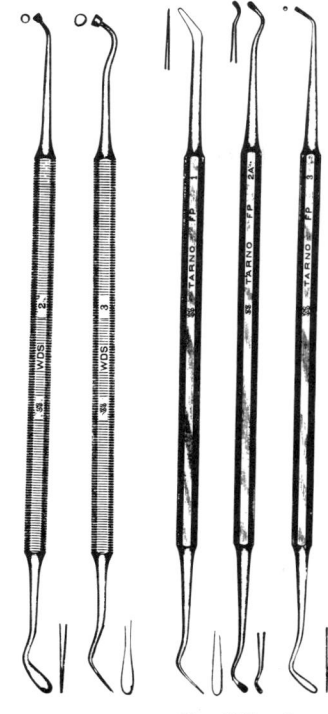

For Silicates

Figure 16-40 | A. Double-ended explorers with various tine designs. B. Operating pliers. (*Courtesy of Clev-dent, Division of Cavitron Corp.*)

Figure 16-41 | Plastic instruments for inserting materials into cavity preparations in teeth. Those used for silicate cement should never be placed in an open flame. (*Courtesy of the S. S. White Dental Products International.*)

due of these materials can be removed by first warming the instrument sufficiently in an open flame to soften the material and then by quickly wiping the instrument with a disposable paper towel while the material is still soft.

After using the zinc phosphate cements, there will usually be cement on the plastic instruments. This can be removed easily if the instruments are inserted in a soda solution while the cement is still soft. Hardened cement on the serrated surface of the instrument handle can be removed effectively with a wire brush.

Resin cement, not unlike other dental cements, has no real adhesive quality when subjected to moisture. Therefore, the material can be removed from instruments after they have soaked in water for a period of time. Soaking in water, however, requires more time than if a resin solvent is used.

The zinc oxide–eugenol cements are best removed from instruments by wiping them with a paper towel while the cement is still soft. If this type of cement is permitted to harden on the instrument, it can be removed only by suitable solvents such as chloroform or acetone.

Keeping plastic instruments clean of all residue material is the responsibility of the assistant, and its importance cannot be overemphasized. It is

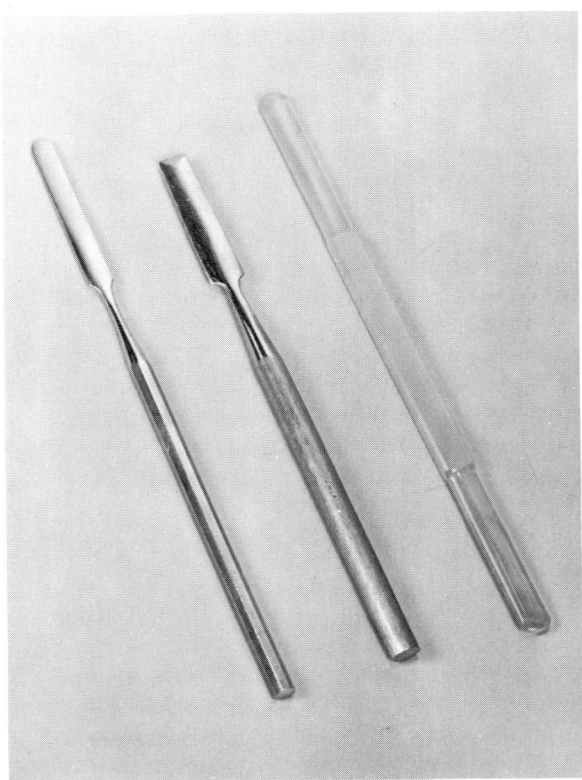

Figure 16-42 | Mixing spatulas. *Left,* flexible-blade spatula. *Center,* rigid-blade spatula. *Right,* agate spatula.

Figure 16-43 | Glass mixing slab for silicate and zinc phosphate cements. The thermometer incorporated into the slab assures that the mixing slab temperature is correct for mixing cements. (*Courtesy of The L. D. Caulk Company, Division Dentsply International Inc.*)

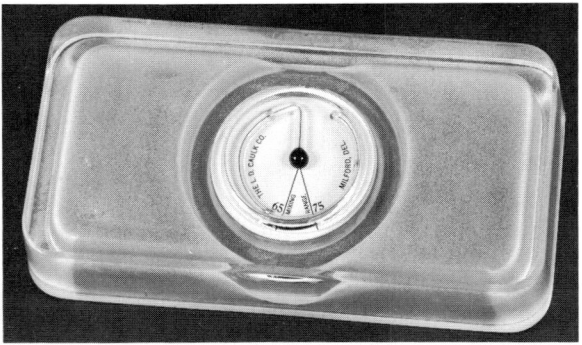

most disturbing to the dentist, and certainly to the patient as well, to see on an instrument materials from a previous operation. Furthermore, bits of hardened cement on these instruments will be incorporated in a fresh mix of cement. This usually is most undesirable and sometimes contributes to the failure of a restoration.

Mixing spatulas are made of stainless steel or cobalt-chromium alloy and have flat, blunt blades, which may be flexible or rigid (Fig. 16-42). The flexible-blade type is used in mixing cement in which pressure is needed during the mixing process, as with zinc phosphate cement. The rigid type of blade is usually of cobalt-chromium alloy and is used for mixing silicate cement, in which case pressure is contraindicated. (Many dentists prefer an agate spatula or one made of plastic for the mixing of this silicate cement.) What has been said regarding the cleaning of plastic instruments also applies to mixing spatulas. Bits of old cement from a previous cement mix must not be left on the spatula, because they will cause undesirable effects in the physical properties and behavior of a future cement mix. An untidy spatula is also evidence in the eyes of the patient of uncleanliness and carelessness.

Glass Slabs

The zinc phosphate cement and silicate cement are mixed on glass slabs. Cements of the zinc oxide–eugenol type are mixed preferably on a paper pad. Using a paper pad for cement mixing is indicated wherever possible, because it eliminates the necessity of cleaning a glass slab. *However, the zinc phosphate and silicate cements always should be mixed on a glass slab* (Fig. 16-43). Putting soda solution on cement to be removed from a glass slab, before the cement has hardened appreciably, will greatly aid in its removal. The assistant should be careful to avoid, as far as possible, scratching the surface of a glass slab. A slab with many scratches should be replaced with a new one. Not only is a badly scratched slab unsightly, but it is also detrimental to new mixes of cement since deep scratches are usually filled with cement particles from previous mixes which may become dislodged and incorporated in a new cement mix; this will result in a change in the physical properties of the cement.

Burnishers

Burnishers are steel instruments (usually stainless) with handles similar to those of the hand cutting instruments but with working points in the shape of balls and "beavertails" of different sizes. These instruments are used primarily to burnish (adapt) the margins of a gold restoration to a better fit.

Amalgam Instruments

Amalgam *condensers* (pluggers), generally made of stainless steel, are used to pack or condense, by hand pressure, amalgam into a prepared cavity in a tooth (Fig. 16-44). They have handles similar to those of the hand cutting instruments, but the working points, called nibs, present flat faces or surfaces which are circular, rectangular, ovoid, or crescent-shaped.

The face of a condenser may be plain (smooth) or serrated. If it is serrated, the assistant must inspect it each time the instrument is used to detect any amalgam stuck or lodged in the serrations. Such bits of amalgam should be removed immediately by brushing with a steel brush. Amalgam that has been allowed to remain and harden on the condenser face may be removed in the same manner. It is important that the assistant understand the seriousness of leaving bits of hardened amalgam on the face of an amalgam condenser. Such bits will surely be incorporated in a subsequent mix while it is being condensed into a cavity, resulting in possible faulty margins and a weakened restoration. Furthermore, this will cause undesirable effects in the carving and finishing of the amalgam.

Amalgam carvers are steel instruments similar to the hand cutting instruments, except that the working ends are of suitable design (displaying curved sharp edges of various radii) to facilitate the carving of fresh amalgam or inlay wax to anatomic form immediately after the material has been condensed into the cavity. These instruments should not be excessively heated, nor should they be used in the carving of plastic temporary filling materials. Such heating will usually ruin the appearance of the instrument as well as destroy its carving edge.

Amalgam carriers are used to convey the fill-

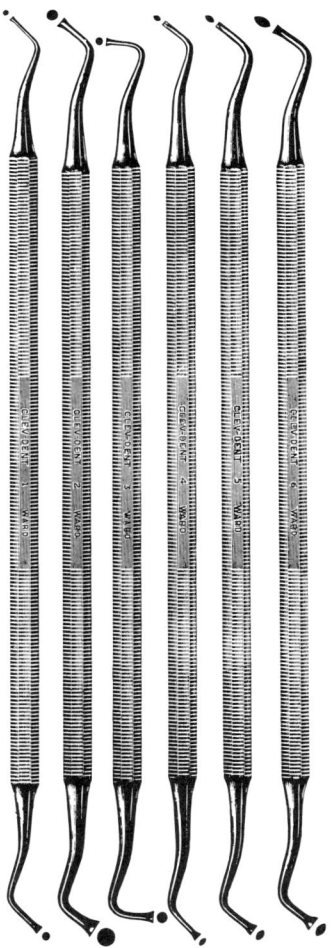

Figure 16-44 | Amalgam condensing instruments. The black markings opposite the ends of the instruments show the shapes of the condensing surfaces. (*Courtesy of Clev-dent, Division of Cavitron Corp.*)

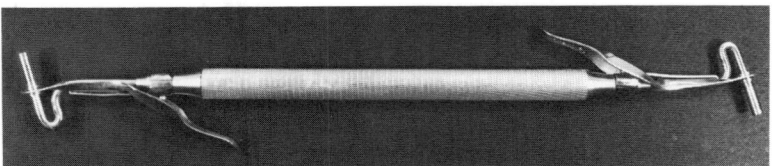

Figure 16-45 | Double-end lever type of amalgam carrier. The ends of the carrier differ in size, thus permitting large or small amounts of amalgam to be transferred.

ing material into cavities and may be of several designs. One is the plunger type, consisting of a tube and plunger with a flexible rod extending the length of the instrument. Another design is the lever type, consisting of a short tube and plunger operated by a lever located very close to the working end of the instrument (Fig. 16-45). The plungers expel the amalgam from the carrying tube. Unless the carriers are kept clean, hardened material will cause them to stick. Heating will soften any hardened amalgam so that it can be expelled and the instrument quickly made ready for use. Hardened bits of amalgam in these carriers may be incorporated in a subsequent filling. This may cause the restoration to fail for the reasons previously given in the section on amalgam condensers.

The *mechanical amalgam mixer* (Fig. 16-46) is designed to triturate (mix mercury and amalgam alloy to produce a plastic mass) amalgam in a small fraction of the time it takes by hand. Hand trituration is accomplished with a glass mortar and pestle but is less convenient and less accurate than mechanical mixing. Instructions that come with the machine should be followed explicitly. It is important that the assistant keep the capsule and pestle clean and free of hardened bits of amalgam. An excellent method of cleaning the mixed amalgam out of all corners of the capsule is to replace the freshly mixed amalgam into the capsule, leaving the pestle out. Then mix (this may be called the mulling operation) again for 1 second. This will gather all the amalgam into one rounded mass and will seldom leave any traces of the fresh mix on the inside surfaces of the capsule and capsule lid. Any remaining traces of the mix in the capsule, capsule lid, or on the pestle should be removed before the amalgam hardens by brushing with a tuft bristle brush. The brush is a conventional prophylaxis tuft bristle brush mounted in a straight handpiece mandrel.

Amalgam *matrix retainers* constitute a group of equipment pieces that are extremely important to the success of the dentist's work. Matrix retainers, with their matrix bands (Fig. 16-47), are mechanical devices designed to retain (contain) amalgam while it is being condensed into a cavity that involves two or more surfaces of a tooth. There are many designs of retainers available, and usually several of them are found in the dental cabinet. The assistant will soon realize which retainer the dentist is likely to use and can thus anticipate his or her need by having it ready.

Commonly used retainers hold thin steel matrix bands of varying shapes and sizes tightly around the tooth. The experienced assistant will learn to assist the dentist by choosing the right band and attaching it to the retainer, ready for application.

A matrix band which has been used several times and which no longer is reasonably smooth should be discarded.

The assistant is urged to provide an area in one of the drawers of the dental cabinet for ma-

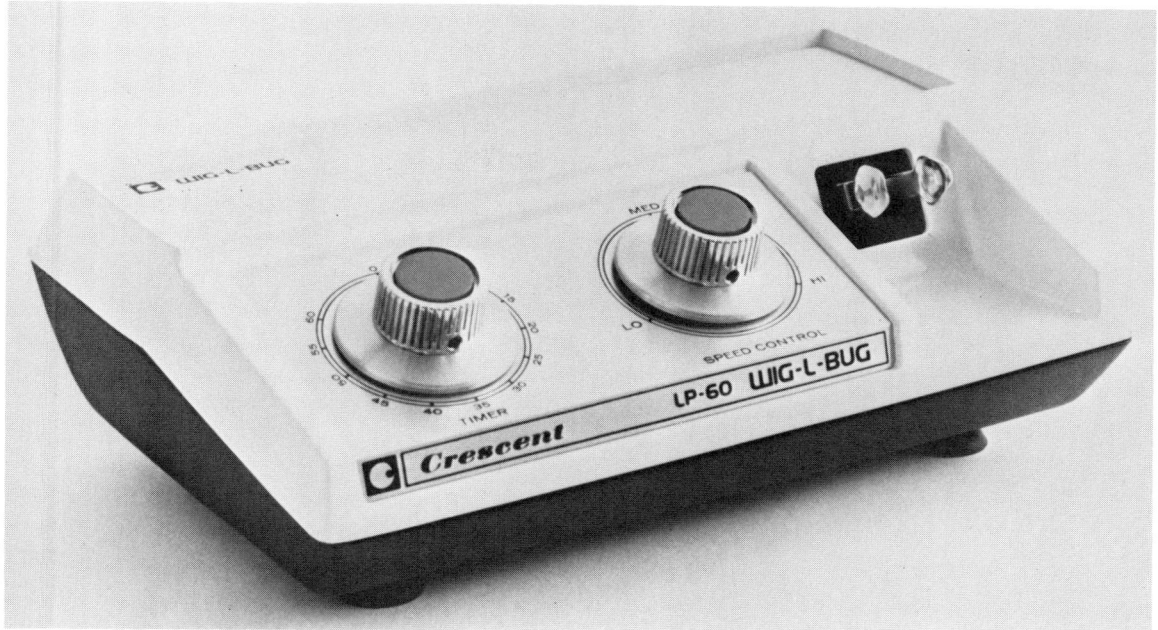

Figure 16-46 | Mechanical amalgamator with variable speed control and timer dials. By using various capsules and variable settings, materials other than amalgam alloy can be mixed. (*Courtesy of Crescent Dental Manufacturing Co.*)

trix retainers and bands in order to facilitate their selection as to size and design. The assistant or the dentist should be able to find the right matrix band at a glance. Divided plastic boxes may be used for keeping different sizes and shapes in an orderly manner.

The matrix retainer and the matrix bands should be sterilized after each use.

Reamers and Files

Reamers and files are part of the armamentarium used in endodontics. They are used along with other specific types of instruments in root canal therapy and should be assigned a specific place in the dental cabinet. The assistant should keep in mind that these instruments are relatively delicate and sharp and should be handled with care. Aseptic technique is extremely important in endodontic procedures, and when these instruments are used, they should be placed on a sterile towel on the bracket table. After use, they are cleaned, wrapped in a towel, autoclaved, and then stored in the towel.

The dental assistant should become thoroughly familiar with the sizes and shapes of these instruments and the proper handling of them during an endodontic operation. The use of endodontic instruments is thoroughly explained in Chap. 24, Endodontics.

Pliers

Pliers in dentistry are not confined to laboratory procedures. The dental cabinet in the operating room should contain several pliers, as illustrated in Fig. 16-48. The assistant will find that in some operations the dentist will use pliers other than

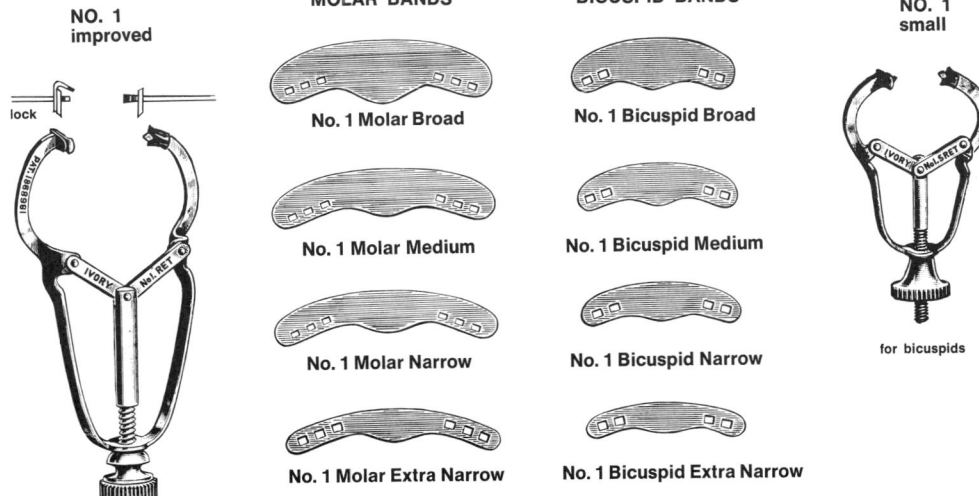
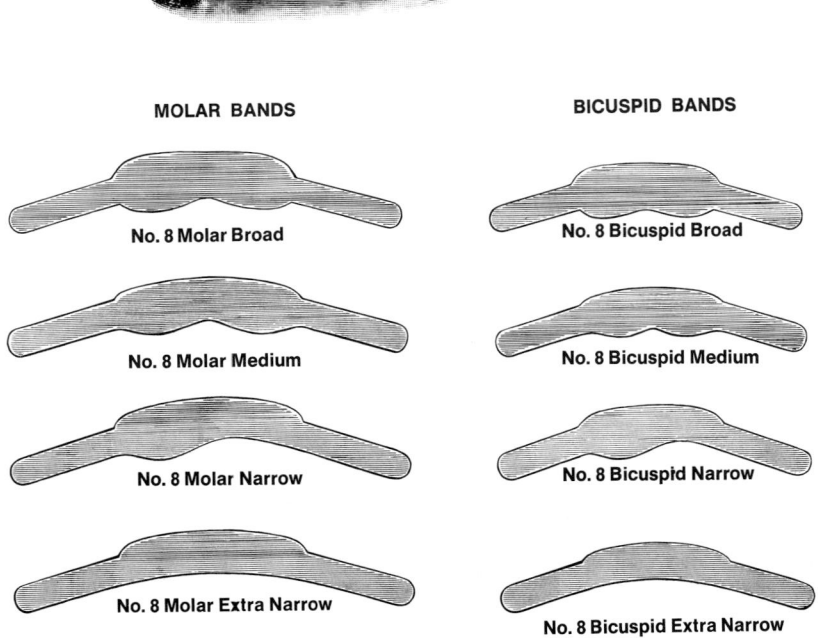

Figure 16-47 | Selection of matrix retainers and bands. Retainers and bands in upper half of illustration are used with two-surface cavity preparations. Those in the lower half are used with more extensive cavity preparations. (*Courtesy of J. W. Ivory, Inc.*)

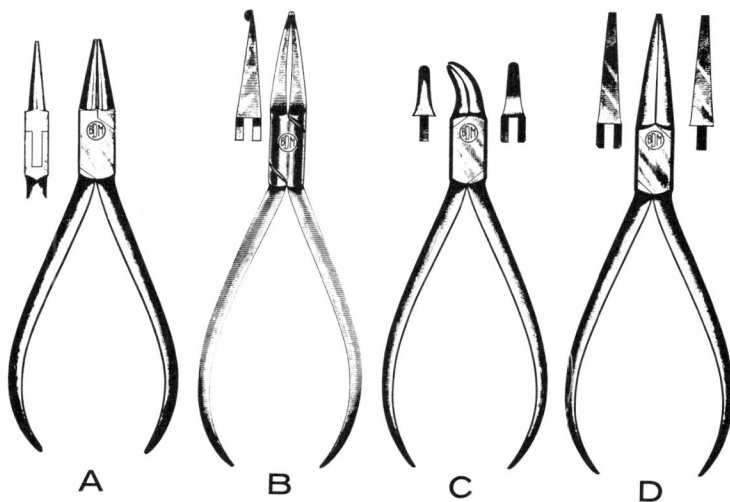

Figure 16-48 | Office and laboratory pliers. A. Round-nose (no. 107). B. Smooth-crown (no. 110). C. Contouring (no. 115). D. Serrated long-nose (no. 121). (*Courtesy of Buffalo Dental Manufacturing Company.*)

the operating pliers. The various beaks on pliers make them adaptable to different procedures, and the assistant must learn the type of pliers required by the dentist for specific operations. Pliers of this type should not be placed on the bracket table, but rather handed to the dentist as needed. Since they do not usually touch mouth tissue, they can be disinfected by wiping with a gauze sponge saturated with a germicidal solution.

The orthodontist uses a wide variety of pliers, and these are usually held in a special rack on the bracket table. Orthodontic instruments (including pliers) are discussed and illustrated in Chap. 27.

Equipment for Condensed Gold

Equipment commonly used by the dentist when restoring teeth with condensed gold includes alcohol burner, annealing tray, gold foil holding instrument, plugger points, and hand mallet (Fig. 16-49). A pneumatic, automatic (mechanical), or electric condenser is often used in lieu of the hand mallet.

The *annealing (degassing) tray,* consisting of a mica plate or an enameled metal tray, is supported by a suitable metallic frame over an alcohol flame. Annealing trays may also be placed over the Bunsen burner, which is often attached to the bracket table of the dental unit. On this tray the pellets of gold are heated. This prepares them for insertion into the cavity in the tooth. The assistant should exercise care to keep the tray surface absolutely clean and free of dust at all times. It is recommended that the tray be kept in a covered box when not in use. If an alcohol lamp is used, the assistant should have the lamp filled with pure alcohol, either methyl or ethyl alcohol, or a combination of the two.

The *holding instrument* and the *pluggers* (Fig. 16-49) have very small faces which are serrated. These instruments are used to condense the gold into the cavity by delivering a force initiated by the hand mallet or a mechanical or pneumatic condenser. These instruments, like the tray, must be kept clean. If a plugger is contaminated (e.g., by the fingers, which could possibly leave an oily film on its face), it should be cleansed by scrubbing with a small brush previously dipped in pure alcohol. Then, if the point is to be used immediately, the alcohol film is burned away by passing it quickly through a flame. If the point is not to be used immediately, the alcohol film will evaporate and leave the instrument clean.

If these precautions involving the cleanliness of any instrument that touches the gold are not observed, the restoration will be a failure because any contamination of the surface of the gold will prevent it from welding (that is, uniting molecularly into one coherent gold mass) as it is condensed under the plugger point. To safeguard the points against contamination when not in use, they are best kept in pockets of a felt roll.

Sterilization of plugger points is not necessary or indicated.

Syringes

Figure 16-50 illustrates three designs of syringes that are used in introducing elastic impression materials into and around prepared teeth. These syringes are used primarily with the "rubberlike" impression materials.

The manufacturer of each type of syringe recommends a specific method for loading and cleaning the syringe, according to the design of the instrument. These syringes are disinfected simply by wiping with a gauze sponge saturated with a germicidal solution. If the syringe used in the office utilizes plastic tips, it is the responsibility of the assistant to have an ample supply of the proper plastic tips available.

Other types of syringes are also used in dentistry. The most common types, the Luer type (glass) and the cartridge type (metal), are illustrated in Chap. 22. The Luer syringe is used primarily for irrigation, while the cartridge syringe is used in the application of local anesthetic.

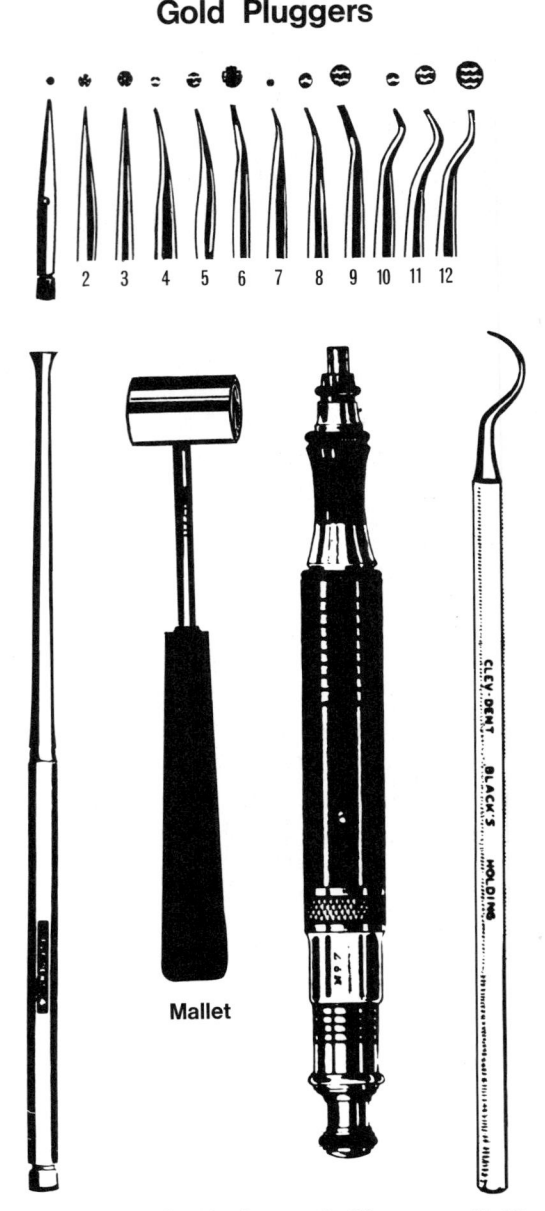

Figure 16-49 | Gold condensing instruments. Pluggers may be placed in handle, automatic plugger, or pneumatic condenser handpieces. (*Courtesy of Clev-dent, Division of Cavitron Corp.*)

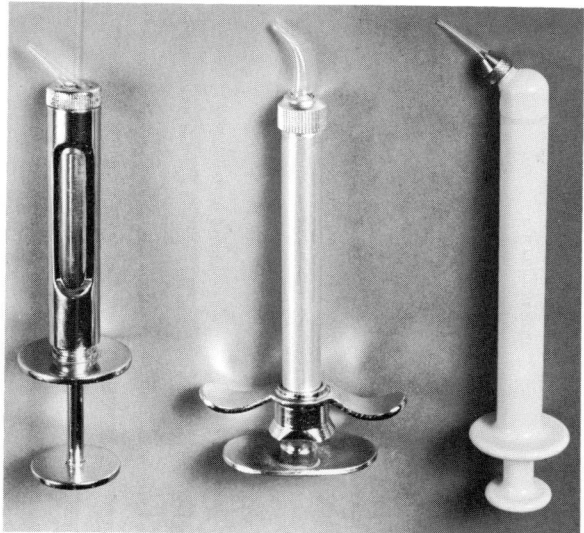

Figure 16-50 | Syringes of various designs, which are used in conjunction with the impression technique utilizing the rubber-like impression materials.

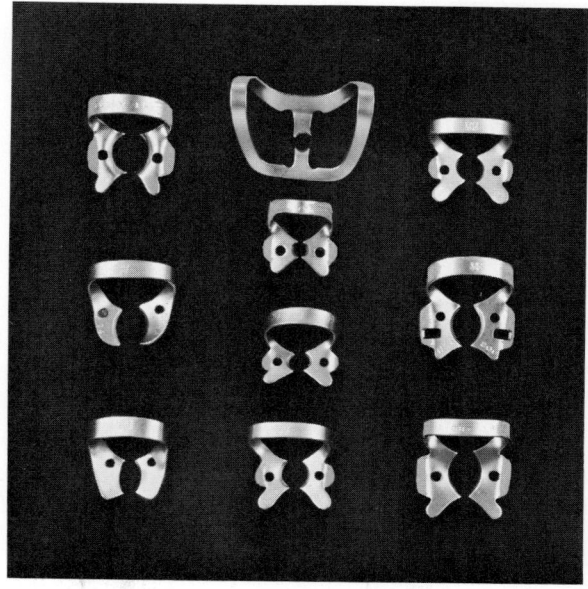

Figure 16-51 | A typical selection of rubber dam clamps including a cervical clamp (*top center*). (*From Sturdevant, Barton, and Brauer (eds.), The Art and Science of Operative Dentistry, Copyright 1968 by McGraw-Hill, Inc. Used with permission of McGraw-Hill Book Company.*)

Rubber Dam Equipment

Equipment used in the application of a rubber dam consists of the rubber dam material, clamps, holder, punch, and forceps.

The *rubber dam* material is applied to the mouth in order to isolate several teeth from the oral environment. The material is supplied in rolls or in precut sheets (5 × 5 in or 6 × 6 in). It is available in light or dark colors and in various thicknesses, thin, medium, heavy, extra-heavy, and special heavy.

The *rubber dam clamp* is placed on a specified tooth to hold the dam in position. There are many different sizes and shapes available (Fig. 16-51). They should be placed in separate receptacles, properly labeled, in the operating cabinet drawer. This will facilitate rapid selection of a clamp.

The *holder* is fastened to that rubber dam material outside of the mouth (Fig. 16-52) and maintains the position of the rubber dam as well as keeps the bulk of the material away from the operative site. Several types of holders are available such as the U-frame type and the clip type.

The rubber dam must have cleanly cut holes punched in it to correspond to the teeth that are to be exposed. A special *punch* is used which is capable of producing holes of various sizes (Fig. 16-53). The instrument has a rotating metal disc with six holes of various sizes and a tapered, sharp-point plunger. The punch should never be closed unless the plunger fits one of the holes exactly; otherwise the holes will not be clean-cut and the rubber dam will be subject to tearing in these areas.

The *rubber dam clamp forceps* (Fig. 16-53) is used to grasp the rubber dam clamp, expand it, and slide it over the tooth. Likewise, it is used to remove the clamp from the tooth.

When the rubber dam is to be in place for a considerable length of time a *rubber dam napkin*

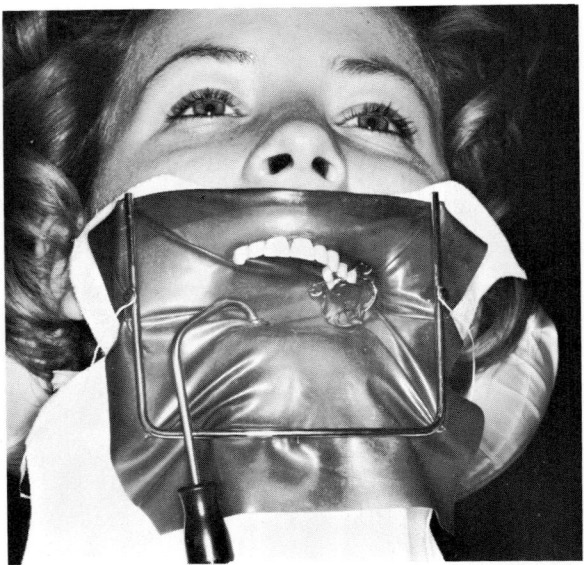

Figure 16-52 | Completed rubber dam in place. Note that frame keeps the dam taut and the operating area free of excess rubber dam material.

STERILIZATION AND DISINFECTION EQUIPMENT

As related in Chap. 7, sterilization and disinfection are two different concepts, and both have a proper place in dentistry. The two procedures are really not interchangeable, and the assistant must be fully aware of the end result of each.

Among the various types of equipment used in sterilization and disinfection are those which accommodate boiling water, steam, dry heat, hot oil, molten metal, glass beads, chemicals, and gas. A description of the various methods as well as the recommended method for various instruments is presented in Chap. 7.

The transfer of infection among dental patients and office personnel must be avoided, and this responsibility rests largely with the dental as-

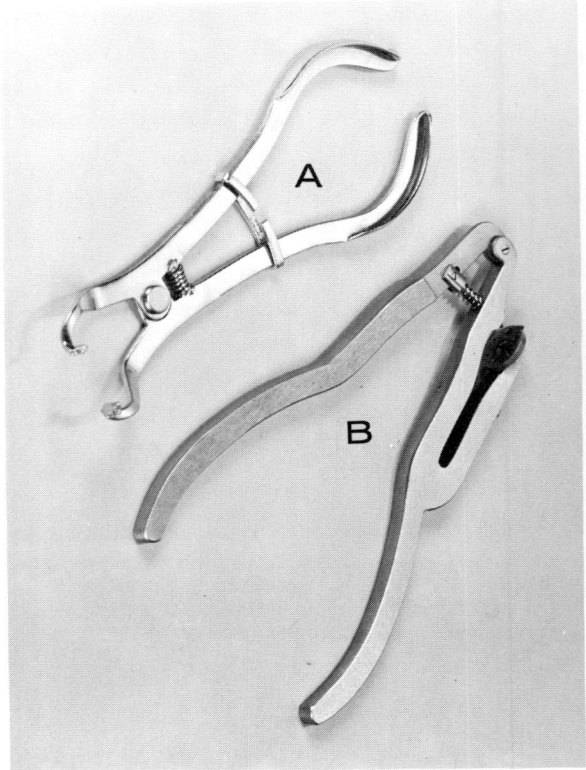

Figure 16-53 | A. Rubber dam clamp forceps for placing and removal of the rubber dam clamps. B. Rubber dam punch for placing various size holes in the rubber dam.

sistant. Information received from the patient and patient appearance do not always ensure the absence of some type of transmittable infection. Proper and complete sterilization or disinfection procedures must always be followed in relation to the use of the various dental instruments and pieces of equipment.

INSTRUMENT SHARPENING

As the hand instruments are used, they become dull and lose their cutting efficiency. It therefore becomes necessary for the assistant to sharpen these instruments. There are several different types of equipment with which dental instruments may be sharpened. These include the mechanical sharpener, sharpening stones that are attached to the handpiece, flat stationary stones, cylinder and tapering cylinder stones, grooved stones, and diamond hones. Every dental office has one or more of these pieces of equipment for sharpening purposes. One type of sharpening equipment may be better suited for a particular group of hand instruments than another, but all will do a suitable job if handled properly.

Mechanical Sharpening

The mechanical sharpener and some handpiece stones have a blade guide which aids in keeping the correct bevel of the cutting edge and the correct angle of the cutting edge to the blade (Fig. 16-54). It is very important that these angles be maintained when sharpening an instrument. Mechanical holders are also available for use with a flat stationary stone to help maintain these angles. When chisels, hatchets, or hoes are sharpened with the aid of a guide, the blade is placed in the middle slot. When angle formers or gingival margin trimmers are sharpened, the blades are placed in the right or left slots of the guide depending on the angle of the cutting edge.

When using a mechanical sharpener with a guide, the instrument to be sharpened should be held with a pen grasp, pressed firmly against the proper slot in the guide, and pressed with light pressure against the revolving wheel. Care must be exercised not to remove too much metal from the blade in sharpening. When the wheel becomes black and dull (clogged with metal particles), it should be cleaned by placing 10 drops of oil on one end of a cotton roll and wiping the running wheel until the film is softened, and then wiping with the dry end of the cotton roll. To prolong the life of the motor of a mechanical sharpener, it should not be running unless actually in use.

The sharpening instruments, used in conjunction with the handpiece, are manipulated and

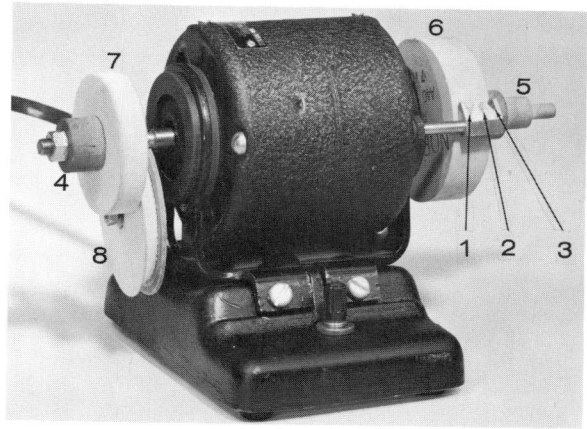

Figure 16-54 | Mechanical instrument sharpener. The sharpener wheel on this instrument sharpener moves backward and forward, enabling the instrument being sharpened to be held in a fixed position. (1) Slot for sharpening left-angle bevels such as angle formers and margin trimmers. (2) Slot for sharpening straight-angle bevels, such as chisels, Wedelstaedts, and hoes. (3) Slot for sharpening right-angle bevels such as angle formers and margin trimmers. (4) Wheel for sharpening spoons or cleaning out margin trimmers for left-angle trimmers. (5) Wheel for sharpening spoons or cleaning out margin trimmers for right-angle trimmers. (6) The sharpening wheel (also used to clean out the inside of Wedelstaedts). (7) Felt wheel for removing bur from instruments after sharpening. (8) Oscillating wheel. (*Courtesy of American Dental Manufacturing Company.*)

cleaned in the same manner as the larger mechanical sharpener.

Hand Sharpening

The stationary stones are commonly called Arkansas stones and can be purchased as a coarse or fine stone. To avoid damage to the cutting edge of an instrument by the creation of heat which will alter the temper of the steel, these stones should be lubricated. Water is adequate for the coarser stones, but oil should be used for the fine stones. In fact, the fine Arkansas stone should never be allowed to dry out and should be covered with a thin film of light oil when

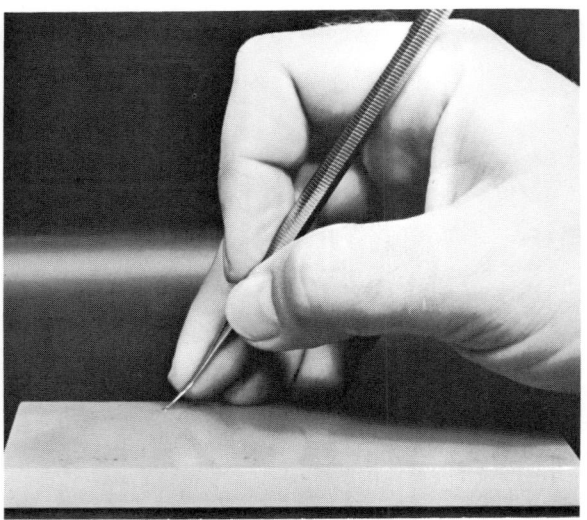

Figure 16-55 | Proper angle of bevel of a chisel to the sharpening stone, proper finger grasp, and proper finger guide for sharpening on a flat Arkansas stone.

stored. These stones may be cleaned with an ordinary cleaning fluid or gasoline.

Sharpening an instrument on an Arkansas stone (Fig. 16-55) may prove disastrous unless a few simple rules are followed: (1) Never sharpen dirty instruments. (2) Before sharpening, establish the proper angle of the bevel and the cutting edge to the sharpening stone. (3) Lay the stone on a flat surface and do not tilt while sharpening. (4) Grasp the instrument firmly so that it will not rotate or change angles while sharpening. (5) Use the third and fourth fingers as a guide along the flat surface or along the stone as a precautionary measure to ensure stability during the sharpening strokes. (Any rolling or dipping motion will distort the bevel.) (6) Do not use a heavy stroke as this tends to create heat and scratch the stone. (7) After sharpening, lightly hone the nonbeveled surface of the cutting edge to remove any metal fragments that may have been created during the sharpening process. (8) Do not do all sharpening on the same area of the stone as this will groove the stone and impair its efficiency and reduce the accuracy of the sharpening procedure.

In sharpening chisels, hatchets, or hoes, the bevel is placed on the stone at the proper angle so that the entire bevel contacts the stone (Fig. 16-55). The instrument is moved back and forth over the stone several times in accord with the previously stated rules. The motivating force should be from the shoulder so that the hand holding the instrument will not change its relation to the plane of the stone during the stroke.

The angle formers and gingival margin trimmers require a little more orientation to the stone because of the cutting edge angle. It may be helpful to use a palm and thumb grasp when sharpening gingival margin trimmers with a 95 or 100 centigrade cutting edge.

Instruments with rounded cutting edges, such as spoons, discoids, and some periodontal instruments, can be sharpened on a flat stone, but a grooved stone is more satisfactory. When the flat stone is used, it involves a rotary movement accompanying a pull stroke to maintain the curvature of the edge. The spoon is placed at the far end of the stone and held so that the handle is toward the operator. As the instrument is pulled along the stone toward the operator, the handle is rotated gradually away from the operator until it is pointing away from the operator at the end of the stroke. The instrument is picked up and placed at the far end of the stone and the motion repeated until the edge is honed (Fig. 16-56A to C). The stone is best held in the hand for this procedure. The inside or flat side of the blade may be sharpened on the edge of the flat stone or with a small-cylinder sharpening stone.

An instrument such as a gold knife is not sharpened along the entire length of the blade bevel. The edge is bibeveled, and continuous sharpening of the entire blade on both sides would soon wear away the thin blade entirely. Therefore, only a very short edge bevel is produced on both sides of the blade by placing the blade at a very acute angle to the flat stone and drawing the instrument toward the cutting edge.

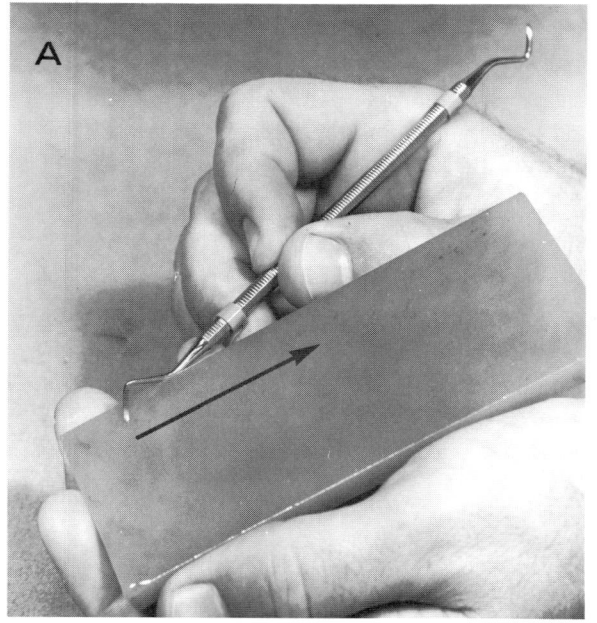
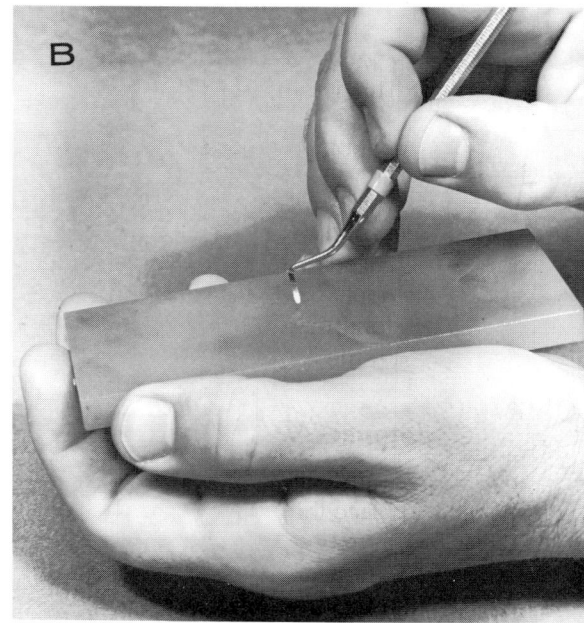
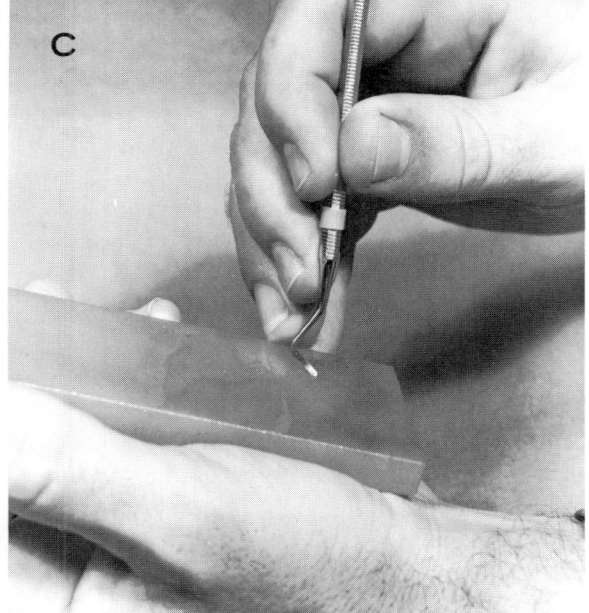

Figure 16-56 | Sharpening a spoon excavator. A. Begin the stroke at the far end of the stone. B. Continue a pull stroke toward the opposite end of the stone while rotating the handle in a direction opposite to the stroke. C. Completion of the stroke and handle rotation. Note that finger guides are used during the entire stroke. (*From Sturdevant, Barton, and Brauer (eds.), The Art and Science of Operative Dentistry, Copyright 1968 by McGraw-Hill, Inc. Used with permission of McGraw-Hill Book Company.*)

(Do not push away from the cutting edge in sharpening.) This is repeated on both sides of the blade.

The diamond hone has grooved and rounded surfaces as well as a straight surface. These surfaces enable easier sharpening of such instruments as scalers and curettes. Since the diamond hone is a so-called stationary stone, the same general rules apply as for the Arkansas stones. This type of stone may be cleaned with a mild detergent and a medium-bristle brush.

Testing Sharpness

To test an instrument for sharpness, hold it in a light grip and place the cutting edge at an acute angle on the thumbnail. When light pressure is exerted, a sharp instrument will dig in while a dull instrument will slide along the thumbnail.

The dental assistant should learn to sharpen instruments under the guidance of the dentist. When proficiency has been attained, then (and only then) the assistant should sharpen instruments when necessary. It is annoying to the dentist to pick up a hand instrument and find it will not do the job because it is dull. The assistant who keeps all hand cutting instruments sharp without being asked to do so is greatly appreciated in any dental office. In order to keep a fine cutting edge and eliminate the excessive loss of metal from the blade, hand cutting instruments should be sharpened at the first sign of dullness. A dull cutting instrument is painful to the patient, annoying to the dentist, and embarrassing to the assistant.

PROSTHODONTIC AND LABORATORY EQUIPMENT

The activities of the dental assistant during prosthodontic procedures are covered in Chaps. 29 and 30. Too often, the instruments and equipment associated with prosthodontics are not kept neat and clean. The assistant must keep in mind that patients do form opinions on the quality of work by the neatness of the surroundings (even though such judgment may be unwarranted).

Equipment pieces that are placed in the patient's mouth or on or around the patient's face should be given the same consideration with regard to sterilization that other instruments placed in the patient's mouth receive. These include metal impression trays, Gothic-arch tracing equipment, facebow, plaster syringe, mold and shade guides, stones or wheels used in denture adjustments, etc. Refer to the principles of sterilization in Chap. 7.

Articulators

In the fabrication of prosthetic appliances and cast restorations, models or casts are made which duplicate the dental arches. These casts

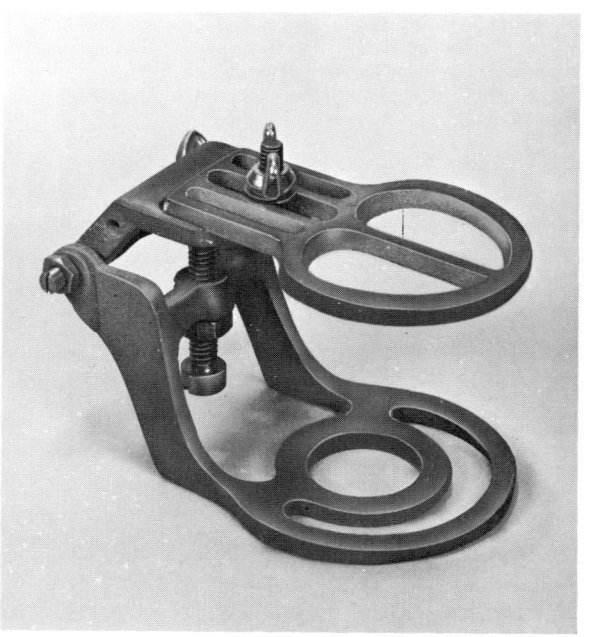

Figure 16-57 | A simple nonadjustable or hinge-type articulator. This type can be opened and closed only and simulates no other jaw movements.

are placed on an articulator which, in turn, simulates the jaw (arch) relationship and movements. Even if an appliance or casting fits the arch or teeth for which it was made, it is unsatisfactory unless it is compatible with the tissues of the opposing arch. If the appliance is too high, the patient cannot close his or her mouth, and if it is malpositioned, the patient cannot chew properly. The articulator helps to properly establish these relationships.

There are many types of articulators available in various sizes, shapes, and complexity. Those used in the processing of inlays, crowns, and bridges are usually small and uncomplicated, while those used in the processing of dentures may be large and complicated when providing duplication of jaw movements. There are two general types of articulators, (1) simple or plain-line, and (2) adjustable. The simple type works as a hinge and allows for only the opening and closing movements (Fig. 16-57) while the adjustable articulators can simulate jaw movements such as lateral and protrusive thrust.

Articulators must be kept clean. After the completion of the case being processed, all traces of plaster, wax, and debris should be removed. Moving parts should be lightly oiled and mounting plates should be covered with a light coat of oil or petroleum jelly. The more complicated the articulator, the more maintenance it must receive.

Laboratory Equipment

Most dental offices have a small laboratory equipped with basic items to perform routine

Figure 16-58 | A well-equipped, well-arranged, neat laboratory. A. Burnout oven. B. Air pressure casting machine. C. Vacuum investing machine. D. Vacuum jar. E. Vibrator. F. Dental lathe. G. Bunsen burners of two different designs. H. Laboratory bench engine, cord arm, and straight handpiece. Ample drawer space allows for storage of items and materials not in use.

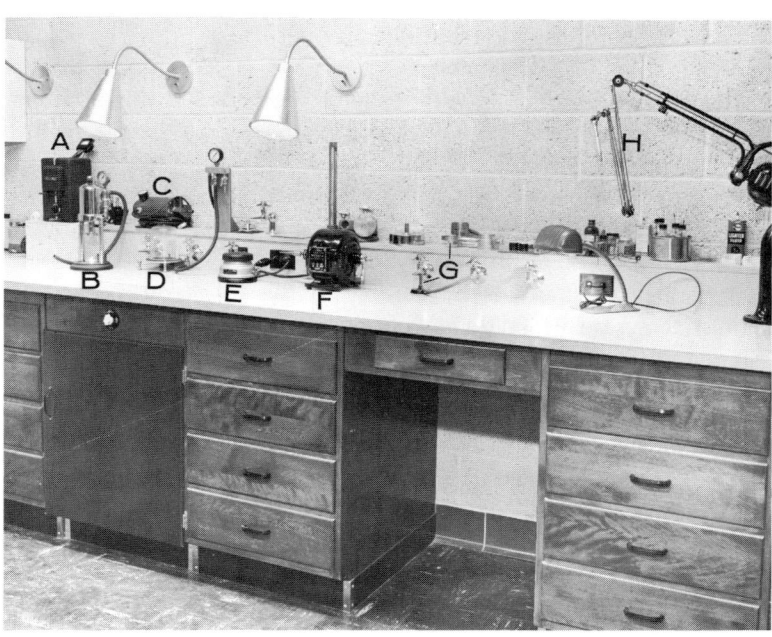

laboratory work (Fig. 16-58). Depending on the type of practice, the dental assistant may or may not be required to perform laboratory procedures.

Laboratory equipment may be divided into heavy and light equipment with the heavy items somewhat stationary. The light equipment is easily moved and includes many hand instruments.

Heavy equipment includes such items as the vibrator, dental lathe, model trimmer, bench dental engine, mechanical investor, inlay furnace, and casting machine. Where appropriate, illustrations and directions for use of these heavy pieces of equipment appear in conjunction with discussion of actual techniques in other chapters of the textbook. However, one such piece of equipment, the model trimmer (Fig. 16-59), warrants additional consideration.

The modern practice of dentistry utilizes models of the dental arches of individual patients for more purposes than the construction of appliances. In many cases, models are used in discussing case presentations with patients and may become a permanent part of the patient's file. Preparation of such models is discussed in Chap. 10. The model trimmer is routinely used to form the art portion of the model, and its proper use and care should be understood.

The model trimmer is essentially a motor-driven abrasive disc which is enclosed in a metal guard which in turn holds a guide table. Materials other than plaster or stone should not be used against the abrasive disc since they will either clog the disc or break off or dull the abrasive particles. When in use, the water wash should always be turned on and after completing trimming a model, the motor and water should be left running until the water flowing from the discharge line is clear and not discolored with gypsum particles.

The guide table on the model trimmer can be adjusted to provide different angle cuts, but basically it should be left perpendicular to the abrasive disc. When using a model trimmer, turn on the motor and then the water before placing the

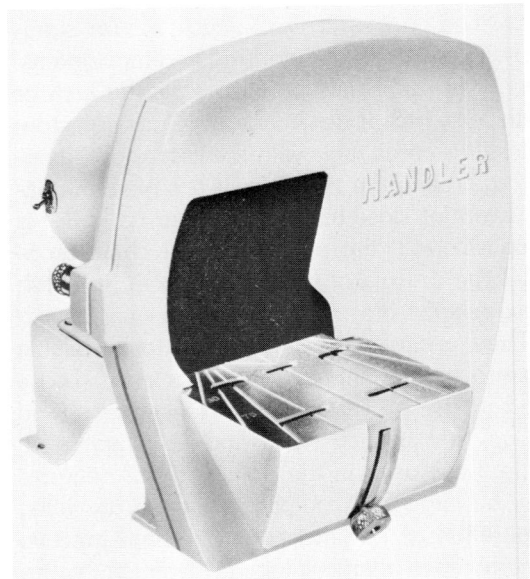

Figure 16-59 | Model trimmer with adjustable calibrated table guide. To trim a plaster or stone model, place it on the table and press lightly against the revolving grinding wheel. The water volume should be small to prevent water from spraying out of the grinding opening. (*Courtesy of Handler Manufacturing Company, Inc.*)

model against the disc. Hold the model firmly with both hands on the platform and press it lightly against the disc. Heavy pressure against the disc is not necessary if the disc is sharp and clean. Care must be exercised not to overcut the art portion of the model or damage the facial surfaces of the teeth. The thickness and form of the art portion of the model are at the discretion of the dentist.

The light equipment includes such items as the plaster bowl, mechanical spatulator, Bunsen burner, balance, articulators, surveyor, water bath, gas-air blowpipe, inlay rings, and an assortment of laboratory knives, pliers, and spatulas. It is important that these items not be scattered around the laboratory but be returned to the correct storage place after being used.

The care of laboratory equipment should also

be the dental assistant's responsibility. This equipment usually does not need as delicate care as some equipment in the operating room. One thing the assistant should always check is that a piece of equipment is not left running when not being used. Each manufacturer supplies maintenance information with the equipment, and the assistant should become familiar with this material and follow the suggestions to preserve the efficiency and life of the equipment.

It cannot be stressed too often that laboratory equipment is just as vital to a productive dental office as the equipment in the operating room. It must be kept clean, and the easiest way to maintain this cleanliness is to clean up each piece of equipment as soon after it is used as possible. This prevents the accumulation of debris which in time will be difficult to remove.

A few helpful hints which the assistant may follow to help in laboratory cleanliness are as follows: (1) Spread paper on workbench tops before using, and after the work is completed gather up this paper along with the debris and dispose of it; (2) clean instruments with wax or any thermoplastic material on them by heating over a Bunsen burner and then wiping with a paper towel; (3) instruments that cannot be heated may be cleaned with solvents; (4) place a paper towel over the vibrator table before use; (5) clean any gypsum product from spatulas, brushes, and mixing bowls immediately after use before the material sets; (6) flush the model trimmer thoroughly with water immediately after use; and (7) place an inlay ring and contents in a pan or bowl of water, rather than in the sink, when securing a casting.

17 | Richard E. Richardson
Oral Diagnosis

OBJECTIVES

Oral diagnosis is the science that deals with patient interviewing, examination, and the gathering of any and all information relative to the discovery and management of disease of the teeth, tooth-supporting tissues, and all related structures of the oral cavity and the head, face, and neck.

The first phase in the treatment of any patient is diagnosis or the determination of the nature of the needs for, and the possibilities of, treatment. This means that a thorough study of each patient must be undertaken before any treatment is begun. Exception to this rule is made in an emergency, but even in these instances time must be taken to explore the background of the complaint and the status of the patient.

Diagnosis is involved with the basic sciences (pathology, anatomy, microbiology, etc.) and with all disciplines of dental practice. No individual treatment plan should be evolved without full consideration of the patient's total problem. Actually, then, diagnosis may be defined as a practical summation and application of all the knowledge that is, or should be, inherent in a total dental-care program.

The dental assistant should understand that dental treatment must be planned and that time must be allotted for the gathering of information for all patients and for special study in many cases. Knowing this enables the assistant to encourage the patient when patience and understanding are needed.

Not all cases are complicated, and in many instances diagnosis will be amenable to quick decisions. Often such decisions will be imperative. Sometimes, however, the real problem will not be disclosed until considerable time has been spent collecting data and information.

The procedures usually employed consist of obtaining information concerning the patient's name, age, address, etc.; taking a dental and medical history, at least in brief; physical and dental examination; radiographs; vitality tests; study casts; blood and tissue examinations; and many other specific tests in certain cases. Not all these procedures are routine, but they are important in a complete dental service.

The ultimate aim of diagnosis is to apply in a practical manner a planned treatment program for the individual patient. The objective is to maintain dental and oral tissues in a state of health, comfort, and useful function.

The procedures in oral diagnosis are designed to protect the patient, the dentist, and supporting personnel from injury or liability relating to treatment and management of the patient, and to result in a better service.

Dentistry should be thought of as a health science and dentists as a part of the health team. Dentists will, in fact, have the opportunity to see and examine patients when early signs of disease can be detected and at a time when a given disease may be amenable to treatment, or they may find some serious, well-established pathology that has not had the benefit of medical treatment. Therefore, there is a natural interrelationship between the dentist and the physician that should be encouraged for the best interests of the patient.

There will be instances in which the dentist will need to confer with the physician prior to proceding with treatment of a patient; some modification of the planned treatment program or some medical consideration may be necessary. In other instances the dentist will discover disease processes that should be referred to a physician for proper medical care. In general, both dentist and physician will have need for each other's cooperation in providing good health care for their patients, and this need is usually recognized and welcomed by all parties.

PATIENT HISTORY

The interviewing of a patient is an important and crucial procedure; it is considered to be standard technique and is, in fact, in some measure, required for all patients. This procedure is known as the *patient history*. The structure of this history taking is fairly uniform in both dentistry and medicine but will vary in details and objectives; its main elements are routine data, chief complaint, history of present illness, past medical and dental history, and family and social history.

The Printed Questionnaire

Someone has said, "Never treat a stranger," and this is indeed a wise injunction. The management and treatment of a dental patient is an extremely personal matter and requires that all who participate in these procedures make every effort to gain the patient's confidence and trust. It is necessary to delve into rather intimate facts regarding the patient because the success or failure of dental care may hinge on such things as attitudes and physical conditions.

From a legal standpoint, the dentist "is expected to know something of the patient." So, aside from the attitude of human concern, it is required that as much information as possible be obtained prior to actual treatment.

Various techniques have been devised to obtain personal information about the patient, but the most successful way to do this is by the use of printed questionnaires combined with an interview by the dentist (Figs. 17-1 and 17-2). In adopting this uniform procedure for all patients, it will be obvious that it is expected of everyone and that the asking of personal questions is not a casual or individual whim. Furthermore, it permits the patient to consider answers

UNIVERSITY OF NORTH CAROLINA
SCHOOL OF DENTISTRY
HEALTH QUESTIONNAIRE

Chart No. _____

Date _____

Name _____

Address _____

Telephone: Residence _____ Business _____

Sex _____ Age _____ Race _____

Height _____ Weight _____

Occupation _____ Marital Status _____

DIRECTIONS

If your answer is YES to the question asked, put a circle around YES.
If your answer is NO to the question asked, put a circle around NO.
Answer all questions. You may comment on answers which require explanation by writing in the space between questions.

#	Question	Y/N
1.	Have you ever been seriously ill?	YES NO
2.	Have you ever been hospitalized?	YES NO
3.	Have you ever had a major operation?	YES NO
4.	Have you been examined by your physician within the last year?	YES NO
5.	Are you being treated by a physician now for any condition?	YES NO
6.	Has there been any change in your general health in the last year?	YES NO
7.	Have you lost weight without dieting in recent months?	YES NO
8.	Have you gained weight in recent months?	YES NO
9.	Have you had any of the following diseases:	
	Rheumatic fever	YES NO
	Arthritis	YES NO
	Diabetes	YES NO
	High blood pressure	YES NO
	Jaundice (yellow skin and eyes)	YES NO
	Tuberculosis	YES NO
	Venereal disease	YES NO
	Heart disease	YES NO
	Anemia (blood low)	YES NO
	Stroke	YES NO
	Infectious hepatitis	YES NO
	Kidney disease	YES NO
10.	Have you ever been told by a physician that you have a heart murmur?	YES NO
11.	Do you ever have asthma or hay fever? (underline which one)	
12.	Do you ever have hives or skin rash?	YES NO
13.	Have you ever experienced an unusual reaction to any of the following drugs?	YES NO
	Aspirin	YES NO
	Penicillin	YES NO
	Iodine	YES NO
	Other (list)	YES NO
	Sulfonamides (sulfa)	YES NO
	Barbiturates (sleeping pills)	YES NO
14.	Are you taking any medicines now?	YES NO
15.	Have you ever experienced an unusual reaction to a dental anesthetic?	YES NO
16.	Do you bleed for a long time when you cut yourself?	YES NO
17.	Do you have frequent, severe headaches?	YES NO
18.	Do you have any complaints regarding your eyes?	YES NO
19.	Do you have any ear trouble?	YES NO
20.	Do you have frequent colds?	YES NO
21.	Do you have sinus trouble?	YES NO
22.	Do you have any chest pain on exertion?	YES NO
23.	Are you ever short of breath on mild exertion?	YES NO
24.	Have you ever had painful and swollen joints?	YES NO
25.	Has your appetite changed recently?	YES NO
26.	Are there any foods you cannot eat?	YES NO
27.	Have you had epilepsy?	YES NO
28.	Are you excessively nervous?	YES NO
29.	Do you think that your teeth are affecting your general health in any way?	YES NO
30.	Are you dissatisfied with the appearance of your teeth?	YES NO
31.	Are you worried about receiving dental treatment?	YES NO
32.	Do you have difficulty in chewing your food?	YES NO
33.	Do you have any sensitive teeth?	YES NO
34.	Have you had a toothache recently?	YES NO
35.	Do you have bleeding gums?	YES NO
36.	Have you ever had a severe sore mouth?	YES NO
37.	Is it difficult for you to open your mouth?	YES NO
38.	Does your jaw click when you chew?	YES NO
39.	Are you a mouth breather?	YES NO
40.	Do you have frequent canker sores or cold sores?	YES NO
41.	Have you ever had any injury to your face or jaws?	YES NO
42.	Have you ever had surgery or x-ray treatment for a tumor, growth or other condition in your mouth or on your lips?	YES NO
43.	Are there any other significant medical problems?	YES NO
44.	Do you have any lesions (sores) elsewhere?	YES NO
45.	Would other members of your family answer any of the above questions "Yes"?	YES NO

SUMMARY STATEMENT

carefully and to be prepared for further explanation, if necessary. These questionnaires provide a framework for the actual interview of the patient by the dentist. The interview becomes an opportunity for the establishment of the favorable patient-dentist relationship so essential to the delivery of quality dental care.

It is best that all persons who are capable be allowed to fill out the printed questionnaire unassisted, for this, of itself, affords some obvious, or subtle, evaluation of the patient; also, there is more of a sense of privacy which promotes a feeling of confidence and a willingness to fully cooperate. However, some patients will seek assistance or may be incapable and will need help. One advantage of having a separate routine data form (Fig. 17-2) from the personal or health questionnaire is that the clerk-receptionist can check basic information without violation of the privacy of information relative to the patient's health status.

Routine Data

Certain information, such as full name, addresses, telephone numbers, occupation, birth date, family status, who will pay, best time for appointments, etc., may be referred to as basic, or *routine, data*. This information, accurately and completely gathered and kept up to date, is vital to the successful management of a practice. Where do you go when it becomes urgent to contact a patient on short notice only to discover that current information is inaccurate? The best time to obtain such information is immediately and constantly (Fig. 17-2). It is wise to make notations and corrections of any new such data as it becomes available and to recheck it frequently. The detail and extent of the information required in individual offices will vary widely, but it is conceivable that almost any given point of knowledge could, under certain circumstances, be crucial to the effective or pleasant delivery of dental service.

Chief Complaint

Most patients will have some prime reason for making the initial contact with a particular dentist, and most will hope that the dentist, or a thoughtfully concerned staff person, will listen to this *chief complaint*. The prospective patient may not have a "complaint" as such, but there will be a reason for seeking care. The chief complaint may be acute, such as a toothache, or long-range, such as the desire for the best possible dental care.

It is rather important that the chief complaint, or perhaps more appropriately, the reason for requesting treatment, be recorded in the patient's own words. It is a mistake to edit or alter the way a patient states the need for treatment. The patient's use of words may reveal a great deal of information that could influence the approach to a plan for treatment or to the actual treatment. An individual who wants "all my teeth pulled" may know what is best, but, on the other hand, if some other course of treatment would be wiser and feasible, the proper approach to this patient may mean the difference between success and failure. By the same token, the patient who wants "the best possible dental care" may or may not be fully informed, and the approach to this person may be to truly provide such care or, unhappily, to discover that the statement is mostly "just talk."

Special consideration must be given persons who are in pain or who have had some accident. Many will profess emergency need; some will be "crying wolf"; all will deserve considerate attention and reassurance with appropriate care as early as the condition demands.

History of Present Illness

This heading implies more of a medical component, but the parallel is apropos to dentistry.

Figure 17-1 | Patient health questionnaire. (*Courtesy of the University of North Carolina at Chapel Hill, School of Dentistry.*)

PRIVATE DENTAL SERVICE
UNC SCHOOL OF DENTISTRY
UNIVERSITY OF NORTH CAROLINA AT CHAPEL HILL
CHAPEL HILL, NORTH CAROLINA 27514

| CHART NUMBER |
| DATE (Month, Day, Year) |
| REVIEWED BY |
| For Office Use Only |

1. PATIENT DATA

1.1 NAME (Last, First, Middle)	1.2 TITLE (Circle One) MR. MRS. MISS DR.	1.3 SEX (Circle One) MALE FEMALE
1.4 ADDRESS (Street No. & Name or Box No. & Route)	1.5 DATE OF BIRTH	1.6 MARITAL STATUS (Circle) SINGLE MARRIED OTHER
1.7 CITY, STATE, ZIP CODE	1.8 PHONE - HOME	1.9 PHONE - BUSINESS
1.10 PERMANENT ADDRESS (If different from 1.4 above)	1.11 CITY, STATE, ZIP CODE	
1.12 SOCIAL SECURITY NO.	1.13 OCCUPATION	1.14 IF STUDENT, NAME OF SCHOOL
1.15 NAME OF COMPANY	1.16 ADDRESS (City, State)	

PERSON TO BE NOTIFIED IN CASE OF AN EMERGENCY.

1.17 NAME (Last, First, Middle)	1.18 PHONE NUMBER	1.19 RELATIONSHIP
1.20 ADDRESS	1.21 CITY, STATE, ZIP CODE	

2. FINANCIAL DATA

2.1 Does the patient have health care insurance which provides dental benefits? (Circle One) YES NO
If answer is "YES", the patient should contact our insurance office at the end of today's appointment. One of the receptionists will be happy to direct you to the insurance office.
NOTE: The Insurance Office will file insurance claims in behalf of the policy holder; however, filing of claims does not relieve the patient and/or the person responsible for payment of the account. Payments received from an insurance carrier will be credited as payment on account.

PERSON WHO AGREES TO ASSUME RESPONSIBILITY FOR PAYMENT OF PATIENT'S ACCOUNT.

2.2 NAME (Last, First, Middle)	2.3 TITLE (Circle One) MR. MRS. MISS DR.	2.4 RELATIONSHIP TO PATIENT
2.5 ADDRESS	2.6 CITY, STATE, ZIP CODE	
2.7 PHONE NUMBER	2.8 OCCUPATION	2.9 NAME OF COMPANY
2.10 BUSINESS ADDRESS	2.11 CITY, STATE, ZIP CODE	

3. MISCELLANEOUS DATA

3.1 NAME OF PATIENT'S PRESENT DENTIST	3.2 PHONE NUMBER
3.3 ADDRESS	3.4 CITY, STATE, ZIP CODE
3.5 NAME OF PATIENT'S PHYSICIAN	3.6 PHONE NUMBER
3.7 ADDRESS	3.8 CITY, STATE, ZIP CODE

3.9 Has the patient ever been treated here or in the Student Clinic? (Circle One) YES NO
3.10 If "YES", when was the last time? (month and year)
3.11 Is patient's dental problem the result of an accident? (Circle One) YES NO
3.12 Is patient being referred by the above dentist or physician for a specific dental problem? YES NO
3.13 What is the nature of this problem? Describe.

4. PAYMENT DATA

NOTE: Statement is payable in full not later than fifteen days after mailing of same unless prior written payment arrangements have been made with the Business Officer.

NOTE: It is the policy of the Private Dental Service to make a charge for cancelled or broken appointments unless patient gives twenty-four advance notice.

I hereby give permission to the University of North Carolina, School of Dentistry, to perform any indicated dental treatment, dental operation, or other dental procedure on myself after I have entered myself for dental procedures other than diagnostic.

I also give permission to the University of North Carolina School of Dentistry or anyone authorized by it to make and use photographs of myself or reproductions thereof, for any educational purpose.

(adult)   Signature_____

Early attention to some acute complaint is often necessary, but some information about the complaint is important and usually a few specific questions will be sufficient for a start and will help to identify the degree of urgency. "How long has it been hurting," "when does it hurt," etc. The dentist may have to go into the history of the present illness to some depth prior to taking action.

Past Medical and Dental History

The taking of a past medical and a past dental history may be separate in form, but actually they are developed together, the printed questionnaire having questions of both natures (Fig. 17-1).

The printed questionnaire provides the introduction for frank discussion between patient and dentist in an effort to bring to light and action any existing conditions, medical or dental, that might influence the outcome of dental treatment. A sick person—that is, one who has some deviation from normal to the extent that it affects or may affect that person's well-being—may present problems which influence dental care. Furthermore, the presence of an infectious disease might jeopardize the well-being of the dental-office staff.

Medical findings may be minor or major and must be dealt with accordingly. Simple oral ulcers, minor allergies, slight physical weakness, and conditions of similar impact may present some inconveniences but probably do not present major problems in dental treatment. However, a history of rheumatic fever may be a critical factor for the patient, and some medical consideration prior to treatment is mandatory. So-called brittle diabetics pose real problems in providing long-range, durable dental care. The patient who is "difficult to handle" may be hyperthyroid and unable to "take it easy." A patient who has a severely decompensated heart will need special care and attention by everyone in the dental office. Furthermore, it is the dentist's legal as well as professional business to elicit such knowledge of a patient and proceed with due care.

Some patients may present histories of diseases that could endanger the health of the dentist, the staff, and other patients. Hepatitis is a realistic example of a disease that may be transferred from one person to another, and special care must be exercised when treating a patient who has had this disease. Meticulous attention to the principles and techniques of sterilization and disinfection is always imperative; the possibility of cross-infection by many diseases is ever-present and must be guarded against (see Chaps. 6 and 7).

A dental history can be extremely significant in many instances, and the proper use of such information may be important in the delivery of dental care. A person who has been pleased with previous dental care probably will be a cooperative patient; one who is busy complaining about various previous dental experiences may present some difficulties in treatment. People who, having had few dental-care needs, present with extensive breakdown require a good measure of study and establishment of the question, Why? Histories of orthodontics, periodontal therapy, accidents, or unusual experiences may alert special considerations in treatment planning.

Probably one of the greatest benefits of careful, concerned, and tactful patient history taking is that it tends to develop confidence, trust, and appreciation on the part of the patient. Such attitudes go a long way toward promoting effective treatment.

Family and Social History

It may be that knowledge of health and physical factors in a patient's close relatives is not vitally

Figure 17-2 | Routine patient data questionnaire. (Courtesy of the University of North Carolina at Chapel Hill, School of Dentistry.)

significant to the patient's dental treatment, but, as a health service, the dentist tries to be alert to familial tendencies in health factors. Family histories of chronic illnesses such as diabetes, heart disease, cancer, and other diseases establish greater probabilities for the tendency of these conditions to reappear in subsequent generations, and the dentist can maintain a higher degree of suspicion with such patients. Indeed, the appearance of any chronic disease may create problems in maintaining continuing oral health.

The dentist has a right to know something of a patient's social history, and this kind of information may require considerably more tact to acquire. To repeat, as with all the factors in a patient's history, the best way to get this is to have a routine whereby all patients are expected to give such information as is proper for the dentist to know; this is best done with the printed questionnaire. Factors such as where a patient has lived in the past, marital status, use of tobacco or alcohol, activities, interests, etc., may have direct importance in treatment planning and management. For example, regardless of whether a patient is anxious to disclose the marital status or not, there are a number of legal complications that could arise out of not knowing who is responsible for decisions or for payment. Likewise, in the case of a minor, it is vital to know who is the head of the household in which the child resides. Other considerations arise when the patient is routinely involved in contact sports: provision of preventive aid such as a mouth guard or delay of any expensive fixed anterior restorations might be a consideration.

PATIENT EXAMINATION

While the assistant is not expected or permitted to make diagnoses, it is well to understand all aspects of a thorough examination of the patient and to be alert for any information about the patient that might be significant.

The examination often is uncomplicated and

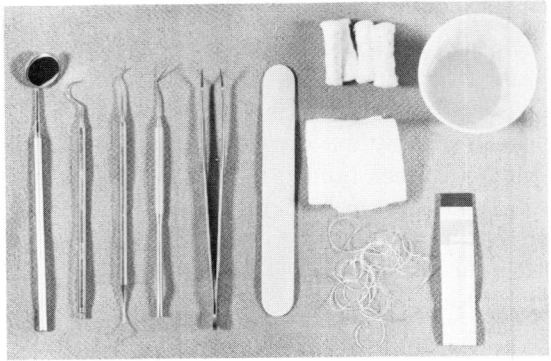

Figure 17-3 | Instrument tray setup for the patient examination.

relatively simple, but it should be thorough and, in some instances, can be quite involved and time-consuming. Attention to details will make this procedure efficient and effective. The actual instruments and materials for a routine examination are fairly well standardized and include a dental mirror, two explorers, dental pliers, periodontal probe, wooden tongue blade, 2 × 2 in guaze squares, cotton rolls, dental floss, articulating paper, and a cup for waste (Fig. 17-3).

Physical Examination

Pulse Rate and Blood Pressure

It is an established fact that many people have high blood pressure, and many of them are aware of it and may be under treatment for this unfortunate condition. Some people are aware of having the condition but are not complying with medical advice and care. Many people are unaware that they are hypertensive because the condition may be present without marked symptoms. Untreated high blood pressure can and does shorten the lives of its victims. High blood pressure can be treated with great benefits for the patient. Many people have cardiac conditions of a serious nature. Patients who have car-

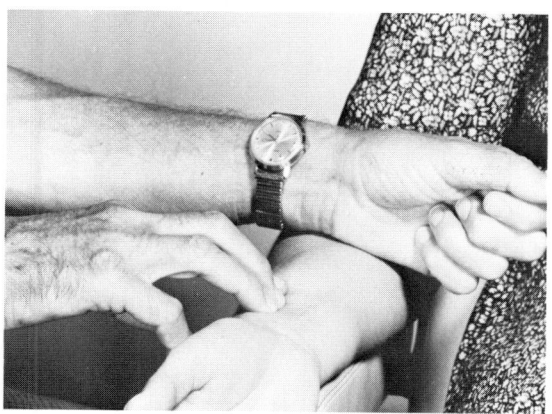

Figure 17-4 | Taking the patient's pulse rate.

diovascular diseases present serious responsibilities for the dentist, and the existence of such conditions must be established and managed in a proper manner. The taking of pulse rate and blood pressure has come to be routine for all patients, and the assistant can be of great service in these procedures. When the patient is first seen and prior to subsequent operation, pulse and blood pressure can be taken and recorded in the

Figure 17-5 | Taking the patient's blood pressure.

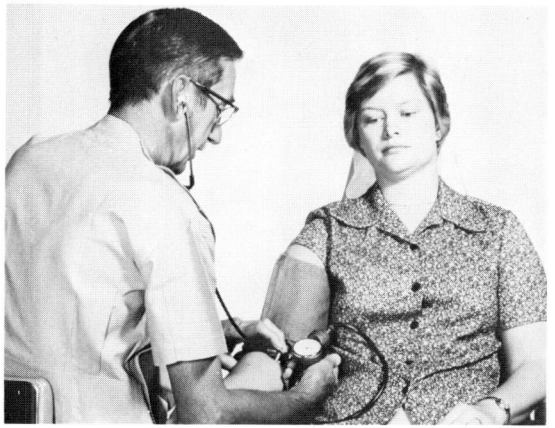

chart quite easily by the assistant; the patient will appreciate this service.

The patient is seated comfortably, semireclining, and allowed to rest from any immediately preceding exertion or excitement. The pulse is taken by placing the tips of the first three fingers on the radial artery (Fig. 17-4). The pulse must be plainly felt and an accurate count made, preferably for a full minute, but a lesser time may be used and a calculation for 1 minute made. Pulse rates of from 60 to 80 beats per minute are generally thought of as being normal.

In taking the blood pressure, the forearm should be slightly flexed and supported so that the upper arm is on a level with the heart. The deflated cuff is placed snugly around the bare upper arm with its lower border 1 to 1½ in above the bend in the arm; the tube should be slightly to the inside of the arm. The bulb and pressure instrument is attached to the tube and the screw valve closed. The earpieces of the stethoscope are placed comfortably in the ears and pointing forward. The radial pulse is felt for; then smoothly and fairly quickly the cuff is inflated until the pulse disappears. The pressure is increased about 20 mm higher. The bell of the stethoscope is placed over the brachial artery, which is usually at the crease of the arm slightly toward the body; the bell should not touch the cuff. The screw valve is released slightly so that the pressure falls about 2 to 3 mm/second (Fig. 17-5). The first tapping sound that is heard is read from the instrument as the systolic pressure. As the pressure falls, the sound will become muffled and then disappear. The reading at the point of disappearance is the diastolic pressure (see also Chap. 21).

The systolic pressure results from the contraction of the heart and peak blood pressure; diastolic pressure results from relaxation of the heart and lower blood pressure. These readings are recorded systolic/diastolic, as, for example, 120/70. Individual normal blood pressures vary widely, but readings over 150/90 generally are considered to warrant further checking and possibly medical consultation. The dentist will establish policy as to whether the assistant should inform the patient as to pulse and blood pressure findings or not. Questionable readings should be repeated.

General Appraisal

Much information about a patient is available by careful observation while preparing for the formal examination. The way a person walks, dresses, talks, and acts may convey positive facts important to communication and management. Emotional states, nutritional status, obvious signs of bodily weaknesses or illness of a significant nature may be readily observable. The understanding of a patient's attitudes and limitations begins with initial contacts, and success or failure may be dependent, in large measure, upon how well this is accomplished.

Head, Face, and Neck

The formal examination begins with direct observation of the head, face, and neck (Fig. 17-6). Information available by this technique covers a wide range of possibilities, and any deviations from normal are carefully noted. Eyes that are abnormally bulging may indicate serious thyroid disorder; yellowish color of eyes or skin may be an indication of liver disease; scars may result from accidents or operations for removal of growths; deviation from normal shape may represent actual pathology or developmental variation; a flushed complexion may signify a blood/vascular problem; there are many other possibilities.

The temporomandibular joint (jaw hinge) is an important part of the dental mechanism and is examined by palpation over the joint while the patient makes opening and closing movements of the jaw (Fig. 17-7). Abnormalities of this joint may present serious complications for both patient and dentist in achieving satisfactory results

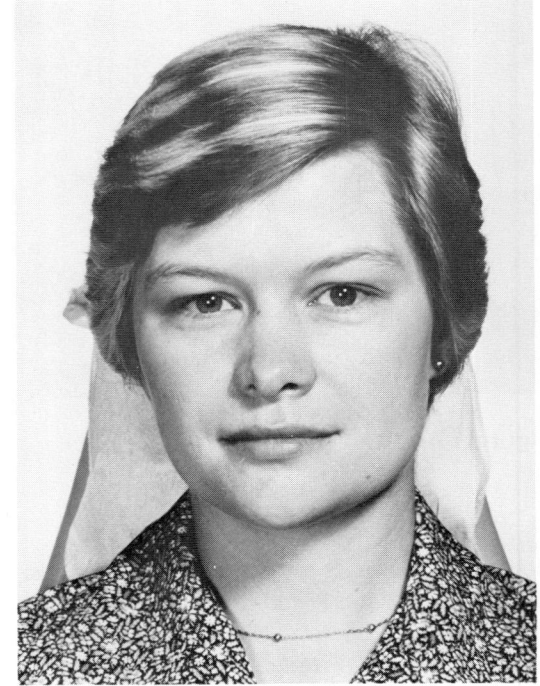

Figure 17-6 | Direct observation of the patient's head, face, and neck.

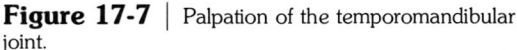

Figure 17-7 | Palpation of the temporomandibular joint.

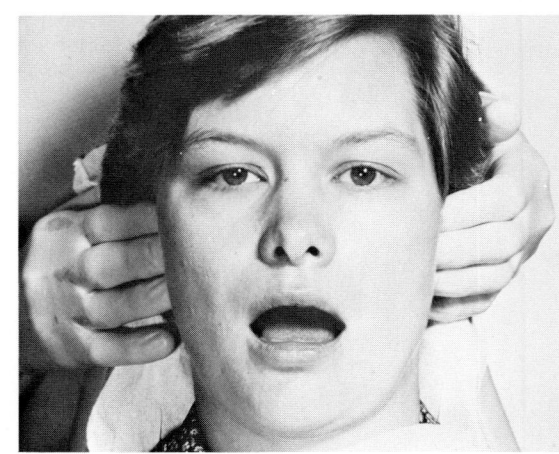

of dental treatment, and any such condition must be noted at the outset.

There are many lymphoid glands in the neck area, and they may be involved in infections of the oral area or may become tumorous. Careful palpation of these glands should be routine (Fig. 17-8A and B). Just below the cricothyroid cartilage ("Adam's apple") on both sides of the trachea lies the thyroid gland; examination of the gland (Fig. 17-9) is a real service to the patient, for any observed enlargement would indicate the need for early medical examination.

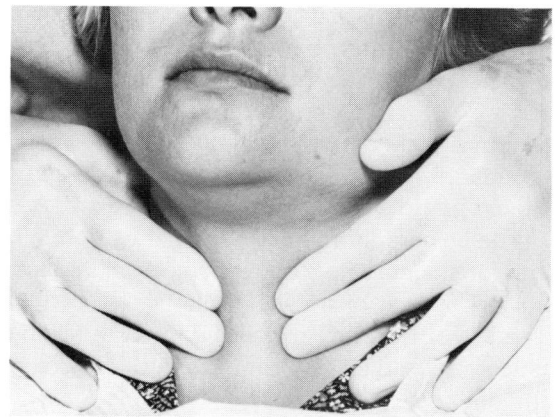

Figure 17-9 | Palpation of the thyroid gland.

Figure 17-8 | Palpation of lymph glands of the neck.

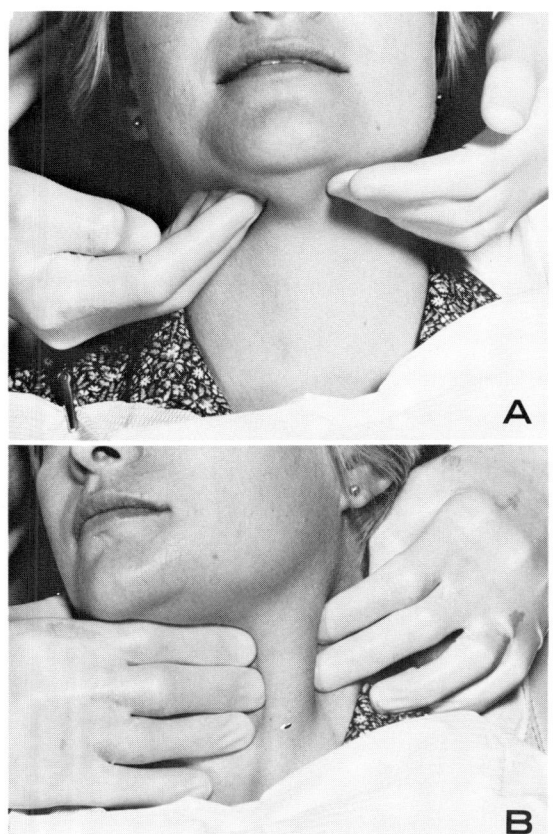

Intraoral Structures

A careful, detailed, and systematic examination of the tissues inside the mouth is important, for many significant changes are possible. The examination begins with a look at the lips at rest (Fig. 17-10). The lips normally are smooth, pale pink in color, and with fine vertical lines. Changes in the surface of the lips are readily observable and range from acute to chronic in

Figure 17-10 | The patient's lips at rest.

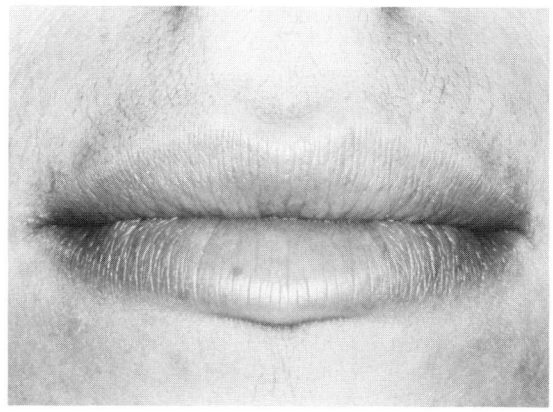

Chapter Seventeen | Oral Diagnosis | 329

young to older people with varying importance. These changes may be briefly annoying, such as the fever blister, or of serious import, such as thickened and hardened areas that may represent malignant growths. Changes such as color, ulceration, surface thickening, deep fissures, etc., should be noted.

The lips are thoroughly palpated with thumb and forefinger to note any stiffening or lump formation or lack of muscle control (Fig. 17-11). The lips are everted or reflected and the lining mucosa observed for any changes in color, smoothness, or softness (Fig. 17-12).

General observation of the teeth in a closed position with the lips retracted is made to note their arrangement, numbers, condition, and the way the lower teeth meet the uppers (Fig. 17-13A and B). Preliminary examination of the gingivae or gums is also noted. Similar observation is made with the teeth wide apart. Detailed examination of teeth and gingivae will be done later.

The cheeks are retracted, one side at a time, and both visual and digital examinations are made (Fig. 17-14). These tissues are smooth, pink, and moist. Faint impressions of where the tissues normally lie against the teeth may be seen. An important structure is a papilla opposite the upper second molar through which opens Stensen's duct; this duct carries salivary fluid from the parotid gland. The gland lies over the posterior border of the ramus of the mandible and can be massaged from the outside to produce an observable flow of clear salivary fluid. If this fluid is cloudy or otherwise changed, some infection or chronic change in the gland may be present.

The palate is seen by having the patient's head tilted upward and backward and with the use of a mirror (Fig. 17-15). The surface of the hard palate is firm, pink, and irregular and exhibits a number of anatomic landmarks. The soft palate is to the posterior and is thin and movable (Figs. 17-15 and 17-19). Changes in the palate may be seen as injuries, acute ulcers, and chronic changes which could represent cancerous development.

The tongue is an important and interesting structure and one with which the dentist must constantly deal. The tongue has long been regarded as highly significant from a diagnostic standpoint. Color and surface changes may reflect systemic or bodily changes, and it is a site of

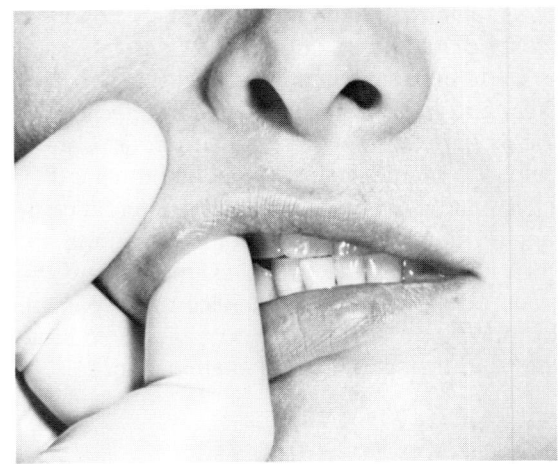

Figure 17-11 | Palpation of the lips.

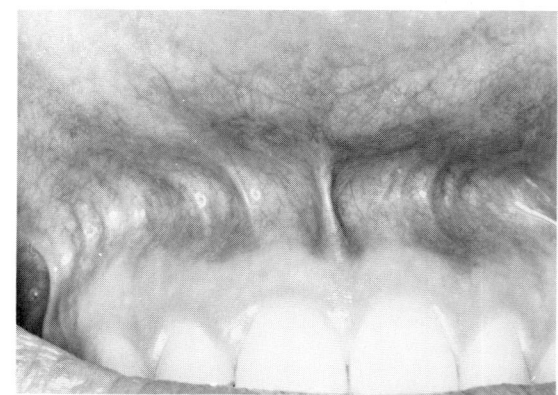

Figure 17-12 | Lining mucosa of the lips.

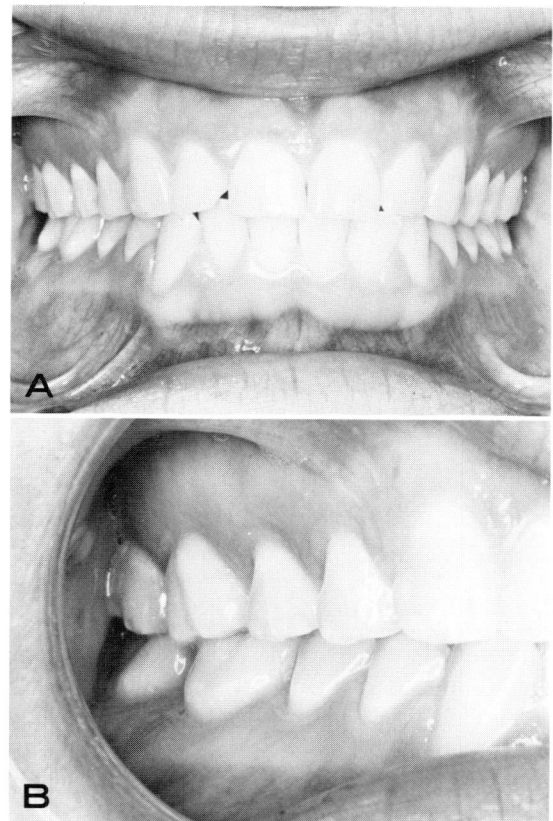

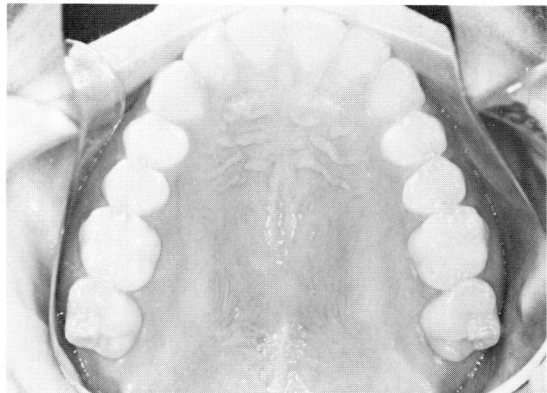

Figure 17-15 | The hard palate and a part of the soft palate.

injuries, ulcerations, and tumorous changes. The tongue is observed in a relaxed position, lifted to see underneath, and pulled forward and to each side with a gauze square to see the sides and base (Figs. 17-16 to 17-18). The tongue is also palpated with thumb and finger for softness and pliability.

When the tongue is elevated, the floor of the mouth may be observed and palpated. This area

Figure 17-13 | Teeth in the naturally closed position.

Figure 17-14 | Lining mucosa of the cheeks.

Figure 17-16 | The tongue in a relaxed position.

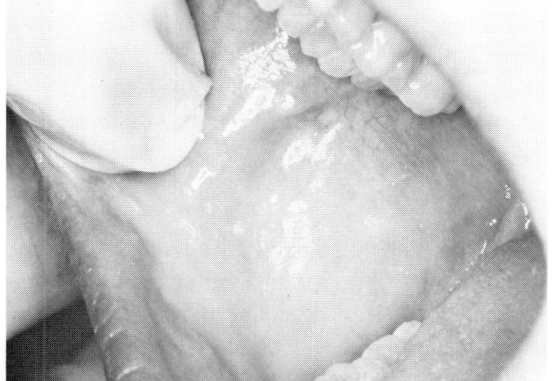

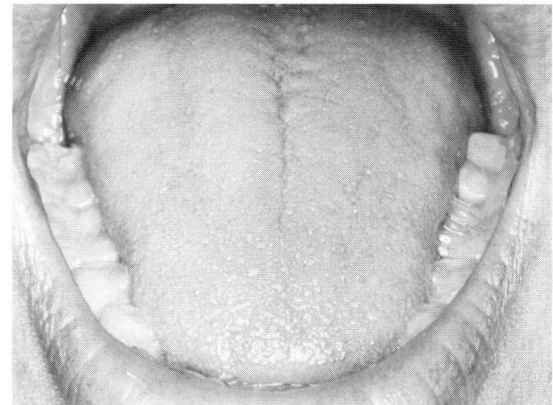

Chapter Seventeen | Oral Diagnosis | 331

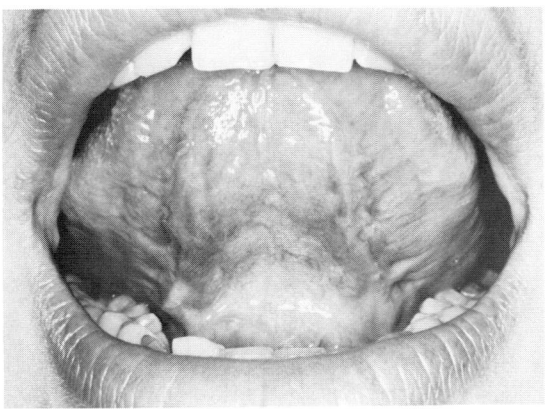

Figure 17-17 | The tongue elevated to show the undersurface.

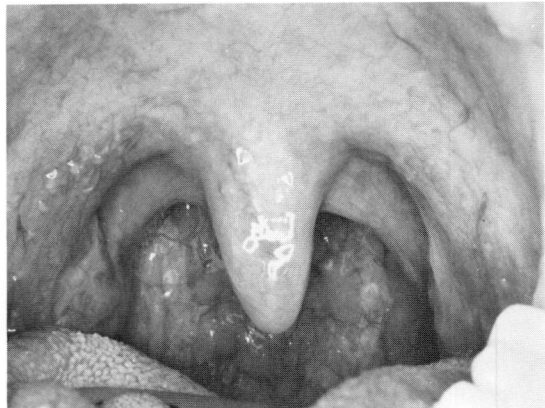

Figure 17-19 | The soft palate and oropharynx.

presents many notable anatomic landmarks that are usually hidden from view. Changes in this area can be significant and important.

The oropharynx (Fig. 17-19) is the back of the mouth and part of the throat and is easily observed. The tonsils are seen, and the tissues in this area manifest changes associated with respiratory infections.

Figure 17-18 | The tongue pulled forward and to the side to show the side and base.

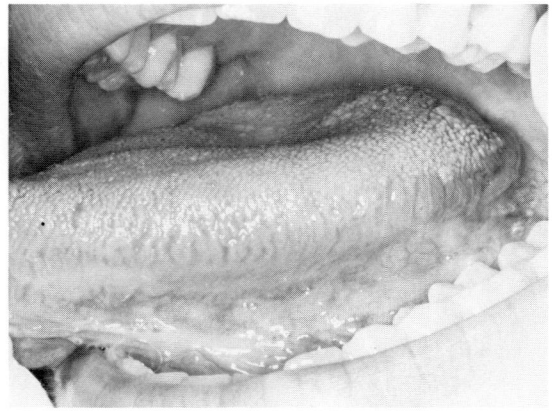

Dental Examination

The patient interviews and physical examination are conducted at the outset of patient relations so that full knowledge as to if, when, and how to treat the patient may be established prior to any actual treatment. When the dental examination begins, concentration centers about the conditions that create the need for dental treatment and the development of treatment recommendations. The thoroughness of dental care is related to the thoroughness of the examination of the dental structures and mechanisms.

In addition to the standard examination tray (Fig. 17-3) there should be available proper radiographs, preferably a full-mouth series and a panoramic film (Figs. 18-10 and 18-38), and a set of study models (Fig. 17-20). Other special instruments and materials may be ultilized.

Periodontium

The structures that support the teeth include the gingivae, the periodontal ligament, and the supporting bone and are collectively known as the *periodontium* (see Chap. 5). These periodontal tissues must be maintained in a healthy state be-

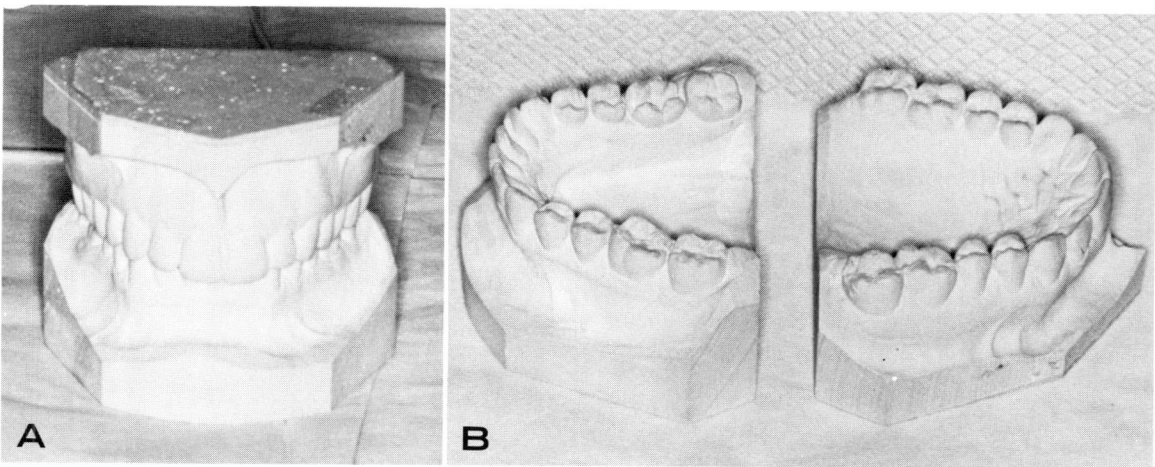

Figure 17-20 | Study models.

cause they provide the foundation for the teeth. Chronic disease affecting these tissues may result in ultimate loss of the teeth.

The gingivae are examined for color, size, texture, and bleeding tendency. Slight changes may be evidence of the beginning of significant disease states either local or systemic. The gingivae are normally pale pink, firm, slightly stippled on the surface, and just fill the spaces between the teeth. There is a crevice or sulcus that surrounds each tooth between the tooth and the free margin of the gingiva (Chap. 5). Excessive depth of this sulcus indicates the presence of periodontal disease (Chap. 25) and is discovered through measurements with a calibrated probe (Fig. 17-21).

Figure 17-21 | Use of the periodontal probe to measure sulcular depth.

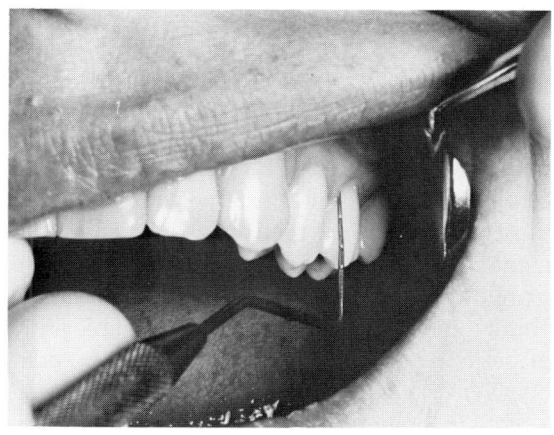

The teeth are examined carefully for the accumulation of deposits such as plaque, calculus (tartar), and stains. The presence of dental plaque is assessed by specific techniques (see Chap. 19) and is essential to the determination of the patient's home-care effectiveness. Such accumulations are believed to promote periodontal disease.

The contacting relationship of the teeth of the opposite jaws on closure is known as *occlusion*. The careful study of how the teeth of the opposing arches relate in contact is important and can be quite complicated, but a thorough analysis of these factors and correction of abnormalities are essential to long-range dental health. The

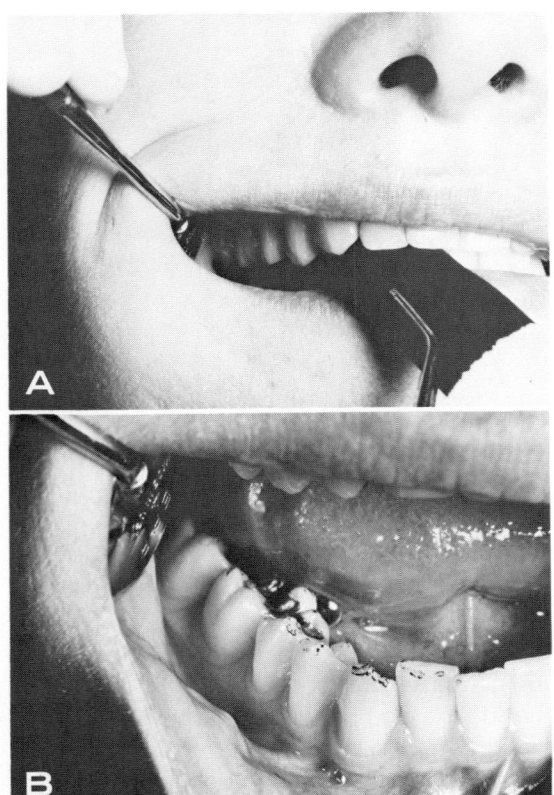

Figure 17-22 | Indication of occlusal contacts by use of articulating paper.

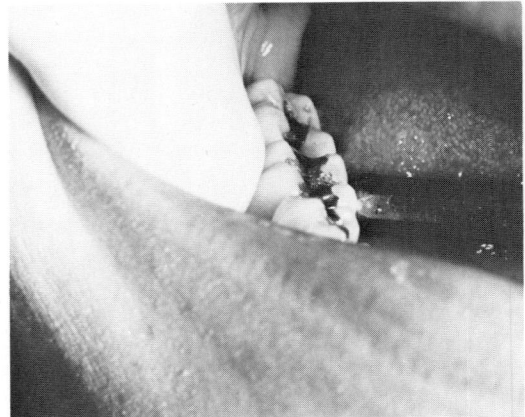

Figure 17-23 | Detection of tooth mobility.

examination consists of precise direction of the patient in opening, closing, and lateral tooth-contact movements of the jaws and observation of tooth relationship during these exercises. Often there are interferences in the interdigitation of the teeth, and these can be seen by the use of articulating paper which will produce marks on the teeth at the points of contact (Fig. 17-22A and B). The presence of occlusal disharmonies can result in damage to the periodontium, abnormal tooth wear patterns, or temporomandibular joint problems with severe discomfort to the patient and difficulties in providing satisfactory dental treatment.

There is some normal movement of teeth in their sockets under pressure, and this can be demonstrated. However, such movement is slight and not normally noticeable. When gross movement by pressure on teeth can be demonstrated, undesirable disease is present. Detection of tooth movement can be done with the fingers, but it is best to use a finger and a hard instrument (Fig. 17-23).

It is important that records of these findings be made; an example of a periodontal charting is in Fig. 25-8. A discussion of the assistant's role in periodontics will be found in Chap. 25.

Teeth

The teeth are examined for number, size, shape, color, structure, caries, restorations, tenderness, traumatic injuries, poor interproximal contacts, etc. The details of tooth examination can be almost limitless and call for a wide variety of instruments, equipment, and materials, for there are many tests that will yield important information about tooth conditions. Routinely, a simple array of basic materials and instruments will be adequate (Fig. 17-3).

Prior to the detailed clinical examination of the

teeth it is best to make a full series of periapical radiographs and, if possible, a panoramic film (see Chap. 18). These films are essential to the discovery of interproximal and periapical disease and faults as well as of more extensive abnormalities of the dental mechanism.

It is desirable to have a set of study models or casts of the patient's dentiton available (Fig. 17-20A and B). These models are prepared from impressions of the patient's teeth by pouring in dental plaster or artificial stone and finishing neatly to produce accurate reproductions of the patient's teeth and adjacent structures (see Chap. 10).

As the examination of the teeth proceeds, a detailed chart of all findings is developed (Fig. 17-24). There will be variations of dental charting in almost every dental office, but the basic principles are the same for all, and they are quite important. Entries on a dental chart should be limited to actual findings, and they should be neat, clean, accurate, brief; they should be in a standard code and of a type to be clearly recognizable by any informed dental person; once the chart is complete, there should be no subsequent changes. Some charts include both periodontal findings and the tooth chart (Figs. 21-5 and 25-8).

The teeth are identified individually and counted and their size and shape noted. This procedure is important in that missing teeth must be identified and the effect of their absence on the remaining dentition evaluated; size and shape will have influences in cases where orthodontic treatment or prosthodontic restorations are required.

Color and structure of the teeth will convey much information as to the health and past history of the teeth. The presence of discoloration may indicate that existing restorations are deep and that overlying tooth structure is weak; the presence of caries may be evidenced by color change; a tooth that has been severely damaged by trauma or disease can show a general darkening of color which may signify that there has been irreversible damage to the dental pulp with destruction of vascular circulation and sensitivity—a so-called nonvital or dead tooth. Structural abnormalities may result from congenital conditions, disease, faults of formation, or trauma. Fractures of teeth are carefully noted.

For the detailed examination of the teeth specific requirements are recognized. Good light and visibility are essential. It is wise to reserve a set of examining instruments for these procedures alone. The explorers, mirrors, probes should be in perfect condition and undamaged by heavy usage. The surfaces of the teeth should be clean and dry; in some practices a preexamination prophylaxis is routine. At least, the teeth should be cleared with floss if any debris at all is present and also irrigated and thoroughly dried. Teeth carefully isolated with cotton rolls and dried will reveal defects much more readily than when covered with moisture. Careful sliding of a sharp explorer over the surfaces of the tooth will help to identify defects such as caries, faulty restorations, and subgingival calculus (Fig. 17-25). Direct vision and a dental mirror with reflected and transmitted light will often reveal even slight defects and early pathology.

Tenderness and possible disease of the supporting tissues of individual teeth often can be located by careful, light tapping on the teeth with a blunt metal instrument such as the butt end of a dental mirror handle. Careful use of floss between the teeth may reveal marginal overhang of restorations or early interproximal caries; it will also help to determine whether interproximal tooth contact is adequate or not.

Abnormal wear of tooth surfaces may have important significance. As an individual ages, various evidences of tooth wear patterns are more or less expected. However, some wear patterns of the chewing surfaces of the teeth may indicate functional tooth interferences or general wear caused by bruxism. Unusual wear patterns on the facial surfaces of the teeth may indicate improper brushing habits resulting in a notching of the teeth.

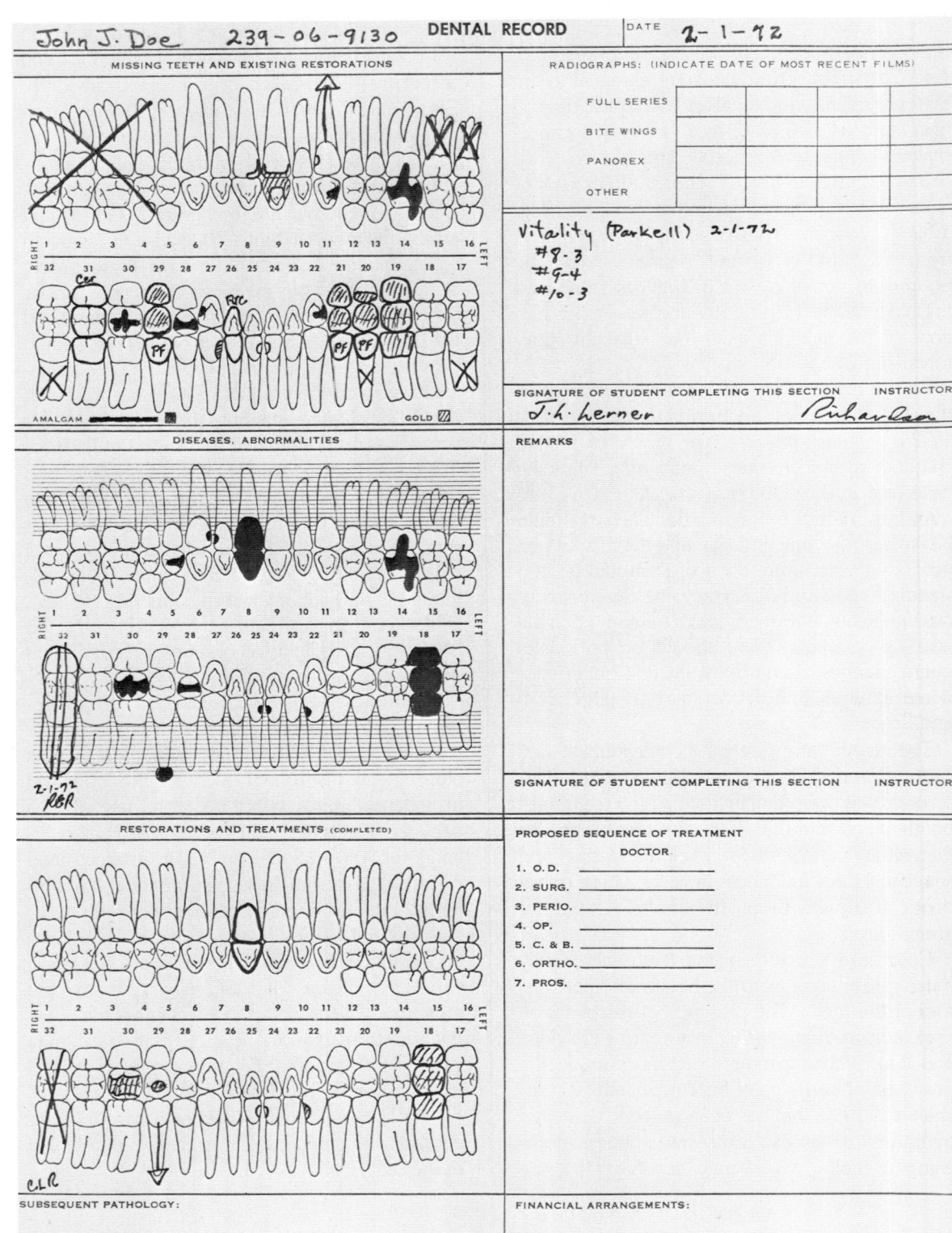

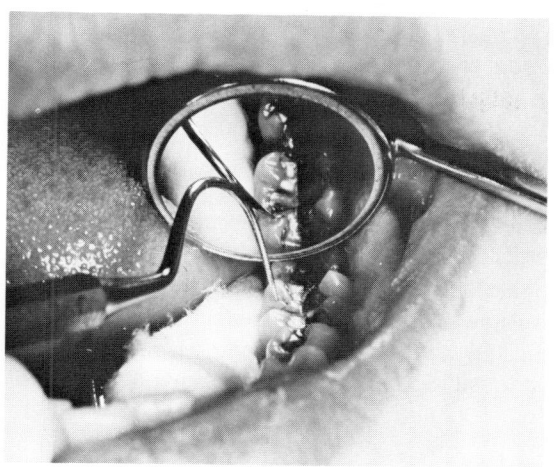

Figure 17-25 | Use of the dental explorer.

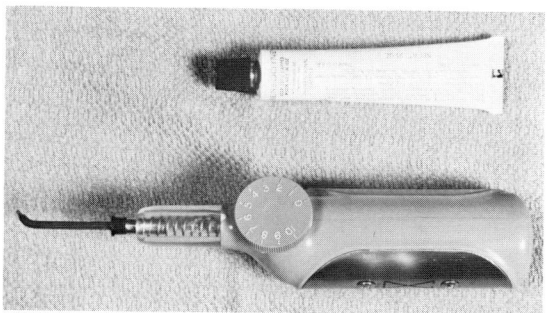

Figure 17-26 | Electrical pulp tester, and toothpaste used for contact medium.

An important aid in the dental examination is the procedure known as *pulp testing*. Pulp testing is done whenever there is a question as to the health of the dental pulp. There are various tests involved in this procedure. Heat and cold may be applied to teeth in the form of hot gutta-percha, ice, or ethyl chloride-soaked pellets. Electrical impulses from an electrical pulp tester applied to a tooth can give much information as to the status of the dental pulp (Figs. 17-26 and 17-27). Chapter 24 carries a fuller discussion of these techniques, but, to emphasize the importance of a precise technique of electrical pulp testing, certain rules must be followed. One can test the instrument by placing its point on one's own skin and observing the impulse. The teeth to be tested must be isolated with cotton rolls and thoroughly dried. The point of the instrument should carry some contacting medium such as toothpaste. The patient should be given a nonfrightening explanation of what is to occur; use words such as tingling, tickling, warm, etc. Arrange with the patient to signal with a hand when the tooth sensation is first felt. A control tooth (one that is not in doubt) is tested first to obtain base-line information relative to the patient's reaction. The instrument tip must contact healthy, dentin-supported enamel and not a restoration or the gingiva. The strength of the impulse is *gradually* increased until the patient gives the signal. The level at which the patient first feels the impulse is carefully noted in the record for each tooth tested.

Figure 17-27 | Tooth contact of electrical pulp tester point with toothpaste.

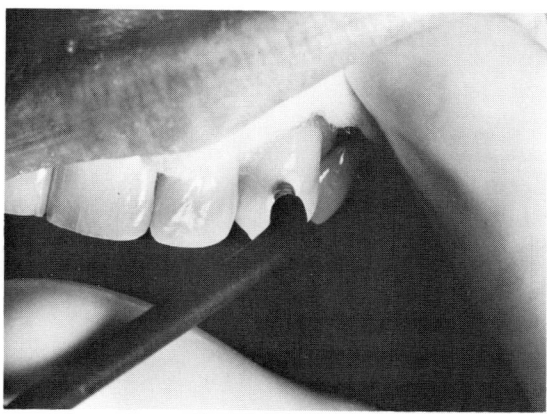

Figure 17-24 | Dental chart.

ADDITIONAL EXAMINATION PROCEDURES

There are many examination procedures that may be necessary or desirable in particular situations; some are used routinely and others in special situations or as clinical findings might indicate.

The use of disclosing tablets or solutions to evaluate the presence of plaque on the teeth and caries activity tests have come to be routine procedures in developing the patient's preventive care program; discussion of these important techniques will be found in Chap. 19.

Routinely, in root canal treatment procedures, it is necessary to obtain material from the root canal, put it in a culture medium, and incubate it for a given period of time. This procedure is an indication as to whether the root canal is sterile or not. The dental assistant will have an important responsibility in the management of the culture and its incubation (see Chap. 24).

Other bacteriologic studies may be desirable and may be carried out in some dental offices or material may be sent to a pathology laboratory for reports. Smears or samples taken of material from suspected lesions such as candidiasis, tuberculosis, actinomycosis, and other disease states can be examined for positive identification.

The dentist may find that the history and clinical examination will indicate that various blood studies or tests will be necessary. If there is a history of prolonged bleeding, there are tests that will determine if an actual bleeding problem might follow a surgical procedure. One of the signs of serious blood cell disorders, the leukemias, may be changes in the gingival tissues which could be observed by the dentist before the disease has been discovered; blood cell counts are essential for this diagnosis. Constant pallor of the skin and oral tissues may suggest one of the anemic diseases; hemoglobin and red blood cell counts may confirm such a suspicion.

The serologic test for syphilis may be indicated. There are many disease states that require blood examination for positive identification. The dentist is in an important position to aid in the early detection of these conditions. These patients are usually referred to a physician for evaluation and determination of the tests required. In some practices the dentist may be able to have the tests done in a pathology laboratory.

A patient may be suspected of having diabetes mellitus, and a diagnosis may be made through various blood and urine tests. Such tests will not commonly be done in the dental office, but there are screening tests for diabetes that may be in use there and which can be a good basis for referral to a physician. The control of diabetes is essential for the patient and is also important for the long-range success of dental care.

Patients may present in the dental office with severe infections that require the use of antibiotic drugs. Sometimes an infection will be resistant to a given antibiotic, and tests may be made that can show which antibiotic is best for the specific organism involved.

When a patient has a lesion or growth that has persisted over an extended period of time, it is important that such a condition be positively identified. There is the possibility that a malignant condition exists. The most dependable way to make a positive diagnosis of such changes is by taking a section of tissue from the lesion or growth and having it examined by a qualified oral pathologist; this is known as a biopsy. Another, less dependable examination in this situation is a cytologic smear. These procedures are discussed in Chap. 8. The assistant will have the responsibility for management of the materials and equipment for these tests and for forwarding of the specimens to the pathologist.

The procedures cited are not the only procedures with which the dentist may become involved, but they are the most likely ones, and the assistant would do well to be as familiar as possible with the mechanism and significance of such tests and examinations.

USE OF DIAGNOSTIC FINDINGS

Treatment Planning

It is logical that the detailed development of diagnostic procedures and materials is to serve the purpose of determining a patient's need for treatment and how that need can be met. From all the information gathered, the dentist will, by careful analysis, develop a treatment plan.

The assistant does not make diagnoses or develop treatment plans, but it is important for him or her to understand the process in order to be knowledgeable when discussing procedures with patients. The assistant will be constantly close to the patient and will often have to provide encouragement and explanation in varied situations.

Generally speaking, the aim in treatment planning is to restore and maintain the patient's entire dental function as perfectly as possible, where need exists. This usually involves more than just meeting some immediate need. The real significance of oral diagnosis is that not only existing disease and problems be identified but that the possibility of such development in the future be anticipated. Many patients present with very involved needs, and it will require the cooperation and understanding of everyone in the practice to help these patients develop the confidence they need to accept proper treatment.

Treatment planning frequently permits optional courses of treatment with the ultimate goal being full care. At other times limited treatment is all that is practical. Whatever is done should be based on the best procedure for a particular case.

In general, a patient's immediate needs must be met first. This often takes the form of emergency care. No matter what the procedure, a history and examination must be done first to be certain that there are no contraindications for that treatment.

At the outset the principles and practice of preventive dentistry should be presented so that the patient can participate in making dental treatment successful.

Surgical procedures are usually done prior to restorative treatment. Nonuseful wisdom teeth and hopeless teeth are eliminated as early as possible. Teeth that require root canal treatment are also attended to as early as possible.

The health of the supporting tissues must be established as soon as possible through the preventive program or actual periodontal therapy if this is necessary. It is quite clear that even if teeth are perfectly sound their foundation or support must also be sound. Response of the tissues to such treatment is a strong clue as to whether the teeth can be maintained or not.

Individual teeth having defects should be reconstructed, in whatever is the most effective material, to the original or normal contours and support. The complexity of this ideal depends upon the individual situation. There may be general rules for certain procedures, but they can be highly variable.

Where the patient has some serious malalignment or has lost functional teeth, orthodontics may be an important consideration in the long-range success of dental care. Usually the possibility of such need is given careful consideration and development prior to major replacement of missing teeth or involved final restoration of individual teeth.

If teeth are lost, they usually should be replaced, and this may require fixed prosthodontics, called bridgework, or removable prosthodontics, called partial or full dentures. In any case the aim is to restore the dental arches to their original anatomy and function as completely as possible.

Once dental treatment and restoration is complete, the long-range maintenance of health and function becomes the objective. Periodic recall and reevaluation is essential for complete and successful care. The operation of an effective recall system is an integral part of a first-class dental practice and should be one of the satisfactions of participating in this important health service.

Patient Consultation

The science of oral diagnosis is the basis for dental care and, when it is applied effectively, it provides for the accumulation of evidence and knowledge necessary for the development of proper treatment. Not all patients will accept the concept of total dental care; some cannot for very real reasons. However, every patient has a right to gain full understanding of the recommendations that will be made.

A consultation between the dentist and the patient, where the factors involved can be fully explained, works to the mutual advantage of both. The dentist has the opportunity to present the philosophy of full care, to relate the problems to the patient, and to explain any options that are possible. Patients have uncertainties and doubts that need to be resolved prior to initiation of treatment. The patient will have questions and will appreciate consideration and willingness to discuss them in a reasonable manner. Most people will want what is best for them and will discover that fine dental care is attainable when the priorities can be made clear. Practically everyone will appreciate careful diagnostic procedures and considerate discussion of the need for and management of any proposed treatment.

Failures in dental treatment will almost always be related, at least in part, to a lack of pretreatment preparation and full communications between the dentist and the patient.

Records

The assistant will surely be involved and be an important person in every step in the process of accumulation of patient information. The preparation of written records, instruments, materials, aids, etc., should be done by precise and meticulous techniques in order that the end products are clear, accurate, and complete. This informational material will be critical to the effective delivery of care at the decision-making stage and throughout treatment.

The diagnostic data will be continuously important to continuing care and evaluation. Therefore, all of this related matter should be carefully stored, preserved, and updated at every opportunity. Pretreatment information should be constantly and readily available. Therefore, original histories, examination findings, study models, radiographs, and all other records and reports should be systematically and safely filed with clear and accurate identification.

18

Stephen R. Matteson
Dental Radiology

ROLE AND PRACTICE OF RADIOLOGY IN DENTISTRY

The dentist must make the correct diagnosis before he or she can properly treat a patient. The clinical oral examination and the radiographic information are carefully considered before developing a treatment plan. Radiographs are films obtained by directing x-rays through portions of the patient to be studied onto the film. The various structures of the patient will absorb the x-rays differently, with bones and teeth absorbing more rays than the soft tissues. The distribution of x-rays on the film produces an image which represents a shadow of the anatomy of the patient.

Radiographs are essential because they permit the dentist to examine areas inside the teeth and jaws which cannot be seen any other way. Many carious lesions, periodontal defects, and jaw diseases can be detected only by the use of radiographs.

Good-quality radiographs of the oral structures are required for each patient to permit visualization of the structures in and surrounding the oral cavity. The properly trained dental assistant will obtain these radiographs in the dental office, and this will be one of his or her most important duties.

An important principle in dental radiographic practice is that the necessary diagnostic information be obtained for each patient with the least irradiation of the patient. This is accomplished in two ways. First, the attending dentist decides the number, type, and frequency of films to be taken. This decision is made according to the diagnostic needs of the individual patient. Radiographs should not be taken according to any regular schedule, such as a full series every 5 years or bitewings every 6 months. All patients must be evaluated for their specific needs and the least number of films taken to satisfy those requirements.

Secondly, after radiographs have been ordered by the dentist, the dental assistant must make every effort to use good radiographic technique and careful darkroom procedures. This will prevent the needless retaking of films and avoid unnecessary radiation exposure to the patient.

RADIATION PHYSICS

Electromagnetic Radiation

Radiation physics is the science of the laws, forces, and general properties of radiation. X-rays are a form of energy which are generated in the dental x-ray tubehead. They are a type of electromagnetic radiation, as are visible light, ultraviolet radiation, radar, and radio and television waves. The principal characteristics of all electromagnetic radiations are:

1. They travel at the speed of light (186,000 mi/second).
2. They are pure energy and contain no mass or weight. These radiations do work without the movement of any matter or mass. For example, light from a bulb illuminates an area with only light energy coming from the light bulb. This is in contrast to a situation in which work is done by moving matter with weight, an example of this being the hammering of a nail into wood with a hammer. Here, the work is accomplished by moving the hammer, which has mass or weight, through a distance to hit the nail. Electromagnetic radiations are energy only, and no mass is transferred from one area to another to do work.
3. They travel through space in wave motion as transverse waves. Think of a length of rope being held by two people. As they shake the rope, a wave will travel from one end to the other. If the two holders walk forward with the waves moving along the rope, this will demonstrate transverse wave motion. Electromagnetic radiations travel in this same manner. The difference between various electromagnetic radiations is determined by the wavelength of the radiation. The wavelength is the distance between successive peaks along the wave (Fig. 18-1). The shorter the wavelength, the more penetrating the radiation will be. Light energy is not very penetrating and can penetrate only thin objects like a sheet of paper. The wavelength of light is relatively long compared to that of x-rays. X-rays have a shorter wavelength and are able to penetrate substances such as teeth and bones.
4. There are electric and magnetic fields associated with the radiations. These properties are responsible for the name electromagnetic radiation. The electric and magnetic fields are present around the wave as it travels through space.

X-rays were discovered in 1893 by Professor Wilhelm von Roentgen while experimenting with a cathode ray tube in his darkened laboratory. Unknown to him, this apparatus was emitting x-rays. He observed that a piece of cardboard coated with phosphorescent material glowed during the use of the equipment. The x-rays were hitting the coated cardboard causing it to glow. He realized he was observing an unknown ray, and through a series of experiments demonstrated most of the basic properties of x-radiation. He learned that the x-rays could

Figure 18-1 | Wave motion. Electromagnetic radiations travel through space in the form of wave motion. The wavelength (λ) is the distance between the peaks of successive waves.

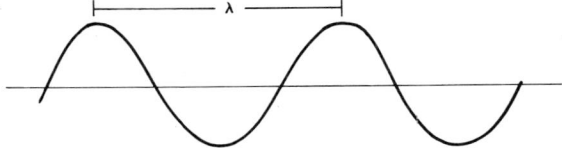

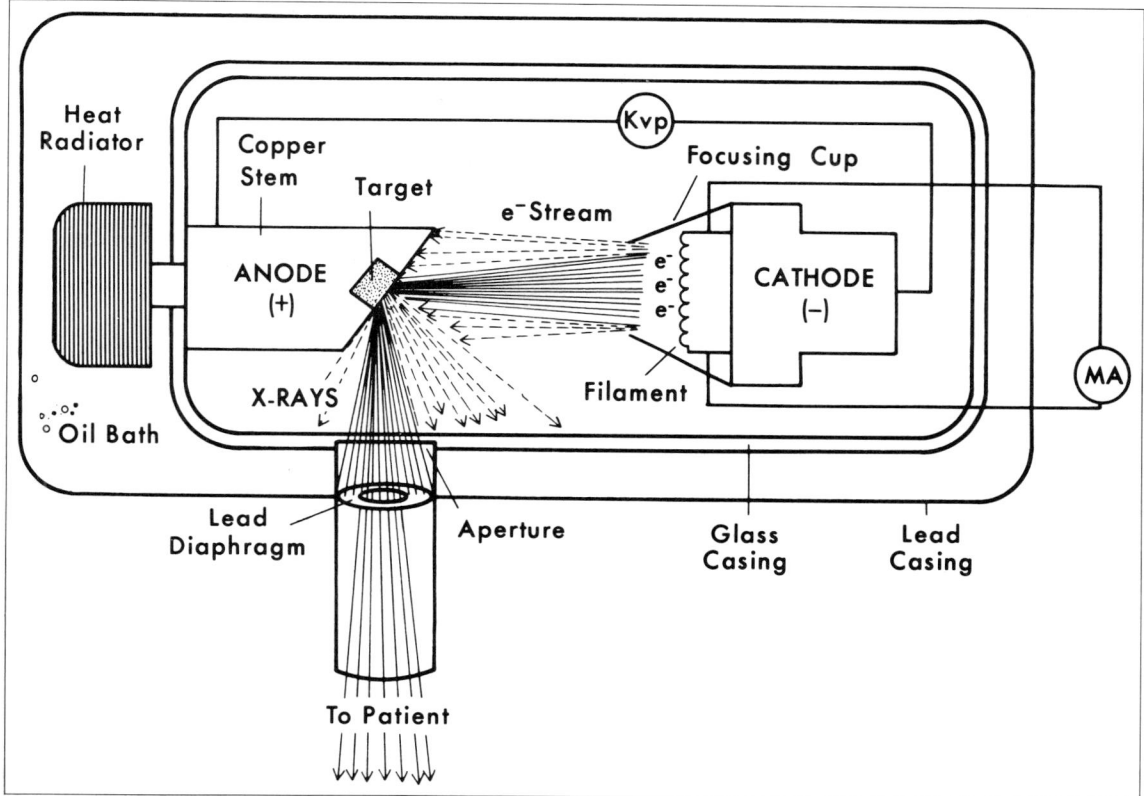

Figure 18-2 | Diagram of x-ray tube. High-voltage circuit (kVp) develops the voltage potential between the cathode (−) and anode (+). Low-voltage circuit (mA) is connected to the filament on the cathode and controls the number of electrons released.

penetrate substances such as wood. One of the earliest radiographs ever taken was of his wife's hand. Within several years x-rays were being used for medical and dental diagnostic purposes.

X-Radiation

X-rays have the following properties which make them very useful in the practice of radiology:

1. They can affect a photographic plate and can be used to make radiographs.
2. They can cause certain chemical crystals to give off light. Not only is this the property that led to the discovery of x-rays, but this is used in the construction of the intensifying screens in panoramic cassettes in dental radiography.
3. They have a short wavelength which permits the penetration of soft tissue and bone. The wavelength of the x-rays used in dentistry is 0.5 to 1 angstrom unit (Å) (one angstrom equals one hundred-millionth of a centimeter).

X-Ray Generation

X-rays are generated in a dental x-ray tube (Fig. 18-2). The tube is enclosed in the tubehead of the x-ray machine which is encased by metal shielding that prevents the leakage of radiation. The internal parts of the x-ray generating tube are:

1. *Cathode:* the negatively charged component which contains a filament wire coil made of tungsten.
2. *Anode:* the positively charged component containing a target area made of tungsten.
3. *Focal spot:* the small area on the target to which the electrons are directed.
4. *Focusing cup:* the negatively charged metal cup adjacent to the cathode.
5. *Aperture:* the opening in the glass envelope for the exit of x-rays.
6. *Copper heat radiator:* the device used to dissipate heat created during the generation of x-rays at the anode.

Two electrical circuits control the x-ray generation by the tube:

1. High-voltage circuit, connected to the anode and cathode. This determines that the cathode is negatively charged and the anode is positively charged. This circuit establishes a peak or maximum voltage potential between the cathode and anode from 65,000 to 90,000 volts [65 to 90 kilovolt peak (kVp)].
2. Low-voltage circuit, connected to the filament of the cathode. This circuit provides 10 to 15 milliamperes (mA) of electrical current and is a factor controlling the amount of radiation produced.

X-rays are generated when the two electrical circuits are simultaneously activated. As current passes through the filament of the cathode, the coil wire filament is heated to a high temperature. Due to a process termed *thermionic emission*, the heating of the filament results in electrons being given off by the wire. The current in the low-voltage circuit determines the quantity of heat in the filament and therefore the number of electrons that are given off by the filament. An increase in current will result in the release of more electrons.

The voltage, or electrical pressure, between the negatively charged cathode and positively charged anode is determined by the high-voltage circuit. The electrons given off at the cathode are negatively charged. With both circuits activated, the electrons which are emitted from the filament are attracted to the positively charged anode at a rapid rate of speed. The focusing cup directs the electrons toward the focal spot on the target of the anode. The kilovoltage in the high-voltage circuit, measured as peak kilovoltage (kVp), determines the speed that the electrons travel to the focal spot. The higher the kVp setting, the faster the electrons will move.

When the electrons hit the tungsten metal of the focal spot, they are stopped rapidly and absorbed there. It is this rapid braking of the electrons that results in the generation of x-rays, and this process is called the *Bremsstrahlen* (rapid-braking) reaction. Rays are produced in all directions from the target, but only those passing through the small opening in the glass case (aperture) are permitted to pass toward the patient.

The penetrating ability of the x-rays produced will vary and depends upon the voltage in the high-voltage circuit. With increasing kilovoltage, the electrons will be attracted to the anode with more force and will travel at a greater speed. The resulting x-rays produced at the target will be of smaller wavelength and be capable of penetrating substances more easily.

A considerable amount of heat is also generated at the target due to the electrons hitting the focal spot. The copper stem radiator serves to dissipate the heat from the target by conducting it to the oil bath surrounding the glass case for this purpose.

DENTAL X-RAY MACHINE OPERATION

Dental X-Ray Machine

Figure 18-3 illustrates a dental x-ray machine. The x-ray generating tube is incorporated into

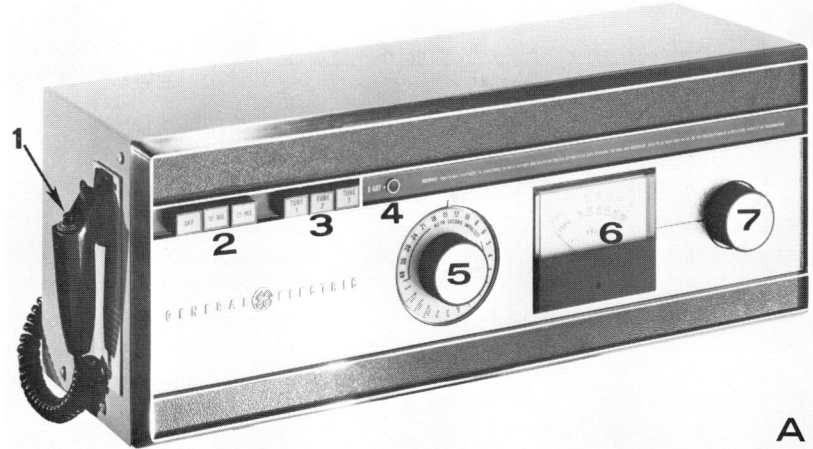

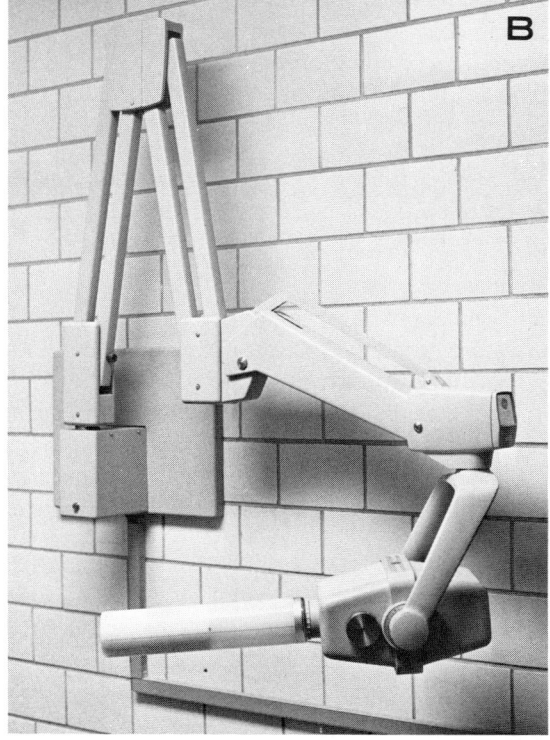

Figure 18-3 | Dental x-ray machine. A. Control panel: (1) exposure button, (2) mA setting and on-off switch, (3) tubehead selector, (4) x-ray exposure light, (5) time setting, (6) kVp meter, (7) kVp control. (*Courtesy of General Electric Company.*) B. Tubehead and flexible arm on wall.

the dental tubehead. This is attached to a tube arm to provide the maneuverability necessary to position the x-ray cone properly during the exposures. The illustrated machine is turned on by depressing the milliampere setting of 10 or 15 mA. Other manufacturers may provide a separate on-off button. The tubehead selector buttons permit the selection of individual tubeheads when more than one radiographic cubicle is controlled by one control panel. The time setting is determined by turning the dial to the correct number of impulses (one-sixtieth of a second). The kVp is set by adjusting the control knob and reading the setting on the kVp meter. Radiation is produced by the machine only when the exposure button is depressed. This button is termed a *dead man switch* because after the button is pressed, only one exposure will occur until the button is completely released. Additional exposures will occur by pressing the button again from its resting position. The x-ray exposure light will remain on only while x-rays are being generated. The operator must keep the exposure button completely depressed until the exposure light goes off by itself. If the operator removes his or her finger from the button before the entire preset exposure has occurred, the resulting radiograph will be underexposed and too light. An example of proper technique settings using a 16-in long cone are 80 kVp, 15 mA, and 24 impulses for the maxillary anterior area using ultraspeed film. If a shorter cone is used, the time setting will be reduced.

Effects of Technique Factors on the Film Image

Milliamperage, Time, and Kilovoltage

The image density or amount of film blackening is determined by both the milliampere and time settings. The effect of these factors can be compared to the lens opening and time setting of a camera. The mA control on the x-ray machine determines the amount of radiation per unit time delivered at the end of the cone. This is similiar to the lens opening of the camera which determines the amount of light allowed to reach the photographic film per unit time. The time setting on the x-ray machine establishes the length of time that the x-rays will be allowed to pass from the end of the cone. Similarly, the time setting on the camera determines the length of time the lens will be open and permit light to reach the film. The combination of these two factors establishes the quantity of x-rays delivered at the end of the cone for each exposure.

The kVp also has a relationship with the density of the film image. A decrease of 10 kVp, e.g., 90 to 80 kVp, will result in a decrease in film density or lighter film by approximately one-half.

The contrast of the film image is determined by the kVp setting. *Contrast* is the distinction between the white and black shadows on the film. Images with high contrast demonstrate sharp distinction between white and black areas on the film and are produced when using lower kVp settings (65 kVp). Low-contrast images are produced by higher kVp settings and show more grey intervals between the white and black shadows. The dentist will determine the kVp setting by judging whether high- or low-contrast images will provide the needed diagnostic information for the individual patient.

Effects of Distance on Film Image

The density of the film image is also affected by the distance from the x-ray target to the film. The correct technique factors are established using a cone of specific length. The settings must be adjusted if a cone of different size is put on the machine. The effect of distance on film density follows the inverse square law which states that the intensity of the beam of x-rays varies inversely as the square of the distance from the x-ray source (target) to the film. Think of a beam of light from a flashlight shining on a wall. As the flashlight is moved away from the wall, the brightness of the light on the wall decreases. As the flashlight is moved closer to the wall, the brightness increases. The same principle applies to the beam of x-rays. If the x-ray cone is positioned too far from the face of the patient, the image on the film will be too light. The inverse square law also defines quantitatively the change in intensity of the light or x-ray beam at various distances. If the distance is doubled, the intensity of the beam will be reduced by 4 (distance squared).

RADIATION BIOLOGY

Radiation biology is the science that deals with the effects of radiation on living tissues. Some of the x-rays from an x-ray machine pass through the patient to form the image on the film. Some of the x-rays are stopped in the tissues, and the interaction between the x-rays and tissue cells may result in a harmful effect.

X-rays can cause tissue damage because they are a form of ionizing radiation. Ionization is the dissociation of a substance into its constituent ions in a solution. An example of ionization is the dissociation of salt (sodium chloride, NaCl) when dissolved in water. The sodium ion (Na$^+$) with a positive electrical charge is separated from the choride ion (Cl$^-$) with a negative charge. These charged atoms are called ions, and the process is ionization. X-rays cause ionization of the atoms within the cells and tissues of the body, and this can result in permanent damage to the tissues.

Cells and tissues are composed of a high percentage of water (H$_2$O). The ionization of water results in the formation of chemical substances called radicals, e.g., hydrogen peroxide, H$_2$O$_2$. These radicals cause chemical damage in the cells and tissues, and this is a basic mechanism of radiation tissue damage.

Certain cells in the body are more sensitive than others to x-ray damage. Rapidly dividing cells which are increasing their numbers are more subject to radiation damage. These cells are not mature functioning cells. Examples are immature blood cells in the bone marrow and basal cells in the skin. Fully mature cells with specialized functions are more resistant to radiation damage. These cells are not dividing rapidly. Examples of these are muscle, nerve, and mature circulating blood cells. The cells in an embryo are especially sensitive to radiation because they are growing and dividing so rapidly. For this reason, the abdomen of a pregnant female should not be exposed to any x-radiation unless for absolutely necessary medical purposes.

X-rays may cause either an immediate or delayed effect. Immediate radiation effects usually result from exposure to relatively large doses of x-rays such as those used in radiation therapy. Skin reddening is an example of an immediate effect of higher doses of radiation. Examples of delayed effects are early aging of the tissue and the development of certain forms of cancer. These later effects do not become evident until many years following the exposure to the x-radiation.

Radiation damage can be cumulative with each additional exposure. Unfortunate early dentists who held dental films in their patients' mouths during the exposure of the film developed skin cancer of their fingers. This was caused by many successive exposures to the then-used higher doses of radiation.

Most of the damage caused in cells and tissues by low levels of radiation is repaired by the usual healing process. The repair may not be complete, however, and nonreplaceable cells may be killed or altered in form or function. Somatic radiation effects are those directly effecting the tissues of the exposed individual. Genetic effects are those which result from the exposure of the reproductive cells of an individual. These effects are seen on the offspring of the exposed individual. Immature reproductive cells can be sensitive to x-radiation, and all reasonable efforts should be taken to avoid unnecessary exposure to the reproductive regions of the dental patient.

In the area of the head and neck, the thyroid gland in the neck and the lens of the eye are especially sensitive to radiation, and all reasonable efforts to minimize exposure to these two areas should be made when taking dental radiographs.

RADIATION PROTECTION

Both primary and secondary radiation are important in radiation safety. *Primary radiation* is the original beam of x-rays that exit from the end of the cone. This beam of x-rays passes outward from the target in the tubehead in an expanding cone shape. This beam can be considered the useful x-rays which actually exit from the end of the cone. The cone shape of the x-ray beam can be demonstrated by observing a beam of light from a flashlight. This also is cone-shaped and increases in size as the light passes from its source. *Secondary radiation* is the radiation resulting from the interaction between the x-rays in the primary beam and the substances in the path of the primary beam. This can also be termed *scatter radiation*. During the exposure of patients, secondary radiation scatters throughout the entire room in all directions, and this is the reason that the dental assistant should stand behind an x-ray barrier during patient exposures.

Any exposure to radiation carries some small risk of biologic damage. Therefore, the basic principle to be followed in radiologic practice is that both the patient and the operator should be exposed to the minimum of x-radiation during the radiographic examination.

Patient Protection

The dental patient will be exposed to the least amount of x-radiation if the assistant follows these rules:

1. *The use of proper collimation.* The collimator is a lead disc with an opening in the center located in the dental x-ray cone which limits the size of the beam of radiation to a diameter determined by state law, e.g., in North Carolina 2¾ in at the surface of the patient's face. The collimator prevents the primary x-ray beam from being larger than necessary to cover the dental-size film.
2. *The use of aluminum filtration.* A disc of solid aluminum is placed in the dental x-ray cone in a position such that the entire field of x-rays must pass through it. The aluminum metal serves to selectively remove from the beam x-rays which have low penetrating power (long wavelength). These radiations would only be absorbed by the soft tissues of the patient and would contribute nothing to the film image because they are unable to reach the film. The thickness of aluminum filter used is determined by state law; e.g., North Carolina requires 1.5 mm of filtration below 70 kVp and 2.5 mm of aluminum above 70 kVp.
3. *The use of high-speed film.* Ultraspeed film (D-speed film) permits the use of lower levels of radiation compared to those required with slower, less sensitive films. The ultraspeed film is the most common film used in dental practice today.
4. *The use of a protective lead apron.* When placed over the chest and lap of the patient during the exposure of intraoral radiographs, a lead apron will reduce the amount of scatter radiation reaching the reproductive areas of the patient. During panoramic exposures the apron should be placed over the patient's back because the x-ray beam passes behind the patient's head.
5. *The use of long, lead-lined, open cones.* These reduce scatter radiation when compared to the pointed plastic cones.
6. *The use of film-holding devices.* Several different types of film holders are available which position the film in the mouth. Film holders eliminate unnecessary radiation exposure to the patient's fingers.
7. *Care in procedures.* The use of proper darkroom and radiographic techniques will eliminate the need of retaking radiographs because of avoidable errors.

The protection of the patient from any radiation other than that required to expose the film directly is the responsibility of the dental-office staff. Efforts in this cause will lead to obtaining the maximum diagnostic radiographic information using the least possible amount of radiation.

Operator Protection

The dental-office staff should be alert to the possible hazards of radiation exposure to themselves and to the need to conduct the radiographic examination in a manner to prevent any avoidable exposure. The operator should be located behind a lead barrier during the exposure of each radiograph. A leaded glass window is built into the lead barriers to permit the operator to observe the patient during the exposure. If a lead barrier is not available, the radiographer should be located no closer than 6 ft behind the head of the patient. The operator should *never* stand in the path of the primary x-ray beam, hold a film in the patient's mouth, or hold the machine tubehead during the exposure.

Film badge monitoring systems are available for detecting radiation to the operator. The badge is worn in the dental office and will detect the amount of radiation reaching office personnel. These are sent to the film badge company on a regular basis, and a report is returned indicating the radiation that has reached the film badge. The radiographic techniques of those persons whose badge report is positive can then be reviewed so that corrective measures can be taken.

The National Committee on Radiation Protection restricted the maximum permissible whole body dose for persons working around x-ray machines to a yearly dose of 5 rem or 0.1 rem/week. The 13-week dose is limited to 3 rem. The maximum accumulated dose may be calculated by use of the formula $5(N - 18)$, where N is the age in years and is greater than 18. For example, the maximum accumulated dose for a 35-year-old person may be figured as $5(35 - 18) = 85$. Therefore, a person working around x-ray equipment should not receive more than 85 rem as a maximum accumulated dose by the age of 35.

DENTAL FILM

Intraoral films are designed to be placed within the mouth while the exposure is being made. They are wrapped in a light-proof packet consisting of white moisture-proof paper that encloses the film. Sheets of protective paper surround the film and a sheet of lead foil behind the film prevents x-rays from scattering back against the film. Intraoral films are made in three types: (1) periapical, (2) interproximal, or bitewing, and (3) occlusal.

The periapical film is designed to show the apexes of the teeth and the surrounding bone. These films are made in three sizes: the 1.2 or standard periapical film ($1^1/_4 \times 1^5/_8$ in); the 1.1 used for many anterior views ($^{15}/_{16} \times 1^9/_{16}$ in); and the 1.0 or child-size film ($^7/_8 \times 1^3/_8$ in). The 1.2- and 1.1-size periapical films are used for adults and older children while 1.0 is mainly used with smaller children.

Bitewing, or interproximal, films may be obtained in three sizes: 2.1 ($^{15}/_{16} \times 1^9/_{16}$ in); 2.2 ($1^1/_4 \times 1^5/_8$); and 2.3 ($1^1/_{16} \times 2^1/_8$ in). Bitewing films are characterized by a tab which is used to hold the film in proper position by the occlusion of the teeth. These radiographs are used to detect interproximal caries, examine the crest of the alveolar ridge, and determine the relationship of permanent tooth buds to the deciduous teeth.

The occlusal film ($2^1/_4 \times 3$ in) is used to show large areas of the maxilla or mandible to examine large pathologic areas, impactions, supernumerary teeth, jaw fractures, and foreign bodies.

Extraoral films are used in dentistry for radiography of the jaws, facial bones, temporomandibular articulations, and facial profile. These films are supplied in light-tight boxes in various sizes. The most commonly used sizes in dentistry are 8×10 in or 5×7 in.

In the dental office, the stock of unexposed films should be stored in a cool place and be used by the expiration date stamped on the box. The supply of films currently in use may be stored in a lead dispenser easily accessible for immediate use. After each exposure, the films should be placed in a lead receptacle for protection against any radiation.

The speed of the film is determined by the sensitivity of the film emulsion. The more sensitive the emulsion, the less radiation that is required to expose the film. Ultraspeed film (speed D) should be used for all dental examinations. Slower-speed films such as radiatized film will result in higher doses of radiation to the patient.

PHOTOCHEMISTRY

A radiographic image is obtained in two steps. The film emulsion is affected by the ionizing radiation such that a latent image is created. This image is not visible on the film until the emulsion is treated with processing chemicals, the developer and fixer.

The dental film consists of a cellulose acetate base which is coated on both sides with a gelatin emulsion containing silver halide crystals. These chemical crystals are affected by the x-rays when the radiograph is exposed.

The developer solution contains two reducing agents, hydroquinone and elon. These in combination cause the exposed silver halide crystals in the film emulsion to turn black. Sodium carbonate is also added to soften the emulsion, allowing the developer to reach the silver halide crystals. The sodium carbonate also maintains the alkaline conditions necessary for the development reaction. One other ingredient is included, sodium sulfite, which inhibits oxidation of the developer.

The fixer solution acts to remove those silver halide crystals that have not been exposed to x-rays. This principal action is caused by the sodium thiosulfate (hypo). Potassium alum is added to reharden the emulsion, and acetic acid maintains the acidic condition necessary for the fixing reaction.

The films are washed for 30 seconds after contact with the developer to prevent developer solution from contaminating the fixer. After the fixing step, the films are washed for 20 minutes to remove all fixer from the film surface. Inadequately washed films can turn brown and become opaque after a period of time.

DARKROOM

Darkroom Equipment

Each office requires a darkroom closed from any outside illumination in order to unwrap and process films without exposing them to light. All potential sources of light leakage into the darkroom should be adequately sealed so that when the assistant is inside with the lights off, no light can be seen from outside the room.

It is necessary for each office to maintain a system to prevent the accidental exposure of films in the darkroom. When the assistant is unwrapping any films in the darkroom, a sign or light must indicate to office staff outside the darkroom not to enter. If the darkroom door is opened while films are being unwrapped, all unprocessed films will be ruined by light exposure. Items of equipment required in the darkroom are:

1. *Developing tank* (Fig. 18-4). The tank is made of stainless steel and consists of three compartments. The large center area contains running water for washing the films. The outside two compartments are for developing and fixing solutions. A drain is present in the bottom of the water bath allowing circulation of the water. Openings with stoppers are located in the inner walls of the side compartments to allow the emptying of the developer and fixer into the center compartment. When

Figure 18-4 | Developing tank. Water circulates throughout large tank. The developer and fixer compartments are placed into the sides of the main tank. (*Courtesy of General Electric Company.*)

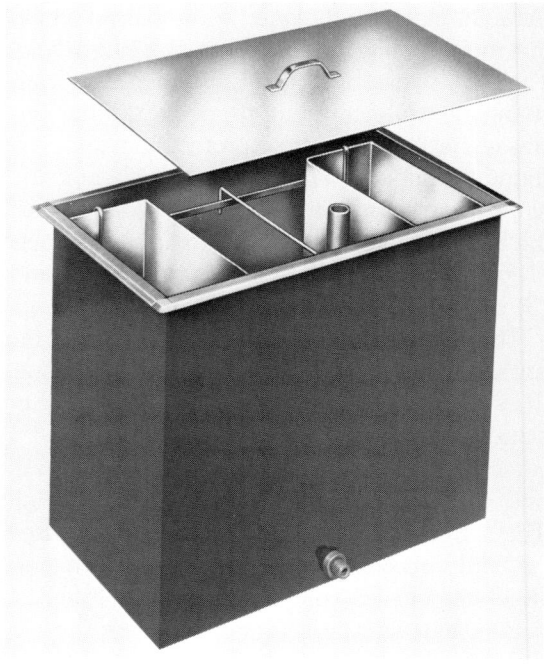

the solutions require changing, the stoppers can be removed simply, and the chemicals drained. A close-fitting tank lid is kept in place at all times except during the actual use of the tank to prevent decomposition of the solutions.
2. *Mixing valve.* A mixing valve is a plumbing fixture installed so that the hot and cold water pass through it on the way to the developing tank. An adjustable dial enables the dental assistant to control the temperature of the water and processing solutions usually at 68°F.
3. *Safelight.* This is a special light fixture installed in a darkroom that gives off a faint light. A special filter, usually the Wratten B or its equivalent, and a 15-watt bulb are used. The safelight allows enough light for the dental assistant to see in the darkroom but not enough to expose the film. The safelight should be installed at least 4 ft from any unwrapped dental film. The *penny test* can be used to check the darkroom for leakage of light to the area where films are unwrapped: A coin is placed on an unwrapped film and placed on the counter top where films are placed on racks for processing. The coin and film are left undisturbed for 1 minute in the darkened darkroom with the safelight on. The film is then processed, and if any image is visible, the light is fogging the film either from outside the room or from an improperly installed safelight.
4. *Interval timer.* This timer is a special clock that enables the dental assistant to time accurately the films being processed. Films are placed in the developer and fixer for precise periods of time; for example, developer for 4½ minutes, fixer 10 minutes, and wash for 20 minutes if the temperature of the solution is 68°F. The timer can be set for the proper length of time, and a bell will ring at the end of that period. The assistant is able to be outside the darkroom and return at the sound of the bell to place the films into the next stage of development (Fig. 18-5).
5. *Film racks.* These are metal holders with clips for the films. With the films attached, they are placed into the processing solutions (Fig. 18-6).
6. *Thermometer.* A floating style thermometer is used to measure the temperature of the developing solutions.

Darkroom Procedure

The following orderly procedure should be followed by the dental assistant when processing radiographs:

1. Wipe all saliva from the film packet after it has been removed from the patient's mouth. Otherwise, the moisture will cause the layers of paper inside the packet to stick to the film.
2. Check the temperature of the developing solutions and establish proper developing time using the time-temperature chart.
3. Set the interval timer to the time indicated for development.
4. Organize the films on the film racks and record the rack number used for each patient. This will permit proper identification of the films after the processing is completed.
5. Working with only the safelight on, unwrap the film packets and *securely* clip the films onto the film rack. If the film is not firmly held by the clip, it can be lost in the developer fixing tank (Fig. 18-7).
6. Place the film rack with the films attached into the

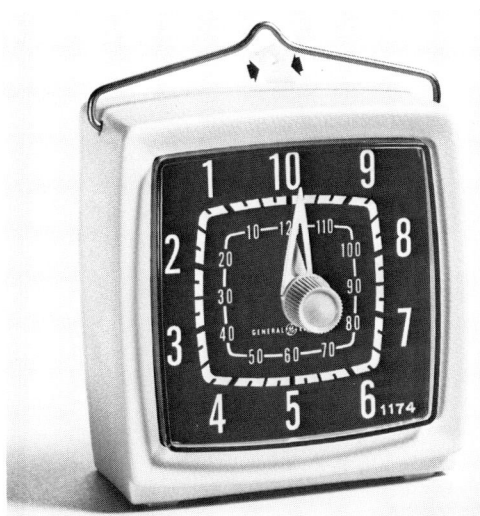

Figure 18-5 | Interval timer. Preset desired time by turning knob counterclockwise. The large numbers indicate the minute setting. When films are placed in the developer, the start lever (arrows) is cocked to start the time running. (*Courtesy of General Electric Company.*)

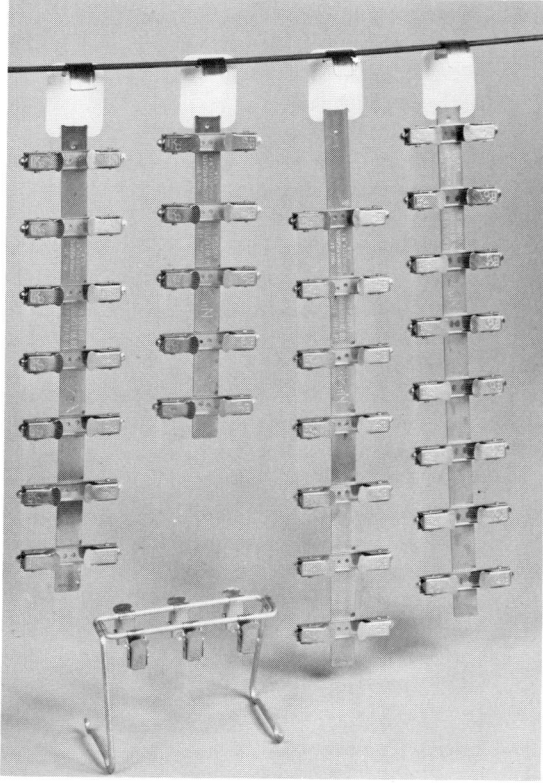

Figure 18-6 | Film racks. The white plastic tags are used to number the racks. This aids in identification of patient's films. (*Courtesy of Eastman Kodak Company.*)

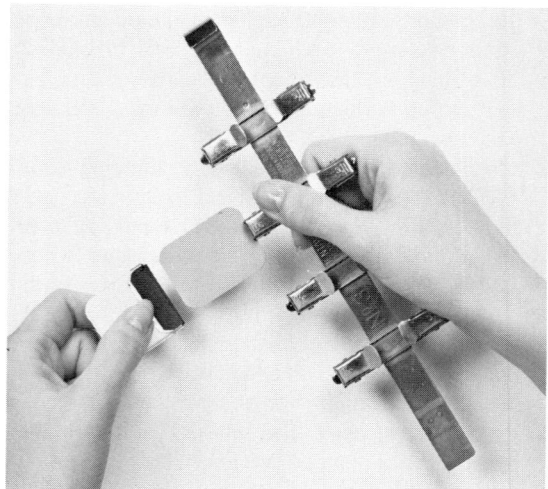

Figure 18-7 | Film placement on rack. Films must be firmly held by clip on the rack, or they can fall into the processing tanks. (*Courtesy of Eastman Kodak Company.*)

developing solution, being sure all the films are completely covered by the solution. Start the interval timer running.

7. At the sound of the timer bell indicating the proper development time has elapsed, remove the film rack from the developer, rinse for 30 seconds in the water, and place the rack in the fixer. Again be sure the films are completely immersed in the processing solution. Set and start the interval timer for 10 minutes.
8. After fixing is complete, place the film racks in the running water for 20 minutes. Hang the racks to dry after the washing is completed.

These procedures are illustrated in Fig. 18-8.

Automatic Processing

Automatic processing equipment is available which will process dental radiographs (Fig. 18-9A). These processors contain tanks for developer, fixer, and water. A series of rollers conveys the films through the chemicals to a drier (Fig. 18-9B). The completed films are available in 4 to 5 minutes. The routine maintenance of these machines is very important, and the cleaning of rollers and changing of solutions must be completed according to the manufacturer's recommendations. The solutions used for automatic developing machines are designated as rapid processing (R.P.) chemicals.

Film Mounting

After the films are processed and dried, they are prepared for the dentist by placing them in

Figure 18-8 | Procedure for film processing. (*Courtesy of Eastman Kodak Company.*)

Manual Processing KODAK Intraoral Dental X-ray Film

GENERAL RULES

Correct manual processing makes a definite contribution to the quality of a radiograph. It is also a fact that properly processed film requires only the minimum of exposure. The importance of correct processing cannot be overemphasized. The three fundamentals for good processing are fresh solutions, adequate equipment, and a standardized method.

This chart describes and pictures the basic steps in correct time-temperature processing.

Timer and Thermometer. Both must be accurate and in good working order. It is essential to use them routinely.

Safelight. A lamp in good condition should be located at least 4 feet from the working surface. Use KODAK Safelight Filters, KODAK WRATTEN Gelatin Filter Series 6B, for extraoral dental x-ray film, a KODAK Safelight Filter, Type ML-2 (Light Orange) for intraoral dental x-ray films. A 15-watt bulb is required for all dental x-ray films (KODAK Single-Coated Medical X-ray Film—Blue Sensitive requires a 7½-watt bulb at a distance of 4 feet).

Chemicals. In preparing solutions, follow directions on the packages exactly. Maintain levels of the solutions in the tanks with proper amounts of replenishment solutions. The solutions must cover the top films on the hanger. KODAK Dental X-ray Developer is recommended for the times in the chart below. KODAK Liquid X-ray Developer and Replenisher or KODAK Rapid X-ray Developer can also be used, but under controlled processing conditions there may be some differences in speed, contrast, and gross fog.

Film Handling. Handle film carefully when attaching it to a hanger to avoid finger marks or abrasions. Be sure films do not touch tank walls, films, or another hanger.

1 STIR SOLUTIONS
Dilute developer and fixer solutions as directed on the container. Stir to equalize both the temperature and the distribution of the chemicals in the solution. Use a separate paddle for each solution. Note: Stir gently. Do not whip.

2 CHECK TEMPERATURE
Check temperature of developer with an accurate thermometer.

3 SET TIMER
Set the timer for recommended development time based on temperature of the developer. Do not start the timer until after Step 5.

DEVELOPMENT TIMES	
65°F (18.5°C)	6
68°F (20.0°C)	5
70°F (21.0°C)	4½
72°F (22.0°C)	4
75°F (24.0°C)	3
80°F (26.5°C)	2½

4 LOAD FILM HANGER
Remove films from packets and attach carefully to a multiple-clip hanger, such as the KODAK Dental Processing Hanger, No. 4S. Avoid finger marks, scratching, or bending.

5 IMMERSE FILM IN DEVELOPER
Completely immerse the film in the developer. Do it smoothly and without pause to prevent streaking. Start timer.

6 AGITATE FILM
Immediately raise and lower hanger (agitate it) several times so that the film surfaces are thoroughly bathed to remove air bubbles.

7 RINSE THOROUGHLY
When the timer bell rings, remove hanger from the developer. Place film in rinsing section for 30 seconds with clean running 60°–80°F water. Lift from rinse and drain into wash tank. Do not drain back into developer tank.

8 FIX ADEQUATELY
Place film in the fixer solution. Agitate the hanger vigorously. Generally, film should remain in fixer for twice the time required to "clear" it. See specific instructions for fixing times. Do not view film before it is cleared.

9 WASH COMPLETELY
Place film in the washing compartment. Wash for at least 20 minutes in running water. Eight volume changes per hour are recommended.

10 DRY
Suspend hanger from drying rack in dust-free area. Use fan to accelerate drying. When dry, remove films from hanger and mount.

EASTMAN KODAK COMPANY • RADIOGRAPHY MARKETS DIVISION • ROCHESTER, NEW YORK 14650

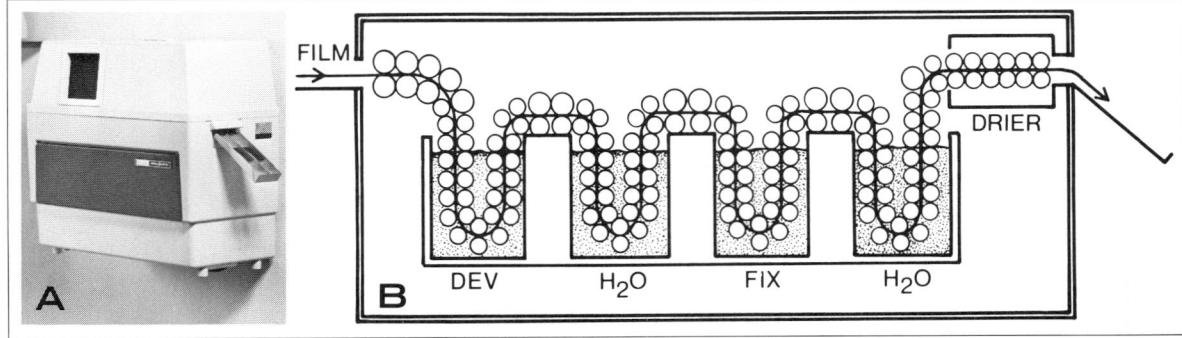

Figure 18-9 | A. Automatic processor. This processor is equipped with a light-tight hood which permits the processing of films in lighted areas. (*Courtesy of General Electric Company.*) B. Diagram of functional components of automatic processor. The film passes through the developer, fixer, water wash, and drier and is processed in 4 to 5 minutes.

film-viewing mounts. Each dental office will stock mounts with the proper number and size openings for the selection of radiographs that the dentist prefers. A variety of styles are available from several manufacturers. One standard adult mount accommodates 4 bitewing films and 14 periapical films (Fig. 18-10).

Films can be mounted in two ways, and the dental assistant will be instructed by the individual dentist which method is used in that office. Each intraoral film is stamped in the corner with an embossed dot by the manufacturer. The convex or raised side of the dot will always be located on the side of the film adjacent to the teeth, while the concave side of the dot will always be located on the side of the film toward the palate or tongue. This dot is used to correctly orient the film in the viewing mount.

The films can be placed in the mount so that it will appear to the viewer that he or she is looking at the front of the patient. This will locate the patient's right on the observer's left. With this perspective, the raised (convex) side of the dot will be toward the front of the mount (Fig. 18-10).

The films can also be placed in the mount such that the viewer will be looking at the teeth from the lingual side. This will place the patient's right on the viewer's right. With this persepective, the concave side of the dot is placed toward the front of the mount.

Film mounting is a very important procedure and must be done without error. The dentist must be able to rely on the dental assistant to place the films correctly in the mounts because decisions will be made from the radiographs regarding the location of caries and other dental disease.

INTRAORAL TECHNIQUES

Principles of Shadow Casting

Intraoral films are obtained by placing the film packet inside the mouth of the patient and directing the x-ray beam through the structures to be examined. A *shadowgram,* or composite shadow, of the teeth and supporting structures is produced on the film. The objective of the dental assistant is to provide a radiographic image of the patient which is accurate and free of distortion. To obtain this goal, procedures should be followed which will result in the radiographic

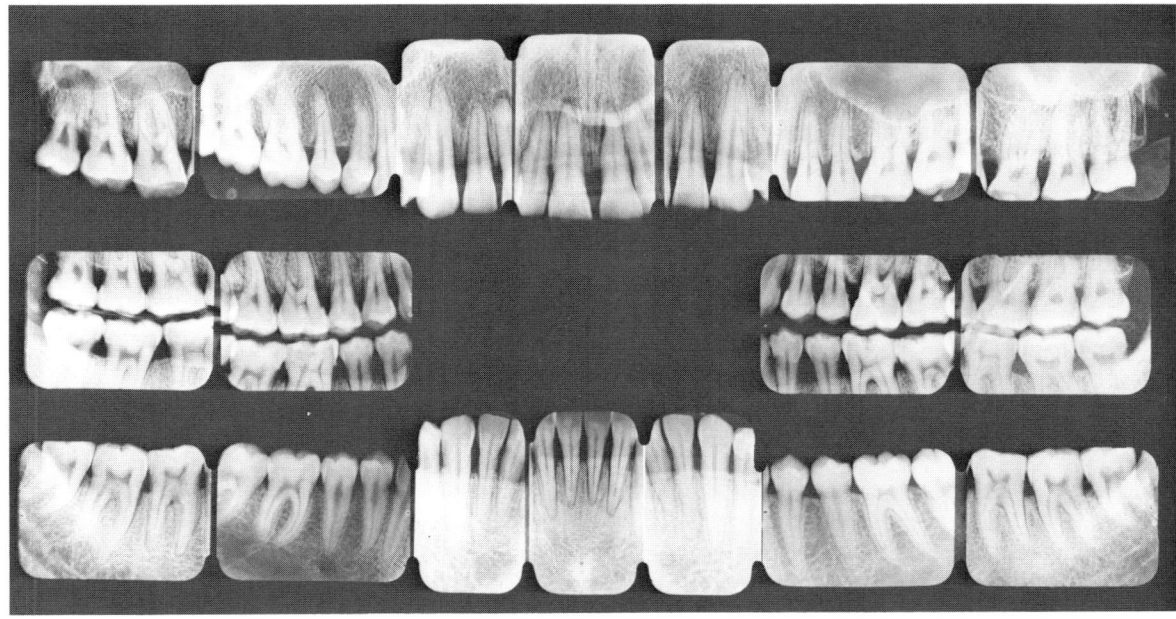

Figure 18-10 | Mounted complete full series of radiographs.

image exhibiting sharpness of detail, accurate size, and freedom of distortion.

Sharp images are seen when the edges of the teeth and bones are clearly seen on the film. The sharpness of these structures is controlled by three factors: the size of the focal spot on the target in the x-ray tube, the distance between the teeth and the film, and the distance between the x-ray source and the teeth.

A smaller focal spot results in images with improved edge sharpness. With a larger focal spot, the x-rays originate from a broader area and will be less parallel to each other. This results in a blurring of the edges of the teeth on the film. To illustrate this point, think of a flashlight beam shining past a hand and producing its shadow on a wall. The edges of the shadow will be sharp. If two flashlights are used instead of one, and both beams of light are directed past the hand onto the same spot on the wall, the edge of the shadow will not be as sharp. This is because the source of light is spread across a larger area. The same principle applies to the focal spot from which the x-rays originate, and the larger the focal spot, the more blurred the edges of the teeth will be. The size of the focal spot in dental x-ray machines is controlled by the manufacturer.

Image sharpness is also affected by the distance from the film to the teeth. As this distance increases by moving the film away from the teeth, there will be less sharpness of the image. Think of the shadow of the hand against the wall again. As the hand is moved farther from the wall, the edge sharpness is reduced, and the edges become more blurred. Therefore, there is an advantage to placing the film as close to the teeth as possible.

The third factor affecting image sharpness is the distance between the x-ray source or target and the teeth. As this increases by placing a

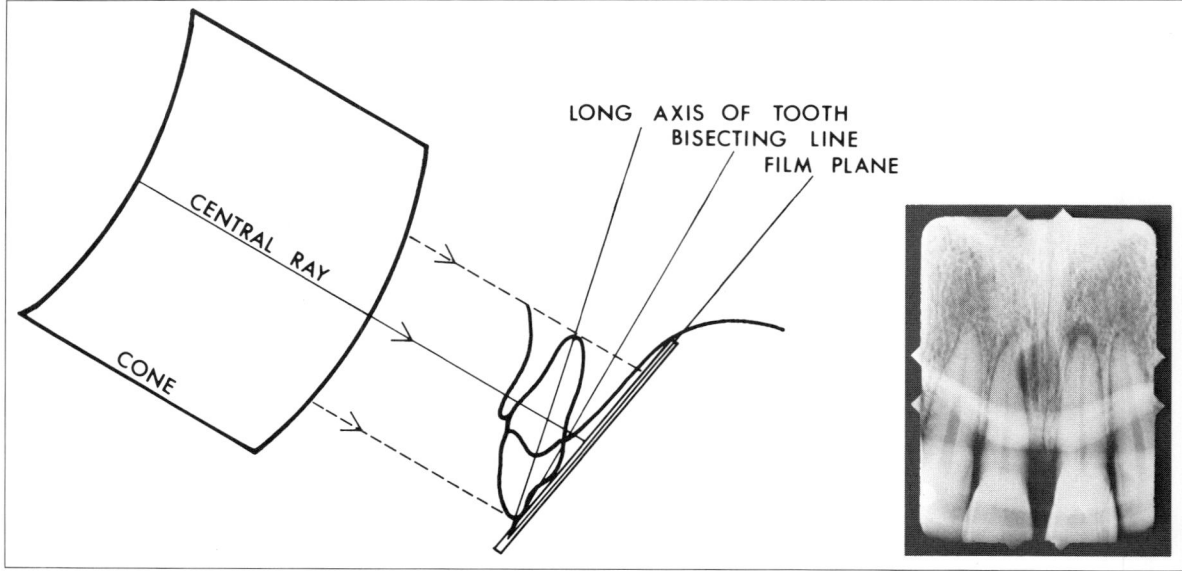

Figure 18-11 | Theory of vertical angulation in bisecting-angle technique. The central ray is directed at a right angle to the bisector of the angle formed by the film plane and the tooth plane. Radiograph on right shows teeth with normal length.

longer cone on the x-ray machine, the x-rays that reach the patient will be more parallel to each other and will result in a sharper image. For this reason, the 16-in cone is recommended for dental radiography.

The size of the teeth on the film image is important and should be as close to the true size of the teeth as possible. This is accomplished by placing the film as close to the teeth as possible. Think of the shadow of the hand on the wall again. As the hand is moved away from the wall, the shadow of the hand gets bigger. Similarly, as the film is moved away from the teeth, the size of the teeth will increase. This is another advantage of placing the film as close to the teeth as possible.

Image distortion occurs when the images of the teeth are not in proper proportion. If when making the hand shadow, the hand is tilted, the shadow will be distorted compared to the flat-plane profile of the hand. Tooth images in proper proportion will be obtained by placing the film parallel to the teeth being studied and directing the x-ray beam at right angles to both the long axis of the teeth and the film. This principle is applied in the paralleling periapical technique.

Intraoral Techniques

The three most commonly used introral films are the periapical, the bitewing, and the occlusal. The periapical film demonstrates all of the crowns and roots of the teeth with the structures surrounding the root apex (periapical). The bitewing film shows the crowns of the maxillary and mandibular teeth. The occlusal film shows a larger area of the maxilla or mandible for special examinations. Two intraoral radiographic techniques are available to obtain the periapical films,

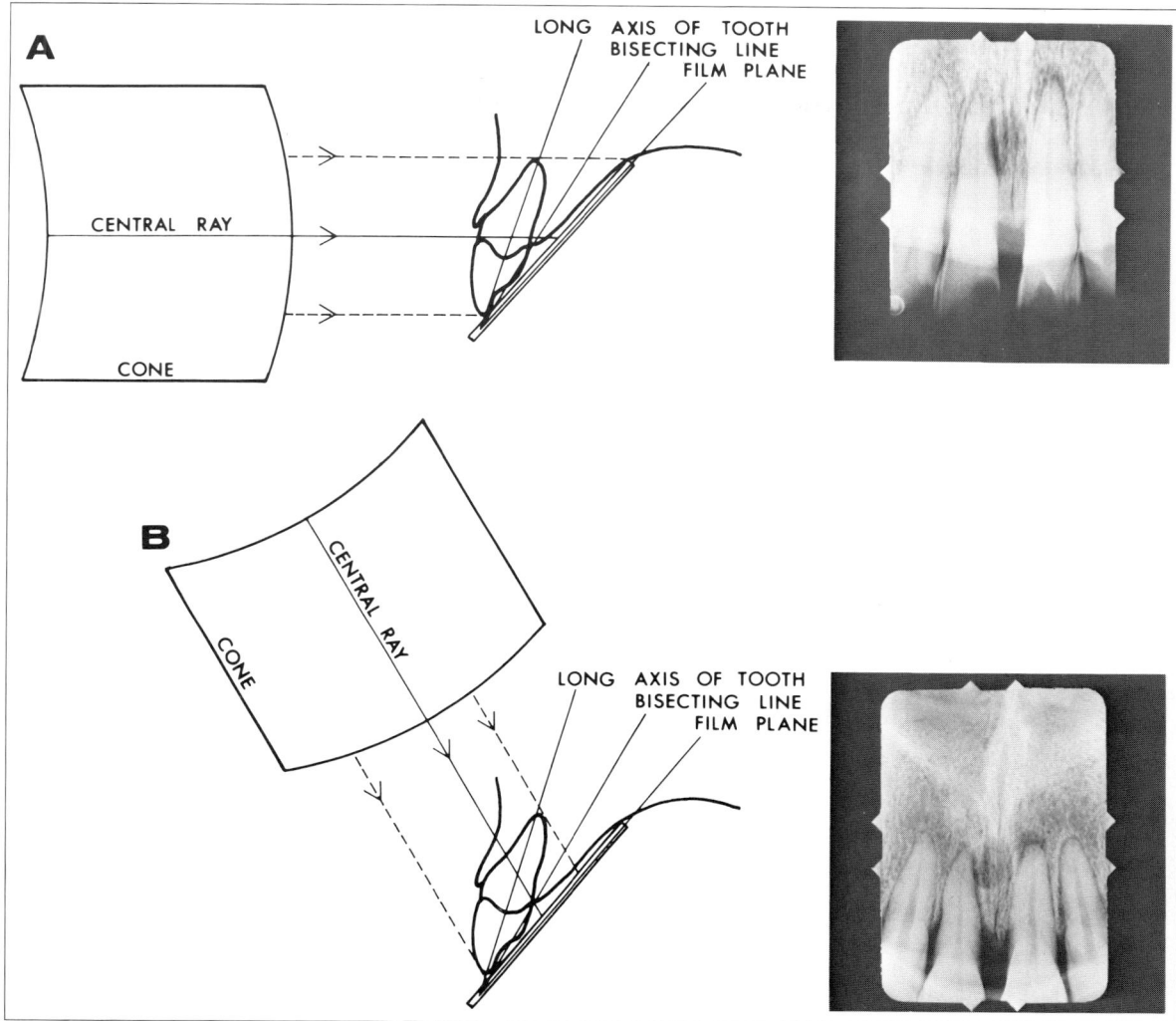

Figure 18-12 | Results of errors in vertical angulation. A. Vertical angulation is not steep enough. Radiograph on right shows elongated teeth. B. Vertical angulation is too steep. Radiograph on right shows foreshortened teeth.

the bisecting-angle and the paralleling techniques.

Bisecting-Angle Technique

The bisecting-angle technique was introduced by Cieszynski in 1907 when he applied the "rule of isometry" to the vertical angulation used in dental radiography. An angle is formed at the intersection of the tooth plane and the film plane. This rule states that the central ray should be projected at a right angle to the bisector of that angle (Fig. 18-11). The resulting images are accurate in size but are distorted. If too steep a vertical angle is used, the resulting tooth images will be foreshortened. If the vertical angle is not steep enough, the resulting tooth images will be elongated (Fig. 18-12).

The patient's head must be positioned carefully when using the bisecting-angle technique. When taking radiographs of the maxillary arch, the head should be positioned with the sagittal plane perpendicular to the floor and the occlusal plane of the maxilla parallel to the floor. When obtaining radiographs of the mandibular teeth, the occlusal plane of that arch should be parallel to the floor. The film packets should be located in the mouth of the patient for each projection to obtain a good representation of the areas being examined.

The usual full series of intraoral radiographs consists of 14 periapical and 2 or 4 bitewing radiographs. The following general principles apply to the structures which must be seen in the complete series. Each tooth apex must be seen at least once with ¼ in of bone beyond the root apex. Each interproximal surface must be seen clearly at least once. The density of the films should be correct and not be too light or too dark. The teeth should not be foreshortened or elongated.

Size 1.2 films are used for all periapical projection with the bisecting-angle technique. There are various methods for holding the films in the patient's mouth. The previously used technique of having the patient hold the film with a finger or thumb has been discarded due to the unnecessary radiation exposure of the fingers. The Snap-A-Ray (Rinn Corporation, Elgin, Ill.) is a convenient method for film holding for the bisecting-angle technique (Fig. 18-13). The film is placed lengthwise at the anterior projection end of the holder for all of the central incisor and canine lateral projections. The film is grasped sidewise by the movable sections of the holder so that when the patient closes on the bite plane, the film will be properly positioned for the posterior film.

The task of completing each radiographic projection can be divided into two basic steps—packet placement and cone alignment. See Figs. 18-14 and 18-18 for the maxillary and mandibular central incisor radiographs. The film packet is placed directly against the lingual side of those teeth with the midline of the film adjacent to the interproximal space between the central incisors. The vertical angulation is established by directing the central ray at a right angle to the line bisecting the angle formed by the tooth plane and film plane. The horizontal angu-

Figure 18-13 | Snap-A-Ray film holder. A. Anterior projections. B. Posterior projections.

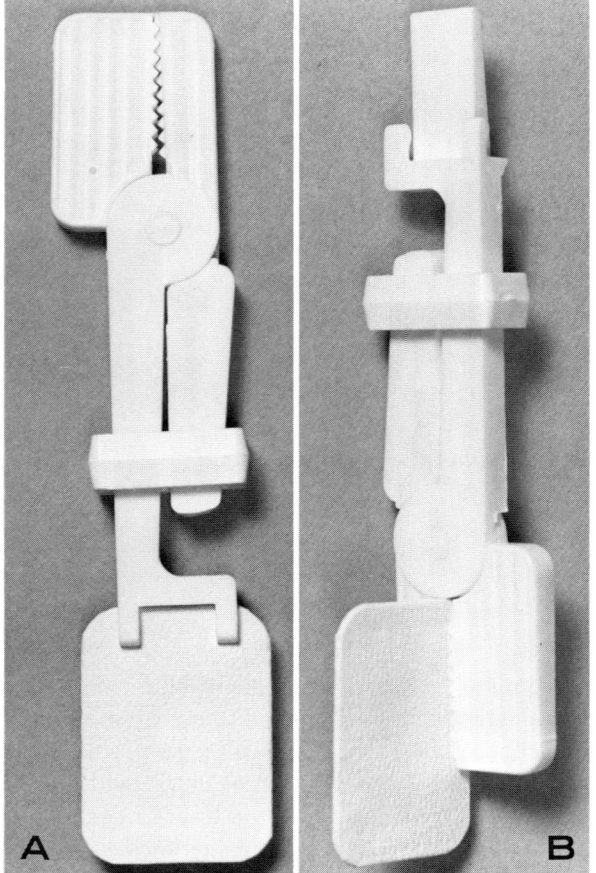

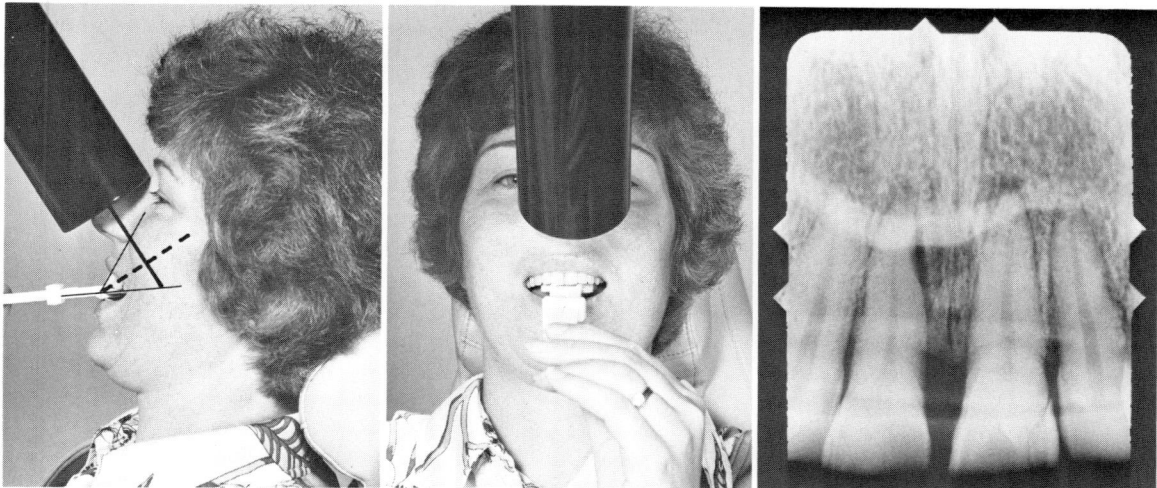

Figure 18-14 | Bisecting-angle technique—maxillary central incisor.

lation is established by directing the central ray through the interproximal space between the central incisors. Finally, the cone should be adjusted to be sure that all the film packet will be covered with radiation in order to prevent cone cutting.

See Figs. 18-15 and 18-19 for the lateral incisor-canine radiographs. The film packet is placed directly against the lingual side of those teeth so that the interproximal space will be projected along the vertical midline of the film. The vertical angulation is established by directing the

Figure 18-15 | Bisecting-angle technique—maxillary lateral incisor and canine.

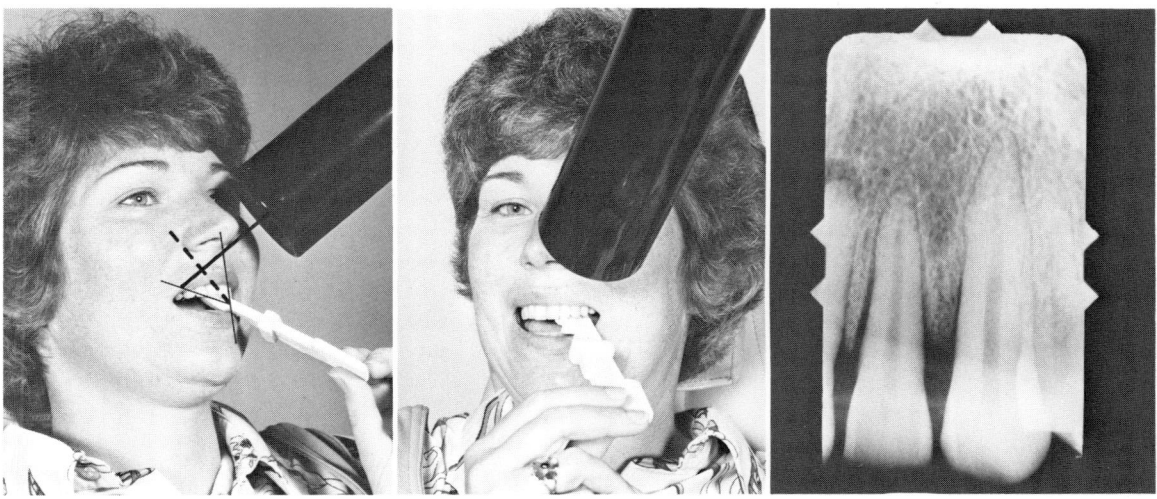

Chapter Eighteen | Dental Radiology | 359

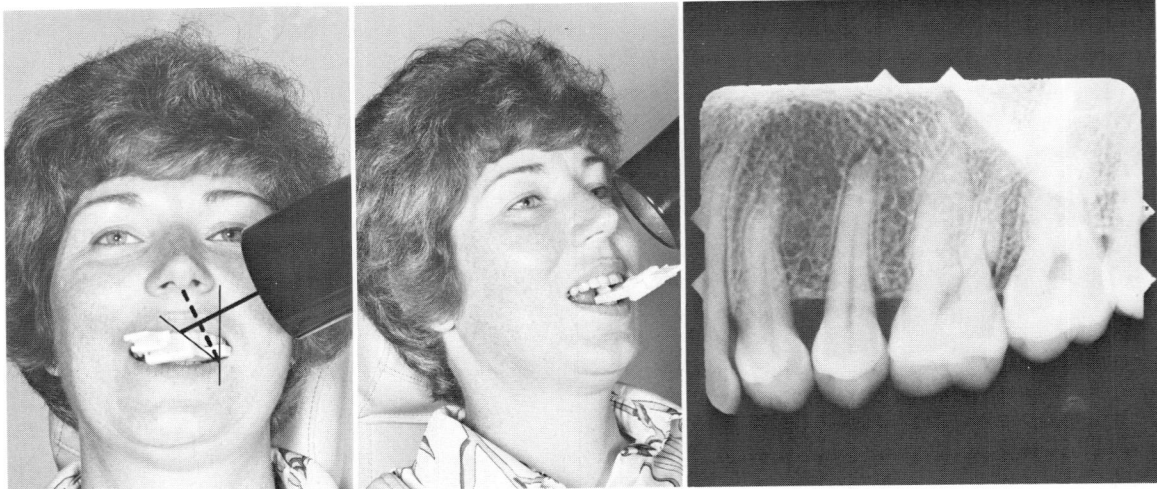

Figure 18-16 | Bisecting-angle technique—maxillary premolar.

central ray at a right angle to the line bisecting the angle formed by the tooth plane and film plane. The horizontal angulation is established by directing the central ray through the interproximal space between the lateral incisor and canine. The cone is adjusted to cover the entire film with the beam of radiation.

See Figs. 18-16 and 18-20 for the premolar projections. The film packet is placed directly against the premolar and molar teeth with the

Figure 18-17 | Bisecting-angle technique—maxillary molar.

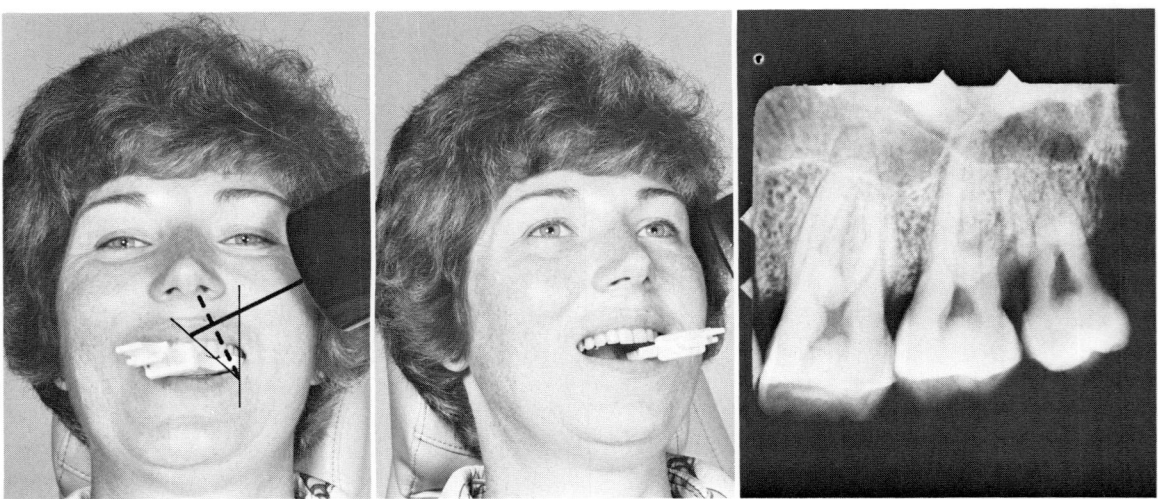

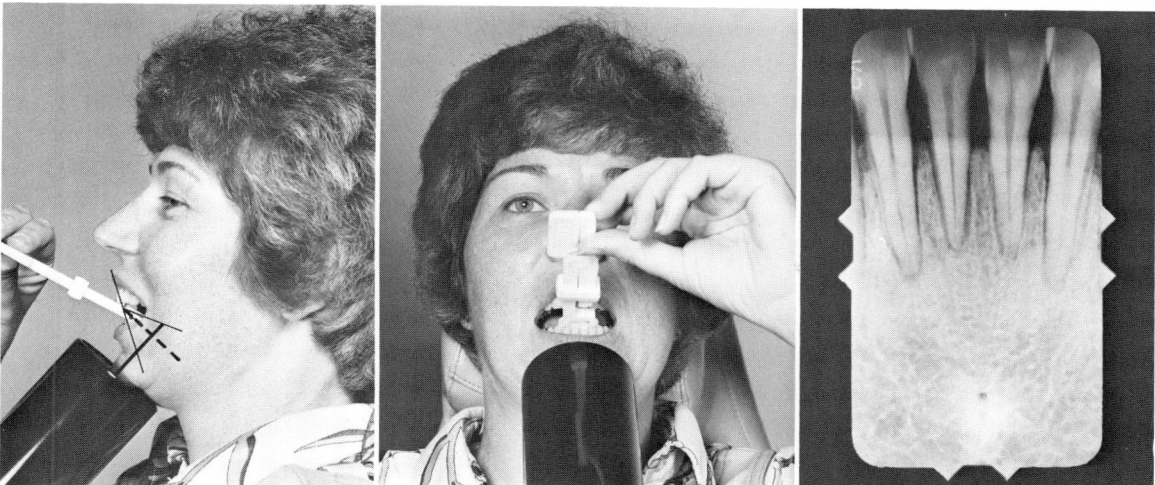

Figure 18-18 | Bisecting-angle technique—mandibular incisor.

mesial edge of the film adjacent to the center of the canine. The vertical angulation is established by directing the central ray at a right angle to the line bisecting the angle formed by the tooth plane and film plane. The horizontal angulation is established by directing the central ray through the interproximal space between the second premolar and the first molar. The cone is adjusted to cover the entire film with the beam of radiation.

See Figs. 18-17 and 18-21 for the molar pro-

Figure 18-19 | Bisecting-angle technique—mandibular lateral incisor and canine.

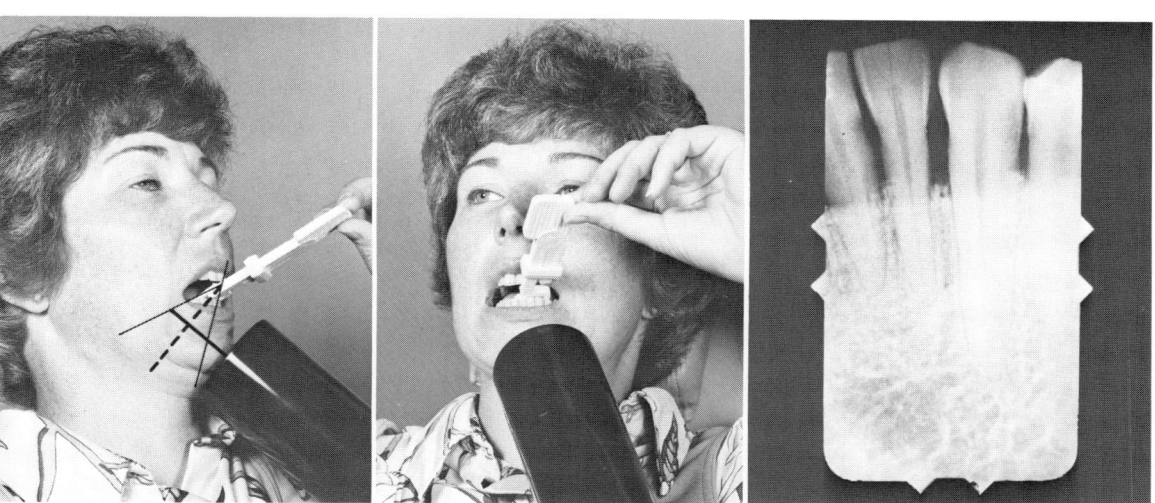

Chapter Eighteen | Dental Radiology | 361

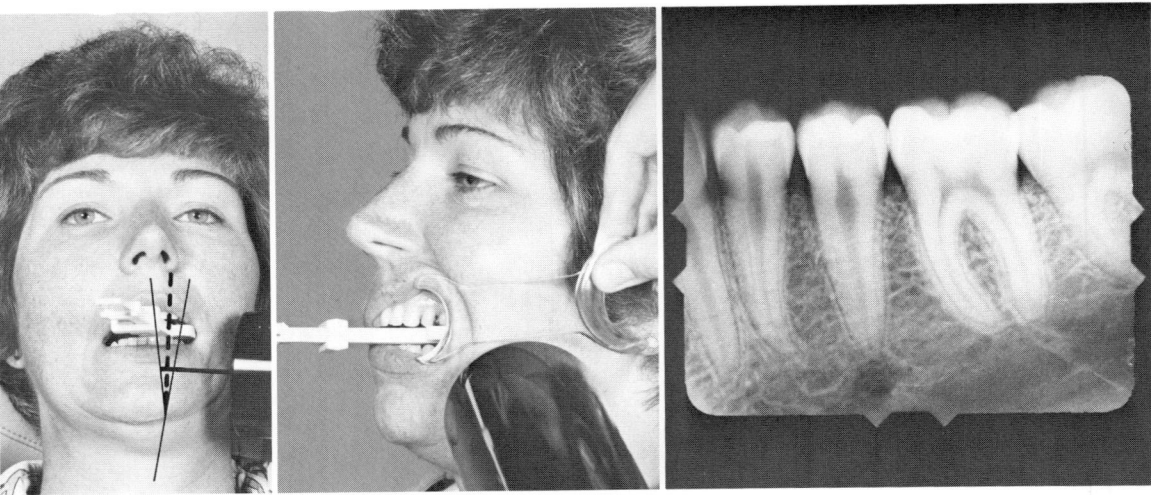

Figure 18-20 | Bisecting-angle technique—mandibular premolar.

jections. The film packet is placed against the molar teeth with the mesial edge of the film no farther forward than the middle of the second premolar. The vertical angulation is established by directing the central ray at a right angle to the line bisecting the angle formed by the tooth plane and film plane. The horizontal angulation is established by directing the central ray through the interproximal space between the first and second molars. Finally, the cone is ad-

Figure 18-21 | Bisecting-angle technique—mandibular molar.

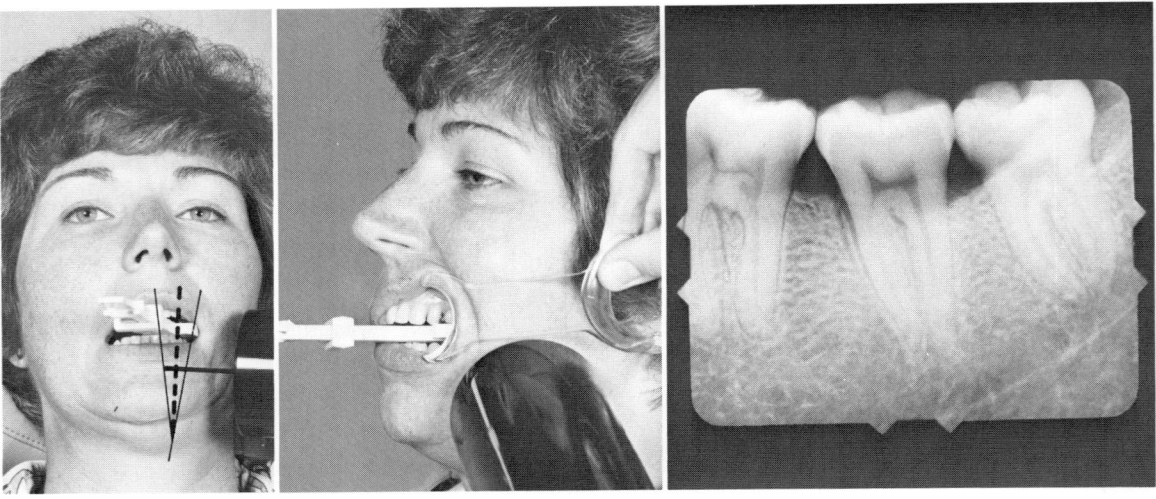

justed to cover the entire film with the beam of radiation.

The bisecting-angle technique satisfies the shadow-casting principle of image sharpness by placing the film directly against the teeth. Image distortion does occur but can be minimized by using a 16-in cone. A major disadvantage of the bisecting-angle technique occurs in the maxillary molar radiograph. Because of the steep vertical angle required, the shadow of the zygomatic arch is projected downward and is superimposed over the roots of the molar teeth. This significantly reduces the diagnostic use of this film. Also, image distortion occurs frequently in the maxillary lateral incisor-canine radiograph due to bending of the film because of the shape of the palate.

Paralleling Technique

The paralleling technique was introduced by Fitzgerald in 1947. This method was developed to improve the distorted images and superimposition of the zygomatic arch over the maxillary molar roots which are inherent with the bisecting-angle technique.

Both packet placement and cone alignment are different than those used in the bisecting-angle technique. The long axis of the film packet is placed parallel to the long axis of the teeth. This provides the name of the paralleling technique. The vertical angulation is established by aligning the central ray at a right angle to the film plane (Fig. 18-22). A 16-in-long cone must be used with this procedure.

Several types of film holding devices are available for correctly holding the film packet. The styrofoam Stabe holder (Greene Dental Products, Inc., San Fernando, Calif.) is a convenient disposable film holder which is simple to use and avoids the necessity of sterilizing the holding instruments. Other devices available are the Rinn instruments (Rinn Corporation, Elgin, Ill.) and the Precision instruments (Isaac Masel Co., Philadelphia, Pa.). These two devices include an indicator for the positioning of the x-ray cone. The paralleling technique will be described and illustrated using the Stabe holder, but the same basic

Figure 18-22 | Theory of vertical angulation in paralleling technique. The central ray is aligned at a right angle to the film plane.

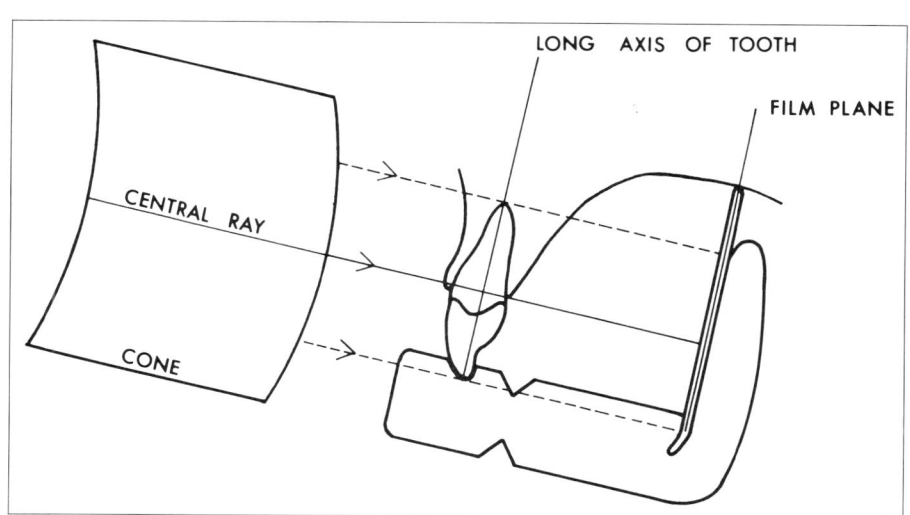

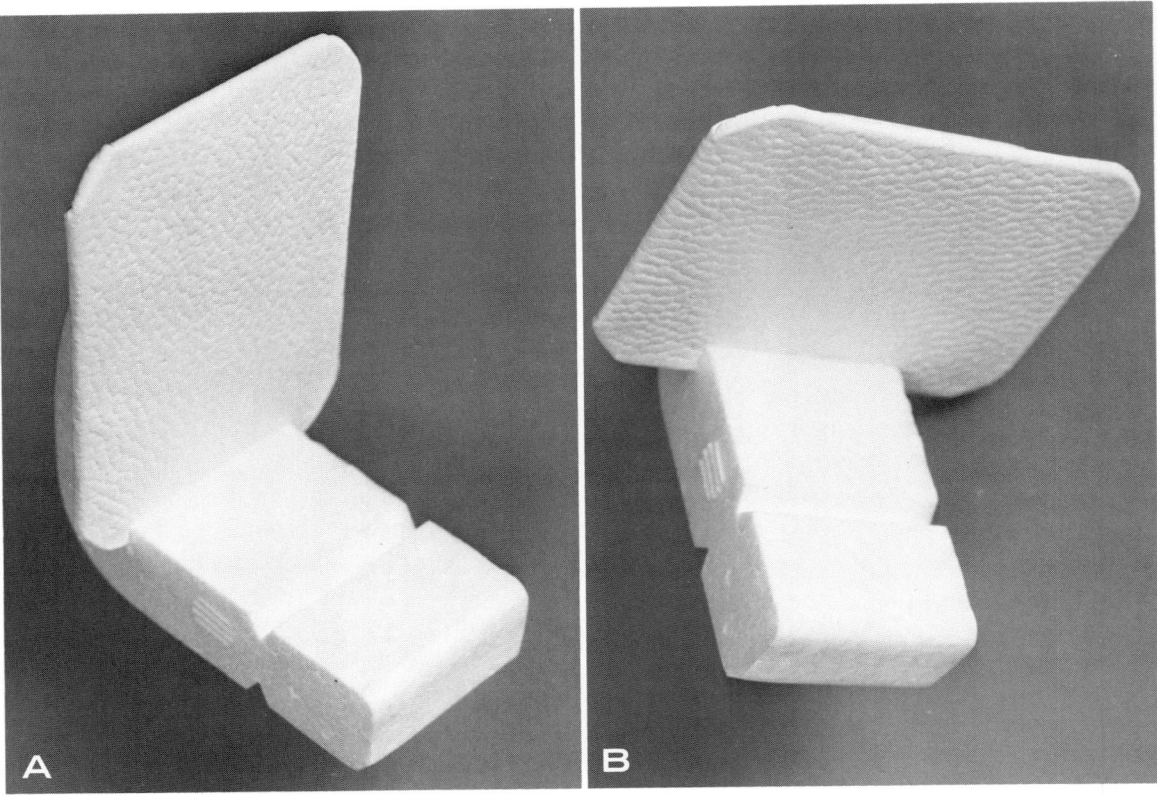

Figure 18-23 | Stabe film holder. A. Anterior projection. B. Posterior projections.

principles apply to the other types of film holders.

The usual full series of radiographs consist of 14 periapical films and 2 or 4 bitewing films. For the central incisor and all premolar and molar projections 1.2-size film is used. For the mandibular central incisor and the four lateral incisor–canine radiographs 1.1-size film is used. The narrower film is used for these five projections because it can be positioned parallel to the teeth more easily than the 1.2 film. For the anterior radiographs, the film is firmly positioned in the slot of the Stabe with the short dimension of the film in the slot. For posterior radiographs, the long dimension of the film is placed into the slot of the Stabe (Fig. 18-23).

See Figs. 18-24 and 18-28 for the maxillary and mandibular central incisor projections. The film packet is positioned away from the teeth with the patient closing on the outer end of the Stabe. The packet is aligned so that the interproximal space between the central incisors will be projected onto the vertical midline of the film. To align the cone, the vertical angulation is established with the central ray perpendicular to the film plane. An imaginary T is formed between the film packet and cone. The horizon-

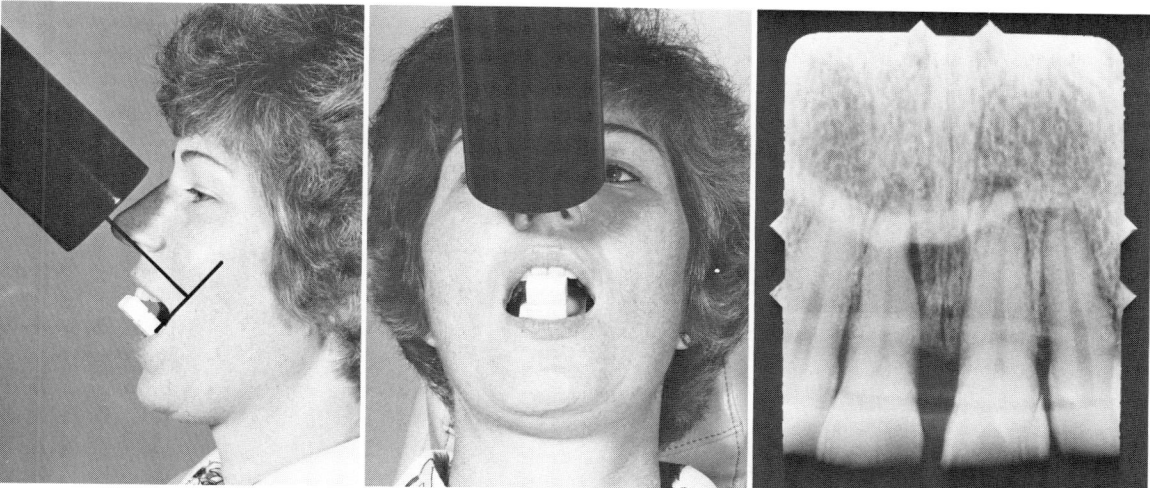

Figure 18-24 | Paralleling technique—maxillary central incisor.

tal angulation is established by directing the central ray through the interproximal space between the central incisors. To prevent cone cutting, the cone is adjusted to be sure that the entire film packet will be covered with the x-ray beam. For maxillary radiographs, the bottom edge of the cone is positioned evenly with the lower edge of the Stabe. For mandibular radiographs, the top edge of the cone is aligned with the top edge of the Stabe.

Figure 18-25 | Paralleling technique—maxillary lateral incisor and canine.

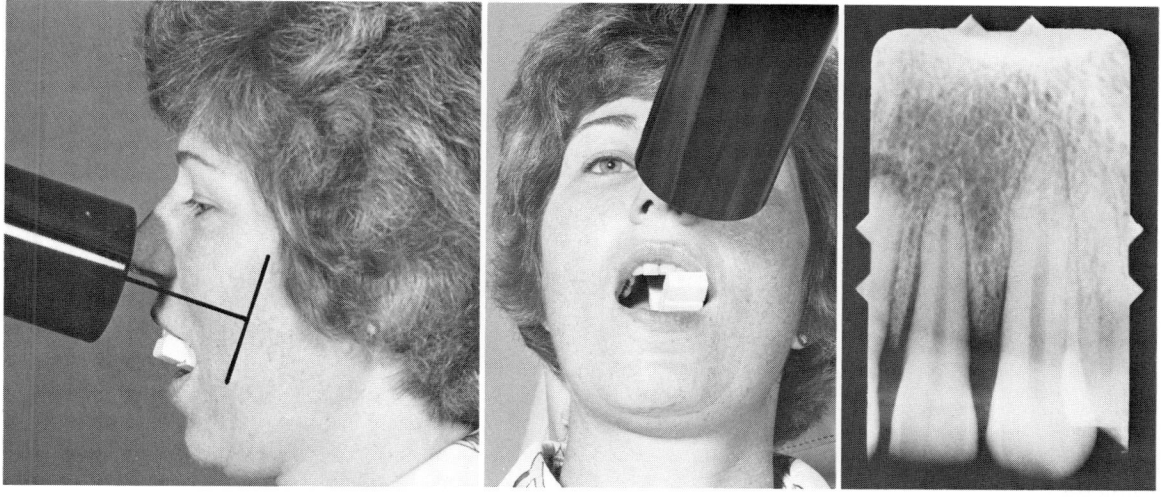

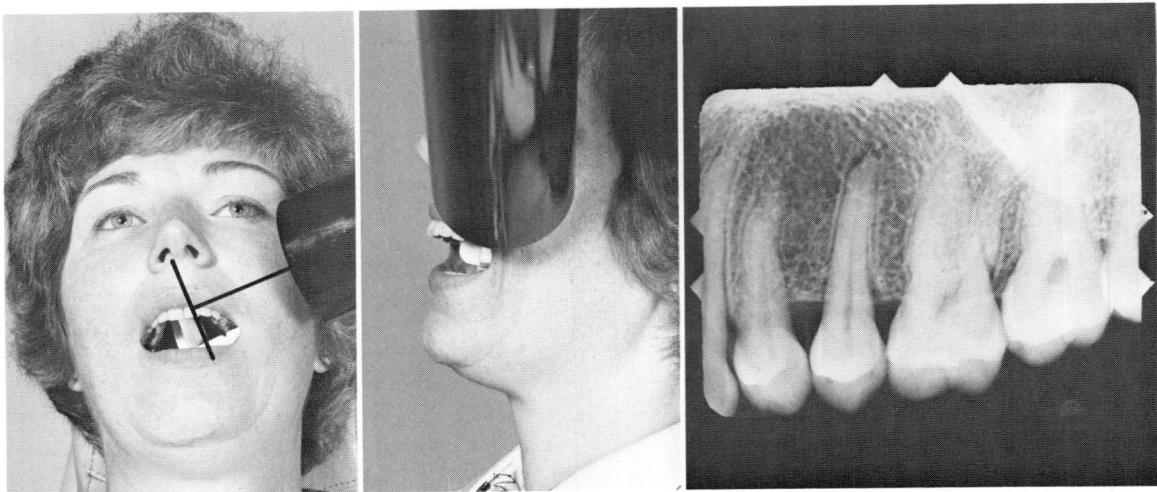

Figure 18-26 | Paralleling technique—maxillary premolar.

See Figs. 18-25 and 18-29 for the lateral incisor and canine projections. The 1.1 film is used. The film packet is positioned away from the teeth with the patient closing on the outer end of the Stabe. The packet is aligned so that the interproximal space between the lateral incisor and canine will be projected onto the vertical midline of the film. To align the cone, the vertical angulation is established with the central ray at a right angle to the film plane. The hori-

Figure 18-27 | Paralleling technique—maxillary molar.

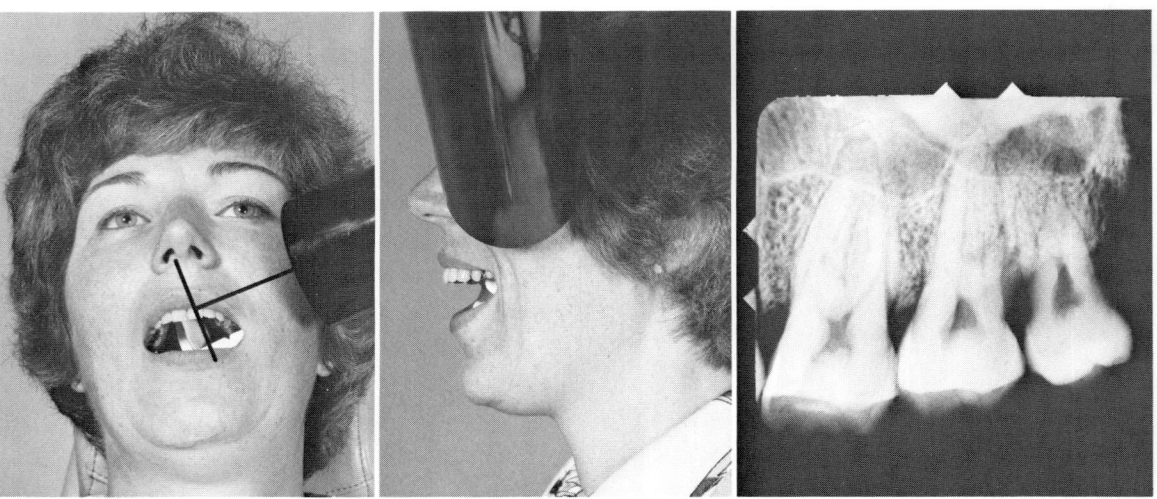

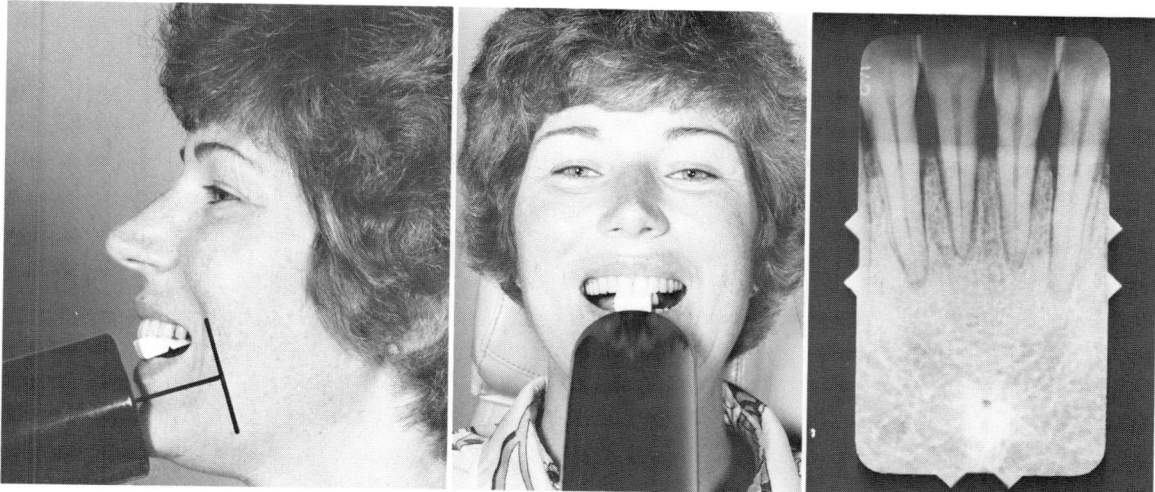

Figure 18-28 | Paralleling technique—mandibular central incisor.

zontal angle is established by directing the central ray through the interproximal space between the lateral and canine. Finally, the cone is adjusted to cover the entire film with the beam of radiation.

See Fig. 18-26 for the maxillary premolar projection. The film packet is positioned away from the premolar and molar teeth with the top edge of the film in the center of the palate, and the mesiodistal axis of the film parallel to the arch

Figure 18-29 | Paralleling technique—mandibular lateral incisor and canine.

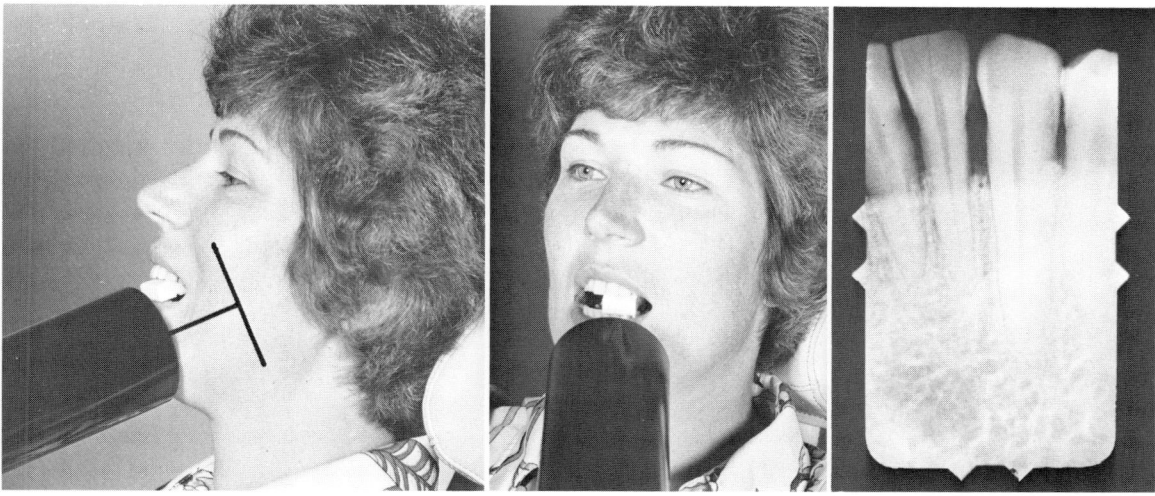

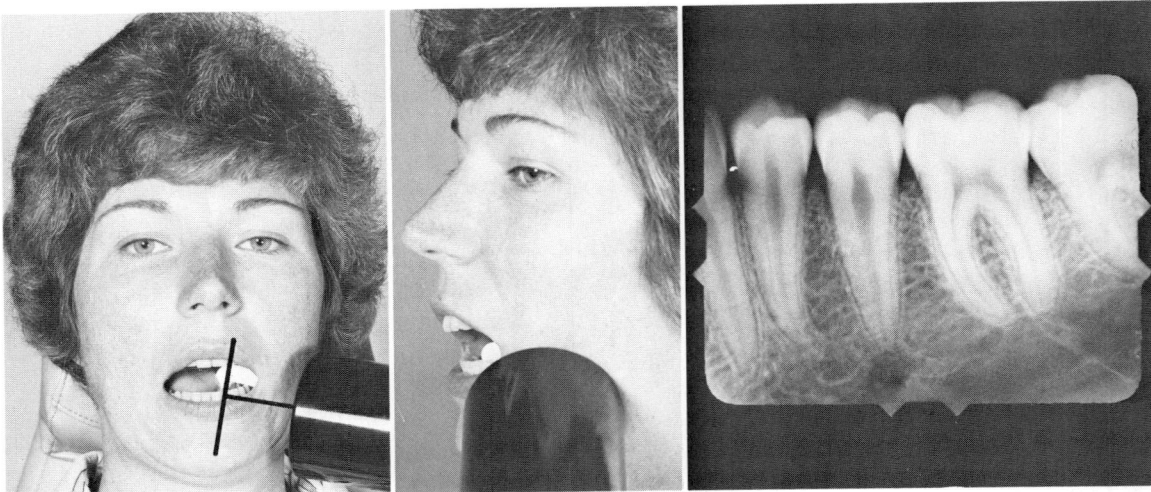

Figure 18-30 | Paralleling technique—mandibular premolar.

being studied. The mesial edge of the film is even with the middle of the canine. To align the cone, the vertical angulation is established with the central ray perpendicular to the film plane. The horizontal angulation is established by directing the central ray through the interproximal space between the second premolar and first molar. The cone is adjusted to cover the entire film with the beam of radiation.

See Fig. 18-27 for the maxillary molar projec-

Figure 18-31 | Paralleling technique—mandibular molar.

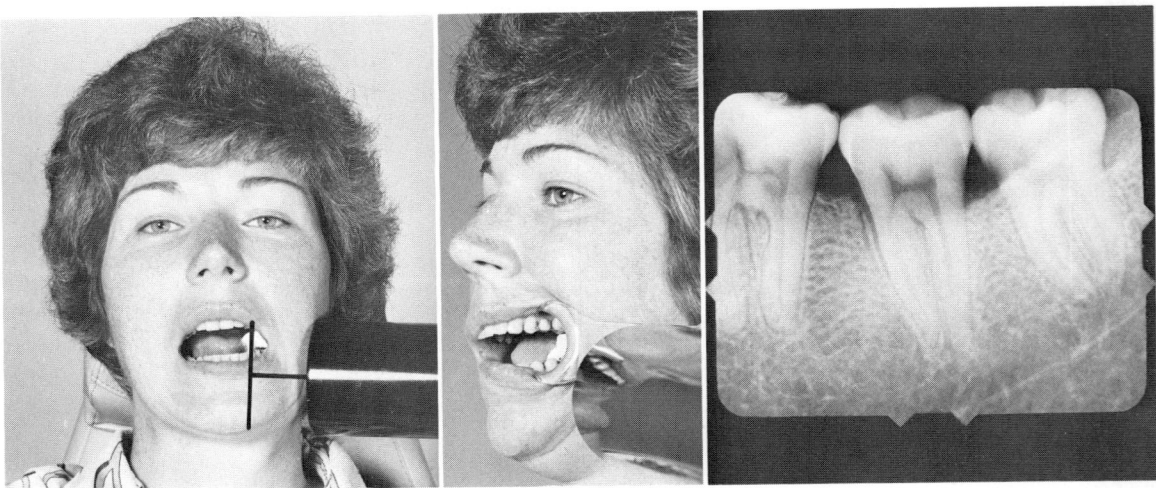

tion. The film packet is positioned away from the teeth with the top edge of the film in the center of the palate and the mesiodistal axis of the film parallel to the arch being studied. The mesial edge of the film is even with the center of the second premolar. To align the cone, the vertical angulation is established at a right angle to the film plane. The horizontal angulation is established by directing the central ray through the interproximal space between the first and second molar.

See Fig. 18-30 for the mandibular premolar projection. The end section of the Stabe is removed at the slot to permit the film to be positioned adjacent to the premolar and molar teeth. The mesial edge of the film is even with the middle of the canine. To align the cone the vertical angulation is established at a right angle to the film plane. The horizontal angulation is established by directing the central ray through the interproximal space between the second premolar and first molar. The cone is adjusted to cover the entire film with the x-ray beam.

See Fig. 18-31 for the mandibular molar projection. The end section of the Stabe is removed at the slot to permit the film to be placed directly against the molar teeth. The mesial edge of the film should be located no farther forward then the middle of the second premolar. To align the cone the vertical angulation is established at a right angle to the film plane. The horizontal angulation is established by directing the central ray through the interproximal space between the first and second molars. The cone is adjusted to cover the entire film with the beam of radiation.

The paralleling technique satisfies the shadow-casting requirement of obtaining distortion-free radiographic images because the film plane is parallel to the long axis of the teeth. Also, the central ray is parallel to both the teeth and film. However, this technique does not completely satisfy the shadow-casting requirement of image sharpness because the film is not immediately adjacent to the teeth in some projections. This deficiency is corrected by increasing the x-ray

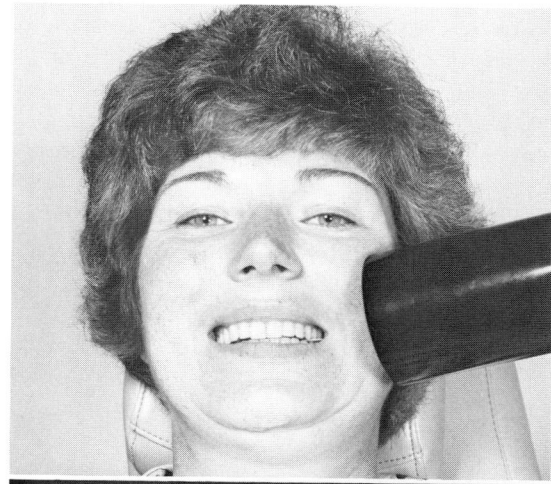
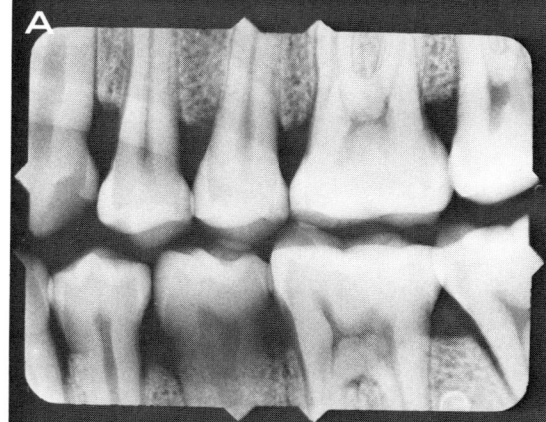
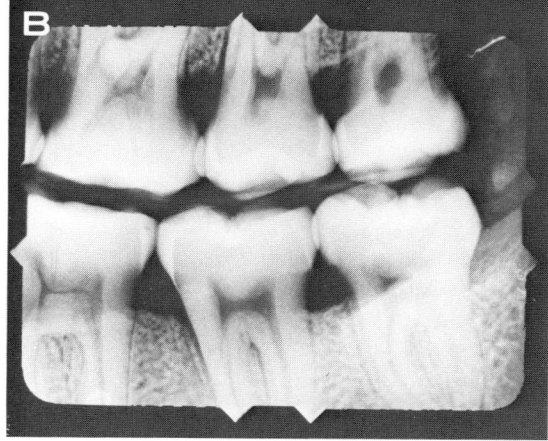

Figure 18-32 | Bitewing technique. A. Premolar bitewing. B. Molar bitewing.

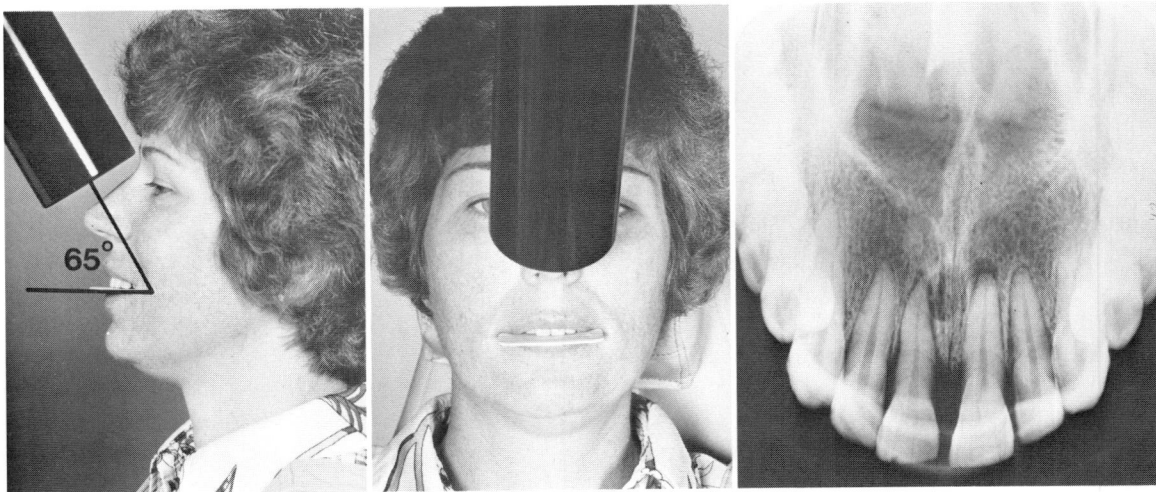

Figure 18-33 | Maxillary topographic occlusal technique and film.

source to tooth distance, and for this reason the 16-in long cone is required.

The maxillary lateral incisor-canine and molar radiographs obtained using the paralleling technique are superior to those obtained using the bisecting-angle technique. The lateral incisor-canine film can be obtained without bending of the film corners which is commonly done with the bisecting-angle technique. In the maxillary molar radiograph, the vertical angle used in the

Figure 18-34 | Mandibular topographic occlusal technique and film.

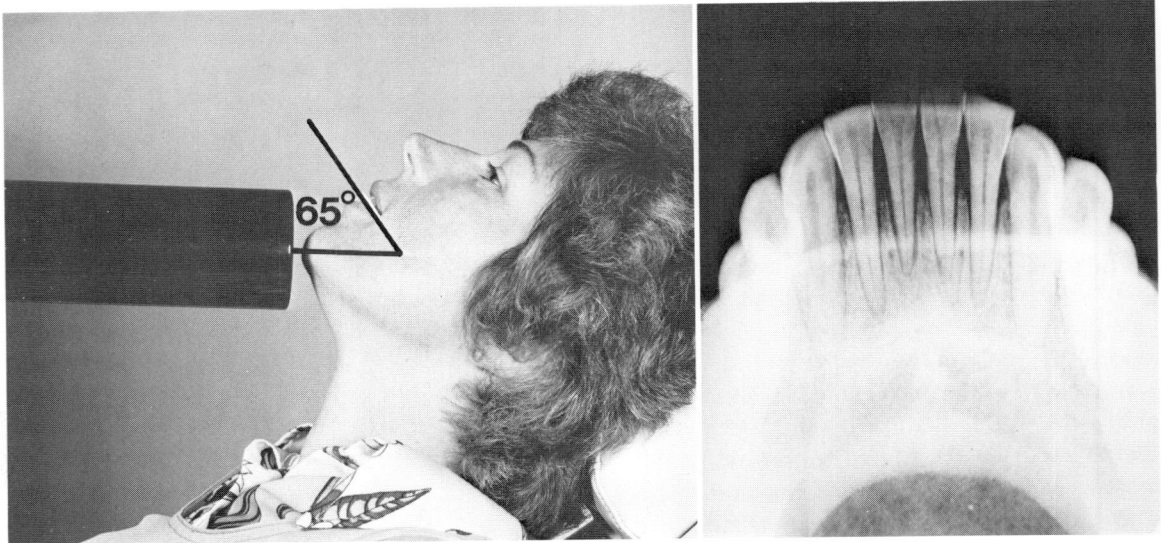

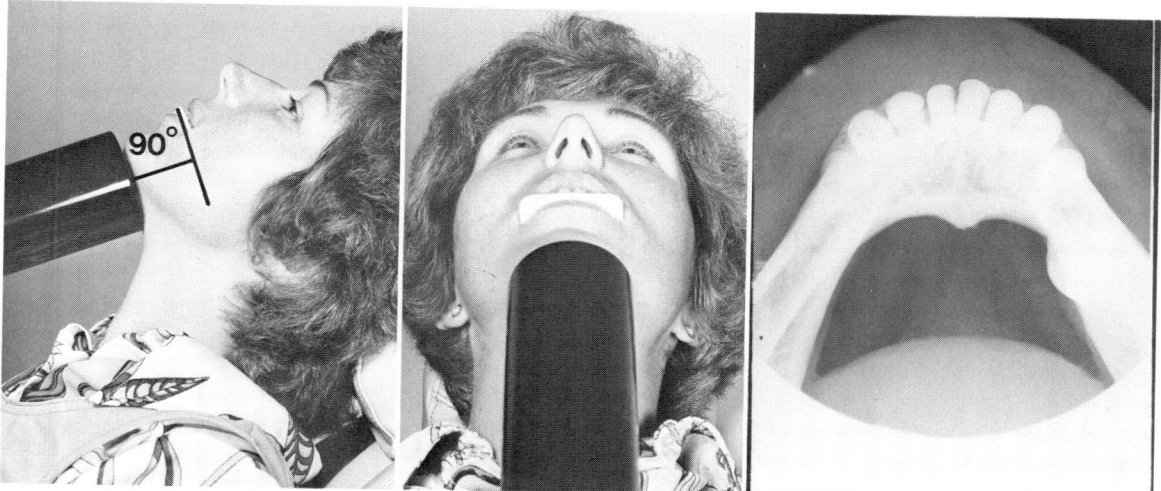

Figure 18-35 | Mandibular cross-sectional technique and film.

paralleling method projects the image of the zygomatic arch upward and provides a better view of the maxillary molar roots.

Bitewing Technique

The bitewing radiograph shows the crowns of both maxillary and mandibular teeth from the distal half of the canines to the distal surface of the third molars. Interproximal caries can be discovered using this radiograph and the status of the alveolar crest of the bone between the teeth can also be evaluated.

For the bitewing examination, 2.0, 2.1, 2.2, or 2.3 films can be used, and the film size will be determined by the age and size of the patient.

A bitewing tab is attached to the film to provide the means for the patient to hold the film in place. A smaller film is selected for the child patient, and one bitewing film is taken on each side of the mouth. For the adult patient, at least one premolar bitewing is obtained on each side. If all the molar interproximal spaces are not shown adequately, molar bitewings are also taken.

The patient's head is positioned with the occlusal plane parallel with the floor for all bitewing films. The premolar bitewing film packet is placed with one-half of the film adjacent to the mandibular crowns. Care must be exercised to be sure that the occlusal plane will be symmetrically located along the longitudinal midline of the film. The mesial edge of the film is placed in the center of the mandibular canine. The patient is instructed to close firmly in his or her natural occlusion on the bite tab. The cone is aligned with a vertical angulation of +10 degrees (aiming downward). The horizontal angulation is established to pass directly through the interproximal space between the second premolar and the first molar. The cone is adjusted to cover the entire film with the x-ray beam.

The molar bitewing packet is placed with the mesial edge of the film no farther forward than the middle of the second premolars. The vertical angle is +10 degrees, and the horizontal angle is directed through the interproximal space between the first and second molars. The cone is adjusted to cover the entire film with the x-ray beam.

The resulting radiograph should demonstrate

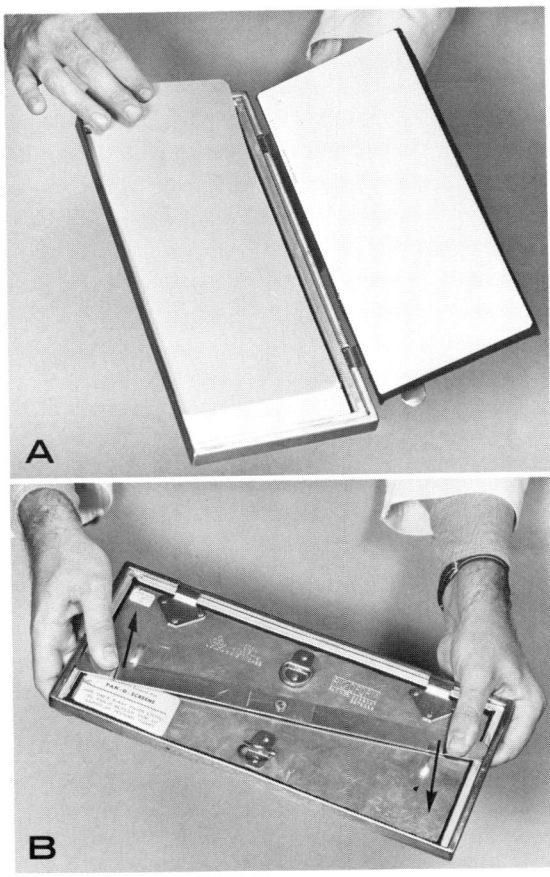

Figure 18-36 | Panoramic cassette. A. Film loading. B. Locking cassette.

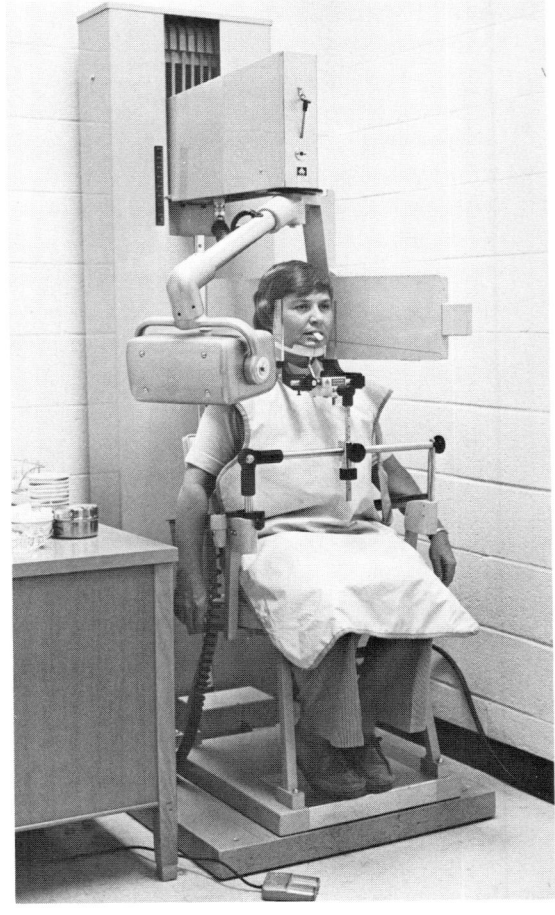

Figure 18-37 | Patient positioning for Panorex radiograph.

the interproximal surfaces of the teeth clearly with no overlapping (Fig. 18-32).

Occlusal Technique

The occlusal radiograph shows a larger area of the maxilla or mandible and is used for special patient examinations. A 3.4-size film is used. Two types of occlusal techniques are available—the topographic and cross-sectional.

The topographic occlusal technique is used in both the maxilla and mandible. See Fig. 18-33 for the maxillary topographic projection. The patient is positioned with the sagittal plane perpendicular to the floor and the occlusal plane parallel to the floor. The packet is placed in the mouth with the stippled side of the film facing upward. The distal edge of the film should be against the anterior edge of the mandibular ramus. The cone should be aligned along the sagittal plane of the head at +65 degrees (aiming downward)

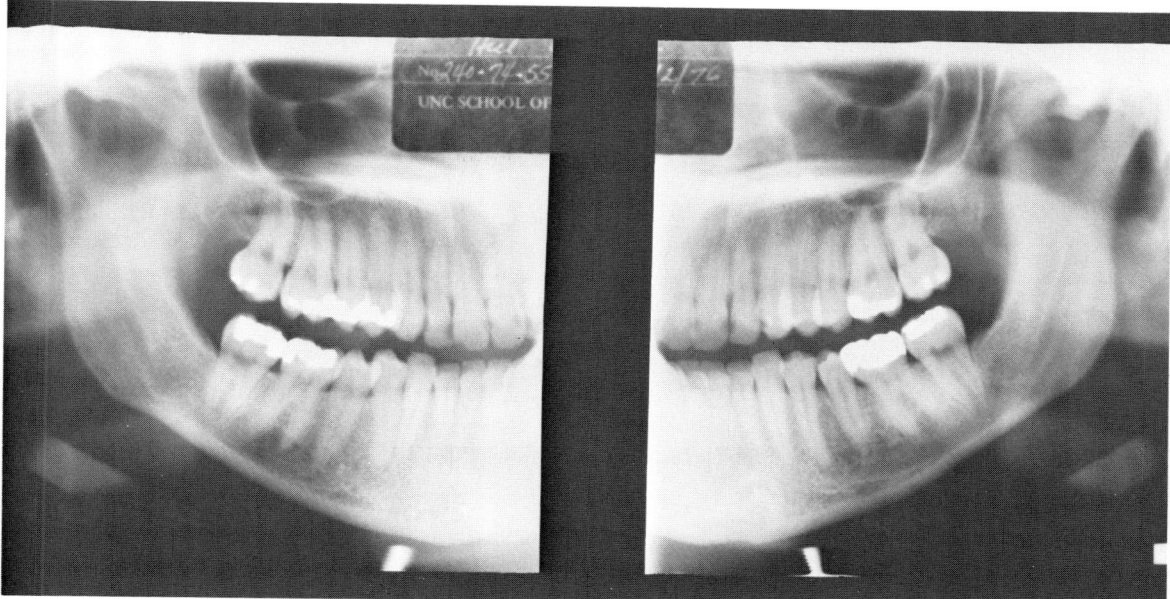

Figure 18-38 | Panorex radiograph.

and should be adjusted so that the entire film is covered by the x-ray beam.

See Fig. 18-34 for the mandibular topographic projection. The patient is positioned with the sagittal plane perpendicular to the floor. The packet is placed with the stippled side of the film downward and with the distal edge against the mandibular ramus. The cone is aligned along the sagittal plane at −65 degrees (aiming upward) to the occlusal plane and so as to cover the film with the x-ray beam.

See Fig. 18-35 for the cross-sectional occlusal projection which is normally used only for the mandible. The packet is placed with the stippled side toward the x-ray tube and with the distal side of the film against the mandibular ramus. The cone is aligned along the sagittal plane of the patient and at a right angle to the film. The cone is also adjusted so as to cover the film with the x-ray beam.

PANORAMIC RADIOGRAPHY

A panoramic radiograph is obtained by using special x-ray equipment which moves the film and x-ray tubehead around the patient. A 5 × 12 in film is used and placed into a cassette (Fig. 18-36). The cassette is a special film holder which contains intensifying screens. These screens enhance the effect of the radiation by changing the x-ray energy into light. This permits the exposure of the film with less radiation dose than would be used if no intensifying screens were employed.

See Fig. 18-37 for the patient positioning during exposure of a Panorex radiograph. The patient's head should be extended upward and the chin tipped downward. During the exposure, the x-ray tubehead passes behind the patient and the film passes in front of the head. The panoramic radiograph shows the entire facial area and is used for patient screening, evaluation of oral pathology and injuries, and the examination of children (Fig. 18-38).

BIBLIOGRAPHY

Christensen, E. E., Curry, T. S., III, and Nunnally J.: *An Introduction to the Physics of Diagnostic Radiology,* Lea & Febiger, Philadelphia, 1972.

Crandell, C. E.: *Dental Radiology for Auxiliary Personnel,* University of North Carolina Press, Chapel Hill, 1972.

Eastman Kodak Company: "X-Rays in Dentistry," Radiography Markets Division, Rochester, N.Y., 1972.

Ennis, L. M., Berry, H. M., and Philips, J. E.: *Dental Roentgenology,* 6th ed., Lea & Febiger, Philadelphia, 1967.

Frommer, H. H.: *Radiology for Dental Auxiliaries,* The C. V. Mosby Company, St. Louis, 1974.

de Lyre, W. R.: *Essentials of Dental Radiography for Dental Assistants and Hygienists,* Prentice-Hall, Inc., Englewood Cliffs, N.J., 1975.

Stafne, E. C., and Gibilisco, A.: *Oral Roentgenographic Diagnosis,* 4th ed., W. B. Saunders Company, Philadelphia, 1975.

Wuehrmann, A. H., and Manson-Hing, L. R.: *Dental Radiology,* 4th ed., The C. V. Mosby Company, St. Louis, 1977.

19

William R. Stanmeyer
Preventive Dentistry

BASIC KNOWLEDGE

Philosophy of Dental Care

The American Dental Association Board of Trustees has approved a statement of philosophy aimed at all dentists providing dental care to the American public. It states in part that "the natural dentition should last a lifetime and that the profession now has the scientific knowledge to recognize and control disease. . . ." In the past several years, most dentists have changed the character of their practices from one which was almost totally treatment-oriented to one which places prevention as the preferred solution for almost every problem of dental disease. From a purely professional standpoint, prevention or bacterial control of dental diseases should be the prime objective of therapy; these preventive procedures should not be denied to any adult or child who has normal abilities of comprehension. From the patients' standpoint, their efforts along with the dentist's and the dentist's staff will result in keeping teeth for a lifetime, minimizing the need for dental care, keeping the cost of care low, and remaining comfortable with good oral health and good general health as it is affected by dental health.

What is Preventive Dentistry?

The term preventive dentistry is a widely misused term. Almost everything dental personnel do is prevention. A good soft-tissue and hard-tissue examination is prevention; proper restoration or replacement of teeth is prevention; endodontics and orthodontics are prevention; even surgery is prevention when the spread of infection from a nonrestorable tooth is controlled. The scaling and polishing of teeth is prevention, and the protection of the patients and yourself from excessive radiation when taking x-rays is prevention. For purposes of containment, this chapter will be confined to the primary control of dental caries and periodontal disease caused by the accumulation of bacteria on the teeth and soft tissues.

Dental Disease: An Infection

Dental disease (caries and periodontal disease) is an *infection*. The cause of this infection is a bacteria capable of degrading sucrose to produce a sticky, mucilaginous, tenacious mass on areas of the teeth not usually reached by persons untrained in tooth-cleaning techniques. This mass contains millions of bacteria capable of producing acids of sufficient strength to initiate decalcification of the tooth or of producing bacterial by-products that irritate the soft tissues initiating an infection of the soft tissues. This gelatinous mass is called *plaque*.

To a large extent the *rapidity* with which plaque forms, the *frequency* with which bacteria in the plaque insult the tooth and soft tissue, and the *length of time* the insult lasts depends on the patient's eating habits. Gustafsson (1954) has shown that if the patient eats foods containing sucrose only at mealtimes, the tissue will not be insulted nearly as much as with a person who is a frequent snacker. In the same light, the individual who eats sucrose-containing foods that are sticky and adhere tenaciously to the teeth will have more disease than the person whose sucrose is in liquid form and is rapidly cleared from the mouth. Still a third factor must be taken into consideration. The fact remains that two individuals with the same amount of plaque who eat the same diet may have different degrees of the disease, whether it be caries or periodontal disease. This may be attributed to the patient's resistance to the disease.

Dental Disease: A Multifactorial Process

The cause and extent of dental disease is due to multiple factors—bacteria, diet, susceptibility. Orland's (1955) studies with germ-free animals have shown that bacteria alone will not cause dental disease. They also show that sucrose in the absence of bacteria will not cause dental disease. It takes certain bacteria plus certain foods to cause caries or periodontal disease, but even then whether the patient gets the disease, or what type of disease, or how severe the disease depends on his or her resistance or susceptibility to it. Paul Keyes (1969) has graphically shown this symbiosis, and his scheme is shown in Fig. 19-1 with some modification.

The concept that dental disease initiation is multifactorial in nature has lead to the conclusion that a successful preventive dentistry program must also be multifactorial in nature.

A Brief History of Preventive Dentistry

Prevention in dentistry is not new. Aristotle has been quoted as saying that sweet figs sticking to the teeth cause cavities. W. D. Miller (1890) was one of the first researchers to propound the

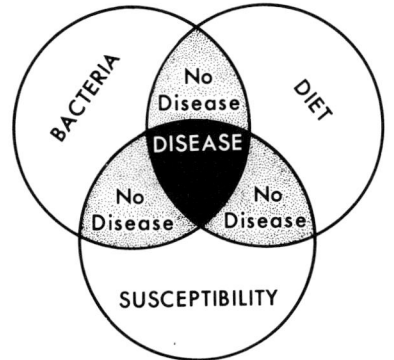

Figure 19-1 | Dental disease is multifactorial in etiology. It requires bacteria plus a diet which supports bacterial growth plus tooth or soft-tissue susceptibility to the disease.

theory that there was an interaction between carbohydrates and bacteria to form acids which decalcified enamel (bacteria + food → acids → decay). His theory was supported and enlarged upon by G. V. Black (1909), who described plaque and how this mass of bacteria sticking to the teeth around the gum line and in between the tooth caused cavities and gum disease. As more and more scientists became interested in dental research, they first attacked the problem of disease prevention from the part of Miller's formula that dealt with food.

Hanke (1933) and the Chicago Research Study Club placed a number of children on a controlled diet and showed they could get a significant drop in dental disease. Herman Becks (1950) and Philip Jay (1959) controlled carbohydrate input on selected patients with a major caries problem and were able to control the disease. This research in dietary input showed that disease control could be obtained from diet, but it was an impractical approach to dental caries control for the entire population. Research interest, however, did not lag and began to zero in on plaque itself. Stephan (1966) measured acid changes in plaque after eating and also measured the rapidity and extent of acid production when various foods were consumed.

Fluorides: Systemic

In the mid 1940s research efforts and money were attracted to the finding that the element fluoride when ingested in controlled and minute amounts could make the tooth much more resistant to the attack of plaque bacteria. Fluoride was added to communal water supplies in the amount of 0.8 to 1.2 ppm (parts per million) The amount of fluoride added to the water was based on the mean average temperature of the community and was found to reduce dental caries by about 60 percent. This material is called systemic fluoride because it is ingested and transmitted to the teeth through the body's fluid transport systems. It does its greatest good from birth to 12 years, the time interval during which the crowns of first molars start to calcify until at 12 years the crowns of the third molars are calcified. Once teeth have erupted, the effects of systemic fluoride are greatly reduced. Communal water fluoridation is relatively inexpensive, 10 to 15 cents per year per person, when compared to the needless destruction of teeth and the cost of treatment when infected. Water fluoridation is accepted worldwide and endorsed by the World Health Organization. It has been hailed as the most effective, most practical, most convenient, and most economical means for the partial reduction of dental caries. It has been so widely acclaimed that several states have passed laws making it mandatory for communities within the state to fluoridate their water supplies. Nutritional biochemists have determined that the element fluoride is necessary for the normal growth and development of all calcified tissue and that those persons who lack fluoride in their diets are malnourished and have calcified tissues less able to resist insults from their oral environment. Fluoride has been classified as an essential mineral nutrient.

About 95 million Americans receive fluoride from artificially fluoridated water supplies and another 5 million from naturally fluoridated supplies. Small towns, rural homesites, and some communities with outright opposition to placing fluoride in the water supply compose the other 110 million people in America who do not receive the benefits of systemic fluoride. These people can be provided with fluoride benefits by their dentist. The dentist needs to procure a sample of the patient's water supply, have it analyzed (many state public health departments provide this service on a no-cost basis), and then prescribe a systemic fluoride supplement to be taken on a daily basis. Systemic fluoridation is also important from the standpoint that it has been estimated that only 40 percent of the United States population visit the dentist once per year, and many of these visits are for minimal or only crisis care. The discovery of the benefits of systemic fluoridation has been hailed as the greatest discovery in dentistry in the last four decades, and it has been estimated that aside from the benefits received by each individual, if we could increase the number of children who drank fluoridated water by 50 million, it would be equivalent to educating 17,600 dentists (French, 1975).

Fluorides: Topical

The partial success of systemic fluorides led to continued research for alternate methods of administrating fluoride either to supplement the action of systemic fluoride or to provide some anticariogenic effect by applying fluorides topically to the teeth. We must remember that the effectiveness of systemic fluoridation is limited almost entirely to the tooth calcification period but results in a lifetime of tooth resistance. To improve on the 60 percent effectiveness of systemic fluoridation and in an attempt to provide the tooth with a resistance factor that it did not derive from fluoride availability during calcification, several compounds were developed to apply topically on the clinical crown of the tooth at periodic intervals. How well these compounds work is still a matter of research, but it is generally agreed their full potential has not been completely defined. Topical fluorides presently available for professional use are sodium fluoride (NaF) 2 percent, stannous fluoride (SnF_2) 8 percent, and acid phosphate fluoride (APF) 1.23 percent fluoride (*Federal Register*, 1974). These fluorides are available in liquid or gel form, and their methods of office application are similar. In each instance the teeth are first cleaned and thoroughly polished with a commercially available polishing agent. The teeth are then air-dried and kept dry with cotton rolls. In the case of NaF the teeth are painted until they are visibly wet and then allowed to air dry for 3 minutes. When SnF_2 or APF are used, the teeth are kept continuously wet for 4 minutes. During the period of fluoride application with all three compounds, the solution should be introduced to the interproximal surfaces by gently working unwaxed dental floss through the contact points and around the proximal surfaces. It is important that the teeth be kept free of saliva during the entire topical application procedure.

When using SnF_2 and APF the topical application is given and repeated at regular recall visits established by the dentist. With NaF there are some slight differences. Immediately after the teeth are cleaned and dried, the NaF is applied for 3 minutes. The patient is reappointed for two more visits about a week apart. At these subsequent visits the fluoride is applied again but is not preceded by a prophylaxis. Another difference is that the first series of applications is given at 3 years and then repeated at 7, 11, and 13 years, whereas with SnF_2 and APF the patient is treated at each recall visit. Conclusions to be drawn from the use of topical fluorides are that they all will reduce the caries incidence about 30 to 40 percent and that the choice of fluorides used in the office will depend on the preference of the dentist. Following office-applied topical fluorides, patients should be urged to use an ADA approved dentifrice containing fluoride on a daily basis.

In a recent report by Paul Keyes (1975) the statement was made that theory and experimental and clinical evidence indicate that the potential of fluoride therapy to prevent and control dental disease is far greater than that presently attained by conventional preparations and when conventional methods of application are used. He claims that infrequent (only at regular recall periods) topical application of fluoride gives a slight reduction in the rate that teeth infected with plaque are invaded. Ira Shannon (1974) contends that patients who are classified as advanced-risk patients should have daily or almost daily topical applications of fluoride home-administered. An advanced-risk patient is one who lives in a community having fluoridated water who still has cavities; a patient who has root surfaces exposed because of periodontal disease; a patient undergoing orthodontic treatment; a patient with rampant or excessive caries;

and those patients who have salivary gland dysfunction or low salivary flow rates. Still another advanced-risk patient is a patient about to receive radiation about the head and neck for the control of pathogenic tumors. New compounds in the form of oral rinses and fluoride gels to be used in a mouthpiece or on a toothbrush at home are becoming available with increasing frequency. Several fluoride compounds can now be made available to the patient by prescription for home use. These are (1) sodium fluoride, 0.2 percent pH 7 aqueous solution for use as a rinse once a week; (2) sodium fluoride 0.05 percent pH 7 aqueous solution for use as a rinse once a day; and acid phosphate fluoride 0.02 percent pH 4 when used as a rinse once a day. These compounds are constantly undergoing review by the Food and Drug Administration, and it is suggested that current information on acceptable products be obtained by writing the Council on Dental Therapeutics, American Dental Association. These home-administered products can be in the form of mouth rinses, gels that can be placed in mouth guards, gels that can be brushed on the teeth or rubbed on the teeth with fingers or gauze, or special toothpastes. Most of these products' manufacturers recommend that the material be used at bedtime after cleaning the teeth and rinsing the mouth. The fluoride gel, rinse, or paste should be kept in contact with the teeth for at least 1 minute after which the individual expectorates but does not rinse.

Plaque Control

In the middle 1950s the dental-research pendulum began to swing again; the major bacterial entity which causes plaque to form was identified. Since medicine has been able by means of vaccines and inoculation to control certain bacteria or viruses and their by-products, research was undertaken to explore the fields of chemotherapy—to find a chemical or other agent that would either kill or inactivate the bacteria and their by-products that cause dental caries and periodontal disease. Criteria established for such an agent were that it could not harm the soft tissues or teeth; it would not sensitize the patient; it would not cause the bacteria to become resistant; it would not permit an overgrowth of other organisms; and it would not cause any unfavorable side effects. Many agents have been tested, but each agent thus far has fallen short in one or more of these criteria.

Present thinking is that the odontopathic infection can be prevented or controlled by merely keeping the bacteria from establishing colonies on the tissues where they do their harm—the teeth and soft tissues surrounding the teeth. This can be done mechanically with the toothbrush, dental floss, and other adjuncts that are presently available. It involves, however, developing a capability in the patient to recognize the presence of plaque and be able to identify it on all surfaces of all teeth. The patient must be then provided with the proper instrumentation and knowledge of how to remove these bacteria on a once a day basis.

Prevention of Dental Disease: A Multifactorial Process

One of the shortcomings of many preventive dental programs in the past is that prevention or control has been attempted by trying to control only *one* of the causative factors. For example, *rigid* control of the diet will in fact greatly reduce the number of organisms that cause dental disease, but for most patients this is impractical. To attain control in this manner the patient must usually be hospitalized initially, and then remain under rigid supervision for long periods of time. Diet is very important in the overall problem, but it probably will not be successful when used as the only means of attack. Systemic fluorides which increase the resistance of the tooth to plaque insults have proven to be about 60 percent effective, but any attempt to increase this degree of success by adding more fluoride may produce irreversible harmful effects in the tooth structure during its calcification stages. Topical fluorides are an attempt to provide the tooth with a decrease in susceptibility to bacterial insult after the teeth have erupted into the mouth. They provide additional protection but like control of diet are only partially successful.

Plaque control, the complete removal of bacterial plaque from the teeth on a daily basis, is still a third approach to dental-disease control. In theory, if a patient each day were able to interrupt the colonization of odontopathic bacteria, he or she would have no bacteria caused infections. This works with many patients who are taught how to recognize and remove plaque, but, as before, a single approach to disease control is not the most effective manner to control dental disease.

Dental disease is the result of many factors—bacteria, diet, and resistance; its cause is multifactorial. The prevention or control of the disease, therefore, is best accomplished by a multifactorial approach; an approach that involves bacterial removal, decreasing the susceptibility of the tissues by fluorides, good nutrition, and evaluating the diet in terms of those foods that contribute to bacterial growth and activity.

DEVELOPING A PREVENTIVE DENTISTRY CONTROL PROGRAM

Your concern when providing instruction in preventive dentistry is to provide the patient with

1. Skills to remove plaque
2. The urge to sustain these skills for long periods with minimum supervision

It is not enough that the patient merely learn facts. For years people have been warned that smoking is injurious to their health, but sales of tobacco have not declined. People know that seat belts should be fastened before their automobile is set in motion. If they were examined on their knowledge in this area, almost everyone would answer correctly even though they don't use the knowledge correctly. In teaching preventive dentistry the same factors apply. It is not enough that patients know how dental disease occurs or understand the importance of diet and nutrition; there must be a change in habits that initially brought about the disease factors.

Motivation: Satisfying a Need

Changes in habits come about because patients either like what they are doing or because of some factor that is important to them. What may be logical to you may have no meaning to your patient. Health-product advertising long ago abandoned approaches to the public that were aimed at the logic of good health. Most dentifrice advertisements are directed toward attracting a desired friend with a beautiful smile or not offending a friend because of bad breath. Some are aimed at a person's ego wherein he or she acquires wisdom to impart to the children or family. They aim their appeal at what they think is important to the buyer.

In preventive dentistry much the same is true. It is not enough to teach the causes of dental disease and to demonstrate to the patient the techniques of its control. The preventive assistant must appeal to a felt need of the patient in order that what is learned can be used to satisfy something the patient feels is important and which will hopefully result in a habit pattern. The chapter on applied psychology and its approach to patient–dental assistant relationships is of utmost importance in developing a successful program in preventive dentistry. Of particular importance is an understanding of Maslow's (1954) hierarchy of needs and its two basic rules (Fig. 19-2):

1. A satisfied need does not motivate.
2. Higher levels of need do not emerge until lower levels are satisfied.

Maslow teaches that there are basic needs that make people do things. It may be an inborn need like the need for food and water (physio-

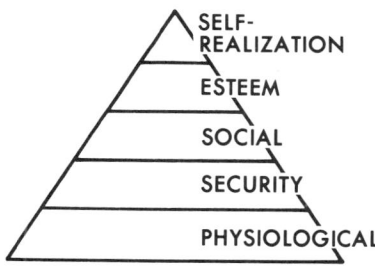

Figure 19-2 | Maslow's hierarchy of needs. Higher levels of need do not forcefully emerge until lower levels are satisfied.

logic needs); protection from economic or physical peril (security needs); the need for love, friendship, or understanding (social needs); the need for attention from others or having a status in life like others (esteem); and last, a desire to be the absolute tops in a certain role (self-realization).

Patients will respond to a need they feel. In the dental office the areas most productive are social and esteem needs. In general the physiologic and security needs are usually satisfied in our society, and self-realization needs are unobtainable. Commercial advertising of dental products recognizes this, and most of the appeals are aimed at making friends by not having bad breath (social needs) or by having teeth that are as white and sparkling as a roommate's (esteem needs).

It is important to seek the kind of need to which the patient may respond. Obviously you would not teach preventive dentistry techniques when a patient has a toothache (physiologic need). In Maslow's hierarchy, higher needs do not emerge until lower needs are satisfied. In the same vein of thought, a dental assistant would not appeal to the security level if the patient had financial security, friends, and the patient's place in life was a happy one. Rule number one states that a satisfied need does not motivate.

Some generalities in directing an appeal to the social level can be made. With most adolescents an appeal to the social level stands a good chance of being successful. Most young people are searching for their place in life, trying to change from their reliance on their parents to independence. They move out of the restrictive atmosphere of their homes to the challenge of the world. They meet new people, change their life-styles and will respond to a suggestion that good oral health, clean teeth, and clean breath will help them achieve their aims (social needs). Most females attempt from adolescence onward to be attractive to men and to be admired by other females; an appeal to their esteem needs might very likely be successful, provided that lower levels of need have been met.

It is important to realize that since every person is different and may respond differently to the same appeal, it is probably of foremost importance to first rule out those level of appeals that you know will *not* work for a specific patient. These levels of need may overlap, and once a lower need is satisfied the next higher need doesn't always emerge. Your ability to listen to the patient, to communicate with the patient, to create a situation of high trust in an adult relationship is most important.

Remember that your logic in having a plaque-free mouth is to have a disease-free mouth; unfortunately, this is not the logic that most patients respond to, and an attempt to achieve success through this approach can be disappointing. You must, through communications with your patient, find out what is important to him and then by showing him how he can satisfy his needs, achieve success. Communications is first a listening process. Find out your patients' beliefs, values, and myths about dental care and his level of understanding of the values of oral health. There are barriers to listening, such as assuming you know what the other person is thinking and feeling, as well as your preoccupation with your own problems. You must avoid causing anxiety and placing the patient on the defensive.

Most people when they seek dental care are anxious about what is going to happen. This anxiety has been built up from past experiences, pain, and fear; they enter the office apprehensive, fearing an injection, the sound of the drill, the odor, and are just waiting to get hurt. Such people are tense and frightened. They are also preprogrammed to be passive, sitting in the dental chair while the dentist fills a tooth or the dental hygienist cleans their teeth. The dental office reeks of treatment to be provided to a passive patient. The treatment room is a barrier to communications. This atmosphere is contraindicated in preventive dentistry, where patients cannot be passive. Their education must not rely on a flow of words, images, or information; they must get actively involved; they must participate; and there must be a change of attitudes, habits, and behavior.

Cassidy (1968) has outlined the stages people go through in making a decision. First, they must become *aware* that dental disease is an infection that can be minimized or prevented. Second, they must show an *interest* in it and want to know how it could affect them. Third, they get *involved*. They are taught the etiology of dental disease and the recognition of plaque in their own mouths and techniques of the removal. Fourth, they become *active* by developing skills that clean their teeth thoroughly each day with frequent assessment or evaluation of their results. Fifth, a habit is formed, and it becomes as integral a part of their daily routine as eating, sleeping, and working.

CHARACTERISTICS OF GOOD INSTRUCTION

Once a patient becomes aware of the dental-disease control program and shows an interest in it, the dental assistant should be aware that an invitation to teach has been received. How the patient is taught is directly related to the ultimate success of the program. It's not how long you spend, but how well you spend your time.

There are four basic fundamentals in teaching:

1. Small step size
2. Active participation by the learner
3. Immediate feedback
4. Self-pacing

Small Step Size, Active Participation, Immediate Feedback

Small step size means optimal step size. You should not go too fast or too slow, but at a pace that you think the patient can handle at one time. How much you can teach the patient at one step depends on such things as present knowledge, skills, dexterity, and interest. It also depends on what you require of the patient in terms of dexterity before you proceed to another step. For example, if a patient has never flossed before and has difficulty placing the floss between the upper anteriors, wrapping it around these teeth, and then scraping off bacteria by a pull toward the incisal edge, it would be folly to proceed and teach him how to hold, place, and manipulate floss between lower molars. Patients will vary in their learning capabilities because of factors influencing them outside of the dental office—a sick baby, an upcoming examination, a parking ticket—and this message must be received by the dental assistant and the step adjusted accordingly. The step size can be determined by *active participation* and *immediate feedback*.

In active participation the patients are no longer passive. They are not sitting there listening to you or watching you demonstrate on models the technique of plaque removal. Patients get involved in what is going on. They try to reproduce in their mouths what you have demonstrated to them up to this time. In teaching a tooth-cleaning technique you might proceed in this manner: After having selected a proper toothbrush for the technique you intend to teach, you would demonstrate on a model the placing of the brush and the motion in which the brush should be moved. Then have the patients look into a mirror and you place the brush at the proper angle on the teeth, where it is easy for them to see. While you are doing this, you must explain the reason for the brush angulation. After brush placement, the brush is now moved in the proper direction for plaque removal. While you are still holding the brush at proper angle, ask patients to lightly grasp the brush with you and place it in motion. Take your hand away. Have the patients stop the motion and remove the brush. Now have the patients replace it in the same area and go through the motions with no help from you. As the patients do this, you are getting *immediate feedback* and can decide if the patient's dexterity, skill, and knowledge are sufficient to proceed. If you are satisfied, proceed to other areas in the mouth, helping in brush placement and brush movement until you are satisfied that with further practice the patients will accomplish what you desire. It is always best to start in those areas of the mouth most easily seen by the patients—the facial surface of upper and lower teeth. Once these techniques are understood you can proceed to the lingual surfaces and make changes in brush angulations to suit each patient's dental-arch conformation. From the active participation and with immediate feedback, the step size for a visit can be determined. One other factor must be taken into consideration and that is the pace with which the patients learn and their desire to proceed.

Self-Pacing

For example, let us assume that you have taught a patient how to hold dental floss, place it between the upper anterior teeth, and scrape off the bacteria. The patient now demonstrates for you by placing the floss between the upper anterior teeth and flosses properly. The patient then asks if she can try placing the floss between the molar and premolar teeth. Don't turn her off! She wants to learn more; she is receptive. She should be allowed to learn at her own rate and explore what has been taught to her, and permitted to overcome her difficulties. She should be allowed to proceed at a pace she sets for herself, but you should always remember that doing something once does not mean the patient has learned it. You, therefore, should decide how far and how fast to proceed, encouraging the patient to learn at a self-determined pace but not to proceed at a rate that would be overwhelming.

STEP-BY-STEP DENTAL-OFFICE PREVENTIVE DENTISTRY PLAN

A preventive plan in a dental office should consist of three separate and distinct segments. The number of visits in each segment depends on the educational step size and the patient's ability to develop dexterity; this also relates to your ability to communicate with, teach, and motivate the patient. The time between segments is related to the patient's ability to develop a level of proficiency required by yourself and to the time required by nature to form plaque that can be visualized by the patient after its removal. Each segment should have objectives that must be achieved before moving to the next-higher segment.

Segment 1

The objectives of this segment are

1. To teach plaque recognition
2. To teach techniques of plaque removal

This segment is completely variable in the number of visits required; it may be as little as one or as many as five. The time between each visit may be as short as 1 day but not to exceed 7. The number of visits will depend entirely on how quickly the patient gets involved, and the time between the visits is related to how frequently you desire feedback after the patient has practiced at home those things you taught in the office. The outer limit is 7 days, because you must assure yourself that the patient is not inflicting self-injury or developing a technique contrary to that originally presented.

Step 1: Preventive Philosophy of Dental Care

Early in the first visit of segment 1 a philosophy of dental practice should be read and given to the patient. This philosophy in many offices is presented to the patient at the very first visit with the dentist prior to starting preventive dentistry education. In some offices it may be sent to the patient through the mail so that the patient will understand that he or she will be taught how to become actively involved with dental health. A sample philosophy follows:

Dental disease (cavities and gum trouble) is the most universal of all diseases. It is a disease that begins early in life, gets progressively worse with age, is accumulative, irreversible, and does not heal itself. It is a disease the results of which can affect oral health, general health, social acceptance, and good looks. It is also a disease that we now know can be *minimized* or *prevented*.

In the past, most patients sought dental care either when they knew they had troubles or on a routine basis to let the dentist find, repair, and treat disease that had already occurred. This was expensive, time-consuming, and a needless destruction of teeth and soft tissues during the disease and treatment process. Today we feel that the repair or replacement of a tooth, the cleaning of teeth, or the treatment of gums is not an end in itself. Decay will recur, as will gum disease, unless we teach you how to recognize and eliminate the factors in your mouth that cause it.

Goals

Would you agree that these are our goals?

1. To keep you attractive
2. To keep you comfortable
3. To keep your own natural teeth the rest of your life
4. To minimize the need for dental care
5. To keep dental bills as low as possible

To achieve these goals, you, the patient, are more important than the dentist. The dentist can treat you and even help you minimize disease but he or she cannot *prevent* the disease from occurring unless you take the leading part. The first step in accepting you as a patient is to look at you as a total patient. What are your needs both education-wise and treatment-wise that will offer you good oral health in the future?

A detailed diagnosis of these needs is most important since we will try to project for you the condition of your oral health 5, 10, or 20 years from now. We will try to teach you everything that you need to know about the present condition of your mouth, why it is in this condition, and what you and I can do to make it and keep it healthy. Our first appointments will be devoted to this end, since it is most important that we both agree on what we are trying to do, and you will understand the tremendously important role *you* play in achieving our goals.

Emergency problems will be cared for first; then we will proceed in an orderly manner teaching you or treating you in a sequence that fits your individual needs. I'm certain that we will have a pleasant relationship together and that I can help you to understand how you may achieve good oral health for the rest of your life.

Step 2: Presentation of Objectives

Inform your patient that when you are through with this segment he or she will be able to recognize the areas of the mouth where infection is occurring (plaque recognition) and will know how to clean these bacteria from the teeth and gums (plaque removal).

Step 3: Caries Activity Test

There are a number of tests available, but none of them are reliable for caries activity. They either measure the number of bacteria (*Lactobacillus acidophilus*) in a specific quantity and dilution of saliva or measure the number of acid-forming organisms in the saliva as determined by growing them in a medium to which a color indicator has been added (Snyder's test; Alban's test; Sim's test, Grainger test). Of these the Grainger test (1965) removes a sample of bacteria from the facial surfaces of the upper right and lower left molar and premolar teeth by rubbing these surfaces with a cotton swab. The swab is then inserted into Grainger's medium (a modification of Snyder's medium) in a small test tube, rotated several times, and then broken off leaving the infected cotton in the medium. The infected tube is incubated for 48 hours at 37.5°C, and the amount of acid formation can be determined by the use of a potentiometer or an inexpensive colorimeter. Patients with a high caries potential or whose diet is high in retentive carbohydrates produce changes that indicate large quantities of acid formation. In preventive dentistry, such a test is an invaluable motivational tool to demonstrate to patients the bacterial factors present in the mouth that cause dental disease, or the need for diet modification to reduce the food supply to the bacteria.

Step 4: Plaque Index

The plaque index should record plaque accumulations on all areas of all the teeth. It should also provide a score that can be easily interpreted by both patient and teacher. Since most plaque is on the gingival half of the tooth, this area should be given special consideration. The index should provide a quick and simple measuring tool for both the patient and teacher, and it serves as a motivational factor by measuring accomplishments and setting goals for achievement. Figure 19-3 illustrates an index called the plaque control record, developed by O'Leary et al. (1972). Techniques of using this record follow:

1. Have patient rinse.
2. Disclose plaque using a disclosing agent.
3. Have patient rinse.
4. Dry maxillary arch with air syringe.
5. Record any plaque seen on distal, facial, mesial, or lingual surface by blocking out the area on a record.
6. Dry mandibular teeth and proceed as before.
7. Cross out missing teeth.

Now count the number of teeth present and multiply by 4 (number of surfaces recorded for each tooth). This gives the total number of tooth surfaces observed for plaque. Now count the number of surfaces that have plaque; divide this number by the total number of surfaces. This figure is a plaque score that can be plotted on a graph that can be used as a plaque control record. If this decimal score is multiplied by 100, it will be converted into percent.

$$\frac{\text{Number of surfaces with plaque}}{\text{Total number of tooth surfaces}} \times 100$$
$$= \text{percent plaque source}$$

As the plaque score is recorded at subsequent visits, both you and the patient can visualize the progress being made. The plaque control record shows when plaque-removal technique instruction should be repeated or will show patterns of plaque accumulation which may require special techniques or additional armamentaria for removal.

Step 5: Tour of Mouth and Self-Examination Methods

The patient is shown in the mouth what you were recording in step 4. This is best accomplished by you pointing to plaque on facial surfaces of teeth while the patient observes in a mirror. The patient should now be provided with an intraoral mirror so that the lingual, distal, and interproximal surfaces can be observed. The mirror best suited for this purpose is a Floxite dental reflector (Fig. 19-4). This highly polished reflector permits patients to retract the cheek while looking at the distal and interproximal surfaces of the upper and lower teeth when viewed from the facial and to retract the tongue while looking at the same surfaces from the lingual. While taking this tour, it may be beneficial to point out restorations, malaligned teeth, inflamed soft tissues, and teeth needing restorative care. This is probably the first time your patient has really "seen" his or her teeth, and it provides first-hand information to relate to when you or

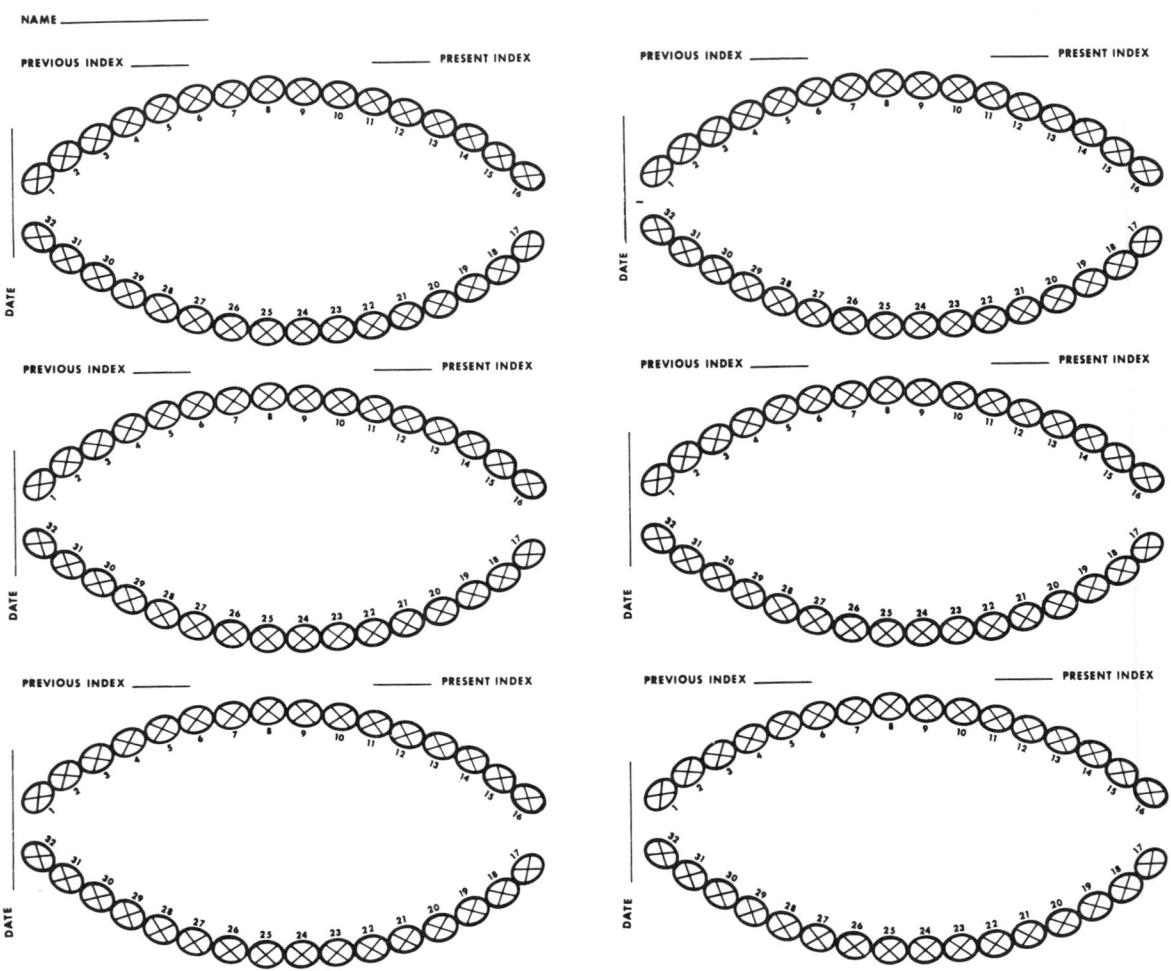

Figure 19-3 | Plaque control record. This record tells the dentist at a glance how the patient is progressing in plaque control and if there are problem areas that require special patient instruction. The record is also a good motivational tool to illustrate progress to the patient.

your dentist talks about dental health and the need for dental care or when your patient reexplores at home his or her own mouth. After you have shown the patient plaque, ask him or her to demonstrate to you how to place the mirror to see plaque on the various areas of the teeth (active participation). As the patient places the reflector and retracts the tongue or the cheek, you get immediate feedback and can determine whether or not your patient requires further help from you or whether with a little practice at home reflector placement can be improved.

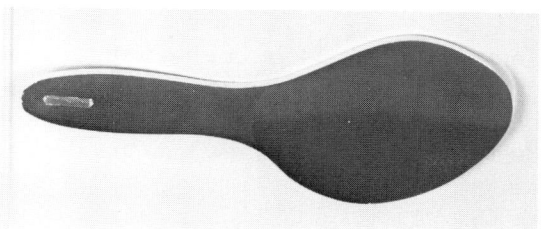

Figure 19-4 | Floxite reflector. This aid permits the patient to view distal and lingual surfaces of teeth while retracting the tongue or cheek.

Step 6: Etiology of Dental Disease

The patient has seen disclosed plaque on his or her teeth. It now becomes important to relate what the patient has seen to its potential in the disease process. This has best been explained in the chapters on microbiology, dental pathology, and nutrition. You are urged to review these chapters in order that you can present to your patient the interrelations of bacteria in plaque and their ability to produce acids of such pH as to invade the tooth or to produce toxins or enzymes which initiate a gingivitis, the precursor of periodontal disease. A simple diagram (Fig. 19-5) may assist you in your presentations. Your explanation should be aimed at the educational level of your patient and at no time should you attempt to convince your patient of how knowledgeable you are. Choose your words wisely, keep it short but thorough; attempt to elicit participation by your patients by interposing questions on matters that have already been taught.

Step 7: Phase Contrast Microscopy

The techniques of preparing a bacterial specimen for your patient to view under the phase contrast microscope have been discussed in the chapter on microbiology. This step is a motivational step, and each movement should reinforce the fact that dental disease is an infection caused by bacteria that have formed colonies on the teeth. To enhance this point, the slide, transport medium, and cover glass should be brought to the patient. With the patient looking in a hand mirror, scrape plaque from a tooth and immediately place it in the transport medium on the slide. Tease the material, place the cover glass over the specimen, press and dry, all in the patient's view. Let the patient accompany you to the microscope and watch you place the slide on the stage, focus and then view the sample with you. At this point let the patient pick out on a sample bacterial plaque age chart (see "Microbiology") the type and age of bacterial plaque being viewed. This once again is *active participation,* and you get an *immediate feedback* of understanding. Phase contrast microscopy is a valuable motivational tool for at this time the patient sees those bacteria that you have described as being the causative factor of dental caries or gingival irritation.

Step 8: Tooth-Cleaning Techniques, Oral Physiotherapy

There is a difference between tooth brushing and tooth cleaning. Almost everyone brushes

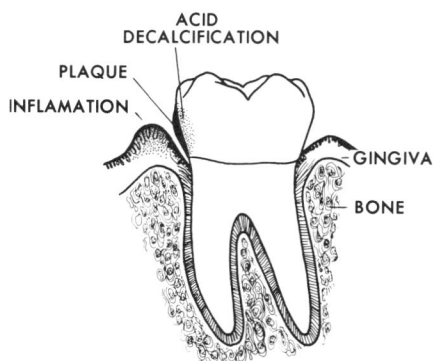

Figure 19-5 | A simple diagram drawn for all patients and given to them when they leave the office explains how plaque causes cavities and periodontal disease.

their teeth, but most people do not clean them. The term tooth brushing in itself means cleaning the tooth with a brush, and this is impossible when only a brush is used. A brush will clean facial, lingual, and occlusal surfaces but cannot clean the proximal surfaces; dental floss must be used for these surfaces. The function of oral physiotherapy is to (1) clean plaque, bacteria, and stains from all surfaces of the teeth; (2) stimulate the soft tissues; (3) replace fluorides that are lost from the tooth surfaces to saliva. Basic armamentaria for plaque and bacteria removal are a toothbrush, dental floss, and a disclosing agent. Since plaque is invisible without being disclosed, these agents should be used at an interval established with your patient to detect plaque while it is immature and able to be removed by the brush and/or floss. A dentifrice is not necessary for plaque removal but is a part of stain control. When first teaching plaque removal techniques, it is a good idea to not use a dentifrice; all dentifrices contain a detergent which will take the color out of stained plaque so that it can't be visualized, thus giving the patient a false sense of accomplishment.

If teeth are cleaned well, other tooth coverings which may cause loss of esthetics, malodorous breath, or dental disease will also be removed. These coatings are generally classified as materia alba and food debris. Materia alba is a soft white mixture of salivary protein, bacteria, and cellular debris. This material can adhere loosely to plaque, teeth, restorations, and the gingiva and can act as an irritant to the tissue. Food debris, another coating, usually becomes liquified by bacterial enzymes. It can supply a continuous source of food to bacterial plaque and is in itself a cause of halitosis. Materia alba and food debris can be removed by rinsing, the action of saliva, the tongue and muscles forming the oral cavity, and by water sprays. Uncalcified plaque requires the mechanical action of a brush and floss for removal. Stains require the abrasive component found in a dentifrice, and calculus or calcified plaque must be removed in a dental office.

The Toothbrush

There are numerous toothbrushes on the market differing in head design, hardnesses, number of bristles, bristle material and design, and handle design. This is one of the few tools that dentists can guide their patients in buying, and yet most patients are never given this information and buy a toothbrush because its color matches the decor of their bathroom.

The ideal toothbrush (Fig. 19-6) has been described as having the following specifications: plain, straight handle $7/16$ in in width; three rows of bristles with six tufts of bristles per row; bristles should be of high-quality nylon with 80 bristles per tuft and $11/32$ in long (this provides a *soft* classification to brush); each bristle should be tapered to 0.007 in in diameter and be rounded and polished and have a flat trim. Some toothbrush manufacturers even go so far as to take the glaze off the side of the nylon bristles to provide a cleansing action that is normally found only in natural bristles.

When you prescribe a toothbrush for a patient another point to consider is the head size. A toothbrush may have most of the characteristics of an ideal brush, but its head size and design must be taken into consideration. In general it is

Figure 19-6 | Head design of a toothbrush with "ideal" specifications.

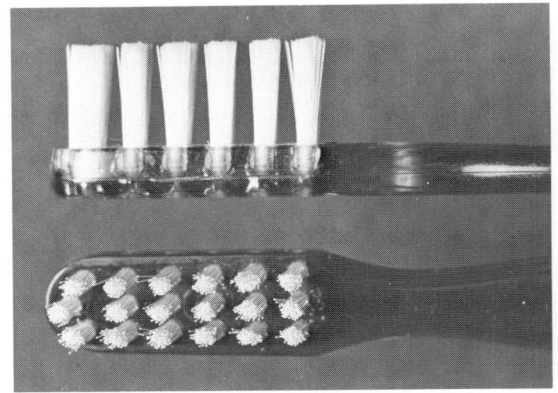

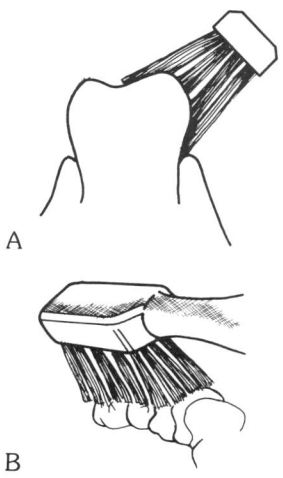

Figure 19-7 | Bass technique. A. Proper placement of bristles into sulcus of posterior teeth. B. Position of brush on several posterior teeth. The movement of the head is in a *vibratory* horizontal motion.

desirable to use the largest brush that will fit the dental arch. You can determine this by placing your finger on the facial surfaces of the upper posterior teeth and finding how much room is present between the buccal muscles and bony structures proximal to the posterior tooth.

Figure 19-8 | Bass technique. Brush position and bristle placement for lingual surfaces of anterior teeth. The movement is either vibratory or slightly circular.

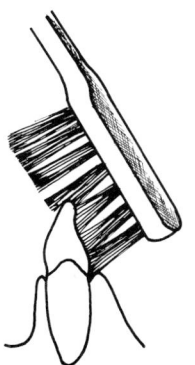

Techniques

There are many techniques of tooth brushing, but the four to be described are the easiest taught and will effectively do the job of removing bacteria from the teeth.

Bass Technique (1954)

In this technique the bristles are placed at 45 degrees to the long axis of the teeth with the bristles gently pushed in between the teeth and under the gums (Fig. 19-7). The brush is then vibrated in a horizontal motion. The motion should not be of such magnitude that the bristles are dislodged from the sulcus. The vibratory motion is stopped, the bristles are moved and replaced in a new area, and vibratory motion is repeated. This should be done for all facial and lingual areas of the teeth. For cleaning the lingual surfaces of the upper and lower anterior teeth, the bristles of the tip of the brush are guided from the incisal third toward and inserted into the sulcus where a small circular motion is employed (Fig. 19-8).

Press-Roll Technique

The roll technique may be used in all mouths but is most appropriate where there is a minimal change in the normal dentogingival relationship. The bristles are placed well upon the attached gingiva at a 45-degree angle (Fig. 19-9). The sides of the bristles are *pressed* against the tissues and then *rolled* incisally or occlusally against the gingiva and teeth, with pressure against them at all times. The motion should be confined to the movement of the wrist and can be compared to turning a key in the lock of a door. This technique stimulates the vascular system of the attached and free gingiva and does an excellent job of polishing the teeth. For cleansing the lingual surfaces of the upper and lower anterior teeth, a digging motion is used (Fig. 19-10).

Charter's Technique (1948)

The bristles are placed at right angles to the long axis of the teeth with the points of the bristles in contact with the tooth surfaces (Fig. 19-11). Then with gentle pressure the bristles are forced between the teeth with care taken not to pierce the gum. When the brush is in place, the brush is given several slight rotary or vibratory movements. This causes the sides of the bristles to come in contact with the free gingiva producing a massage of these tissues. The brush is removed and reinserted in same area, and the process is repeated. This assures a cleansing action of the tooth and stimulation to the gums. You must be sure to proceed around the dental arch on the facial and lingual surfaces, inserting the bristles into each interproximal space.

Scrub Technique

This procedure requires no manipulation of the brush within the oral cavity. The brush is used as a scrub brush, the bristles pushed against the teeth and moved in every direction. Parfitt (1963) claims this method can result in damage to the teeth and tissues if a toothbrush containing other than soft bristles is used or if the patient uses a dentifrice with a coarse abrasive. It is usually prescribed for children who are too young to master a more sophisticated technique, and they are told, after disclosing, to brush the red off.

The occlusal surfaces in all techniques are best cleaned by forcing the bristles perpendicularly into the pits and fissures and then vibrating the brush to physically remove bacteria and debris from these areas. The placement and action should be repeated using different angles of mouth entry.

For many patients a combination of techniques should be taught. All patients should begin by cleaning the occlusal surfaces and then, upon your evaluation of needs, be taught one or more of the aforementioned techniques.

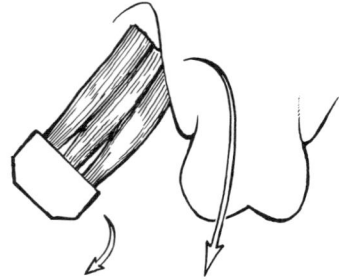

Figure 19-9 | Press-roll technique. From this initial position bristles are pressed laterally against the soft tissues and then rolled over the tissues and teeth.

The toothbrush can clean only the facial, lingual, and occlusal surfaces of teeth; it cannot clean the interproximal surface even with Charter's technique. We must now go to the second part of the basic armamentarium, dental floss, to clean the interproximal surfaces.

Dental Floss

The function of dental floss is to *scrape* plaque and bacteria from the teeth. To accomplish this objective the dental floss should be unwaxed and preferably unbonded. Manufacturers have produced waxed floss for years and, in the past few years, bonded unwaxed floss. This has been

Figure 19-10 | Press-roll technique. Brush position for cleaning lingual surfaces of the anterior teeth.

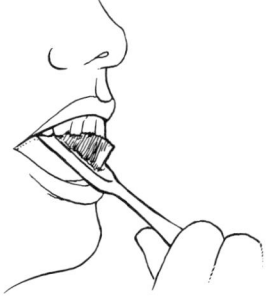

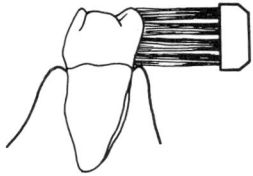

Figure 19-11 | Charter's technique. Bristles are placed perpendicular to teeth and then gently pushed into the interproximal spaces taking care to not injure the gums. A circular movement cleans the teeth and stimulates the soft tissues.

done to meet a market demand because unwaxed floss is a little more difficult for the patient to use and will tear if a tooth contains an inadequate restoration, calculus, a cavity, or anything but a clean, smooth surface. Waxed and bonded floss minimizes this problem of tearing but may be covering up the need for dental treatment.

The first lesson in teaching use of dental floss is how to hold it. About 18 to 20 in should be removed from the spool. One end of the floss is anchored on the middle finger of the left hand and the remaining floss wound on the middle finger of the right hand. This is done so that as a tooth is flossed, the floss can be unrolled from the right finger and taken up on the left finger making a clean piece available. Now the index fingers are placed on the floss not more than $1/2$ in apart (Fig. 19-12). With fingers in this position all the lower teeth may be flossed.

With the two index fingers in place, the floss is pulled so that the $1/2$ in between the index fingers is taut. A slight sawing movement is used to ease the floss through the contact point until it falls into the interproximal space. The first phase of flossing is then complete, and the patient may relax. In the second phase of flossing, the floss is *gently* worked to a position under the gum. Then it is wrapped around the tooth with both hands pulling in the same direction; keeping pressure on the tooth, the floss is pulled up toward the biting edge *scraping* the tooth clean. When it is clean, it will have a squeaky sound. This is repeated on the proximal surface of the adjacent tooth. At first, flossing may be awkward and slow if the patient has never done it before. Proceed slowly until you are assured that the patient, with practice, can develop the dexterity required (small step size).

To teach the patient to hold the floss properly for use in the upper arch, have the patient first proceed to the point where the floss is wrapped around the middle fingers with the index fingers $1/2$ in apart on the floss. Then have the patient remove the right index finger and replace it with the right thumb (Fig. 19-13). Keeping the thumb on the outside of the teeth, the patient can ease the floss between any of the teeth on the right side of the mouth—wrapped around the tooth as before, pulled tight, and then pulled toward the biting surface. For the left side, the left thumb is used.

Adjuncts to Tooth Cleaning

Dentifrices

Dentifrices can be classified as plain or therapeutic. A therapeutic differs from a plain dentifrice in

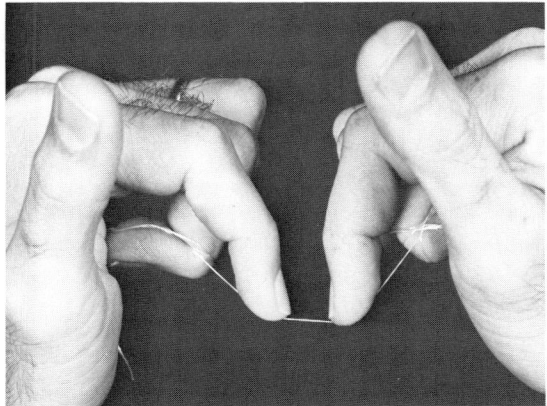

Figure 19-12 | Finger position for flossing lower teeth.

that it has incorporated into its formula fluorides which are not bound to the abrasive component and are available to the teeth. The function of a dentifrice is to clean and polish the teeth and to provide fluorides lost from the teeth. It should also provide a feeling of oral cleanliness and leave a pleasant taste sensation in the mouth after use. Even though a dentifrice should not be used when teaching plaque recognition and removal techniques, it is an important adjct in controlling stains and polishing the teeth; it may be introduced to the oral-hygiene regimen as learning progresses.

Almost all dentifrices contain the following ingredients:

Ingredient	Function
Abrasive	Cleans and polishes
Foaming agent	Helps in cleaning
Humectant	Keeps dentifrice from drying out
Binding agent	Gives dentifrice body
Water (except in powders)	Bulk
Flavor	
Sweetening agent	
Alcohol (in liquid dentifrices)	

The abrasive agents in various dentifrices have different hardnesses and particle sizes based on their claims to remove stain or polish teeth. None of the abrasive agents used will injure the enamel, but any of them with sufficient hardness and particle size to remove stain are capable of cementum abrasion. The American Dental Association (ADA) classified dentifrices several years ago in the order of their abrasiveness (Fig. 19-14). It must be remembered that there are no governmental controls over plain dentifrices since they are classified as cosmetics and their formulas may change from month to month. Therapeutic dentifrices have more stable formulas which cannot be changed. The most guarded secret of all dentifrices is their flavor. When your patient asks you, "What dentifrice should I use?", you must take into consideration

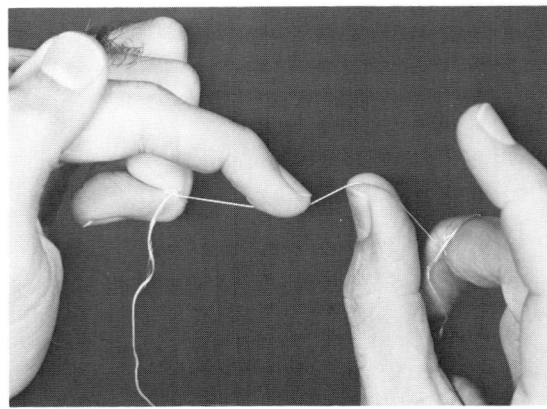

Figure 19-13 | Finger position for flossing upper teeth. When the right thumb is placed under the floss, teeth on upper right side can be flossed. The left thumb is used when flossing upper left side.

whether or not he or she requires one for its effectiveness against caries (coronal or root); for sufficient abrasiveness to remove a stain factor; and if cementum is exposed, if the particle size is too large or the abrasive too coarse.

Water Irrigation Devices

These are devices to direct a stream of water between the teeth either as a steady or pulsating stream. The Council on Dental Materials has stated that these devices may be useful as an adjunct to the toothbrush in removing loose oral debris and improving oral hygiene.

Interdental Stimulators.

Several companies produce devices intended to be placed between the teeth with pressure on the papilla to stimulate gingival tissue. Some of these are rubber tips in a separate handle or on the end of a toothbrush which are intended to be placed between the teeth and moved with a rotary action. Others are pyramidal pieces of soft wood that are pushed into the interproximal

Name	Abrasive Index
T Lak	20
Thermodent	24
Listerine	26
Pepsodent	26
Amm-i-dent	33
Colgate MFP*	51
Ultra-Brite	64
McLeans — Spearment*	66
McLeans — Regular*	70
Pearl Drops	72
Crest — Mint*	81
Close-Up	87
Crest — Regular*	95
Plus White	110
Phillips	114
Plus White Plus	132
Vote	134
Sensodyne	157
Iodent #2	174
Smokers	202

*Approved by the ADA as a therapeutic dentifrice.

Figure 19-14 | Comparison of dentin abrasiveness of several dentifrices. Those marked * are approved by the ADA as therapeutic dentifrices for the control of dental caries. They have stable formulas; the others may change.

space and used with a pumping action, and still others are special small brushes that can be placed between the teeth (Fig. 19-15).

Floss Threaders and Holders

A floss threader is a device to thread floss interproximally when it cannot be taken through the contact point. It is an essential adjuct for patients with fixed bridges and orthodontic appliances (Fig. 19-16).

With a small number of your patients, holding the floss and taking it through the contact point is an unobtainable objective. A device illustrated in Fig. 19-17 may assist these patients. It has its disadvantages in that the floss cannot be wrapped around the tooth. Another disadvantage is that once this floss is between the teeth it must be removed through the contact again. It frequently will "hang up" causing discomfort and frustration to your patient. It is recommended for use only when you feel that finger flossing is an unobtainable technique.

Mechanical Devices for Plaque Removal

Figure 19-18 is an example of a device that can be used on areas of the teeth from which plaque is difficult to remove with a toothbrush. The holes at either end are tapered so that a round wooden toothpick can be forced in. With about 1½ cm sticking out, the wood is softened in water and splayed by crushing it between the upper and lower anterior teeth. It is then used perpendicular to the tooth in an erasing motion. Some toothbrushes now come with such a hole in their handle.

Electric Toothbrushes

Some reports contend that these devices are better than hand brushes, but others show little or no differences. Initially, the electric brush may do a better job but, within a short time span, the novelty has worn off, and the hand brush is just as good. All advocates of the use of the electric toothbrush agree that the user must have proper instruction in its use to make it effective.

Mouthwashes

Unfortunately, mouthwashes are frequently advertized to the public to imply their worth in disease prevention or control of mouth odors. Most of these claims should be viewed with caution. Their use should be confined to that of a pleasant-tasting solution adding to the comfort of the patient but considered to have a very limited function.

Reprints

There are a number of inexpensive reprints available to give your patients to read at home. Some of these are directed at understanding plaque; others on how caries or periodontal disease starts; some are on nutrition; some are aimed at the young patient, while others at the more mature person. The ADA has an excellent selection and publishes a catalog once a year.

Sometime during this first segment the patient should be encouraged to keep a diet diary which will later be evaluated from a nutritional and dietary standpoint and its relation to caries and periodontal disease. This is usually accomplished in segment 3 of the program; the details of dietary evaluation are discussed in the chapter on nutrition.

As the patient is dismissed at the end of each visit of this segment 1, the points covered during the session should be thoroughly reviewed, and at departure the patient should be given the brushes, floss, and adjuncts to use in practice while at home.

This series of visits concludes segment 1. The time limit between segments 1 and 2 should be 4 to 7 days. This provides the patients with time to develop skills.

Segment 2

Segment 2 involves both the dental assistant and someone licensed to do an oral prophylaxis. This segment is usually a one-visit segment. The objectives of this visit are (1) to review plaque recognition; (2) to review plaque-removal techniques; (3) oral prophylaxis; (4) fluoride treatment.

Plaque Recognition

During segment 1, as a preventive dentistry therapist you demonstrated plaque in your patient's own mouth. As this present visit proceeds, someone in your office will remove from your pa-

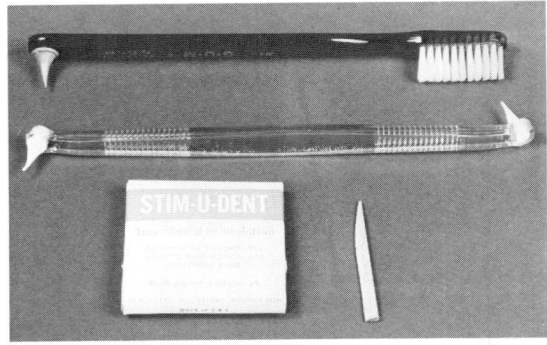

Figure 19-15 | Several types of interdental stimulators. *Top,* rubber tip on toothbrush handle; *middle,* plastic holder with rubber tip on either end; *bottom,* soft wood stick shaped to be pushed interproximally for free gingival stimulation.

tient's teeth the plaque and stains which the patient was not able to remove because of its tenaciousness or calcification with age. The patient will leave the office plaque free after this visit. It is important, therefore, that you are absolutely positive that the patient can recognize plaque on

Figure 19-16 | Devices which can be threaded with dental floss to clean under bridges or orthodontic appliances.

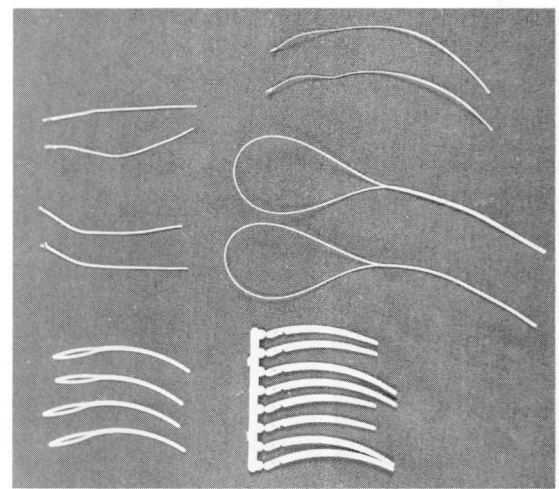

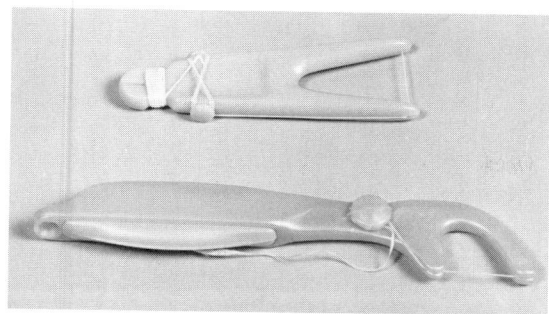

Figure 19-17 | Some patients may require help in holding dental floss. There are many such devices on the market; two are illustrated.

all surfaces of all the teeth. This can be accomplished as follows: Have the patient chew a disclosing tablet and gently rinse. Then provide a face mirror and ask the patient to point out plaque to you. With this mirror, plaque should be visible on the facial and mesial surfaces of all posterior teeth and on all surfaces of the anterior

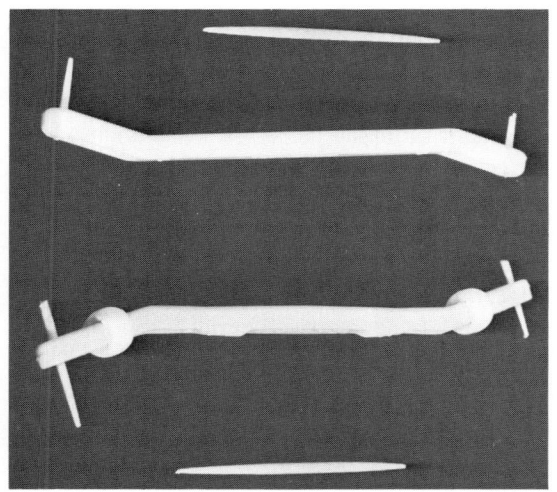

Figure 19-18 | An important adjunct to the toothbrush and dental floss is a device to hold a rounded wooden toothpick. When moist and softened it can be used to "erase" plaque missed by the brush and floss in hard-to-reach areas.

teeth except the lingual. If this inspection is performed satisfactorily, provide the patient with an intraoral mirror (Floxite reflector, Fig. 19-4) and point to a tooth on which you recognize plaque on the distal surface and ask "Does this tooth have plaque on it?" If the answer is "Yes," say, "Where?" and have the patient point it out. Use the same technique where plaque is on a lingual surface; to be absolutely certain of plaque recognition, point to a tooth without plaque and ask the same question. If the patient responds that the tooth is plaque free, you are certain that you have accomplished the first objective.

Oral Physiotherapy Techniques

Now have the patients demonstrate for you all the techniques of plaque removal that were taught in segment 1. As you get immediate feedback you can make any necessary minor adjustments in tooth brushing, flossing, or the use of adjuncts provided. The patient is now sent to the dentist or dental hygienist for a dental prophylaxis.

Home Instruction

When the prophylaxis is complete, the patient should be returned to you, given a disclosing tablet, and allowed to rinse. Let the patient look at all surfaces of all teeth to see what a clean, plaque-free mouth looks like. Explain again that as plaque forms, it is immature and is very easy to remove on a daily basis. During the period between this and the next visit, the patient should be instructed to continue to clean the teeth at least once a day and to check the thoroughness of the cleaning with a disclosing tablet. If the patient sees any plaque, it should be removed at once.

Fluoride Treatment

The patients should now be provided with a topical fluoride treatment; the types of fluoride available and methods of office application have previously been discussed. Your dentist will determine if your patient is advanced-risk patient and, if so, will ask you to instruct the patient in the more frequent use of home fluorides.

This concludes segment 2 of the preventive dentistry program. The time limit between segments 2 and 3 is critical and should be not less than 7 days nor more than 21 days. The length of time permits plaque bacteria to colonize if not removed, but not to calcify.

Segment 3

Even though plaque-forming bacteria are on the teeth immediately after an oral prophylaxis, it takes about 3 days before they can be visualized. Then because of the logarithmic reproduction of these bacteria, the colonies grow rapidly if left undisturbed and by the seventh day can easily be seen. The start of segment 3 should be delayed until this time so that if tooth-cleaning techniques and plaque recognition were initially inadequately learned, you will have a visible plaque base from which to continue your teaching. Plaque at this stage can still be easily removed by the patient. If the start of segment 3 is delayed beyond 21 days and the plaque has not been removed by the patient, it may have become tenaciously attached to the teeth or calcified so that it will once again require professional removal.

The objectives of this segment are to teach the patients self-evaluation techniques; to provide the patients with nutritional guidance; to evaluate their diet as it relates to dental disease; and to establish a recall schedule suited to the needs of the patients.

Self-Evaluation

When the patient returns 7 to 21 days following the end of segment 2, provide the armamentarium that was originally issued with the exception of a disclosing tablet. Ask the patient to clean the teeth and to call you when finished. A time limit of 10 to 15 minutes should be set. This is considered a reasonable length of time that a person will periodically devote to maintaining oral health. The patient should be left alone in the preventive dentistry room. At the end of the agreed-upon time, you should reappear, ask the patient to disclose the plaque, and evaluate the plaque-removal technique. If the patient sees any plaque, she should be told to try to remove it. As before, provide another 5 minutes without your presence in the room.

Upon return to the room you will be faced with three potential situations.

1. Patient may say she is plaque free and when you do a new plaque index, you may find that she is plaque free.
2. Patient may say that she is plaque free except for one or two areas where she recognizes plaque but can't remove it with the techniques and armanentarium provided. This, too, is a success in that she knows plaque is present. This may require a slight modification of technique or the introduction of an additional adjunct for the particular problem.
3. Patient may say she is plaque free and when you do a plaque index, you may find that she is not plaque free and requires further help.

At this time it is important to not recriminate against such patients but to proceed in an orderly, friendly, helpful manner to find out why this patient has not met your criteria. This situation might be easily corrected by changing to a disclosing tablet that has more blue in it, or is a deeper red, or even to a Plak Lite (Fig. 19-19), where plaque fluoresces a yellow color. Also check the mirror surface and placement and the reflection of light from source to mirror surface to tooth surface. You might check the distance from the light and mirror to the teeth the patient is trying to see. In most instances a little understanding of the patient's problems and tolerance on your part in retraining will achieve the objective you and your patient are striving to attain.

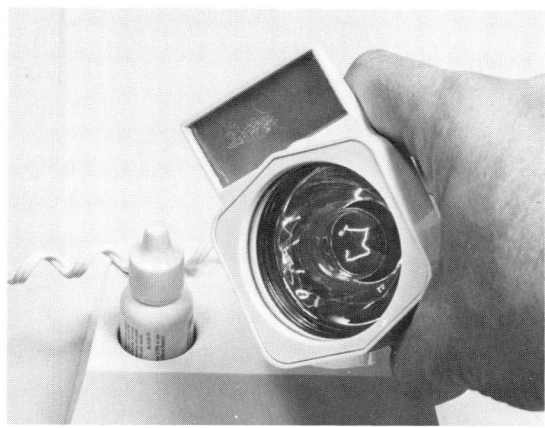

Figure 19-19 | The Plak Lite uses an ultraviolet light plus a fluorescent dye to disclose plaque.

Home Schedule

During this self-evaluation visit a home self-evaluation schedule is set up for the patient. The patient is told to remove plaque from the teeth at least once a day and that brushing, flossing, and the use of other adjuncts do not all have to be done at the same time. It isn't necessary to use a disclosing tablet daily but the patient should evaluate plaque-removal abilities at least once a week and follow the same procedures just completed in the dental office.

Diet Evaluation

The remaining portion of this visit is used in nutritional guidance and dietary counseling which is described in the chapter on nutrition.

Recall

The patient is dismissed, and an appointment is made for reevaluation of plaque removal and for patient remotivation in 1 month. The same procedures of self-evaluation are followed at this visit as were followed during the segment 3 visit. The patient may have further questions at this time and may also be seeking a word of encouragement. At the end of this appointment another meeting is scheduled for 3 months. Once again the same procedures are followed as before, and a plaque index is taken from which the patients' progress can be determined. New brushes, floss, and other items that require replacement should be reissued. Four to six months will have elapsed since the program was started. At this time most patients will have reached a plateau that they are content to live with. In many patients it will be a plaque-free mouth; in others it may range from 60 to 90 percent of plaque-free tooth surfaces. In almost every patient the mouth will be maintained at a cleaner level than before the program started. Depending on the extent of behavioral modification and the habit pattern formed, a recall schedule may now be set at intervals of from 2 to 12 months. There are other factors which may have an effect on the recall schedule, but plaque-removal abilities should play a major part in establishing a recall schedule appropriate for each patient. At each subsequent recall, the time interval between visits may be changed to suit the needs of the patient.

BIBLIOGRAPHY

Bass, C. C.: "An Effective Method of Personal Oral Hygiene," *J. La. State Med. Assoc.,* **106:**103–104, 1954.

Becks, H.: "Carbohydrate Restriction in the Prevention of Dental Caries Using the L.A. Count as One Index," *J. Calif. Dent. Assoc.,* **26:**53, 1950.

Black, G. V.: "Some Problems in Dentistry Which Should Have Further Development or a Wider Diffusion of Practical Information," *Ill. State Dent. Soc. Trans.,* pp. 134–140, 1909.

Cassidy, R. J.: "A Model of Professional Policy Orientation and Patient Communication," in *The Curators, University of Missouri: Motivation in Preventive Dentistry,* Columbia, 1968, pp. 131–184.

Charters, W. J.: "Proper Home Care of the Mouth," *J. Periodontol.,* **19:**136, 1948.

Food and Drug Administration, U.S. Department of Health, Education, and Welfare: *Federal Register,* **39**:94, Tues., May 14, 1974, p. 17215.

French, N.: "Perspective on Prevention," *J. Am. Coll. Dentists,* **42**:98–106, 1975.

Grainger, R., et al.: "Swab Test for Dental Caries Activity," *J. Can. Dent. Assoc.,* **31**:515–526, 1965.

Gustafsson, B. E., et al.: "The Vipeholm Dental Caries Study," *Acta Odontol. Scand.,* **11**:232, 1954.

Hanke, M. T.: *Diet and Dental Health,* The University of Chicago Press, Chicago, Ill., 1933, part II, pp. 75–193.

Jay, P., Beeuwkes, A. M., and MacDonald, H. B.: *Dietary Program for the Control of Dental Caries,* The Overbeck Co., Ann Arbor, Mich., 1959.

Keyes, P. M.: "Present and Future Measures for Dental Caries Control," *J. Am. Dent. Assoc.,* **79**:1395–1404, 1969.

————, and Englander, H.: "Fluoride Therapy," *J. Am. Soc. Preventive Dent.,* Jan./Feb., 1975, p. 17.

Maslow, A. H.: *Motivation and Personality,* Harper & Row, Publishers, Incorporated, New York, 1954.

Miller, W. D.: *The Micro-Organisms of the Human Mouth,* S.S. White Dental Mfg. Co., Philadelphia, 1890.

O'Leary, T. J., Drake, R. B., and Naylor, J. E.: "The Plaque Control Record," *J. Periodontol.,* **43**:38, 1972.

Orland, F. J., et al.: "Experimental Caries in Germfree Rats Inoculated with Enterococci, *J. Am. Dent. Assoc.,* **50**:259–272, 1955.

Parfitt, G. J.: "The Cleansing of the Subgingival Space," *J. Periodontol.,* **34**:133–139, 1963.

Shannon, M. W., and Shannon, I. L.: "Control of Decalcification in Orthodontic Patients by Daily Self-Administered Application of a Water-Free 0.4% Stannous Fluoride Gel," *Am. J. Orthod.,* **66**:275–279, 1974.

Stephan, R. M.: "Effects of Different Types of Human Foods on Dental Health in Experimental Animals," *J. Dent. Res.,* **45**:1551, 1966.

20

William R. Stanmeyer
Nutrition

INTRODUCTION

Food is more than just something to eat! The first five words in Nizel's (1972) textbook on nutrition in preventive dentistry are "We are what we eat." It is almost inconceivable that in a country like ours where the availability and variety of foods are almost unlimited that a large percentage of our population is eating diets lacking in one or more essential nutrients. Many of our people eat food to satisfy their hunger needs and never stop to think that our bodies are made up of billions of cells and that each cell requires specific foods to live, reproduce, and function. Denial of essential foods to these cells causes them to function beneath their capacity, to transfer their function to some other overworked cell, or to die; this results in early aging of tissues, loss of resistance, increase in susceptibility to disease insults, and possibly symptoms of a disease. It is true that today, in our country, we are not confronted with as much clinical evidence of malnutrition (rickets, pellagra, beriberi) as we were 50 to 70 years ago. Our knowledge of nutritional biochemistry and the availability of care has increased so that these clinical symptoms are diagnosed early and treatment is provided before the condition becomes irreversible. It is important to understand, however, that clinical evidence of the disease is one of the *last* symptoms to occur. Prior to having symptoms, there have been more subtle changes that have taken place in the tissues and, prior to that, histochemical changes have occurred at the cell level which might have been detected in the blood and lymph nutritional transport systems. Scurvy, for example, just doesn't occur spontaneously; it is preceded by all the aforementioned changes. When it is detected clinically, it is an advanced, not the first, symptom of the disease.

Your *diet* is what you eat and drink. The amount and balance of what you eat provide nutrients for cellular and body functions. This is called *nutrition*. Diet is concerned with what you take into your mouth; nutrition is concerned with the utilization of what you eat to provide growth, maintenance, repair of tissues, and energy requirements.

Sir William Osler once stated that the oral tissues were a mirror of general health. The dentist and dental auxiliaries are in a unique position in that they see patients who have dental disease but may have no immediate reason to see their physician. Because of the universality of dental disease, dentists see many more physically "well" patients than the medical doctor. The dentist also sees children during adolescence who are otherwise healthy but are going through one of the greatest periods of growth and development. The dentist, therefore, has the responsibility to recognize and recommend to the patients any dietary or nutritional conditions that might affect general health and urge them to see a physician if treatment other than that of a dental nature is considered necessary.

Figure 19-1 (Chap. 19) emphasized the multifactorial aspect of dental disease. It is interesting to note in the figure that two of three circles—diet and susceptibility—are concerned with what one eats (diet) and with resistance or susceptibility to disease (nutrition). There is no doubt that in the prevention of dental disease, diet and nutrition are just as important as plaque control. The greatest advancement in preventive dentistry has been made in the area of susceptibility, in that when the mineral nutrient fluoride is added to an individual's diet in minute quantities during the time when tooth calcification is occuring, the incidence of dental caries can be reduced by as much as 60 percent. Fluoride has been classified as a nutrient essential for good bone and tooth calcification.

As discussed in Chap. 19, the oldest dental research can be related to the diet circle (Fig. 19-1) in that Aristotle is purported to have said that sweet figs sticking to the teeth is a cause of dental cavities. When W. D. Miller gave dentistry a theory of dental caries (bacteria + food → acids → tooth → cavity), most of the research starting in the 1920s involved diet and nutrition because of the complexity of the bacterial component. Hanke (1933) showed that children who benefited from nutritional guidance had fewer carious teeth than those without guidance. Becks (1950) and Jay (1959) were two of the first dentists who treated patients with rampant caries by dietary control. Stephan (1966) and Bibby (1975) presented much research on those foods that were conducive to the formation of oral disease. The Vipeholm dental caries study by Gustafsson (1954) gave us new insight into the effect of frequency by eating and retentiveness of foods on dental caries, and Nizel (1972) through research and his writings has tied together the science and practice of nutrition in preventive dentistry.

These are just a few who contributed immeasurably to the knowledge of prevention of dental disease through diet and nutrition.

FOOD IS MORE THAN JUST SOMETHING TO EAT

There is no one perfect food. Good nutrition requires a mixture of foods from plant and animal sources to provide about 45 to 50 nutrients essential at the cellular level. Each nutrient can be placed in a broad category and classified as

Carbohydrate
Fat
Protein
Vitamin
Mineral
Water

Of these nutrients, some can be stored in the body and released for use when required, while others must be eaten on a daily basis because the excess nutrient ingested in each day is excreted.

FUNCTIONS OF FOOD

The body is analogous to a machine; it is a human machine. The foods that we eat are converted to body tissues and energy. Our bones, muscles, nerves, and skin are all products of cells that required food to form them; the repair of these tissues when they are injured depends on food. The food we eat also maintains a constant body temperature, the proper relationship of acids and bases, and a constant internal and external cell pressure to allow assimilation of nutrients and excretion of waste products by each cell. Food regulates such body processes as calcification, enzymatic and hormonal systems, oxidation and reduction processes, and solvent capabilities. Finally, food provides energy for the body to breathe, to circulate blood, to stay alive, to receive nervous stimulation, and to work. Food enables us to perform various types of work, whether it be mechanical (heartbeat, walking), electric (nerve impulses), chemical (cellular reproduction or repair), or biologic (growth). Each nutrient has a specific job and functions in combination with all other nutrients, and without a balance of food required by cells to perform these functions, the general body will operate on a less efficient basis, age early, and eventually die. You are what you eat, and food is more than just something to eat.

CARBOHYDRATE NUTRITION

Carbohydrates are important foods in that they are our major source of *energy*. Of our daily requirement of calories (cal), about 45 to 75 percent comes from carbohydrates in one form or another. It has been calculated that 1 g of carbohydrate provides 4 cal.

Carbohydrates can be classified as monosaccharides, disaccharides, or polysaccharides. The monosaccharides contain one sugar molecule, and there are three important ones: glucose (dextrose), fructose, and galactose. Disaccharides contain two sugar molecules, and three important ones are sucrose (table sugar) lactose (milk sugar), and maltose (malt sugar). Polysaccharides contain many sugar molecules, and three important ones are starch, cellulose, and glycogen. Of all these carbohydrates only two are found in the body. Glucose is found in the bloodstream, and glycogen is found in the liver and muscle. Glycogen is the storage form of glucose, and glucose is the only carbohydrate the body can use quickly. To use other carbohydrates, it must first break them down to glucose.

The body requires glucose for energy; for utilization by the nervous system; as an energy source for oral and intestinal bacteria; to stimulate some bacteria that synthesize vitamins B and K; as an aid in the oxidation of fats; to save the use of protein as an energy source; as an aid in collagen formation; to be converted into body fat; and to make food more palatable.

Another important carbohydrate is cellulose. Cellulose is indigestible because the body has no enzyme to break it down. This fact makes it very important to the gastrointestinal tract in that its bulk, when in the small intestine, causes a rhythmic expansion and contraction of the intestine called *peristalsis*. This moves the bolus of food through the small intestine toward elimination at a rate which will allow assimilation of the nutrients into the bloodstream and lymphatic system and eventually to the cells that use them.

CARBOHYDRATES AND DISEASE

Carbohydrates are necessary for energy, but the pattern of carbohydrate consumption has been changing. Many years ago most of our carbohydrates came from the polysaccharides in the form of starch, and less than 5 lb per person of sucrose was consumed per year. Latest figures indicate that the average American now consumes 120 lb of sucrose per year per person.

Much of the sucrose is in the form of "hidden sugar" added by the manufacturers to such products as packaged cereals, candy and gum, soft drinks, dairy products such as chocolate milk and ice cream, pies, cookies and cakes, jams and jellies, canned fruits, vegetables, and meats, peanut butter, mayonnaise, and even products like antacids and vitamin tablets. The United States government laws on labeling require the manufacturer to indicate the contents of each product on the label. If you are not sure of what you are eating, read the label.

Studies with germ-free animals have shown that the bacteria associated with dental caries (*Streptococcus mutans*) best utilize sucrose to form plaque. These bacteria produce an extracellular enzyme which forms plaque and hastens sucrose fermentation. The fermentation of sucrose in the plaque forms lactic, pyruvic, acetic, proprionic, and formic acids of such strength that they break down the enamel and eventually cause cavitation. Some bacteria in this plaque produce enzymes and toxins which attack the periodontal tissues to cause periodontal disease. The carbohydrate sucrose, therefore, is probably the single most important etiologic factor in dental caries and periodontal disease.

Sucrose is called a plaque-conducive food. The amount of plaque formed and the *activity* of the bacteria within the plaque are not dependent on the refinement of sucrose. What is important is the *frequency* with which it is ingested and the *retentiveness* of the form in which it is eaten. For example, sucrose (table sugar) in a cup of coffee will not produce plaque activity as long as toffee candy because the toffee candy sticks to the oral tissues longer and feeds the bacteria for a much longer time. However, drinking a sweetened drink at frequent intervals, particularly between meals, is just as bad as eating a single piece of candy or cake during the same time interval. The amount of sucrose, also, is not as important as the frequency and retentiveness. Small amounts in the mouth will cause the same plaque activation as larger amounts. When doing a dietary evaluation for a patient, one of the things to search for in the diet is the form of sucrose and the time when it is consumed; one then attempts to have the patient make substitutions for sucrose consumption at those times that it does the most harm.

Sucrose has also been associated with other diseases. A high intake of sugar-containing foods reduces appetite for other foods which are required. Recently, it has also been shown that increased sucrose intake results in an increased level of blood triglycerides in some individuals, and this has been associated with atherosclerosis. Still another disease associated with sucrose intake is diabetes mellitus. Sucrose does not cause this disease, but sucrose intake must be controlled because persons with this disease have too little insulin to take glucose out of the blood.

LIPID NUTRITION

Lipid or fat nutrition provides an important source of energy. One gram of fat provides nine calories. Lipids are important components of cells and membranes, act as a cushion for vital organs, and maintain body temperature. Fats are usually associated with high-quality protein and provide fatty acids which are necessary for normal growth of the body and good condition of the skin. A very important function is that they act as a solvent and carrier for vitamins A, D, K, and E and permit these vitamins to provide cellular nutrition by way of the lymphatic system.

Fatty acids are classified as fully saturated, found in animal fats; monounsaturated, found in olive oil, beef, lamb, and poultry fat; and polyunsaturated, found in vegetable oils. Certain cardiovascular diseases like atherosclerosis are associated with the deposits of fats, such as cholesterol, in blood vessels; high cholesterol levels are frequently associated with high ingestion of saturated animal fats. A physician will frequently suggest the use of polyunsaturated fatty acids to control high levels of blood cholesterol as a preventive measure for a heart attack.

PROTEIN NUTRITION

Proteins are nutrients required by the cytoplasm and nuclei of every cell and by all regulatory systems such as the hormonal and enzymatic systems. They are essential for growth and repair of tissues and in the form of antibodies provide resistance to disease. In instances where energy requirements are not met from other sources, protein can even supply energy. One gram of protein supplies four calories.

Proteins consist of approximately 20 amino acids. Of these amino acids 12 can be synthesized by the body and are called *nonessential dietary amino acids*. The other 8 amino acids cannot be made by the body and are classified as *essential amino acids*; these must be supplied by the diet. Protein is found in both animal and plant foods, and these foods contain both essential and nonessential amino acids. Animal proteins that contain all eight essential amino acids are called complete proteins. No one plant food contains all eight amino acids, and they, therefore, are called incomplete proteins. Diets should contain mixtures of animal and plant foods to get all the essential amino acids. A person on a vegetarian diet must eat a *variety* of vegetables to be sure to get the necessary amino acids for cell and glandular functions.

The amount of protein required a day varies with the life stage and physical well-being of an individual. During periods of growth 2.2 g of protein are required for each kilogram of body weight (1 kg = 2.2 lb). In adults the requirement is reduced to 0.8 g/kg. During many sicknesses, protein needs are increased, but in some diseases, such as liver and kidney disease, protein input must be restricted. This is because one of the end products of protein breakdown is nitrogen, and the liver and kidneys are important organs in protein utilization and excretion.

VITAMIN NUTRIENTS

Vitamins are organic compounds whose function is to activate body processes. The best sources of vitamins are in a balanced diet. Vitamins have no caloric value, and their importance is based on the fact that they assist in the metabolism and absorption of food nutrients and in changing the chemicals of food into the chemical components of body tissues (see Table 20-1). These compounds are classified in terms of their solubility; those that are soluble in fats are vitamins A, D, K, and E, and those that are water-soluble are vitamins B and C. Fat-soluble vitamins can be stored in the body, whereas water-soluble vitamins cannot, and the diet must contain adequate amounts on a daily basis.

Vitamin A

Vitamin A is a fat-soluble vitamin essential for growth, vision, and a healthy skin. Deficiencies of this vitamin result in night blindness which is an inability of the eye to adapt quickly from bright light to dim light, such as in going from the bright outside into a dimly lit movie. This vitamin is also involved in the health of all tissues of epithelial origin. The health of the skin depends on vitamin A, as does the formation of tooth enamel which is of epithelial origin. It has been shown in animal research that deficiency of vitamin A at the time enamel is forming results in a tooth less resistant to oral disease when it erupts into the mouth. All glandular function is dependent on adequate amounts of vitamin A, because all glands are of epithelial origin. Of particular importance in dentistry is salivary gland function, and research has repeatedly shown that there is

Table 20-1 | Summary of the Function, Source, and General Deficiency Effects of Vitamins

Vitamin	Fat-soluble	Water-soluble	Function	Source	Deficiency effects
A	×		1. Formation of visual purple 2. Differentiation of epithelium 3. Bone remodeling 4. Eye function	Preformed: fish fat and fish liver Carotene: fruits and vegetables green or yellow in color	1. Night blindness 2. Epithelial changes in glands, skin, and mucous membranes 3. Lowered resistance 4. Retarded growth
B_1 (Thiamine)		×	1. Utilization of carbohydrates 2. Coenzyme	Yeast, whole wheat, enriched cereals, breads, liver, beef, dried peas, nuts, and beans	1. Polyneuritis (beriberi) 2. Tiredness, loss of appetite, irritability
B_2 (Riboflavin)		×	1. Utilization of carbohydrates 2. Catalysis of oxidation-reduction reactions in tissues	Milk, liver, cheese, eggs, leafy green vegetables	1. Glossitis 2. Angular cheilosis 3. Dermatitis
Niacin		×	1. Carbohydrate metabolism 2. Muscle and nerve function	Whole grain cereals, liver, yeast, meat, legumes, and nuts	1. Pellagra 2. Diarrhea 3. Dermatitis
B_6		×	1. Assistance in protein and amino acid metabolism 2. Red blood cell regeneration 3. Nervous tissue function	Liver, whole grain cereals, legumes, meat	1. Dermatitis 2. Irritability 3. Cheilosis 4. Glossitis
Pantothenic acid		×	1. Release of energy from carbohydrates 2. Hemoglobin formation	Liver, eggs, whole grain cereals, legumes	1. Dermatitis 2. Infertility 3. Retarded growth
Biotin		×	1. Activation of enzyme systems	Liver, milk, eggs, yeast	1. Dermatitis 2. Lassitude 3. Muscle pain
Folic acid		×	1. Manufacture of blood cells	Glandular meats, yeasts, leafy green vegetables	1. Anemia
B_{12}		×	1. Blood formation	Liver, eggs, milk, cheese, and fish	1. Anemia
C (Ascorbic acid)		×	1. Function of cellular elements of all tissues 2. Phagocytosis 3. Prevention of anemias 4. Cell division 5. Collagen formation	Citrus fruits, peppers, parsley, turnips, greens, broccoli, spinach, cabbage	1. Capillary fragility 2. Impaired wound healing 3. Swollen, inflamed gums 4. Lowered resistance 5. Lassitude and loss of appetite
D	×		1. Absorption of calcium and phosphorus	Fish liver oils, fortified milk	1. Rickets 2. Osteomalacia
E	×		1. Stability of membranes	Cereals, meat, butter, fish	
K	×		1. Blood coagulation	Green vegetables, egg yolk, soybeans, liver	1. Prolonged clotting time

a direct correlation between salivary flow and the amount of dental decay.

The recommended daily dietary allowance (RDA) of vitamin A is 5000 IU. (An IU [international unit] is the amount of a vitamin that produces a specific effect and is a measure of potency of the substance.) This vitamin can be stored in the body, and a diet containing 20 to 30 times the RDA ingested for long periods of times can result in some toxic symptoms. There are two main sources of vitamin A. The first is preformed vitamin A and is found in such animal foods as fish fats. The second source is found in plant foods having a deep-yellow or green pigment. This is called carotene and is converted in the body to vitamin A. See Appendix for major sources of this vitamin.

Vitamin D

Vitamin D is a fat-soluble vitamin having the function of controlling intestinal absorption of calcium and phosphorus and the mineralization of bone and teeth. Deficiencies of this vitamin result in rickets or osteomalacia. This is the most toxic of all vitamins. The RDA is 400 IU, and quantities above that amount should be taken by prescription only. The amount of vitamin D in natural foods is small, but because of the direct correlation between calcium, phosphorus, and vitamin D, it is usually added to milk, which is one of the best dietary sources. When more nutrients are added to a food than are usually found in the food (such as vitamin D to milk), it is called *fortification*.

Vitamin K

Vitamin K is a blood-coagulating vitamin. This vitamin is synthesized by the body in the small intestine; green leafy vegetables are excellent dietary sources. Diets should be supplemented with vitamin K only when patients are on prolonged antibiotic or salicylate therapy, or when suffering from some disease which inhibits intestinal production of the vitamin. In the dental office it may be prescribed presurgically for patients who have demonstrated prolonged blood-clotting times and hemorrhagic tendencies.

Vitamin E

This fat-soluble vitamin has been called the vitamin looking for a disease. It is considered to be essential in the diet, but its exact role is unknown. It is known that it readily accepts oxygen, which may protect those body compounds that could be destroyed by oxygen; because of this property it is said to have antioxidant properties. It is found in large quantities in whole grain cereals, in green leafy vegetables, meat, and butter. Vitamin E is considered nontoxic to human beings, unlike the other fat-soluble vitamins.

Vitamin B

Vitamin B is a water-soluble vitamin and, with the exception of vitamin B_{12} which the body stores, must be consumed on a daily basis in the diet. Vitamin B is not a single vitamin but at least 11 separate vitamins with similar functions. Vitamin B_1 (thiamine), vitamin B_2 (riboflavin), niacin, pantothenic acid, and biotin have the principal function of releasing energy from carbohydrates. Folic acid and vitamin B_{12} have as their principal function the catalysis of red blood cell formation to prevent anemia. Vitamin B_6 is not a single substance but a group of interrelated pyridoxines and has both an energy-releasing function and an antianemic function. The last 3 of the 11 vitamins in the vitamin B complex, para-aminobenzoic acid, choline, and inositol, have not been classified for human need.

Because of the close relationship of these vitamins, a deficiency of a single one of them is rarely seen. Deficiencies of the complex are seen clinically as neuritis, apathy, fatigue, weight loss, glossitis (color and topographic changes), fissured or macerated corners of the mouth, red and swollen oral mucous membranes, dermatitis, poor wound healing, and anemia.

The vitamin is found in whole natural plant and animal foods, brewer's yeast, pork, liver, beef, whole wheat, and enriched cereals and breads. Cooking in water causes a loss in food vitamin B content because of its water solubility. The amount of loss in food will depend on the amount of water used and how long it is cooked; fresh freezing of vegetables has only a small effect on its loss in potency. Probably the greatest loss of vitamin B occurs during the milling process of grains; approximately one-half of the B_6 content is lost. The germ and bran of the cereal contain almost all of the vitamin B complex and during the milling process these are removed, leaving the endosperm which is mostly carbohydrate with a small amount of protein. Much of the vitamin B removed during the milling process is added back to the flour after milling. This is called *enrichment,* and many breads and flours sold in our supermarkets bear this label.

Vitamin C

Vitamin C is a water-soluble vitamin sometimes called ascorbic acid. It must be supplied to the body regularly because it is not stored. Good sources of vitamin C are citrus fruits, peppers, parsley, turnip greens, and such leafy vegetables as broccoli, cabbage, and spinach (see Appendix). We are one of the few animal species that cannot synthesize vitamin C. When it is lacking from the diet, clinical symptoms occur rather slowly; the end result of vitamin C deficiency is scurvy and possibly death. Early deficiencies can be detected, if suspected, quite easily by measuring blood plasma concentrations. As deficiency symptoms progress, anemia, lowered resistance to infections, swollen and bleeding gums, and capillary fragility evidenced by easy bruising and petechial hemorrhages in the skin occur. Oral manifestations have been listed as enlarged gingivae with a bluish red color that bleed easily; necrotizing ulcerative gingivitis

Table 20-2 | **Mineral Nutrients**

Essential macrominerals	Essential microminerals (trace elements)
Calcium	Iron
Phosphorus	Fluorine
Magnesium	Copper
Sodium	Zinc
Potassium	Iodine
Sulfur	Cobalt
Chlorine	Manganese
	Molybdenum
	Selenium
	Chromium

may be a complicating factor. The recommended daily dietary allowance for vitamin C is 45 mg. Some investigators, however, have recommended a daily intake of from 2 to 10 g claiming this amount will diminish one's susceptibility to upper respiratory and other infections. The efficacy of such a dosage has never been proved, but it is known from studying blood plasma and urinary excretion levels that during any stress situations there is a need for higher input of this vitamin. It has been demonstrated that wound healing following surgery is enhanced, in that the wound heals much faster with less pain and danger of infection, when the patient's diet is supplemented by vitamin C.

MINERAL NUTRIENTS

The minerals can be classified as macrominerals or microminerals depending upon the amounts found in the body. The macrominerals, present in relatively large amounts in the body, must be supplied by the diet at levels of 100 mg or more a day. Microminerals, sometimes called trace elements, must be supplied by the diet at levels of a few milligrams or less per day. Seven macrominerals and ten trace elements are considered essential for humans. Table 20-2 lists these minerals and classifies them as essential macrominerals or essential microminerals. All of the listed elements are essential for good nutrition and good cellular metabolism. In this chapter, however, only the minerals calcium, phosphorus, fluoride, iron, and iodine will be discussed.

Calcium and Phosphorus

These two minerals make up most of the skeletal structure and are the most abundant minerals in the body. About 99 percent of the calcium is found in the bones and teeth with about 1 percent in the soft tissues and blood. In like manner, 70 to 80 percent of the phosphorus is stored in the bones and teeth and the remaining percent in the soft tissues. Both of these minerals give rigidity to the bones and teeth but have some dissimiliar functions also.

Calcium is important to the cardiovascular system in that the rhythmic beat of the heart depends on the proper ratio of calcium to sodium, potassium, and magnesium. Calcium is also essential in the blood-clotting mechanism. Another important function is that when calcium levels of the blood are low, the irritability of the nervous system is increased, causing tetany or cramps in muscles. Calcium is also an important factor in activating certain enzymes.

Phosphorus has a major function in providing quick release of energy to the muscles when stimulated as well as being an essential component of compounds found in the nucleus and cytoplasm of every cell. Phosphorus also helps in the absorption and metabolism of glucose and glycogen to supply energy demands of the body. Still another function is that it acts in blood and saliva as a buffer so that the acid content of blood and saliva varies only within very narrow limits. Meats, fish, eggs, legumes, and some fruits provide good sources of phosphorus, while milk and milk products are excellent sources of calcium (see Appendix).

Fluoride

Fluoride has been classified as a mineral nutrient essential for the proper calcification of bones and teeth. It is a trace element required in very small amounts in the diet. The research that led to the discovery that fluorides, when in the diet during tooth-crown calcification at levels of 0.8 to 1.2 parts per million (ppm), reduced dental caries by 50 to 60 percent has been hailed as the greatest accomplishment in dental research in the past 40 years. About 100 million persons in America now drink water from community sources which have been fluoridated or from natural sources where the content of water fluoride has been controlled.

The protective action of fluoride was discovered as a result of research that was investigating the reasons for a condition called mottled enamel. This is a condition which results in hypoplastic enamel formation with clinical symptoms of pitted malformed enamel with a brownish discoloration. The etiology of this condition was the ingestion of fluorides above 1.5 ppm for long periods of time during enamel calcification. Dietary fluoride during enamel formation and calcification should be carefully adjusted so that the patient gets enough fluoride for optimal calcification of bones and teeth but not so much fluoride to cause mottled enamel or more serious general-health symptoms.

When the patient in your office is a young child, his or her source of drinking water should be investigated. If the child is not on a source of supply containing optimal qualities of fluoride, sufficient amounts should be provided in his or her diet. This is done by having a sample of the home water supply analyzed for fluoride content and then providing the child with sufficient fluoride on a daily basis to approximate 1 ppm. Table 20-3 outlines the method of calculating the required adjusted allowances. The addition of fluoride to a patient's diet must be done by prescription. Once you have determined the fluoride content of the patient's drinking water, your dentist will write a prescription with instructions on how to add the additional fluoride to the diet.

Iron and Iodine

Iron is present in the red blood cells as hemoglobin which is an important carrier of oxygen in all fundamental biologic processes. Iron deficiencies are more common during pregnancy, the menopause, and in children 6 months to 1 year of age. In an infant the deficiency is usually of dietary origin, while in the adult it may be caused by diet or abnormal blood loss. Good sources of iron are beans, beef, liver and other organ meats, seafood, egg yolk, and soybeans.

The thyroid gland has the greatest concentration of iodine. The secretion of this gland is called *thyroxine* and is 65 percent iodine. Its function is to regulate the *metabolism* of the body. Deficiencies of iodine in the diet result in goiter or some other functional or structural change in the body. Good sources of iodine are available in seafoods. In those sections of the country where seafoods are not readily available

Table 20-3 | Fluoride Adjusted Allowance*

Water fluoride, ppm	Adjustment, mg NaF/day	Allowance, mg F/day
0.0	2.2	1.0
0.2	1.8	0.8
0.4	1.3	0.6
0.6	0.9	0.4

* From *Accepted Dental Therapeutics*, 35th ed., American Dental Association, Chicago, 1973–1974, p. 241.

Table 20-4 | Food and Nutrition Board, National Academy of Sciences—National Research Council Recommended Daily Dietary Allowances,[1] Revised 1974
(Designed for the maintenance of good nutrition of practically all healthy people in the U.S.A.)

	Age, yr From up to	Weight, (kg)	Weight, (lb)	Height, (cm)	Height, (in)	Energy, (kcal)[2]	Protein, (g)	Fat-soluble vitamins Vitamin A activity, (RE)[3]	Vitamin A activity, (IU)	Vitamin D, (IU)	Vitamin E activity,[5] (IU)
Infants	0.0–0.5	6	14	60	24	kg × 117	kg × 2.2	420[4]	1400	400	4
	0.5–1.0	9	20	71	28	kg × 108	kg × 2.0	400	2000	400	5
Children	1–3	13	28	86	34	1300	23	400	2000	400	7
	4–6	20	44	110	44	1800	30	500	2500	400	9
	7–10	30	66	135	54	2400	36	700	3300	400	10
Males	11–14	44	97	158	63	2800	44	1000	5000	400	12
	15–18	61	134	172	69	3000	54	1000	5000	400	15
	19–22	67	147	172	69	3000	54	1000	5000	400	15
	23–50	70	154	172	69	2700	56	1000	5000		15
	51+	70	154	172	69	2400	56	1000	5000		15
Females	11–14	44	97	155	62	2400	44	800	4000	400	12
	15–18	54	119	162	65	2100	48	800	4000	400	12
	19–22	58	128	162	65	2100	46	800	4000	400	12
	23–50	58	128	162	65	2000	46	800	4000		12
	51+	58	128	162	65	1800	46	800	4000		12
Pregnant						+300	+30	1000	5000	400	15
Lactating						+500	+20	1200	6000	400	15

[1] The allowances are intended to provide for individual variations among most normal persons as they live in the United States under usual environmental stresses. Diets should be based on a variety of common foods in order to provide other nutrients for which human requirements have been less well defined. See text for more detailed discussion of allowances and of nutrients not tabulated.
[2] Kilojoules (KJ) = 4.2 × kcal.
[3] Retinol equivalents.

or where the soil is deficient in iodine, iodine is readily available as iodized salt at the grocery store and should be used instead of plain salt in seasoning foods.

RECOMMENDED DIETARY DAILY ALLOWANCES (RDA)

The Food and Nutrition Board, National Academy of Sciences–National Research Council has developed over the years a recommended daily dietary allowance intended to provide guidelines for selected essential nutrients to be adequate in the maintenance of good nutrition in persons in the United States. These allowances are intended to provide for individual variations among most normal persons as they live under usual environmental stresses. Table 20-4 lists the essential nutrients required to promote normal growth and development and to satisfy the physical, mental, and physiologic needs of an individual in good health. It is to be noted that guides are provided for different age periods, for men and women, and for females during pregnancy and lactation. For example, during these periods in a woman's life, the recommended daily dietary allowances are increased for calories, protein, most vitamins, calcium, phosphorus, iodine, iron, magnesium, and zinc. There may be other circumstances during a female's life when increases in specific nutrients may be desirable, such as when taking birth control pills. Mead Johnson and Company (1972), one of the manufacturers of these pills, has recommended the need for increased vitamin B and C as well as zinc to maintain nutritional balance. With any unusual medication or condition, the physician should be consulted.

The Recommended Daily Dietary Allowances is an excellent source of information for the use of the specialist nutritionist. In the dental office,

Water-soluble vitamins							Minerals					
Ascorbic acid (mg)	Folacin,[6] (µg)	Niacin[7], (mg)	Riboflavin, (mg)	Thiamin, (mg)	Vitamin B_6, (mg)	Vitamin B_{12}, (µg)	Calcium, (mg)	Phosphorus, (mg)	Iodine, (µg)	Iron, (mg)	Magnesium, (mg)	Zinc, (mg)
35	50	5	0.4	0.3	0.3	0.3	360	240	35	10	60	3
35	50	8	0.6	0.5	0.4	0.3	540	400	45	15	70	5
40	100	9	0.8	0.7	0.6	1.0	800	800	60	15	150	10
40	200	12	1.2	0.9	0.9	1.5	800	800	80	10	200	10
40	300	16	1.1	1.2	1.2	2.0	800	800	110	10	250	10
45	400	18	1.5	1.4	1.6	3.0	1200	1200	130	18	350	15
45	400	20	1.8	1.5	2.0	3.0	1200	1200	150	18	400	15
45	400	20	1.8	1.5	2.0	3.0	800	800	140	10	350	15
45	400	18	1.6	1.4	2.0	3.0	800	800	130	10	350	15
45	400	16	1.5	1.2	2.0	3.0	800	800	110	10	350	15
45	400	16	1.3	1.2	1.6	3.0	1200	1200	115	18	300	15
45	400	14	1.4	1.1	2.0	3.0	1200	1200	115	18	300	15
45	400	14	1.4	1.1	2.0	3.0	800	800	100	18	300	15
45	400	13	1.2	1.0	2.0	3.0	800	800	100	18	300	15
45	400	12	1.1	1.0	2.0	3.0	800	800	80	10	300	15
60	800	+2	+0.3	+0.3	2.5	4.0	1200	1200	125	18[8]	450	20
80	600	+4	+0.5	+0.3	2.5	4.0	1200	1200	150	18	450	25

[4] Assumed to be all as retinol in milk during the first six months of life. All subsequent intakes are assumed to be one-half as retinol and one-half as β-carotene when calculated from international units. As retinol equivalents, three-fourths are as retinol and one-fourth as β-carotene.
[5] Total vitamin E activity, estimated to be 80 percent as α-tocopherol and 20 percent other tocopherols. See text for variation in allowances.
[6] The folacin allowances refer to dietary sources as determined by *Lactobacillus casei* assay. Pure forms of folacin may be effective in doses less than one-fourth of the RDA.
[7] Although allowances are expressed as niacin, it is recognized that on the average 1 mg of niacin is derived from each 60 mg of dietary tryptophan.
[8] This increased requirement cannot be met by ordinary diets; therefore, the use of supplemental iron is recommended.

M _____ Diet Evaluation Summary _____
       (patient)   (Date)

Food Groups	1st day	2d day	3d day	4th day	5th day	Average per day	Recommended Amounts			Difference
							Child	Adolescent	Adult	
Milk Group (Milk, Cheese)							3 to 4 servings	4 or more servings	2 servings	
Meat Group (meat, fish, chicken, egg, dried peas, or beans)							2 or more servings			
Vegetable-fruit group Total servings (Including those rich in Vitamin C & Vitamin A)							4 or more servings 1 serving daily 1 serving every other day			
Bread-cereal group Enriched or whole grain							4 or more servings			

Sweets intake

Form	When eaten	1st day	2d day	3d day	4th day	5th day	Total number of exposures
Sugar in solution	During meal						
	End of meal						
	Between meals						
Solid and retentive sweets	During meal						
	End of meal						
	Between meals						
						Grand total	

Department of Preventive Dentistry
School of Dentistry   Dr. _____
The University of North Carolina
at Chapel Hill

however, the use of *food guides* in a diet evaluation form (Fig. 20-1) is an important tool to help communicate information regarding the types and amounts of foods required daily to supply the necessary nutrients in adequate amounts for good nutrition. Food guides also help in that many people think in terms of food rather than nutrients and these guides help in selecting the kinds and amounts of food to be included in the daily diet. The guide most universally used in the United States contains four food groups—milk group, meat group, vegetable-fruit group, and bread-cereal group. The vegetable-fruit group has two subgroups which record those fruits and vegetables that are high in vitamin C and vitamin A content. These four food groups form the protective or foundation foods. If two servings of the milk group, two servings of the meat group, four of the vegetable-fruit group, and four of the bread-cereal group are eaten daily, the individual will receive approximately 1250 calories and 75 to 100 percent of all other major essential nutrients except iron.

MILK GROUP
(TWO SERVINGS A DAY)

The milk group provides two-thirds of the daily calcium, one-half of the riboflavin (B_2), and one-quarter of the daily protein needs. It is low in ascorbic acid (vitamin C) and iron. These foods may be taken as whole or evaporated milk, butter, yoghurt, dry milk, cheese, or ice cream. Milk from which the fat has been removed should be fortified with vitamins A and D; otherwise, it has the same nutrient value as whole milk. A serving is 8 oz of milk or a 1 in cube of cheddar cheese. A dish of 8 oz of ice cream is equal to one-half serving, and one-half cup of cottage cheese is equal to one-third cup of milk.

Figure 20-1 | Diet evaluation summary.

Different allowances of the nutrients found in this group are required during certain age periods (childhood and adolescence) and by females during pregnancy and lactating periods. Additional sources of calcium other than milk and milk products can be found in the Appendix.

MEAT GROUP
(TWO SERVINGS A DAY)

The meat group supplies protein, niacin, iron, some vitamin A, thiamine (B_1), and riboflavin (B_2); the cost of foods in this group is not related to their food value. These nutrients are found in beef, lamb, veal, pork, fish, poultry, eggs, nuts, and dried beans or peas. The last two sources are a most economical source of protein, but because they are incomplete proteins must be eaten with a mixture of vegetables or with small amounts of meat. For example, chili con carne, franks and beans, pea soup and ham are economical as well as good sources of total protein.

A serving is 2 to 3 oz of meat that is lean and cooked with all fat, gristle, and bone removed. A small amount should be eaten with each meal. Also, 2 eggs, 1 cup cooked dried beans or peas, or 4 tablespoonsful of peanut butter can be counted as a serving.

VEGETABLE-FRUIT GROUP
(FOUR SERVINGS A DAY)

One of the four servings a day of this group should be a food high in vitamin C, because vitamin C is a water-soluble vitamin and the body is incapable of storing it. This group contains such vitamins as A and C and almost every other nutrient even though they may be present in small amounts. The vegetable-fruit group also provides sensory pleasure when eating and, because it is the primary source of indigestible cellulose, regulates the alimentary excretory process. This group contains very few calories

FOOD INTAKE DIARY

of: _____
(Name)

For the five days (include one weekend day or a holiday)

_____
Dates (period covered)

Instructions

1. Please record in detail everything you eat or drink. This includes between-meal snacks, candies, gum, as well as regular meals.
2. The following should be included:
   a. The kind of food.
   b. The approximate amount in household measures, 1 cup (8 oz).
   c. The preparation (raw, cooked, fried, etc.).
   d. The order in which they are eaten at the meal.
   e. The number of teaspoons of sugar or sugar products eaten as well as milk added to cereal, beverages or other foods.
3. Particular information is essential on the time and frequency that between-meal snacks are eaten.

First Day

Food: Quantity: Prepared:

Breakfast

Between Meals
(Indicate time)

Lunch

Between Meals
(Indicate time)

Dinner

Between Meals
(Indicate time)

Fifth Day

Food: Quantity: Prepared:

Breakfast

Between Meals
(Indicate time)

Lunch

Between Meals
(Indicate time)

Dinner

Between Meals
(Indicate time)

Section on Preventive Dentistry   School of Dentistry   The University of North Carolina at Chapel Hill

(215 per pound) and is an important group for persons who are overweight.

Color is a guide to the nutrient value of foods in this group; the deeper the color, the more the nutrient value. Using this rule of thumb, carrots have more nutrients than corn, and spinach is better than celery.

A serving is considered to be one-half cup of the fruit or vegetable eaten or a portion as it is the custom to eat—an apple, a half grapefruit, an orange, a banana.

Two vitamins found in this group are of particular importance and are listed as subgroups within the group. These are vitamins C and A. Vitamin C recommended daily dietary allowance is 45 mg. This is best supplied by a serving of citrus fruit, mangos, cabbage, cole slaw, collards, broccoli, strawberries, peppers, potato, tomato or tomato juice, watermelon, or asparagus. Vitamin A is found in carrots, greens, broccoli, apricots, watermelon, squash, pumpkin, and sweet potato. (See Appendix for foods high in vitamins C and A.) For a more complete listing of the nutritive value of most foods you are referred to *Composition of Foods; Agriculture Handbook No. 8,* U.S. Department of Agriculture. It may be purchased from the U.S. Government Printing Office, Washington, D.C., 20402.

BREAD-CEREAL GROUP (FOUR SERVINGS A DAY)

This is the energy group. It is the most economical source of nutrients in our diet and as much as 50 percent of the daily energy needs come from breads and cereals. The whole grains of wheat, rice, corn, rye, oats, and barley provide not only energy but also are a good source of vitamin B and iron. When these grains are milled to provide flour to suit our acquired oral tactile sense,

Figure 20-2 | Food intake diary.

most of the nutrients found in the bran and germ of the grain are removed. The U.S. Food and Drug Administration has set standards for the amount of iron and vitamin B that must be added to the milled flour for it to be labeled *enriched.*

A serving is one slice of bread, one-half cup of cereal, grits, macaroni, rice, or spaghetti. Nizel (1972) has recommended that an individual should have bread or cereal at each meal and at some meals both; milk at each meal for children and at two meals for adults; vegetable-fruits at each meal and meats or a source of protein at each meal. This balance of a diet would provide all the nutrients required at the cellular level and all the energy for physical, mental, and physiologic function.

DIET EVALUATION

In the prevention of dental disease, diet and nutrition have an importance equal to plaque control. To evaluate patients' diets requires techniques of interviewing, teaching, and counseling and must be related to patients' *problems* which they *participate* in solving and to a diet which is *personalized* to their own food preferences. Dietary evaluation begins with an assessment of the patients' health history to ascertain whether a nutritional inadequacy can be attributed to a dietary deficiency or a systemic disorder. In the dental office we most usually are concerned with the former resulting from a lack of knowledge or poor eating habits. The first step in dietary evaluation utilized the skills of *interview.* A food intake diary (Fig. 20-2) should be provided to the patients, and they should be asked to record in detail everything they eat or drink for 5 days. It is important that they include the approximate amount, how it was prepared, and the order in which it was eaten. For example, it would be improper to write "sandwich, drink, and dessert" for lunch. The type of sandwich should be described in detail, i.e., one-quarter lb hamburger on hamburger bun with mayonnaise, slice of tomato, lettuce, and piece of cheese; iced tea with sugar; chocolate sundae. If soft drinks are consumed, the quantity and brand name should be added. If a salad is part of a meal, it is necessary to know if it was a gelatin salad, fruit salad, or tossed salad. Even the type of fruit and contents of the salad should be recorded. The time of eating all between-meal snacks should be indicated, and such items as chewing gum, breath mints, medicine, vitamins, lozenges, snacks, and drinks should be time-related.

When patients are reappointed, the meeting should take place in a consultation room not a dental operatory. The dental operatory is a treatment room, and from past experience patients expect to be passive there while you do something for them. In providing patients with a dietary evaluation, you must make them be aware of their problems, participate in their solution, and prescribe a diet for themselves which they will agree to eat. They must do something; they must get involved. The dental operatory, therefore, places the dietary evaluation therapist at a psychologic disadvantage.

The patients should be put at ease and talked to on their level. Listen to them; don't cut them off. Through *interviewing* techniques get as much information about their daily routine and the underlying reasons for this routine. Make them feel important and talk with them; not at them. You must have the patient's confidence, because the basis of this session is truth.

When you reach a point where you feel you have accumulated sufficient information to help your patients make intelligent decisions about changes in their diet, you must switch from interviewing to *teaching* techniques. They may already know many facts about nutrition, diet, and their relationship to general and oral health. If this is so, reinforce this knowledge; if not, provide them with a brief but understandable explanation of which nutrients are found in each of the food groups and the function of these nutrients in maintaining their health and well-being.

Using many of the same techniques as were used in motivation for plaque control (Chap. 19), emphasize these nutrient functions toward reasons that are important to the patients. Proceed slowly and invite questions; get patients involved in their learning process because they will learn best when they become participants in this process. When you have transmitted to them what you want them to know about nutrients, the next step in dietary evaluation is *counseling*.

Place the diet evaluation summary form (Fig. 20-1) and food intake diary (Fig. 20-2) in front of the patients and have *them* transpose from their food intake diary to the evaluation form the record of the foods they said they ate during the 5-day period. For example, if on the first day of keeping the diet diary they list their food intake as below, the food intake should be recorded on the Diet Evaluation Summary as indicated. Help them by suggesting the group to which the food belongs and whether or not credit should be given for a full or partial serving. When all foods from the diary have been recorded, total each group separately and divide by 5 to obtain the "average" number of servings per day. When this has been completed, have the patients record under "difference" the discrepancy between their average intake per day and the recommended number of servings per day. You have now reached a critical point in this session in that your patients have been shown deficiencies in their way of life. Do not criticize; do not create a situation wherein the patients may become antagonistic or rebellious; do not deflate their egos. Make it clear that this session is to help them toward good health and emphasize their assets and the good points of their diet. Many patients will become defensive and state that the week their food intake was recorded was an unusual week not at all typical of their normal diet. Agree with them but suggest that the session continue and that if they wish to repeat the process during a "normal" week, you will do so in the future.

The tone of the session now reverts to the

First Day

Food	Quantity	Prepared	Group
Breakfast			
Grapefruit	½	Fresh	1 mark vegetable or fruit (vitamin C)
Eggs	2	Fried	1 mark meat
Toast and jelly	2		2 marks bread-cereal
Milk	1 glass		1 mark milk
Between meals (indicate time)			
10 A.M. coffee—sugar			
Doughnut	1		1 mark bread-cereal
11 A.M. gum	1 stick		
Lunch			
Cheeseburger	1		1 mark meat; ½ mark milk
Roll	1		2 marks bread-cereal
Tossed salad, lettuce, oil dressing			1 mark vegetable or fruit
Iced tea—sugar			
Between meals (indicate time)			
2 P.M. apple			1 mark vegetable or fruit
3:30 coke			
Dinner			
Carrot salad	1	Fresh	1 mark vegetable or fruit (vitamin A)
Steak	8 oz	Broiled	2 marks meat
Potato	1		1 mark vegetable or fruit
Asparagus	½ cup		1 mark vegetable or fruit
Coffee—sugar			
Between meals (indicate time)			
10:30 milk,	1 glass		1 mark milk
apple pie	1 piece		1 mark bread-cereal
			1 mark vegetable or fruit

teaching component once again. Early in the preventive dentistry visits you had taught the patients the interrelationships of bacteria, resistance, and diet (Chap. 19). It now becomes necessary to single out those foods in the diet that are particularly conducive to plaque formation—sucrose and in some instances retentive forms of the monosaccharides. The process of dental-disease infection should be reviewed, as should the fact that among all foods sucrose is most responsible for plaque formation and for activation of bacteria within the plaque. This activation produces those substances which infect the teeth with their acids or the soft tissue with their toxins and enzymes. To make this explanation more meaningful to the patients they should be told that sugar in solution and sugar in a solid or retentive form causes bacterial activity of varying lengths and, therefore, insults to the tissue for varying periods of time. They should be informed that sucrose may be a source of quick energy and calories but that it has no other nutritive value. It is frequently consumed in such quantities that other more nutritious foods are not eaten which could result in a nutritional deficiency.

The patients are asked to return to the food intake diary and circle in red all foods containing sucrose and those monosaccharides that are retentive—dried figs, dates, raisins. Help them to recognize not only the obvious sources of sugar in coffee, tea, and soft drinks, but also those hidden sugars in such foods as presweetened cereals, chewing gum, breath mints, desserts, canned fruits and juices, cookies, cakes, pies, antacids, crackers, and snack foods. Now have your patients go back to the diet evaluation summary and with each sugar input place a mark in the proper box after first determining whether it was sugar in solution or in a retentive form and if it was eaten during the meal, at the end of meal, or between meals. The sweets intake of the previous sample diet would be recorded as follows:

First day

Food	Quantity	Prepared	Group
Breakfast			
Grapefruit	½	Fresh	
Eggs	2	Fried	
Toast and (jelly)	2		1 mark, retentive sweets, during meal
Milk	1 glass		
Between meals (Indicate time)			
10 A.M. coffee—(sugar)			1 mark, sugar in solution, between meals
(Doughnut)	1		1 mark, retentive sweets, between meals
11 A.M. (gum)	1 stick		1 mark, retentive sweets, between meals
Lunch			
Cheeseburger	1		
Roll	1		
Tossed salad, lettuce, oil dressing			
Iced tea—(sugar)			1 mark, sugar in solution, end of meal
Between meals (Indicate time)			
2 P.M. apple			
3:30 (coke)			1 mark, sugar in solution, between meals
Dinner			
Carrot salad	1	Fresh	
Steak	8 oz	Broiled	
Potato	1	Baked	
Asparagus	½ cup	Steamed	
Coffee—(sugar)			1 mark, sugar in solution, end of meal
Between meals (Indicate time)			
10:30 milk,	1 glass		
(apple pie)	1 piece		1 mark, retentive sweets, between meals

Add the total number of exposures in each category. Then multiply the total number of exposures of sugar in solution by 20 minutes. Do the same for solid and retentive sweets, but multiply by 40 minutes. When these two time totals are added together, you can provide an approximate but meaningful number of minutes that the patients insulted their oral structures through their diet and which in most instances provided no nutritive input to their health. For example, on the sample presented there were four sweets intakes in solution and four retentive sweets intakes. According to our formula $4 \times 20 = 80$ minutes of plaque activity caused by sweets in solution and $4 \times 40 = 160$ minutes of plaque activation caused by solid and retentive sweets, or a total of 240 minutes (4 hours) on this day in which the teeth and soft tissues were being insulted by bacterial action. You are now ready to proceed to the next stage in dietary evaluation by writing a *diet prescription.*

DIET PRESCRIPTION

Food habits are acquired through the years in almost an unconscious manner. They are the total sum of cultural, social, and economic influences as well as emotional and physiologic experiences. Add to this a person's attitudes, likes, and dislikes, and you must realize that providing the patient with a preprinted unpersonalized diet recommendation won't usually work. The diet recommendations must be *personalized* and must contain foods that the patient will eat. The patient is the best person to do this. Fig. 20-3 is an example of a diet prescription which patients must fill out with your help.

Have them write down under "Continue Eating" those foods that contributed to good nutrition from *their* food intake diary. Next have them refer to the diet evaluation summary and in those groups where a deficiency occurred, choose foods of their liking that satisfy the nutrient requirements of the food group. At this point you might help them by suggesting foods about which they might not have nutritional knowledge. For example, if they were deficient in the vitamin-C group and don't like citrus fruits, you might explore their likes or dislikes of such foods as brussel sprouts, cabbage, broccoli, cauliflower, lamb, liver, parsley, or tomatoes, all of which are good sources of vitamin C. The Appendix contains lists of foods high in vitamin C, vitamin A, and calcium. It also contains a list of hidden sugars as well as snack suggestions from which your patients may select foods they will eat. Have them record under "Improve the Quality of Your Diet" by adding the foods that supply the food group nutrients which they like and will agree to eat. In the next step have them record those foods that they are willing to give up under "Eliminate the Following Decay-Producing Foods Found in Your Diet." These are in most instances those between-meal snacks that are solid and retentive sweets. Many patients at this point are unwilling to completely eliminate all disease-producing or nutritionally unimportant foods from their diet, and when this occurs, it is better to develop a less than ideal diet prescription than one that they won't follow when they leave.

Your patients have now provided you with a listing of those foods that they eat and are nutritionally important and a list of those foods that were not in their food intake diary, but which they like and which would fulfill the requirements of the *Recommended Dietary Daily Allowances.* Using these foods as a nucleus, have your patients now write out breakfast, lunch, and dinner menus. These menus are *personalized;* they meet *their* needs; they provide solutions of *their* problems.

An additional responsibility and need you must fulfill is that of substituting for the undesirable snack food that your patients have agreed to eliminate from their diet with a snack food that is acceptable. The after-school snack, coffee

An Evaluation of Your Diet and Nutritional Status Suggests	A Suggested Menu to Suit Your Individual Tastes and Dental Needs
Continue eating:	Breakfast
Improve the quality of your diet by:	or
	Lunch
Eliminate the following decay producing foods found in your diet:	
	or
Use the following substitutes:	Dinner
a. Raw fruits, grapefruit, oranges, peaches, pears, pineapple, tangerines.	
b. Raw vegetables, carrots, celery, cucumbers, lettuce, salad greens and tomatoes.	or
c. Unsweetened fruit juices, tomato or vegetable juices.	
d. Milk.	Extras
e. Cheese, hard or soft varieties (Cheddar, cream or cottage).	
f. Nuts, all kinds.	
g. Combinations of above.	

Figure 20-3 | Food intake instruction for better oral health.

break, and television commercial lull are examples of habit patterns brought about by our social and cultural development. Another similiar habit pattern is gum chewing. In most instances the habit or desire is too ingrained to eliminate completely, and the solution depends on substitution. With gum chewing, the use of a sugarless gum is usually a readily acceptable solution.

With other snacking, suggestions of suitable substitutes should be provided to the patients, and they should be allowed to choose those snacks which are pleasing to them (see Appendix). Lists of nonsucrose foods, such as raw fruits and vegetables, unsweetened fruit juices, and in some instances artifically sweetened soft drinks, milk, cheese, nuts, or combinations of these, should be given to them for home reference. Such a list will go a long way in helping them solve their between-meal snacking problem.

Dietary evaluation doesn't stop with this visit. As with plaque control, modification of habits is not a dental problem but a psychologic one. Long-term motivation with behavioral change depends on solving problems that are important to the patient (see Chap 19). Each time the patients return for restorative care or for a recall appointment, they should not only be evaluated for plaque control but also should be questioned about changes in their dietary habit patterns. They should be made to *feel* your interest in their general and oral health. Once a high-trust–low-fear relationship is established and the patients' visits to you are on an adult-to-adult relationship rather than a treatment–passive patient relationship, you will have made an immeasurable contribution to your patients' total health care.

BIBLIOGRAPHY

Becks, H.: "Carbohydrate Restriction in the Prevention of Dental Caries Using the L. A. Count as One Index," *J. Calif. Dent. Assoc.,* **26:**53, 1950.

Bibby, B. G.: "The Cariogenicity of Snack Foods and Confections," *J. Am. Dent. Assoc.,* **90:**121–132, 1975.

Gustafsson, R., et al.: "The Vipeholm Dental Caries Study," *Acta Odontol. Scand.,* **11:**232, 1954.

Hanke, M. T.: *Diet and Dental Health,* The University of Chicago Press, Chicago, Ill., 1933.

Jay, P., Beeuwkes, A., and Macdonald, H.: *Dietary Program in the Control of Dental Caries,* The Overbeck Co., Ann Arbor, Mich., 1959.

Mead Johnson and Company: "Oral Contraceptives and Your Nutrition," 1972, p. 406.

Nizel, A.: *Nutrition in Preventive Dentistry: Science and Practice,* W. B. Saunders Company, Philadelphia, 1972, pp. 3, 27.

Stephan, R. M.: "Effects of Different Types of Human Foods on Dental Health in Experimental Animals," *J. Dent. Res.,* **45:**1551, 1966.

21

Matthew T. Wood

First Aid

INTRODUCTION

The dental office is not usually thought of as a place where emergency conditions may arise which could be vital to the subsequent welfare of a patient's total health. However, it is a fact that unforeseen problems do arise and accidents do occur wherever people assemble. Regardless of how serene and tranquil the environment of a dental office may seem, an emergency situation may arise which will require immediate recognition and prompt action if an unfortunate outcome is to be avoided.

It has been reported that the incidence of emergencies in the dental office is increasing due to several factors that possibly did not exist in the past. The use of ultraspeed rotary instruments for routine operations has often set the stage for a variety of mishaps which may not only be injurious to the patient but which may also endanger the dentist or the dental assistant. There are an increasing number of elderly patients in the average dental practice who are often more susceptible to stressful situations than younger patients. Common drug therapy, which by design is meant to be helpful, is capable of producing hidden side effects that may result in reactions of a serious nature when the patients are subjected to routine dental procedures. By the very nature of many dental practices, patient appointments are quite lengthy due to necessity for accomplishing a complex treatment program; this may overtax the patient's ability to remain comfortable throughout the procedure (McCarthy, 1965).

The concept of first aid in the dental office is

not a new subject by any means and there is often a narrow border line where first aid ends and bona fide medical treatment begins. Due to increasing claims of negligence in emergency situations and the moral obligation of the dental team to be prepared to manage their patients in the best possible manner, it is mandatory that dental personnel be knowledgeable of the prevention, differential assessment, and proper treatment of emergency states.

Increased utilization of ancillary personnel in the dental office has placed the responsibility for an awareness of emergency problems squarely on the shoulders of the dental assistant. It is the purpose of this chapter to clearly define the role of the dental assistants in such problem situations so they may be better prepared to cope with needs as they arise.

GENERAL CONSIDERATIONS

First aid is the emergency care, given an injured or sick individual, which is intended to be a helpful or preventive measure until the services of the dentist or of a physician can be obtained. Every dental assistant should know the principles of first aid and must be prepared to offer competent assistance to a needy individual. Although each episode presents its own unique problems, there are some general considerations which apply to practically all situations. A thorough understanding of the following rules before trying to master more specific first-aid or emergency treatment is recommended.

1. Seek the aid of the dentist or a physician immediately or as soon as possible.
2. Remain as quiet and calm as you can during an emergency. Carry out your first-aid procedures quickly but do not rush around in a frantic manner.
3. Do not waste valuable time looking for first-aid materials and items that are not readily available; do the best you can with what is at hand.
4. Keep the patient lying down in a comfortable position, the head level with the body, until the seriousness of the condition is determined.
5. Appraisal of signs and symptoms of asphyxiation (impaired breathing), hemorrhage (serious bleeding), shock, and circulatory disorders are most important since these conditions may require supportive breathing from a mechanical source or other prompt actions to maintain life.
6. Tight clothing about the patient's neck, waist, and legs should be loosened.
7. Never administer liquids by mouth to an unconscious patient since the swallowing mechanism is not efficient. It is of the utmost importance to maintain a patent airway and at the same time prevent aspiration of liquids.
8. Treat injuries in order of their importance: first, asphyxiation; second, hemorrhage; third, shock.
9. If the patient is vomiting, turn the head to one side to prevent choking.
10. Do not touch an open wound with bare hands unless the emergency requires you to do so.
11. Try to maintain the body temperature of the patient within relatively normal limits.
12. Do not attempt to move an emergency patient unless it is of absolute necessity.
13. Do your utmost to keep the patient as comfortable as possible, to minimize pain, and to reduce anxiety.
14. Most important of all, realize that it is best to defer any definitive treatment until you are sure of the primary problems.

In general, it is not wise to try to perform or administer treatment which is beyond your knowledge and training. Subsequently in this chapter, you will find information which may enable you to go somewhat beyond the ordinary limits of first-aid treatment (Bureau of Naval Personnel, 1955).

PREVENTIVE MEASURES

In 1967, a report was published which furnished information relative to the safety of the practice of dentistry and the mortality rate in dental offices in a specific geographical area. This report made several constructive recommendations toward the management and prevention of emergencies and deaths in the dental office. Of more importance, the report reflected a significant and apparent unpreparedness of some dentists to treat emergencies. It was noted that members of the dental team should be made more aware of the possibility of complications due to foreign-body accidents, drug reactions, anaphylactic shock, management of the airway, and cardiopulmonary resuscitation (Bell, 1967).

General Care of the Patient

Prior to rendering initial dental treatment to a new patient, or treatment to a former patient seeking treatment following a lengthy absence from the dental office, information should be sought relative to general health status. It is unwise to assume that background information about the patient is unnecessary even though you may be knowledgeable of the patient as a friend or from other nonprofessional contacts.

Without exception, a definite routine whereby the patient is received into the practice should be established, primarily to ensure proper management and treatment of the patient's physical problems.

History

Each patient in the dental office should, by standard procedure, be required to answer certain questions relative to medical history. If the patient is to undergo any operative procedure which will require the use of a local or general anesthetic, there is absolutely no excuse for this information not being available. If the patient is not an adult, the information should be obtained from the parents prior to performing any procedures.

There are several ways the information desired may be obtained, but the most efficient manner seems to be by the utilization of a printed form (Fig. 21-1). After completion of this form, it should be reviewed for preliminary evaluation. Questionable points should be reviewed further in a more specific manner to determine if the dentist should proceed or is willing to accept the responsibility for the patient's welfare. In the event a question does arise which is beyond the capabilities of the dentist to assess, the patient should be told and the matter referred to a physician for clearance (McCarthy, 1967b).

Arterial Blood Pressure

Screening dental patients for hypertension should be adopted as routine function of a modern dental practice. The data gained during periodic checks should be recorded and therefore become an important body of information in the dental record. It is well documented that hypertension, often an undiagnosed disease, is a primary cause of premature death. Hypertension can lead to stroke, kidney failure, and congestive heart failure and may be a major risk factor in coronary artery disease. Hypertension is easy to detect, diagnose, and treat in most instances. The resulting proper control of hypertensive patients greatly decreases the levels of morbidity and mortality (Berman, 1976).

The systemic arterial blood pressure reflects cardiac output and peripheral resistance of the circulatory system. It is measured by an indirect means utilizing a sphygmomanometer which is composed of a blood pressure cuff and a manometer. A stethoscope is also utilized for the purpose of hearing the blood flow within the artery while the sphygmomanometer is operating. This method is termed *recording blood pressure by auscultation* (Fig. 21-2).

The systolic pressure is that pressure when the heart is in the pumping phase of the beat, and the diastolic pressure is considered to be that pressure when the heart is at rest. The systolic pressure is recorded first, and the diastolic pressure is recorded last. For instance, when the systolic pressure measures 120 mm and the diastolic pressure measures 80 mm, the patient's

Date **3 Aug 1970**

Mr. **John M. Daniels** Home phone **942-6312** Office phone **942-1468**
Date of birth **9 Jan. 1920** Age **50** Home address **902 Hickory Court** City **Dray, N.C.**
Marital status **M** Spouse's name **Bess M. Daniels** Referred by **self**
Your occupation **clerk** Employer **Dow's Dept. Store**
Employer's address **102 Main Street** City **Dray, N.C.** Years with firm **12**
Spouse's occupation **housewife** Employer ———
Employer's address ——— City ——— Years with firm ———
Person financially responsible **John M. Daniels** Relationship to you ———
Billing address **902 Hickory Court** City **Dray, N.C.** Zip code **27614**
Your physician **Dr. M.I. Fleming** Phone **942-6235** Dental insurance? **No**
Former dentist **Dr. I.F. McGee** Address **302 Branch St., Dray, N.C.**
Your children's names and ages ———

Please "X" each circle if the answer is "yes." Leave blank if "no."

- ☒ Do you prefer to save your teeth
- ☒ Is your general health good

On your previous dental visits . . .
- ☒ Were you given a local anesthetic
- ☒ Were X-rays taken
- ○ Were home instructions given
- ○ Were regular preventive visits made
- ☒ Was there a history of dental decay
- ○ Were there any special problems:
- ○ ———

Is there a sensitivity in your mouth to . . .
- ○ Heat ○ Sweets ☒ Chewing
- ☒ Cold ☒ Biting ○ Previous injury

Do you have a history of . . .
- ○ Nail biting
- ○ Hard swallowing
- ☒ Mouth breathing
- ○ Biting hard objects

Have you had . . .
- ☒ A recent physical exam
- ○ Any heart problems
- ○ High blood pressure
- ○ Low blood pressure
- ○ Circulatory problems
- ○ Nervous problems
- ○ Radiation treatments
- ○ Pain in region of ears
- ○ Excessive bleeding
- ☒ Bleeding gums
- ☒ Food collect between teeth
- ○ Fluoride treatments
- ○ Tooth sensitivity tests
- ○ Allergy to local anesthetics
- ☒ Allergy to antibiotics
- ○ Any other allergies:
- ○ ———

- ☒ Tonsils out
- ☒ Adenoids out
- ○ Anemia
- ○ Arthritis
- ○ Asthma
- ○ Cerebral palsy
- ☒ Chicken pox
- ○ Chronic sinus
- ☒ Diabetes
- ○ Epilepsy
- ○ Malignancies

- ○ Mastoid/ear infection
- ☒ Measles
- ☒ Mumps
- ○ Nephrosis
- ○ Rheumatic fever
- ☒ Scarlet fever
- ○ Thyroid
- ○ Tonsilitis
- ○ Tuberculosis
- ○ ———
- ○ ———

Please describe any current medical treatment, including drugs, impending operations, pregnancies, or other information the doctor should be aware of:

Receives insulin daily

Signature **John M. Daniels**

FORM AQT   COPYRIGHT 1966 BY BLANCHARD & ASSOCIATES • BOX 11701 • PALO ALTO • CALIFORNIA

Figure 21-1 | General information and health questionnaire. (*Courtesy of Blanchard and Associates, Palo Alto, Calif.*)

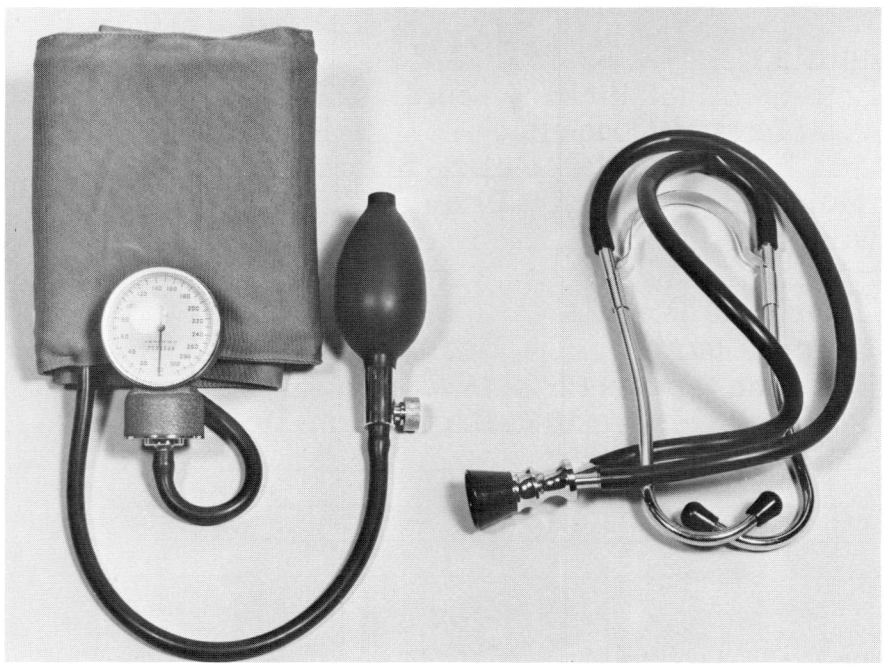

Figure 21-2 | Sphygmomanometer and stethoscope.

blood pressure is recorded as 120/80, which is within the normal range.

The arterial blood pressure can be recorded when the patient is seated in the dental chair. The upper arm should be bare where the blood pressure cuff is to be placed; the forearm should be slightly flexed and supported on the dental-chair arm rest at the same approximate level as the heart.

The deflated blood pressure cuff is applied snugly to the upper arm approximately 2 in above the antecubital fossa. The cuff is inflated, and a preliminary systolic blood pressure reading is taken by palpation by placing two fingers over the radial artery. After the cuff pressure has been rapidly released, it can be noted when the pulse reappears, and this is called the *palpatory systolic pressure* (Fig. 21-3). Next the stethoscope is placed over the brachial artery, and the cuff is inflated to 30 to 40 mm of mercury higher than the previously recorded palpatory systolic pressure. The cuff is gradually deflated at a rate of 2 to 3 mm of mercury per second.

When the first sound is heard through the stethoscope, it is noted as the systolic blood pressure. As the cuff continues to deflate, a muffled sound is heard just before the sound disappears and should be considered as the diastolic pressure (Fig. 21-4).

Blood pressures should be recorded at least on an annual basis, and any deviation from the normal range for a patient should be noted. The patient should be made aware of the condition and referred to his or her physician for appropriate treatment. It is important to impress upon the patient the importance of an appointment with their physician and to find out if indeed the appointment was met (Chue, 1975).

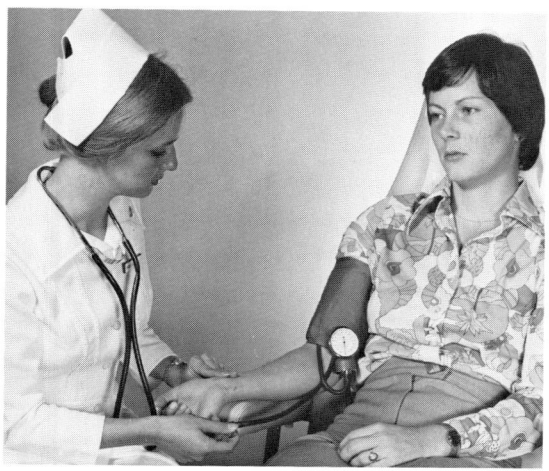

Figure 21-3 | Recording palpatory systolic pressure.

Records

Prior to performing definitive treatment, it is wise to have a written record of at least the areas in the oral cavity to be operated on; it is best to chart the condition of all the structures in the oral

Figure 21-4 | Recording blood pressure by auscultation.

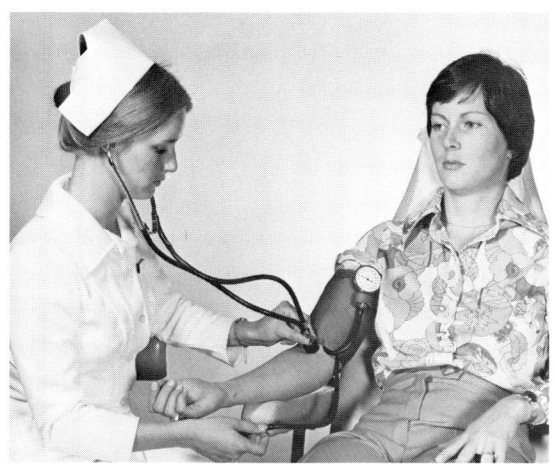

cavity (Fig. 21-5). It is the duty of the dental assistant to assist the dentist in accurately recording this information in a legible and understandable fashion.

Radiographs

Radiographs show conditions that may exist that are not apparent on visual examination and provide the dentist with vital information. In many dental offices, it has become the delegated responsibility of the dental assistant to produce radiographs of acceptable quality and quantity. When operative procedures are instituted without radiographs of good quality, proper concern for the patient has been disregarded and the stage is set for possible unpleasant situations.

Operating Environment

When a patient is receiving dental treatment, what is seen, heard, or smelled during the treatment session may precipitate an unpleasant experience due to needless apprehension. The patient may be considered to be a captive person and is very subject to the power of suggestion. All members of the dental team, through action and words, should refrain from any activity which might cause the patient to be apprehensive.

Dental instruments, such as the syringe and needle used in administering a local anesthetic, should be kept from the sight of the patient in a discreet manner. This is especially important with suture needles and extraction forceps.

In case of profuse hemorrhage from a dental procedure, try to aspirate the oral cavity prior to allowing the patient to rinse or use the cuspidor. Also, when the napkin about the patient's neck becomes stained or an excess of soiled gauze sponges collect, they should be discarded.

In electrosurgical procedures, from which unpleasant odors may result and be a problem, proper and careful manipulation of the high-volume evacuation equipment will aid greatly in

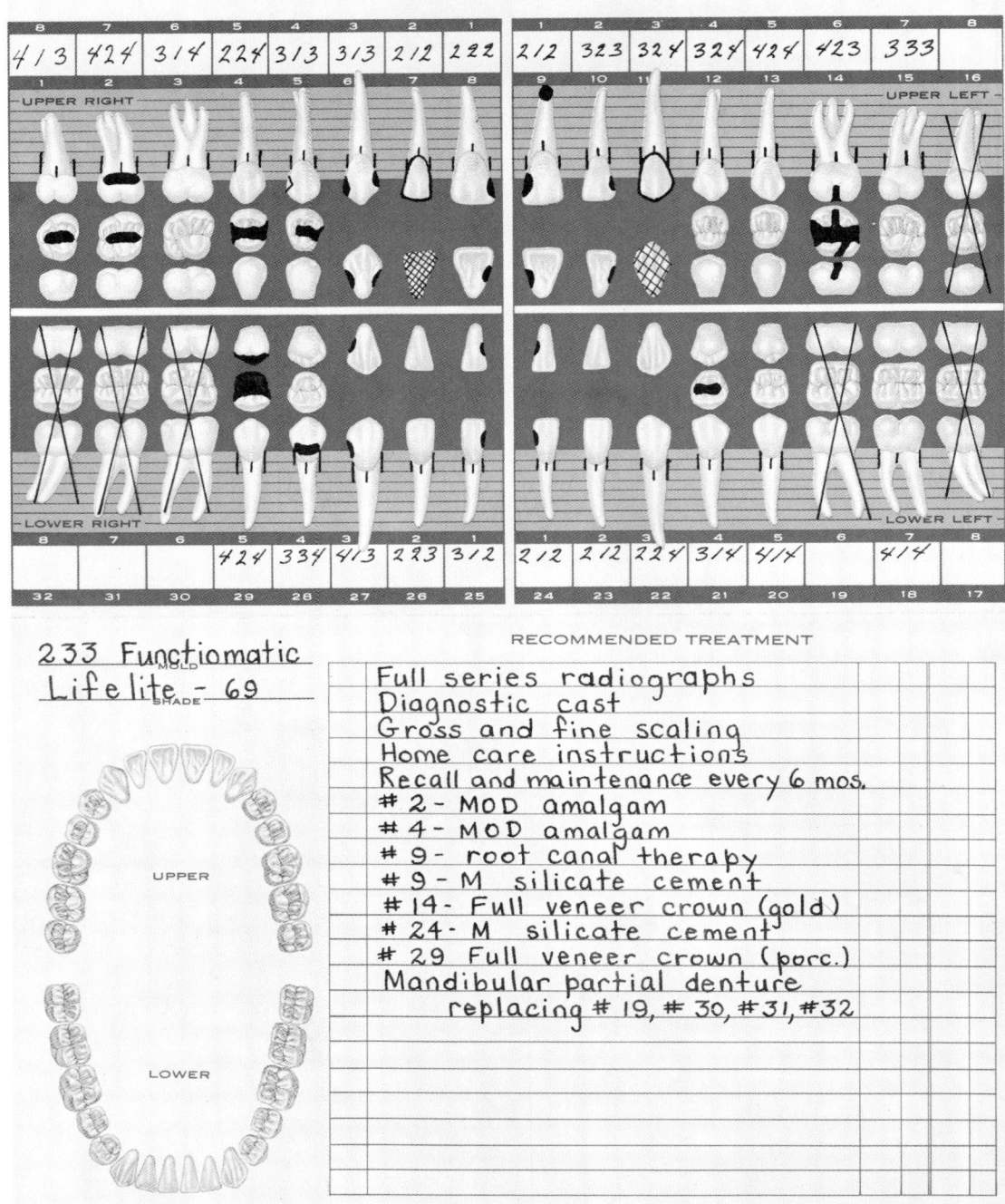

Figure 21-5 | Charting of patient's oral condition. (*Courtesy of Blanchard and Associates, Palo Alto, Calif.*)

the reduction of the odor. At times it may be in order to offer the patient a face mask.

Thoughtless statements made by the members of the dental team during treatment may serve to complicate or hinder an already delicate situation. Statements should not be forewarning of what is to come, but rather should be reassuring. Conversation should prepare the patient with a reasonable explanation of what the nature of the treatment is to be and some idea of how it will be accomplished. It is well established that fear may be reduced in almost any situation when the nature of the problem is reasonably understood.

Always refrain from statements such as these in the presence of a patient:

1. Doctor, where in the world is all this blood coming from?
2. This is the same procedure that caused Mrs. Smith to faint the last time.
3. Did you see that tooth break into three pieces?
4. Oh, I believe you slipped and cut her tongue.
5. Should I have sterilized that instrument before you used it?

In every instance try to reduce apprehension by treating the patients as you would like to be treated (Sheppard, 1965).

Premedication

At times preoperative medication of patients with sedatives is necessary in order to accomplish proper treatment. Premedication is usually indicated when apprehension on the part of the patient is very apparent, or the patient's physical condition dictates the use of drugs. Drugs that may be employed range from mild to extremely potent, depending upon the requirement of the individual patient. The manner in which a patient reacts to a drug may depend on that person's physical and mental condition at that particular time.

Although it is not the duty of the dental assistant to prescribe, dispense, or administer drugs to a patient, it is important that the assistant be aware of several guidelines that should be followed for premedicated patients:

1. Patients who receive premedication should be accompanied by another individual.
2. On arrival at the office, premedicated patients should be received as promptly as possible.
3. Patients who are to receive premedication on arrival at the dental office should receive this drug promptly so as to allow sufficient time for the drug to accomplish its purpose prior to treatment.
4. After a treatment has been completed, premedicated patients should remain in the dental office until it is deemed safe for them to leave by themselves or with the individual who accompanied them.
5. At all times patients receiving drugs should be observed closely and not be left unattended.

Housekeeping

In a busy dental office, efficient organizational routines and habits are absolutely essential. Every item should be in its proper place. Without a doubt, the reduction of "clutter" will aid in the prevention of office accidents. A few suggestions are listed below that may be thought provoking in meeting this goal:

1. Do not leave a dental handpiece hanging over a patient, as it may fall and cause injury to the patient or a member of the dental team.
2. Scatter rugs about the office that a patient or office personnel may slip on should be avoided.
3. An open flame used in a dental procedure should not be held over the patient unless the patient is draped with a proper protective apron.
4. Caustic medicaments such as phenol, acids, or bleaching agents should not be used without draping the patient.
5. Protective glasses to be worn by members of the dental team should be readily available during certain procedures.
6. Sharp-edged or pointed instruments should never be placed near the patient's eyes.
7. The rest room should not become a storage area

for inflammable cleaning agents, caustic, or poison materials since unattended children may tend to investigate these.
8. Proper maintenance of instruments and items with movable parts will allow for these specialized pieces of equipment to function at an optimal level.
9. In laboratory procedures, never take shortcuts at the expense of safety.
10. When patient procedures are completed, restore order to the operatory so that subsequent operations may be carried out efficiently.

PREPAREDNESS FOR EMERGENCIES

Countless hours of training are necessary for the dentist and assistants to learn and become proficient in the numerous and skillful procedures they are required to perform during the course of a routine day in a dental office. By constant practice and setting certain routine standards, the dental team may establish a performance level that results in precise and efficient treatment.

Keep in mind that emergencies are not planned in advance, but occur without warning. When they do occur, the very nature of the situation requires that they be approached with the same finesse and confidence as a routine dental operation. To do this, it is necessary that the dental-office emergency routine be well established and practiced.

Importance of the Assistant

It is not uncommon for a dental assistant to be the first one of the dental team to recognize the early stages of a stressful situation. One reason for this is that often the dental assistant is alone with a patient while the dentist is in another operating room attending to the needs of another patient. Second, a reaction to a local anesthetic, thoughts of a dental procedure, or reaction to a subtle suggestion may be delayed until after the dentist has left the operating area.

It is not expected that the role of the dental assistant during emergency situations should be that of a physician or a medically trained nurse, but it is expected that the assistant be competent to render services in such a manner as to aid the patient in those things which will sustain life in a critical situation (Hooley and Conn, 1966).

Alertness, Awareness, and Responsibility

Only by close observation and careful attention to the more obvious signs and symptoms may a dental assistant realize what is about to take place. Tactful questions directed to the patient may elicit important information relative to the reason for expressed discomfort. In turn, these clues also may offer the key to the prevention of a more stressful episode.

It is the responsibility of the dental assistant to summon the dentist immediately and in a manner so as not to alarm the patient. Actions of a comforting and firm nature may reassure such patients that they are in good hands.

On arrival of the dentist, the signs and symptoms should be expressed clearly and concisely in order to expedite the initiation of necessary treatment (Webster and Wood, 1965).

EMERGENCY ARMAMENTARIUM

Every dental office should have available supplies of drugs, instruments, and equipment which are primarily designated for emergency use. These items should be located in proper and readily accessible places at all times so that they may be located quickly; time is of the essence!

Organization

The emergency armamentarium should be organized in such a manner that it is relatively compact and easily identified (Fig. 21-6). It is unwise to keep these supplies and instruments, particularly the more important ones, loosely arranged in a drawer or cabinet since they may be difficult to locate quickly.

All items that go to make up the emergency armamentarium must be labeled or tagged with information pertinent to their use. Labeling serves as an immediate reference index for obvious reasons.

It is important to remember that some emergency items may have a shelf life which is critical to the potency of a drug or the sterility of an instrument. This requires that the unused or seldom-used items be routinely checked and periodically updated to ensure their reliability (Kruger, 1968).

As previously mentioned, the training of a dentist or a dental assistant by no means qualifies him or her as being as competent or qualified as a physician in dealing with the more complicated medical problems that may arise. For this reason, it is necessary for the dental office to have established procedures for obtaining assistance from physicians and medical facilities in emergency situations. Everyone in the dental office should be aware of these arrangements, and the telephone numbers and addresses of the physicians and medical facilities should be available in an easily visible location on the emergency kit and near the telephone (Fig. 21-7) (Webster and Wood, 1965).

Equipment

Equipment items included in the emergency armamentarium which are of the greatest importance are those associated with the treatment of respiratory difficulty. In cases of respiratory embarrassment, it is necessary to have available a convenient source of oxygen and an apparatus for its administration under pressure (Fig. 21-8). The administration of oxygen, a life-preserving gas, is often the primary and most important definitive treatment that may be necessary for the simpler as well as the most complicated emergencies (Webster and Wood, 1965; Hooley and Conn, 1966). A thorough knowledge of the operation of the equipment and patient management,

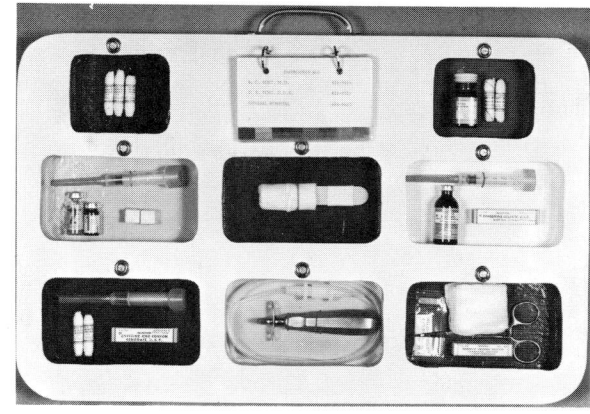

Figure 21-6 | Office emergency kit. (*Courtesy of University of North Carolina, Chapel Hill, N.C.*)

as suggested by the manufacturer, are essential; these procedures should be instituted with confidence and efficiency.

Oxygen-inhalation equipment requires periodic checking and maintenance to ensure its ability to function at all times. The following checklist is suggested:

1. A reserve cylinder of oxygen should always be on hand.
2. The face mask, manual resuscitator bag, and flexible rubber tubing should be free of holes, deforming bends, and dust.
3. The equipment should have a flowmeter and a reducing gauge which can deliver a constant flow of oxygen from the cylinder to the mask.

Other equipment may include a sphygmomanometer and a stethoscope for determining blood pressure.

Instruments

The emergency kit includes a variety of instruments. The selection of these instruments depends upon the types of emergencies for which preparedness is intended. Generally speaking, there is a need for several 2-ml or 3-ml syringes; needles for intravenous and intramuscular injections; tongue depressors wrapped in gauze and tape; needles and suture material; rubber tubing; cricothyreotomy needle; hemostats; metal saw blade; and sterile gauze sponges. Additions to this list, such as an oropharyngeal airway tube (Fig. 21-9), may be made according to the wishes of the individual dentist.

Drugs

Certain categories of drugs, ointments, and medicaments must be readily available. A suggested list of drugs and indications for their use will be described later under treatment procedures.

Regardless of which drugs are selected for use, it is recommended that they be packaged in containers that are easily handled. Liquids or solids that must be dispensed from large or cumbersome containers could delay administration. Drugs in small containers such as Carpules, ampules, and capsules are simpler to administer (Webster and Wood, 1965). (See also Chap. 9, under "Emergency Drugs.")

TREATMENT OF EMERGENCIES

The dental team will be well advised to prepare and rehearse emergency procedures. A simulated emergency drill may answer some of the following questions:

1. Who brings the emergency kit?
2. In what order does the secretary place calls when necessary?
3. Is the assistant capable of loading syringes from ampules or vials?
4. Who puts on the blood pressure cuff?
5. Who operates the oxygen-inhalation equipment?
6. Who does closed chest massage?

If the answers to these questions are not clear, it is obvious that members of the team do not know how to perform their assignments. It should be remembered that once a reaction has

```
         FOR EMERGENCY ASSISTANCE
                   CALL
B. R. WILLIAMS, M.D.           936-4225
S. N. HOLOMAN, D.D.S.          936-1992
GENERAL HOSPITAL               936-1871
```

Figure 21-7 | Available medical contacts.

occurred, attention must be focused on the existing condition of the patient and an appropriate treatment must be administered (Costich, 1966).

Respiratory Difficulty

This type of distress is almost always very important and may indicate serious condition of the patient. Respiratory embarrassment in the dental office may be associated with the swallowing or aspiration of a tooth fragment, cotton, crown, inlay, vomitus, or piece of impression material and may lead to partial or complete respiratory obstruction.

Diagnosis

With a partial obstruction, the patient will usually gag or cough and demonstrate by outward signs that something is lodged in the throat. In instances of a more complete obstruction, there may be noisy breathing or absence of breathing, straining of muscles of the neck and chest, and cyanosis of the skin and mucous membranes. In case of a complete obstruction, the patient may be very violent and almost uncontrollable in an attempt to gain a source of oxygen, and shortly may lose consciousness.

Treatment

When there is partial obstruction, coughing or gagging may cause the object to be expelled. It

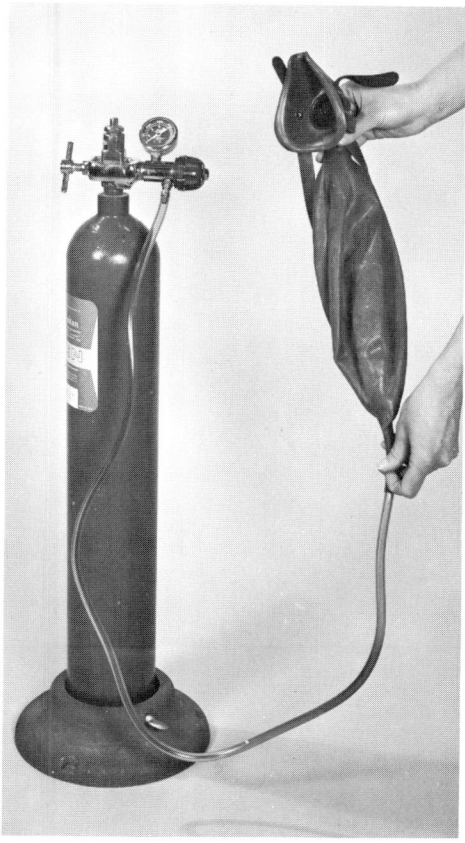

Figure 21-8 | Oxygen-inhalation equipment.

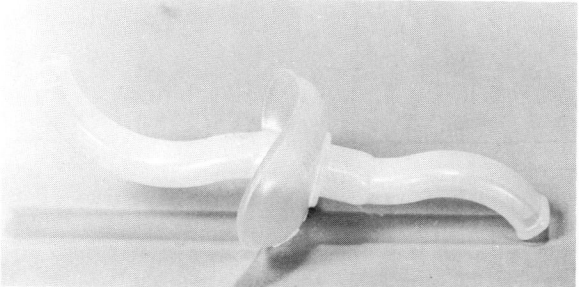

Figure 21-9 | Oropharyngeal airway tube.

of the airway, there are only a few minutes during which treatment must be accomplished, if irreversible brain damage or death is to be prevented. The following steps are recommended:

1. Place patient in supine position.
2. Open patient's mouth, extending the neck and forcing the mandible and tongue forward to facilitate and open airway path.
3. Attempt manually to remove the obstruction.
4. If the object cannot be removed, resort to mouth-to-mouth resuscitation, administration of oxygen with inhalation equipment, or the Heimlich maneuver in an attempt to afford normal respiration.
5. Failure to restore chest movement necessitates immediate surgical opening of the airway by a tracheotomy procedure (Berlove, 1959).

Methods of Resuscitation

There are several accepted methods for offering respiratory support during respiratory distress. They are mouth-to-mouth breathing, utilization of oxygen-inhalation equipment, the Heimlich maneuver, and surgical approaches for creating an airway.

Mouth-to-Mouth Breathing

Mouth-to-mouth resuscitation is recognized as an excellent method for the administration of

may be necessary to have the patient bend forward with head between the knees and to pound on the back to initiate coughing as a means of expelling the foreign object. If the obstruction is to be removed manually, have the patient lie back with the head dropped sharply down and the tongue and mandible extended forward. Use of the fingers, instruments, or suction may be of aid in this situation. Persons who have apparently swallowed objects or aspirated foreign bodies should be referred to a physician for proper management.

When there is severe or complete obstruction

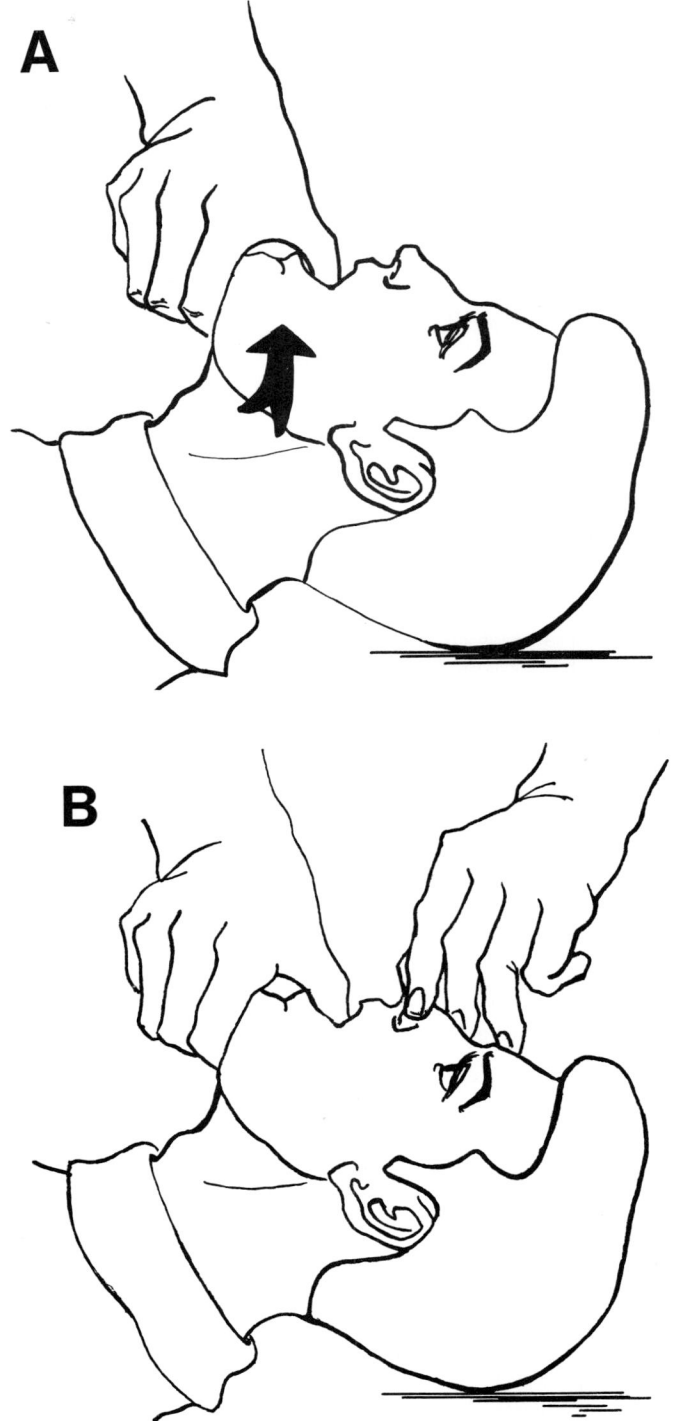

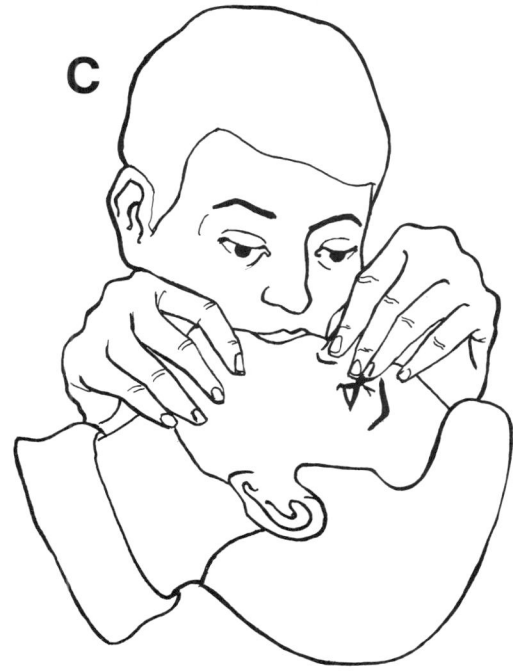

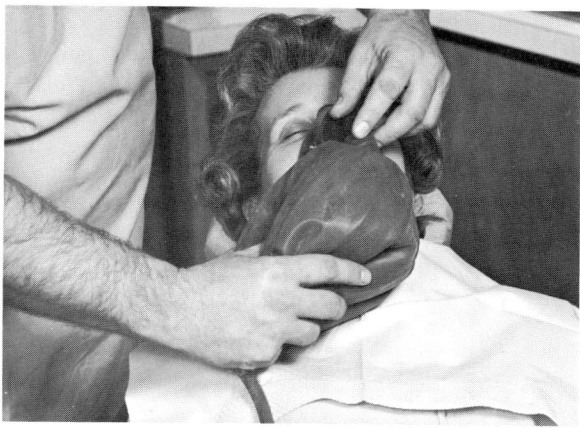

Figure 21-11 | Application and manipulation of oxygen mask and bag.

emergency artificial respiration. The following steps are recommended (Fig. 21-10):

1. The nostrils are pinched closed and the head is stabilized by placing one hand in the corner of the mouth and lifting.
2. The lower jaw and tongue are maintained in an elevated position by placing the thumb of the other hand in the corner of the mouth and lifting.
3. After taking a deep breath, the resuscitator opens his or her mouth widely and makes a seal over the patient's open mouth and blows forcefully until a normal chest rise is apparent. This cannot occur if the airway is totally obstructed.
4. Next, the resuscitator withdraws and allows the patient to exhale. At the same time the resuscitator takes another breath. The patient's lungs should be inflated at the rate of 10 to 12 times per minute for an adult and approximately 20 times per minute for a child (Cole and Puestow, 1965).

Figure 21-10 | Mouth-to-mouth resuscitation.

Oxygen-Inhalation Equipment

Inhalation equipment is most useful for many emergencies that may occur in the dental office. Proper utilization of the equipment will allow the administration of supplemental oxygen with positive pressure. The following steps are recommended (Fig. 21-11):

1. The mask should be fitted and held tightly over the patient's mouth and nose with one hand.
2. The flowmeter is adjusted so as to deliver a flow of 5 to 10 liters of oxygen per minute to the patient's lungs.
3. The movement of the patient's chest is observed as an indicator of a patent airway. Also the color of the skin and the pulse rate are noted.
4. If necessary, increased chest movement may be accomplished by applying intermittent pressure to the rubber bag at the rate of 18 to 20 respirations per minute until normal breathing is restored (Hagen, 1965).

Heimlich Maneuver

Aspiration of an object is most likely to occur during inspiration, or otherwise the object would not be resting over the laryngeal opening. It is therefore logical to assume that the patient's lungs are partially expanded at the moment of aspiration. A technique which would forcefully compress the residual air in the lungs would increase the air pressure in trachea and larynx and hopefully loosen or eject the lodged object. The following steps are recommended:

1. In a position behind the patient, wrap your arm around the waist making a fist with one hand, the thumb side against the abdomen and slightly above the patient's navel. While grasping the fist with the other hand, press rapidly and strongly into the abdomen in an upward thrust, forcing the diaphragm superiorly in an effort to expel the object (Fig. 21-12).
2. If the patient is on the floor, place the person face up and assume an astride position about the patient's hips. With one hand on top of the other in the middle of abdominal region slightly above the navel, press the abdomen with a sudden upward thrust (Fig. 21-13).
3. If possible, a second person on the emergency team should be available to assist in the removal of the ejected object from the patient's oral cavity with their fingers (Heimlich, 1974).

Emergency Tracheotomy

Hopefully, the need for a tracheotomy or cricothyreotomy in the general practice of dentistry will be exceedingly rare. This surgical means of establishing an airway serves as a last resort for saving a patient's life. Consideration of the circumstances and a prior knowledge of the anatomic structures in the area of the operation are a must before performing this procedure. The following steps are recommended (Fig. 21-14):

1. Locate the interval between the cricoid and the thyroid cartilage by palpation with the index finger while the patient is in a supine position if possible.
2. Insert the tracheotomy trocar and tube into the trachea. Penetration of the posterior tracheal wall with a subsequent esophageal fistula must be avoided. The proper design of the trocar may serve to prevent this from occurring.

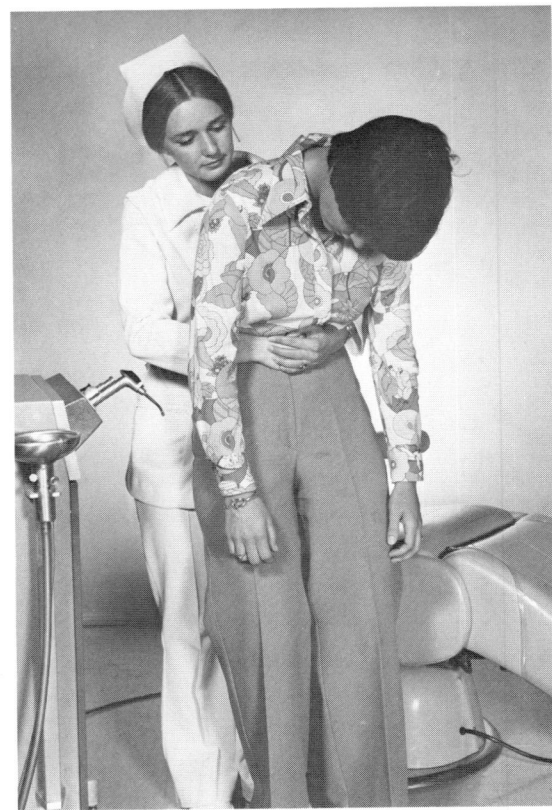

Figure 21-12 | Heimlich maneuver from standing position.

3. Devise a method to attach a rubber tube from the oxygen equipment to the inserted tube to offer a higher concentration of oxygen when deemed necessary.
4. Call medical aid at once to administer supportive care when this procedure has been performed on a patient (Webster and Wood, 1965).

Neurogenic Shock

Neurogenic shock or fainting is certainly one of the most common emergencies that occur in the dental office. It may be precipitated by numerous factors acting on the nervous system, either by direct or psychologic influences. Pre-

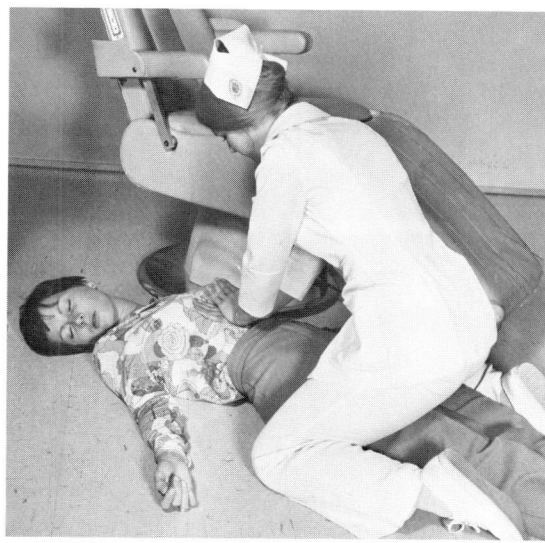

Figure 21-13 | Heimlich maneuver from supine position.

vention of neurogenic shock can best be secured by establishing rapport with the patient prior to the performance of dental procedures so as to reduce fear and apprehension factors. A patient who presents a history of fainting episodes in the dental office may likely be a candidate for premedication to reduce nervousness, to elevate the pain threshold, or to reduce anxiety and fear. Typical dental etiologic factors that may lead to neurogenic shock are:

1. The mere thought of the treatment to be rendered
2. Sharp pain
3. The sight or insertion of a needle during anesthetic administration
4. The sight of blood
5. Uncomfortable environment such as a poorly ventilated room during course of treatment

Neurogenic shock or primary shock is due to a decreased amount of blood in the area of the brain as a result of the dilation of capillary beds and blood vessels in the peripheral parts of the body. Although fainting, in most instances, is a relatively simple problem to manage, it should be recognized as a possible forerunner of a more complicated emergency. The condition of the patient may range from slight disorientation to unconsciousness.

Diagnosis

The patient may express a sensation of general weakness and light-headedness; there may be nausea followed by vomiting; dilation of pupils, pallor, and increased perspiration are usually noted; and the pulse may be rapid and thready (Fig. 21-15).

Treatment

When neurogenic shock is evident, specific management should be initiated. The back of the dental chair should be lowered so that the head is slightly lower than the rest of the body. A patent airway should be maintained and supplemental oxygen may be administered. It is well to monitor and record the blood pressure and pulse rate during the stressful period. Drug therapy suggested is to crush an ampule of aromatic ammonia and allow the patient to inhale intermittently the escaping vapors. Also one teaspoonful of spirits of ammonia in one-half glass of water may be drunk by the patient. Remember, *liquids should not be offered to a patient that is not fully conscious.* As the patient shows signs of returning to normalcy, allow him or her to remain in a reclined position for 10 to 20 minutes or longer; assure such patients they will be all right (Kinney, 1965).

Anaphylactic Shock

Anaphylactic shock is an allergic reaction and is precipitated when an incompatible drug is introduced into the body. The reaction that results is due to the liberation of histamine in the blood

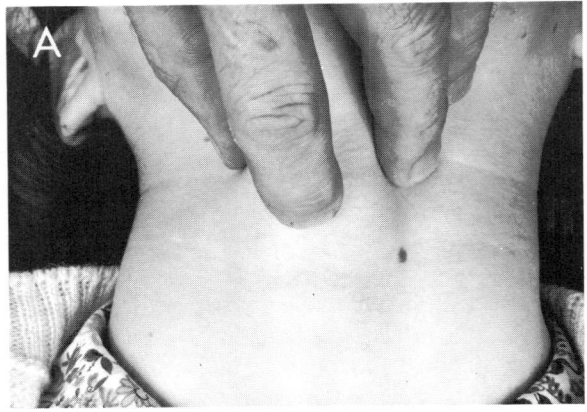
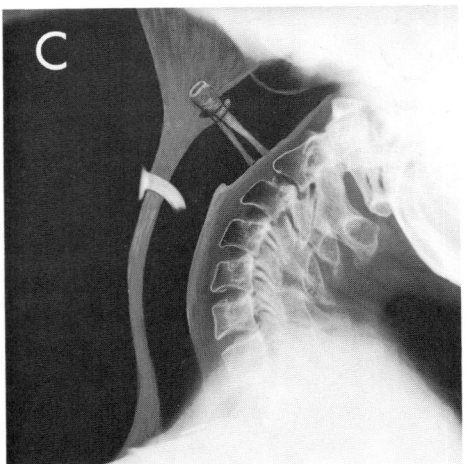
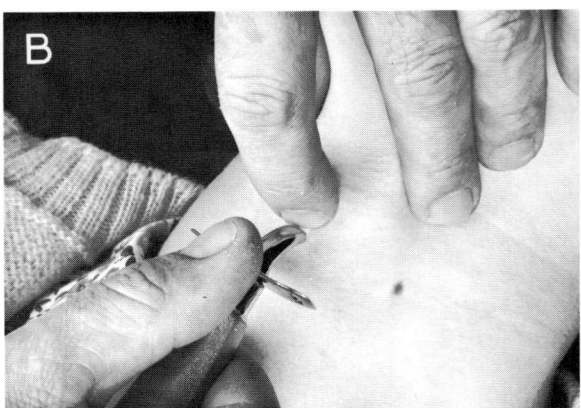
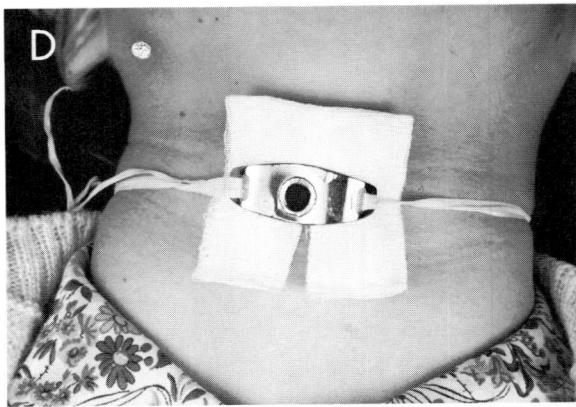

Figure 21-14 | Emergency tracheotomy. A. Palpation of cricothyroid cartilage and stabilization of trachea. B. Insertion of cricothyreotomy cannula. C. X-ray of cricothyroid cannula inserted in proper position. D. Cricothyroid cannula stabilized in trachea. (*Courtesy of Dr. M. E. Chapin, Chapel Hill, N.C.*)

vessels producing an unfavorable antigen-antibody reaction.

In the dental office, local anesthetics and penicillin are two types of agents that are most likely to produce anaphylactic shock.

Due to the possibility of the death of a patient who suffers a true anaphylactic shock, it is of primary importance to have, in advance, a thorough medical history and a record of any past experiences that might indicate the existence of an allergic state.

Anaphylactic shock caused by the administration of a local anesthetic is usually characterized by a rapid onset of observable signs and symptoms. The major systemic problem is one of circulatory collapse with a marked fall in blood pressure with a weak or imperceptible pulse. The condition of the patient may range from mildly

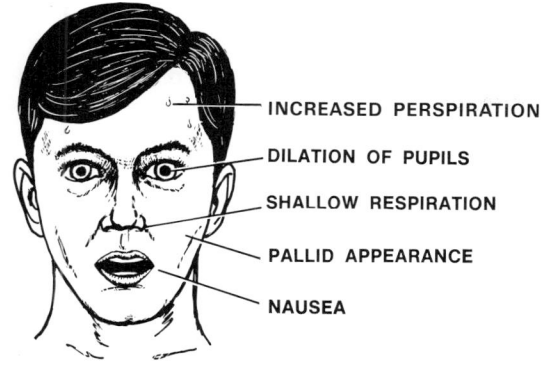

Figure 21-15 | Visual manifestations of shock.

expressed discomfort to unconsciousness. This type of shock is seemingly very similar to neurogenic shock, but the underlying causes are quite different. Only by careful differential diagnosis may the proper treatment be instituted.

Diagnosis

In the less severe cases, the patient may exhibit signs of itching, impaired respiration due to bronchospasm, urticaria, and a rash along with other signs and symptoms previously discussed.

Treatment

The patient should be placed in a horizontal position with the legs slightly elevated. The drug of choice to combat anaphylactic shock is 1:1000 epinephrine. This drug has a direct and opposite effect to that of the histamine which has been liberated. It should be administered as a subcutaneous injection of 0.5 ml per injection. A patent airway should be provided and respiration maintained with oxygen under pressure. A physician should be called as soon as possible. In the event the patient does not improve in a few minutes, administration of the sympathomimetic agent (epinephrine) should be repeated (Laskin, 1964).

Circulatory Difficulty

Circulatory difficulty may occur during or shortly after the administration of a local anesthetic injection. The circulatory embarrassment is thought not to be due to the nature of the anesthetic agent, but rather to apprehension, fear, or poor technique employed during administration.

The actual mechanism of this emergency is a vasovagal reflex which is triggered by a state of restlessness. The reflex causes the vasodilation of many peripheral blood vessels and capillary beds. In turn there is a reduced flow of blood to the brain. This type of distress is usually one of the more severe types of problems that may be associated with syncope (fainting). To avoid this kind of problem care should be exercised not to inject anesthetic solutions into blood vessels, or pass the needle through a muscle. Injections should not be made rapidly, but slowly, to reduce unwarranted pain and discomfort.

Diagnosis

The patient may exhibit a temporary hyperemia of the skin, sweating, and lowered blood pressure. The vermilion border of the lips may be cyanotic. In general, the same signs and symptoms as for neurogenic shock are apparent. Consciousness may or may not be lost.

Treatment

The head should be lowered by tilting the dental chair into a horizontal position to improve the blood supply to the head. The administration of oxygen or inhalation of aromatic ammonia will serve as a simple remedy and is usually very effective.

In severe situations when consciousness is lost and does not return with the above treatment, 500 mg (7½ grains) of caffeine and sodium benzoate should be administered intramuscularly to stimulate the heart. A physician should be called at once to offer more experienced medical assistance (Webster and Wood, 1965).

Cardiac Emergencies

A heart attack in the dental office, regardless of the circumstances, is a most frightening and serious medical problem. Frequently the onset of angina pectoris may be sudden or unsuspected unless a history of previous attacks has been noted. When a patient is known to have had previous attacks, a medical consultation is desirable before any dental procedures are performed. All dental treatments should be postponed for at least 6 months after an original acute attack.

Angina pectoris is a painful condition resulting from an existing known or unknown heart disease. The pain experienced is directly related to the collapse or occlusion of one or several blood vessels that supply the tissues of the heart. Emotional factors may bring on an attack of angina. The attack may last for a few minutes or persist for a longer period.

Diagnosis

The patient may appear deathly pale and perspiration may be severe. There is substernal (chest) pain which may radiate to the left arm or left side of the neck. A feeling of numbness may be experienced in the areas to which the pain radiates. The pulse may be weak and rapid along with an altered blood pressure, depending upon the magnitude of the problem.

Treatment

With the onset of the signs and symptoms and mild substernal pain, one or two tablets of nitroglycerin, one two-hundredth grain, should be placed under the patient's tongue. Relief should be obtained in 2 to 3 minutes. For more severe episodes and when nitroglycerin does not relieve the pain, an amyl nitrite pearl may be crushed under the patient's nose in a piece of gauze so that the patient may inhale the vapor. Both nitroglycerin and amyl nitrite act as vasodilators. Oxygen administration may also be employed as a supportive measure. When the pain subsides, the patient should remain quiet and be placed in a slightly reclined position. A physician should be summoned as soon as possible (McCarthy, 1967a).

Diabetes Mellitus

Prior to performing dental procedures, it should be determined if the patient is a known diabetic. If the history does reveal diabetic problems, the dentist should consult with the physician in charge. Knowledge of this condition realized in advance will provide valuable information for the treatment of an episode related to this disease. It is advisable that diabetics' dental appointments be arranged 1 to 2 hours after breakfast and insulin administration when the blood-sugar level should be relatively normal.

There are two possible complications that should be easily recognized by the dental team; they are *insulin shock* and *diabetic coma*.

Insulin Shock

This complication is a result of either an excessive amount of insulin secreted or an overdose of insulin prior to the dental appointment. Excess insulin in the circulation serves to promote a lowered blood-sugar level which sets the stage for the distress.

Some of the early signs and symptoms noted with this condition are expressed weakness, sweating, and general discomfort; the patient may appear nervous and have a pallid complexion. It is not uncommon for the patient to experience short periods of unconsciousness and convulsions. The episode may come on quite quickly when the dentist is performing a feared or dreaded operation.

The diabetic patient may often be able to forewarn the dentist of an impending attack. It is advisable to immediately give to the patient several cubes of sugar or a cup of sweetened juice. Either one of these will serve to balance the diminished blood-sugar level. If the patient should lose consciousness, dextrose U.S.P., 50 percent, or 0.5 to 1 mg of Gulcagon may be administered intravenously. Of course the patient's physician should be contacted as soon as possible for subsequent or more definitive treatment (Costrich, 1966).

Diabetic Coma

A diabetic coma results from a condition known as hyperglycemia (increased blood-sugar level) due to insulin deficiency. Hyperglycemia is due to the fact that there is a depression of carbohydrate metabolism in the body resulting from the lack of insulin which is necessary for normal function. A diabetic coma usually requires several hours or even days before the patient is comatose, while in the case of insulin shock, the onset is rapid.

The patient may complain of excessive thirst and general weakness; drowsiness, stomach pains associated with nausea, and vomiting may also be noted. In addition, the eyes may appear sunken in the face and the face may appear flushed. There is also a marked odor of acetone or fruity odor of the breath.

On recognition of this condition a physician should be called with admission of the patient to a hospital in mind. The main needs of the patient are insulin and intravenous fluids immediately or as soon as possible. The patient while in the dental office should not be left alone and should be kept as comfortable as possible (Laskin, 1964).

Epileptic Seizures

Epileptic seizures are one of the most feared convulsive states and are very frightful experiences when completely unanticipated. Fortunately less than 1 percent of the population of the United States suffers from this malady. The epileptic condition may be due to either genetic or acquired factors.

Due to the fact that this condition seems to reflect a real or psychic social stigma, many patients are reluctant to supply information for the dental team that would be extremely helpful in case of a seizure during a dental appointment.

In cases where a patient fractures anterior teeth due to seemingly ridiculous reasons, presents evidence of scars on the tongue, or severe gingival hyperplasia not due to local causes, a history of epilepsy would not be too surprising.

Epilepsy is a neurologic disorder of an intermittent nature. The convulsions are believed to be caused by a sudden and excessive release of cerebral energy. The seizure may actually appear as a combination of sensory disturbances, loss of consciousness, and convulsive movements.

Diagnosis

Hopefully, the patient will know when an attack is imminent and will warn the dentist so that precautionary measures may be taken such as allowing the patient to rest and having the assistant quickly obtain emergency equipment. One of the first signs will be that of a warning aura and cry, followed by frothing at the mouth and convulsion.

Treatment

The patient should not be restrained entirely, but rather placed on the floor away from surrounding objects so as to reduce the risk of injury. It is advisable to attempt to wedge a padded tongue depressor between the patient's teeth to prevent biting of the tongue during the convulsion (Fig. 21-16). Loosen all the patient's restrictive clothing. When the patient exhibits respiratory problems, it is possible that the tongue has

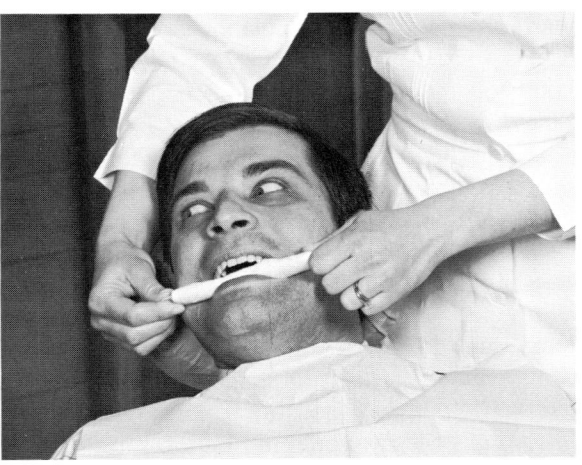

Figure 21-16 | Prevention of tongue biting during an epileptic seizure.

fallen posteriorly and is obstructing the airway. Care should be taken to pull the tongue forward and administer oxygen. An oropharyngeal tube may greatly aid in holding the tongue forward (Fig. 21-17). The patient's physician should be notified at once (Webster and Wood, 1965).

Figure 21-17 | Maintaining a patent airway during an epileptic seizure.

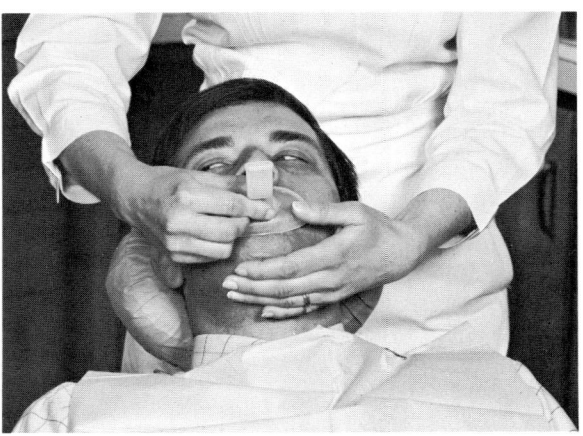

Dislocation of the Mandible

This emergency does not commonly occur in the dental office, but presents an unusual problem when it does. Wide opening of the mouth for gargling, yawning, or fatigue due to lengthy operative procedures may precipitate this stressful situation. The true etiology is the incoordination of muscle action that guides the movement of the condyle.

When the condyles are dislocated, the patient may seem relatively unconcerned if it has happened several times previously. Quite an opposite reaction may be exhibited when the patient first realizes that the jaws cannot be closed. Usually the episode is not as painful as it is frightening, although some pain may be experienced with the muscle spasm that is characteristic of this condition.

Diagnosis

There is no problem in determining what has occurred when the jaw is dislocated. The patient in garbled language usually tries to explain that the teeth cannot be brought together. This is quite apparent with the mandible immobilized in a wide-open position.

Treatment

The individual who is to reduce the dislocation should at all times protect the fingers from a power closure of the jaw during the reduction procedure. The best way to do this is to wrap both thumbs with a towel or gauze prior to placing them in the oral cavity. When attempting the reduction, stand in front of the patient and place the thumbs along the buccal aspect of the mandibular second molars. The mandible should then be grasped firmly underneath with the fingers and forced downward and backward (Fig. 21-18). The jaw should snap into place relatively easily if the dislocation has not persisted too long. In some instances, it may be necessary to resort to general anesthesia or muscle relaxants to afford a reduction. The only precautionary measure necessary for a patient to follow after a simple dislocation is to avoid opening too wide for several days (Irby and Baldwin, 1965).

Hemorrhage from Lacerations

Hemorrhage regardless of where or when it occurs must be considered an emergency. Whether the hemorrhage site presents a serious problem or not, most patients will consider bleeding to be abnormal and it will be alarming.

Instruments used in dental procedures may be the cause of a soft-tissue laceration. The accident may be due to the inability of the patient to hold the tongue aside, poor retraction techniques by the dental assistant, or the careless or unavoidable manipulation of the instrument by the dentist. It is not uncommon for the patient to unknowingly bite or chew either tongue or lip while anesthetized. The traumatization may take the form of an abrasion, a cut, or a puncture.

Since soft tissues in and about the oral cavity have a rich blood supply, bleeding may be profuse even though the injury is not too serious. The usual results of the injury after the hemorrhage has ceased will be swelling, discoloration, and impaired function for several days.

Diagnosis

Bleeding is, of course, a sign that tissues have been injured. It is well to examine the injured area carefully to determine if it will be necessary to ligate a vessel, suture the laceration, or merely resort to topical medication, or subject the area to pressure.

Treatment

Initially, a sterile gauze pad should be placed under pressure over the injured area. This is very effective in checking capillary bleeding. The use

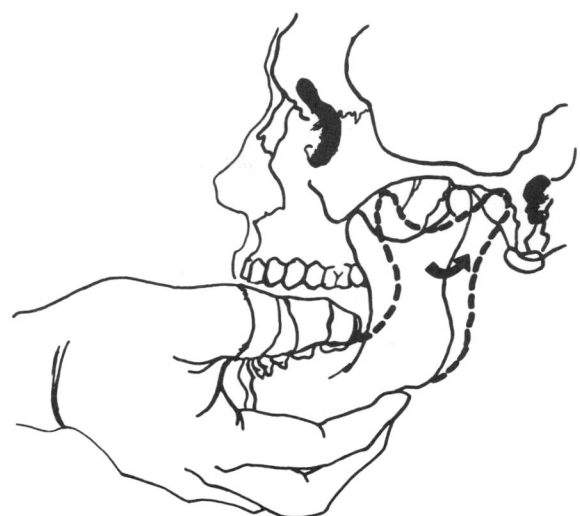

Figure 21-18 | Reduction of dislocated mandible.

of a sterile gauze pad moistened with epinephrine hydrochloride (1:1000 solution) will greatly aid in the control of more profuse bleeding. When the laceration is deep and involves a vessel it should be clamped and sutured with subsequent closure of the tissue with several sutures. In case of deep wounds, caution should be taken to eliminate any foreign particles such as amalgam or calculus. The seriousness of the wound will determine the postoperative follow-up (Berlove, 1959).

Injury to the Eye

With the routine use of high-speed rotary instruments in the practice of dentistry it is not uncommon for particles of teeth and restorations to lodge in the eyes. Also, there is the hazard of such things as bits of calculus, instruments, and caustic medicaments causing eye injury.

Regardless of how slight an eye injury may seem, it should be considered serious until proved otherwise. Daily preventive measures should be practiced to avoid exposing a patient to the possibility of such injury. It is well to ask the patient to close both eyes or offer a protective shield when a risk is apparent. Prevention not only should be practiced with the interest of the patient in mind, but also adequate protection should be a rule with the members of the dental team.

In the event of an injury, first aid should be rendered keeping in mind that impairment of vision can result from fumbling or inexpert attempts to remove foreign objects.

Management

When foreign objects are a problem the following suggestions should be followed:

1. Do not allow the patient to rub the eye.
2. Do not press against the eye, or manipulate it in a manner to cause additional irritation.
3. For foreign objects that are seemingly embedded in the eye, apply a loose bandage and refer the patient to an ophthalmologist.
4. To clear the eye of extremely small objects, wash the eye with copious amounts of water while holding the eyelids apart.
5. When foreign objects are not apparent on the surface of the eye, the lids may be retracted and removal attempted with a small twist of cotton or the corner of a clean tissue (Fig. 21-19).
6. When chemicals are the source of injury, flush the eye thoroughly with water, bandage loosely, and contact an ophthalmologist.

Falls and Resulting Injuries

Volumes have been written on the hazards of waxed floors, loose lamp cords, and frayed edges on rugs which may cause a person to lose balance and fall, with resulting injury. One of the most common places in the dental office for such accidents is around the dental chair. Many times patients have been allowed to leave the chair while they still felt faint. Sometimes, a sudden rise from a reclining position in the dental chair may result in dizziness. The footboard on a dental chair can also be hazardous when the patient rises. It is well, therefore, to assist a patient from the chair, both as a courtesy and to prevent an accident. If such an accident does occur, it is well to recognize the symptoms of various injuries and to know the first-aid measures which are necessary.

Fracture

A fracture may be defined simply as a break in a bone. The discussion here will be limited to the broad classification of simple and compound fractures.

In a simple fracture the bone is broken, but the skin remains intact. The compound fracture is characterized by puncture of the skin usually by one end of the broken bone. Improper management of a simple fracture may result in a compound fracture, which is more vulnerable to infection.

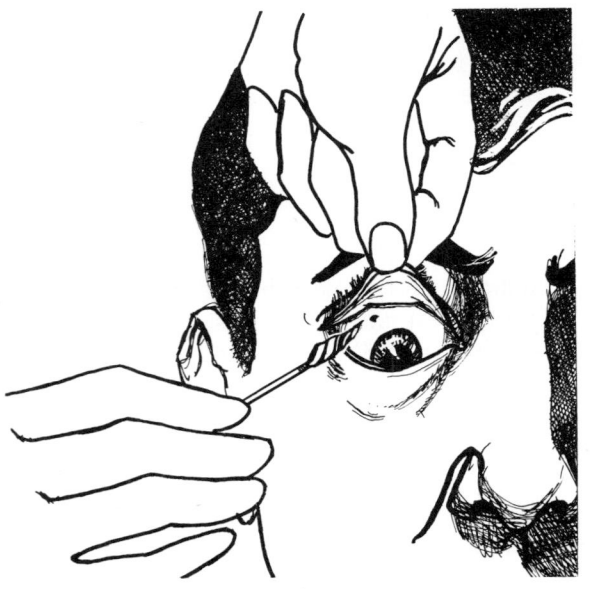

Figure 21-19 | Removal of foreign body from eye.

The symptoms of a fracture generally follow a pattern. A compound fracture is determined easily, since the bone can be seen projecting through the skin at the location of the break. A simple fracture may be more difficult to recognize, since the bone may be split lengthwise without a separation of the two broken ends.

The patient may hear or feel the bone snap, and there usually will be pain and tenderness at the point of the break. Pain is the most pronounced symptom, and, in most cases, there will be limited use of the injured part. Gentle palpation of the area with the fingers may reveal a lump or asymmetry at the point of the fracture. It is well to compare the injured part of the body with a similar area on the opposite side to see if there is any deformity.

If a fracture is suspected, do not disturb the injured part. A physician should be called for examination and for proper care. If there is a compound fracture with bleeding, place a sterile gauze compress over the wound, and apply a tourniquet if gross arterial bleeding occurs. A patient with a fracture may go into shock, and if this occurs, the previously described procedures for shock should be followed.

Sprain

These injuries occur in the joints and are the result of a sudden, violent force exerted either directly or indirectly to the part. The injury is either a partial or complete tear of the supporting ligaments of the joint that is caused by a forced movement beyond the normal range. When such forced movement occurs, the ligaments and perhaps a bone become involved.

The symptoms of a sprain may be similar to those of a fracture or a dislocation. There usually is severe pain and a rapid swelling of the joint, and the patient will be unable to use this area without increasing the pain. Discoloration, due to internal bleeding, may not be observed immediately, but it will last for several weeks.

If there is any doubt in the dental assistant's mind as to the nature of the injury (whether it is a sprain, dislocation, or fracture), it always should be treated as a fracture. The general first-aid treatment for a sprain is:

1. Elevate the part by placing it in a sling or by propping it up on a folded coat, blanket, or pillow.
2. Use cold applications on the area. This may be accomplished by applying an ice pack or cold, wet towels or by holding the part under cold, running tap water. These cold applications should be continued for a few hours or until a physician sees the injury.
3. If the sprain is severe, the patient should not use that part of the body until it has been examined by a physician.

Bruise

A bruise usually is caused by a blow to some part of the body. The blow causes a rupture of the small blood vessels under the skin, and as the blood oozes from the broken vessels into the tissues, it causes swelling and discoloration. The skin may or may not be broken, but if there is a break in the skin surface it should be cleansed thoroughly and treated as any other open wound.

It is not usually necessary to give first-aid treatment for bruises. Cold applications, immediately placed, will help to prevent discoloration, keep down the swelling, and relieve the pain to a certain extent.

Dislocation

A bone that gets out of place with its commuting bone in a joint is dislocated. When dislocation occurs there usually are torn ligaments, blood vessels, and nerves and often a fracture of a part of the bone. Pain frequently is very intense in any dislocation, and there usually will be a marked deformity of the joint. By gentle palpation of the injured joint and a similar joint on the opposite side of the body, it is quite evident that a bone is out of place. Marked swelling will occur rapidly, and the patient may go into a state of shock. There is usually a complete loss of movement of that portion of the body.

Reduction of the dislocation should not be attempted by a first-aider, and the patient should be seen by a physician as soon as possible. Inexperienced help may cause further injury to the blood vessels, muscles, tendons, and nerves around the joint. The patient and the injured part should be made as comfortable as possible. Cold compresses may be applied to the area to help relieve pain and prevent swelling. Treat the condition of shock if it occurs; a mild pain-relieving drug may be indicated. A physician should be called as soon as possible.

BIBLIOGRAPHY

Bell, W. H.: "Emergencies in and out of the Dental Office: A Pilot Study in the State of Texas," *J. Am. Dent. Assoc.,* **74:**778–783, 1967.

Berlove, I. J.: *Dental-Medical Emergencies and Complications,* The Year Book Publishers, Inc., Chicago, 1959.

Berman, D. L.: "Why Dentist Must Screen Patients for Hypertension," *Dent. Survey,* 59–63, May 1976.

Bureau of Naval Personnel: "Standard First Aid Training Course," 1955.

Chue, P. W. Y.: "The Clinical Measurement of Arterial Blood Pressure," *Dent. Medicine,* 30–35, June 1975.

Cole, W. H., and Puestow, C. B.: *First Aid, Diagnosis and Management,* 6th ed., Appleton Century Crofts, New York, 1965.

Costich, E. R.: "Special Issue: Emergencies in the Dental Office," *Dent. Practice,* **4:**3–18, 1966.

Hagen, J. O.: "Oxygen Therapy, Blood Pressure and Pulse Determination, and Venipuncture Technique," in *Dent. Clin. North Am. Index 1963–1965,* W. B. Saunders Company, Philadelphia, 1965, pp. 769–778.

Heimlich, H. J.: "Pop Goes the Café," *Emergency Med.,* 154–156, June 1974.

Hooley, J. R., and Conn, R. D.: "A Simplified Approach to the Treatment of Medical Emergencies in the Dental Office," *J. Am. Dent. Assoc.,* **73:**77–83, 1966.

Irby, W. B., and Baldwin, K. H.: *Emergencies and Urgent Complications in Dentistry,* The C. V. Mosby Company, St. Louis, 1965.

Kinney, W. B.: "The Treatment of Shock as It Relates to the Practicing Dentist," in *Dent. Clin. North Am. Index 1963–1965,* W. B. Saunders Company, Philadelphia, 1965, pp. 779–787.

Kruger, G. W. (ed.): *Textbook of Oral Surgery,* 3d ed., The C. V. Mosby Company, St. Louis, 1968.

Laskin, D. M.: "Emergency Treatment of the Dental Patient: Part I, A Guide to Hospital Dental Procedures," American Dental Association, Chicago, 1964, pp. 43–44.

McCarthy, F. M.: "Pretreatment Physical Evaluation in the Dental Office," in *Dent. Clin. North Am. Index 1963–1965,* W. B. Saunders Company, Philadelphia, 1965, pp. 545—555.

———: "Heart Attack," *J. South. Calif. Dent. Assoc.,* **35:**490–491, 1967a.

——— (ed.): *Emergencies in Dental Practice,* W. B. Saunders Company, Philadelphia, 1967b.

Sheppard, G. A.: "Legal Aspects of Dental Emergencies," in *Dent. Clin. North Am. Index 1963–1965,* W. B. Saunders Company, Philadelphia, 1965, pp. 803–821.

Webster, W. P., and Wood, M. T.: "Dental Assisting, Course III, Preclinical Sciences," University of North Carolina, Chapel Hill, 1965.

22

Cecil R. Lupton

Anesthesia and Pain Control

INTRODUCTION

The abolition of pain during dental procedures has been the most significant contribution to the advancement and acceptance of dentistry as it is currently practiced.

There have been many materials and techniques developed that have advanced dentistry to its present state; without local anesthesia, sedation, and general anesthesia, their contributions would be insignificant. Inherited attitudes, cartoons, and comedy routines still portray the dentist as a purveyor of pain rather than a reliever or preventer. This unfortunate public attitude can only be overcome by the dentist in the daily conduct of his or her practice; selecting and administering anesthetics and other drugs that allay the fears and apprehensions of the patients. In this respect, we, the dental staff, are the best resource for public relations.

HISTORY OF ANESTHESIA

A dentist, Dr. Horace Wells, is credited with being the first individual to use a general anesthetic for an operation. In 1844, he used nitrous oxide to allay pain while removing a tooth. It is generally accepted that Dr. Crawford Long and Dr. W. E. Clark from Georgia used ether to perform operations prior to 1844. Their mistake was that they did not publicize the event, and Dr. Wells is generally credited as being the first to use a general anesthetic.

The advancement of the total field of surgery and dentistry, as we know it today, can be directly related to the above events. The first local anesthetic used was cocaine, a naturally occurring product that was obtained from plants. Its toxicity, addictive qualities, and attendant complications caused a justifiable reluctance by the dentist to use the anesthetic as a routine measure for dental procedures. Procaine was synthesized by Einhorn in 1905, and since the trade name Novocain was used, this is the usual name for a local anesthetic when referred to by the public. Since 1905, the production of procaine, adjunctive additions (epinephrine, etc.), and the discovery of new anesthetics has brought us to the present state of the "routine" use of local anesthesia for dental procedures. These are still drugs; they are a material foreign to the body and in that context should not be administered without knowledge of their possible adverse effects on local tissue and of possible systemic reactions.

The development of general anesthetics since the Horace Wells and Crawford Long era has been primarily by the medical profession. Presently, there are indications that the use of general anesthetics by the dental profession is increasing. No doubt, the use of nitrous oxide has had a tremendous resurgence in the dental profession. It is classed as a general anesthetic; it should not be used as such because of side effects. With proper application, it is an excellent analgesic modality.

Sedation techniques in the dental office have reached a popular and public acceptance level. Drug developments and teaching of such techniques have made this a daily practice in many dental offices.

Sedation cannot take the place of local anesthesia as it does not block sensory nerves. Sedation must be supplemented with local anesthesia to obtain the desired cooperation from the patient. The attempted use of sedation to overcome the lack of ability to properly administer local anesthesia is a trap that must be avoided by the dentist. Sedation is an adjunct, not a replacement, for local anesthetics.

ANATOMY, PSYCHOLOGY, AND PHYSIOLOGY OF PAIN

Pain is a protective mechanism for the body. The basic anatomy and physiology involve a sensory nerve that receives a stimulus and reacts by conducting a message to muscle, brain, or other tissue, where a mental and physical response is made. This is a simple explanation of a most complicated process. Much is known about the process, much is being discovered, and yet, the surface is only scratched. How local anesthetics work is still not completely understood.

Teeth and Jaws; Nerve Anatomy

The sensory nerves to the teeth and supporting structures are derived from the fifth cranial nerve, the trigeminal. The trigeminal nerve has three divisions: ophthalmic, maxillary, and mandibular. Generally, the ophthalmic receives stimuli from the upper one-third of the face area; the maxillary from the middle one-third; and the mandibular from the lower one-third. These three main divisions branch to receive stimuli from more well-defined anatomic structures such as individual teeth and their supporting tissues (Figs. 22-1 and 22-2).

Pain Stimuli and Conduction

The objective with local anesthesia is to prevent the conduction of stimuli (impulses) along the sensory nerves to the central nervous system (brain). This is accomplished by placing a local anesthetic solution in an anatomic position so the solution can come in contact with the nerve and alter or block the usual physiologic reaction that takes place during the conduction of the im-

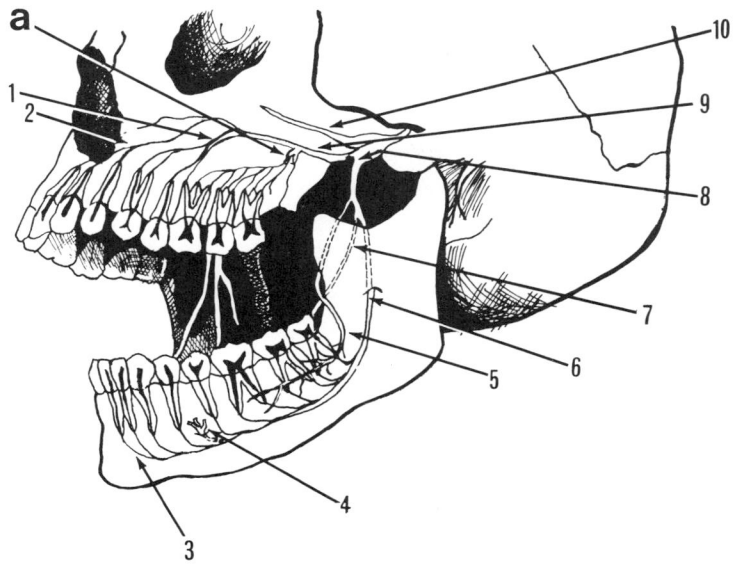

Figure 22-1 | Skull drawing. A. Posterior superior alveolar nerve, (1) middle superior alveolar nerve, (2) anterior superior alveolar nerve, (3) incisive nerve, (4) mental foramen and nerve, (5) buccal nerve, (6) inferior alveolar nerve, (7) lingual nerve, (8) mandibular nerve (third division), (9) maxillary nerve (second division), (10) ophthalmic nerve (first division).

pulse. The nerve end, as in a tooth or the gum, is stimulated sufficiently to start the physiologic reaction in the nerve body. The reaction results in a change in polarity as it travels along the nerve and results in the message being received in the central nervous system. The strength of the stimulus required depends on many factors in each individual patient. Some of these factors are pain reaction threshold, emotional states, physical condition, age, sex, and others. For example, the child that has lost sleep due to a toothache and has been fatigued with a day at school will require a more profound anesthesia to accomplish a dental procedure. Preconceived notions that associate pain with dental procedures will present a patient more difficult to anesthetize. Each situation must be judged individually and treated appropriately.

GENERAL ANESTHESIA

Definition

General anesthesia is the state created whereby the whole body is insensitive to painful stimuli. General anesthesia is accomplished by agents reaching the central nervous system (brain) through the circulatory system. The agents are placed directly in the bloodstream by the injection of a drug in a vein, or they are administered through the inhalation of a gas or vapor and consequently reach the circulatory system through the lungs. Oral intake, injection in muscle tissue, and anal suppositories are other routes used to administer general anesthetics. They are not as easily controlled and efficient as intravenous and inhalation routes and are not used with great frequency. When absorbed, general anesthetics block the painful stimuli at the center where they are received, the central nervous system (brain and spinal cord).

Agents

Ether, halothane, trichloroethylene, and others are some of the volatile agents that are used for general anesthesia. Nitrous oxide, ethylene, and cyclopropane are gaseous agents that are used for general anesthesia. Nitrous oxide will be discussed later under the heading of analgesia. Barbiturate derivatives are intravenous agents used for general anesthesia.

Indications

Very few general dentists use general anesthesia in their offices; many oral surgery practices have a general anesthesia capability. Its use requires more extensive equipment, special training, space, and more personnel than other techniques of anesthesia. General anesthesia is indicated for patients who cannot be managed by less complicated methods. Mental retardation, emotional states, extensive procedures, and the dentist's preference and training are some of the indications for general anesthesia in the field of dentistry. Most general anesthesia is accomplished in a hospital by specialists with special training in that field.

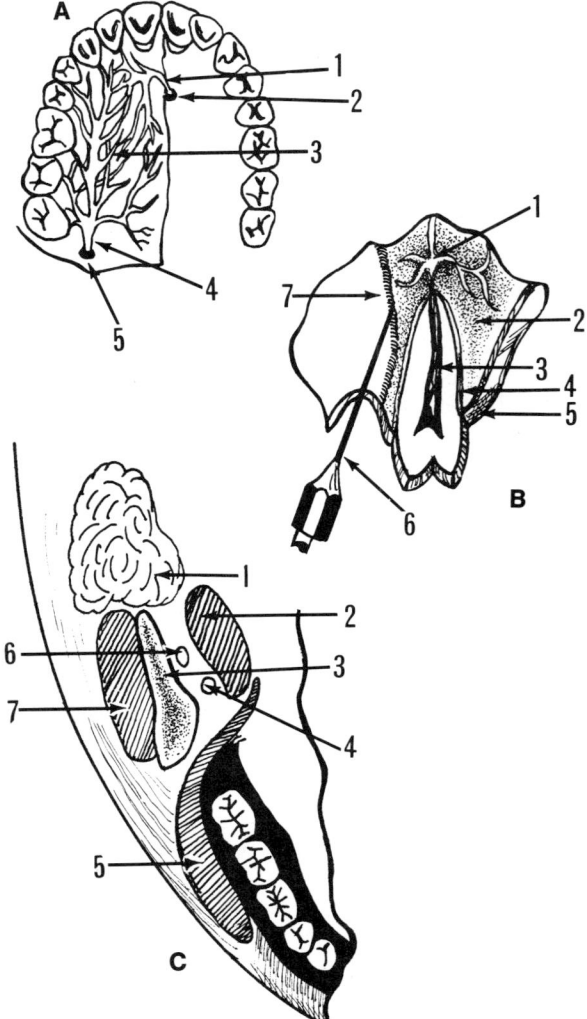

Figure 22-2 | Representative sections of the maxilla and mandible. A. Sensory nerves of the hard palate, (1) nasopalatine nerve, (2) incisal canal, (3) plexus between nasopalatine nerve and anterior palatine nerve, (4) anterior palatine nerve, (5) major palatine foramen. B. Section through region of a maxillary premolar tooth, (1) site of nerve plexus, (2) porous alveolar bone, (3) tooth pulp, (4) periodontal membrane, (5) palatal gingiva, (6) hypodermic needle, (7) periosteum. C. Cross section through the head at a level immediately above the mandibular foramen, (1) parotid gland, (2) internal pterygoid muscle, (3) ramus of the mandible, (4) lingual nerve, (5) buccinator muscle, (6) inferior alveolar nerve, (7) masseter muscle. (*Drawing after H. M. Seldin, Practical Anesthesia for Dental and Oral Surgery, 3d ed., Lea & Febiger, Philadelphia, 1947.*)

LOCAL ANESTHESIA

Definition

The word anesthesia is derived from the combination of two Greek words: *an*, meaning not or negative, and *aisthesis*, meaning sensation. Hence, anesthesia means the loss of feeling or sensation. An anesthetic is administered to accomplish anesthesia. Usually, the word is applied especially to the loss of pain sensation to permit

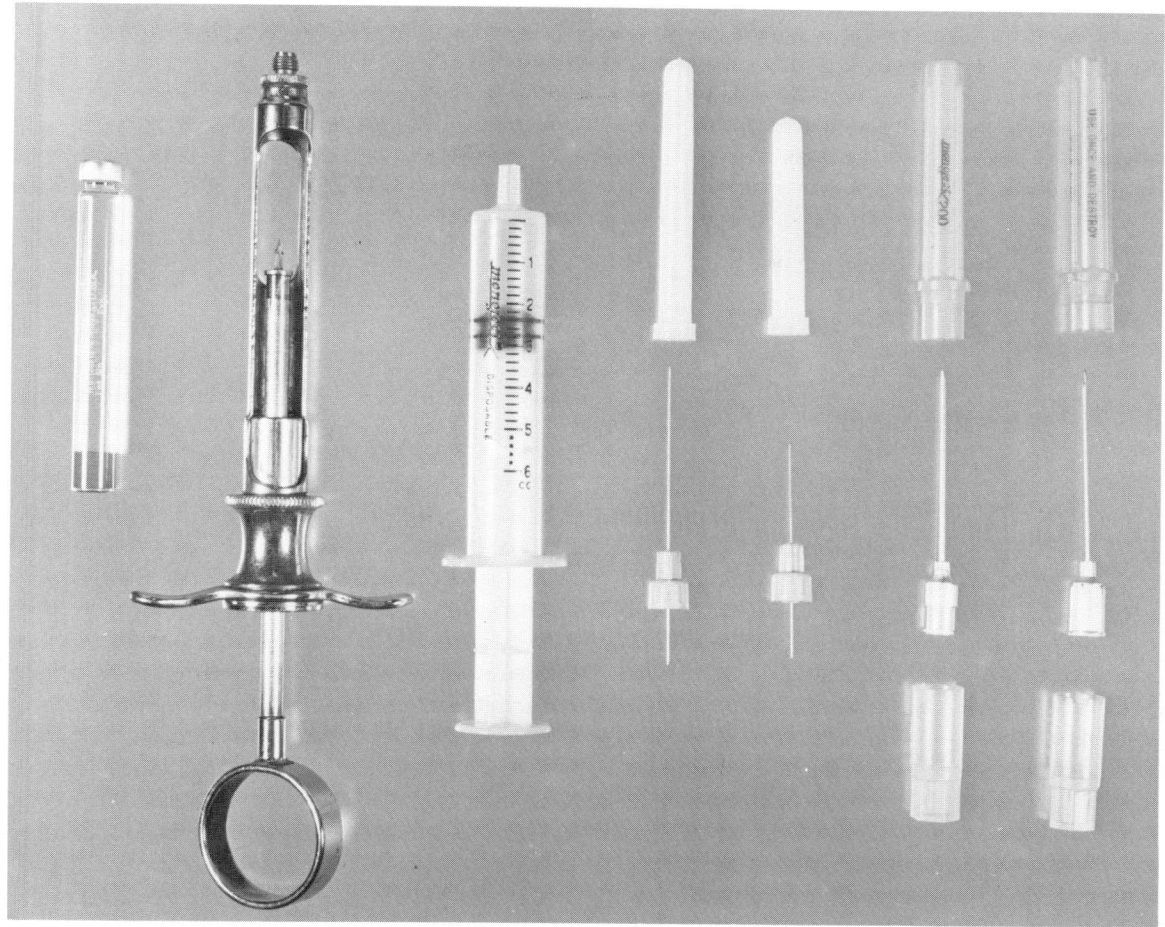

Figure 22-3 | Cartridge of anesthetic, 1.8 ml; cartridge syringe; Luer-Lok syringe; cartridge syringe needles; Luer-Lok syringe needles.

performance of surgery or other potentially painful procedures. Removing caries from a tooth is not generally thought of as surgery; however, it is a cutting procedure in living tissue, and if a strict definition is applied, it could be defined as a surgical procedure. This discussion is primarily concerned with anesthesia of teeth and supporting structures, and the term local anesthesia is applicable. There are many other forms of anesthesia; excellent texts on the subject are available.

Three things are needed to accomplish local anesthesia for teeth and supporting tissues: a solution of local anesthetic, a syringe, and a needle (Fig. 22-3). Someone must give the injection in the correct place, in the correct amount, to prevent the conduction of possible pain stimuli.

Agents

First, consider the chemical solution, the anesthetic. There are many agents available. The

Table 22-1 | Local Anesthetics

Anesthetic agent	Vasoconstrictor concentration usually employed	Relative duration*
Procaine (Novocain) 2%	Epinephrine 1:50,000	Medium
Procaine (Novocain) 4%	Phenylephrine 1:2500	Medium
Tetracaine (Pontocaine) 0.15% with 2% procaine	Levonordefrin 1:20,000	Long
Propoxycaine (Ravocaine) 0.4% with 2% procaine	Levonordefrin 1:20,000	Long
	Levarterenol 1:30,000	Long
Lidocaine (Alphacaine; Doracaine;	None	Medium
Lidocaton: Octocaine; ProLido;	Epinephrine 1:50,000	Long
Xylocaine) 2%	Epinephrine 1:100,000	Long
Mepivacaine 2% (Arestocaine; Carbocaine; Isocaine)	Levonordefrin 1:20,000	Long
Mepivacaine 3%	None	Short
Prilocaine (Citanest Plain) 4%	None	Short
Prilocaine (Citanest Forte) 4%	Epinephrine 1:200,000	Medium

* Durations are variable and classifications are approximate.
SOURCE: American Dental Association, *Accepted Dental Therapeutics, 1977–78,* 1977.

most frequently used will fall in one of two chemical categories: those which contain an *ester* linkage and those which contain an *amide* linkage. Patients who have an allergy to one anesthetic in a group will most likely be allergic to other anesthetics in that group. From an idealistic standpoint, none of the available local anesthetics meet all of the ideal criteria of potency, toxicity, nonirritability to local tissue, nonallergenicity, stability, and others. Time has and will produce anesthetics with properties that enhance their resemblance to the ideal agents. Some of the currently available local anesthetics are listed in Table 22-1.

Most local anesthetics used contain a substance to prolong and enhance the anesthesia for the patient. This chemical is a vasoconstricting agent that constricts the blood vessels in the area to slow the circulatory uptake and transport of the anesthetic. One of the following vasoconstrictors is usually used: epinephrine, norepinephrine, nordefrin (Cobefrin), phenylephrine (Neo-Synephrine), or levonordefrin (Neo-Cobefrin). On occasion, it may be indicated to use an anesthetic without a vasoconstrictor due to the physical condition of the patient or other circumstances. These agents are very potent chemicals and are used in very small amounts in the anesthetic solution. Great care is exercised to prevent injection of the anesthetic, with its vasoconstrictor, directly into the circulatory vessels when administering anesthetics. Undesirable reactions will occur. Other substances are contained in the anesthetic solution to preserve the solution until it is used and make it less toxic to local tissues.

Anatomy; Injection Sites

In the oral cavity, local anesthetic injections are made to block the nerve conduction at a point between the area to be anesthetized and the central nervous system or injected in the area to be anesthetized. These two methods are referred to as *block* and *field,* or infiltration, anesthesia.

In the mandible, the usual injection to anesthetize the teeth is an inferior alveolar block at the point of entry of that branch in the ramus of the mandible (Fig. 22-1). This same injection anesthetizes the lingual nerve that conducts sensory sensation from the anterior one-third of the tongue, the gingiva, and alveolar mucosa on the lingual surface of the mandible. To anesthetize the cheek and lip side of the mandibular teeth, a buccal injection must be given. An alternative to the inferior alveolar block that will anesthetize the premolars, canines, and incisors is an injection in the mental foramen. On occasion, field anesthesia for the incisors is possible. This may not be successful due to the density of bone in the area that prevents diffusion of the anesthetic to the tooth apex.

Maxillary teeth are usually anesthetized by injecting for field anesthesia. A posterior superior alveolar injection is made to anesthetize the third molar, second molar, and part of the first molar (Fig. 22-1). The mesiofacial root of the maxillary first molar is usually supplied by the middle superior alveolar nerve (Fig. 22-1). The middle superior nerve also supplies the premolars. The canine, lateral incisors, and central incisors are anesthetized by field block of the anterior superior alveolar nerve. All of the above injections (maxillary) block sensation in the gingiva and alveolar mucosa of the injected area. Anesthesia of the palatal mucosa and gingiva must be accomplished by blocking the anterior palatine nerve at the greater palatine foramen and the nasopalatine at the incisive foramen (Fig. 22-2). Due to the density of palatal tissue, anesthesia by injecting at the operative site is not as desirable as blocking at the nerve's bony exit. Anesthesia for a single tooth in the maxilla is usually effective by injecting over the apex of the tooth or slightly distal to the apex.

Second (maxillary) and third (mandibular) cranial nerve division blocks are possible and will block all sensation supplied by that particular division (Fig. 22-1). These blocks are made by deposition of anesthetic solution in the area where the nerve exits from the skull. These and other blocks are possible to anesthetize larger areas than described in the preceding paragraphs. They are not generally used in the average dental practice.

Armamentarium and Technique

Anesthetic solution may be purchased in bulk amounts or cartridges. Cartridges are the most convenient and are more expensive. Because of the convenience they are the most frequently used in the practice of dentistry. A syringe to accommodate the cartridge with an appropriate-size needle attached are the items required for dental anesthesia. If bulk anesthesia is used, a Luer-Lok–type syringe with needle is required (see Fig. 22-3). The cartridge syringe should be an aspirating type; that is, negative pressure should be possible in the cartridge prior to injection of the anesthetic. This is to ensure that the solution is not being deposited in a blood vessel. Screw threads, barbs, harpoons, and other techniques are used to allow negative pressure to be placed mechanically on the cartridge. If something works, the specific mechanics are not important. Cartridges of anesthetic are made in two sizes, 1.8 ml and 2.2 ml, and the plungers are color-coded to indicate the vasoconstrictor concentration in that particular manufacturer's product. The needle attached to the syringe should be the appropriate length for the particular injection site; usually 1 in (short) or 1½ in (long). The gauges for intraoral use range from 20 to 30 and are an individual choice. The larger the number, the smaller the needle. A 30-gauge needle is smaller in diameter than a 20-gauge needle. Disposable, presterilized needles are the most popular. When needles are to be reused, they must be properly prepared and sterilized, and sharpness maintained.

With syringe, needle, and cartridge assembled, the injection site must be prepared for injection. The required items are sponges, antiseptic, and optional topical anesthetic. Sterile, cotton-tipped applicators are placed in the solutions, the site dried with a sponge, antiseptic swabbed on the area with the cotton-tipped applicator and, if desired, followed by placement of the topical anesthetic in the area (Fig. 22-4).

At this point, the prepared syringe is made

available to the operator. Remember—once the sterile cotton-tipped applicators have been placed in their respective solutions and removed, they should not be returned to the solutions. They are contaminated and would contaminate the solutions for future use. Following the injection, sterility of the equipment must be maintained as repeated or other injections may be necessary for that patient.

Complications

The most frequent adverse reaction to a local anesthetic injection is fainting. The patient will become pale, clammy, nauseated, and possibly may lose consciousness. The treatment is prescribed in the chapter on first aid. Other more severe physical reactions can occur, the most severe being an acute allergic reaction. The assistant must aid in recognizing an impending reaction and be prepared to assist in treating any adverse situation. Each individual office should have a prescribed plan of action to handle potential problems, at all times, with each individual assigned specific duties. The ultimate is for each office to have the potential to render cardiopulmonary resuscitation.

At the completion of the dental appointment, the assistant should assist in reminding patients not to traumatize anesthetized tissue by biting, pinching, or consuming food that may damage the anesthetized area. The period of "numb feeling" will not last too long, and normal function can resume at that point. This is particularly important for young patients who are not conditioned by previous anesthesia experience.

ANALGESIA

Analgesia is the diminishing of pain perception or pain interpretation without the loss of consciousness. A basic example of an analgesic drug would be aspirin. The ability of the dentist and the dental assistants to apply "psychologic analgesia" in their practice is a very important part of dental practice. Allaying patient fear, projecting an atmosphere of professional confidence, demonstrating office efficiency, and many other techniques can assist in enhancing psychologic analgesia.

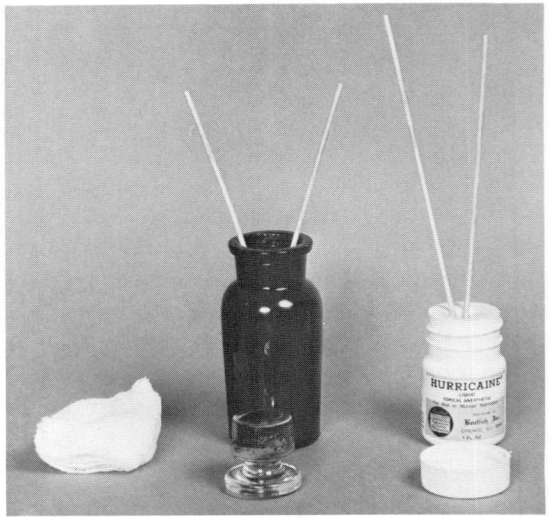

Figure 22-4 | Sponges, 2 by 2 in; antiseptic and topical anesthetic with cotton-tipped applicators.

For office procedures, the usual analgesic drugs used are narcotics and nitrous oxide. These drugs, as previously discussed, have other properties, and these properties should not be ignored during administration. The patient's medical history and current medications will dictate whether these drugs are used and, if used, the appropriate drug for that patient.

The most commonly used natural narcotic analgesics are morphine and codeine. The synthetic preparations most commonly used are meperidine (Demerol) and fentanyl. Individual operators will usually use one of the above as their choice of analgesic, and the assistant should become familiar with the properties of office medications by studying package inserts and texts, and by astute observation of patient reaction during and after administration.

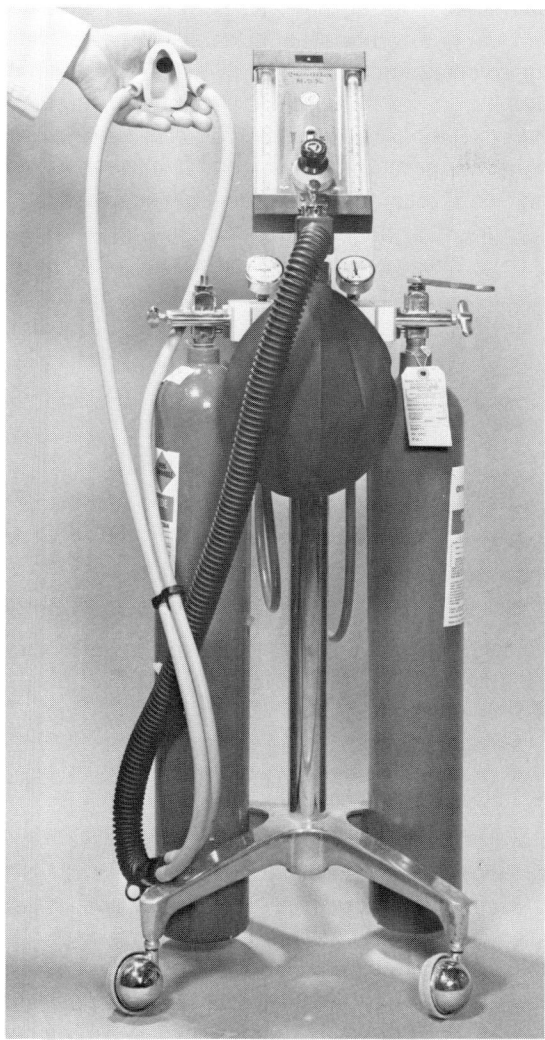

Figure 22-5 | Typical nitrous oxide machine and mask.

As previously cited, nitrous oxide is enjoying a resurgence in popularity for dental procedures. A large number of dental schools are teaching its use and clinical application. It is classified as a general anesthetic, and this fact should not be ignored in its routine use. When used at the proper concentration for analgesia, the drug (gas) is reliable and safe. Many texts will classify nitrous oxide as a sedative (psychosedative). The fact that the pain threshold is altered certainly permits its classification as an analgesic. Use of nitrous oxide requires special equipment that is bulky and requires a continuous supply of drugs (nitrous oxide and oxygen). The assistant must be familiar with the machine's operation and monitor the tanks of nitrous oxide and oxygen to ensure an adequate supply during the procedure (Fig. 22-5). The mask must be cleaned with an antiseptic between patients and its position checked during administration to ensure efficient operation.

The hazards to office personnel of expired and escaping nitrous oxide must be given consideration and appropriate measures to minimize the breathing of significant quantities should be a constant concern.

SEDATION

Sedation is used for the dental patient to relieve apprehension and fear. The techniques and drugs used do not render the patients unconscious, and their protective reflexes remain intact. The patients, at proper levels of administration, will respond to commands by the dentist and assistant and are able to cough, swallow, breath, and maintain all physiologic functions at reduced levels.

Agents

Diazepam (Valium) is one of the most popular agents used. It is currently a most widely prescribed drug by the medical and dental profession; many dental patients are on daily doses of the drug for various dental, psychic, and systemic reasons. It can be used at levels that give profound sedation, muscle relaxation, and an amnesic effect. Patients also enjoy a period of euphoria following the dental procedure and do not usually suffer the "hangover" experienced with some drugs. Diazepam and the barbiturates are generally accepted as the most desirable sedative drugs when all aspects of their action, effectiveness, and undesirable reactions are considered.

The use of hydroxyzine hydrochloride (Vistaril) has wide popularity for the dental patient, especially children. It is generally given by intramuscular injection; intravenous administration is contraindicated. Its antiemetic effect and ability to control anxious, hyperkinetic children make its use popular for this age group when patient management by the drug route is indicated.

The barbiturates are the oldest and probably still the most widely used sedative drugs. There are a wide variety of drugs in this category and they are generally classified as

1. Ultra-short-acting
2. Short-acting
3. Intermediate-acting
4. Long-acting

The short-acting groups, pentobarbital and secobarbital, are usually the barbiturates of choice for dental procedures. The above are generic names, and the brand (proprietary) names available in this and the other three groups are many. Again, review of the literature and the package insert for the brand in office use is indicated.

Narcotics have sedative properties; their use is usually for their analgesic effect or to enhance the sedative effect of some other drugs. Meperidine (Demerol) is usually the narcotic used when a narcotic is chosen for its sedative properties. Meperidine is enhanced in its sedative and analgesic action by the addition of promethazine hydrochloride (Phenergan) to the preparation. Phenergan's antiemetic, sedative, and antihistamine effect makes the combination a better sedative drug than Demerol alone.

Neuroleptic Analgesia

The area of neuroleptic analgesia anesthesia may be classified somewhere between sedation techniques and general anesthesia. Generally, the use of this modality in dental practice is contraindicated unless the dentist has had special training in anesthesia. The patient may be rendered unconscious with the techniques, and constant monitoring with the ability to recognize and correct any adverse reactions is necessary. Neuroleptic analgesia is accomplished with the intravenous use of droperidol (Inapsine) and fentanyl (Sublimaze). The addition of nitrous oxide will give neuroleptic anesthesia. The potency of the individual drugs and especially when combined with one or two others requires special training for their administration.

Drug Combinations

The use of combinations of drugs is to make use of the desired properties of each of the individual drugs or to take advantage of the synergistic action of the combination or to counteract undesirable effects.

One of the basic drug combinations that has withstood the test of time is the one developed by Dr. Niels Jorgensen and appropriately referred to as the Jorgenson technique. The combination is given intravenously by starting with 100 mg of pentobarbital given in gradual increments until light sedation is reached. This is followed with meperidine (25 mg) and scopolamine (0.32 mg) in a separate syringe. The amount of the latter two administered is a percentage of the amount of barbiturates used to obtain light sedation for that individual. For example, if 40 mg of the barbiturate is used to establish base line (light sedation), then 40 percent of the solution of meperidine and scopolamine is given the patient. The assistant may be called upon to assist in calculating the required dosages and should be familiar with any techniques used by the individual dentist.

Other drug combinations have been mentioned, and certainly others will be developed subsequent to this writing. The assistant is reminded to become familiar with those used by the individual doctor and to assist in all aspects legally permissable.

Routes of Administration

In most instances, the most efficient method for administering analgesics and sedatives is by the intravenous route. Immediate effect is obtained, the correct amount to obtain the desired effect for a particular individual is given, and immediate counteractive drugs can be given when indicated. A vein in the antecubital fossa or the dorsum of the hand is the usual area chosen for venipuncture. Some agents cannot be given by the intravenous route because of their physical state, and others cause undesirable reactions within the venous system. Nitrous oxide, being a gas, can only be used by inhalation. Hydroxyzine hydrochloride should not be given in a vein, as the complication of thrombosis and its resultant morbidity incidence is high. The above are two examples, and there are many other possibilities.

The oral route is probably the most frequent route for intraoffice drug administration. It requires no special equipment or preparation and in minimal amounts is probably the safest. The disadvantages are a slow and variable rate of absorption depending on gastric content, condition of the gastric mucosa, and time-consuming dosage adjustment for individual physiology and psyche.

In children and hyperactive individuals, the intramuscular administration may be the best route for administration as opposed to the intravenous or oral. The intramuscular route requires little time, less technical involvement, and generally has less postinjection complications when compared to the intravenous route. Also, the effects of the drug will usually last longer when given intramuscularly. The deltoid, gluteus maximus, or lateral thigh muscles are the usual choices for injection.

Two other routes are possible for giving needed drugs in the dental office: rectal and subcutaneous. These are probably the least frequently used routes for dental patients. The type of drug used would usually dictate the use of this modality.

ASSISTANT'S ROLE IN DRUG ADMINISTRATION

Equipment and Drugs

All equipment for administering drugs must be readily available and in good working order. When indicated, sterility of equipment is of paramount importance. As with local anesthetic needles, most offices use prepackaged, sterile needles and syringes for administration. Many drugs are available in premeasured doses in the syringe with attached needles. If drugs are not used frequently, this is probably the best way to purchase same. Many medications may require refrigeration to prevent deterioration and most are dated. Drugs that have become outdated should not be used under any circumstances. Any change in the usual appearance of the drug is important—color change, precipitate, and foreign material are some of the changes to be checked.

Preoperative Considerations

Prior to preparing the medication, the patient record should be checked for any positive findings in the medical history and possible past record of dental treatment that may preclude or modify the use of the medication. Drugs that may suppress reflex actions of the individual should not be given a patient who does not have an escort home. In such instances, the assistant should check with the patient regarding an escort prior to going into the operatory.

Monitoring

Once the patient is seated and placed in a semi-reclining position, pulse and blood pressure should be recorded. The blood pressure cuff should be left on the patients' arm to allow intraoperative monitoring. All information regarding vital signs before, during, and after completion of the procedure should be recorded in the patient's record.

Drug Preparation and Records

All drugs, including local anesthetics, with name and amount should be recorded. Preparation of the drug for use is the most important part of its administration. The name and amount should be triple-checked. Local regulations regarding qualifications to perform this and other functions by assistants should be checked. Federal and some local regulations require strict record keeping for dispensed drugs. Patient name, drug name, amount dispensed, and date are required by law for many drugs and should be a part of office records in all offices.

Security and Responsibility

All medications and especially controlled substances should be stored under lock and key. Dental offices are prime targets for drug theft, and strict security measures cannot be overemphasized. One individual in each office should have the responsibility for record keeping and security. Divided responsibilities in this area can cause confusion and allegations that should be prevented by specific assignment for these duties.

BIBLIOGRAPHY

American Dental Association, Council on Dental Therapeutics: *Accepted Dental Therapeutics,* 36th ed., American Dental Association, Chicago, 1975.

Bennett, C. R.: *Conscious-Sedation in Dental Practice,* The C. V. Mosby Company, St. Louis, 1974a.

_____: *Monheim's Local Anesthesia and Pain Control in Dental Practice,* 5th ed., The C. V. Mosby Company, St. Louis, 1974b.

_____: *Monheim's General Anesthesia in Dental Practice,* 4th ed., The C. V. Mosby Company, St. Louis, 1974c.

Blakiston's Gould Medical Dictionary, 3d ed., McGraw-Hill Book Company, New York, 1972.

Jorgenson, N. B., and Hayden, J., Jr.: *Sedation, Local and General Anesthesia in Dentistry,* 2d ed., Lea & Febiger, Philadelphia, 1972.

McCarthy, F. M.: *Emergencies in Dental Practice, Prevention and Treatment,* 2d ed., W. B. Saunders Company, Philadelphia, 1972.

23

Cecil R. Lupton
Oral Surgery

INTRODUCTION

Oral surgery is defined as "that part of dental practice which deals with diagnosis and the surgical and adjunctive treatment of diseases, injuries, and defects of the oral and maxillofacial region." This definition was revised and adopted by the American Dental Association (ADA) House of Delegates in October 1976.

Oral surgery is the oldest recognized dental specialty. Dr. Simon P. Hullihen (1810–1857) is credited with being the first man to be designated as an oral surgeon. The list of pioneers and contributors to the advancement of the specialty is too long to relate. Presently, training for recognition as a specialist consists of a minimum of 3 years following attainment of the D.D.S. or D.M.D. degree. A few training programs are offering 5-year programs that include oral surgery specialty training and awarding of a Doctor of Medicine degree.

Surgical procedures may be classified into major and minor surgery. It is difficult to apply strict classification to each individual surgical procedure. Minor procedures are usually those performed in the dental office in a relatively short period of time that do not require professional care and observation in the postoperative period. These procedures would include removal of erupted teeth and some tooth impactions, biopsy, frenectomy, alveolectomy, apicoectomy, and others. Most jaw fractures, orthodontic surgery, correction of atrophic jaws, temporomandibular joint surgery, and many others are major surgery and are performed in

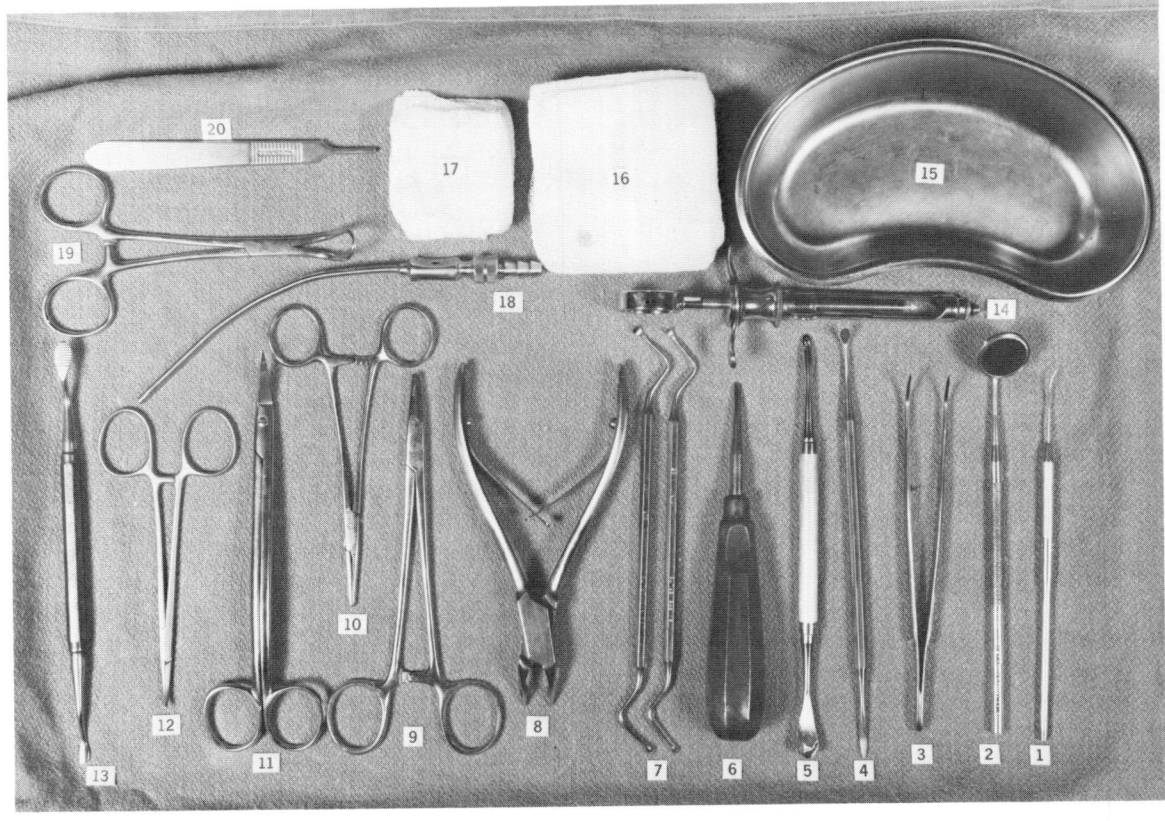

Figure 23-1 | Typical oral surgery basic tray with instrument names. (1) Gilmore probe, (2) mirror, (3) cotton pliers, (4) Woodson plastic instrument, (5) periosteal elevator, (6) straight elevator, (7) curettes, (8) rongeur forceps, (9) needle holder, (10) straight hemostat, (11) scissor, (12) curved hemostat, (13) bone file, (14) aspirating, cartridge syringe. (15) emesis basin, (16) sponges, 3 by 3 in, (17) sponges, 2 by 2 in, (18) suction tip, (19) towel clip, (20) blade handle.

the hospital. Some minor procedures become major when concomitant medical problems are present.

ASEPSIS

Office

Asepsis is important in all dental procedures; in surgical procedures, it assumes the same priority as the operation being performed. All instruments must be sterile, sterile covers must be placed on the patient, the surgeon and assistant must be scrubbed and gloved to prevent contamination and its possible consequences. Ideally, each office will have a standard basic setup of surgical instruments on a tray that is sterilized with sterile covers (towels) for draping included (Fig. 23-1).

Instruments that may be used in addition to those on the basic tray may be stored in sterile

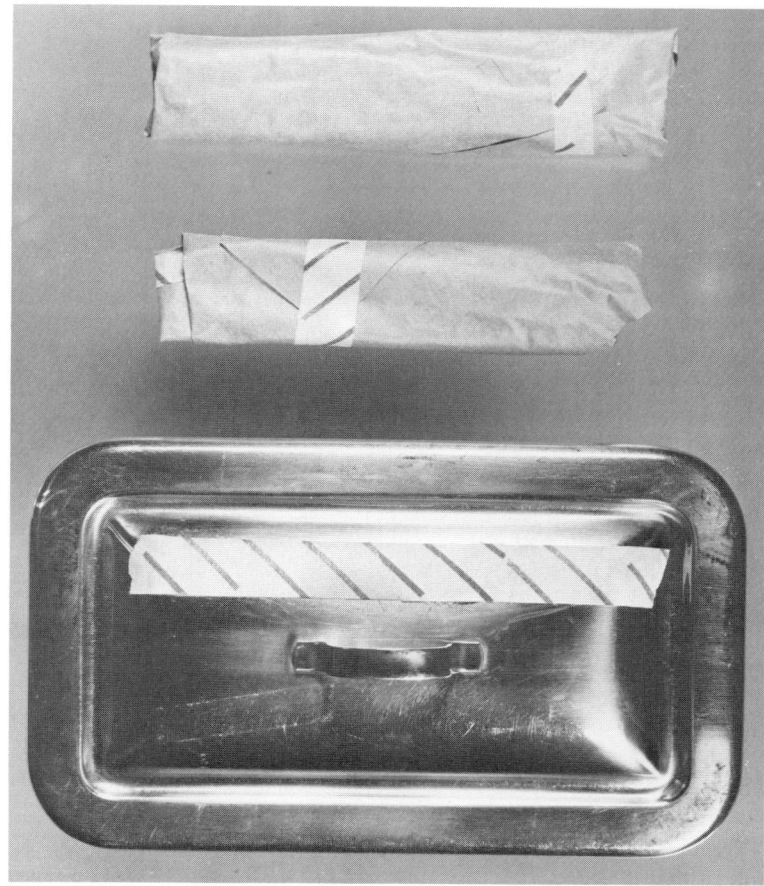

Figure 23-2 | Instrument pan with sterile instruments and wrapped sterile instruments. Both labeled with indicator tape to assure sterility.

containers or wrapped prior to sterilization (Fig. 23-2). Indicator tape to ensure sterilization is advisable; it is easy to confuse instruments that are prepared for sterilization and those that have been sterilized. Any doubt should be eliminated by labeling with indicator tape.

For office procedures (minor surgery), the surgeon and assistant should wear a clean scrub shirt or dress, head cover, mask, and gloves (Fig. 23-3). Once the surgeon and assistant are attired in proper dress, the hands are scrubbed with an appropriate antimicrobial agent and gloves put on. Once this has been accomplished, the hands should only touch sterile surfaces and the patient's oral structures. The hands should not be dropped by the side; keep them up to maintain sterility and to remind other personnel that you should not be contaminated.

Assuming the patient has been seated, properly positioned, medical history reviewed, etc., the patient is now ready to be draped with the sterile covers that are on the tray (Fig. 23-4). The tray covering towel is placed with the upside down on the patient's chest. This may be an appropriate time to remind the patient not to touch this and other sterilized instruments or material. Next, the other sterile cover (towel) is placed on the patient's head and the sterile covers secured. The team and patient are now ready to begin the surgical procedure.

Hospital

If the surgery is taking place in a hospital, the same basic requirements for asepsis still apply. The one major difference will be in operating room attire. Complete scrub suits or dresses replace street clothes, special shoes or shoe covers with grounding strips are worn, and a sterile gown is worn. Different hospitals have different procedures and protocol; the primary objective is the same.

PREOPERATIVE PLAN

Intentionally, asepsis and sterile technique have been discussed prior to the preoperative plan and other surgery topics. Hopefully, this will lend emphasis to asepsis in surgery.

The patient's radiographs should be placed on the view box, patient's record reviewed, and the surgeon reminded of any information in the record that may be pertinent to medication, anesthesia, surgical procedure, or patient welfare. If the assistant is not sure of the operation to be performed or instruments required, the surgeon should be asked for guidance.

Instruments

If teeth are to be removed, indicated forceps are placed with the basic setup. There are a large number of forceps manufactured, and each dentist has favorites. Names or numbers may be used to designate each forceps. Some typical forceps are shown in Fig. 23-5.

Elevators are just as varied in number and style as forceps. They can be classified as *dis-*

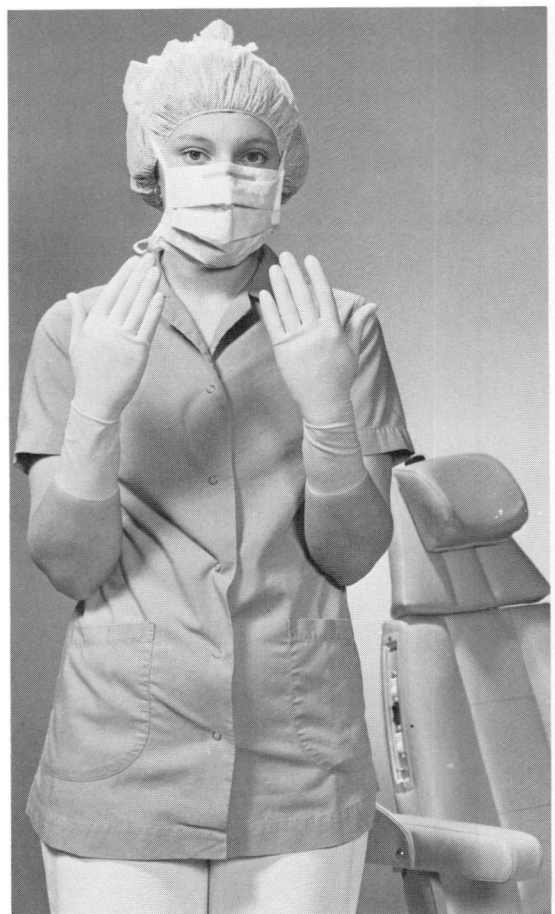

Figure 23-3 | Surgical assistant dress with head cover, mask, scrubbed and gloved.

placing elevators or *lever* elevators. Most are paired instruments, and to differentiate between paired elevators terms such as east and west, right and left, or clockwise and counterclockwise are used. These terms are difficult for the assistant to interpret until surgical experience is gained with the individual operator. Like forceps, elevators have names and numbers, and the individual operator will have certain favorites. A few examples are shown in Fig. 23-6.

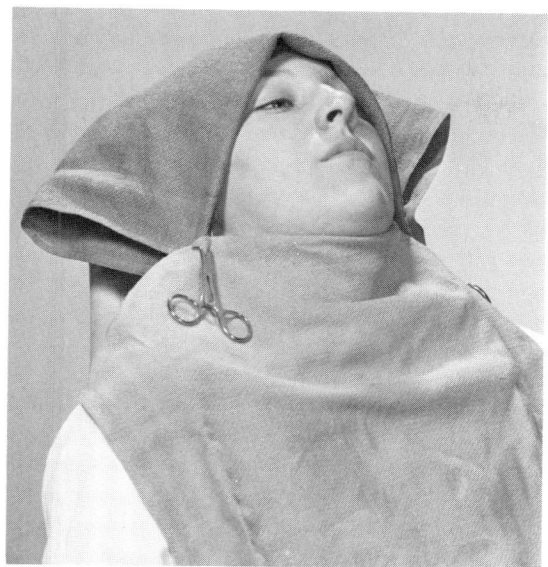

Figure 23-4 | Patient draped with sterile covers.

Mallet and chisels or handpieces with burs are used to section teeth and remove bony structures. Chisel design may be single bevel or bi-bevel, straight, or curved. They must be sharp to accomplish the procedure with efficiency. The assistant is usually called upon to tap the chisel with the mallet to section the tooth or to remove the bony structure. The first experiences with the mallet usually are intimidating; the chisel should be struck with authority and the technique subsequently adjusted by instructions from the surgeon.

Handpieces and burs should be sterile and the bur run in a liquid medium to enhance cutting efficiency, prevent overheating of the tissues, and remove cutting debris; this is accomplished by applying sterile physiologic saline or plain sterile water to the area with a syringe (Fig. 23-7).

Sutures

Sutures are placed with many surgical procedures and may be either an absorbable or non-absorbable type, depending on the surgeon's preference. Suture material is available in many sizes, many different materials, and with different type and size needles. A usual type of suture placed in the oral cavity would be 4/0 black braided silk on a half-circle cutting-edge needle. The size of the material ranges from 3 to 7/0. The size 3 is the largest and 7/0 the smallest.

Needles may be straight, half-circle, half-curved, or many other shapes. They may have a cutting edge, with inside or reverse bevel, or be atraumatic—round and without a cutting edge. The suture material may be purchased in pre-sterilized packages with the needles attached. When purchased in a prepared package, the needle does not have an eye. The suture material is placed in the hollow end and the end crimped by the manufacturer. In this instance, the suture material is said to be *swaged* to the needle.

A practical and economical method of purchasing suture material is to buy it unprepared. The needles are purchased separately and reused. The suture material is purchased by the spool, cut, tied to the needle, wrapped on a sponge or cotton roll, and sterilized for surgical use. Time is required to prepare sutures by this method and may not be economical in some offices. Information on suture material could easily fill a chapter, and such a volume of information is not practical for our purposes. Nonabsorbable (silk, nylon, etc.) suture material must be removed in 5 to 7 days, and patients with these sutures should return for a postoperative appointment.

Anesthesia has been discussed in the previous chapter and is only mentioned here as a reminder for the basic surgical setup.

Vital Signs

The patient's preoperative temperature, pulse, and blood pressure should be recorded prior to the surgical operation. This is important for future reference in the event that abnormal

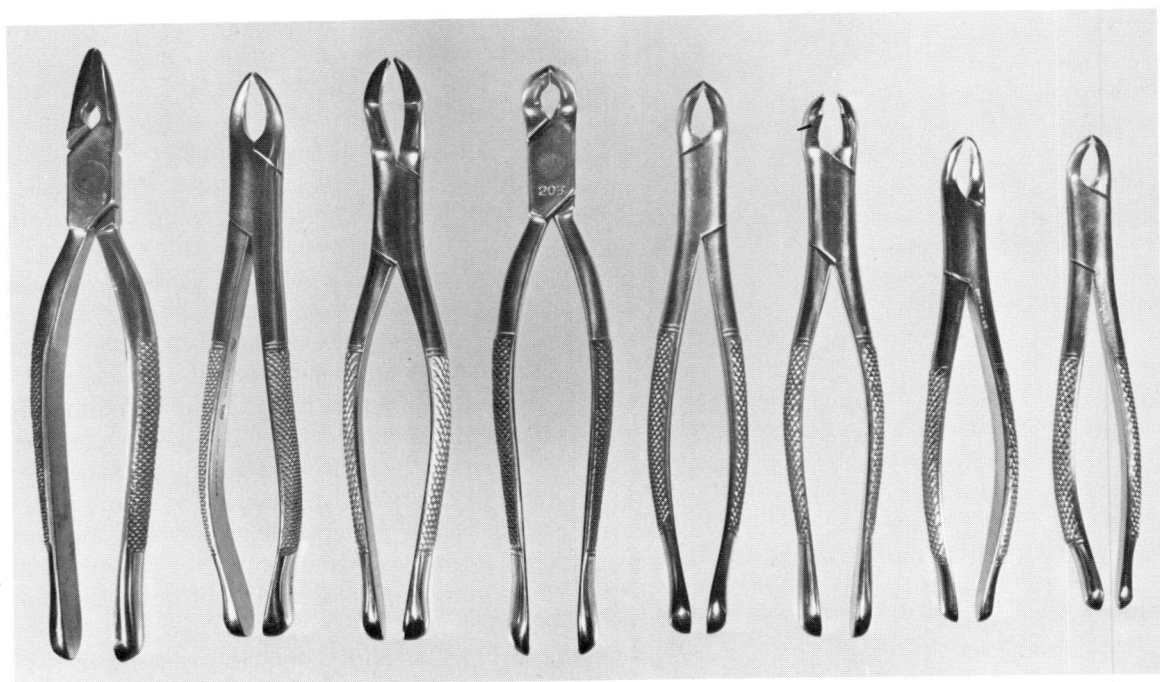

Figure 23-5 | Typical forceps. *Left to right,* maxillary anterior, no. 1; maxillary premolar, no. 150; maxillary molar, no. 4; mandibular anterior, no. 203; mandibular premolar, no. 151; mandibular molar, no. 17; maxillary pedodontic, no. 150S; mandibular pedodontic, no. 151S.

responses occur during the operation or anytime afterward. For instance, the patient may develop a postoperative infection, and the preoperative vital signs could be important in making decisions regarding diagnosis and treatment. Just as importantly, the preoperative vital signs may offer clues to systemic conditions that require medical consultation prior to any treatment. Remember, leave the deflated blood pressure cuff on the arm until completion of the surgery.

OPERATIVE PROCEDURES

The assistant's role during the procedure is to help accomplish same with efficiency and dispatch. Foremost is to maintain a clean surgical area and to afford visibility for the surgeon. It is important to retract the cheek, tongue, or other tissue to afford visibility and access for the surgeon.

A clean site is accomplished with a suction apparatus (aspirator) and retraction with fingers or retracting instruments. On occasion, the aspirator tip may become clogged with clotted blood or other debris. In such circumstances, a stylus or other sterile instrument should be used to clean the aspirator tip. Sterile water or saline may be run through the tip to assist in cleaning. Never, never use the water running in the cuspidor or other unsterilized media to free the clogged instrument.

Instruments should be passed at the surgeon's request and cleaned of blood or other debris as

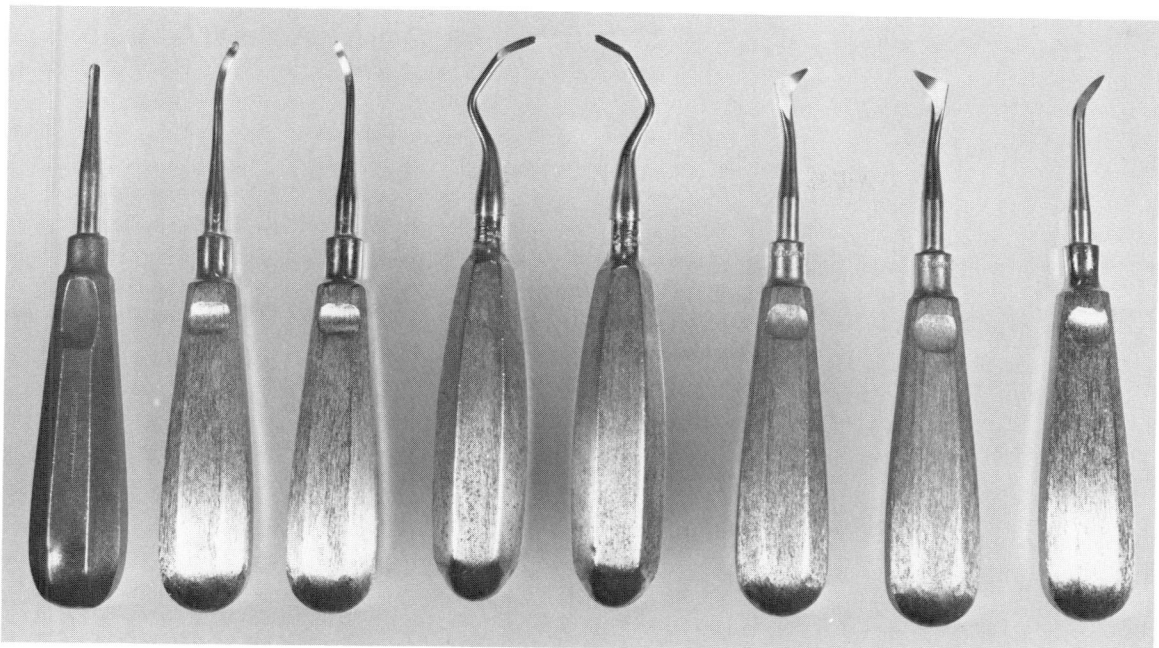

Figure 23-6 | Typical elevators. *Left to right,* straight, no. 40; upper Miller (paired), nos. 73 and 74; lower Miller (paired), nos. 71 and 72; Cryer (paired), nos. 1 and 2; Crane pick, no. 8.

Figure 23-7 | Physiologic saline being applied to the surgical site.

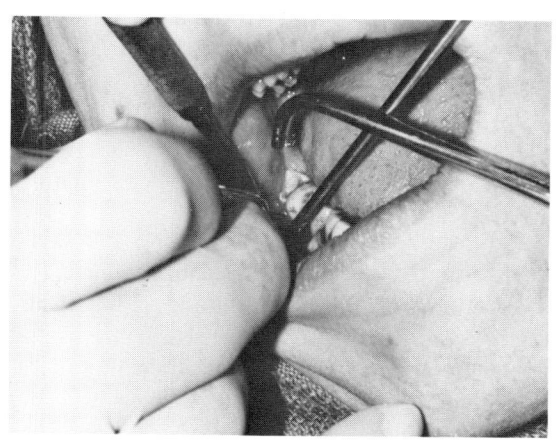

necessary. With experience, the assistant will be able to anticipate instrument needs and pass them to the surgeon as necessary.

With a "third eye" the assistant should observe the patient for any patient reaction that should be brought to the surgeon's attention.

During brief operation interludes, such as changing burs in a handpiece or waiting for supplemental anesthesia, a sponge pack should be placed over the surgical area and the patient allowed to close. Any brief rest is a welcome relief to the patient and should be instituted when possible. Keeping saliva, blood, and other debris evacuated from areas away from the surgical site is comforting to the patient and suppresses the gag reflex and any unnecessary desire to spit.

The patient's lips, the commissure, and other vulnerable anatomic areas should be protected

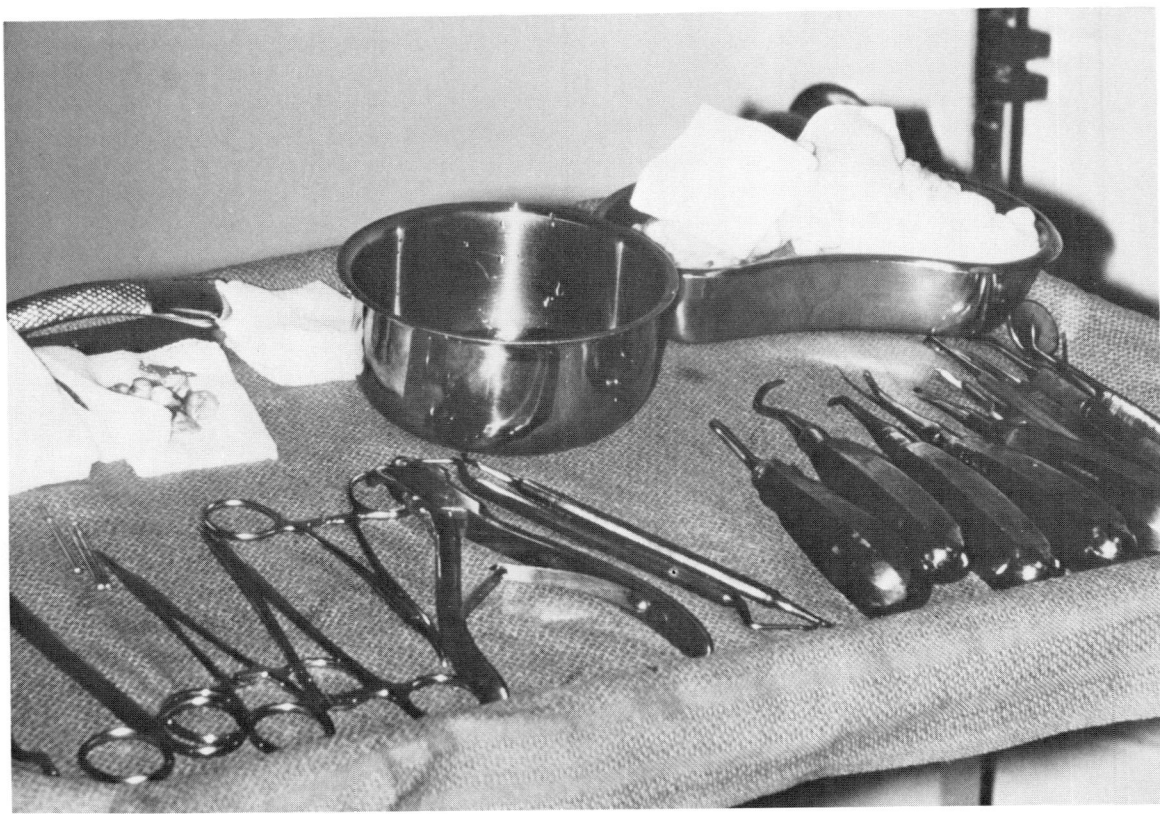

Figure 23-8 | Intraoperative surgical tray.

from trauma from forcep handles and other instrument manipulations.

Instruments are easier to find on the tray if they are replaced in their original order on the tray, and all soiled sponges and debris are placed in an appropriate receptacle (Fig. 23-8).

Any break or breach of the sterile technique should be immediately corrected. If a new sterile tray is indicated, it should be obtained. Torn or cut gloves should be immediately replaced. Dropped instruments are pushed aside with the foot and, if needed, a sterile replacement obtained. When such a break or breach is unrecognized by the surgeon, the assistant should discretely call attention to the fact. If such principles are not adhered to, all previous preparation and concern for asepsis are a waste of time and effort.

POSTOPERATIVE

Upon completion of the procedure, the sterile drapes are removed from the patient's head and chest and placed on the tray to cover the instruments, bloody sponges, and any other items that would be repugnant to viewing by the patient. The patient's face should be checked and any smudges of blood removed with a damp sponge

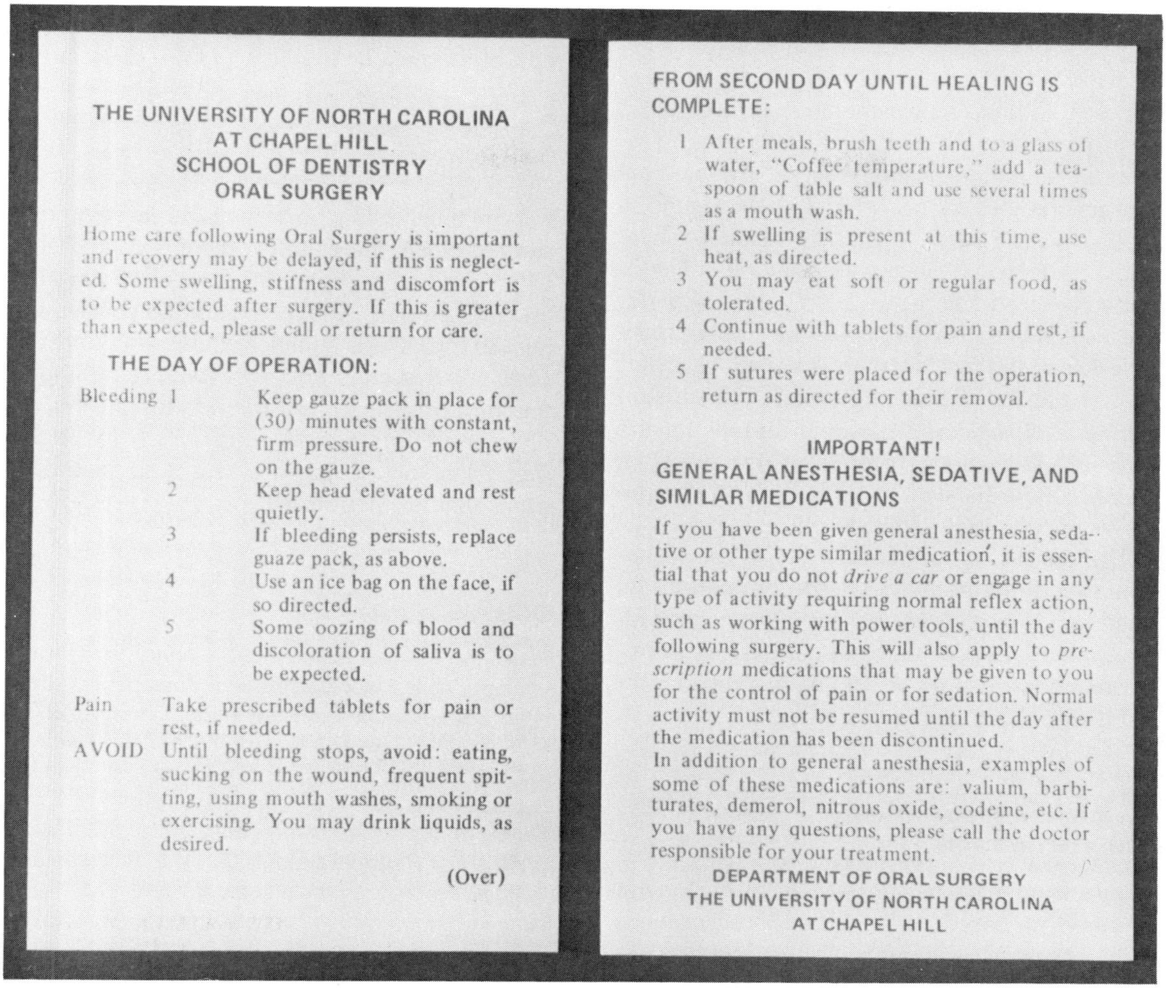

THE UNIVERSITY OF NORTH CAROLINA
AT CHAPEL HILL
SCHOOL OF DENTISTRY
ORAL SURGERY

Home care following Oral Surgery is important and recovery may be delayed, if this is neglected. Some swelling, stiffness and discomfort is to be expected after surgery. If this is greater than expected, please call or return for care.

THE DAY OF OPERATION:

Bleeding 1 Keep gauze pack in place for (30) minutes with constant, firm pressure. Do not chew on the gauze.
2 Keep head elevated and rest quietly.
3 If bleeding persists, replace guaze pack, as above.
4 Use an ice bag on the face, if so directed.
5 Some oozing of blood and discoloration of saliva is to be expected.

Pain Take prescribed tablets for pain or rest, if needed.

AVOID Until bleeding stops, avoid: eating, sucking on the wound, frequent spitting, using mouth washes, smoking or exercising. You may drink liquids, as desired.

(Over)

FROM SECOND DAY UNTIL HEALING IS COMPLETE:

1 After meals, brush teeth and to a glass of water, "Coffee temperature," add a teaspoon of table salt and use several times as a mouth wash.
2 If swelling is present at this time, use heat, as directed.
3 You may eat soft or regular food, as tolerated.
4 Continue with tablets for pain and rest, if needed.
5 If sutures were placed for the operation, return as directed for their removal.

IMPORTANT!
GENERAL ANESTHESIA, SEDATIVE, AND SIMILAR MEDICATIONS

If you have been given general anesthesia, sedative or other type similar medication, it is essential that you do not *drive a car* or engage in any type of activity requiring normal reflex action, such as working with power tools, until the day following surgery. This will also apply to *prescription* medications that may be given to you for the control of pain or for sedation. Normal activity must not be resumed until the day after the medication has been discontinued.
In addition to general anesthesia, examples of some of these medications are: valium, barbiturates, demerol, nitrous oxide, codeine, etc. If you have any questions, please call the doctor responsible for your treatment.

DEPARTMENT OF ORAL SURGERY
THE UNIVERSITY OF NORTH CAROLINA
AT CHAPEL HILL

Figure 23-9 | Typical postoperative instruction card; front and back.

or towel. The patient should remain seated until postoperative instructions are given, indicated prescriptions prepared, and necessary return appointments made.

Histopathologic Examination

Tissue that requires histopathologic examination (biopsy) should have been placed in a specimen bottle at the time of removal or, if not, it should be placed in same at this point. A report sheet to the pathologist accompanies the specimen, and the basic information (patient name, etc.) should be recorded on the sheet by the assistant. It is of utmost importance to be sure that the report and bottle are together. It would be tragic for a patient to receive a diagnosis of a morbid nature that belonged to another patient. A negative report for a patient with a morbid condition would be just as tragic.

Patient Instructions

Brief postoperative instructions regarding the use of cold and heat, replacement of sponge packs, pain medication or other medication, and general care should be given. As stated, these verbal instructions should be brief and then supplemented with a written instruction card or sheet (Fig. 23-9). Most patients will not hear or remember verbal instructions, because of the usual desire at this point to terminate the appointment quickly and the fact that many may still be suffering some anxiety and apprehension. The surgeon will have biologic and personal reasons for the type of instructions given and the assistant should study the written instructions to ensure consistency in that particular office.

The patient should be escorted to the reception area or the escorting person brought to the operatory to accomplish this task. Young individuals and adults who may not comprehend postoperative instructions should have a responsible adult with them during this procedure.

Instrument Preparation and Sterilization

The instruments are removed from the operatory and prepared and sterilized in accordance with accepted standards. The operatory is checked for cleanliness and prepared for reception of the next patient.

COMMENT

For the individual who plans a career in an oral surgery office, there are excellent texts available which will help in preparing for assisting in such an environment. Also, postgraduate courses are available that will enhance knowledge and expertise in this area. The texts that are published for the professional will provide insight into all phases of the specialty and will help in the understanding of many of the surgical procedures that are performed.

BIBLIOGRAPHY

American Dental Association, Council on Dental Therapeutics: *Accepted Dental Therapeutics,* 36th ed., American Dental Association, Chicago, 1975.

Costich, E. R., and White, R. P.: *Fundamentals of Oral Surgery,* W. B. Saunders Company, Philadelphia, 1971.

Dunn, M. J., Booth, D. F., and Clancey, M.: *Dental Auxiliary Practice, Module 5,* The Williams and Wilkins Company, Baltimore, 1975.

Kruger, G. O.: *Textbook of Oral Surgery,* 4th ed., The C. V. Mosby Company, St. Louis, 1974.

24

R. Jack Shankle
Endodontics

During the first half of this century, less attention than today was given to salvaging pulpally involved teeth through endodontic procedures. During the past 25 years there has been a renewed interest in this area of practice. During the mid-1960s the speciality of endodontics was recognized by the American Dental Association, which has resulted in greater emphasis on endodontic procedures in dental education and practice. Teeth heretofore relegated to the surgeon's forceps are now being maintained in a healthy, functioning manner by endodontic therapy.

The dental assistant actively participates in this area of practice, just as in other areas of the practice of dentistry.

GENERAL INFORMATION

Endodontics may be defined as the diagnosis and treatment of the diseases of the pulp and the diseases of the periapical tissues. The latter conditions usually result from a spread of pulp disease from within the pulp cavity.

Some of the more common endodontic procedures are (1) diagnosis, (2) root canal therapy, (3) pulp capping, (4) pulpotomy, and (5) periapical surgery.

THE DIAGNOSIS

The diagnosis of pulpal and periapical conditions precedes treatment. The importance of a correct diagnosis is emphasized; likewise, the role of the dental assistant in diagnostic procedures is important. The patient is in pain, usually, and reassurance by the dental assistant as to a pleasant outcome of an unpleasant situation may be helpful in allaying anxiety.

There are a number of diagnostic methods used in endodontics. Some of the ones commonly employed by the dentist are (1) visual examination, (2) x-ray, (3) vitalometer (electric pulp test), (4) ice, (5) heat, (6) percussion, (7) palpation, (8) mobility test, (9) anesthetic test, (10) transillumination, and (11) release of pressure.

Visual Examination and X-ray

A visual examination of the oral cavity is made in conjunction with tracing the history of the complaint (Fig. 24-1). A radiograph is made early in the appointment period, generally, and developed immediately by the dental assistant for an emergency reading.

Electric Pulp Test

There are a number of different electric pulp testers, and the types found in dental offices may vary. The one used by the author is pictured in Fig. 24-2, and its operation will be discussed, although the operation is similar for all types. Assembly of the apparatus is simple, with little chance for error, as each connection is designed in such a manner as to prevent interchangeability.

Cotton rolls are inserted in the mucobuccal fold, and the teeth which are to be tested are rendered dry with a blast of air. The doctor applies the tooth electrode after a minute droplet of water or toothpaste has been placed on the part that contacts the tooth, and the dental assistant controls the current.

There is a scale on the instrument with numbers ranging from 1 to 14. The button that slides along this scale must be pressed to com-

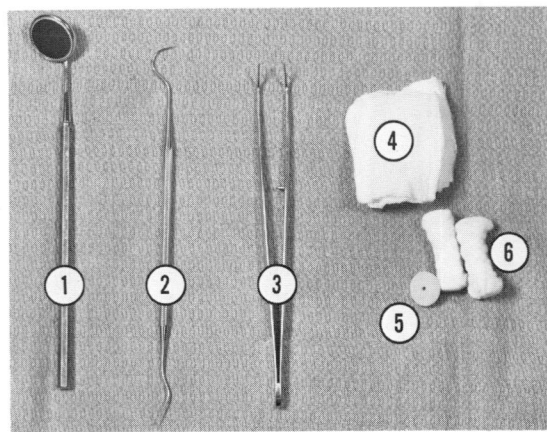

Figure 24-1 | Instrument arrangement for a preliminary examination. (1) Mirror, (2) explorer, (3) pliers, (4) 2 by 2 in gauze, (5) rubber wheel, (6) cotton rolls.

plete the contact. A buzzing sound is heard, as the button is pressed, which assures the dental assistant of a properly functioning apparatus. The current is increased gradually as the button passes down the scale to higher numbers. The patient is instructed to raise a hand whenever a

Figure 24-2 | Electric pulp testing. (1) Water in dappen dish (toothpaste may be used), (2) vitalometer (*courtesy of Burton*), (3) tooth electrode, (4) mirror, (5) explorer, (6) pliers, (7) cotton rolls or 2 by 2 in gauze.

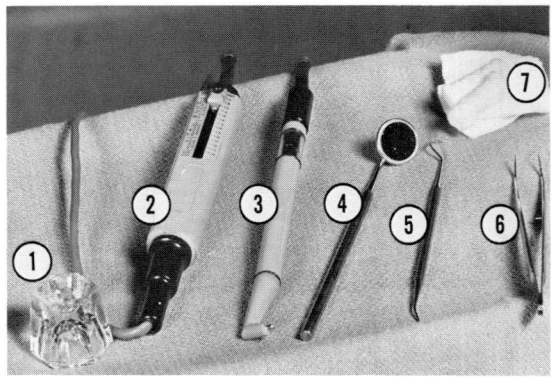

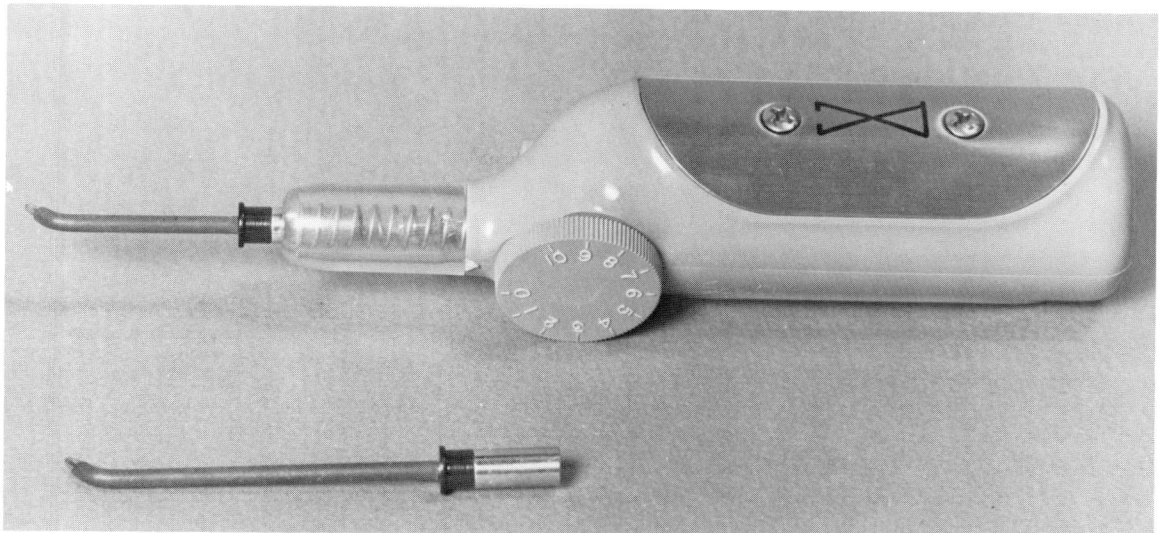

Figure 24-3 | Battery source electric pulp tester. (*Courtesy of Pelton and Crane.*)

sensation is first detected within the tooth. The number at which there is a response is recorded promptly.

The tooth may not respond to the maximum amount of current (no. 14) if the pulp is dead; however, if the pulp is vital, there will be a response early and at a much lower number. The sensation within the tooth created by the instrument may be variously described by different patients. Generally it is a sensation of warmth or glow, although many refer to it as a "tingling" sensation. The patient may be apprehensive about the use of an electrical device for testing tooth vitality; therefore, it is important for the dental assistant to reassure the patient as to safety.

The tooth electrode should be sterilized following its use by (1) autoclaving, (2) boiling water, or (3) cleansing with an accepted germicidal solution. The tooth electrode must be dry before it is used again.

A battery source pulp tester, preferred by many, is shown in Fig. 24-3.

Ice Test

Ice in the form of a stick is applied to the teeth. These ice sticks may be prepared by filling used anesthetic cartridges with water and freezing them. Whenever ice is required for examination, a cartridge is held briefly in the hand to free the ice from its glass compartment. The ice stick then is wrapped in a gauze or facial tissue and passed to the doctor for use (Fig. 24-4).

A frozen stick of carbon dioxide is preferred by some (see Fig. 24-5).

Heat

A small piece of gutta-percha is applied to the end of a plastic instrument and heated until it smokes. This is passed to the doctor for use (Fig. 24-6).

Percussion

Percussion is the tapping of a tooth lightly in order to determine presence of tenderness. A

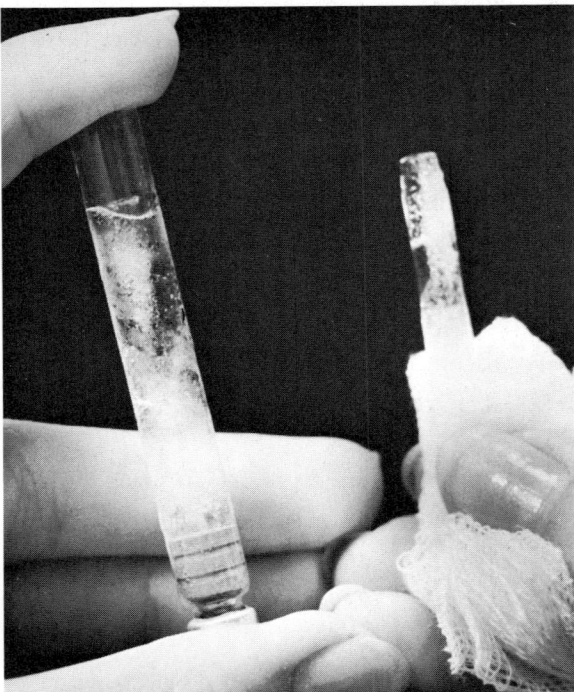

Figure 24-4 | Ice test. (1) Cartridge of ice, (2) ice stick used for vitality test.

finger or instrument handle is used to tap the facial or occlusal (incisal) surface in an effort to elicit pain or to produce an abnormal sound. Pain from percussion is significant of injury to the periodontal membrane. A dull sound signifies destruction to the periodontal membrane, alveolar bone, or both. The opposing teeth as well as adjacent teeth may be percussed in order to compare sensation.

Palpation

Palpation is the application of the fingertips to areas of the mouth in order to detect normal or abnormal tissue. Swelling, pain, and degree of rigidity of tissue are determined by palpation.

Palpation is of particular interest in the diagnosis of periapical disease. The fingers are

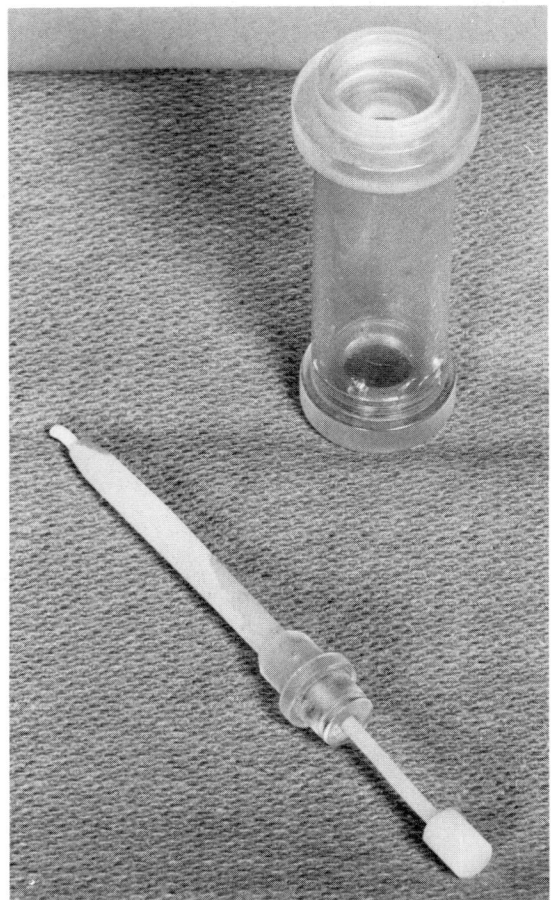

Figure 24-5 | Carbon dioxide may be used for the cold test instead of ice.

pressed gently against the soft tissue overlying the bone and apices of teeth for purposes of comparing the "feel" between abnormal and normal tissue.

Palpation is of value also in determining swelling about the face and in the gland areas.

Mobility Test

Abnormal mobility of a tooth signifies temporary or permanent loss of supporting alveolar bone.

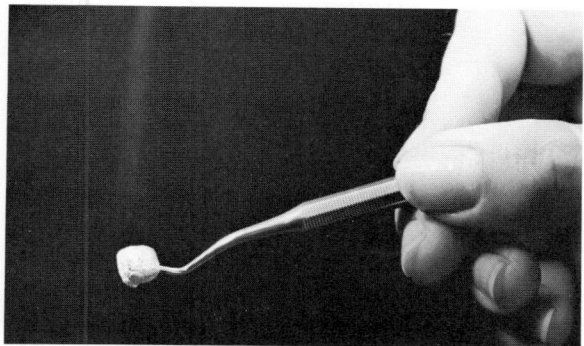

Figure 24-6 | Heat test. Smoking gutta-percha used for vitality test.

Extensive loss of bone causes mobility necessitating endodontic treatment, periodontal treatment, or both. Abnormal mobility generally disappears following root canal treatment, periodontal treatment, or both.

Trauma may result in abnormal mobility also. The mobility test is employed by movement of the tooth or teeth between two fingers or between a finger and the handle of an instrument.

Anesthetic Test

An anesthetic test is rendered to provide a possible diagnosis by elimination. In many instances it is difficult to point to the source of pain in the mouth. A local anesthetic is administered to the tooth or area in question, and this may provide a diagnosis if the pain is eliminated.

The anesthetic test is rarely employed although it is of immense value whenever indicated.

Transillumination

Transillumination is rarely used today in diagnosis. In a darkened room, light is played against soft tissue in order to determine the amount of light that is transmitted through the tissue.

Release of Pressure

This test is used for the diagnosis of fractured teeth. These teeth may not be recognized immediately as being fractured and usually present a history of discomfort brought on by mastication. Occasionally the patient presents a history of long-standing pain and a record of having been to more than one dental office. Fractures may be detected many times after the tooth is thoroughly dried and examined with an explorer and magnifying glasses to improve vision. In cases of severe fracture, pain results upon prying into the fracture line, and one portion of the tooth moving away from the other portion.

The release of pressure test is employed by using a rubber wheel between the occlusal surfaces of the upper and lower teeth. The rubber wheel is inserted, and the patient is requested to close tightly against the rubber wheel and to release suddenly. Pain upon release is significant of possible fracture. This test may be repeated a number of times and on various areas of the occlusal surface of the tooth before pain is elicited.

ROOT CANAL THERAPY

The Rubber Dam

A local anesthetic must be given prior to operating within the pulp cavity of teeth possessing vital pulps. The hole or holes in the rubber dam are made and lubricated by the dental assistant. Generally, the tooth receiving root canal treatment is isolated by a rubber dam; thus only a single hole in the dam is required. The guide shown in Fig. 24-7 is helpful in selecting a site on the rubber dam for punching the hole. A notation must be made of the tooth isolated and the number of the rubber dam clamp used. This information is useful at succeeding visits in preventing loss of operating time, as the hole may be punched in the rubber dam and the

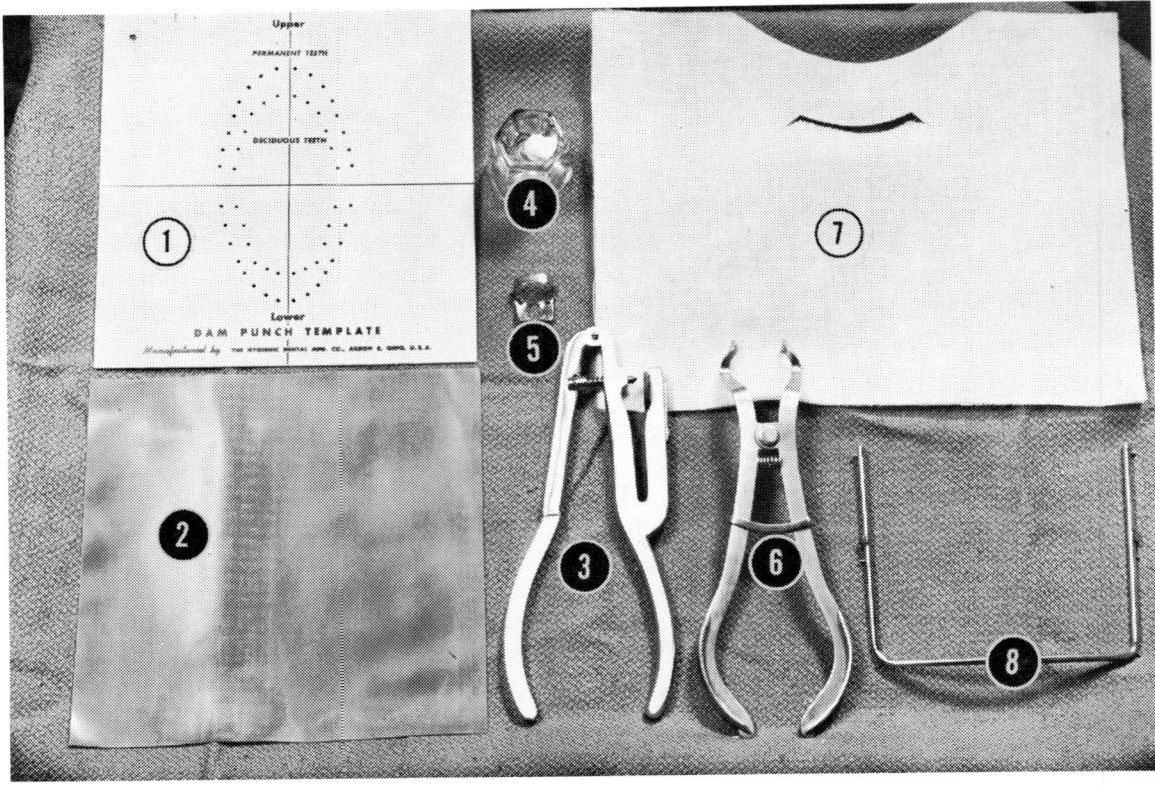

Figure 24-7 | Rubber dam equipment. (1) Guide for punching holes in rubber dam, (2) rubber dam, (3) rubber dam punch, (4) lubricant, (5) clamp, (6) clamp holder, (7) napkin, (8) frame.

clamp made available prior to the dental appointment.

The dental assistant assists the doctor in placing the napkin and rubber dam frame after the clamp has been applied to the tooth. The exposed tooth and the adjacent area are swabbed with a suitable disinfectant, such as untinted tincture of Metaphen, and dried with a jet of air (Fig. 24-8). The doctor now is ready to open the pulp cavity.

Opening the Pulp Cavity

See Figs. 24-9 and 24-10 for typical items that may be required for root canal therapy. The long-handled instruments, viz., mirror, explorer, pliers, excavator, plastic instrument, and scissors, are sterilized by autoclaving, dry heat, or boiling water prior to their use.

Some of these instruments are used in the pulp cavity or contact materials that enter into the pulp cavity. These may be resterilized at the time of their use by immersion in a hot salt or glass bead sterilizer.

The dental assistant should inquire of the doctor as to the type of handpiece and burs necessary for opening into the canal. These are prepared and the stones or burs sterilized, prior to their use, by the dental assistant.

Stones and burs may be sterilized by (1) autoclaving with subsequent storage, until use, in benzalkonium chloride 1:1000 containing a rust inhibitor, or (2) immersing in hot salt or hot glass beads for 10 seconds, just prior to using.

Instruments Used in the Pulp Canal

Broaches are manufactured as smooth and barbed, and in various sizes (Fig. 24-11). The smooth broaches are used as pathfinders in the canal, whereas the barbed broaches are used for removing substances from the canal such as pulp tissue and absorbent paper points.

Reamers are manufactured with long handles, Style D, and with short handles, Style B. The Style D, long-handled reamers are designed for use in anterior teeth, and the Style B, short-

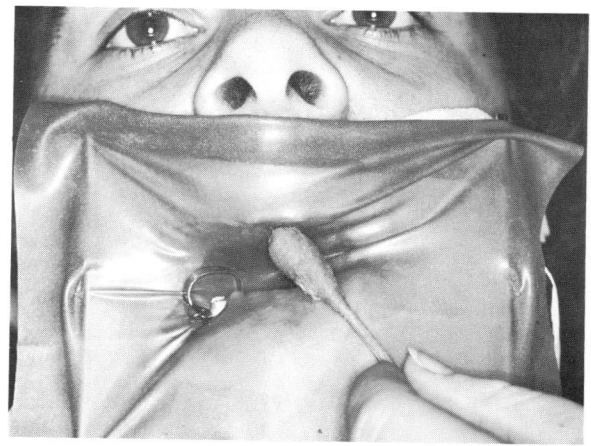

Figure 24-8 | Rubber dam in place. Area is swabbed with a disinfectant.

Figure 24-9 | Typical arrangement of instruments for root canal treatment. Generally this is a tray arrangement in front of the patient. (1) Air and water syringe, (2) high-velocity aspirator, (3) slow-speed handpiece, (4) high-speed handpiece, (5) syringes for intracanal irrigation, (6) stainless steel millimeter gauge, (7) long-handled instruments.

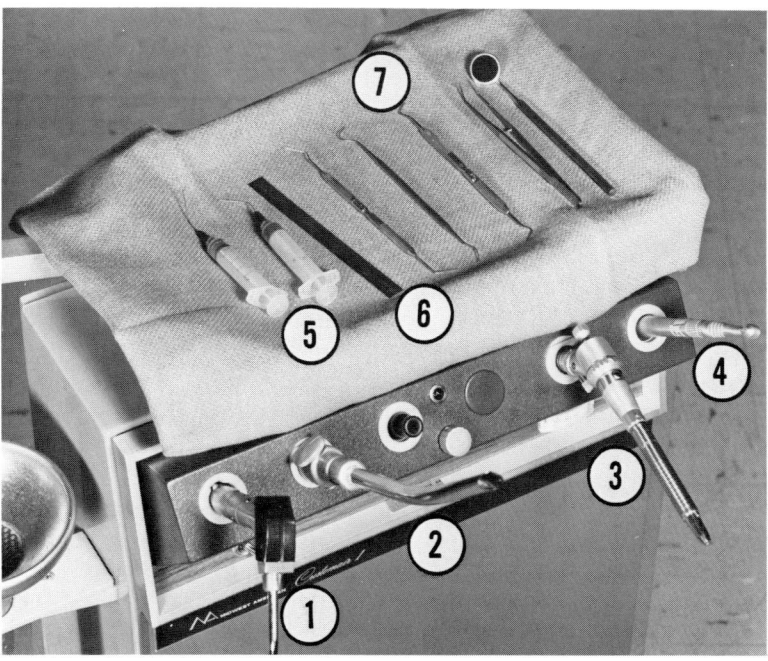

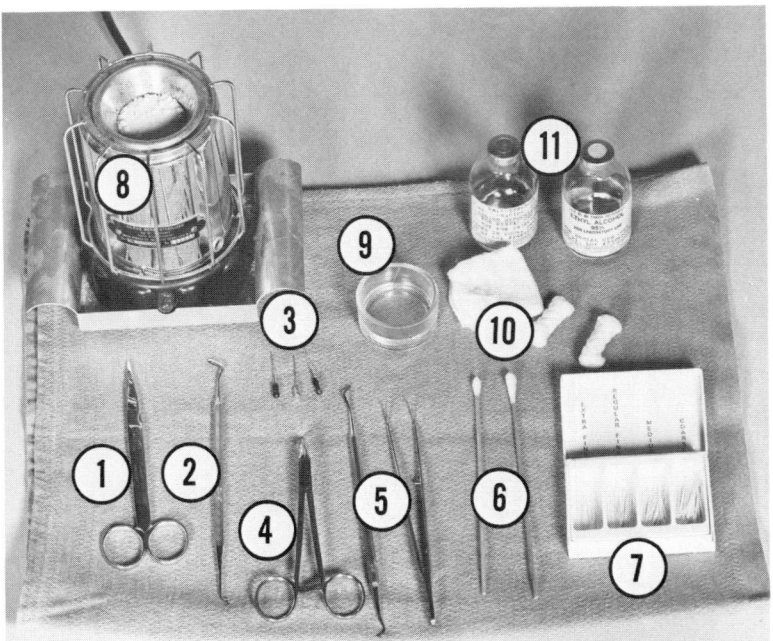

Figure 24-10 | Typical arrangement of instruments and supplies for root canal treatment. Generally these are on a tray readily accessible behind the patient. (1) Scissors, (2) plastic instrument, (3) intracanal instruments (files and reamers), (4) Steglitz forceps, (5) long-handled instruments, (6) cotton applicators, (7) absorbent paper points for intracanal absorption of moisture, (8) hot salt sterilizer, (9) dappen dish with 95 percent alcohol, (10) cotton rolls and 2 by 2 in gauze, (11) sodium hypochlorite and 75 percent ethylene alcohol for intracanal irrigation.

handled reamers are for use in the posterior regions of the mouth. Although long-handled instruments are seldom employed today, a short-handled reamer or file may be used just as effectively as a long-handled instrument for anterior teeth. This simplifies office management by requiring only one-half of the different numbered intracanal instruments. Reamers are made in different sizes, which according to most manufacturers range from no. 10 to no. 100. The sizes advance by five units to size no. 60 and in ten units from size no. 60 to size no. 100. The size is representative of the diameter at the tip in tenths of a millimeter. Size no. 10 is 0.1 mm in diameter at the tip. The next size, no. 15, is 0.15 mm in diameter at the tip. These instruments are designed for the purposes of cleansing and enlarging root canals.

Files correspond in size to reamers as well as being designed with long and short handles. Files serve as instruments for enlarging root canals (Fig. 24-11).

The doctor determines, via measurement, the length of the tooth prior to enlarging the canals. This is done with the aid of a radiograph which is developed as quickly as possible following its exposure. The dental assistant records the tooth length promptly, once the measurement has been established. All reamers and files that are to be used at that appointment are prepared with

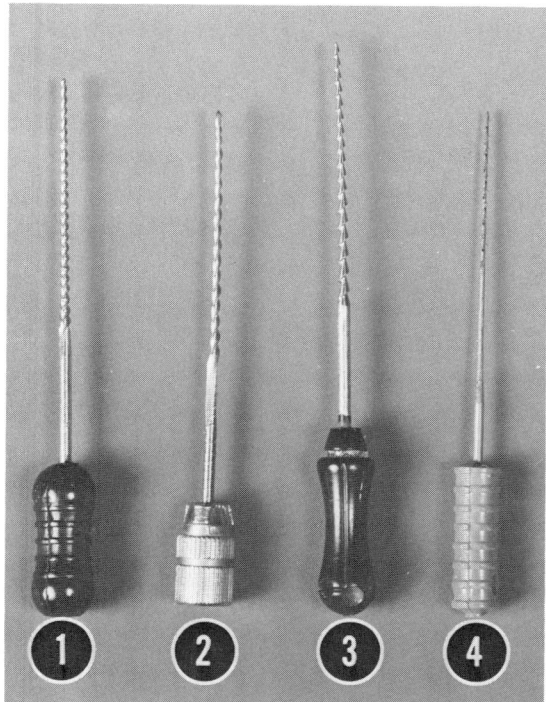

Figure 24-11 | Intracanal root canal instruments. (1) File, (2) reamer, (3) Hedstroem file, (4) barbed broach.

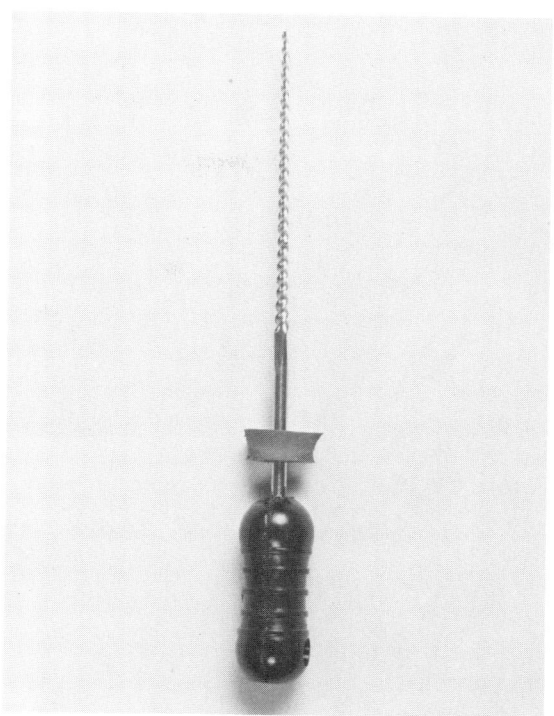

Figure 24-12 | Rubber instrument stop in place. The distance from the rubber stop to the point of the instrument corresponds to the length of the tooth. The rubber is preset by the assistant once the tooth length has been established.

stops which are visible aids in limiting the instruments to the canal during their use (Fig. 24-12).

Absorbent paper points are made in different sizes (Fig. 24-10). Some manufacturers produce absorbent paper points corresponding in size to the sizes of files and reamers. The chief uses of absorbent paper points are (1) drying of the root canal, (2) application of medicaments to the canal, and (3) inoculation of root canal cultures.

The dental assistant should refer to the patient's chart for the tooth length recorded previously and prepare the necessary absorbent paper points in that length by cutting away the small sharp end with scissors (Fig. 24-13).

Broaches, reamers, files, and absorbent paper points are sterilized prior to their application into the root canal. This is accomplished by immersion in a molten metal, a hot salt, or a glass bead sterilizer for a period of 5 to 10 seconds.

Absorbent points may be sterilized and stored, prior to their use, between sterile pieces of gauze or upon the surface of the hot metal, salt, or glass beads of that type of sterilizer. Absorbent points may be obtained from the manufacturer in small numbers, in the individual packets, and presterilized. This eliminates the necessity for chairside sterilization.

Solutions and Medicaments

Irrigation is necessary during the process of enlarging the root canal and at other times when-

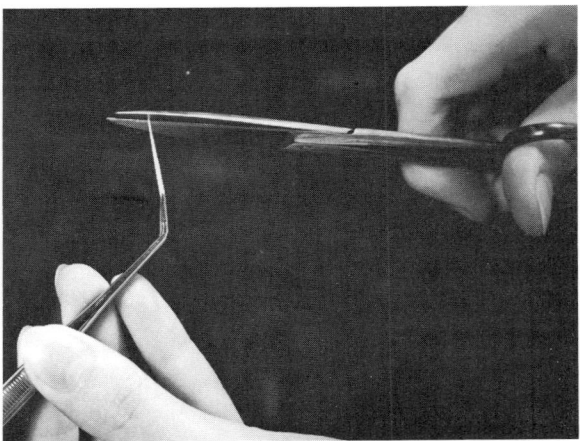

Figure 24-13 | The sharp tip of an absorbent paper point is cut away prior to its introduction into the root canal, thus preventing injury to the periapical tissues.

ever debris or foreign substances are to be removed from the pulp cavity.

Two popular irrigating solutions are sodium hypochlorite and alcohol, used alternately and applied by means of 2-ml Luer-Loc syringes with 23- or 25-gauge blunt needles (Fig. 24-9). The above irrigating solutions should be supplied in amber bottles or stored in a dark place in order to prevent their deterioration from light. Normal saline solution, sterile water, and various other substances may be used for irrigating root canals. The choice of irrigating solutions varies among dental offices.

Hydrochloric acid (HCl) and sulfuric acid (H_2SO_4) have been popular in many offices as solutions that aid in *enlarging* root canals. The dental assistant must use care in handling acid solutions as they are destructive to soft tissues and clothing, as well as to dental instruments. Ethylenediaminetetraacetic acid, abbreviated EDTA, is popular as a solution to aid in enlarging root canals. The pH of this substance is near normal and more desirable therefore than the more caustic agents for use near live tissue.

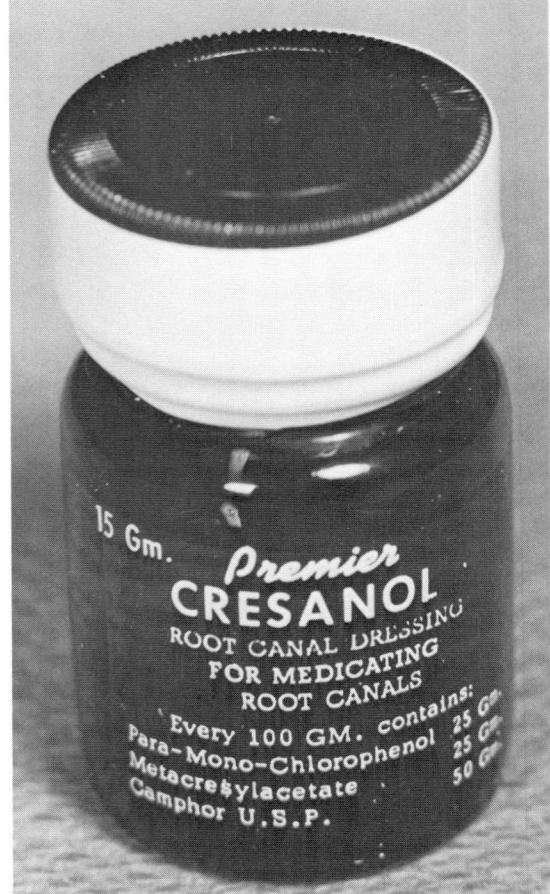

Figure 24-14 | Cresanol (*courtesy of Premier*) is used as an intracanal dressing for medication.

The *disinfectants* used in root canals are generally in the forms of solutions or pastes (Fig. 24-14). These are applied in the chamber of the canal on an absorbent cotton pellet and sealed there for a period of time in order to reduce or prevent the growth of bacteria. There are a number of different disinfectants used in root canals. The disinfectant varies from one office to another and from time to time within the dental office.

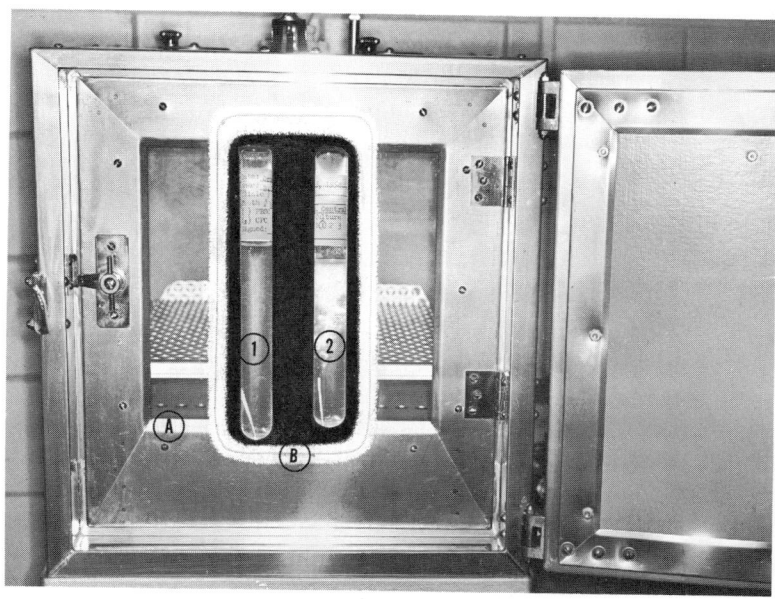

Figure 24-15 | Bacteriology. A. Incubator. B. Culture medium, (1) negative after incubation, (2) positive after incubation. Cloudiness denotes growth of bacteria.

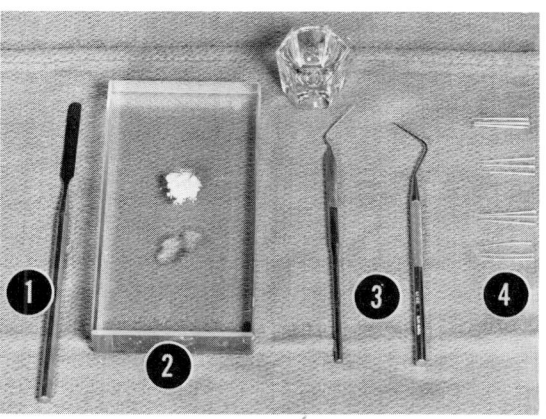

Figure 24-16 | Filling of root canals. (1) Cement spatula, (2) glass slab with cement powder and liquid, (3) root canal spreaders, (4) gutta-percha points in assorted sizes.

Root Canal Cultures

The presence of bacteria within the canal may be detected by means of the culture. A sampling of the canal is introduced into a tube of culture medium and placed in an incubator for a period of time, generally 72 hours to 7 days. The doctor examines the culture for growth of bacteria after this allotted time (Fig. 24-15).

The dental assistant should maintain a supply of prepared culture medium in tubes and under refrigeration. The supply of tubes is dependent upon the extent of the root canal therapy performed in the dental office. The tube is labeled properly prior to the inoculation of the culture or immediately thereafter. The label should have the following information: (1) date, (2) name of patient, and (3) first, second, or third culture taken.

The culture is placed in the incubator following its inoculation from the root canal. The dental assistant must observe the incubator thermometer reading periodically in order that a constant and correct temperature of 37°C (98.6°F) may be maintained.

Filling Root Canals

Root canals are filled generally with gutta-percha, silver points, or a combination of both and with a cementing substance.

A glass mixing slab, or dappen dish, spatula, and a root canal spreader may be packaged in a towel and autoclaved to effect sterilization. Other means of sterilizing these items may be employed in lieu of autoclaving, viz.: (1) The glass slab or dappen dish is rubbed with untinted tincture of Metaphen followed by alcohol, and held over the flame briefly, to hasten drying. (2) The cement spatula and the root canal spreader may be sterilized by immersion in a hot salt or glass bead sterilizer for about 1 minute.

Silver points are sterilized by direct flame or in a hot salt or hot glass bead sterilizer. Gutta-percha cones are sterilized by immersion in Metaphen for 3 minutes and rinsing in 95 percent ethyl alcohol. Drying is accomplished by blotting the cones between pieces of sterile gauze.

Figure 24-17 | A calcium hydroxide–base paste with instrument for application of the paste to an exposed vital pulp.

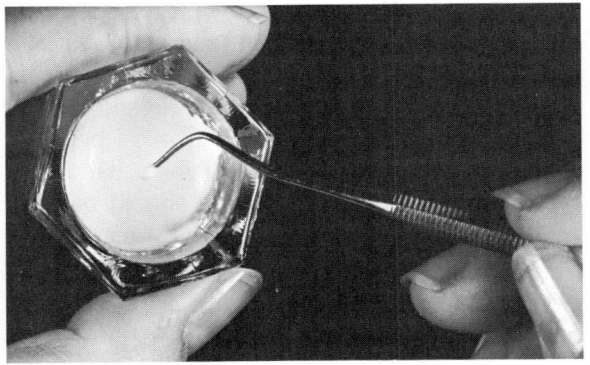

Additional instruments and materials that are used for a root canal filling operation are seen in Fig. 24-16.

PULP CAPPING

A local anesthetic must be given prior to this operation. The rubber dam and rubber dam equipment should be available for use whenever a request is made by the doctor for these items.

The exposure of a vital pulp often warrants pulp capping. The exposed pulp is covered with a layer of calcium hydroxide or a compound containing calcium hydroxide, usually in the form of a paste. This may be prepared by mixing the calcium hydroxide powder with water to the desired consistency (Fig. 24-17). The calcium hydroxide is covered by a layer of free-flowing zinc oxide and eugenol followed by a layer of a more durable cement such as zinc phosphate cement. There are commercial preparations containing calcium hydroxide that are available for pulp capping.

The dental assistant must have available all the materials and instruments necessary for this procedure.

PULPOTOMY

A pulpotomy is an operation in which the bulbous or crown portion of a pulp is removed. The intact pulp is retained in the root canal(s) with the amputated ends covered with layers of calcium hydroxide, zinc oxide and eugenol, and zinc phosphate cement, in that sequence.

Equipment and Materials

The following additional items should be available for use:

1. Round burs, sizes nos. 6 and 8
2. Sharp excavators

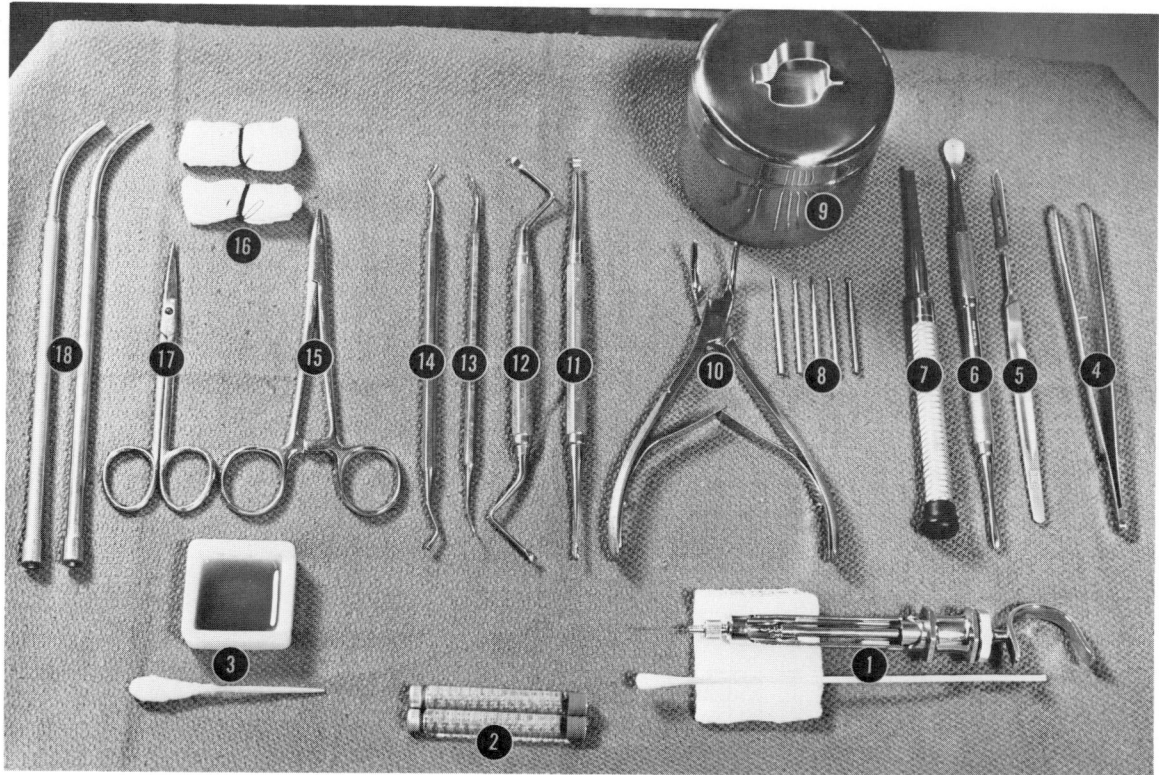

Figure 24-18 | Items used for a root resection. (1) Anesthetic syringe, (2) cartridges of anesthetic, (3) disinfectant that is applied topically prior to injections and subsequent incision, (4) pliers, (5) B-P scapel handle with no. 15 blade, (6) periosteal elevator, (7) bone chisel, (8) burs, (9) container of benzalkonium chloride 1:1000, with sodium nitrite, for storage of burs following their sterilization, (10) rongeurs, (11) straight curette, (12) curved curette, (13) periodontal curette, (14) plastic instrument, (15) needle holder, (16) sutures and needles, (17) scissors, (18) aspirator tip.

3. Irrigation solution of sterile saline, or anesthetic solution in cartridge syringe
4. Cotton pellets of various sizes
5. Calcium hydroxide, paste form or dry powder
6. Slab, spatula, and probe for applying cements
7. Zinc oxide and eugenol
8. Zinc phosphate cement

Refer to Fig. 24-19 for sterilization of instruments and supplies.

PERIAPICAL SURGERY

This is a procedure in which an incision is made and the bone penetrated near the apex of a tooth for the purpose of removing foreign bodies, periapical lesions, a portion of the root end, or a combination of any of these.

An anesthetic is given prior to the operation. The surgical armamentarium should be similar to that shown in Fig. 24-18. The area of the opera-

Item \ Method	AUTOCLAVING	BOILING WATER	DRY HEAT OVEN	MOLTEN METAL, SALT, GLASS BEAD	ALCOHOL & FORMALIN WITH FLAMING	METAPHEN UNTINTED	METAPHEN FOLLOWED BY ALCOHOL	FLAMING	BENZALKONIUM CHLORIDE 1/1000 WITH SODIUM NITRITE
BLADE, SCALPEL	X	X	X	X					
BROACHES			X	X					
BURS			X	X	X				
BURS, SURGICAL	X	X	X	X					*
CHISEL, BONE	X	X	X						
CLAMPS, RUBBER DAM	X	X	X			X			
COTTON PLEDGETS	X			X					
CURETTES	X	X	X						
DAM RUBBER						X	X		
ELEVATOR, PERIOSTEAL	X	X	X						
EXCAVATORS	X	X	X		X				
EXPLORERS	X	X	X		X				
FILES			X	X					
HOLDER, NEEDLE	X	X	X						
MIRROR	X	X	X						
	X	X	X						
PLASTIC INSTRUMENT	X	X	X		X				
PLIERS	X	X	X		X				
PLUGGERS, ROOT CANAL	X	X	X						
POINTS, GUTTA PERCHA						X	X		
POINTS, ABSORB PAPER	X		X	X					
POINTS, SILVER								X	
REAMERS			X	X					
SCALPEL	X	X	X						
SCISSORS	X	X	X		X				
SLAB, GLASS	X						X		
SPATULA, CEMENT	X	X	X	X				X	
SPREADER, GUTTA PERCHA	X	X	X						
SUTURE	X								

*For storage following sterilization

Figure 24-19 | Items used in various endodontic procedures, with methods for their sterilization.

tion in the mouth should be isolated, dried, and swabbed with untinted tincture of Metaphen. The handpiece is sterilized according to the method prescribed by the doctor. The dental assistant should be in position on the opposite side of the chair, and with a surgical aspirator at the time an incision is made. *Care must be exercised in handling the lips and tissues in order to prevent excess trauma that may cause postoperative discomfort to the patient.*

The dental assistant must be certain that the patient has recovered from the operation before giving permission to leave the dental office. The patient should understand all postoperative instructions given by the doctor, and these instructions must be given verbally as well as in writing.

An appointment for suture removal should be made at this time.

Sterilization in Endodontic Procedures

The chart shown in Fig. 24-19 should be used by the dental assistant as a reference for sterilization in endodontics.

BIBLIOGRAPHY

Brauer, J. C., et al.: *Dentistry for Children,* 4th ed., McGraw-Hill Book Company, New York, 1958.

Grossman, L. I.: *Endodontic Practice,* 8th ed., Lea & Febiger, Philadelphia, 1974.

Sanderson, E. S.: "A Note on the Sterilization of Surgical Instruments," *J. Lab. Clin. Med.,* **7:**360–363, 1922.

Sommer, R. F., Ostrander, F. D., and Crowley, M. C.: *Clinical Endodontics,* 3d ed. W. B. Saunders Company, Philadelphia, 1966.

25 | Grover C. Hunter, Jr.
Periodontics

INTRODUCTION

The objective of this chapter is to give the dental assistant a condensed overview of the field of periodontics and to discuss the role of the assistant in this specialty area. Therefore, detailed information on some of the various aspects of periodontal assisting will require supplementation by manuals and other modules of instruction.

Periodontics is that specialty of dentistry which deals with the treatment and prevention of periodontal diseases and abnormalities of the supporting tissues of the teeth. The main reason for tooth loss after age 25 is periodontitis, an inflammatory process affecting the supportive structures of the tooth. Therefore, the objective of treatment is the preservation of the natural dentition in a state of comfort and health for the lifetime of the patient.

PERIODONTAL DISEASE

Even though the teeth themselves may be normal, they may be lost because their supportive structures (gingivae, periodontal ligament and bone) are damaged and diseased. A post in the ground is not very stable once the ground supporting it is lost or washed away. Thus, teeth whose support is hopelessly diseased are just as great a physical liability to the patient as teeth with large carious lesions that have destroyed the pulp and abscessed.

Periodontal disease (*pyorrhea*) is a chronic

inflammatory disease which usually becomes evident by middle age. However, periodontitis may be traced to early gingival disturbances in children, teenagers, and young adults. In modern human beings periodontal disease, like dental caries, is a universal problem. People are now living to an older age, and so it is very important to preserve the foundation of the teeth in a healthy condition. The habits of modern society are not often helpful in assuring periodontal health. Inadequate oral hygiene, soft foods, and faulty diets are contributing factors to periodontal breakdown. The primary cause of periodontal disease, however, is bacterial plaque which adheres to the tooth or to calculus (calcified plaque) on the tooth in vulnerable areas of the soft tissue attachment (refer to Chap. 6).

The damaging condition resulting from the way teeth strike or hit during functional movements of the jaw is called *occlusal trauma*. This may be a secondary contributing cause in periodontal destruction. Nervous habits such as bruxism (clenching and night grinding) in the presence of gingivitis and the beginning deeper involvement of periodontitis may also contribute to accelerated periodontal breakdown.

Gingivitis

Gingivitis means inflammation of the gingivae immediately surrounding the teeth resulting from soft bacterial plaque or calcified plaque (calculus or tartar). The normal healthy gingivae surrounding the teeth are stippled (grainy like an orange peel) (Fig. 25-1), coral-pink in color, and firm. In the anterior region, the marginal gingivae peak to a knifelike edge; in the posterior region, the marginal gingivae are flatter because the underlying bone is thicker faciolingually. In acute gingivitis however, the gingivae become red, inflamed, and lose their grainy (stippled) appearance (Fig. 25-2A). In chronic gingivitis the

Figure 25-2 | A. Gingivitis, edematous. B. Gingivitis, calculus, and associated change in gingival color and contour.

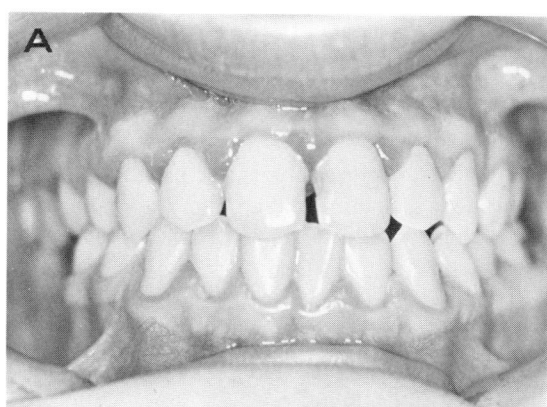

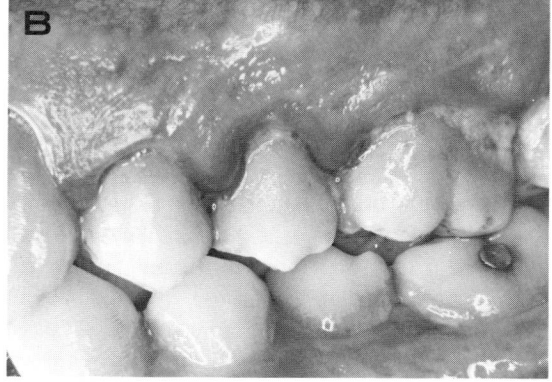

Figure 25-1 | Normal gingival stippling and adequate zone of attached gingiva (masticatory mucosa).

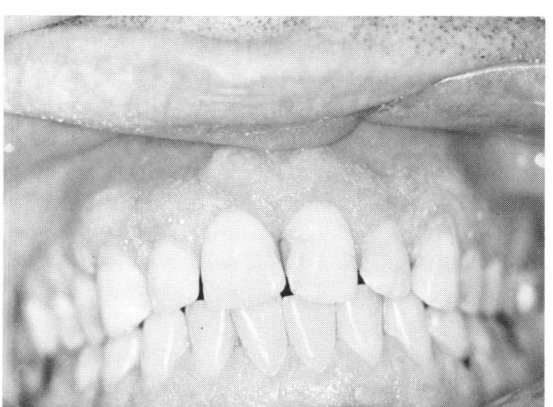

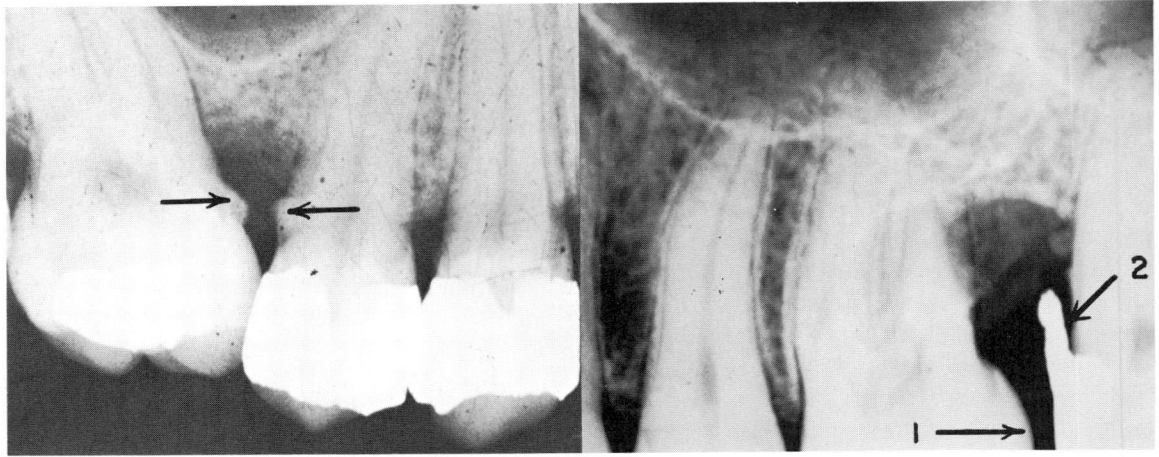

Figure 25-3 | Periodontitis (radiographs). Arrows indicate calculus. (1) Open contact, (2) filling overhang.

gingivae may lose their characteristic form, demonstrate rolled margins, blunting of the papillae (Fig. 25-2B), and become bluish in color (cyanosis).

Gingivitis is most often associated with poor hygiene, i.e., failure of the patient to disrupt and remove bacterial plaque on the tooth itself both above and below the soft-tissue margin. Poorly fitting dental restorations, improper contacts, and food impaction between the teeth (Fig. 25-3) all share in laying the groundwork for inflammatory changes by favoring retention of bacterial plaque.

Systemic conditions, such as blood dyscrasias (leukemias) and vitamin deficiencies, may be predisposing factors promoting gingivitis. In certain nutritional deficiencies, tissue degeneration may be primary and gingival inflammation is exaggerated because of the lowered resistance of the already inflamed tissue. Expectant mothers develop pregnancy gingivitis usually as a result of a temporary hormonal disorder superimposed on a preexisting gingivitis and/or periodontitis.

Periodontitis

If gingivitis is not reversed in its early stages, the inflammatory process may progress to the deeper supporting tissues and cause destruction of bone. Along with this involvement of the supporting bone, the sulcus around the neck of the tooth becomes deeper, and the result is a periodontal pocket. A periodontal pocket is a deepened sulcus (greater than 2 to 3 mm) resulting from the disruption of the attachment apparatus to the root of a tooth. Bacterial plaque cannot be removed effectively by the patient using toothbrush and floss if the sulcus is more than 2 to 3 mm in depth. The resulting condition is called *periodontitis*.

There is a degenerative form of periodontitis in adolescence and early adulthood termed *juvenile periodontitis* (*periodontosis*). It is characterized by incipient to severe bone loss around the first permanent molars and maxillary and mandibular anteriors. Prognosis is poor, since the condition seems not to be associated with local factors which can be controlled by the dentist and patient. The pursuit of systemic factors has not usually proven fruitful in helping the clinician solve this difficult treatment problem.

PROGRESSION OF PERIODONTAL DISEASE

The early lesion of gingivitis (when the bone is not yet affected) is usually reversible to a state of health with minimal treatment and cooperation of the patient with effective oral hygiene. However, once the supportive bone is affected (periodontitis), the progress of the disease is not completely predictable for an individual patient. The initial lesion begins usually in the interproximal sulci between the teeth, which is a difficult area to keep free of bacterial plaque. Sometimes the breakdown is rapid, and sometimes it is a very slow process. Old radiographs are helpful in assessing this time component.

There is a constant microscopic warfare between the causative agents (such as bacteria) and the natural defenses of the body (immune mechanisms). A truce may bring about a situation in which the supporting bone is little affected over the years. When other aggravating factors such as occlusal trauma, bruxism, metabolic disease, poor nutrition, and destructive emotional factors are added to the bacterial component, the destruction may be more rapid. The rapid destructive type of the disease when seen in teenagers and young adults generally indicates a poor prognosis, i.e., the teeth will probably be lost unless the majority of the causative factors can be brought under control. More research is needed to shed light on the unanswered questions of periodontal disease.

MUCOGINGIVAL PROBLEMS

In addition to gingival changes seen in inflammation, there may be noninflammatory conditions or abnormalities, resulting in a loss of attached gingiva (masticatory mucosa). Attached gingiva is that portion of the immovable masticatory mucosa which is firmly bound down by connective-tissue fibers to the underlying bone and periosteum.

When there is not an adequate band of attached gingiva (less than 2 or 3 mm), recession may occur, exposing the root surface. In some anatomic areas of the oral cavity, recession may be accelerated by the pull of frenal and muscular attachments (Fig. 25-4). The vestibular movable mucosa does not provide an adequate barrier to gingival inflammation and trauma.

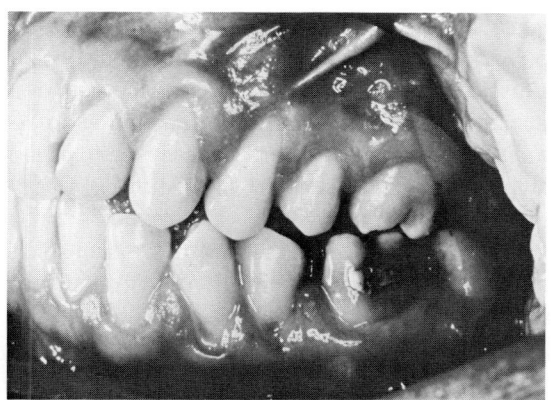

Figure 25-4 | Mucogingival problem. Lack of attached gingiva on facial surface of premolar complicated by frenal pull. (*Courtesy of W. T. McFall.*)

RECESSION

Recession is a pathologic condition in which the gingivae and underlying bone recede from the normal attachment level at the cementoenamel junction of the tooth. It may be induced by gingival inflammation from failure of the patient to remove bacterial plaque or by trauma from an improper toothbrushing technique. The surgical treatment for pocket elimination can also produce areas of recession on teeth.

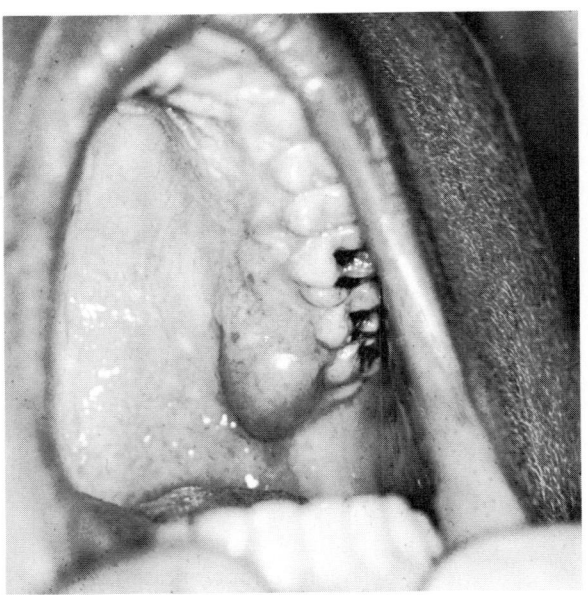

Figure 25-5 | Periodontal abscess.

The exposed cementum and dentin in areas of recession are sometimes sensitive to heat, cold, air, sweets, and acid-type foods. This condition is known as *root sensitivity*. Desensitizing agents such as topical fluorides are used to treat these exposed root surfaces.

Figure 25-6 | ANUG (Vincent's infection).

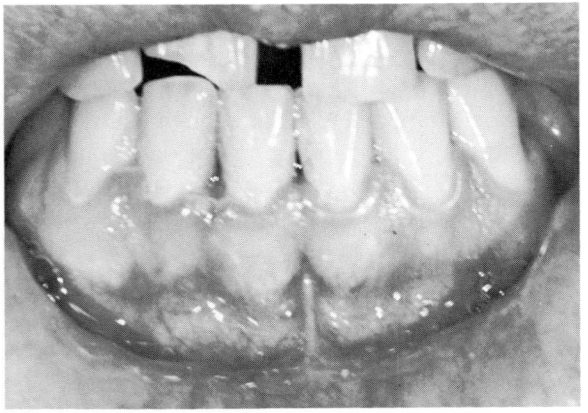

PERIODONTAL ABSCESS

A periodontal abscess is a localized acute inflammatory reaction in a periodontal pocket (Fig. 25-5). It may drain spontaneously through the orifice of the pocket or point through alveolar bone if the orifice is occluded. In multirooted teeth, the furcal area between the roots is a favored site for abscess formation. Occlusal trauma is sometimes a contributory factor in triggering the abscess, especially in teeth with mobility. If drainage cannot be established by instrumentation through the orifice of the pocket, treatment is incision and drainage.

ACUTE NECROTIZING ULCERATIVE GINGIVITIS (VINCENT'S DISEASE)

This gingival infection is perhaps as old or older than recorded history. It was not until the end of the nineteenth century that a French physician named Vincent isolated the bacteria associated with the infection. For a more detailed discussion of the microbiology of this condition, consult Chap. 6.

Clinically a more descriptive term is *acute necrotizing ulcerative gingivitis* (ANUG). This infection seems to favor the gingival extensions (papillae) which lie in the interproximal spaces between adjacent and contacting teeth (Fig. 25-6). The odor of the infection is sometimes quite foul and definitely detectable within conversational range. Poor oral hygiene seems to be one of the most important predisposing causes of the condition, and meticulous oral hygiene is of paramount importance in its treatment. Other predisposing causes seem to be fatigue, anxiety, dissipation, and poor and inadequate diet. During World War I many of these predisposing factors were present among soldiers living in trenches, resulting in many outbreaks (epidemics). The term *trench mouth* originated from these findings. There is little or no evidence to support transmission of the disease from one person to another.

EXAMINATION AND CHARTING

The periodontal probe is a blunt-ended, slender instrument calibrated in millimeters and is one of the most important diagnostic tools in identifying periodontal abnormalities. There are several types of periodontal probes on the market, each having its own limitations and usefulness (Fig. 25-7). Slender probes are used to measure accurately pocket depths, while heavier probes may be used to identify bone topography (sounding) during periodontal surgery.

The dental assistant will need to know the symbols used by the dentist or periodontist in recording the patient's existing periodontal condition. Furcal problems, degrees of mobility of the teeth, poor interproximal contacts, overhanging restorations, mucogingival abnormalities, and occlusal discrepancies will need accurate recording (Fig. 25-8). In addition a recording of periodontal pocket depths will be required on each tooth, three on the facial and three on the lingual or palatal aspects (Fig. 25-9).

A bacterial plaque index is useful in obtaining an objective evaluation of the patient's efforts at daily oral hygiene. The assistant will need to identify and record on the plaque chart the surfaces of the teeth where plaque is present. For more detail on plaque scoring, consult Chap. 19.

INITIAL PREPARATION

Initial preparation refers to removal of local factors such as bacterial plaque, calcified bacterial plaque (calculus), planing of the root surfaces, smoothing down rough restorations and gingival overhangs so that plaque control by the patient can be efficient. The assistant's role here is principally aspiration and curette sharpening for the operator. The response of gingival tissues to initial preparation is often very dramatic (Fig. 25-10).

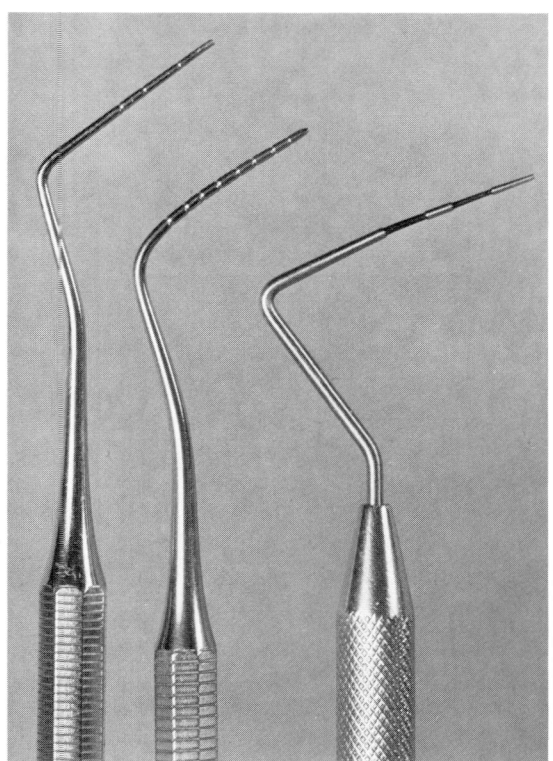

Figure 25-7 | Periodontal probes (*from left:* Premier O–Michigan; Williams; Hu–Friedy CP-12).

INSTRUMENT SHARPENING

During initial preparation, curettes are the hand instruments most frequently used by the operator. A curette is an instrument with a double-edged cutting blade and is used to remove deposits beneath the gingival margin, plane the root surface, and remove the epithelial lining on the soft-tissue side of the pocket (gingival curettage).

Many methods and devices have been utilized to effect and ensure the sharpness of both edges of the curette blade. A medium-grit, flat sharpening stone, comfortable in size to handle, is selected. It must be a stone that permits sterilization along with the curettes so that sharpening can occur when needed during scaling procedures. A sharp curette is an efficient instrument and reduces the operator's chair time.

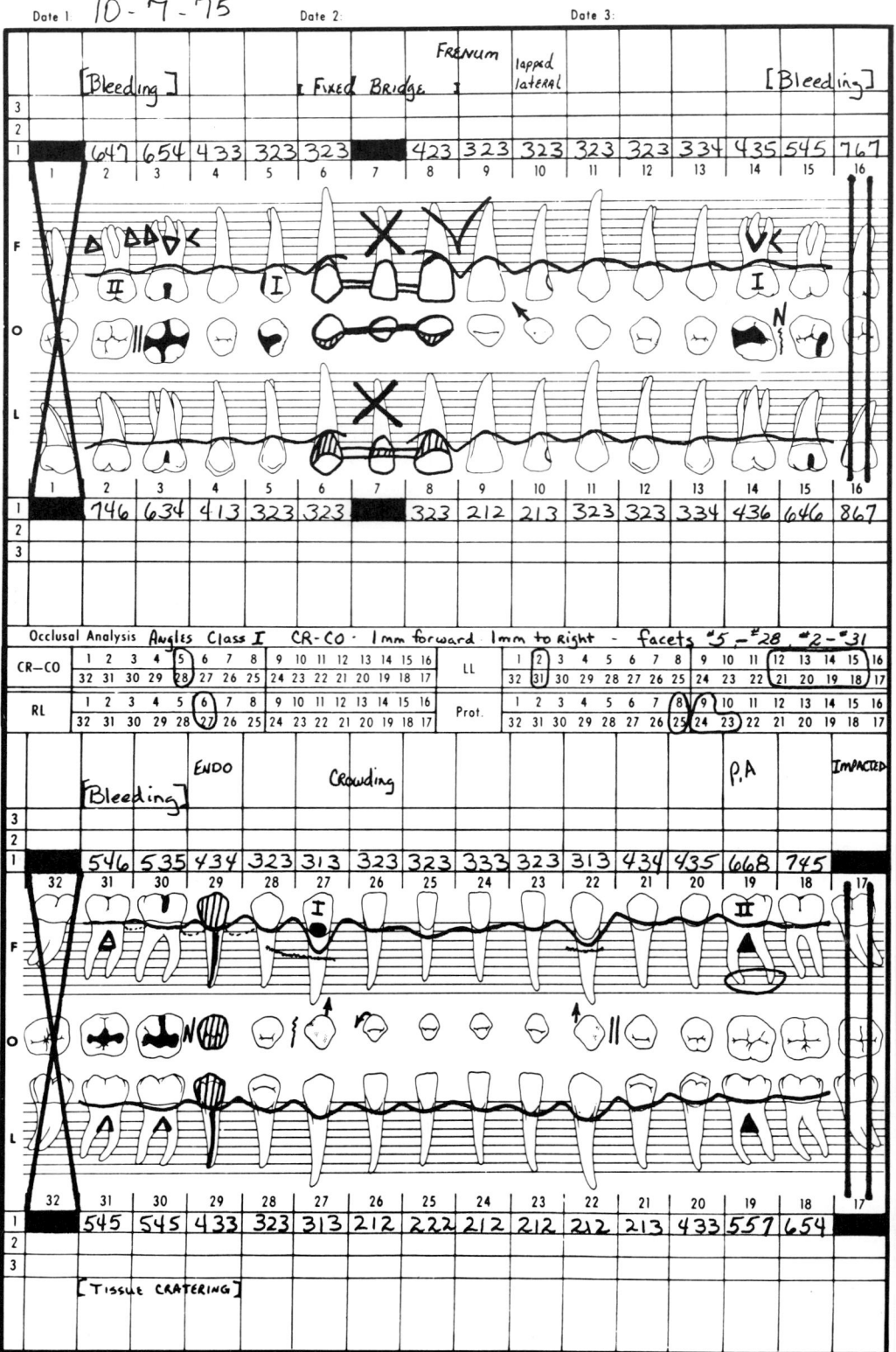

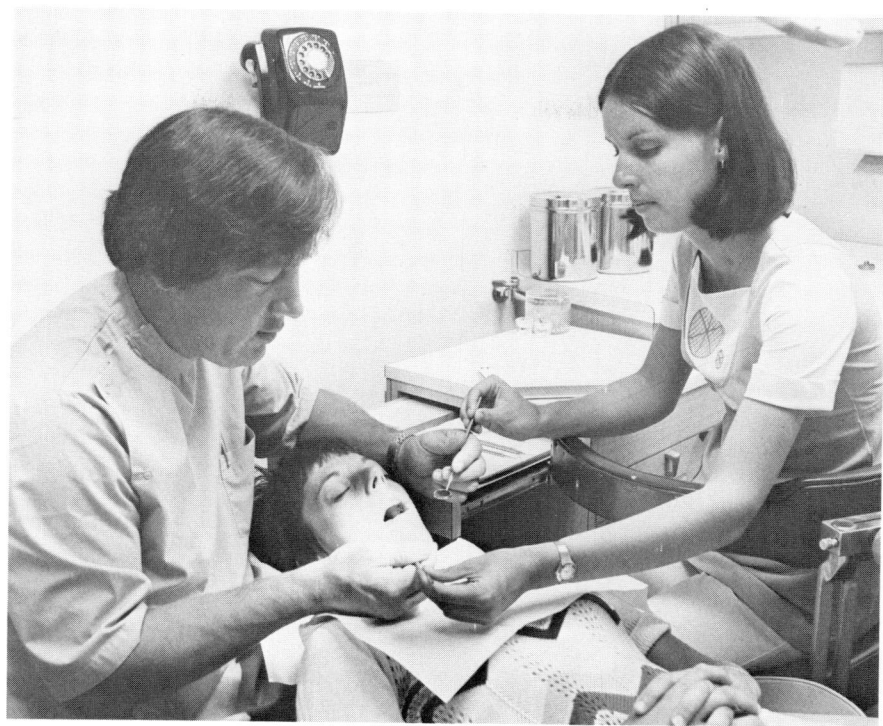

Figure 25-9 | Assisting with periodontal examination and charting. (*Courtesy of L. H. Hutchens.*)

The key surfaces of the curette are the face and lateral surface. The junction of these is the working edge, the angle being 70 to 80 degrees. The instrument is braced in the right or left hand, and the free hand is used to move the stone up and down along the lateral surface (70 to 80 degrees), starting at the heel and working toward the tip. Sharpening is accomplished primarily on the downstroke. The number of strokes required depends on how dull the instrument is. If the instrument is kept in good condition, generally 10 to 20 light strokes are sufficient to restore a sharp

Figure 25-8 | Periodontal chart. (*Courtesy of the Department of Periodontics, University of North Carolina at Chapel Hill, School of Dentistry.*)

edge. The stone is moved with several light strokes at the correct angle (Fig. 25-11A) and can be tested for sharpness by scraping the fingernail (Fig. 25-11B). For sterility reasons, this type of test cannot be used when the curettes are being sharpened at chairside during scaling and curettage procedures. The correct angle of stone to blade will ensure that the width of the blade is not reduced during the sharpening procedure.

Periodontal surgical knives must also be sharpened after each surgical procedure and prior to sterilization. These may be sharpened on a flat stone, by the technique similar to sharpening a pocket knife. Many of the periodontal surgical knives were originally designed for gingivectomy and gingivoplasty procedures. These procedures have given way largely to flap

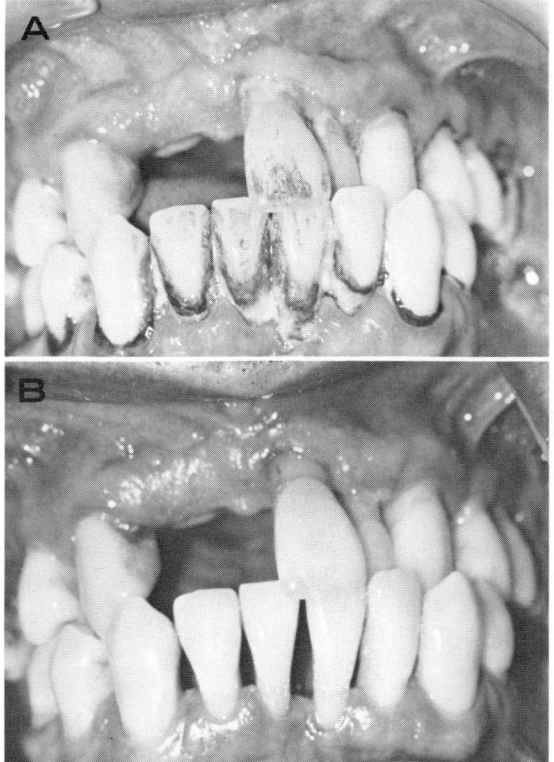

Figure 25-10 | Initial preparation. A. Before scaling and root planing. B. After scaling and root planing. (*Courtesy of W. T. Baldock.*)

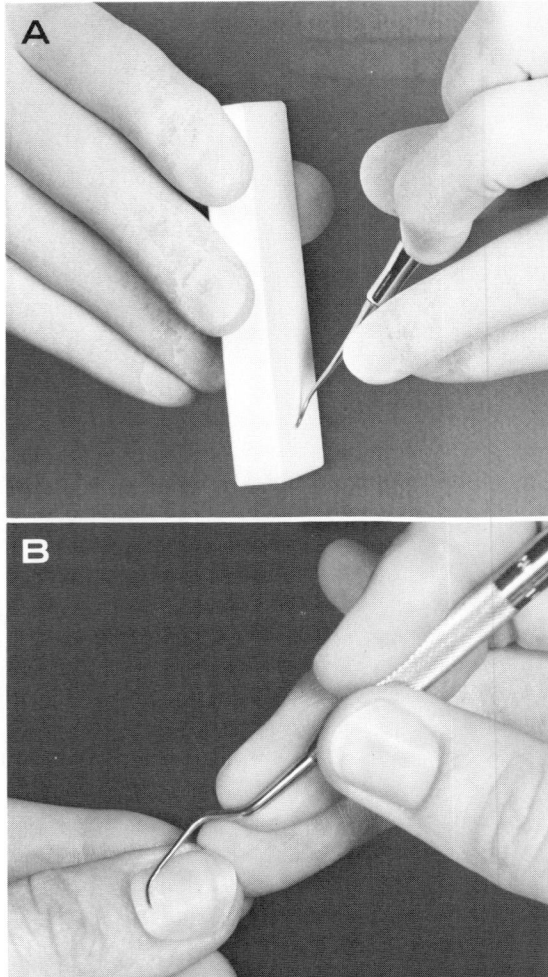

Figure 25-11 | Sharpening curettes. A. Correct angulation of blade with sharpening stone. B. Testing for sharpness of cutting edge. (*Courtesy of R. Cray.*)

surgery and the consequent use of disposable blades. This trend has tended to reduce the time needed to keep the regular periodontal knives in top condition.

ULTRASONIC INSTRUMENTS

Most dental offices utilize ultrasonic as well as hand instruments to remove stains and deposits on teeth (Fig. 25-12). The principle of such instruments is the utilization of ultrasound waves to vibrate the accretions off the teeth. To reduce heat generation, a constant flow of water through a tube onto the tip of the instrument produces an aspiration problem for the operator, thus requiring adequate suction.

The assistant may be required to set up the in-

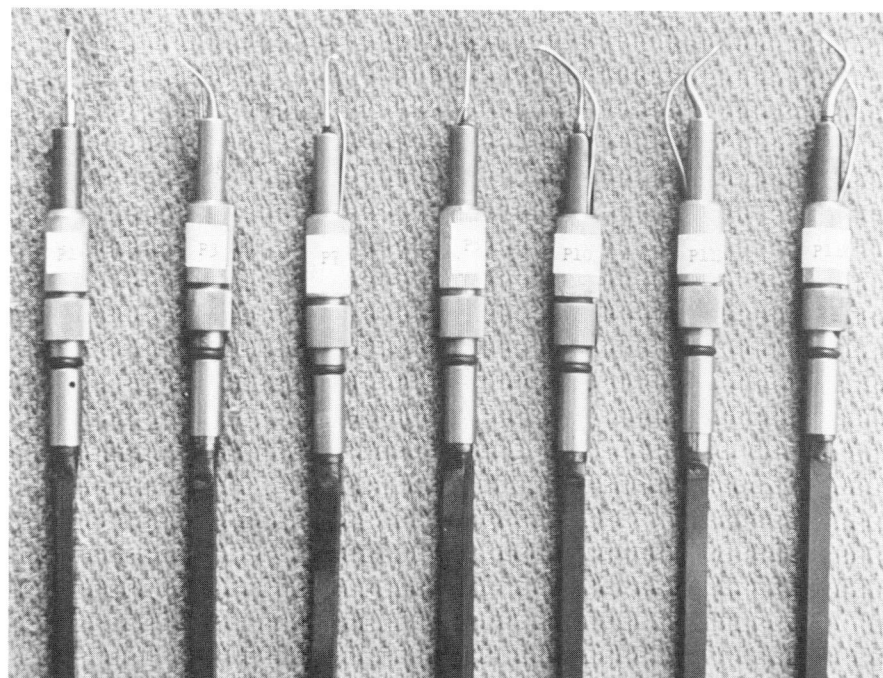

Figure 25-12 | Cavitron inserts and tips. (*Courtesy of B. Green.*)

strument, place the insert into the water line, tune the instrument (frequency), and adjust the power (amplitude) and the flow of water onto the tip. The main concern of the assistant will be to assure adequate suctioning of water and saliva for the operator.

After use, the ultrasonic inserts and tips will need to be disassembled, cleaned, reassembled, and sterilized for the next time they are to be used.

OCCLUSAL ADJUSTMENT

One of the procedures most often needed in the treatment of advanced periodontal disease is occlusal adjustment. The purpose of occlusal adjustment is to eliminate destructive forces which produce damage to the supporting tissues (periodontal ligament and bone). This is accomplished by reshaping the teeth in such a way as to eliminate prematurities and interferences during the functional excursions of the mandible.

One of the methods utilized in recording functional tooth contacts requires the use of both hands of the operator (Fig. 25-13). The assistant is needed to keep the ribbon or articulating paper between the teeth for accurate registration of occlusal contacts. The occlusal surfaces of the teeth must be kept dry to assure accurate markings. Also unusual wear areas (facets) on teeth cannot be seen clearly except in a dry field.

Selective grinding is accomplished by the use of rotary stones. The assistant will need to become familiar with the armamentarium which the operator utilizes for this procedure.

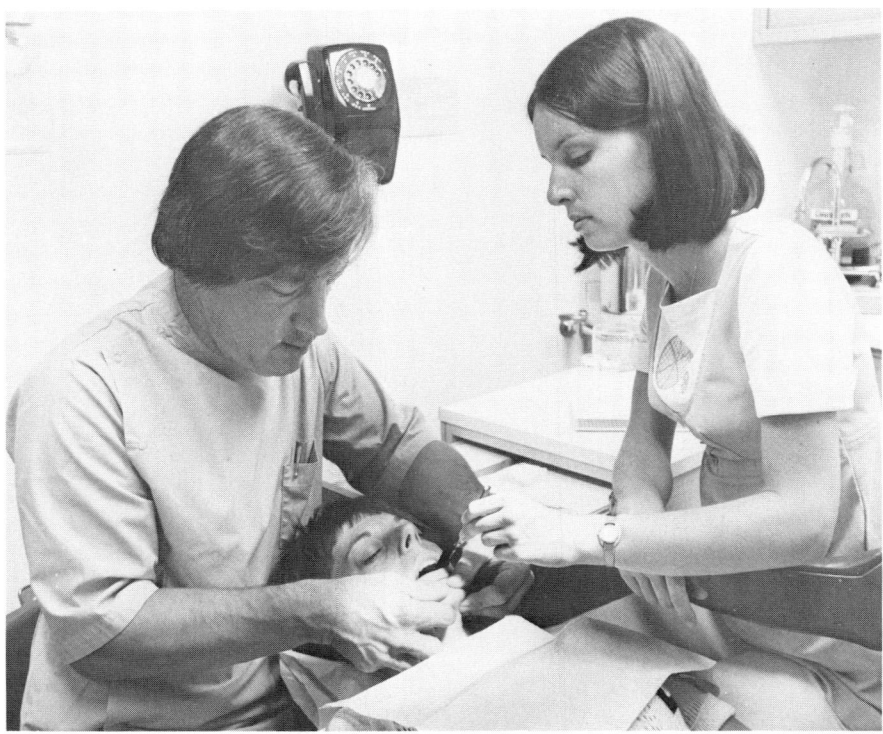

Figure 25-13 | Dental assistant holding articulating paper between the patient's teeth during occlusal adjustment.

PREPARATION FOR SURGICAL PROCEDURES

The assistant will need to have a routine established for preparing the patient for surgery, such as taking base-line blood pressure and pulse readings, draping the patient, obtaining the sterile surgical tray setup (Fig. 25-14A and B), and maintaining a sterile technique. Following the surgical procedure, scrubbing the chair, unit, and cleaning instruments for sterilization will be required. For more detail, consult Chap. 23.

PERIODONTAL SURGERY

Surgical procedures are performed to eliminate periodontal pockets and to correct deformities of the supporting tissues resulting from the disease. The patient is then able to maintain healthy tissue by routine oral-hygiene performance.

Surgical procedures are also performed to correct mucogingival problems and to provide sufficient crown length for restoring crowns of teeth that are severely decayed or fractured below the gingival margin.

Types of surgical procedures in periodontics can be classified as follows:

1. Curettage
2. Gingivectomy and gingivoplasty

Figure 25-14 | A. Periodontal surgical tray setup: mucogingival surgery. B. Periodontal surgical tray setup: osseous surgery.

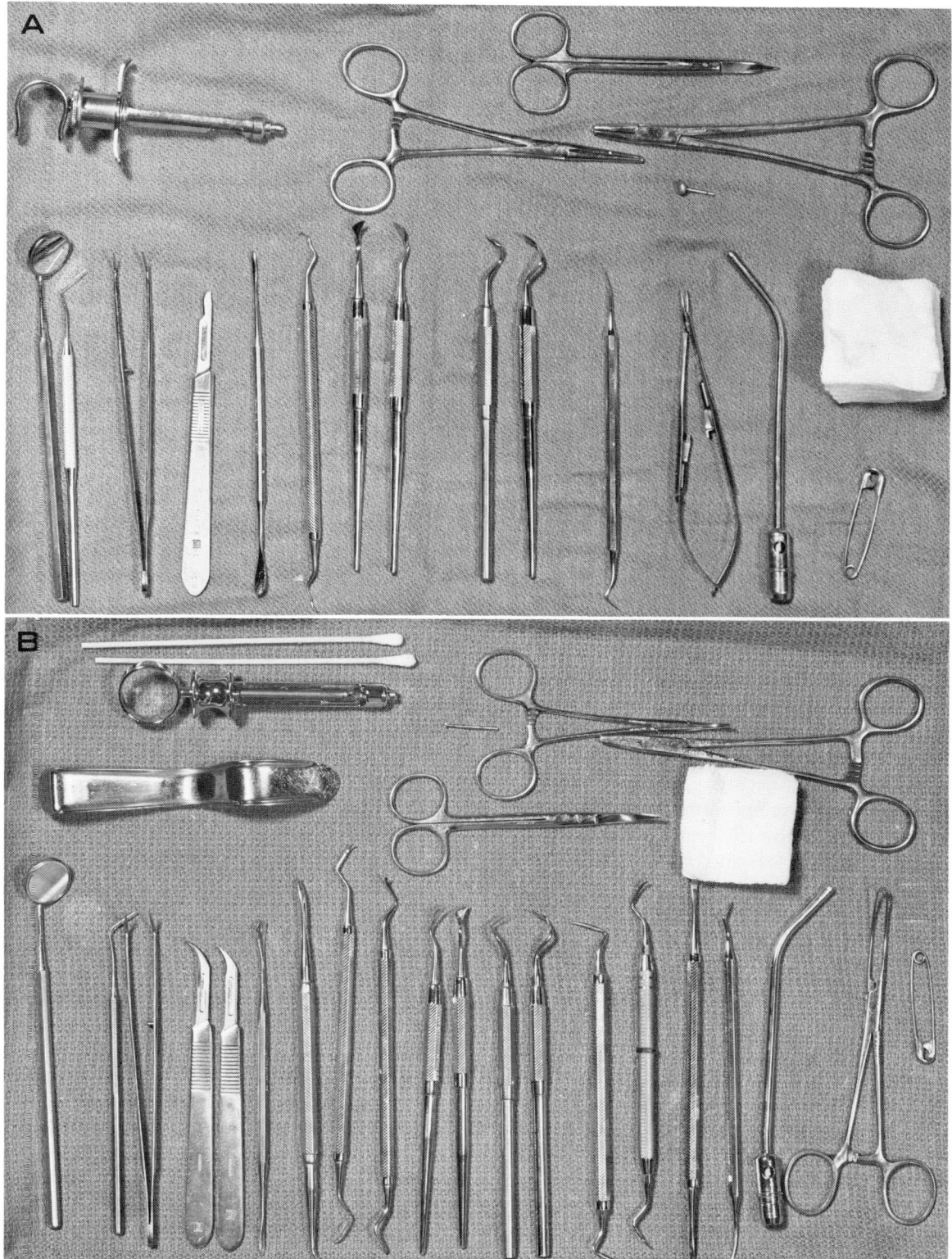

3. Mucogingival surgery
   a. Free-gingival graft
   b. Pedicle graft
   c. Frenectomy (vestibular extension)
4. Surgical correction of osseous defects
   a. Osteoplasty and ostectomy
   b. Bone implants
   c. Intramarrow penetration
   d. Root amputation and hemisection

Curettage (Gingival)

Curettage is the scraping of the soft-tissue wall of the pocket in order to remove the ulcerated epithelium and granulomatous tissue (Fig. 25-15). This procedure is indicated for correction of gingival inflammation (gingivitis) in which the pockets are suprabony (above bone).

Gingivectomy and Gingivoplasty

Gingivectomy means the resection of the gingivae for the elimination of suprabony pockets. There must be enough expendable attached gingiva to permit this procedure. So the indications for gingivectomy are limited to the gingival pocket, the walls of which have a large amount of attached gingiva.

Gingivoplasty refers to the reshaping of the gingival architecture to a more physiologic form to permit better cleansing by the patient. Gingivoplasty may be performed by scraping with a periodontal surgical knife or by a rotary diamond stone using sterile water as a lubricant (Fig. 25-16A to E).

Mucogingival Surgery

Mucogingival surgery is utilized to correct abnormalities of the soft-tissue attachment to the bone and teeth, such as recession, inadequate zones of attached gingiva, frenal and muscular pull on the attachment, and inadequate vestibular depth.

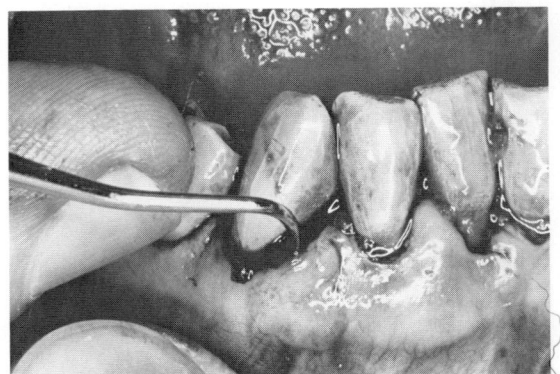

Figure 25-15 | Gingival curettage. (*Courtesy of B. Green.*)

Free-Gingival Graft

This is a plastic-surgical procedure to gain attached gingiva. The donor site is usually the palate in the area of the premolars and molars. Special precaution in the use of the suction is needed during the graft removal to prevent the free graft from being suctioned. The free graft must be kept moistened with sterile saline water on a sterile gauze sponge until it is placed at the recipient site and sutured.

Pedicle Graft

A pedicle graft is a plastic-surgical procedure involving a recipient site and a donor site. The donor site is contiguous with the recipient site, and the graft when freed still maintains its blood supply. The term first used for this procedure was the *lateral sliding flap*. This procedure is more predictable in covering roots than is the case with the free-gingival graft.

Frenectomy

Frenectomy is the surgical resection of the frenal attachment and may be accompanied by vestibular extension to provide a deeper vestibule. Since the return of the frenum may reoccur with

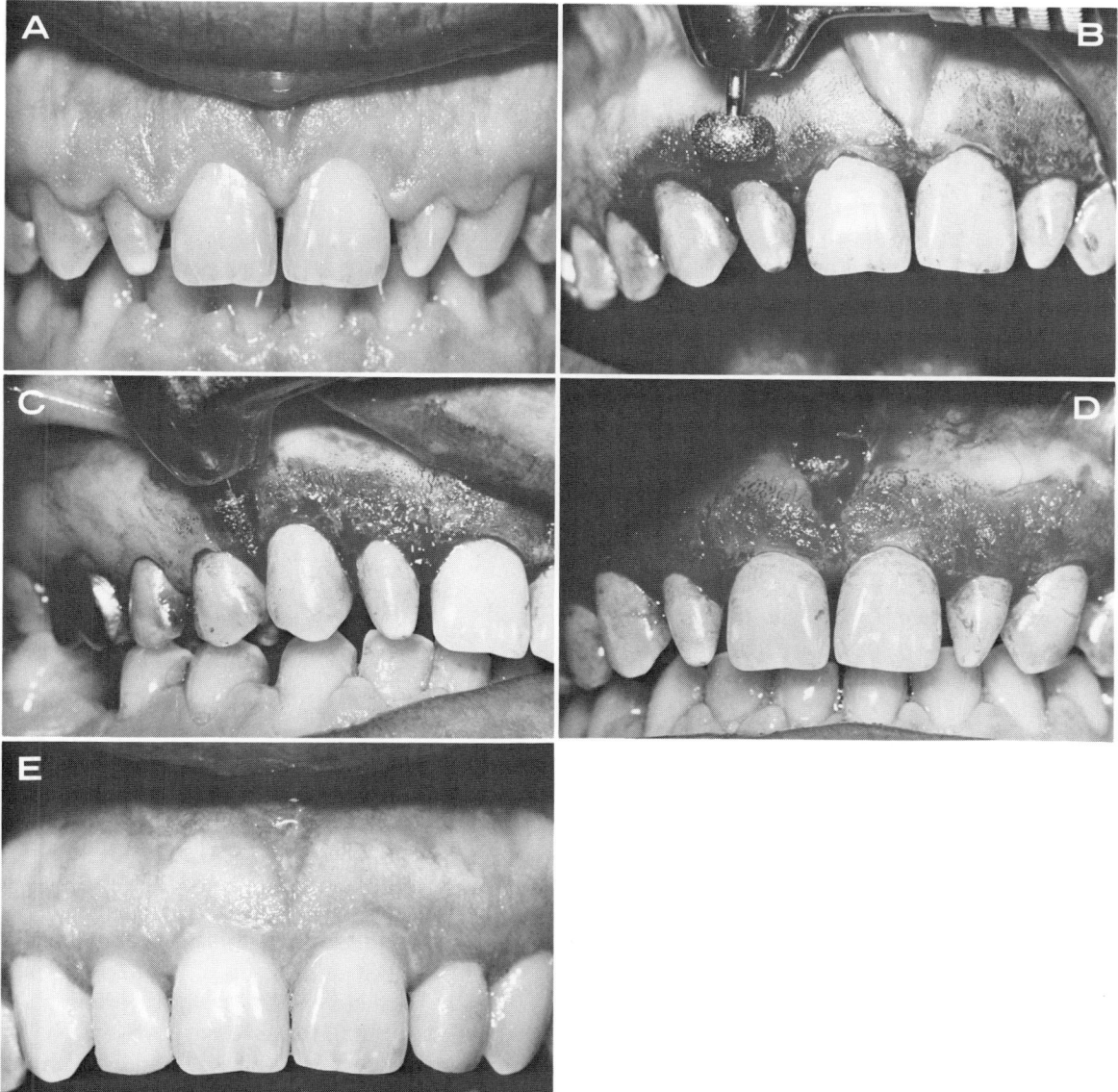

Figure 25-16 | Gingivoplasty procedure. A. Gingival hyperplasia. B and C. Recontouring gingivae with rotary diamond stones. D. Gingival architecture after recontouring. E. Gingival healing following gingivoplasty. (*Courtesy of D. Simpson.*)

time, a free-gingival graft is usually performed at the same time to prevent this from occurring.

Surgical Correction of Osseous Defects

Osteoplasty and Ostectomy

In recent years various techniques have been developed for the correction of bony defects resulting from chronic periodontal disease. If the bony defects are mild such as shallow interproximal craters, then reshaping of the bone by diamond stones or burs is performed. This procedure is called *osteoplasty*. If the defects are larger, more bone must be removed or resected to correct the abnormal architecture; this procedure is called *ostectomy*.

All the surgical approaches to correct bony architecture involve a soft-tissue flap approach. A periodontal flap results from the surgical separation of the gingivae and mucosa from the teeth and underlying bone (Fig. 25-17). Flaps may be full thickness or partial thickness, the difference being that the thin connective-tissue covering over the bone and teeth (periosteum) is not disturbed in the partial-thickness flap. Aspiration of saliva and blood must be downstream, so to speak, in order not to damage the flap in any way while helping to retract the tissue for the operator. The operator must have a clear view of the field at all times (Fig. 25-18).

Bone Implants

Sometimes periodontal disease results in deep vertical defects in the bone, which are not ideally correctable by osteoplasty and ostectomy because too much bone would be removed and poor overall bony architecture would be the result. These vertical defects vary in shape, depth, and topography. They also may be narrow or broad, or circumferential (circling the tooth). Generally the narrower the defect with a greater

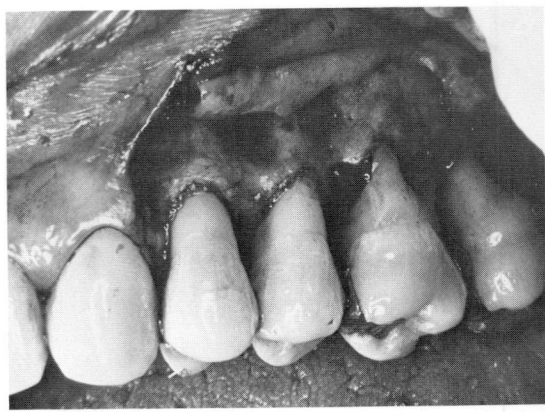

Figure 25-17 | Flap turned and retracted: maxillary area. (*Courtesy of B. Green.*)

number of walls, the better the chance for success with a bone implant.

There is a recipient site for the bone implant and a donor site. The donor site of the bone implant that is most frequently utilized is the tuberosity of the maxilla. Cancellous bone seems to give better results than cortical plate. Another donor site in the same individual (autogenous graft) which has been employed is the marrow of the iliac crest (hip bone). Special precaution in aspiration must be employed to prevent the donor tissue from being suctioned and lost.

Bony implants from donors other than the patient have been utilized, but these implants are not as predictable because of the rejection phenomenon. Human tissues other than bone have also been utilized to fill bony defects, but these are still in the experimental stage.

Intramarrow Penetration

There is some clinical evidence that healing of an osseous defect is promoted by penetrating the walls of the defect with a small, round surgical bur in several locations. This technique is often employed in the case of implants or where no implant is used.

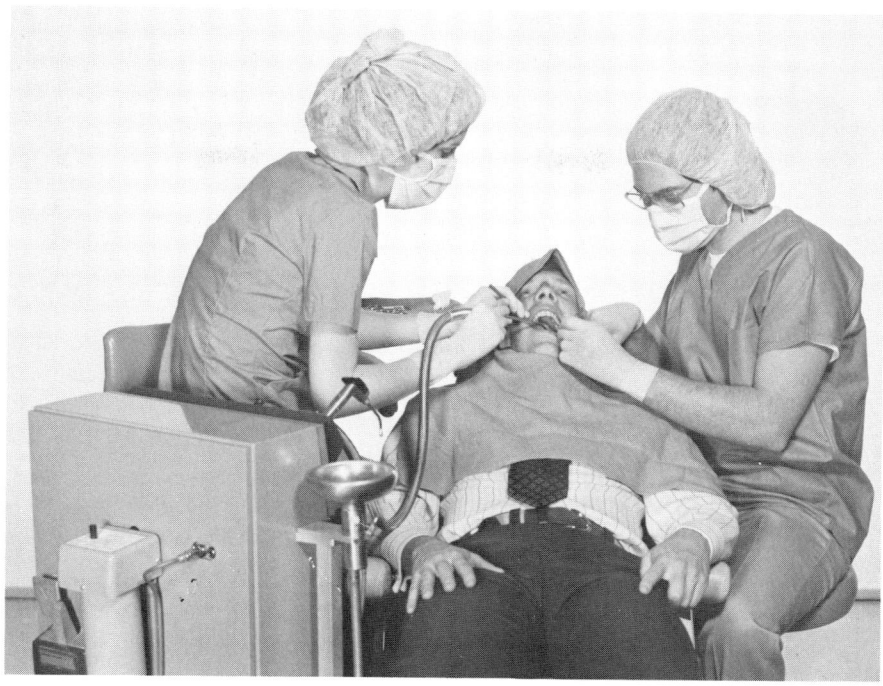

Figure 25-18 | Dental assistant aspirating during a surgical procedure.

Root Amputation and Hemisection

Where the osseous (bony) lesion has penetrated the furcal areas of multirooted teeth, sometimes the correction of the defect is facilitated by root amputation or hemisection. Root amputation means the surgical removal of one or more roots of a multirooted tooth at the interradicualr area. Hemisection means sectioning the crown of a multirooted tooth in half faciolingually, thus creating two separate crowns. Root amputation is employed primarily for maxillary molars, and hemisection for mandibular molars.

TERMINATION OF SURGICAL PROCEDURES

The assistant will need not only to keep the field dry but to assist the operator in suturing by holding the tissue in place and being ready to cut the suture when the operator indicates to do so. Suction should not be applied to the suture material or to the needle before the suture is tied.

When the suturing procedure is completed, a suitable periodontal dressing is mixed. The dressing may be a eugenol or a noneugenol type. Both types of dressing powder and liquid or pastes are mixed similarly, and rolled into thin ropes (Fig. 25-19). The teeth are then dried with a sterile sponge, and the roll of dressing is applied at the crest of the flap (gingival-tooth junction) and pressed gently interproximally all along the area of surgery (facial and lingual or palatal). The facial and lingual parts of the dressing should be pressed so as to connect interproximally. The dressing should not extend beyond the mucogingival junction, and should not cover any portion of the occlusal or incisal surfaces of

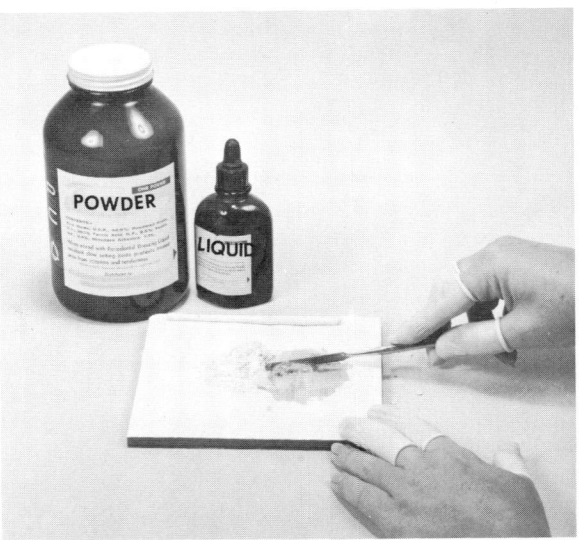

Figure 25-19 | Dental assistant mixing periodontal dressing.

the teeth. The width of the dressing should be about 8 to 10 mm.

The primary purpose of the periodontal dressing is to protect the surgical wound and provide for patient comfort. The dressing also protects the sutures from displacement and aids hemostasis.

In some offices, enough dressing is mixed at the beginning of the day to last for the entire day's surgical requirement and stored in a refrigerator. Each time there is a need for a dressing, a small amount is removed from storage and heated under running hot water and kneaded until manageable for placement.

POSTOPERATIVE INSTRUCTIONS

The operator usually prescribes analgesic medication for several days to allay pain and discomfort. The operator will also instruct the patient what to expect and when to telephone if discomfort should arise. The assistant may be assigned the task of giving the postoperative instructions. Special dietary instructions may be furnished the patient along with a prepared handout on oral-hygiene instructions.

POSTOPERATIVE CARE

At the first postoperative appointment (5 to 7 days), the surgical site is cleansed with 2 percent hydrogen peroxide solution. After having the patient rinse with a mouthwash, the dressing is gently loosened by easing a blunt scaler or curette between the apical portion of the dressing and the tissues, both facially and lingually. Cotton pliers can then be used to remove the facial and lingual segments of the dressing. Care must be exercised to be sure that the dressing has not engaged a suture.

Once the dressing (bandage) has been removed, the sutures are cut with surgical scissors and removed with tissue forceps or cotton pliers. At this time the dentist will examine the surgical site and determine the need for the assistant to place another periodontal dressing. Generally with osseous procedures at least two or three postoperative visits will be required.

ORAL PHYSIOTHERAPY (POSTSURGICAL)

In some offices the dental assistant is expected to teach preventive measures and give oral physiotherapy instructions (refer to Chap. 19). When the patients are surgically treated periodontal patients, modifications of techniques of cleaning will be needed. Surgical corrections, especially osseous procedures, leave the tissues at a lower level, creating wide-open spaces interdentally which may require the use of adjunctive cleaning aids in addition to the toothbrush and regular-sized unwaxed floss. An interproximal brush and larger-sized dental floss may be required to clean these interproximal areas effectively.

CLINICAL PHOTOGRAPHY

The use of clinical photographs as part of office records has been increasing for a number of reasons, the primary one being case documentation and case evaluation. If the assistant has already learned or is willing to learn how to use a clinical camera and take acceptable photographs, the benefit to the dentist will be great. This skill frees the operator from having to do two jobs at the same time (patient management and taking photographs), and helps preserve the chain of sterility.

Keeping a log of photographs taken, mailing films for processing, identifying them on return from the processor, and filing them in correct sequence in a specially designed notebook for housing films would be a great aid.

Peer review of treated periodontal cases in study clubs is greatly facilitated by good clinical photographs and is a superb learning device. In some periodontal offices the entire staff, including other health professionals, participate in a weekly study group. This type of activity promotes mutual harmony and teamwork as well as allaying boredom.

OFFICE SUPPLIES

At designated intervals clinical supplies will require an inventory using a minimum-maximum system to determine the need for reordering. For periodontics such supplies would include polishing agents, staining tablets, toothbrushes, floss, and surgical items such as blades, sutures, and periodontal dressings.

PERIODONTAL MAINTENANCE

There are few periodontal patients sufficiently motivated to achieve such efficiency and perfection in daily oral hygiene that they no longer require periodic help from the dentist. Therefore recall maintenance for most patients is needed to ensure continuous periodontal health. Some patients require help with a greater frequency than others. The degree of help needed determines both the recall interval, and the length of the appointment.

In some offices the assistant is assigned the task of evaluating the oral-hygiene performance of the patient at each recall appointment. In some group practices, this may well be one of the major assignments for one of the assistants employed by the group.

Setting up a recall system and monitoring it may also be an assignment for the dental assistant. Since each office handles the recall system differently, this will probably be an on-the-job skill to be acquired.

The specialty of periodontics is requiring more skills of the dental assistant, as this type of practice is continuously becoming more complex and as states amend their laws regulating the practice of dentistry.

Periodontists are associating together now in partnerships and group practices and are employing several assistants as well as other health-professional personnel. Office manuals are in common use, and the practice of cross-training within an office is beneficial for all concerned.

BIBLIOGRAPHY

Allen, D. L., McFall, W. T. Jr., and Hunter, G. C., Jr.: *Periodontics for the Dental Hygienist,* 2d ed., Lea & Febiger, Philadelphia, 1974.

Glickman, I.: *Clinical Periodontology,* 4th ed., W. B. Saunders Company, Philadelphia, 1972.

———— and Smulow, J. B. *Periodontal Disease,* W. B. Saunders Company, Philadelphia, 1974.

Goldman, H. M., and Cohen, D. W.: *Periodontal Therapy,* 5th ed., The C. V. Mosby Company, St. Louis, 1973.

Grant, D. A., Stern I. B., and Everett, F. G.: *Orban's Periodontics,* 3d ed., The C. V. Mosby Company, St. Louis, 1968.

Prichard, J. F.: *Advanced Periodontal Disease: Surgical and Prosthetic Management,* 2d ed., W. B. Saunders Company, Philadelphia, 1972.

Stone, S., and Kalis, P. J.: *Periodontics, Module 6, Dental Auxiliary Practice,* M. J. Dunn, series ed., The Williams and Wilkins Company, Baltimore, 1975.

Ward, H. L., and Simring, M. (eds.): *Manual of Clinical Periodontics,* The C. V. Mosby Company, St. Louis, 1973.

26

Benjamin R. Baker

Pedodontics

INTRODUCTION

Within the memory of many, the child in the dental office was said to be recalcitrant, unmanageable, unprofitable, and unwanted. The child was tolerated in the dental office as a necessity in order to retain the parents as patients. As a result, a generation or two ago dentistry for children was sadly neglected by the rank and file of the dental profession. Luther Burbank many years ago stated, "If we paid no more attention to our plants than we have to our children, we would now be living in a jungle of weeds" (McBride, 1937). It is fortunate that this attitude of 40 years ago does not exist predominately today in the profession. The efforts of early pioneers in dentistry for children prevailed, and today pedodontics is a recognized dental specialty. The child of today and tomorrow can receive dental care which will allow development and maintenance of dentition in optimum condition. This security is due to the courage and convictions of progressive individuals in the dental profession.

The development of pedodontics, like all dental specialties, occurred as a result of a definite need. The compilation of standards and requirements in pedodontics grew out of the trials and errors of actual practice. The early didactic and clinical courses of study consisted of a patchwork of scattered lectures in the schools which saw a need for dental students to have some information about children's teeth.

The emergence of pedodontics from the "ugly duckling" stage began on a national scale with the announcement by the Council on Dental

Education in 1942 that dentistry for children should be taught in all dental schools.

HISTORY

Pedodontics is a new field as compared to older specialties such as oral surgery and orthodontics. However, there have always been a few dentists who championed its cause. Prior to 1900 there was little material in the dental literature oriented toward the child. Dr. Evangeline Jordan was the first pedodontist of record in the United States. She opened an office shortly after 1900 in Los Angeles. The first dental school to offer a course in pedodontics was the Dental Dispensary at Tufts University in Boston. The first dental student in pedodontics was Dr. H. C. Pucket, who enrolled for the Tufts course of study in 1919. It was through this man's efforts that the modern approach to dentistry for children was begun.

Many advances followed the establishment of a pedodontic course at Tufts, but only a few schools offered instruction in this area. In 1927 the American Society for the Promotion of Dentistry for Children was founded. The efforts of this agency caused many schools to take heed of the need for a separate course in the dental curriculum. However by 1935 it still was not given proper prominence, and lectures in pedodontics in the majority of dental schools were delivered by the various departments of operative dentistry, prosthetics, surgery, and others as the need arose (Hogeboom, 1939).

Thus in the years prior to World War II the position of pedodontics was one of little emphasis in the dental profession. From its early organized efforts in 1927 the teaching of pedodontics has grown faster than any other specialty in dentistry. Today every dental school offers a separate undergraduate course in pedodontics. This has been realized through the efforts of the early leaders. The growth and activities of the American Society of Dentistry for Children, the recognition of pedodontics as a dental specialty, the high standards which the American Board of Pedodontics has maintained, and the influence of the American Academy of Pedodontics have collectively resulted in the elevation of the standards of dental practice for children.

DEFINITION

What is pedodontics? What is involved in the practice of pedodontics? Must pedodontics be limited to the specialist? The answers to these questions will provide the student of dental assisting with an insight into one of America's greatest problems in dentistry. The subsequent pages of this chapter deal with the many aspects of pedodontics and its service to the dental health of children.

The following definition of pedodontics has been approved and is currently accepted to consider the scope of service expected of the pedodontist:*

Pedodontics is that area of dental practice which is limited to the treatment of children; dynamic organisms which undergo periodic change in physical, mental and emotional growth.
To provide a program of complete oral health care during this developmental period, the specialist must possess the knowledge and skill to:
Diagnose and manage abnormal behavior patterns;
Perform restorative technics peculiar to the child patient;
Direct surgical procedures necessitated by anomalous and traumatic conditions;
Perform pulpal therapy peculiar to primary and permanent teeth;
Diagnose and treat a variety of congenital and developmental anomalies;
Give special emphasis to accepted preventive procedures.

* Definition and statement presented by representatives of the American Board of Pedodontics, American Society of Dentistry for Children, and American Academy of Pedodontics, at the Second Conference on Dental Specialties and Specialization, Chicago, Sept. 7 and 8, 1960.

Pedodontics is, then, the general practice of dentistry limited to children. It includes all the ramifications and underlying problems of a growing organism. The primary objective of pedodontics is to provide complete, comprehensive dental services. This may also be applied to dentistry in general as well, but, in relation to the child, it cannot be assumed that service may be of lesser quality because the primary teeth are in the mouth for a limited number of years and will be replaced. Any dental service for a child must be performed with the highest standards of quality. After reading the above definition the student might conclude that children's dental services should be limited to the specialist in pedodontics. Nothing could be further from the truth. The child patient must be treated by the general practitioner. The various reasons for this are explained below. The dental assistant should be aware of pedodontic services in case of electing to devote a career to a pedodontic practice. In future years dental assisting may also be divided into specialties. For these reasons also it is important to know specialties of dentistry in detail.

NEED AND DEMAND FOR PEDODONTICS

Few children escape dental-health problems. Dental decay is the most prevalent disease of humankind. It affects 95 percent of the human race. The teeth of children under 14 years of age are decaying six times as fast as they are being filled, and many preventable deformities of the teeth and the oral complex develop every year. It is not remotely possible for specialists in pedodontics to provide for the dental service for all children. In point of fact, with the current rate of attack and dental personnel availability to combat dental disease in children, it is questionable whether the profession as a whole can meet the impending problem. The existing backlog of unmet dental needs in the United States is so great that it is difficult to describe it to the public in meaningful words. The following statistics may serve to describe the problem as it relates to children.

In 1967 there were some 74 million children in the United States under age 19. This figure is projected to increase to 98 million by 1985. Among this increasing number of younger children 50 percent will have decayed teeth by age 2. The average child upon entering school has three decayed teeth, and between ages 5 and 9 children average three unfilled decayed teeth. A student reaching high school at age 14 typically has eleven decayed, missing, or filled permanent teeth (Galagan et al., 1964).

In the ages from 6 to 11 children develop carious teeth at the rate of 1 per year. This increases to 1½ in the period between 12 and 15 years. Decay accounts for 75 percent of the tooth loss for children in the 15-to-24-year-old group. One out of every two children needs orthodontic care, and periodontal diseases of the gingivitis type occur in a major portion of the child population. The dental literature relating to these problems increases with every publication. The challenge to dentistry today to meet these needs is greater than ever before. This is a challenge which cannot be met by the profession alone. As long as a victim of dental disease does not get professional care, the conditions requiring treatment become more complex and the patient moves closer to a point of no return (Galagan et al., 1964).

The efforts of organized dentistry to meet this need and the emerging governmental participation are placing dental care for children in the prime position of consideration. It can therefore be seen that the colossal proportions of dental needs of children and the universality of the problem relative to the dental-disease attack rate place an unparalleled demand upon the dental profession. The family dentist must treat as many children as time and preparation will allow. The dentist should do everything possible to propagate the principles of prevention so that children whose dental needs are met may remain so.

Socioeconomic and Federal Influences

The historical experience of dental service and dental demand by the public offers some interesting data to supplement the rationale for dental service for children. Demand for service in the future will increase even though the current population increase is mild. More people will be able to afford dental service, and an increasing public awareness of health needs and the benefits of a healthy body and a healthy dentition will bring more demand for service. In most middle-class families health insurance is one of the top priorities for money designation in the family budget. In addition, prepaid dental programs affect several million people in the country at present, and these are increasing each year as companies and industrial concerns include these items in fringe benefit programs. Many people will receive dental services through these mechanisms who would otherwise not receive them at all (McCaslin, 1968; Brown, 1974; Rose, 1975).

Other factors leading to the increase of numbers of people who seek dental treatment are the many federal programs which have a dental-service component (McCaslin, 1968). Congress has had numerous major bills related to the need for and implementation of a national health insurance. All of these bills have as a basic component some form of dental benefits, and all of them begin with treatment for children (Klebe, 1976). While congress has not made a final decision relative to what specific type of national health insurance it will enact into law, it can be reasonably concluded that before the end of the decade of the seventies a federal program of national insurance with a component dental service for children will be a reality. There is a unanimous feeling within the profession of dentistry and among the lawmakers who sponsor health insurance that the dental-health problems in the United States may best be met through a massive assault on dental disease by primary care for children. In this way dental health in the future may be brought under control and maintained. The solution is simple in statement but not so easily accomplished.

If it is accepted that a shortage of dentists exists and the ability of the dental profession to relieve the shortage is questionable, other methods of meeting the potential demand for services must be explored. The greater utilization of the trained assistant, with greater latitude in duties, has been suggested as one method of providing needed services. The assistant must, therefore, look to future training in the area of pedodontics for a significant role in the provision of dental services (Brown, 1974).

With the need for dentistry in the United States as it has been demonstrated in such staggering proportions, it should be easy to recognize that all of dentistry must be responsible for dentistry for children. The combined efforts of the dental profession in concert with organized labor, insurance companies, and the state and federal governments must place dentistry for children in the forefront of the programs of a health-conscious nation. With this realization the subsequent pages of this chapter will serve to provide the student dental assistant with a better understanding of pedodontic dental service.

THE PRIMARY DENTITION

Description

In order to discuss the growth and development of teeth and to understand them properly, the dental assistant should become familiar with a few basic terms and factors. Human beings are provided with two sets of teeth. These are the *primary* (deciduous) teeth and the *permanent* teeth. The first set of teeth are called the baby teeth by most people. The correct name for these teeth is the primary or deciduous dentition. Deciduous comes from the Latin *decidere*, meaning to fall off. The process of eruption and shedding gives the baby teeth their technical name. Permanent teeth are known as *succe-*

daneous teeth from the Latin *succedere*, meaning to follow after. One usually thinks of a newborn child as being toothless or without teeth. Tooth formation begins within the first 2 months of pregnancy, and the process of development and maturation of the primary and some of the permanent teeth occurs during the final 7 months of pregnancy. Thus at birth the child has within its jawbones 20 primary teeth which are almost entirely formed with the exception of the completed roots (Brauer et al., 1964).

The mouth is divided into four areas or quadrants, each of which represents one-quarter of the dentition. These are the maxillary right and left quadrants and the mandibular right and left quadrants. The teeth in each quadrant have the same names. The right and left maxillary quadrants and the right and left mandibular quadrants make up the upper and lower dental arches.

Beginning with the tooth adjacent to the midline of the face the primary teeth are positioned in the following order. The first tooth is the central incisor. The second tooth is the lateral incisor. These are used for cutting food. The third tooth from the midline is the cuspid (canine), which is used for tearing food. The fourth tooth from the midline and the fifth tooth from the midline are the primary first and second molars. These teeth are used for grinding food. Figures 26-1 and 26-2 are illustrations of the primary dentition of a 4-year-old. The primary teeth have been designated alphabetically to further identify them. This is to facilitate dental service on a universal basis so that there is a single nomenclature. Beginning with the upper right second primary molar, the maxillary teeth are identified as "A" through "J" respectively. Beginning with the lower left second primary molar the mandibular primary teeth are identified as "K" through "T" respectively (Fig. 26-3).

Importance

The practice of dentistry in the past and the lack of knowledge of the value of the primary teeth

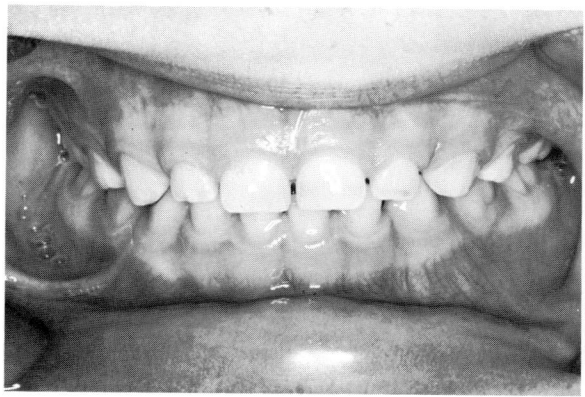

Figure 26-1 | The primary dentition of a 4-year-old boy.

have contributed to the mutilation of countless dentitions. Old wives' tales and ignorance of the uses of the primary teeth have been explained with the typical comment that since the baby teeth will be replaced it is not necessary to be particularly zealous in their care. This is untrue. There are several very vital functions associated with the primary teeth which individually are reasons sufficient to retain the primary teeth until they are naturally lost by exfoliation. Collectively, the reasons are absolute in providing the optimum oral health for the patient.

There are several reasons why the primary teeth are important to ensure dental health throughout life. The primary teeth are necessary for the proper mastication of food. The period in life when nourishment is most important is during a child's growing stages. If the teeth of a child are decayed and infected, the child may not be able to do an adequate job of chewing foods essential to normal growth and development. Even though the primary teeth will be replaced by the permanent teeth, some of them must be retained through age 12 and sometimes longer. Twelve years of function for a tooth represents approximately one-sixth of a person's life. Untreated carious primary teeth can cause

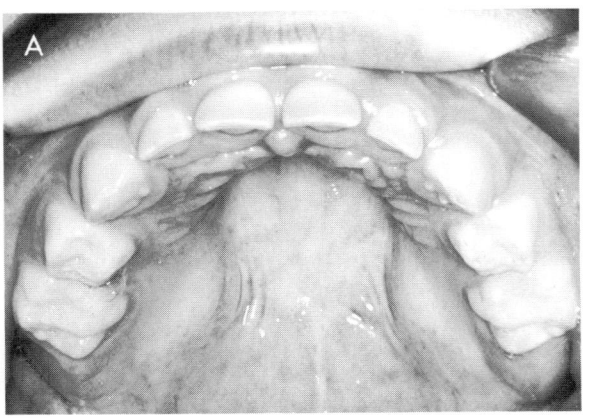

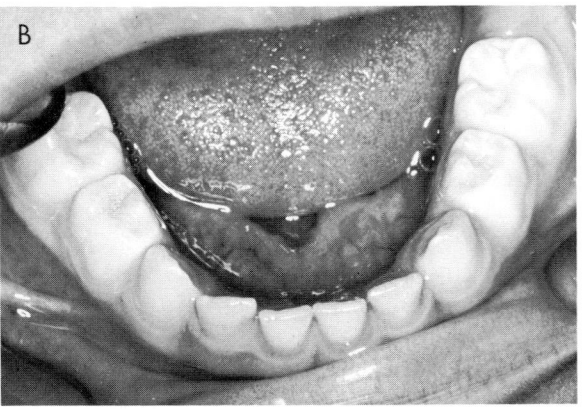

Figure 26-2 | Intraoral view of the primary dentition. A. Maxillary arch. B. Mandibular arch.

pain and greater infection. This can lead to other health complications of a general nature and specifically may damage developing permanent teeth which are in the underlying tissues of the jaws.

The primary teeth in the jaws serve to reserve space for 20 of the permanent teeth. They also aid in the development of the jaws through function. During the preschool years the primary teeth are essential to the development of proper speech. The tongue uses the lingual surface of the upper anterior teeth for the correct production of many sounds and words. If those primary teeth are prematurely lost due to trauma or neglect, it is difficult for the child to learn the correct pronunciation of certain words and sounds. Children are also acutely aware of their social environment, and the untimely loss of teeth, anteriors particularly, may produce self-consciousness as well as more severe psychologic feelings of inadequacy.

The premature loss of primary teeth in any area of the dental arches may result in space loss by the movement of adjacent teeth into the empty space. This will result in inadequate room for permanent teeth to erupt to their proper position. An orthodontic problem is the end result.

The prevention of dental complications through adequate care of the primary teeth is one of the most important services in dentistry. Therefore, the value of the primary teeth is not limited solely to a temporary functional purpose in the early childhood years. The care and guidance of the dentition must begin at the earliest possible age and be continued throughout adult life. The dental assistant who is knowledgeable in these areas and in the reasons for pedodontic dental service not only renders the dentist an invaluable service but also contributes generously to the health of the dentist's family of patients.

Eruption

The first teeth to appear (erupt) in the jaws are the lower central incisors. They usually erupt between the sixth and eighth months after birth. Not all children will erupt teeth during this given period or in the same order. It is not uncommon for some children to be 8 to 10 months of age before their first teeth appear in the dental arches. In general the lower teeth erupt before the same upper teeth, and girls have a tendency to erupt teeth earlier than boys.

After eruption of the lower central incisors the upper central incisors come in during the next 3 to 4 months; the upper lateral incisors follow closely behind the centrals. Approximately 1 month after the upper laterals erupt the lower lateral incisors appear. Thus after the first anterior tooth appears, there are successive eruptions of the upper and lower anterior teeth over a period of 6 months until all eight incisors are in the mouth by age 10 to 12 months.

Subsequent to the incisors' eruption, there is a quiescent period where no further teeth appear for a time. At about 15 to 17 months of age the first primary molars begin to appear in both dental arches. The child may experience some discomfort from these eruptions due to the broad occlusal surface which causes greater difficulty in breaking through the soft tissue which lies over the dental ridges.

As the first primary molars appear in the dental arches, there is a space between the lateral incisors and the first molars. This is the space reserved for the eruption of the primary cuspid (canine) teeth. The child is usually 20 months old when this occurs. Finally, the primary second molars appear in the mouth between ages 24 to 30 months; with the eruption of the second molars the full complement of 20 primary teeth is completed (Schour and Massler, 1940; Salzmann, 1957; Meredith, 1946).

The eruption of teeth in a child can be difficult or unremarkable. The eruption of teeth is not usually accompanied by any significant disturbance. "Teething" is a physiologic process, and there is no specific reason to explain why one child may be irritable during this period and another is not. In children who seem to have eruption problems there may be some irritability during meals and excessive drooling. There is very little which can be done to speed up the eruption of teeth although the normal eruption of teeth may be aided by chewing on teething rings, teething biscuits, toast, a cloth which will not shred, and other aids. Pacifiers as teething aids are not recommended since deleterious habits may result from this use. Chewing on hard objects does act to help the tooth pierce the soft tissue overlying the tooth. There is no definitive evidence that tooth eruption causes high temperature, sniffling, colds, or diarrhea. If these health problems accompany teething, they are likely due to other causes. The energy involved in the eruption of a tooth can, however, lower a baby's resistance, and if the teething aids are unclean, infection can result. If a child exhibits pain from teething, gum massage with the ball of the finger can relieve the discomfort. Some dentists prescribe mild topical anesthetics. Judicious use of aspirin can also relieve pain of tooth eruption. Sustained difficulty of teething with associated pain and other complications should be treated by a pediatrician with the suspicion of other causes for the distress (Spock, 1957; Burket, 1957).

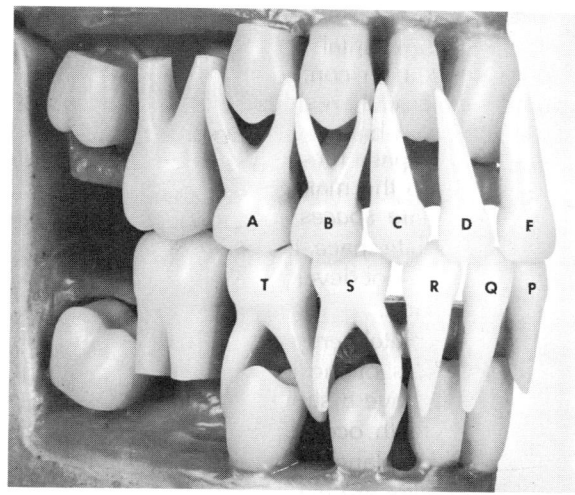

Figure 26-3 | Antomic wax carvings of the upper and lower right quadrants of the primary dentition. The teeth are lettered according to the universal system for identification of primary teeth.

Occlusion

When all the primary teeth have erupted, there will be interdentation around 2½ to 3 years of age. That is, the occlusion or *bite* is established. The mandibular dental arch will occlude within the maxillary arch throughout the entire arch.

The primary dental arches usually show very little variation in conformation. In other words they are generally ovoid, and there may or may not be spaces between each tooth. Most arches will have a space mesial to the maxillary cuspid and distal to the mandibular cuspid. These are called *primate spaces*. Some children will not have a primate space. If none is present at age 3, the child will not develop a primate space in primary dentition.

In a completely erupted primary dentition the distal surfaces of the upper and lower second molars will have a straight terminal plane since these two teeth occlude in an end-to-end relationship. This plane will remain constant until the second molars are exfoliated. There are factors which can cause the plane to become uneven. These are certain oral habits like thumb-sucking and tongue-thrusting or interproximal decay of teeth which will cause the adjacent teeth to drift into the carious area, or the adjacent teeth may collapse toward each other. The position of the primary teeth in the arches is usually perpendicular to the occlusal plane. There is very little overbite, and as the child grows in age, the wear of the primary teeth may yield even less overbite. This will depend to a great extent upon the types of foods which are eaten. If coarse foods are a steady diet, then more wear will occur (Moyer, 1963).

The occlusion of a child which is established at age 3 will remain stable until age 6 when the primary teeth begin to exfoliate and the permanent teeth are ready to begin the process of eruption (Marks, 1968).

THE CHILD FROM 2 TO 6

By the time a child reaches the end of the second year, all the primary teeth usually have erupted. Within the next 6 months the primary dental arches become stable, and the teeth are in occlusion. There will be little change in the dental situation from a developmental point of view until the child reaches 6 years of age. The period between ages 2 and 6 is a dynamic time in the child's life. If the child's dentition is to be kept in a sound condition, it is important to begin regular visits to the dentist when all the primary teeth are in occlusion. A good rule of thumb is to bring the child for a first visit around the time of the third birthday. It is rare to have complicated dental problems develop prior to age 3 if the child is healthy and the child's diet is adequate. However, any problem which a parent perceives as unusual or different should be seen by the dentist regardless of age.

Beginning a child's visits to the dentist with a pleasant experience is most desirable. Dental-decay problems which manifest before the age of 3 are almost routinely the fault of improper diet and improper home care. Therefore when a youngster of 2 years of age presents with these problems, one cannot expect enthusiasm about what seems to be an unpleasant experience. The maturational level and social adjustment level of the 2-year-old is such that a negative reaction to any type of dental treatment is likely. This is a period in which orientation is in an oral phase. It is a period characterized by trust versus basic mistrust (Callahan, 1964). Any threat to security, especially in the oral area, can be cataclysmic, and the child may react with basic mistrust in all subsequent visits to the dentist. Unless the child exhibits some real dental problem, the age of 3 is early enough for a first dental-office experience. It is, however, a good plan to have the child of 2 accompany mother on her visits to the dentist. The child should be allowed to watch the parent being examined, radiographed, and other various procedures. This is a method of introduction to the office for the child, and it must come directly from the child, that is, the child must want it. When the child becomes familiar with the surroundings in the office, examination at age 3 will be easier. If the parent is a poor patient, this method of introduction to the dental office is contraindicated. Little eyes and ears see and hear more than adults realize. For this reason a negative experience by parents in this instance will prejudice the child at a later age. This applies to conversation about dentistry at home. One should always avoid negative terms like bad, hurt, pain, and shot in conversations which the 2-to-6 age group can hear.

The 3-year-olds are imaginative creatures and love play. These children can be reasoned with to a degree, but they are possessive. They undergo constant struggle which revolves around what they can accomplish or achieve. They are in a period of rapid fluctuation of extremes and interaction with others. They have a rather rigid pattern of life and may become upset with anything that diverges from their pattern of activity. It is important to be tolerant yet firm with this age group. The 3-year-olds will try to please, and they will cooperate frequently if good reason can be shown to them. The best approach for handling this age is moderation and holding the middle ground (Callahan, 1964).

The 4-and-5-year-old period is one of initiation and identification with something. During this period children are developing a sense of grammar and proficiency in speech. Their developmental stage is at a point where they can begin to form concepts of things. They constantly imagine things and are known as incessant questioners. The preschool children are at a time when they begin to compare realistically to their position in life, and they begin to see just how small they are in the area of things. It is a time when they need and want to understand everything affecting them in situations. Bigness is important to them in comparing themselves to others and things (Ilg and Ames, 1955).

The assistant should be aware of these factors. Many of the children in a dental practice will have their first experience with operative dentistry during this age. It is therefore important for the assistant to learn to relate to children at their own levels. Cooperation in dental appointments of this age group depends upon understanding how they view the staff. It is important to let the child participate. If initiative is removed, the child may become resistive or even recalcitrant and react violently. The child can distinguish between truth and falsehood. If a dentist or assistant tells an untruth to a child about the appointment procedures, the child will not forget it, and resultant negativism will be justified.

The typical reaction of normal 2-to-6-year-old youngsters is generally good when the correct approach is used. The dentist and assistant represent authority figures to them, and they also represent the unknown. The children's reactions to authority and to the unknown are typical and should be expected. These are negativism, anger, resistance, panic, violence. The personalities of the staff should be such that these reactions do not anger them. Rather, they must be tolerant of these expected reactions. Understanding of young children and their various reactions is fundamental to successful children's dentistry. The dentist and assistant who know these natural reactions of children can treat them better. Those who ignore these concepts and force the child without explaining may precipitate severe problems in subsequent appointments. It should be remembered, however, that when the child's dental condition dictates a dental procedure, it should be done. No one can expect to guide a child through life with the exclusion of all but pleasing experiences. Young children are malleable and generally make ideal patients when treated with firmness and respect.

THE CHILD FROM 6 TO 12— MIXED DENTITION

The time in a child's life when both primary and permanent teeth are present is known as the *mixed dentition* period. The mixed dentition begins with the appearance of the first permanent molars. With the arrival of these four first permanent molars the critical process of changing from the primary dentition to the permanent teeth begins. It is a critical time because of the possibilities for development of malocclusions with their associated orthodontic problems.

Between the age of 6 and 12 it is extremely important to have close supervision of the dentition by the dentist, as this is probably the most important period in the healthy transition of the child's mouth and teeth. During this span of years all the primary teeth are exfoliated and replaced by the permanent teeth. After age 12 there are eight more permanent teeth which appear. These are the second permanent molars and the third molars or wisdom teeth. Thus by ages 18 to 20 all 32 permanent teeth have made their appearance in the dental arches. The processes of exfoliation of primary teeth and their replacement with permanent teeth are explained in the following paragraphs.

The sequence of eruption of permanent teeth seems to be more important than the time of eruption since eruption of certain permanent teeth may lead to difficulties of proper tooth position in the arches.

The first permanent teeth to appear in the jaws are the four 6-year molars. It has been stated that these are the most important teeth in the dental arches. They come in behind the second primary molars, and they do not have a primary tooth predecessor. They serve as the foundation about which the permanent dental arch forms, and their position determines the basis for the proper permanent dentition bite or occlusion (Moyer, 1963). In addition, they are the most important chewing teeth. Any alteration in a child's mouth which causes an adjusted position of the 6-year molars can lead to malocclusion. Therefore, the problems of heredity, deleterious habits, decay, and improper dental care can be the cause of poor occlusion beginning at an early age.

When a permanent tooth is fully formed and ready to erupt, the primary tooth will loosen and be shed in order to provide the space for eruption of its successor. Shedding (exfoliation) of primary teeth occurs as a result of the process of resorption (dissolving) of the primary tooth root until it no longer has support in the bone and soft tissues of the jaws. Thus the tooth finally just wriggles out.

The first primary teeth to loosen and drop out are the lower central incisors. This occurs at about age 6. The lower permanent central incisors are followed by the upper permanent central incisors. The lower lateral incisors also appear at this time. The upper laterals erupt a little later to complete the incisor group. Thus during the period from age 6 through age 8 all the primary incisors are lost and replaced by the permanent successors. The sequence of eruption of permanent teeth corresponds to that of the primary teeth. That is to say that mandibular teeth precede the maxillary teeth.

Following the eruption of the incisor group there is a short span of time when no further teeth are lost. Then between ages 9 and 10 the primary cuspids in the mandible are lost, and the mandibular permanent cuspids appear. It is not uncommon for some first bicuspids to appear around 10 years of age. In the period between ages 10 and 11 the bicuspids appear following the exfoliation of the primary molars. In the twelfth year the maxillary primary cuspids are replaced by the permanent cuspids, and all the primary teeth have been exfoliated. The second permanent molars appear, and all the permanent teeth are in the mouth with the exception of the wisdom teeth (Hurme, 1949; Salzmann, 1957).

It has been stated previously that the mandibular teeth generally erupt prior to their maxillary counterparts. The sequence of eruption of permanent teeth for each arch is as follows: In the mandible the first molars (19, 30)* erupt first with the central incisors (24, 25) at about the same time or close behind. These are followed by the lateral incisors (23, 26), the cuspids (22,

---

* These numbers in parentheses and in all such instances following refer to the universal tooth-numbering system for permanent teeth (Fig. 26-4).

27), the first bicuspids (21, 28), the second bicuspids (20, 29), and finally the second permanent molars (18, 31). In the maxillary arch the first permanent molars (3, 14) appear first followed by the central incisors (8, 9) and the lateral incisors (7, 10). The first bicuspids (5, 12) and the second bicuspids (4, 13) follow the lateral incisors. The cuspids (6, 11) next erupt with the second permanent molars (2, 15) appearing last. Figure 26-4 illustrates the primary and permanent dentition as they are graphically shown on a patient chart.

Between the ages of 6 and 12 the child develops into a little adult. If the dentist has been visited on a regular recommended basis since the child was 3, there will be a minimum of resistance and management. Restorative dental service is not such a significant problem for this group. When children have not been to the dental office prior to ages 6 to 12, rather disconcerting problems can manifest themselves. In the population today it is uncommon for a child to have a first visit to the dentist at such a late stage of life. It is important for the dentist or the assistant to be an effective communicator with all children in order that dental service may be provided with the greatest facility. In the paragraphs below some insight is given into certain patterns of behavior which are important to know and recognize in children.

Behavior Patterns

The 6-year-olds of today have had some experience away from the home in nursery school, kindergarten, and the first grade. These are social forces which influence their personality, and they begin to reflect these in their desire for outside activities. Their friends take on greater importance. In situations like visits to the physician and dentist they may manifest fear of the appointment. They may ask questions which have an underlying fear of blood or of being alone. Their vocabulary has increased so that there are questions asked especially as they relate to what is to

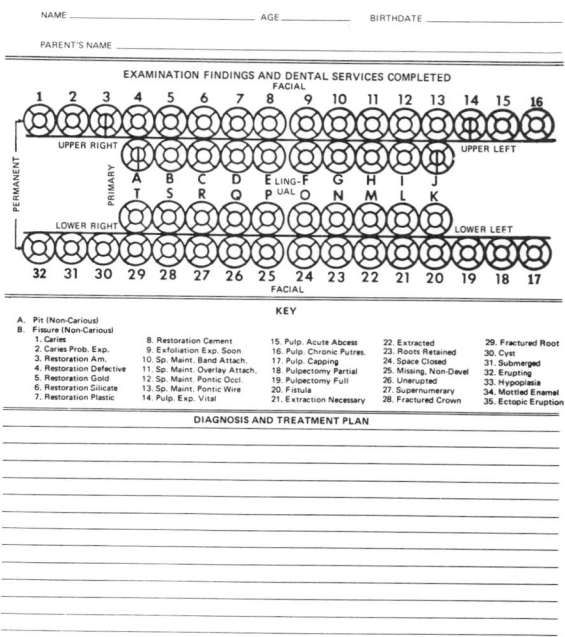

Figure 26-4 | A pedodontic patient chart which illustrates the universal numbering system for primary and permanent teeth. The permanent teeth number 1 through 32 while the primary teeth are symbolized by letters "A" through "T." Each system begins with the upper right teeth and ends with the lower right teeth.

be done to and for them. Appointments for dental service during times when they are accustomed to other more enjoyable pursuits may reflect in recalcitrance. It is not wise to chastise a 6-year-old with ridicule. A negative response will often result instead of a yielding one (Ilg and Ames, 1955).

The 7- and 8-year-olds respond in a similar manner to the 6-year-olds. The social sense is becoming stronger as they feel greater comfort in their surroundings. Bigness and smallness of size are important facets of their personality and self-appraisal. The assistant should try to find some favorable aspect of smaller children in this age group. The 8-year-olds are emerging into a decided same-age, same-sex period. It is a time characterized by struggles with the parent of the same sex and deep attachment to the parent of the opposite sex. The assistant may see problems in this age at appointments where the conflicting parent brings the child.

As children move on into ages 9, 10, and 11 the above characteristics continue. The outside world revolves around children of the same age and sex. These years are the period in which learning occurs with the greatest rapidity. Play is of prime importance to them because it is their refuge where they can retreat to overhaul their egos. It is also a period where mastery of self and things occurs. There will be great pride exhibited in their ability to develop skills. They may become deeply interested in the way ancient cultures developed, and they become devoted to informative periodicals like the *National Geographic*. It is an age of development of interests in athletics and in things mechanical. The interests of the child in the preadolescent years of today are far more sophisticated than those of 20 to 30 years ago because of the emergence of new educational systems, automation, space research, and better media of communication. The dental assistant should be acutely aware of the interests and likes and dislikes of this age group. Dental appointments as they relate to establishing communication with the patient should be centered around these areas (Ilg and Ames, 1955; Callahan, 1964).

The 12-year-old is on the threshold of adolescence. This is the period when the child is beginning to undergo physiologic and social revolution. It is a time when greater expectations from parents occur. It is the beginning of total revamping of personality. This is a period of extreme hypersensitivity especially in relations with others. It is also a period of extreme hypersensitivity in fitting what is expected with what has gone before. These children want to be recognized as adults with extra privileges but shirk adult responsibilities which parents insist accompany adult privilege. It is a time when the utmost importance is to keep identity with something. Group status is of paramount importance. There is tremendous group activity and attachment, and the 12-year-old will often react violently to comments attacking the group. These are the areas of personality of the child which begin at age 12 and continue with increasing intensity through the adolescent years (Callahan, 1964).

Dental assistants cannot be practicing child psychologists and know intimately all the traits and characteristics of every age of the child. The foregoing are only brief introductions to the child patient. However, if the assistant applies a knowledge of certain signal points in the child's personality, it is of considerable value to the dentist in maintaining cooperation and congeniality in the office.

The dynamic period of the child's life from ages 6 through 12 is often the period when most dental problems are manifested. It is a period in which parents and the dentist must do everything possible to maintain the integrity of the dental arches. As the child enters this age group, the majority of parents assume that all the primary teeth will soon be lost. This process does begin at age 6; however, the last primary tooth to be exfoliated is not lost for another 6 years at age 12. The value of primary teeth and the necessity for their maintenance in a healthy condition have already been discussed in this chapter. In the following paragraphs some elaboration is given to maintaining the integrity of the dental arches when certain primary teeth have been prematurely lost or compromised by decay, trauma, or other dental problems.

PEDODONTIC PROCEDURES

The treatment of children in dental offices can be one of the most rewarding and enjoyable experiences in a dentist's professional life, or the bane of existence. There is no secret to successful handling of a pedodontic dental service. Children are similar to adults in that each has a unique personality, which should be respected. In order to properly care for children it may often be necessary to develop flexibility so that adequate care may be accomplished. This is constantly done for adult patients and simply needs application on the appropriate level of the child to ensure success. It is of paramount importance to be frank and truthful in all expressions for pedodontic treatment. Honesty in dealing with children, especially in answering their questions, will cultivate more respect and admiration than any other method of dealing with them. Conversely, devious means and trickery to accomplish treatment for children create distrust and management problems for subsequent sessions which may escalate into major proportions.

There is probably a greater percentage of dentists and dental auxiliaries who are afraid of children than there are children who are afraid of dentistry. Most children fear the unknown of the office rather than the people in it. Those who recognize this fact make children's dentistry a refreshing break in the day's appointment schedule. Good dentistry requires enthusiasm. Enthusiasm produces earnestness and sincerity, and from this manner patients are convinced that they are in good hands. An enthusiastic dentist will have great self-confidence and limitless capability (Summers, 1961).

There are no special equipment requirements to provide dental service for children. Good dental service can be rendered with the routine equipment of the dental office. The services for children are the same as those for adults. There are some alterations in procedures, but the equipment and instruments are exactly the same. Children must be examined and radiographed for diagnostic purposes. They receive restorative dentistry, prosthetic dentistry, oral surgery, and preventive dentistry, all of which are common adult dental services. Children may also receive interceptive orthodontic services which are not commonly offered to adults.

Every dentist and every auxiliary person should know that the child's future dental health depends upon the care of the primary teeth.

They should recognize the profound impact it has upon appearance, speech, personality, and happiness. Proper treatment of children also lays the foundation for the future adult patient in the office. For these reasons it is essential to provide a comprehensive service for children. In the final pages of this chapter the various procedures for treatment of children are briefly discussed.

The First Appointment

It is recommended by many in the profession that the child should be examined in the dental office around the age of 3. This is not a steadfast rule since dental caries and other problems may become manifest prior to this time. Parents therefore should bring the child in for a first visit when they are suspicious of a problem or when they see any black or brown area on the teeth which cannot be removed by brushing (Summers, 1961).

At the appointed time for the child the assistant should bring the patient from the reception area and into the operatory. It has been determined in specialty practices of pedodontics that more can be accomplished for the child in the absence of the parent. Therefore the parents are requested to remain in the reception area (Demeritt, 1967). The child will have had limited experience with the office and will have no knowledge of what to expect. In view of this fact the reactions and deportment of the normal child will reflect largely education, training, and discipline in the home. These reactions may give the assistant a keen insight into the parental type at an early time in the patient's treatment.

The examination of a child patient is not limited merely to the teeth and the oral cavity. The dentist will need a minimum of armamentarium for this appointment. The responsibility of the assistant in this appointment is to act chiefly as a recorder for the dentist and indicate the findings on the patient's chart at the appropriate place.

In the examination of the child the hands are examined first for evidence of habits. The facial profile is recorded as it may indicate tooth positions before the inside of the mouth is seen. The relationships of the jaws are noted. The child is checked for mouth breathing. The tongue is then examined to see its size, shape, and condition and whether it is tied down by the lingual frenum. While the mouth is open and the tongue is out, the dentist may also see the tonsils and the condition of the throat. During this time the child should be complimented often for cooperation to further establish rapport. The occlusion is checked by having the patient open and close several times. This may reveal the early development of malocclusions and deviations of the jaws which are recorded.

The final area to be examined should be the teeth and gingiva. The dentist will systematically review the dentition, one tooth at a time, as the assistant continues to record the findings as well as to assist in maintaining a clear field in which to conduct the examination. Upon completion of the examination the records are reviewed, and the parent is brought into the operatory where the findings are related and demonstrated in simple language. At the completion of the explanation of the condition of the child's dental condition the dentist will explain and recommend the necessity for adequate radiographs to ensure good treatment and comprehensive diagnosis. If the parent agrees to this necessary service, the radiographs are taken (Summers, 1961).

Radiographic Service

The radiographic examination of children may often require some deviation of procedure such as variation in size of intraoral film or in the method of film placement to accomplish adequate records. The fundamental principles of roentgenology are always followed, however. The angulation of the cone of the machine and the head positions have been discussed elsewhere in this book.

In recent years new techniques have emerged in radiographic service. Some of these are quite amenable to the radiographic dental service for children. The panographic film which is an extraoral procedure is becoming more extensively used especially with the very young patient where there is considerable difficulty in securing clear intraoral films. Many areas also use lateral jaw film exposures in combination with some intraoral film for the radiographic survey. The lateral jaw procedure with regular periapical film exposures of the anterior segments are recommended by many for the preschool child (Indiana University School of Dentistry, 1960). Exposure of films in children for this series follows the same principles as that for adults.

A radiographic series for the child who can easily tolerate an intraoral film consists of ten periapical films and two bitewings or a panographic film and two bitewing films (University of North Carolina School of Dentistry, 1968). The film size used for children should be what the child can tolerate. Generally, the small size film, type 0, will be used until the eruption of the first permanent molar. Thereafter type II film should be used. In no case should the two types be mixed as this will provide problems in mounting the films later. There are several aids which may be utilized in taking radiographs for children. The edges of the film may be bent to prevent their digging into soft tissue. This effort does not tangibly alter the quality of the films since the bent-edge areas are overlapped by other films in the series. Commercial aids such as film holders and bite blocks are extremely useful. Other aids are the use of hemostats as film holders, holding the edge of the film with the finger, and biting on the finger to position it. In smaller children it is sometimes necessary to have the parent sit in the dental chair with the child in his or her lap and hold the film in position. The assistant should never hold the radiograph for exposure. The dangers of radiation are obvious as the contraindication for this.

In the management of children during the radiographic survey there are certain aids which have proved useful for patient cooperation. The assistant should know these and use them as

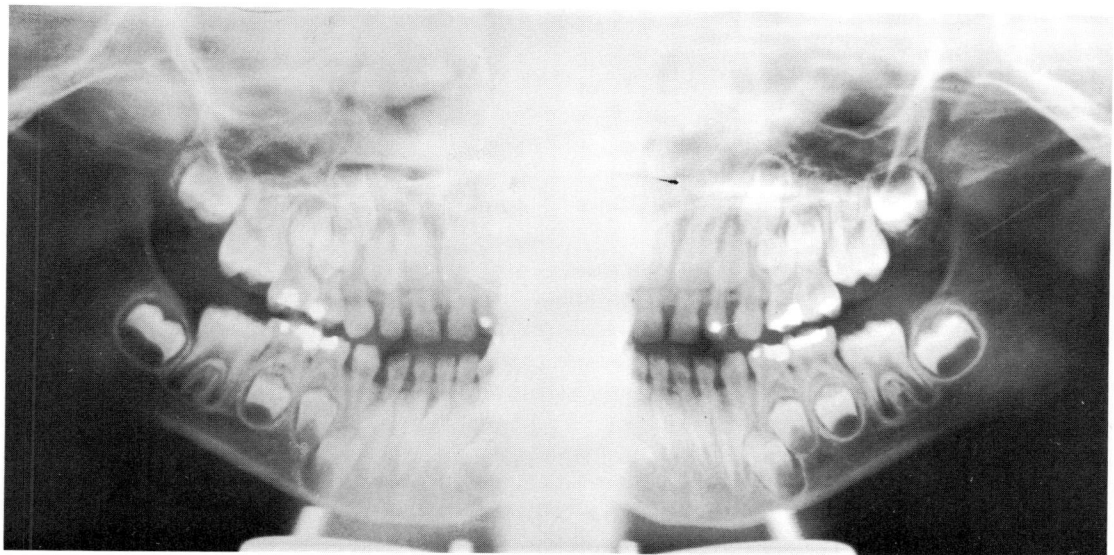

Figure 26-5 | A Panorex radiograph of a 5-year-old child. Notice the developing permanent teeth in the jaws.

they ensure greater quality of films and gain the confidence of the patient, which creates a cooperative attitude.

The child should be addressed by its given name, using positive language. Use language that the child can understand in the explanation of the procedure. Keep up a constant flow of conversation in which praise, flattery, and the interests of the child are used. Exclusion of parents from the area will help produce greater cooperation. When the film is placed in the child's mouth, it should be exposed immediately and removed. This requires that the timing be set prior to placement and the angulation of the cone of the machine established as closely as possible in advance so that only minor adjustment is necessary. Often the child will gag to test the operator and avoid the series of films. This should not be a deterrent. Simply instruct the child to breathe through the nose and insist on continuing. When a true gag reflex is triggered with the film, the use of topical anesthetics in the gag reflex area is useful. If these techniques are unsuccessful, an extraoral series may be indicated. Upon development of the radiographs they are read and interpreted by the dentist. At a later date the patient is reappointed for the consultation appointment. Figure 26-5 illustrates an exposed Panorex film.

Consultation Appointment

The economics of successful dentistry for children and the comprehensive care of children's dental needs are dependent upon the presentation of a treatment plan to the parent. In this appointment, which is the second appointment for the child, all the diagnostic information of the first appointment is utilized in presenting the dental treatment plan to the parents. The doctor will have a detailed outline of the projected treatment with an estimate of the time required for each appointment and the number of appointments necessary to complete the service. A total cost is included. During the presentation it is important for the doctor to have the undivided attention of the parents. Often this is difficult to obtain. One of the chief distractions at this time is the small child who constantly competes for the parent's attention. This situation may be avoided by having the assistant remain in the room to keep the child occupied.

In general there are two areas where consultations are presented. These are in the operatory where the dental service is accomplished or in the doctor's private office. There are advantages and disadvantages to either area. The important factor in this instance is that both the doctor and the parent should be comfortable during the treatment-plan explanation, and all the materials for adequate explanation and demonstration should be at hand. The psychology and rationale of the case presentation appointment have been covered in Chap. 3. The choice of area for case presentation is individual in nature. Therefore each dentist should establish through experimentation which setting is most effective.

The consultation appointment for pedodontics is a wonderful opportunity for individual dental education. Every dentist and dental auxiliary who participates in the appointment should be aware of this fact and utilize it to its full potential. It is essential that the attention of the parent be held. It is wise to begin the conversation by thanking the parent for giving his or her time to hear about the necessary dental treatment and the dental future of the child. The value of complete dental health is emphasized through the practice of dental-health principles. Emphasis is placed upon the fact that complete dental health is an individual commodity which cannot be bought. The dentist can restore a mouth to health, but it cannot be sustained without cooperation from the patient. The dentist will inform parents of times in which they may provide education for correct oral habits. Mothers are the chief instrument for continued oral care. Suggestions are offered by the dentist to take advantage of the desire of the child to please by using these learning times of the child's life to teach fundamental health principles. This is followed by the admonition to set a good example. Correct oral care if reinforced by planned conversation between parents or other adults within the hearing of the child. This indirect learning has a dramatic impact on the child (Summers, 1961). Information is related to the parent on the subject of dentifrices, toothbrushes and brushing technique, fluoride treatment, diet, and the value of the primary teeth and their retention until natural loss. This information which is given to parents at the consultation can often be the most beneficial factor which the parent receives from the office.

When the information period is completed the doctor will review the clinical findings of the child. These are correlated with the radiographic findings to provide a thorough review of the patient's dental status and needs. A definitive treatment plan for correction of problems is discussed and is based upon the needs. It is wise to have available more than one method of treatment to accomplish the desired end. The doctor will make every effort to convey the dental needs in a clear, concise, and simple manner. Major effort is devoted to avoiding confusion and misunderstanding. It is relatively easy to detect confusion, and when this is evident, a review is indicated.

After the presentation of needs and the means of correction has been provided, the necessary appointment time is discussed. This is followed by financial arrangements for the service. Compensation for dental service to children has long been the great deterrent for many dentists. This is caused by the misconception of the public that the primary dentition is a temporary dentition and will be replaced. The difficulty of overcoming the reticence of parents to invest in dental health of the primary teeth because of the temporary teeth misconception is the reason for the failure of many dentists to provide proper care for children. The value of the primary teeth does not need further discussion at this point. It is sufficient to point out that care of these teeth is necessary.

The cost of dental service to children should

be based upon the same rationale as service to adults. The time of the dentist is the only element upon which to base a fair and equitable compensation for service rendered. The cost of operating a dental office remains the same regardless of the patient who receives service in a given amount of time. When the dentist presents the plan for treatment of a child to reasonable parents who care, they will expect to pay for the service received (Brauer et al., 1964). For this reason, a comprehensive consultation appointment in which the needs of the patient are explained is the foundation of good dental service. When treatment is provided without comprehensive planning, explanation, and financial arrangements, the only one who suffers is the dentist.

In many offices today the auxiliaries are given the responsibility of making the financial arrangements and the appointment schedule. This is a good practice, but the personnel must be well trained for this purpose. The demand for dental service in the United States is increasing on a day-to-day escalation basis. In the near future most or even all of the responsibilities of the consultation appointment may fall within the scope of the dental auxiliary. This is currently being done in many sophisticated offices. Here again it should be emphasized that the dentist must delegate responsibilities which do not require a dentist's special talents. The emergence of the multifunctioning auxiliary into more professional aspects of the profession is nowhere better applied than in the consultation appointment.

Operative Dentistry

Operative dentistry for the child is technically identical to that for the adult patient. That is, the basic procedures of cavity preparation, pulp protection, and insertion of restorative materials are the same. The responsibilities of the assistant for these items do not differ from adult procedures. There are certain modifications inherent in the child patient which must be considered. These are the morphology of the primary teeth and the considerations of a growing and changing dentition. Unless allowances are made for these variables in dentistry for children the dentist is doing a distinct disservice to the patient and to the dental profession. Dentistry for children is therefore based upon factors which not only include mechanical findings but developmental, physiologic, and maturational aspects as well (Brauer et al., 1964).

There are a number of areas which must be recognized in effective dental procedures for children. One of the chief items is centered around the preparation for the procedure. It is of the utmost importance to be thoroughly prepared for the appointment prior to seating the patient. The modern concept of teamwork dentistry is brought into play here probably more so than in adult appointments. It is important to provide the highest quality of service in the minimum amount of time in treating children due to their attention span. The longer a child must sit in the patient chair for treatment the less cooperative the child will be toward the end of the procedure. Preplanning by the auxiliary and fingertip access of the complete armamentarium for a particular procedure are essential to successful procedures for children.

In general, restorative dentistry on the child patient in an office which follows the teamwork dentistry concept, wherein the auxiliary is fully utilized, consists of the following. The armamentarium is set up for the procedure before the patient is seated. The assistant will bring the patient to the patient chair. Parents are routinely requested to remain in the reception room. Once the patient is seated, the assistant does not leave the child's side. When the dentist is seated for the operation, the patient will be anesthetized with a local anesthetic. Although most children do not differentiate between pressure and pain in operative procedures for the primary teeth, it is advisable to administer a local anesthetic routinely to avoid the possibility of pain especially for deep carious removal and in Class II preparations. Generally, it is not necessary or advisable to premedicate children except in severe management problems and in the very young child. As part of the maturation process, the normal child should learn that anxiety-producing situations can be dealt with. After administration of the anesthetic the rubber dam should be placed. The obvious advantages of the rubber dam are discussed in Chap. 28. In addition, for the child it serves as an aid in management and excludes the tongue from the operative area. The author has found the rubber dam to be one of the most effective methods of maintaining a clear field in which to operate. A heavy-texture rubber dam is recommended (Brauer et al., 1964). Often the child will also need a mouth prop to aid in holding the mouth open for operative access. The preparation of the tooth follows the principles of using proper coolants and evacuation technique and visual access which are so important in teamwork dentistry for preferred dental operations. Upon completion of the preparation the assistant will flush the cavity and dry it. This is followed by the application of sedative bases and cavity liners of the operator's choice. The matrix is placed for condensation. For the placement of the restorative material in children, the spot-welded matrix has been shown to be a very efficient and effective matrix. Insertion of the restorative material is accomplished by continued cooperation between the dentist and the assistant using a minimum of instrument exchanges. When possible, the assistant should place the restorative material in the tooth at the direction of the dentist. The dentist's responsibility thereafter is proper condensation. When the restorative material has been properly condensed, the excess is removed, and the operator begins to carve and refine the contours to proper proportions as the assistant maintains a clear field to work in and makes available instruments for exchange. When the restoration is complete, the rubber dam is removed. The occlusion may be checked for high spots with articulation paper by the assistant. The patient is then dismissed with an appointment for the next procedure. In several states many, and in some cases all, of these functions may be delegated to the assistant. The trained assistant should know the state law and encourage the dentist to allow the full range of delegable functions to be exercised under the law.

Silver amalgam is the material used for most primary restorations. In recent years composites and resins have been used successfully for a more cosmetic and esthetic result. These materials work well for anterior restorations and fractured permanent incisors. They are often used in conjunction with the acid-etch technique of restoring teeth. There is no indication for composites to be placed in the posterior Class II preparations due to the wear factor which will close spaces in proximal restorations. Figure 26-6 illustrates dental restorations of high quality which have been placed in the primary teeth.

Pulp Therapy

The term pulp therapy applies to the treatments accorded to teeth which have deep carious lesions, vital pulp exposures from caries or trauma, mechanical pulp exposures, and root canal treatment of nonvital teeth. The specific treatment in each instance depends upon the particular involvement of the tooth in question. The procedures may be listed as pulp capping, indirect pulp capping, pulpotomy, and pulpectomy (Grossman, 1962). In dentistry for children wide use of pulp therapy procedures may be employed. In order for an insulted pulp to recover and remain vital there are certain factors which must be considered clinically. These are aseptic technique and clinical management. Histologically, successful pulp therapy is dependent upon vitality and a rich blood supply to the affected tooth. In children the resorptive process which the primary tooth undergoes constantly provides a rich blood supply. Young permanent teeth where the roots are incomplete are another instance of good blood supply to teeth in the child. The efficacy of pulp therapy to keep teeth vital is

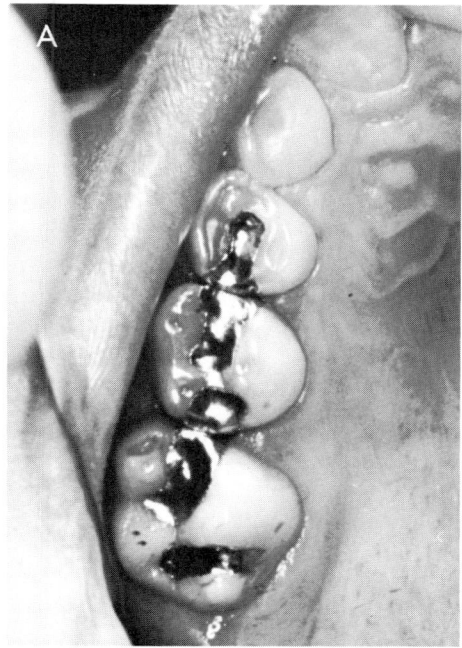

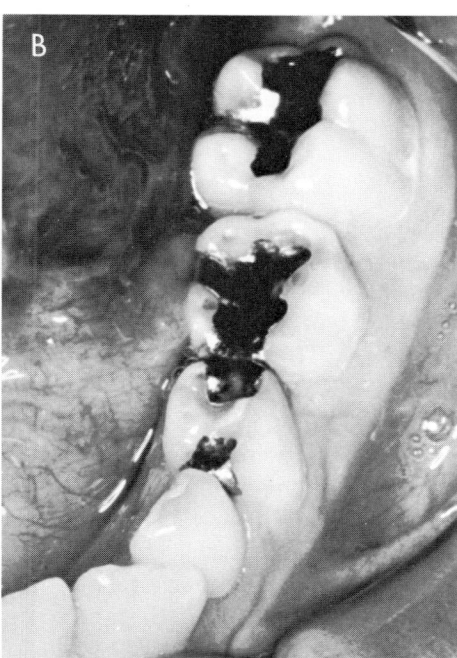

Figure 26-6 | Silver amalgam restorations which have been inserted in primary molar teeth and the first permanent molar teeth. A. Maxillary restorations. B. Mandibular restorations. Photographs were taken 1 year after insertion and polish.

unquestioned since success will ensure keeping the tooth rather than extraction. In some instances as in root canal treatment and certain forms of pulpotomy the pulp is lost, but the tooth remains in the mouth.

Pulp Capping

Pulp capping is the protection of a small exposed healthy pulp by means of an antiseptic or sedative medicament which encourages the pulp to recover and maintains its vitality (Grossman, 1962). The pulp cap procedure is indicated in exposures which occur as a result of excavation of deep carious lesions or in accidental mechanical exposure. Often a child will move causing the rotating bur to accidentally penetrate too deep and expose a pulp horn. The pulp cap procedure consists of overlaying the exposure with a calcium hydroxide product which seals the exposure. This is followed by placing a restoration. The calcium hydroxide seems to cause a reaction in the adjacent pulp tissue which results in sealing of the exposure site by the laying down of a secondary layer of dentin. In all cases the pulp cap is an added procedure to an appointment for restorative dentistry. The function of the assistant when this technique is indicated is to provide the necessary materials, mix them, and make them readily available to the dentist in a minimum amount of time. The assistant should refer to Chap. 12 for further knowledge of dental cements.

Indirect Pulp Capping

The most common type of pulp exposure is that which results in the removal of the last layer of carious dentin in a tooth preparation. In recent years the practice of indirect pulp capping has become widely used. This is a technique in which the last remaining layer of carious dentin is left in the tooth to prevent pulp exposure. This layer is overlaid with a medicament of either zinc oxide and eugenol or calcium hydroxide. The tooth is then sealed with a temporary restoration for a suitable period of time. During the recuperative period the medicament sterilizes the remaining decay and encourages a sclerosing-type reaction of the affected underlying dentin. At a later appointment the temporary restoration and medicament are removed, the dry sandy caries is removed, and the treated area is examined for exposure. If there is no exposure, the tooth is then filled with a permanent restoration. The indirect pulp cap may be done in a routine operative procedure as is done in the pulp cap procedure. It may also be done as a caries control technique when all carious areas in a child are grossly excavated and temporarily filled with zinc oxide–eugenol to remove the active caries process (Starkey, 1968). The responsibilities of the assistant in this procedure are preparing the materials and assisting in the insertion. In many states the assistant may insert the temporary filling material.

Pulpotomy

Occasionally a tooth will be vitally exposed with an exposure site too large to use the pulp cap procedure. This most often occurs in deep caries excavation but may occur in fractured teeth as a result of trauma. In these instances it is necessary to remove the coronal portion of the pulp under aseptic conditions and place the medicament in direct contact with the remaining pulpal tissue. If the tooth is to remain vital, a calcium hydroxide preparation is placed against the remaining pulp tissue and supporting base cements are used to seal the area from oral fluids. After a suitable waiting period of 6 to 8 weeks a dentin bridge will be evident directly under the calcium hydroxide medicament. When the dentin bridge can be identified a permanent restoration may be placed on the involved tooth. Vital pulpotomies are limited to the permanent teeth.

In recent years the use of formocresol as the medicament for pulpotomies has become widespread. Formocresol does not react on pulp tissue to create a secondary dentin bridge as in the case of calcium hydroxide. It fixes the remaining pulp tissue with ultimate fibrosis of the pulp tissue. The result is that the tooth remains in the arch with a fixed pulp. The technique for this procedure is identical to the calcium hydroxide technique. Only the choice of medicament differs. The assistant must be familiar with these two methods of pulpotomy in order to function properly with the dentist upon the occasion of their use. Formocresol pulpotomy currently is limited to large cariously exposed primary teeth. There is no precedent for its use in permanent teeth at this time (Starkey, 1968). Pulpectomy is not widely practiced in primary teeth due to the tortuous root canal configuration which makes hermetic seal of the canals impossible (Shiere, Frankel, and Fogel, 1961). However, many dentists today perform root canal therapy on primary teeth. The only difference between root canal work for primary teeth and for permanent teeth is that the primary root canal filling material must be resorbable so that as the primary tooth root resorbs, the material in the canal will do likewise. Therapy for permanent teeth is covered in Chap. 24. of this book.

Prosthetics for Children

In the growing child the premature loss of primary teeth can be ultimately catastrophic in that it can create orthodontic problems, speech problems, masticatory inefficiency, cosmetic detriments, and in some cases psychologic disturbances (Lindahl, 1961). In view of these factors primary teeth which have been prematurely lost must be replaced with prostheses to eliminate or at least minimize these problems before they arise. Prosthetic service for children may be of the fixed crown and bridge type or the removable type. The indications for each of these depend upon the dental age of the child and the estimated length of time expected for the child to keep the appliance. It is better to use fixed prostheses where possible since after cementation they are not removed and essentially become a functional part of the dentition. Unfortunately all prematurely lost primary teeth are not indications for fixed prostheses. For instance in children where teeth are lost which will have a permanent replacement within 2 years it is economically unfeasible to place a fixed bridge. For these patients a removable partial denture, or a nonfunctional space maintainer, is the treatment of choice. Conversely in children who are quite young, between the ages of 18 months and 4 years, a fixed bridge is the only logical choice as the child will need to keep it for several years. In addition young children who cannot understand reasons for a prosthesis will not tolerate a removable appliance. In the preschool child the fixed bridge to replace prematurely lost teeth is the treatment of choice (Brauer et al., 1964). Often there is an economic factor and patients elect the removable partial denture.

Regardless of the type of appliance which is ultimately placed in a child's mouth, it must be designed and constructed so that adjustments for growth are included in the product. In the case of fixed bridges which extend across the midline of the face a pin and sleeve must be built into the bridge to allow for unimpeded growth in the midpalatine suture. Figure 26-7 is an illustration of a bridge for a child in which a growth factor pin and sleeve have been incorporated in the appliance. It is not necessary to include an expansion factor in fixed appliances which do not cross the midline. Figures 26-8 and 26-9 are examples of unilateral fixed bridgework for children. Fixed prostheses in children are most commonly referred to as functional space maintainers. This is due to the fact that they maintain space for the developing permanent successor in the edentulous area as well as provide function for chewing (Brauer et al., 1964).

Removable prostheses are also space maintainers which provide function as well. A removable partial denture may be in combination with a preventive orthodontic appliance for minor tooth movement. Removable prostheses are for

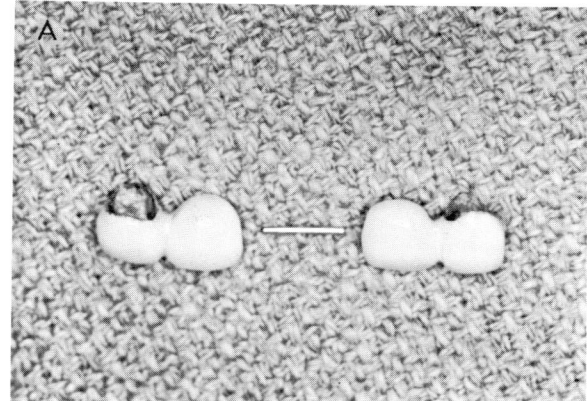
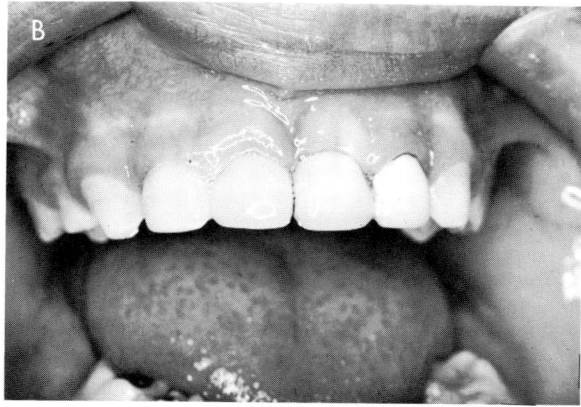

Figure 26-7 | A porcelain-fused-to-metal anterior bridge in the primary dentition. A. The bridge segments before cementation; notice the pin addition for the midline which provides for uninhibited natural growth of the maxillary segments. B. The bridge after cementation. (*Courtesy of the University of North Carolina at Chapel Hill, School of Dentistry, Department of Pedodontics, Chapel Hill.*)

esthetic and speech purposes or space-maintaining purposes. There are various designs for these appliances. In the lower arch the best design seems to be the cast partial denture framework with processed acrylic (Fig. 26-10). The cast partial in the lower arch must make allowances in the anterior lingual area for the eruption of the permanent anterior teeth. This is accomplished through relief areas in the waxup

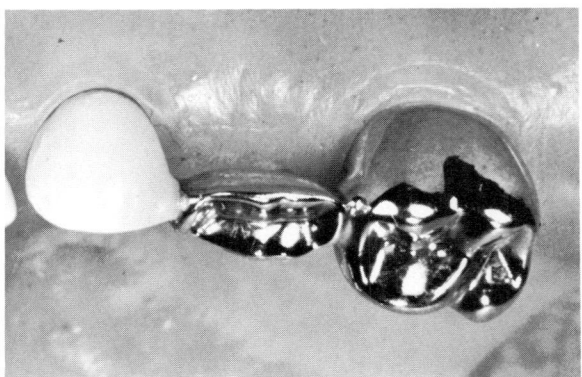

Figure 26-8 | A maxillary cast gold fixed space maintainer with processed resin facing on the anterior retainer. This appliance maintains space created by the premature loss of the first primary molar.

of the framework which will allow a space between the lingual tissue and the tissue surface of the appliance (Fig. 26-11). In many instances an all-acrylic appliance is fabricated without the lingual bar (Fig. 26-12). These appliances are easily broken but will function well for the specific purpose. They are also easy to adjust. As the

Figure 26-9 | A mandibular distal shoe space maintainer. The appliance protects space created by premature loss of the second primary molar. In addition it preserves the integrity of the position of the first permanent molar.

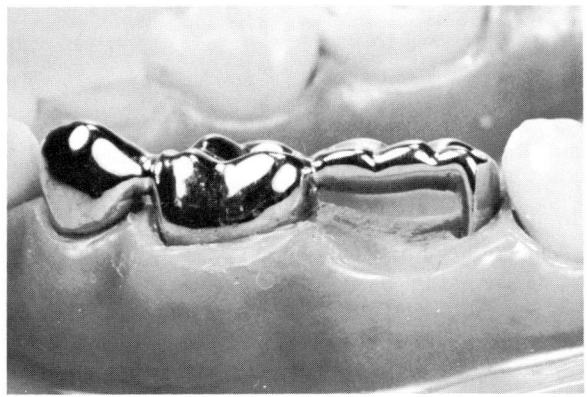

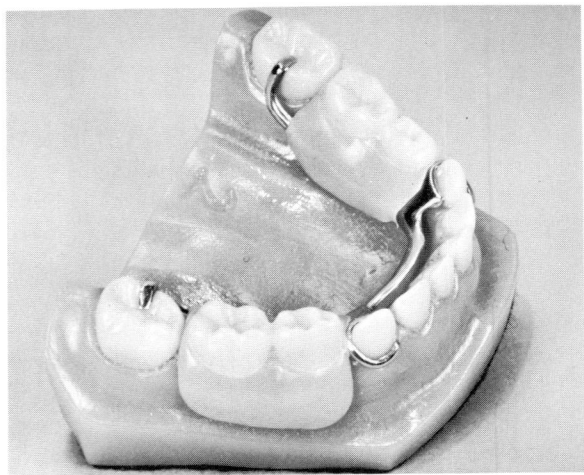

Figure 26-10 | A mandibular cast framework partial denture suitable for the primary and mixed dentition.

permanent teeth erupt it merely requires the removal of enough of the partial denture to allow unimpeded eruption. It is not necessary to include expansion devices in partial dentures as they are removable and do not tie the teeth down. It is, however, recommended that the

Figure 26-11 | The lingual bar area of a cast framework partial denture. Notice the significant relief area which provides space for uninhibited eruption of the permanent central and lateral incisors.

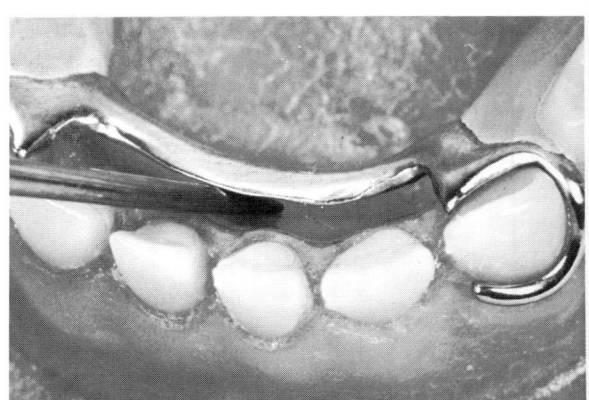

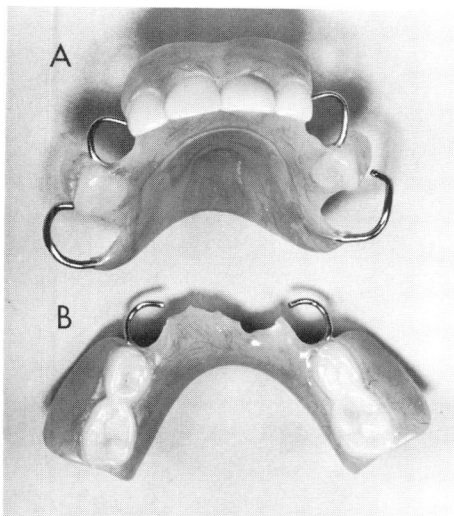

Figure 26-12 | Illustrations of all-acrylic partial dentures for children. A. Maxillary partial denture. B. Mandibular partial denture. Retention clasps are fabricated from chrome-cobalt wire.

clasp arms on the facial aspect of the cuspids be removed in partials where clasps are used to gain retention on the cuspids (Lindahl, 1961).

In posterior teeth which are compromised by decay to the extent that a crown is necessary for restoration there are two choices available. These are the cast gold crown and the chrome steel crown. The cast gold crown is unequivocally the best because of its tissue tolerance and accuracy in adaptation. However, there are occasions where it is not economically feasible to use cast gold in the primary dentition such as an early exfoliation time of the tooth in question. Every patient may not be able to afford the cast gold crown, which is of necessity more expensive. The emergence of the chrome steel crown for pedodontic service has been a valuable contribution in recent years (Starkey, 1968). Appointments for the fabrication of a chrome steel crown have the same armamentarium and assisting requirements as cast crown or bridge preparation appointments. Figure 26-13 is an

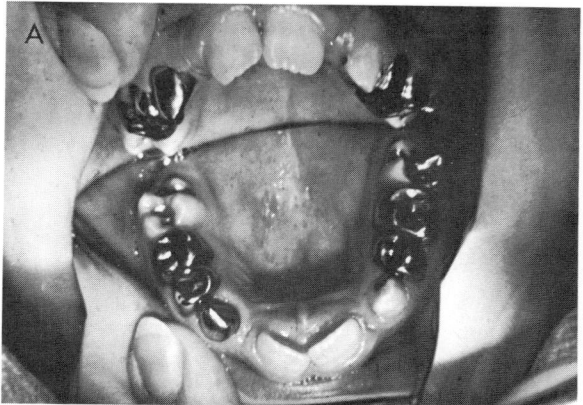

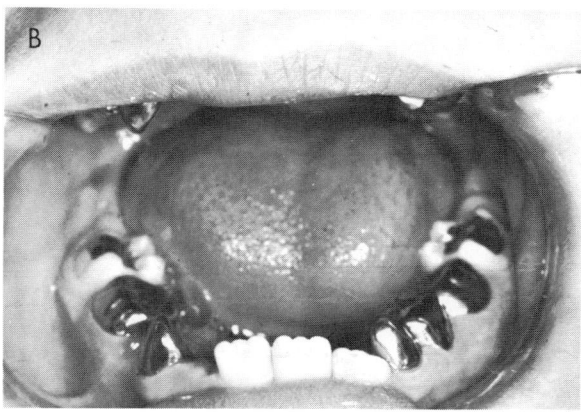

Figure 26-13 | Chrome steel crowns used in rehabilitation of a young patient with rampant decay. A. Maxillary arch. B. Mandibular arch. (*Courtesy of Dr. George Lyman.*)

example of chrome steel crowns which have been placed in a young child.

Fractured Young Permanent Teeth

When a traumatic accident causes the loss of a portion of a young permanent tooth the remaining tooth structure must be protected in order that it may recover from the insult. In appointments for treatment of fractured permanent teeth a definite sequence of events must be fol-

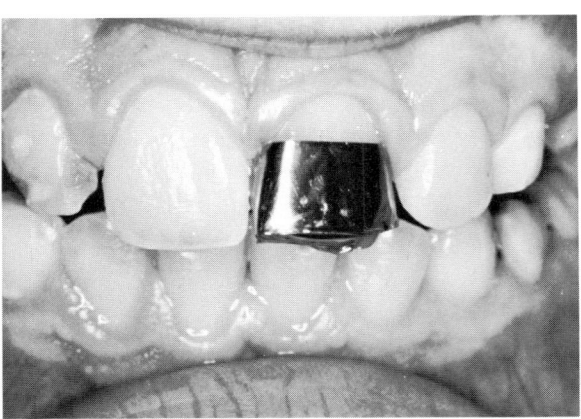

Figure 26-14 | A protective temporary coverage for a fractured permanent incisor. Orthodontic band material is used for the protective crown which is cemented with sedative cement.

lowed. The doctor will determine the extent of the damage to the tooth through means of manipulation, clinical examination, and radiographs of the affected area and that of the teeth with which the injured tooth occludes. The dentist will determine whether the fractured crown has a pulpal exposure and if the root has been fractured. When there is a significant amount of mobility, the tooth will be stabilized to ensure reattachment in its correct position. If the tooth does not have a vital exposure of the pulp, a sedative cement is placed upon the exposed dentin to allow the tooth to recover. This essentially is identical to the procedure for indirect pulp capping. If an exposure exists, the current thought is to effect a calcium hydroxide pulpotomy to secure a secondary dentin bridge. Direct pulp caps for exposed fractured teeth are not indicated since the oral fluids have already contaminated the pulp and the prognosis of a dentin bridge is poor. If the contact areas of a fractured tooth are lost as a result of the fracture, it is of the utmost importance to restore contact with a temporary splint. This may be in the form of orthodontic band material, self-curing resin temporaries, or chrome steel crowns (Marks, 1968). Figure 26-14 shows a protective cover for a fractured incisor. The assistant should be familiar with all the above-named procedures for treating fractured incisors since they are only adaptations of procedures already discussed. Restoration of fractured teeth after recovery from traumatic injury follows the crown and bridge preparation for abutments and cementation. In recent years the acid-etch technique for restoring fractured incisors of less destructive nature has emerged. This is a simple restorative procedure which involves a minimum removal of tooth structure followed by treatment of the freshly prepared enamel with phosphoric acid or citric acid for 1 to 2 minutes. The preparation is then thoroughly flushed with water and dried. A frosted appearance of the enamel treated with the acid is indicative of the etching which provides microscopic retention areas for the restorative material. Sockwell (1976) indicates that most composites and resins will adhere to the small retentive area to provide a permanent restoration in these small fracture problems.

Figure 26-15 | An acid-etch stabilizing splint for protecting subluxated teeth. It is also used for stabilizing luxated teeth which have been reimplanted. (*Courtesy of Dr. Joe Camp.*)

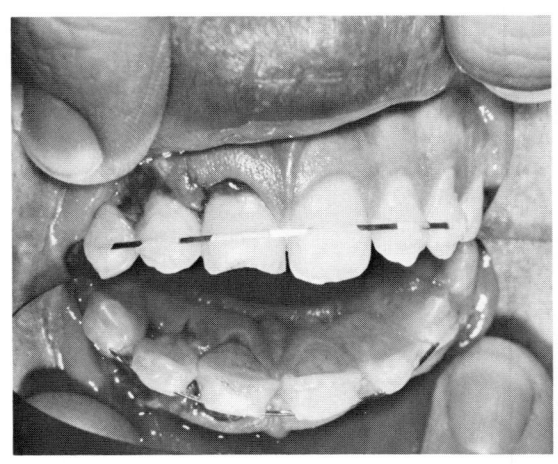

The acid-etch technique may also be used to stabilize subluxated teeth by etching several teeth adjacent to the subluxated teeth and flowing acrylic resin onto the areas which may be united with an orthodontic wire. Figure 26-15 illustrates this method of splinting teeth for stabilization.

Occlusal Sealants

Dental decay in molar pits and fissures produces much of the operative work that is required in children's teeth. While fluoride is known to be effective in reducing decay on smooth surfaces and in the interproximal surfaces of teeth, its effect of reducing incidence of decay is not as great in the occlusal pits and fissures of primary and permanent teeth. The inability of the usual prevention measures to dramatically reduce the incidence of decay on these surfaces is recognized by the dental profession to be a major factor in new caries incidence in children (Merrill, 1973). Recently, after many years of research and experimental work, new substances called sealants have been introduced for dental use in filling pits and fissures without cutting tooth structure. Sealants are materials which adhere to the enamel surface and prevent fluid and food debris exchange in the area underlying and the oral environment.

In the 1950s the acid-etch technique was introduced as a method of increasing the adhesion of acrylic resins (Buonocore, 1955). The etching technique removes the outer inert layer of enamel and exposes the underlying fresh enamel surface. The new surface has a greatly increased area due to the creation of microscopic fissures and grooves in the enamel. These areas provide mechanical locks for the resin sealants to flow into for greater retention (Sockwell, 1976). The promising results of research efforts in developing an occlusal sealant that was effective led to the commercial development of pit and fissure sealants which were advertised as the replacement preventive measure for the prophylactic odontotomy. Many general practitioners and pedodontists now use this technique as a preventive measure in the care of children's teeth.

The clinical procedure for occlusal sealant application consists of a series of treatment steps. The teeth are identified for the treatment. The teeth are thoroughly cleaned, rinsed, and dried. Cotton rolls are applied either with a cotton roll holder or individually as the dentist chooses. The teeth are then thoroughly dried, and an application of phosphoric or citric acid follows to remove the inert enamel layers and provide a greater retentive surface through etching. After a suitable waiting period which is precisely timed, the treated teeth are rinsed with a flow of water. The oral evacuator then removes all etchant, water, and saliva from the teeth. Dry cotton rolls are again placed, and the conditioned occlusal surfaces are dried with the air syringe. The sealant which has been prepared to the manufacturer's direction is applied to the teeth. This is usually done with a fine camel's hair brush. The sealant is allowed to polymerize in a dry field according to the manufacturer's instruction. This is an especially responsible duty for the assistant. Some of the sealants are autopolymerizing, and some require the exposure of ultraviolet light to polymerize. After the sealant is hardened and set, any excess is removed, and the occlusion is checked with articulating paper. If high spots are evident from the articulating paper, the dentist will reduce these with a finishing bur. The resultant shield of sealant over the pits and fissures provides a preventive service to the patient without the cutting of the tooth structure. This preventive tool has proved to be effective for up to 2 years with current materials. Future research may provide a permanent sealant for occlusal pits and fissures of molar teeth in children. (Merrill, 1976). The dental assistant functions in this appointment by maintaining a clear, dry field for the dentist and providing another pair of hands in the procedure to further facilitate in saving time and the correct execution of the service.

BIBLIOGRAPHY

American Dental Association: "Dental Health Program for Children," *J. Am. Dent. Assoc.,* **74:** 330–338, 1967.

Brauer, J. C., et al.: *Dentistry for Children,* 5th ed., McGraw-Hill Book Company, New York, 1964, pp. 69–103.

Brown, W. E., et al.: *Oral Health, Dentistry, and the American Public,* University of Oklahoma Press, Norman, Okla., 1974, pp. 287–322.

Buonocore, M. G.: "A Simple Method of Increasing Adhesion of Acrylic Filling Material to Enamel Surfaces, *J. Dent. Res.,* **34:**849–853, 1955.

Burket, L. W.: *Oral Medicine,* 3d ed., J. B. Lippincott Company, Philadelphia, 1957, pp. 417–419.

Callahan, J. D.: "Emotional Problems of Childhood," paper read before the American Academy of Pedodontics, St. Louis, 1964.

Demeritt, W. W.: Personal communication, 1967.

Diefenbach, V. L.: *Summary of Recent Legislation Affecting Dentistry,* U.S. Government Printing Office, 1967, pp. 620–654.

Galagan, D. J., et al.: "Dental Health and the Need for Prevention," *Symposium on Applied Preventive Dentistry,* Washington, 1964, pp. 1–7.

Grossman, L. I.: *Endodontic Practice,* Lea & Febiger, Philadelphia, 1962, pp. 94–129.

Hogeboom, F. E.: "The Past, Present and Future of the A.S.P.D.C.," *Rev. Dent. Child.,* **6:**3, 1939.

Hurme, V. O.: "Ranges of Normalcy in the Eruption of Permanent Teeth," *J. Dent. Child.,* **16:**11, 1949.

Ilg, F. L., and Ames, L. B.,: *The Gessell Institute's Child Behavior,* Harper & Row, Publishers, Incorporated, New York, 1955, pp. 40–44.

Indiana University School of Dentistry: *Radiographic Survey for the Pre-School Child,* 1960.

Klebe, E.: "National Health Insurance," brief no. IB73015, Library of Congress, May, 1976.

Lindahl, R. L.: *Dental Clinics of North America,* W. B. Saunders Company, Philadelphia, 1961, pp. 649–661.

McBride, W. C.: *Juvenile Dentistry,* Lea & Febiger, Philadelphia, 1937.

McCaslin, A. J.: "Implications of Federal Legislation on the Practice of Dentistry for Children," unpublished paper, University of North Carolina School of Dentistry, Chapel Hill, 1968.

Marks, S. C.: Personal communication, October 1968.

──────: Development of Occlusion," lecture series given at University of North Carolina School of Dentistry to graduate pedodontic students, Chapel Hill, 1966.

Meredith, H. V.: "Order and Age of Eruption for the Deciduous Dentition," *J. Dent. Res.,* **25:**43–66, 1946.

Merrill, S. A.: "Methods of Evaluating Pit and Fissure Sealants," master's thesis, Department of Pedodontics, University of North Carolina School of Dentistry, Chapel Hill, 1973.

Moyer, R. E.: Personal communication, 1976.

──────: *Handbook of Orthodontics,* 2d ed., Year Book Medical Publishers, Inc., Chicago, 1963, pp. 51–120.

Rose, T. A.: "Health Care Reports 1975," Blue Cross and Blue Shield of North Carolina, 1975.

Salzmann, J. A.: *Orthodontics—Principles and Prevention,* J. B. Lippincott Company, Philadelphia, 1957, pp. 169–245.

Schour, I., and Massler, M.: "Studies in Tooth Development: The Growth Pattern of the Human Teeth," *J. Am. Dent. Assoc.,* **27:** 1778–1793, 1940.

Shiere, F. R., Frankel, S. N., and Fogel, H. R.: "Pulp Therapy for Primary and Immature Permanent Teeth," in *Dental Clinics of North America,* W. B. Saunders Company, Philadelphia, 1961, pp. 639–648.

Sockwell, C. L.: Personal communication, 1976.

Spock, B.: *Common Sense Book of Baby and Child Care,* Duell, Sloan & Pierce, Inc., New York, 1957, pp. 238–245.

Starkey, P.: "Dentistry for Children," paper read before the North Carolina Society of Dentistry for Children, November, 1968.

Summers, F. W.: "Dentistry for Children," paper read before the Kansas Society of Dentistry for Children, Kansas City, Mo., May 1961.

University of North Carolina School of Dentistry: "Clinical Procedure for Undergraduate Students in Pedodontics," Chapel Hill, 1968.

27
Robert M. Nelson
Orthodontics

INTRODUCTION

Every general practitioner is involved to varying degrees in either orthodontic prevention or minor orthodontic procedures, and it is the purpose of this chapter to serve as a reference and to provide a basic knowledge of terminology and orthodontic objectives. The word orthodontics is derived from the Greek prefix *orthos,* meaning straight, and *odont,* a Greek word for tooth. Orthodontics may be defined as that branch of dental science and arts which deals with the recognition, prevention, and treatment of conditions involving irregularities of the teeth, jaws, and face and their influence on the physical and mental health of the individual. The following is a list of the most important goals that orthodontics strives to achieve:

1. To maintain or establish (insofar as is possible) a normal functioning occlusion of the dentition
2. To improve, if possible and necessary, the facial esthetics of a patient to the extent that it is influenced by the dentition and supporting skeleton
3. To eliminate etiologic factors that may disrupt the normal growth and development of the dentofacial complex
4. To diagnose and correct conditions that fall within the field of preventive orthodontics
5. To serve with oral and plastic surgeons as part of a team in the rehabilitation of severe oral and facial anomalies (deformities)

It is evident from this list that the field of orthodontics includes a broad spectrum of dental and facial problems. To understand many of these problems a basic knowledge of growth and development is essential. Orthodontics by its very nature must take into account not only the immediate dental condition, but the individual's dentofacial complex through the entire period of growth and development and maturation. While it is quite true that a great number of orthodontic problems are of local origin, some are influenced by systemic conditions in which overall growth, nutrition, and health play a major role. A vivid example of a systemic condition that hampers orthodontic treatment occurs in patients taking the drug Dilantin for epilepsy. In these patients the gingival tissues undergo an abnormal increase in growth (hyperplasia). This condition may create a space between the teeth and thereby prevent them from moving together. The orthodontist finds it difficult to close such spaces. Thus, general health is an important factor in the successful treatment of an orthodontic case. Likewise, good oral and dental health are necessary prerequisites.

ETIOLOGY

Etiology as it pertains to orthodontics is the science of finding the cause of the dentofacial deformity. It is most important to know the etiology of the orthodontic problem, since if the cause is still exerting its influence at the completion of mechanical treatment, it is quite likely that there will be a relapse toward the original deformity.

The etiology of dentofacial deformities falls into three general categories involving (1) genetic origin, (2) systemic influences, and (3) local oral influences. Each of these causes will be discussed briefly.

Genetic Origin

Since the teeth and jaws are of different genetic origin, the following abnormal conditions are possible:

1. Small jaws and larger-than-normal teeth
2. Large jaws and smaller-than-normal teeth
3. Normal-sized jaws and teeth either too small or too large
4. Normal-sized jaws and teeth in the maxillae either larger or smaller than the teeth in the mandible
5. Abnormal anterior-posterior relationship of dental arches in respect to their bony bases (maxillae and mandible)
6. Abnormal relationship of the maxillae and mandible to each other
7. Abnormal relationship of the maxillae and mandible in reference to cranial base
8. Any combination of the above

Facial and palatal clefts are two additional abnormalities which can be of genetic origin. The severity of the cleft determines the extent of the associated dental malocclusion.

Supernumerary teeth may be found in any area of the dental arch and are of genetic origin. If they form early during the primary dentition, they may force the permanent teeth to erupt into unnatural positions. Supernumerary teeth may develop after the permanent dentition has erupted, and their growth sometimes jumbles the dental arch.

Congenitally missing teeth are also of genetic origin and may be responsible for some orthodontic problems. Missing teeth may create spaces, permitting the drifting of teeth adjacent to the space. This may result in collapse of the dental arch (Fig. 27-1).

Any significant alteration—morphology of jaws and teeth, position of jaws and teeth, timing and direction of eruption and exfoliation of teeth—can result in an orthodontic problem.

A large tongue may also present an orthodontic problem, since excessive pressure may be directed to the teeth and thereby force them off their bone support. The reverse may also be true; a small tongue generally allows the dental arch to collapse lingually. The muscles in the cheeks and lips also influence the position of the teeth. Consequently, the teeth are in some balance with the forces exerted by the tongue

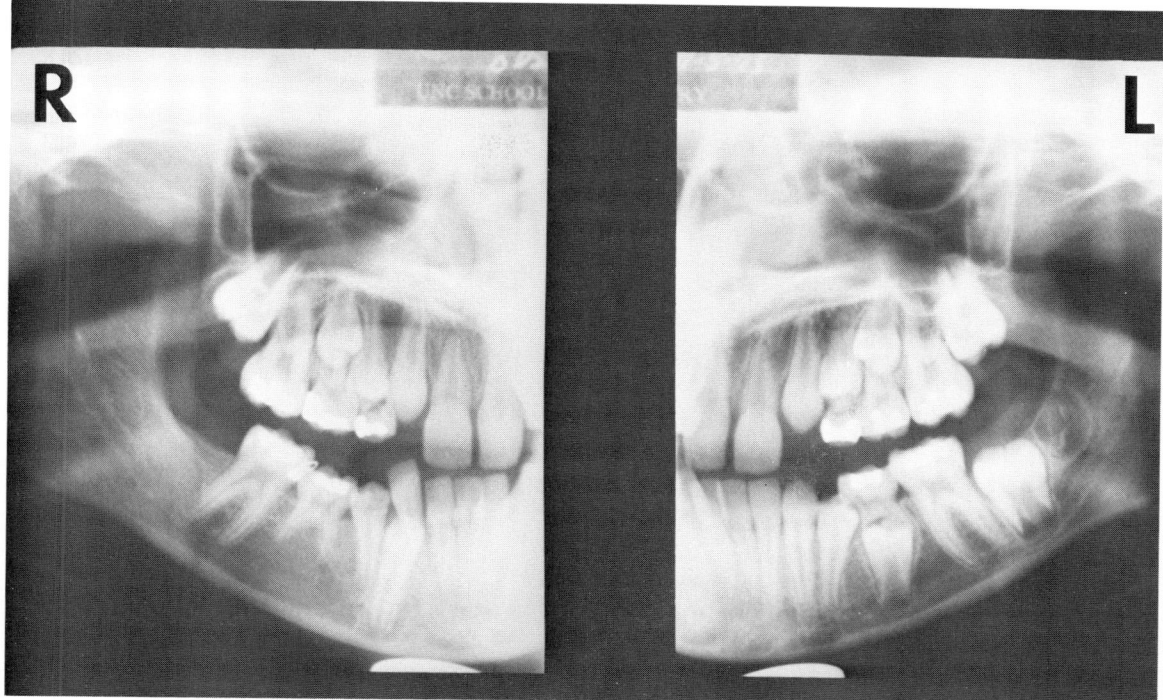

Figure 27-1 | Panorex of 12-year-old girl showing the following conditions: Upper right third permanent molar missing, upper right and left permanent laterals missing, upper left third permanent molar missing, abnormal development of lower left third molar, blocked lower left first bicuspid, impacted lower right cuspid, missing lower right second bicuspid, missing lower right second and third permanent molars.

internally and by the cheek and lip muscles externally.

In addition to the size of the tongue affecting the occlusion, any aberration in its attachments may also be detrimental to the dental arches. The most obvious aberration is a short lingual frenum (tongue-tie), which may lead to a detrimental tongue postural habit during speech and swallowing.

The lips and their development are also factors in dental-arch function. For example, if the upper lip is too short, it may not support the dental arch anteriorly, and forward tipping and drift of the anterior teeth may occur.

Clefts of the lip and/or palate are almost always associated with extensive orthodontic problems.

Systemic Influences

Infectious diseases, nutritional deficiencies, and endocrine disturbances may influence the health of the dentofacial complex and directly or indirectly alter the development, eruption, or caries index of the dentition. Any of the factors cited may lead to the loss of one or more teeth or affect the occlusal pattern and, accordingly, present an orthodontic problem requiring correction.

Local Oral Influences

Orthodontic problems of a local origin are mainly due to the following factors:

1. Early or delayed loss of deciduous teeth
2. Early or delayed eruption of permanent teeth
3. Loss of permanent teeth as a result of caries or periodontal disease
4. Infections of periodontal tissues
5. Local cysts and growths
6. Injuries
7. Habits
8. Enlarged tonsils leading to poor tongue habits
9. Bruxism and traumatic occlusion
10. Congenitally missing teeth (although genetic in origin)
11. Presence of supernumerary teeth (although genetic in origin)

Early loss of deciduous teeth usually results in the drift of teeth adjacent to the missing dental unit, leading to less space for the permanent teeth with a possibility of jumbling.

Delayed loss of deciduous teeth may result in a deflection of the permanent tooth during eruption. The same condition may result from an early eruption of a permanent tooth.

Loss of permanent teeth allows adjacent teeth to drift into abnormal positions.

Infections in the gingiva and alveolar bone may lead to the loss of a tooth or teeth, and without proper prosthesis or space maintenance, drift of the adjacent teeth may take place.

Local cysts or growths of the soft or hard tissue may create pressure on the teeth and move them; this may necessitate the removal of one or more teeth.

Injuries, either superficial or in the nature of fractures of the bones, may likewise result in loss of teeth and subsequent drift of adjacent ones.

Habits are of particular importance to the orthodontist in that they present the greatest chance of failure in treatment. There is little that the orthodontist or general practitioner can do about habits directly, since their elimination is almost entirely dependent on the active cooperation of the parent and patient. This is discussed further on in this chapter under "Preventive Orthodontics."

Enlarged tonsils may force the tongue to assume a more forward position and thereby initiate an unnatural force on the anterior teeth during swallowing and speech.

Bruxism (grinding of teeth) and traumatic occlusion, besides being abrasive to the teeth, may lower the level of bone support, with subsequent loss of teeth; or it may cause jumbling or intrusion of posterior teeth, resulting in closure of the bite.

Congenitally missing teeth and supernumerary teeth were discussed above, under "Genetic Origin."

DIAGNOSIS

Diagnosis in orthodontics is the art of determining what is wrong with any patient and describing how the patient varies from the ideal, dentofacially. It involves an orderly listing of the symptoms or conditions, in a system called a classification, which makes it easy to describe or evaluate for the record the particular condition or problem. The classification also is an aid in making a differential diagnosis, i.e., differentiation between two diseases or conditions that have similar symptoms or patterns but may require a different treatment. A correct diagnosis is the first step necessary in the successful treatment of any case.

Occlusion and Malocclusion

These are terms designating the relationship of teeth to each other. Occlusion is the contact relationship of the teeth of the mandibular arch with

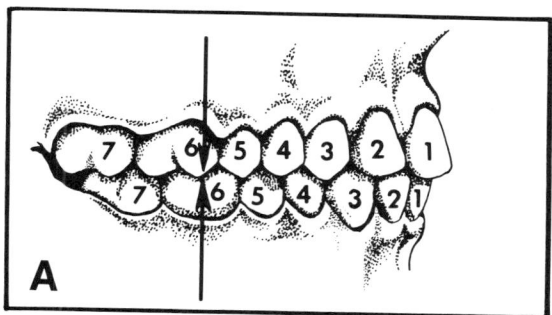
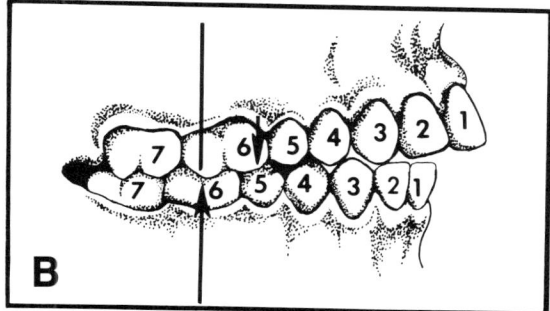
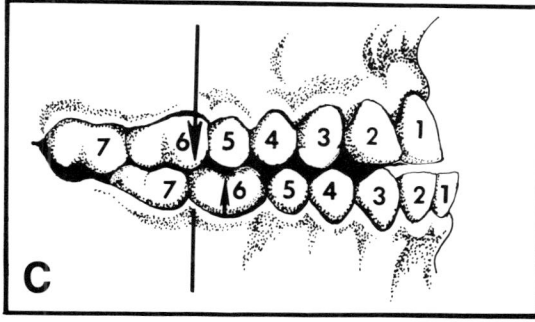

Figure 27-2 | A. Normal molar relationship (Angle Class I). B. Distal molar relationship (Angle Class II). C. Mesial molar relationship (Angle Class III).

those in the maxillary arch. Malocclusion is any deviation from normal occlusion.

Normal or ideal occlusion is the occlusion intended by nature (Figs. 27-2A and 27-3A). In normal occlusion all the teeth of the maxillary arch are in maximum contact with all the teeth of the mandibular arch. The upper anteriors should overlap the incisal edge of the lowers by approximately 2 mm, and they should be in front of the lower anteriors and in passive contact with them. The upper posteriors should interdigitate with the lowers and should be one cusp buccal to them. The lower first permanent molar is one cusp mesial to the upper first permanent molar. The upper first permanent molar has its mesial buccal cusp articulating in the buccal groove of the lower first permanent molar.

Centric occlusion and relation should be the same and is realized when the teeth are in maximal contact and the heads of the condyles are in the most retruded unstrained position in the glenoid fossae.

Classification of Malocclusion

The following classification of malocclusion was formulated by Dr. Angle, and it is generally accepted: Angle Class I presents a molar relation where the mesiobuccal cusp of the maxillary first permanent molar articulates in the buccal groove of the mandibular first permanent molar, as in Fig. 27-2A, however, some teeth are either jumbled, spaced, tipped, blocked out, or rotated. In such cases the maxillae and mandible are in correct relationship with each other and with cranial base, i.e., they are in a straight-line profile of the face (Figs. 27-3B and 27-4E).

Distocclusion (Angle Class II) presents a condition in which the mesiobuccal cusp of the upper first permanent molar articulates between the lower second bicuspid and the mesiobuccal cusp of the lower first molar, and the chin appears weak (retrognathic) (Figs. 27-2B, 27-3C, 27-5E, and 27-6E).

Mesiocclusion (Angle Class III) presents a condition in which the mesiobuccal cusp of the upper first permanent molar articulates between the distobuccal cusp of the lower first molar and the mesiobuccal cusp of the lower second molar. The chin is usually prominent, giving a "jutt-jawed" appearance (prognathic) (Figs. 27-2C and 27-7E).

The teeth in any of the latter classifications can be spaced, jumbled, rotated, or missing, thereby

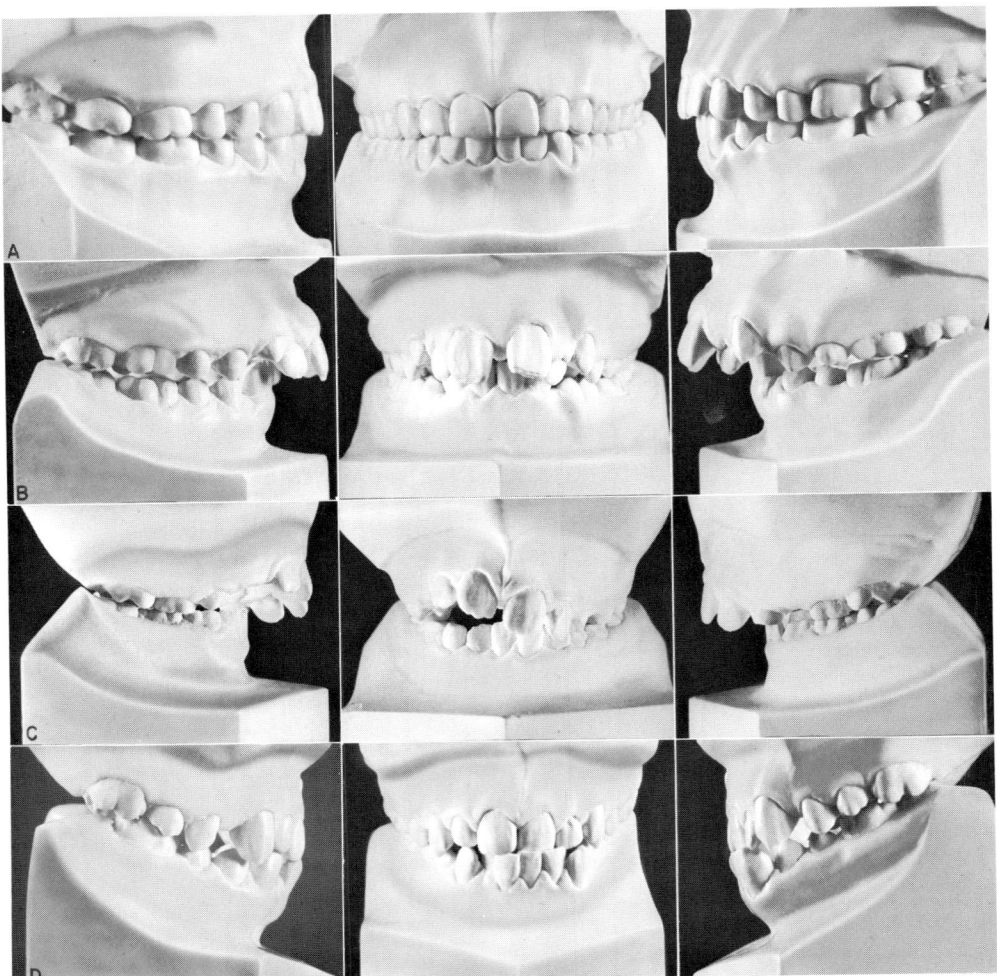

Figure 27-3 | A. Normal occlusion. B. Angle Class I malocclusion, with mesial drift of all posterior teeth blocking out lower cuspids with extreme protrusion of upper anteriors, presenting as well a deep overbite. C. Angle Class II malocclusion, with an extreme open bite on upper right side due to thumb sucking. D. Angle Class III malocclusion with anteriors on the left side being more typical of this type of occlusion.

complicating the condition. In addition to these classifications, a few conditions warrant further comment. In crossbites, the anteriors, or the posteriors, or both may be involved. The upper anteriors may be lingual to the lowers, or the upper posteriors may be lingual to the lowers (Fig. 27-8).

Open bites can involve both the anteriors and the posteriors. In the anterior region an open bite presents a vertical space between the maxillary

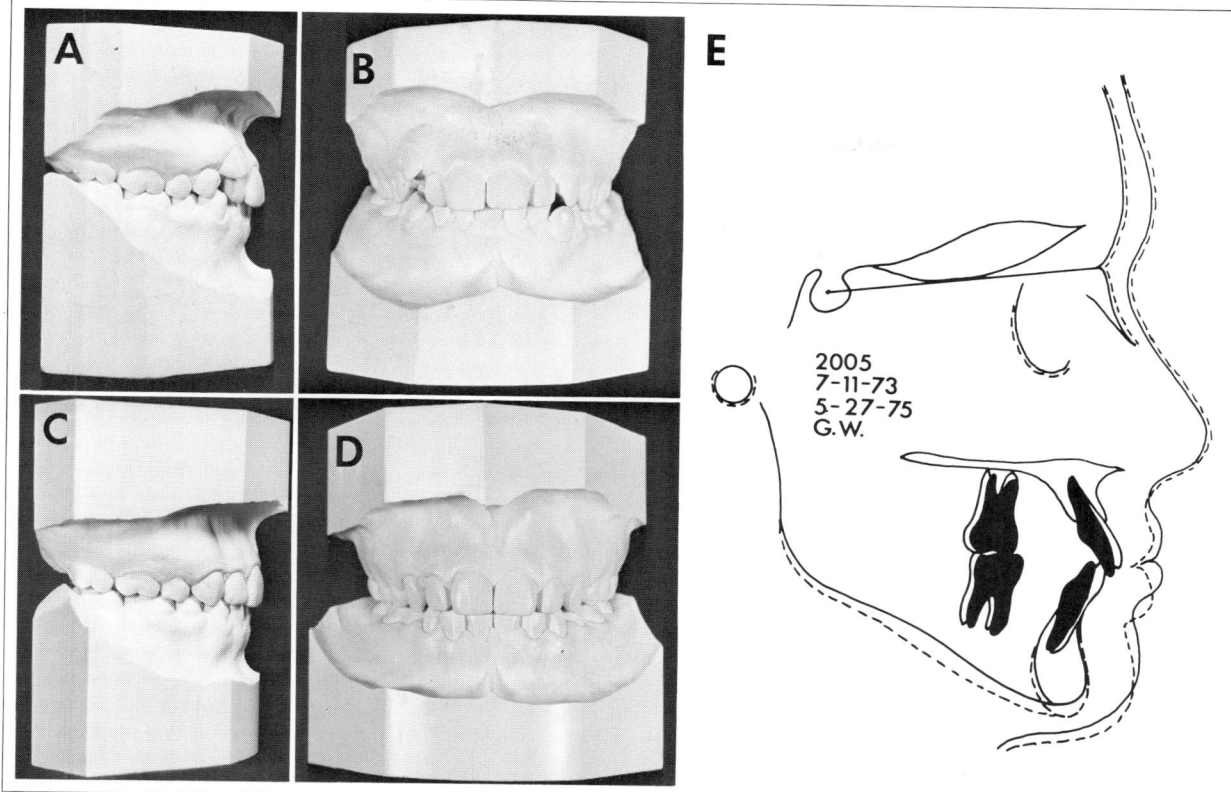

Figure 27-4 | Class I malocclusion jumbled anteriors. A. Right side before treatment. B. Front view before treatment. C. Right view after treatment D. Front view after treatment. E. Superimposed tracings; numbers indicate treatment time and patient's identification. Solid lines and white teeth are before treatment dotted lines and solid black teeth are after treatment.

incisal edges. It may be due to a tongue thrust or a thumb-sucking habit wherein the anteriors have been intruded. It also can be due to overeruption of posteriors (Fig. 27-8).

Closed bite is a condition where there is a greater-than-normal overlapping of the anteriors. This can be the result of the overeruption of the anteriors or a gradual intrusion of posteriors or their lack of sufficient eruption (Fig. 27-3B).

DIAGNOSTIC AIDS

In the past, a diagnosis was limited to a visual examination of the patient. However, the orthodontist now has many valuable diagnostic aids which permit the elimination of guesswork in treatment planning. These diagnostic aids are as follows: (1) records of history and examination of patient; (2) radiographic records—full-mouth, periapical, bitewings, panoramic, cephalometric

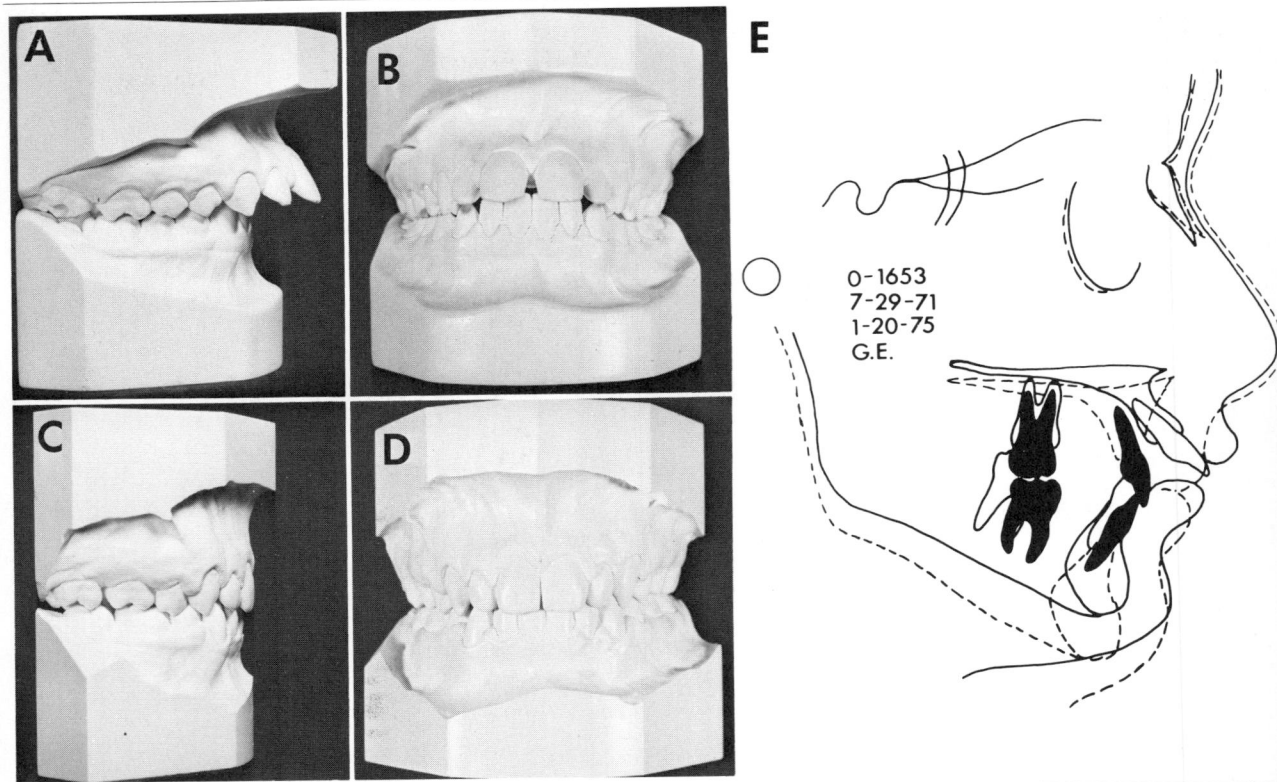

Figure 27-5 | Class II, division 1 malocclusion. A. Right side before treatment. B. Front view before treatment. C. Right side after treatment (four first bicuspid extraction case). D. Front view after treatment. E. Superimposed tracings; numbers indicate treatment time and patient identification. Solid lines and white teeth are before treatment; dotted lines and solid black teeth are after treatment. Note change in soft-tissue profile.

headplate; (3) dental models; and (4) photographs, both facial and intraoral.

Records of History and Examination

Written records are always important; in orthodontics, they are essential. A history of the patient should always include the age, sex, weight, and height. It should list childhood diseases and injuries and record any indications of hereditary tendencies pertinent to growth and development. The body height and weight indicate the overall growth tendency of the individual, and this combined with information on the statural growth of parents and other relatives gives a basis for evaluating the growth potential of this individual. Likewise, an appraisal of the patient's dentofacial growth and comparison with parents and relatives of similar appearance might give an indication of the dentofacial growth potential of this patient. A family history of an anomalous tooth condition, such as missing permanent teeth, should suggest a check of the patient's intraoral x-ray films for a similar condition.

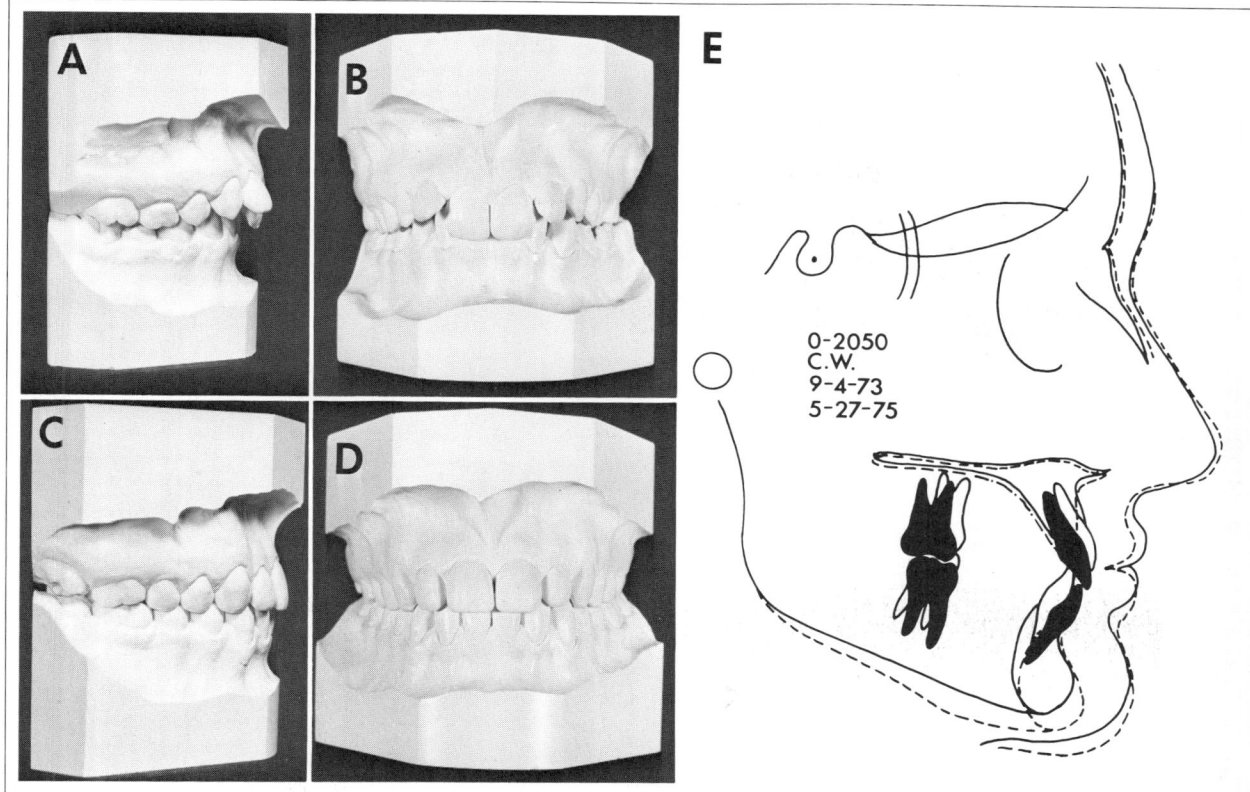

Figure 27-6 | Class II, division 2 malocclusion. A. Right side before treatment. Note blocked out maxillary lateral. B. Anterior view before treatment. C. Right side after treatment. D. Front view after treatment. E. Superimposed tracings; numbers indicate treatment time and patient identification. Solid lines and white teeth are before treatment; dotted lines and solid black teeth are after treatment.

Radiographic Records

Intraoral films are an indispensable aid in making a diagnosis when orthodontic treatment is being considered. Extraoral headplate films are used commonly, and when indicated, temporomandibular joint films are employed.

Intraoral Films

If the orthodontist or general practitioner is going to band and move teeth, it is necessary to know the condition of the teeth and their surrounding tissues. Caries must be eliminated, and any pathology of the gingiva must be treated before any appliances are to be placed. The films are examined for the presence of any pathologic condition of the supporting tissues and bone of the face and for the size, shape, and position of unerupted teeth, missing teeth, and the presence of supernumerary teeth. Often the dentist is plagued by teeth that seem to resist all efforts to move them. In such cases an x-ray examination of the periodontal membrane in its entirety

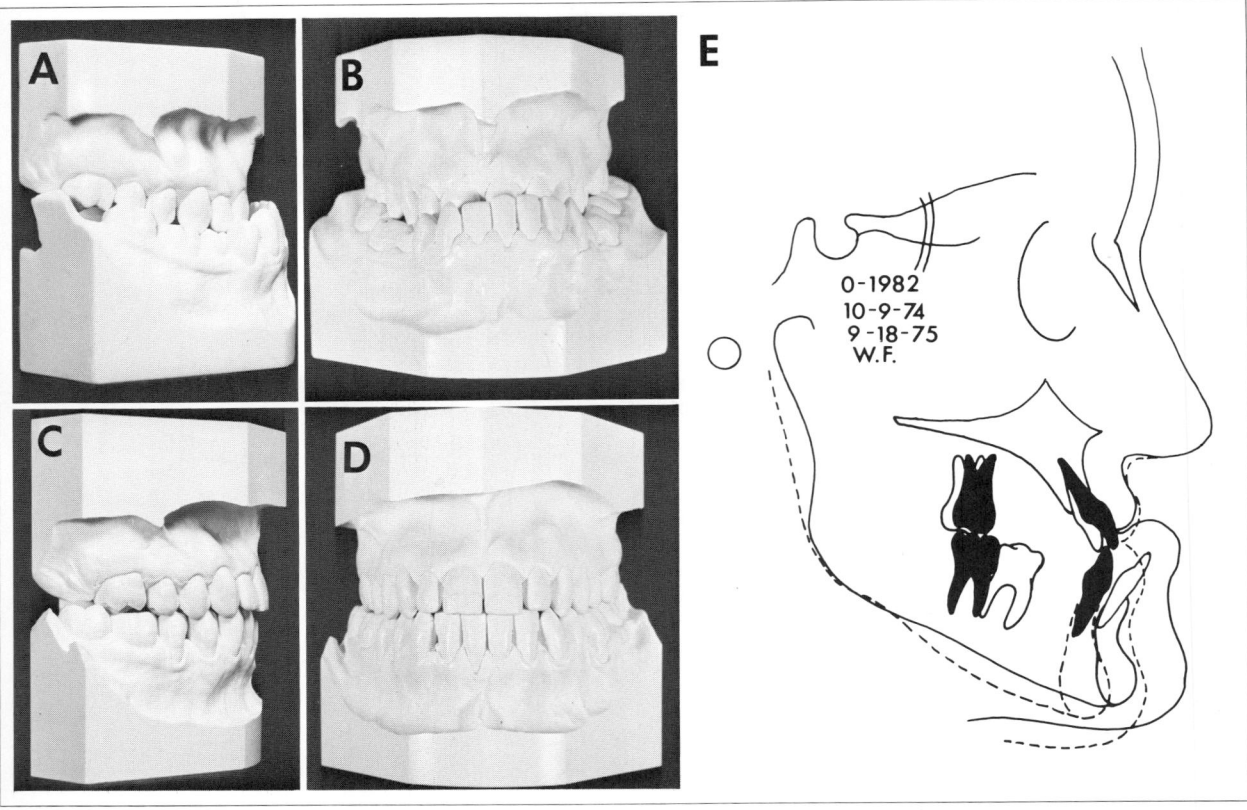

Figure 27-7 | Class III surgical case (adult). A. Right side before treatment. B. Anterior view before treatment. C. Right side after surgery and treatment. D. Front view after surgery and treatment. E. Superimposed tracings; numbers indicate treatment time and patient identification. Solid lines and white teeth are before treatment; dotted lines and solid black teeth are after surgery and treatment. Note the amount of distal placement of mandible through surgery.

about the root will help determine if ankylosis may be the cause.

Extraoral Films

The panoramic film is particularly helpful in showing the overall relationship of the teeth of both dental arches to each other and the presence of pathology of bone not visible in periapical films (Fig. 27-1). The cephalometric headplate films show the bones and teeth of the head in profile, thereby making it possible to measure the relationship of the skeletal maxillae and mandible to the rest of the skull and to each other. It also is possible to determine the relationship of the teeth to each other and their relative position in the jaws that support them. These measurements then are compared to standards based on normal individuals. By evaluating these conditions the dentist is able to determine what areas should be corrected, and what movements of the bones and teeth would be necessary to

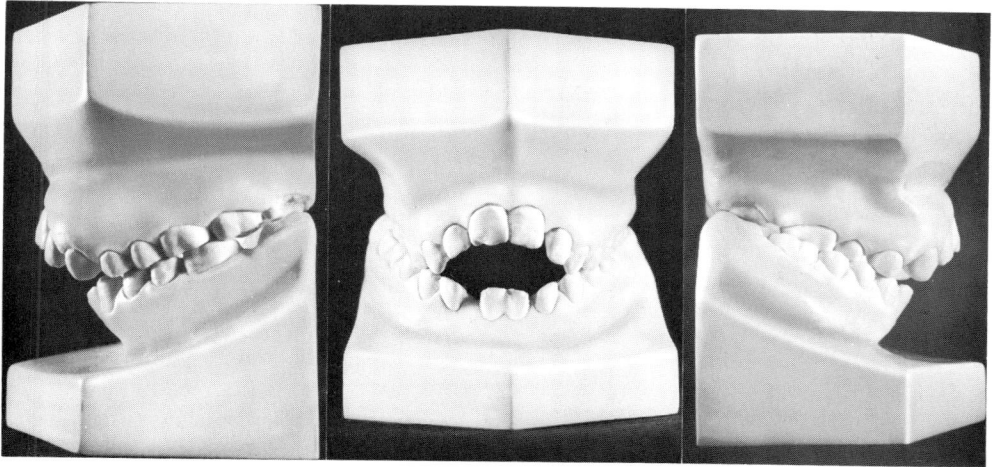

Figure 27-8 | Angle Class I malocclusion, with anteriors with an extreme open bite due to tongue thrust; the right side presents a crossbite in the posterior region.

complete treatment. Cephalometrics therefore makes it possible to classify the skeletal components of a patient's face as we do the dentition and soft-tissue profile.

Frequently it is necessary to determine the cause of an unnatural mandibular movement or position, and the temporomandibular joint films are of diagnostic value in determining the etiology. (Cephalometrics as a diagnostic tool will be discussed in greater detail later in this chapter.)

Models

Plaster models of the patient's dental arches and their supporting tissue provide an important source of information from which the dentist or orthodontist can make a diagnosis. These models permit the study of the denture (teeth and arch relationships) from every angle, since the tongue and cheeks are eliminated. Accordingly, it is easier to view rotated, malaligned, tipped, oversized, and undersized teeth or to visualize the fact that some are missing. From a model it is customary to determine arch-length adequacies or deficiencies. This is important in children from 7 to 14 years of age when there is an exchange of dentition from primary to permanent.

With a duplicate plaster model it is possible to cut off the teeth individually and mount them in wax, leaving out teeth that are to be extracted (if this is part of the treatment plan) and thereby place each tooth in correct position relative to other teeth and to the basal bone. The orthodontist can then determine the direction and amount of all tooth movements necessary for the results desired.

Photographs

Originally, orthodontics emphasized ideal occlusion as its goal; however, there now is an additional goal which is to achieve the best possible esthetic correction of the teeth and face. Profile photographs are a record of the facial type, and they assist the dentist in determining the plan of treatment. The soft-tissue profile is classified, as are the dentition and bone structure of the face (maxillae and mandible), in addition to determining whether the lips are too full (convex) or too weak (concave) with respect to the rest of the face. Photographs show the soft-tissue contours that in effect mask the bone structures beneath them. The before-and-after photograph is the best means of demonstrating to the parents of a prospective patient the child's esthetic problem and the orthodontist's ability to treat a similar case.

PREVENTIVE ORTHODONTICS

Preventive orthodontics implies the application of any dental procedures that are necessary to maintain the health of the teeth and surrounding tissues and to maintain normal occlusion. Education of the patients as to the care of the primary and early-erupting permanent teeth is one of the principal methods available to the profession in the approach to preventive orthodontics.

Perhaps the most important factor in preventive orthodontics is good restorative dentistry. Furthermore, the maintenance of space following the early loss of primary teeth by the use of space maintainers, partial dentures, or orthodontic appliances also permits the retention of good arch form and function. The time of loss of the primary or early permanent tooth also is important. The dentist must determine in each instance if a temporary or more permanent replacement for the lost tooth or teeth should be made.

Preventive orthodontics by definition pertains to Class I cases since by definition Class II and Class III cases usually are not treated early in a preventive approach. The general practitioners and pedodontists should refer the Class II and Class III cases to the orthodontist, who may intercede early in an attempt to correct molar relationships early in Class II cases and may place a chin cap (Fig. 27-9C) on Class III cases in order to slow mandibular growth. Therefore nearly all preventive cases are Class I cases, and they come under consideration for treatment with the beginning of the mixed dentition or when there has been early loss of deciduous teeth. If it is determined by the dentist that space can be lost in the edentulous area, what is called an *arch-length analysis* must be performed, wherein first the length of the dental arch is calculated, and then the size of the permanent teeth to erupt from first permanent molar on the right to first permanent molar on the left and whether there is enough space for the permanent teeth to erupt in good arch form and in proper occlusion. If there is room, a space retainer should then be placed, either a lingual arch or a Hawley removable appliance. If more than enough room is available, it is sometimes possible to recall the patient frequently and observe eruption without the placement of space maintenance.

Another preventive procedure is when primary teeth have been retained beyond the time that they should have been lost (exfoliated). This delay in the loss of primary teeth is usually the result of inadequate root resorption, and this condition may prevent the permanent tooth from erupting properly. Periapical x-ray films taken periodically will show any progressive development of the roots of the permanent teeth and at the same time show the status of resorption of the roots of the primary teeth. If the dentist finds that the roots of the primary teeth are not resorbing properly, extraction of the primary teeth is indicated.

The control of certain habits that are destructive to the dental arch is most important in prevention. Any habit that produces undue pressure on the dental arch will affect it. Thumb sucking is the most common habit that affects occlusion (Fig. 27-8). In many instances the habit does not create great enough pressure to affect the teeth, and in these cases it would not be wise to make an issue of this habit unless it is continued beyond 5 years of age. However, if the habit is destructive and the child is 3 to 4 years of age, it would be best to provide some control of the habit in as pleasant a manner as possible. Antagonism between parent and child should be avoided, for this often provokes the child to a

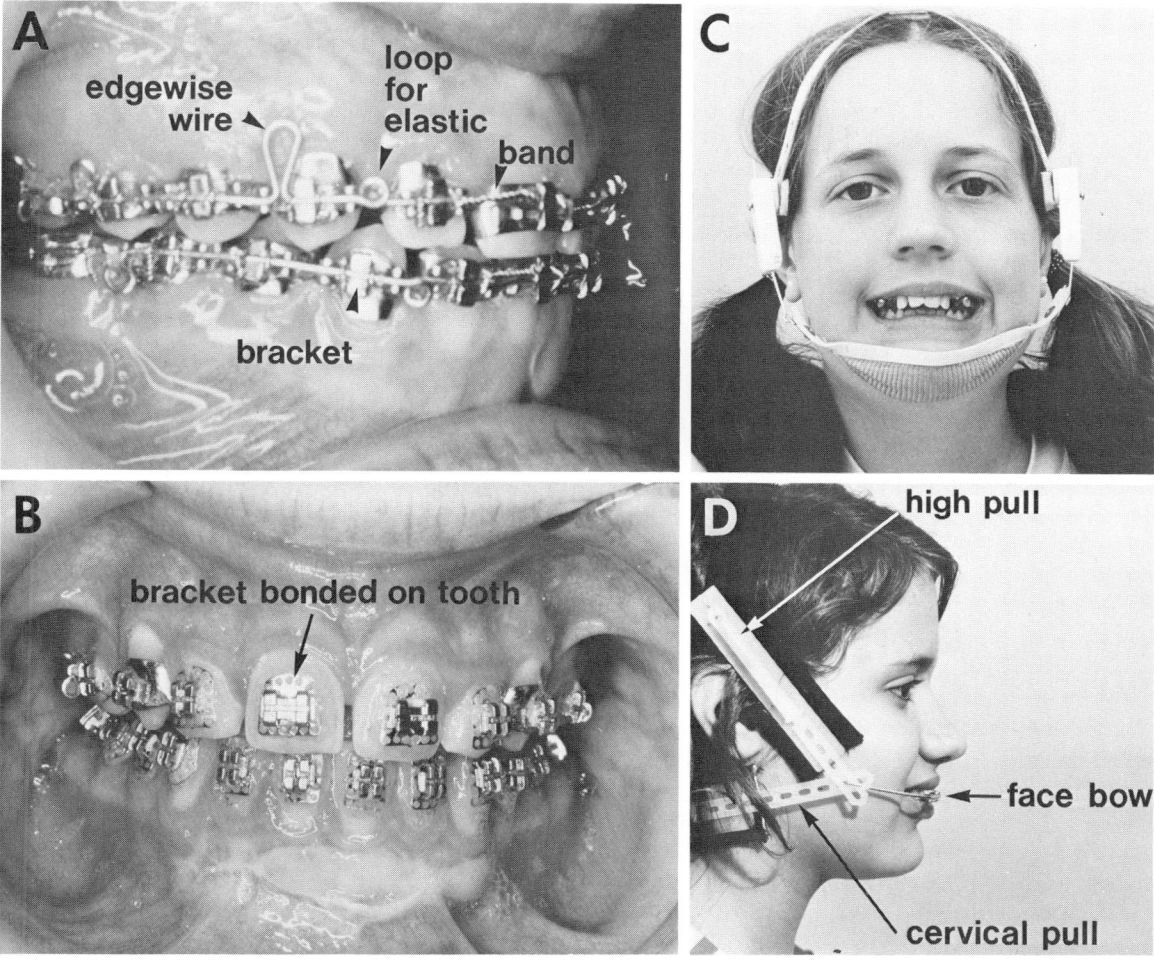

Figure 27-9 | A. Full-banded appliance, with an Edgewise wire in place. B. Brackets bonded directly on teeth. C. Chin cap on patient to restrain growth of mandible. D. Combination headgear which is the use of high-pull along with cervical gear, both of which are attached to a facebow exerting a distal pull on the maxillary first molars, which are fitted with molar bands with buccal tubes into which the inner bow of the facebow fits.

more determined habit. Often all that is necessary is for the dentist to discuss the problem with the child. The child must want to break the habit before success can be attained. If the child seems interested in breaking the habit but is unable to cope with the problem, there are several "reminders" that may be an aid, such as (1) lingual arches with attachments to prevent the placement of the thumb or fingers in the mouth, (2) acrylic plates with the attachments just mentioned, (3) the wearing of thumb or finger guards, or (4) the painting of the thumb or finger with unpleasant-tasting medication as a reminder, always with the child concurring.

Tongue thrusting is equally as destructive to the dentition as is thumb sucking, and is a far more difficult habit to control (Fig. 27-8). Fortunately it is not so prevalent. Most individuals are not aware of their swallowing habits, for this is a reflex and therefore necessitates a concentrated effort to correct. Without control of this habit there is very little hope of a permanent correction of the orthodontic problem.

Postural habits both when awake and while asleep can exert a pressure over a sufficient length of time to affect the dental arch and occlusion. For example, sleeping on one side of the face with the hand, wrist, or arm pressing against the buccal segment of the dentition may force lingually that area of the arch that receives the pressure.

EARLY TREATMENT OTHER THAN PREVENTION

There are several conditions that should be treated early. The following conditions are the most important in this category.

1. Crossbites both anterior and posterior often are associated with convenience bites that may shift the mandible to the right or left when it is a posterior crossbite, or may shift the mandible forward in some anterior crossbites. These convenience bites without correction may lead to a permanent skeletal deformity.
2. Although there is some disagreement on the timing of surgical and orthodontic procedures in cleft lip and palate cases, most dentists agree on early lip closure, and many execute bone grafts in the premaxillary area. Early closure by various soft-tissue grafts of the hard palate is also recommended. Research is also developing methods of expanding the maxillary arch during early infancy.
3. Some patients as early as 4 to 5 years of age exhibit a Class III skeletal relationship where the mandible has overgrown the maxillae arch considerably. These can be helped by the wearing of a chin cap (Fig. 27-9C) with a force that resists forward growth of the mandible. A chin cap can establish a normal relationship of the mandible to the maxillae in approximately 1 year of treatment.

There are other early treatment situations, but the most important have been covered.

ADOLESCENT ORTHODONTIC TREATMENT

The period from 10 to 13 years of age is when the majority of full orthodontic cases begin orthodontic treatment. This is a propitious time for treatment for many reasons. (1) By age 13 most patients have all their permanent teeth except third molars. This makes for accuracy in determining space and in arch-length analysis. (2) If extractions are necessary, the teeth that are to be extracted are fully erupted, which results in less trauma in their removal and maintains a normal alveolar bone level. (3) The orthodontic treatment can be correlated with the patient's adolescent growth spurt which can be utilized to maximize treatment goals. (4) The length of treatment is minimized by starting treatment in early adolescence.

ADULT ORTHODONTICS

Today there is an increased demand for adult orthodontics. Basically adult orthodontics falls into two categories: (1) minor and (2) major.

Minor Adult Orthodontics

Minor adult orthodontics covers those cases where one or several teeth need to be involved in order to correct the problem. The treatment usually can be corrected by either a simple removable or fixed appliance (several teeth being banded). Examples of this type of treatment would be

1. Where a molar adjacent to an edentulous area needs uprighting prior to the preparation of the molar as a bridge abutment. Bridge abutments should be stronger if the abutments are perpendicular to the occlusal plane.
2. Where the malposition or malalignment of one or more teeth is the causative factor for periodontal disease as a result of traumatic occlusion. If there is sufficient space in the arch, it is often simple to correct the malocclusion with either a removable or fixed appliance.

Major Orthodontics

Major orthodontics covers those cases where one or both dental arches will be totally involved during treatment. A fixed appliance is indicated wherein all the teeth are banded and arch wires are used to correct the malocclusion. If the supporting tissues of the teeth are normal and healthy, adult orthodontics can be as rewarding and effective as treating adolescents. However, there is one important difference in treating adults: there will be no further growth to help treatment goals. Therefore, if skeletal relationships are severely malpositioned, surgical procedures along with orthodontic treatment are necessary if ideal function and esthetics are to be attained. Some adults show a greater degree of discomfort with orthodontic tooth movement than do children; probably some of this toleration for pain that children exhibit is due to their desire to please. The dental assistant can be very helpful to both the patient and the dentist in reporting to the dentist any complaints so that the doctor can take whatever steps are necessary. In some instances adults exhibit slower tooth movement due, in all probability, to a lowering of cellular activity that is concomitant with tooth movement.

General Comments on Surgical Orthodontics

In most instances surgical procedures are not initiated until growth is complete for all practical purposes in that portion of the face to be operated on so that further growth does not change the relationship given by surgery. The two most common areas of surgery are (1) the maxillae and (2) the mandible (Fig. 27-7E).

If the maxillae have overgrown forward or vertically, or have not grown enough, they can be moved surgically to correct their position. If the mandible has overgrown, it can be moved back to fit correctly with the maxillae, and if it has not grown forward enough, it can be surgically brought forward.

ORTHODONTIC APPLIANCES

General Comment

Orthodontic appliances are as varied as there are orthodontists to design or construct them. However, there are in general use two main types of appliances, removable and nonremovable. In general, the removable appliance does not use bands on the teeth, and the nonremovable does. This delineation is not totally accurate because one type of removable appliance is a removable lingual arch (Fig. 27-10) which uses molar bands

Figure 27-10 | Model of an upper arch with bands on the first molars and a nonremovable appliance consisting of a labial and lingual arch with finger springs attached. The finger springs are the activating force that moves the teeth with gentle forces.

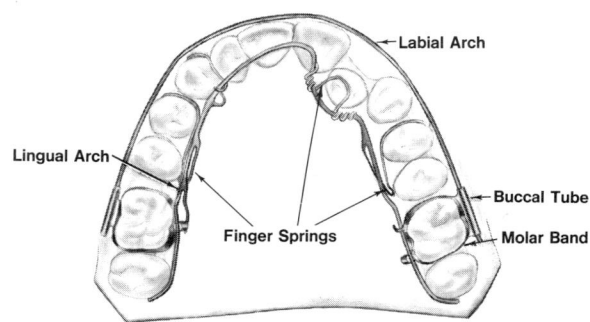

to hold it in place, and there is another, fixed appliance that uses no bands, for the brackets are bonded directly on the teeth (Fig. 27-9B).

Removable Appliances

These appliances are constructed of either acrylic or metal or both and have clasp attachments to hold them in place. They almost always have secondary attachments called finger springs that serve as an adjustable force to move one or more teeth. One type of removable device is a *Hawley* (Fig. 27-11), which is capable of minor tooth movements, mainly tipping, and has wide usage as a retaining appliance, being placed after the removal of a full-banded appliance.

Nonremovable Appliances

These appliances generally have several bands or directly bonded brackets attached to the teeth. They vary considerably in the degree of complexity of their attachments. The most frequently used appliances are (1) light wire–Edgewise, (2) light wire, (3) Universal, (4) twin wire, (5) labiolingual. For an understanding of these techniques it is necessary to read several orthodontic texts wherein several hundred pages serve to give a superficial understanding. All appliances have certain basic parts which will be defined and discussed next (Fig. 27-12).

Bands

These are the preformed metallic attachments that surround the teeth and are cemented in place on the teeth. They have one or more attachments spot-welded to their surface. On the buccal surface of the molar bands are molar brackets or molar buccal tubes which hold the arch wire. All other teeth have bands with brackets welded to the buccal surface. The lingual surface of the molar bands may have tubes for the placement of lingual arches; all

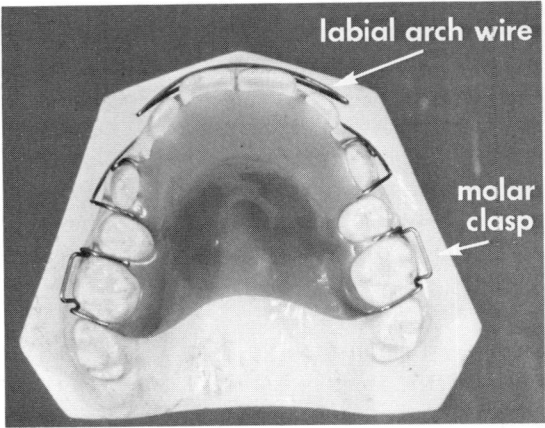

Figure 27-11 | Removable appliance, acrylic with wire attachments. This type of appliance is useful in opening the bite and in limited lingual movement of anterior teeth. It also serves as a retainer.

other bands often have lingual buttons for rotational purposes.

Arch Wires

The main wire is either buccal-labial or lingual. The buccal-labial arch wire usually fits into brackets on each tooth and is ligated into it, and its function is to govern the shape of an arch, level the teeth, and aid in rotations and, depending on type of bracket, can control the long axis position of the teeth (Fig. 27-12). When a lingual arch is placed, its main function is to maintain arch length, or, when auxiliary wires are attached to it, it can effect unit tooth movements (Fig. 27-10).

Brackets

These are attachments welded on the bands, or bonded directly on the teeth. In either instance the bracket transmits the intended force in the arch wire to the tooth itself. Brackets have wings for securely ligating arch wires in their arch-wire slots (Figs. 27-9A and 27-12).

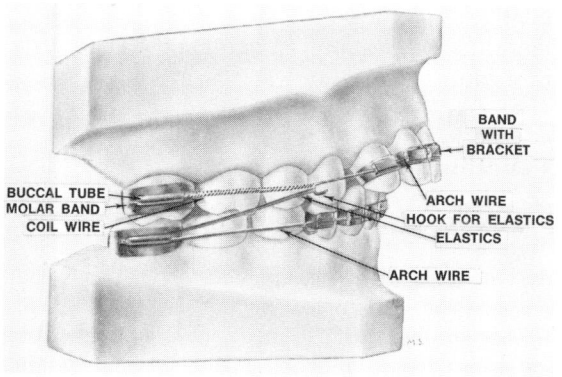

Figure 27-12 | Model of mixed dentition with nonremovable appliance consisting of bands on the first permanent molars and anterior teeth with attachments to secure an upper and lower labial arch wire. The elastic is the main source of force used to move the teeth mesiodistally, while the expansive force is in the arch wire.

Buccal Tubes

Buccal tubes are attachments on molar bands and are the means by which the ends of the labial arch are secured to the molar teeth.

Finger Springs and Coil Springs

Finger springs can be soldered to main arch wires to elicit gentle spring forces to individual teeth (Fig. 27-10). Coil springs are usually placed on an arch wire and are compressed between teeth. They move teeth by the force of the coil attempting to become uncompressed.

Ligature Wire and Separating Wire

Ligature wire is a fine wire that ties the main arch wire into each bracket. Separation wire is a very soft wire that is tied around the contact points of adjacent teeth. By being twisted tightly it creates a force between the teeth, and in several days there is enough space between the teeth for bands to be fitted and cemented accurately.

Elastics

These are rubber bands made especially for orthodontics and are manufactured in various thicknesses and lengths so as to exert whatever force is needed for the movement of teeth. Elastics are the most universally used means of exerting forces between the upper and lower dental arches in order to bring them in correct relationship with each other. Elastics are often used to exert forces within the same dental arch to close space.

In Class II cases, elastics are generally worn from a hook on the maxillary arch wire just mesial to the cuspid bracket and stretched to the buccal tube on the mandibular molar. This will move the maxillary arch distally and the mandibular arch mesially until they are compatible. In Class III cases, elastics are worn from hooks placed on the mandibular arch just mesial to the cuspid bracket and then stretched to the buccal tube on the maxillary molar. This will move the mandibular arch distally and the maxillary arch mesially until they are compatible. Elastics stretching from one arch to the other are called interarch elastics, while elastics used within the same arch are called intraarch elastics.

Extraoral Forces

These are forces that have their source or origin of power for moving teeth or affecting bone from outside the mouth. The most common extraoral forces in use are

1. High-pull headgear
2. Cervical gear
3. Combination of high-pull and cervical headgear (Fig. 27-9D)
4. Chin cap (Fig. 27-9C)

High-pull headgear can be attached directly to molars by way of a facebow and when correctly adjusted, moves molars distally (in the maxillary arch) and keeps the molars from extruding (this is its unique feature). When an intraoral force from molar to anterior teeth is used in conjunction with headgear, it will move the whole maxillary arch distally. When headgear is placed to maxillary molars and used in conjunction with Class III elastics to the mandibular arch wire, the whole mandibular dental arch will move distally. A combination headgear (Fig. 27-9D) which is both a high-pull and cervical pull used at the same time is therefore capable of the same forces as that of high-pull headgear, with the cervical adding additional distal force. Cervical gear is capable of distal forces; however, it cannot exert an intrusive force on upper molars. Chin cap force (Fig. 27-9C) when placed on a young patient with a tendency for overgrowth of the mandible can effect a slowing down of this growth until the maxillae and mandible have a normal relationship anteroposteriorly and can reduce the chances of a Class III case in adulthood.

DUTIES OF AN ORTHODONTIC ASSISTANT

The duties of an orthodontic assistant vary in every orthodontic office. If the orthodontist has just opened a practice and is not very busy, the assistant probably will function as receptionist, chairside assistant, housekeeper, etc. The assistant should be willing to assist in any way possible to help the doctor get the practice started; in time, other office help will be added as the practice grows. The assistant with the proper attitude and industry will be indispensable. In large orthodontic practices there may be a bookkeeping department, one or more receptionists, perhaps as many as eleven chairside assistants, and laboratory personnel. Sickness of any member in the office often requires that someone substitute for that person in order that the office function efficiently. The duties of assistants are limited by law, and they should acquaint themselves with the law regarding these limitations in whatever state they practice. These laws may vary considerably. Therefore, it behooves the dental assistant to be proficient in all or any of the following procedures or duties.

Functioning as a Receptionist

The assistant must be able to

1. Pleasantly greet new parents and patients that walk into the office without an appointment, helping them with whatever questions they ask, knowing what questions should be referred to the orthodontist, and issuing them an appointment.
2. Answer the telephone with an alert and pleasant voice. To make appointments, it is necessary to know most office procedures and the time necessary for each in order to utilize the dentist's time efficiently. In answering complaints, the assistant needs to know what questions or complaints to handle personally and which complaints to refer to the orthodontist. If the orthodontist does not have an office manual outlining everyone's duties and the proper handling of the most common situations, it would be well to encourage constructing one. It is necessary to know how the orthodontist wishes the assistant to handle all parents or patients who call and are worried about appliance breakage, pain, or other problems that occur between appointments. The assistant should know how to answer properly any questions from parents about their financial arrangements or monthly billings. (Parents always feel the office is in error whether this is true or not.) The assistant must know the procedure for arranging a consultation or making appointments with other paramedical or paradental specialists for any patient.

Record Taking

The assistant should know how to obtain and record a medical and dental history of the patient and be able to obtain all diagnostic records, some by assisting the orthodontist. These include (1) all intraoral radiographs or other radiographs taken routinely, (2) photographs of the patient, (3) impressions of the teeth, (4) pouring up, trimming, and finishing models, and

(5) the taking and tracing of cephalometric radiographs. The assistant should know how to keep a daily log of appointments and any financial transactions and how to record in the patient's chart whatever orthodontic procedures were performed during the appointment. Routinely the assistant should inventory instruments and orthodontic supplies (bands, wires, and all similar items). After completing an inventory the next step is to order instruments and supplies when the number of any item falls below a minimum level established by the orthodontist.

Chairside Assisting

The assistant must know (1) how to adjust the dental chair so it will be comfortable for the patient and properly positioned for the dentist for the planned procedure; (2) how to arrange the instruments on the bracket table for the scheduled procedure (see Fig. 27-13); (3) dental anatomy to the extent that separation can be properly placed between the teeth to create room for bands, the proper size of the band for each tooth can be selected, and the procedure for the fitting of bands and assisting the orthodontist in the cementing of bands is known; (4) the technique for the selection and placement of brackets with direct-bonding materials; (5) how to select the proper size of impression tray; how to mix the impression material and assist the orthodontist in the taking of impressions; and how to prepare the patient both mentally and physically for the taking of impressions. The assistant should understand the basic treatment plan for Class I, Class II, and Class III cases and be able to tie in or remove arch wires under the direction of the orthodontist. An assistant should learn the function of each appliance used by the orthodontist. The assistant must understand all types of intraoral forces used by the orthodontist in order to assist in training of the patient in the proper placement of these forces (and the parents also, when necessary). The assistant must know how to assist in the removal of all appliances and how to write a prescription for the construction and repair of all appliances that will be sent to an orthodontic laboratory. In addition it is important to be able to instruct the patient in proper hygiene and care of the dentition and gingiva. The assistant must be aware of the implications of retention in order to instruct and motivate the patient on proper wearing of retainers whether they are Hawleys or positioners. The assistant must maintain a sterile environment for the patient, i.e., sterilize instruments and supplies, and keep the office and equipment as antiseptic as possible.

INTRODUCTION TO CEPHALOMETRICS

Cephalometrics is a radiographic technique used to study growth and development of the dentofacial complex. It is also used as a means to determine anteroposterior relationships of both dental arches and their supporting bony arches to each other and to the anterior cranial base. Lastly, cephalometrics is used to study what changes were accomplished by orthodontic treatment.

First in order to apply the standards used in making an analysis of a patient's headplate x-ray, it is necessary to make a tracing of certain bones of the cranium and face as well as of certain teeth. In order to do this, it becomes necessary to recognize the bones and teeth that appear in a lateral cephalogram (headplate). Figure 27-14 is a tracing in detail of the skeletal anatomy and dentition shown on a radiographic lateral head film of a patient. This should be studied thoroughly. If knowledge of anatomy is not sufficient, refer to any anatomy text and review the bones of the head and in particular any midsagittal drawings. When the assistant is thoroughly familiar with these anatomic relationships, it is possible to trace a headplate. To accomplish this, the headplate film is placed on a view box with a self-contained light source, a

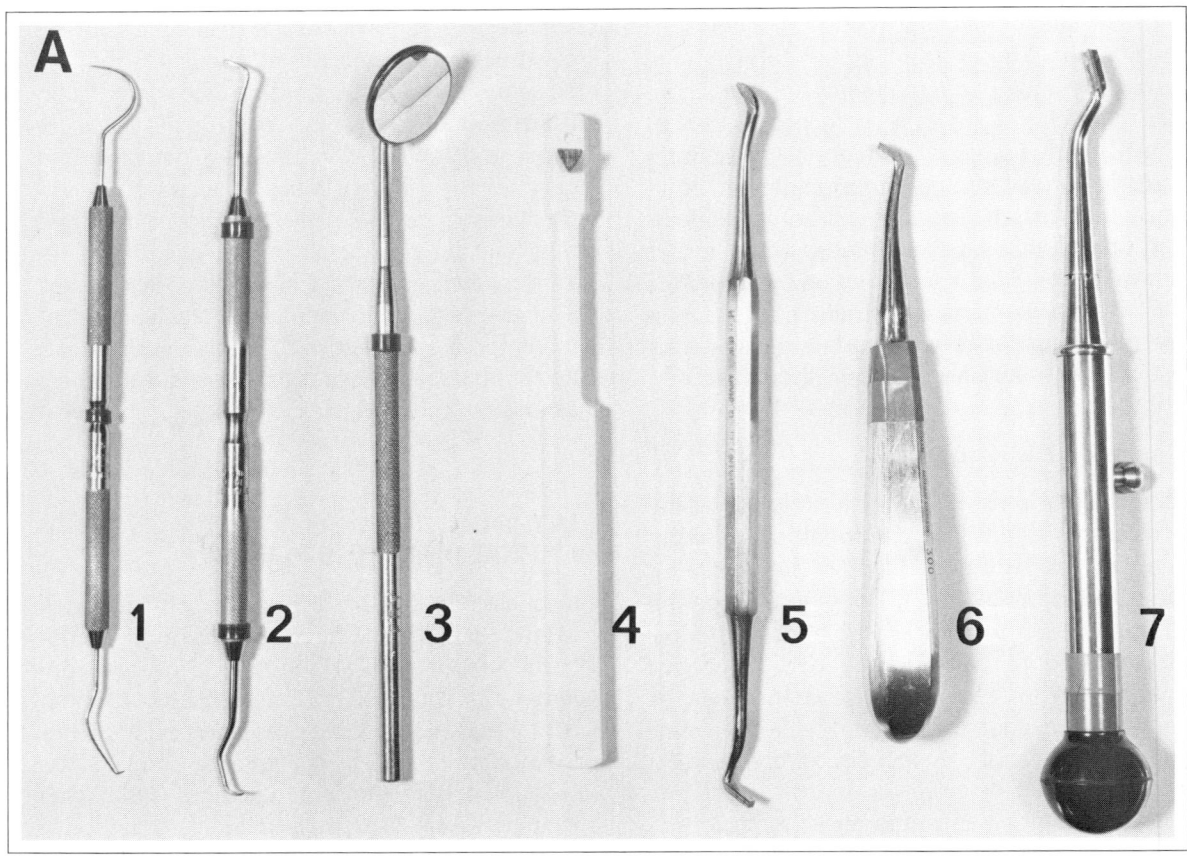

Figure 27-13 | A. Instruments, (1) explorer for testing if cement is firm under bands and for caries, (2) scaler for removing excess cement after cementing bands, (3) mouth mirror for detailed examination of teeth and appliance, (4) band pusher which uses the force of occlusion to seat bands, (5) band pusher which hand pressure to seat bands and adapt, (6) band pusher, (7) Eby band driver, which uses a spring-loaded weight to drive bands into place. B. Instruments, (1) How plier for the placement of bands and arch wires, (2) loop-forming plier for placing loops in arch wire, (3) short-nosed plier for arch forming, (4) long-nosed plier for arch forming, (5) ligature wire cutters. C. Instruments, (1) wire cutters, (2) Edgewise plier for placing torque, (3) arch-forming plier, (4) ligature-tying plier, (5) band-removing plier.

special, clear tracing paper is placed over the film, and a sharp pencil is used to make a more simplified outline of the bones and teeth (see Fig. 27-15). It can be noted that the following bones are outlined:

1. The outer outline of the frontal bone in the area of the forehead and its junction with the nasal bone, N, nasion.
2. The nasal bone.
3. The right and left orbits, with the lowest point designated as O, orbitale.
4. Straight back from N is the sella turcica, which is outlined, the center of which is designated S.
5. Straight back from orbitale (O) is the external audi-

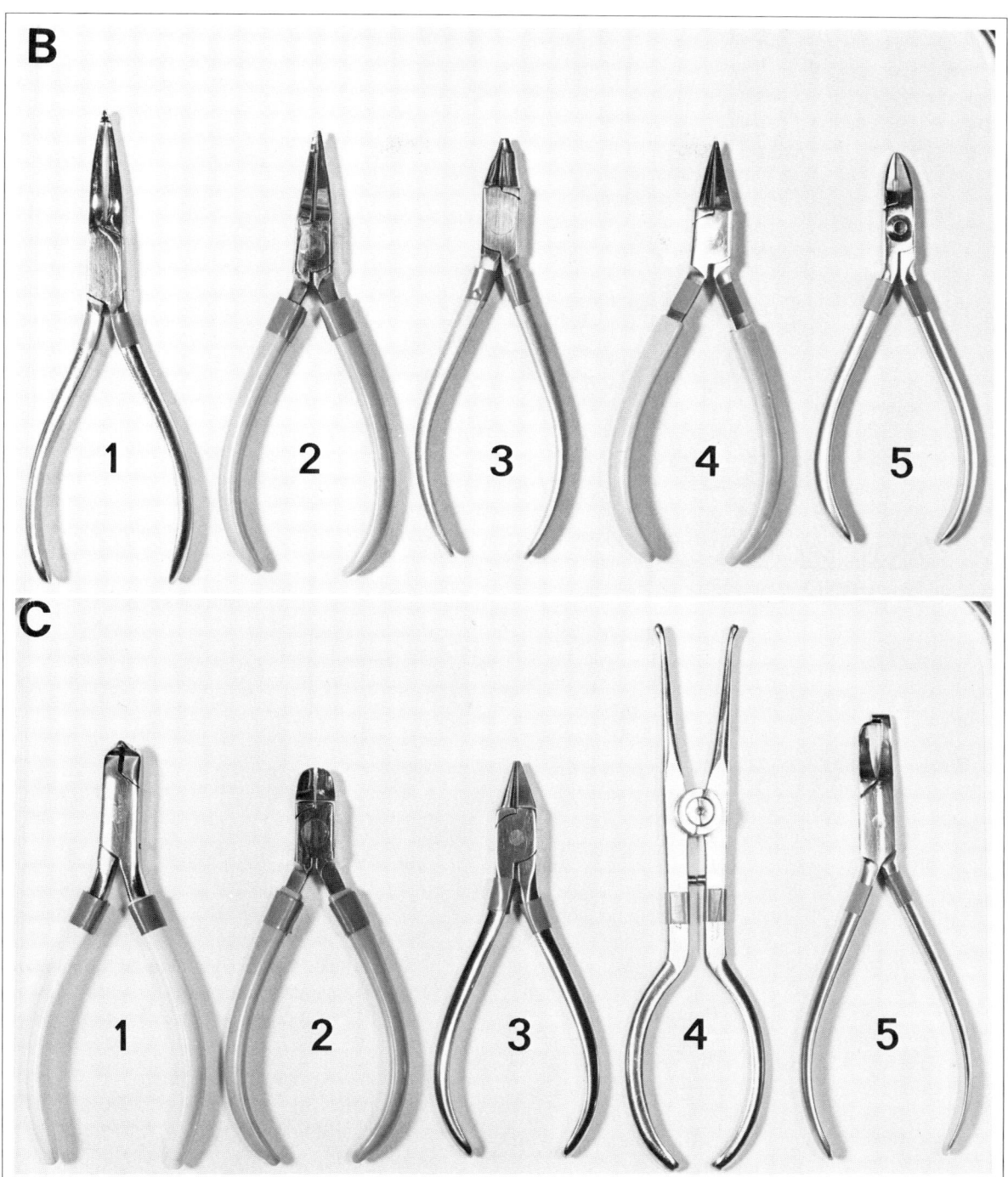

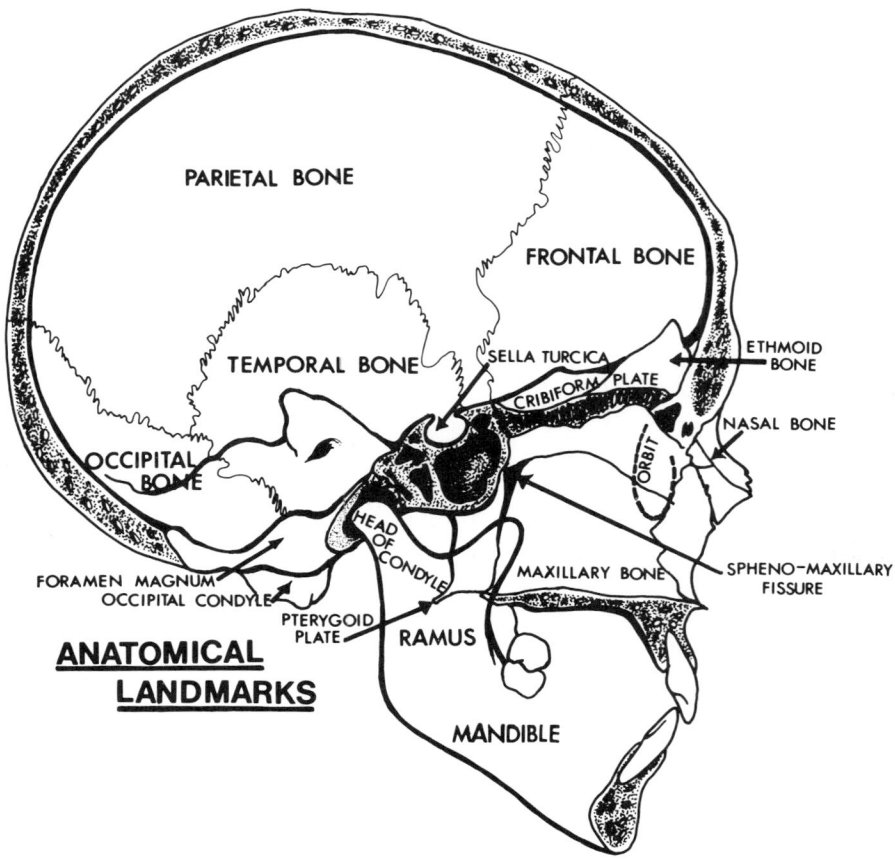

Figure 27-14 | The skeletal anatomy that appears in a lateral cephalometric radiograph.

tory meatus, which usually is indicated by a metal marker on the ear rod (a part of the cephalostat that positions the head in a constant position relative to the film and x-ray source when making the headplate). The upper part of the ear-rod marker is related to the superior point of the external auditory meatus, indicated as P, porion.

6. The maxillary bone, which includes the floor of the nose and hard palate of the mouth. It ends anteriorly as the anterior nasal spine (ANS) and anteroinferiorly forms the alveolar bone that supports the upper central incisor. The anterior alveolar bone beneath ANS shows point A, which is the deepest point of this outline. The maxillary first molar is also traced.

7. Parts of the mandible are also traced; the posterior border of the ramus is traced, as well as the lower border of the mandible and the symphysis (the chin and the alveolar bone that supports the central teeth), and finally the lower incisor. The deepest point on the anterior alveolar bone of the mandible is indicated as point B and the most anterior point on the bony chin is Pg, or pogonion.

The following planes are drawn: (1) from S to N, designated the SN plane, (2) from P to O, designated the Frankfort plane, (3) from G to M, designated the mandibular plane, constructed by drawing a line from the lowest point at the angle of the ramus to the lowest point on the symphysis (bony chin), (4) from N to point A

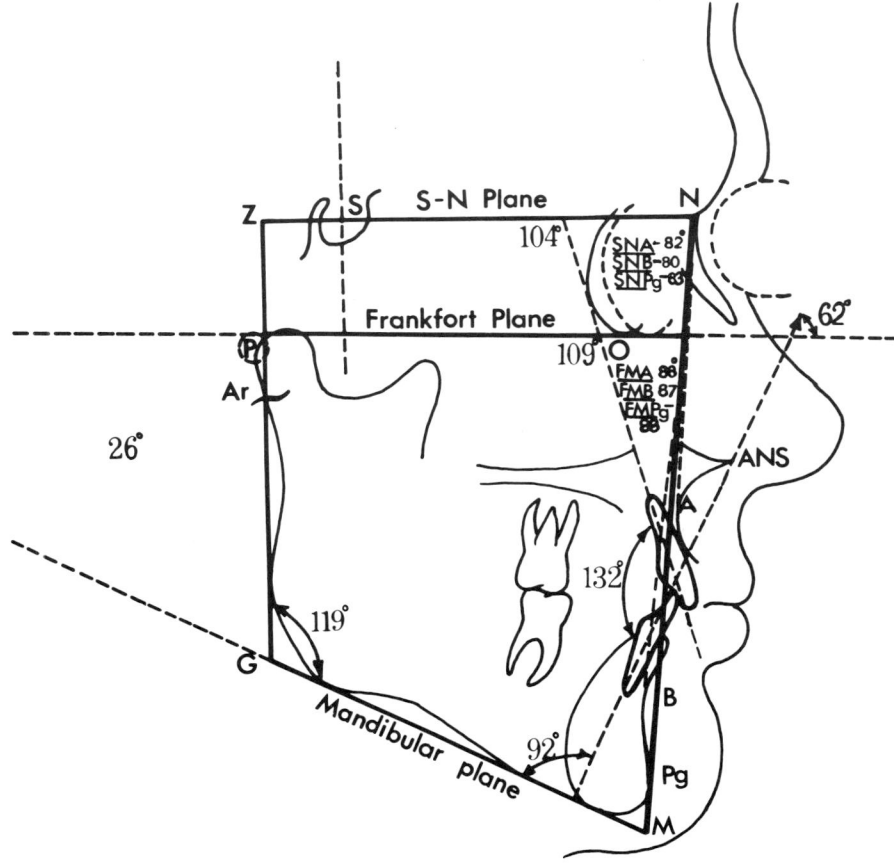

Figure 27-15 | A tracing of a lateral cephalometric headplate with constructions as outlined in the text in "Cephalometrics." The angles written in are ideal standards for 12- to 14-year-olds.

designated the NA plane, (5) from N to point B, designated the NB plane, (6) from N to Pg, designated the facial plane, (7) a plane through the long axis of the upper incisor, (8) a plane through the long axis of the lower incisor.

The following angles are measured with a protractor: (1) SN–NA (SNA angle), (2) SN–NB (SNB angle), (3) SN–NPg angle, (4) Frankfort–NB (FNB angle), (6) Frankfort–NPg (FNPg angle), (7) the angle between the long axis of the upper central and the long axis of the lower incisor, (8) the angle between the long axis of the upper incisor and the SN plane, (9) the angle between the long axis of the lower incisor and the mandibular plane, (10) the angle between the Frankfort plane and the mandibular plane.

The basic meaning of the "ideal" angular readings (see Fig. 27-15) is (1) SNA (80 degrees) measures the anteroposterior relationship of the maxillae relative to the anterior cranial base. If the SNA angle on a patient is 85 degrees, it indicates that the maxilla is forward of ideal. If a patient's SNA is 75 degrees, the maxillae have not grown forward far enough. (2) SNB and SNPg readings indicate the anteroposterior relationship of the alveolar bone and bony chin of the mandible relative to anterior cranial base. For example, the ideal reading for SNPg is 83 degrees; therefore if a patient has a SNPg of 88 degrees, it indicates the mandible has overgrown; and in a patient with a SNPg of 78 degrees the mandible is undergrown. (3) All the angles relative to the long axis of the upper central and lower central are ideal angular relationships of the teeth to indicated planes. (4) The ideal relationship between the Frankfort plane to mandibular plane is 26 degrees. If the reading is appreciably greater, it would suggest that the lower face is growing more vertically than horizontally and if the patient has a weak chin at 12 to 14 years of age, the growth spurt during adolescence will probably not help improve the patient's profile. If this angle is lower than ideal, for example 16 degrees, the mandible will probably grow more horizontal than vertical, and the chin will appear stronger at the end of the growth spurt.

RESPONSIBILITIES

Responsibilities of the Patient

Cleanliness

The teeth are much more difficult to keep clean with the appliances in place, so it is imperative that the patient has established a good pattern of oral hygiene before starting treatment. Neglect of oral hygiene during treatment usually increases the caries index or leads to decalcified areas, and in some cases, may lead to infections about the roots of the teeth. Therefore, cooperation is essential.

Appointments

During the construction of the appliance, one to two long appointments will be assigned to the patient. These in all probability will be spaced rather closely together. Thereafter, the orthodontist will wish to see the patient at 3- to 5-week intervals to make adjustments in the appliance. It is very important that all appointments be kept, since every missed appointment means that the patient has lengthened the time of treatment. Another reason that appointments should not be missed is that if any bands on the teeth have become loose, their detection will be delayed until the next appointment, and damage to the enamel may occur.

Diet

The patient is always instructed that it is essential to have a well-balanced and sufficient diet, for an inadequate diet may cause the gums to become inflamed and swollen and interfere with tooth movement and appliance management. It is equally important that the patient not eat coarse or sticky foods, for these may break or bend the appliance.

The Appliance

The appliance must be kept clean. Elastics, cervical anchorage, or chin cap, when part of the treatment, must be worn at the times indicated by the orthodontist; otherwise the treatment time will be extended. Toying with the appliance should be watched for and discouraged. Patients may distort or break their appliance by manipulation of it with their tongue, finger, or some object such as a pencil.

Responsibility of the Parents

The parent's main responsibility is to maintain the cooperative attitude of the patient, including supervision of the child's oral-hygiene program. The parent should inform the school that the child will be under extensive treatment and will have to have some appointments during school hours. This will prevent undue friction and embarrassment between teachers and patient. They should encourage the child to accept some responsibility in keeping all appointments. This, of course, will depend on the age of the patient.

Responsibility of the Dentist

Before orthodontic work is started, the family dentist should restore the mouth to good health. Then during the treatment he or she should continue to check the patient periodically for necessary dental procedures. The dentist, before starting orthodontic work, has the responsibility of making a careful diagnosis and treatment plan and explaining to the parent and patient what the problem is and what attempt will be made to try to correct it. The doctor should inform these people of their responsibilities and why their cooperation is necessary. If possible, the dentist should explain what might interfere with successful treatment. A clear explanation of their financial obligation and how it is to be managed prevents future misunderstandings.

After treatment has been completed and the appliance removed, the teeth tend to be loose and may drift. Therefore, in most cases it is necessary to place retainers to stabilize the teeth for a period of time.

BIBLIOGRAPHY

Anderson, G. M.: *Practical Orthodontics,* 8th ed., The C. V. Mosby Company, St. Louis, 1955.

Baume, L. J.: "The Biogenesis of the Successional Dentition," *J. Dent. Res.,* **29:**338, 1950.

Finn, S. B.: *Clinical Pedodontics,* W. B. Saunders Company, Philadelphia, 1957.

Graber, T. M.: *Orthodontic Principles and Practice,* 3d ed., W. B. Saunders Company, Philadelphia, 1972.

————, and Swain, B. F.: *Current Orthodontic Concepts and Techniques,* 2d ed., W. B. Saunders Company, Philadelphia, 1975.

Jaraback, J. R., and Fizzell, J. A.: *Technique and Treatment with Light-Wire Edgewise Appliance,* vols. I and II, The C. V. Mosby Company, St. Louis, 1972.

McCoy, J. D., and Shepard, E. E.: *Applied Orthodontics,* Lea & Febiger, Philadelphia, 1956.

Moyers, R. E.: *Handbook of Orthodontics,* Year Book Medical Publishers, Inc., Chicago, 1958.

Salzmann, J. A.: Orthodontics, J. B. Lippincott Company, Philadelphia, 1957, vols. I and II.

Waldo, C. M.: "A Practical Approach to the Problems of Orthodontics," *Am. J. Orthod.,* **39:**322–329, 1953.

28 William D. Strickland
Operative Dentistry

The breadth of the general practice of dentistry requires that the dental assistant be knowledgeable in all treatment procedures accomplished in the total dental care for the patient. Because of the high percentage of operative procedures in general practice and the demands on the operator's time, it is extremely important that the chairside assistant be efficient and effective. Basically, the chairside assistant's primary role is to save the dentist time by doing those procedures which do not require the special skills and talents of the operator. This type of team effort allows the dentist to make optimum use of appointment time, permitting an increase in patient load. In addition, more treatment may be accomplished in a given length of time. Indirectly, other benefits are evident as a result of proper utilization of the chairside assistant. These include increased patient comfort, standardization of procedures which enhance the quality of treatment, better appointment control to eliminate nonproductive time, and the reduction of stress and strain which often lead to physical illness.

DENTAL CARIES AND OPERATIVE DENTISTRY

Dental Caries

Dental caries is a unique disease which affects the calcified tissues of teeth exposed to the oral cavity. People of all ages are susceptible to

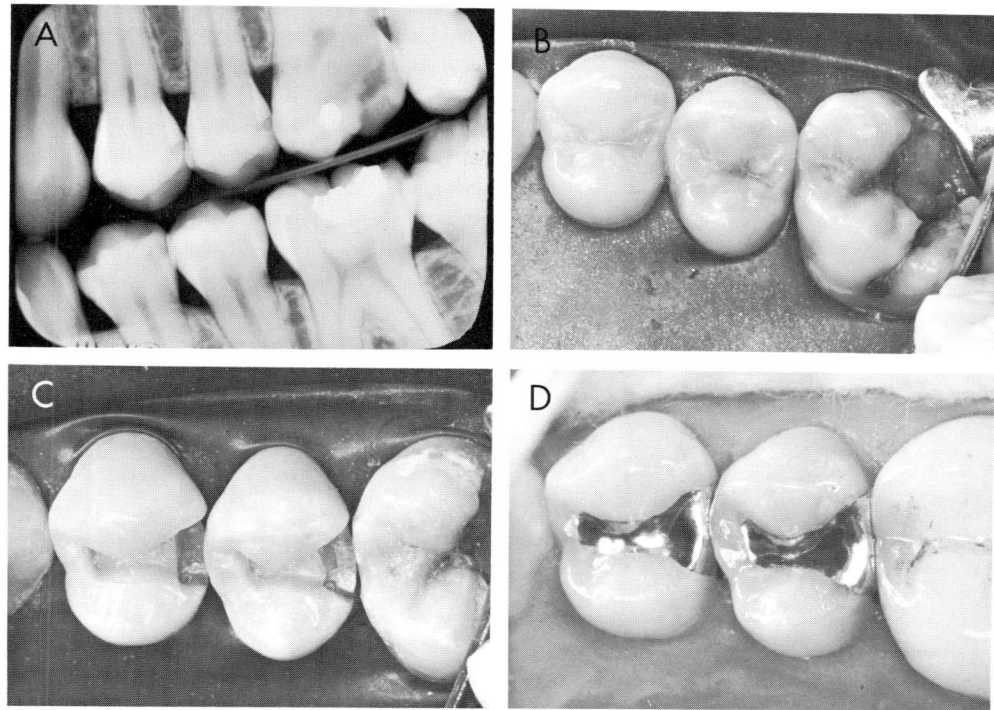

Figure 28-1 | Treatment of caries. A. Bitewing radiograph. B. Teeth prior to cavity preparation. C. Cavity preparations. D. Silver amalgam restorations.

caries, but its rate of incidence is highest in the younger age groups. Historically, treatment has been surgical removal (cavity preparation) and subsequent restoration with one of the various restorative materials (Fig. 28-1). Present-day dentistry now recognizes that a strong preventive dentistry program can significantly reduce the prevalence of caries. Prevention is achieved through patient education as related to proper home care, regular recall examinations, and the early restoration of carious teeth. The student assistant as well as the employed auxiliary should have a complete understanding of the material in Chap. 19. Knowledge of preventive dentistry should provide the auxiliary with the information to properly converse with patients and to function in a preventive-oriented practice in which auxiliaries are delegated patient-education procedures. The role of the auxiliary in preventive dentistry will vary depending on the type of practice and the existing dental laws governing the practice of dentistry in the different states.

Operative Dentistry

Because of the importance of operative dentistry in the total dental and general health of the patient, the following definition is presented to identify the scope of this area of dentistry. Operative dentistry is defined as that *branch or specialty of the science and art of dentistry which deals largely with the diagnosis, prevention, and treatment of diseases of the enamel and dentin of the natural teeth.*

Destruction of tooth structure due to dental caries creates the greatest single need for restoration of teeth; however, other conditions such as erosion, abrasion, and trauma also create the need for operative dentistry. Following the sequence of diagnosis, restorative procedures, and patient education in the area of prevention, maintenance of oral health is the primary responsibility of the patient. It can be stated, then, that the *functions* of operative dentistry are (1) diagnosis, (2) prevention, (3) restoration, and (4) maintenance. It then is not difficult to envision the total importance of operative dentistry to the total health and welfare of the patient. Furthermore, it is not difficult to understand that a dental assistant well trained in all the procedures related to operative dentistry is a valued and essential member of the dentist-assistant team.

OBJECTIVES OF OPERATIVE DENTISTRY

When restoration of a tooth (teeth) is necessary, certain objectives must be fulfilled regardless of the cause for the loss of the tooth substance or the type of restorative material to be utilized. These objectives are (1) to arrest the loss of tooth structure, (2) to prevent recurrence of caries, (3) to restore proper tooth contour, (4) to restore function, and (5) to restore esthetics. Individually and collectively, these objectives require certain knowledge and skills of the dentist which are necessary to restore the tooth to optimum health. It follows, then, that the dental assistant should possess sufficient knowledge of the procedures to be thoroughly efficient in the direct and indirect tasks which relate to the restorative procedure.

Arrest the Loss of Tooth Structure

Often, initial surface caries of the enamel may be treated and controlled before sufficient cavitation occurs to require cavity preparation and restoration. Certainly, whenever possible, this is preferred. Upon examination, when areas of initial caries are detected, the application of topical fluoride, dietary management, and a rigid home-care program may cause these areas to become inactive. The patient must then be scheduled for periodic clinical and radiographic examinations to be certain the disease is under control.

If, however, sufficient cavitation is noted (penetration to the dentinoenamel union) which requires cavity preparation and restoration, the procedure should be accomplished as soon as possible so that the amount of tooth structure removed will be minimal. The tooth requiring a restoration of small size renders the tooth less subject to fracture from occlusal stress; therefore, the life expectancy of the small restoration is longer than that of the restoration of large size.

Prevent Recurrence of Caries

This objective is partially fulfilled by the design of the cavity preparation in that certain rules are followed which place the margins of the restoration in areas which are less susceptible to attack by caries. The outline form of the preparation on the occlusal surface includes all pits and fissures, which positions the cavosurface margin on areas of the tooth which are free of irregularities. Furthermore, any proximal margin is extended beyond the contact areas, which positions these margins so that they may be cleansed during mastication and oral-hygiene procedures.

Once the carious areas are restored, the patient should be reminded that proper home care may reduce (but not alter) susceptibility to caries. In addition, periodic topical fluoride applications seem to be effective in reducing caries. It is also suggested that a reduction of sugars and carbohydrates be a part of dietary control along with a reduction of between-meal snacks.

Once the teeth have been restored the patient must be placed on a regular, periodic recall examination schedule which should include both clinical and radiographic examinations.

Restore Proper Tooth Contour

The value of properly restored tooth form to the future health of the supporting tissues is well recognized. Failure to restore proper contour and contact increases the incidence of periodontal disorders. For example, open or weak contacts occur from incorrect use of matrix bands while incorrect use of interproximal wedges results in gingival overhangs of restorative materials. Such overhangs are significant in incitement of gingival inflammation. This inflammation usually is followed by loss of bone and by pocket formation, destroying the supporting tissues about the tooth. Furthermore, accumulation of food debris in poorly contoured areas often results in failure of the restoration due to recurrent caries.

A high percentage of periodontal problems are related directly to nonphysiologic contours, open or weak contacts, and marginal ridge discrepancies. Obviously, correction can be accomplished only by proper replacement of the restoration.

Restore Function

The natural and proper action of the teeth is dependent on occlusion with teeth in the opposing arch. Without this occlusion the teeth will not perform their individual masticatory functions. It then becomes obvious that when carious teeth are restored, they should be restored to optimal contact with opposing teeth to regain this functional relationship. Usually, when a tooth is in its normal (correct) position in the dental arch, restoration to proper contour will restore the tooth to function. When cast gold restorations are utilized, the dentist has an excellent opportunity to restore malposed teeth to a corrected occlusal plane. Naturally, restoration of function is achieved in the procedure.

Restore Esthetics

Many patients are more concerned about the esthetic quality of a restoration than they are about the expected service of the restoration. However, patient concern about esthetics should not be the governing factor in the choice of restorative materials. Regardless of the restorative material being used, the more nearly the restoration approaches the original form of the tooth, the more pleasing is the final result. However, every effort should be made, particularly in the anterior segments, to obtain as pleasing a cosmetic result as possible. All restorative materials have both good and poor properties. A thorough understanding of the indications and contraindications of the various filling materials is necessary to accomplish restorative procedures that will be both long lasting and esthetically successful.

TERMINOLOGY OF OPERATIVE DENTISTRY

As is true of any profession, dentistry has a language of its own—a language the auxiliary must understand in order to converse with the dentist and the patient. Because reference to teeth, cavity classification, and preparations is made in terms of dental anatomy it is important that a basic knowledge of nomenclature be mastered early in the study of operative dentistry. The following list of definitions provides a foundation in terminology as related to operative dentistry (note Fig. 28-2):

1. *Cavity preparation.* The mechanical procedure required to remove caries and/or existing restorative materials and to properly shape the excavation to receive a restorative material.
2. *Cavity walls.* In all types of cavity preparations, the walls of the cavity take the name of the surface of the tooth toward which they face (e.g., mesial, distal, facial, lingual, and pulpal).
3. *Angles.* When two surfaces meet, they form a line

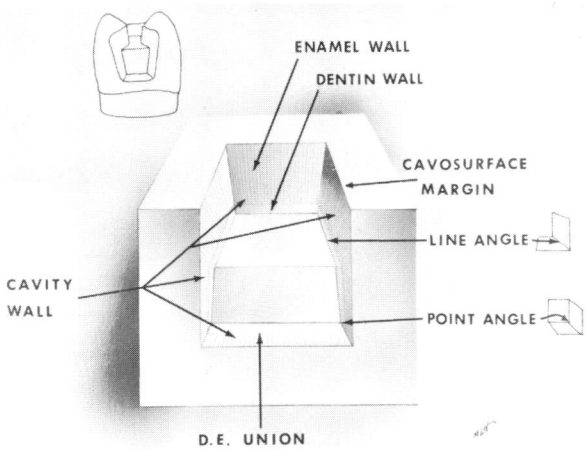

Figure 28-2 | Illustrating terminology used in cavity preparation. (*From Dental Assisting, Course V, Clinical Sciences, University of North Carolina, 1966.*)

which is named for the joining surfaces and which is referred to as a *line angle*. For example, the line formed by the mesial and facial walls would be the mesiofacial line angle. When three surfaces meet they form a *point angle* which is named by combining the names of the joining surfaces (e.g., the junction of the distal, lingual, and pulpal walls forms the distolinguopulpal line angle).

4. *Enamel wall.* That portion of a cavity wall that is enamel.

5. *Dentin wall.* That portion of a cavity wall that is dentin.
6. *Dentinoenamel union.* The line that is formed by the junction of the enamel and dentin.
7. *Cavosurface margin.* The line that is formed by the junction of a cavity wall and the external surface of the tooth.

CLASSIFICATION OF CAVITIES

A classification of cavities is necessary to standardize records during the examination, charting, diagnosis, and treatment of a patient's oral condition. Likewise, communication between dental personnel is facilitated when there is common agreement on cavity classification. One of the prime reasons the dental assistant should be knowledgeable in classification of cavities is that each class of cavity denotes that a certain procedure is necessary to restore the tooth. While each class of cavity demands a different treatment (and instrumentation), it will be noted that certain steps and procedures may be common to all classes. The following classification will help the student understand the assistant's duties relative to operative procedures and to comprehend professional clinics, papers, and journals.

Simple, Compound, and Complex Cavities

The simplest form of cavity classification is according to the *number of surfaces* involved. *Simple cavities* are those occurring on one surface of the tooth. When two surfaces of the tooth are involved the cavity is referred to as a *compound* cavity. When three or more surfaces are involved, the cavity is referred to as a *complex cavity*. See Fig. 28-3. This classification is very generalized but it should indicate to the student that the cavity involving only one surface certainly is less complicated in scope than a complex cavity.

Figure 28-3 | Cavity classification. (1) Simple cavity, (2) compound cavity, (3) complex cavity.

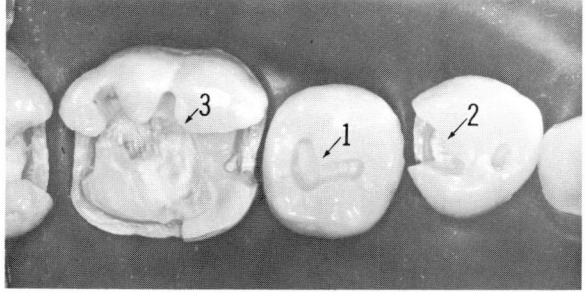

As stated previously, cavities may occur on one or more of the surfaces of the tooth and may be of various sizes ranging from very small to those which include all five surfaces. A second classification uses the names of the involved surfaces (mesial, distal, facial, lingual, occlusal, or incisal). In conversation, a cavity is denoted by naming the surface or surfaces involved such as *mesial* or *distoocclusal*. When writing this classification the first letter of the words naming the surfaces are used as abbreviations, such as M and DO. Note that capital letters are used. Practically all dentists use a number system to identify teeth. When the tooth as well as the involved surfaces are identified, record keeping becomes simple but exact. For example, an entry such as 3-MO-Amal would mean that on the maxillary right first molar a mesioocclusal cavity was restored with amalgam alloy.

Pit and Fissure and Smooth-Surface Cavities

Cavities may be further classified according to the location of the inception of the carious lesion. This classification simply differentiates between *pit and fissure* cavities and *smooth-surface* cavities (Fig. 28-4).

Caries most frequently has its inception in the developmental pits and fissures. Such areas are deeper than the surrounding tooth substance and are almost impossible to thoroughly cleanse, which creates ideal conditions for bacterial plaque formation. Pit and fissure cavities are found in the following locations:

1. Occlusal surfaces of the premolars and molars
2. Lingual pits of maxillary incisors
3. Facial groove and pit of the mandibular molars
4. Lingual groove and pit of the maxillary molars
5. Pits occurring in atypical areas, generally attributed to irregularities during the formation of the enamel

Smooth-surface cavities are found in the following locations:

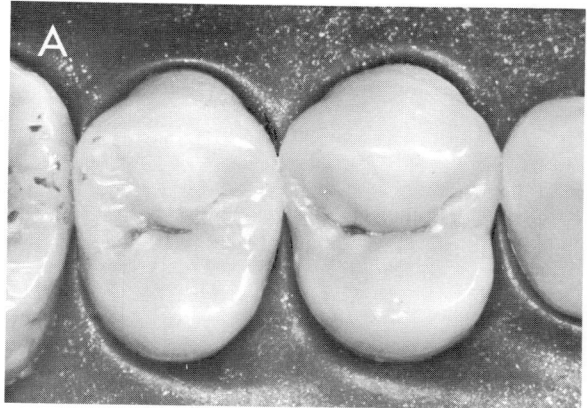

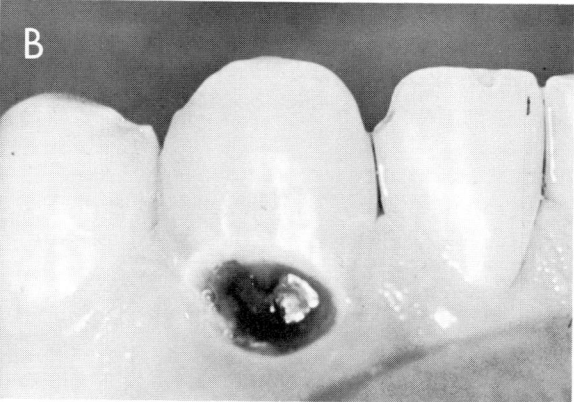

Figure 28-4 | Cavity classification. A. Pit and fissure cavity. B. Smooth-surface cavity.

1. Proximal surfaces of all the teeth
2. Gingival one-third on the facial and lingual of all the teeth

It is difficult to detect initial interproximal smooth-surface caries on posterior teeth because it usually begins just below (gingival to) the contact area where examination with the explorer is virtually impossible. Periodic bitewing radiographs are required to locate these areas. When the teeth are isolated with cotton rolls and dried with air, clinical examination will locate beginning lesions on the facial and lingual of the teeth.

Classification According to Treatment

The following classification is the most widely used, and all cavities may be identified with one of the six classes according to their treatment:

Class I.   All pit and fissure cavities
Class II. All proximal-surface cavities on the premolars and molars
Class III. All proximal-surface cavities on the incisors and canines which do not involve the removal and restoration of the incisal angle
Class IV. All proximal-surface cavities on the incisors and canines which involve the removal and restoration of the incisal angle
Class V.   All gingival one-third cavities
Class VI. All cavities on the incisal edge or the occlusal surface where attritional wear has removed the enamel to expose the underlying dentin

CAVITY PREPARATION DESIGNS

In the preparation of any tooth the dentist must follow certain established rules and base the design of the cavity preparation on biologic and mechanical principles that are of paramount importance in producing good dentistry. It follows, then, that the dental assistant must have a basic knowledge of cavity design in order to properly perform assigned duties. To be completely efficient the dental assistant must anticipate the needs of the dentist and this is possible only by being thoroughly familiar with all types of cavity preparations and the procedures incident to their completion.

Cavity design for a replacement restoration or for the tooth with initial caries is basically dependent upon (1) the location of the caries, (2) the amount and extent of the caries, (3) the amount of lost tooth substance, (4) the restorative material to be used, and (5) the presence of existing restorations in those teeth which need to be refilled due to recurrent caries and/or failure of the restoration from other causes.

One-Surface Cavities

Preparations which are confined to only one surface of the tooth may be designed to receive one of a variety of restorative materials, such as: (1) silver amalgam, (2) gold foil, (3) gold inlays, (4) silicate cement, (5) self-curing resin, and (6) composite resins. Because each restorative material has different physical properties the operator must design the cavity preparation to take advantage of these known properties. In addition, the morphology of the tooth often has an influence on the design of the preparation, regardless of the type of restorative material to be used.

Occlusal-Surface Preparation for Silver Amalgam

This is perhaps the cavity preparation which takes the least amount of the operator's time to complete. Because it is considered a simple cavity and access is usually not difficult, details of cavity preparation which make the difference between a good preparation and a poor one are often overlooked. (It should be remembered that the expected life of a restoration is basically dependent on the quality of the cavity preparation.) The outline form is basically governed by the pit and fissure anatomy on the occlusal surface in that all pits and fissures are removed with the result that the general appearance of the cavity is one of smooth curves rather than sharp angles. As these pits and fissures are removed, the cavity is extended to place the cavosurface margin on relatively smooth tooth structure. Also, the facial and lingual extensions of the preparation do not exceed the position necessary to include the fissure anatomy and/or the existing caries. Should the facial and lingual extensions exceed a point halfway between the central groove and the cusp points, the dentist will usually change the cavity design from a one-surface preparation to a more complex design. The mesial and distal margins are extended only enough to include the caries and remove

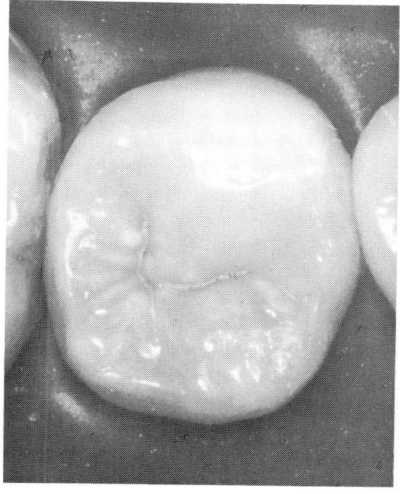 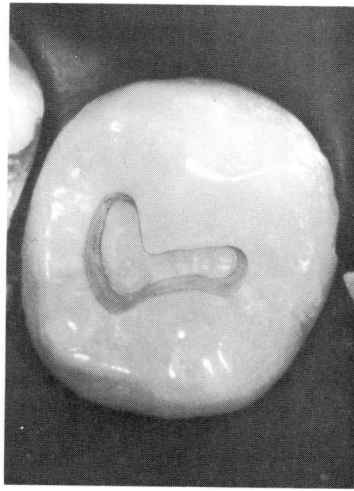

Figure 28-5 | Occlusal-surface cavity preparation for amalgam.

unsupported enamel. The depth of the cavity is established so that the pulpal wall is in dentin—approximately 0.2 mm below the dentinoenamel union. The student should study the cavity preparation in Fig. 28-5 which was prepared as described above.

Facial-Surface Preparation for Tooth-colored Restorative Materials

Usually, the gingival areas of the anterior teeth are restored with one of the tooth-colored restorative materials when the patient is concerned about esthetics. This does not mean, however, that metal restorations cannot be placed in these areas. Restorations in the gingival areas are necessary mainly because the tooth structure is carious or because it has been worn away due to incorrect brushing habits (abrasion). Even though the outline form is relatively simple to obtain (because of the smooth tooth surface) the Class V cavity will often present special problems in preparation and restoration not usually associated with other types of restorations.

The gingival margin is usually positioned just beneath the crest of the free gingival tissue. The mesial and distal margins are extended to include the caries (when metal is to be used as a restorative material these margins are extended to the "corners" of the tooth). Depth of the preparation is approximately 1 mm. Because the cavity walls must follow the direction of the enamel rods they are at 90 degrees to the external tooth surface and diverge outwardly from the pulpal wall. Retention of the restorative material must be provided for by mechanical locks along the incisoaxial and gingivoaxial line angles. Retention may also be established or improved by acid-etching the enamel walls of the preparation. This procedure is described in another section of this chapter. Study of the cavity preparation in Fig. 28-6 should help the student understand the fundamentals of the Class V cavity preparation.

Multiple-Surface Cavities

Whenever caries attacks a proximal surface(s) of posterior teeth, the cavity preparation necessary to include the affected surface must also include preparation of the occlusal surface. Compound and complex cavities may include one or both of the proximal surfaces as well as portions of the facial and lingual surfaces (Fig. 28-7).

Preparation of the occlusal portion of multiple-surface cavities is accomplished using the fundamentals as previously described for one-surface preparations. There are basic differences between the design of preparations when amalgam is to be used and where gold inlays are used. The walls of the inlay preparation must diverge occlusally to provide draw (draft) to the cavity to permit the restoration to be placed en masse, while the walls of the amalgam cavity preparation converge occlusally, providing retention form for the restorative material. Also, a cavosurface bevel is necessary on the inlay preparation to ensure proper marginal fit of the metal to the tooth surface.

In addition, certain other important requirements must be met to fulfill the objectives of cavity preparation. These are (1) sufficient gingival extension to position the gingival wall on sound tooth and out of contact with the adjacent tooth, (2) sufficient facial and lingual extension to position the cavity margins in sound tooth structure and beyond the contact area, and (3) sufficient removal of tooth structure to provide adequate bulk of restorative material. The student must understand the differences in cavity preparation as required for the various restorative materials to effectively assist the operator during preparation procedures.

STEPS IN CAVITY PREPARATION

As with any other technical procedure, cavity preparation is accomplished through a systematic, well-organized approach, with each step performed as nearly perfectly as possible before the next is begun. Situations sometimes occur when the order of steps may be altered; however, if consistent results are to be obtained, it is wise to

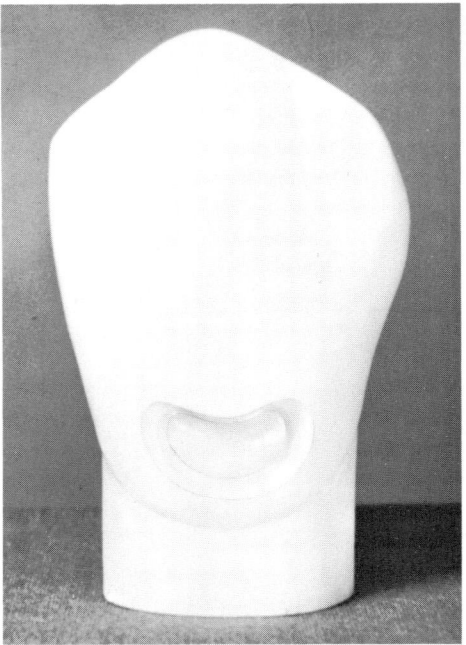

Figure 28-6 | Facial-surface cavity preparation for self-curing resin.

follow the usual sequence. So that the student will fully understand each step of cavity preparation and be entirely capable of performing assigned duties, each step will be briefly discussed. The steps of cavity preparation are as follows:

1. Establishing the outline form
2. Obtaining the resistance form
3. Obtaining the retention form
4. Obtaining the convenience form
5. Removing the remaining carious dentin
6. Finishing the enamel walls and margins
7. Cleansing the cavity

Establishing the Outline Form

Establishing the outline form locates the position of the cavity margins in the completed cavity preparation. Usually the experienced operator will be able to visualize the configuration of the completed cavity before cutting procedures are begun by viewing the extent of the caries in the radiograph, examining the tooth for existing restorations, and noting the position of the soft tissue. While the outline form is somewhat governed by the above, there are some general rules which also dictate the final position of the cavity margin. These are (1) extending the cavity margin to include all pits and fissures, (2) extending all cavity margins until positioned in sound tooth structure, with no unsupported enamel remaining, (3) joining two or more pits and fissures when they are in close proximity to one another, (4) avoiding cusp tips and the eminences of marginal ridges which are subject to occlusal stresses, (5) extending proximal margins to areas accessible to inspection and finishing, (6) extending gingival margins beneath the crest of the tissue when appropriate, and (7) extending the margins to allow sufficient access for proper manipulative procedures.

Many restorations fail due to recurrent caries because the principles of establishing the outline form are violated. Considerable attention to the details in positioning the cavity margins is important in the life expectancy of the restoration.

Obtaining the Resistance Form

Resistance form is obtained by shaping the internal walls of the cavity preparation to enable the tooth to best resist and withstand the stress applied to it during mastication. Because caries or existing restorations, or both, reduce the strength of the tooth, special emphasis is placed on preparing the weakened tooth to withstand not only the vertical forces but also the lateral forces.

There are certain features which when incorporated into the cavity design aid the tooth in resisting the masticatory forces. These include (1) utilization of the box shape with a flat floor which provides a broad base at right angles to the vertical forces of mastication, (2) minimum extension of all cavity walls to retain the strong

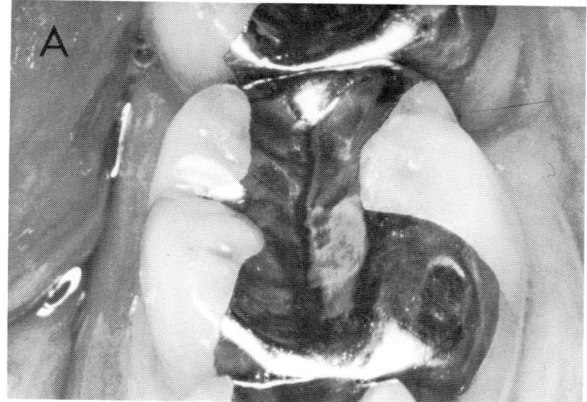
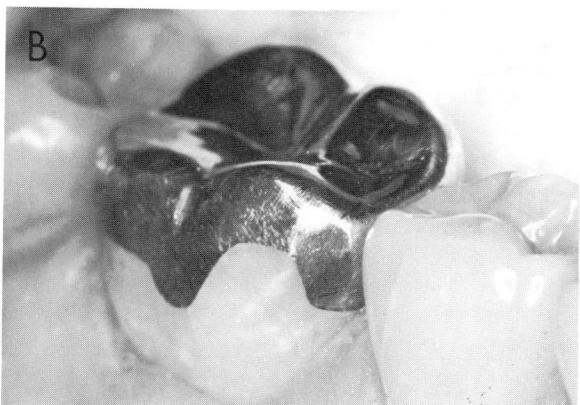

Figure 28-7 | Multiple-surface cavities. A. Amalgam restoration. B. Inlay restoration.

dentin-supported cuspal areas, and (3) inclusion of sufficient tooth within the restoration to prevent or resist fracture of the tooth due to lateral stress.

Obtaining the Retention Form

Retention form is that part of cavity preparation which deals with the provisions for preventing the restoration from being dislodged through tipping or lifting forces. None of the restorative materials presently available to the profession

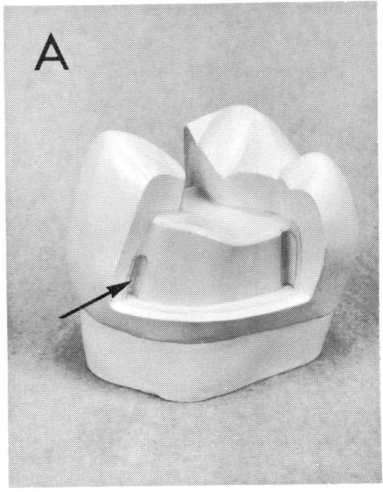
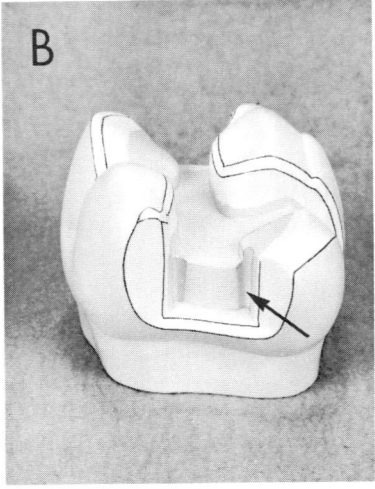

Figure 28-8 | Retention form. A. Retention locks (arrow) in an amalgam preparation. B. Retention grooves (arrow) in an inlay preparation.

have the ability to truly adhere to tooth structure; therefore, some mechanical retention is necessary, even though the filling material is closely adapted to the cavity walls.

Depending on the type of material to be used, certain retentive features are prepared in the tooth structure to enhance the retention of the restoration. Class I cavity preparations for amalgam are four-sided and the convergence occlusally of the facial and lingual walls provides adequate retention form. In Class II cavity preparations for amalgam the facial and lingual walls, both occlusal and proximal, again converge occlusally. This design automatically provides retention for the amalgam alloy. Additional retention is placed in the proximal portion by placing *retention locks* in the facioaxial and linguoaxial line angles. Usually, these locks extend from the point angle to the level of the axiopulpal line angle (Fig. 28-8).

As previously mentioned, cavity preparations for inlays are designed with draw to permit insertion of the inlay. The amount of draw has an influence on the retention form; that is, excessive draw reduces the retentive feature because the walls of the preparation are less parallel. When the clinical crown of the tooth is relatively short, special care is necessary to keep the walls more parallel. As in the amalgam cavity preparation, additional retention is placed in the proximal

Figure 28-9 | Cemented stainless-steel pins provide additional retention for amalgam alloy.

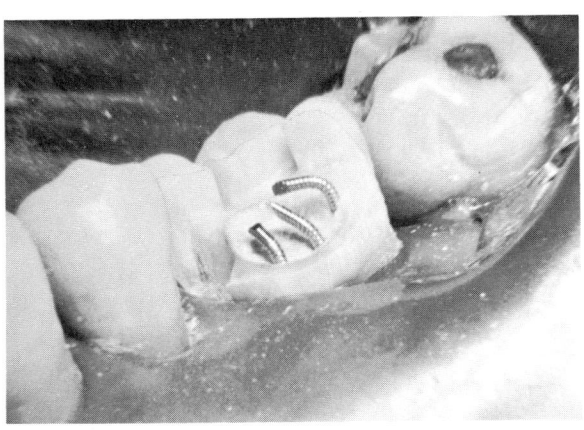

portion in the line angles, with draw, and these are referred to as *retention grooves* (Fig. 28-8).

Often, when most of the tooth crown must be removed in preparation, retention form becomes difficult to obtain. In amalgam procedures, threaded, cemented, stainless-steel or friction-lock pins may be inserted in selected positions around which the restorative material is condensed (Fig. 28-9). When cast restorations are utilized, additional retention is obtained by preparing one or more pinholes which receive wires that are part of the casting and are cemented in the holes in the process of inserting the restoration.

Class V preparations for amalgam, gold foil, silicate cement, composite, and self-curing resins must also include retentive areas for the restorative material. Recall that all the walls in the Class V preparation diverge away from the axial wall, making it essential that mechanical retention be provided.

Obtaining the Convenience Form

Convenience form refers to those considerations which aid the operation, both in cavity preparation and insertion of the restoration. These considerations allow adequate observation, accessibility, and ease of operation. The use of high-speed handpieces has increased the abuse of convenience form because tooth structure removal has been made easy. Slight additional extension of cavity walls is permitted to provide convenient access to remote parts of the cavity preparation. This procedure allows the best visibility and often permits the procedure to be completed without extreme difficulty.

To provide areas to begin the condensation of gold foil, small recesses in addition to the usual retention form are placed in the point angles and are referred to as *convenience points* (Fig. 28-10).

Removing the Remaining Carious Dentin

Removal of remaining caries is that step in cavity preparation in which carious dentin not removed in the preceding steps is removed. In teeth with small carious lesions, the completion of the preceding steps will have removed all the caries when the axial and pulpal walls have been established at their correct position. However, in those teeth with larger cavities, removal of caries should occur in this step. Removal of caries is accomplished using either round burs or spoon excavators or both. Usually, this step of cavity preparation is accomplished with the tooth isolated with the rubber dam. Often, when all the carious material has been removed some stained tooth structure will still be visible. When the dentin has a firm feel with the explorer, removal

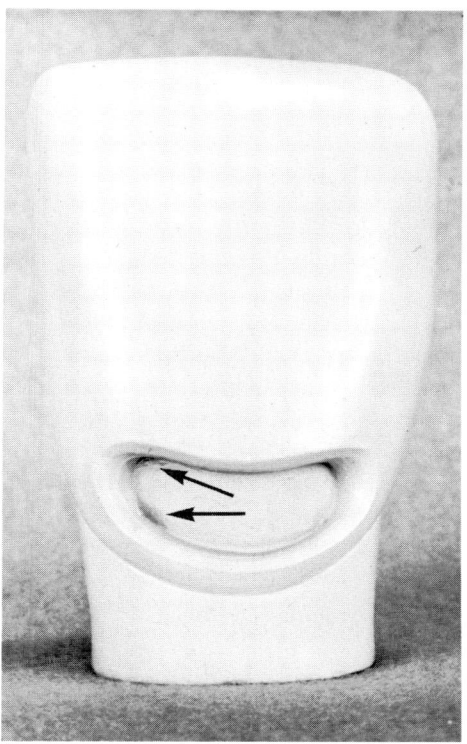

Figure 28-10 | Cavity preparation for gold foil. Note convenience points (arrows).

of tooth structure should cease, even if stained dentin remains.

When a patient presents with many large carious areas, the operator will perform *caries control*. This procedure involves removal of the caries and placement of a temporary restoration, and may or may not include all the previous steps of cavity preparation. The objective in this procedure is to stop the ingress of caries, to place temporary fillings, and to "hold" these teeth until they may be treated individually.

Finishing the Enamel Walls

Finishing the enamel walls, the last *cutting* step in the preparation of the cavity, prepares the enamel walls to effect the best marginal seal possible between the restorative material and tooth structure. With the tooth (teeth) isolated with the rubber dam the operator inspects every portion of the cavity with special attention to the enamel walls. Using carbide burs, diamond stones, or hand cutting instruments, the walls are completed by removing loose or unsupported enamel, or both, to create the strongest possible enamel wall. The strongest enamel walls are those with full-length enamel rods whose ends are supported by sound dentin and which are further supported on the cavity side by shorter rods whose ends are also resting on sound dentin.

Cleansing the Cavity

This is the final step in the preparation of the cavity and includes the removal of accumulated debris, drying the cavity, and final inspection prior to restoration procedures. It is extremely important that all debris be removed from the cavity, especially the margins, because deposits left on them will subsequently dissolve, resulting in a leak which invites recurrent caries.

Flushing the cavity with warm water usually will remove all debris. Stubborn particles of debris can usually be removed with a small cotton pellet, damp with water or hydrogen peroxide. Redrying of the cavity should follow. Once the cavity is cleansed completely, procedures incident to its restoration follow.

The preceding material in this chapter should give the dental assistant sufficient information to be knowledgeable in the fundamentals of operative dentistry. Without this knowledge the dental assistant will be ineffective in assigned duties during chairside procedures. The following material will present those duties required of the dental assistant in the full scope of operative dentistry. Knowledge of operative dentistry principles and mastery of the skills related to chairside procedures permit the assistant to become a valued member of the dental health team.

THE DENTAL TEAM IN PRACTICE

The dental profession well recognizes the value of dental auxiliary personnel, particularly that of the full-time chairside assistant. A part of the dental student education today is training in how to properly utilize a chairside assistant and instruction in the team approach to dental treatment. The concept of teamwork in dentistry is centered on chairside procedures in which the assistant works in close harmony with the dentist to accomplish more and better dentistry with as little stress and strain as possible.

The dental assistant recognizes operative procedures as being divided into three groups of duties, those necessary (1) in preparation for the appointment, (2) during the work-accomplishment phase, and (3) in cleaning up after the work has been done. Because the basis of teamwork is concerned with those duties associated with patient treatment, it is necessary to discuss certain factors which influence the efficiency and effectiveness of the dental team.

Sitting to Work

Teamwork at the chairside cannot be fully developed until both the dentist and the assistant work

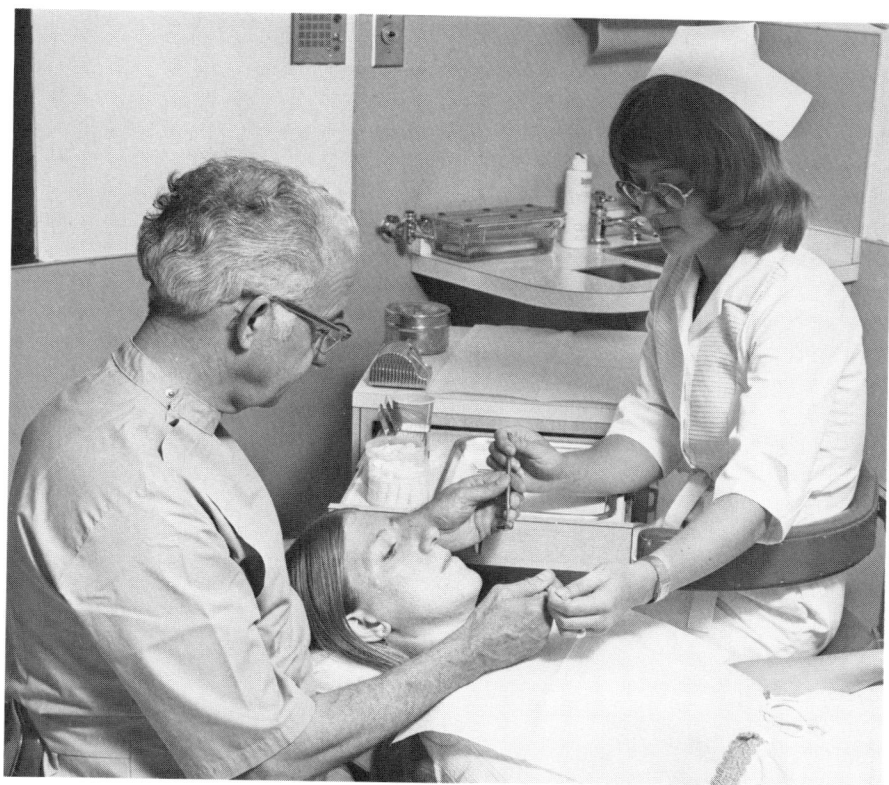

Figure 28-11 | Operator, assistant, and patient properly positioned for sit-down dentistry.

from a seated position and with the patient properly positioned for the team to best approach the work area (Fig. 28-11). The object of having the team sit to work is to reduce tension and body stress during appointments.

Requirements of good posture are that the body be aligned and supported so that the weight is distributed throughout the musculoskeletal system. The operating chair must be designed to permit this type of posture in that it must be fully adjustable for backrest and seat height. First, adjust the vertical height to allow the thighs to be parallel to the floor, the lower legs perpendicular, and the feet flat on the floor. The backrest should be adjusted to a position above the crest of the ilium and below the last rib for proper support to the lower back. The seat should be broader than the posterior anatomy of the person to use the chair. The seat portion of the operator's chair is often contoured for increased comfort. An essential feature of the assistant's chair is a metal footrest (metal ring or platform) which is needed because the assistant normally sits 4 to 6 in higher than the dentist. Without this footrest, the assistant's feet would be improperly positioned and the lower extremities would be in a stressful position due to poor posture.

Also, the chair should be equipped with casters to permit unrestricted mobility about the patient's chair.

Naturally, when the dental team sits to operate, the patient must be reclined sufficiently to place the head at the proper operating level.

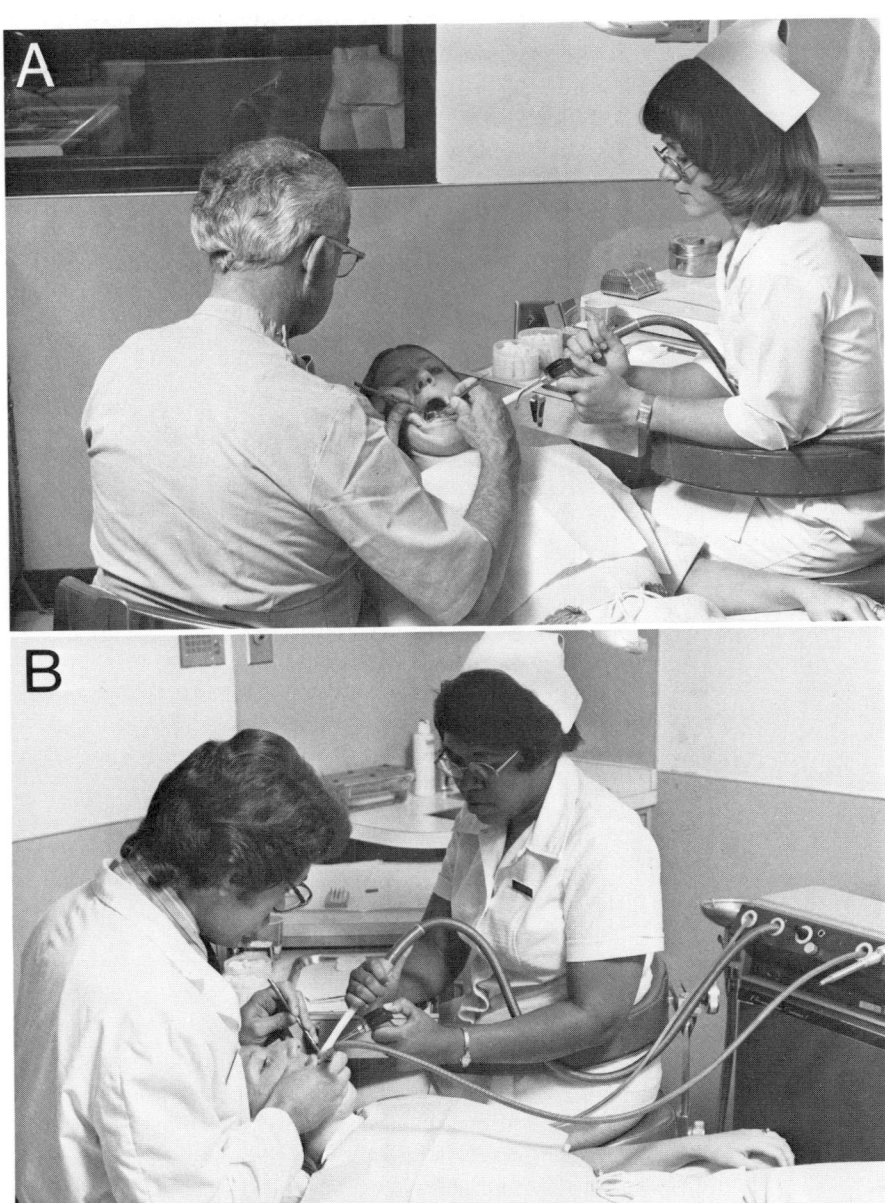

Figure 28-12 | Work positions for the dental team. A. Operator at right front, assistant to patient's left. B. Operator at right rear, assistant to patient's left.

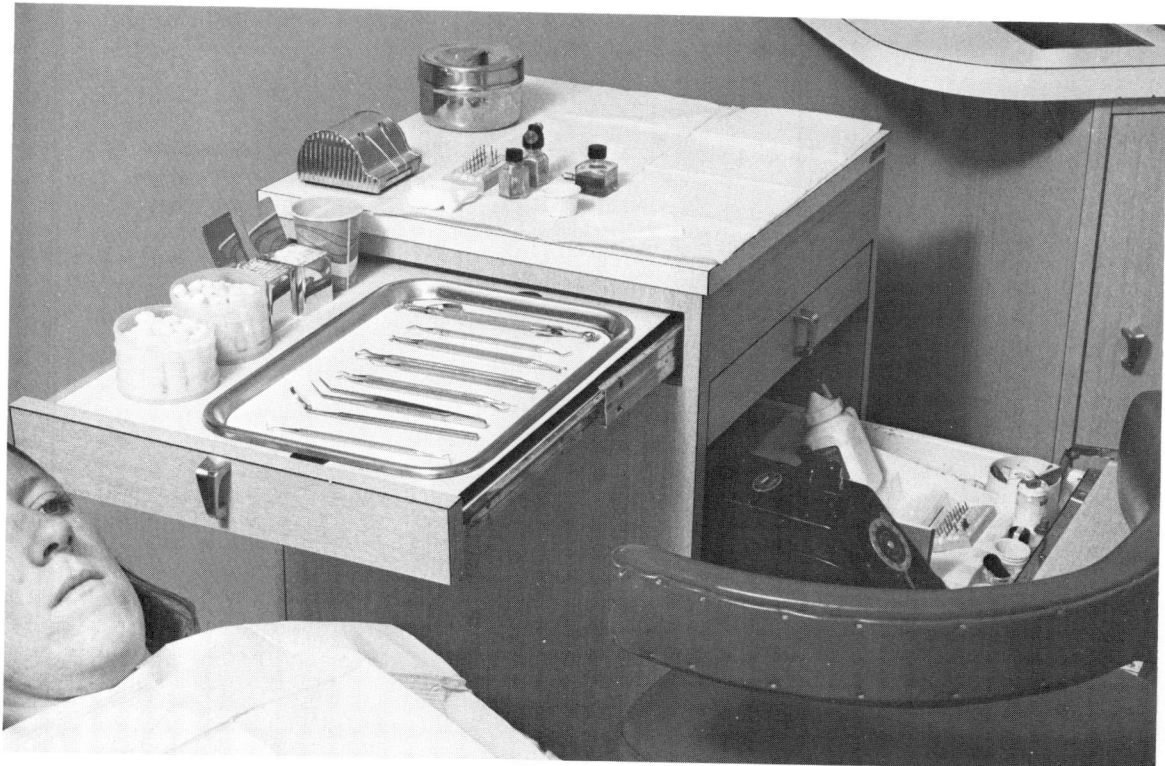

Figure 28-13 | Mobile cabinet in proper position to left rear of patient's chair.

Chair positioning and seating the patient are discussed later in the chapter.

Work Area

Work positions of the dentist and assistant are oriented to the primary work area which is located just in front of the patient's mouth. Depending on the area of the mouth to be operated, the work position should be such that it provides maximum function for the dentist as well as the assistant (Fig. 28-12). Work positions may be oriented by comparing the work area to the face of a large clock with the patient's head being related to the twelve o'clock position. The dentist most often works from a right-rear approach to the patient which is the eleven o'clock position. The second most useful work position for the dentist is a right-front approach, which corresponds to the seven o'clock position. At times, work positions for the dentist may fall between the seven and eleven o'clock positions to make it convenient to work unimpeded; however, a true right-rear or right-front position usually will place the operator in positions to approach any area of the patient's mouth.

The position for the assistant is to the patient's left, facing the patient from the three o'clock position. This position affords the assistant the best access to all instruments and materials with a minimum of movement. Usually, instruments are placed on a tray, either on a tray stand or on a mobile cabinet, and are positioned to the left rear of the patient (Fig. 28-13).

Once an operative procedure is begun, the dentist should not have to reach outside the work zone (that area immediate to the patient's mouth). The domain of the chairside assistant may be divided into a primary and a secondary work circle. The primary work circle includes the tray setup, the unit, and the work zone, all of which are usually within the one to five o'clock positions. All items should be positioned within easy access at comfortable arm's length. The secondary work circle is all the other space in the operatory not included in the dentist's area or the primary circle of the chairside assistant.

Figure 28-14 | Mobile dental cabinet. A. Access to cabinet drawers is to assistant's immediate right. B. Tray setup positioned directly over assistant's lap.

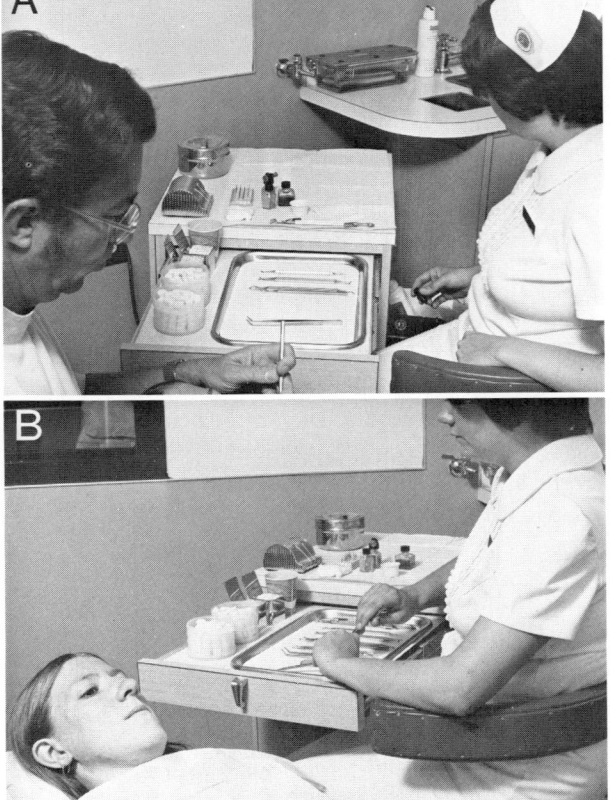

Ideally, a roving assistant should be present and function in the secondary work circle on instruction from either the dentist or the chairside assistant. When there is only one assistant, it is necessary that proper preparation be made prior to beginning the procedure to prevent the auxiliary from having to leave the primary work area.

Mobile Cabinets

The mobile dental cabinet is an improvement in dental operating procedures because it allows the dentist and the assistant to bring the instruments and materials to the chair and unit (Fig. 28-14). In this way any procedure can be performed for any patient without either member of the operating team having to leave the chair. Mobile cabinets also provide a time saving of great value, allow the dentist to see more patients as a consequence, and reduce the number of movements away from the chair for the dentist and the assistant.

In addition, the top of the cabinet may also be used as a setup area which moves the instruments and materials from the patient's view. When tray setups are prepared for all general office procedures, they are particularly valuable because they save so much time and motion for the assistant in the setting-up and cleaning-up phases of the procedure.

Once the auxiliary is seated, the mobile cabinet is moved to the one o'clock position. This position places the tray setup over the assistant's knees, permitting easy access for the assistant and prevents the dentist from reaching to the setup. As long as the chairside assistant is in position, the dentist should never reach for anything; *everything needed is handed by the assistant.*

USE OF ORAL EVACUATOR

One of the primary responsibilities of the dental assistant is the use of the oral evacuator, especially during preparation procedures, to remove water, tooth particles, and saliva from the field of operation. There are other occasions when the evacuator is used to advantage, and these will be mentioned when the various operative procedures are discussed.

The advent of the high- and superspeed handpieces made it necessary to use more water during cutting procedures to flush the area free of debris and to act as a coolant for both the bur and the tooth. Because the saliva ejector does not remove water rapidly and because the patient usually is in a reclined position, the oral evacuator is used because it has the advantage of very quickly removing copious amounts of water, plus solids such as pieces of tooth and old restorations. When the assistant is skilled in the use of the evacuator, the operator can often complete a cavity preparation without annoying or time-consuming pauses.

The proper technique involves first placing a cotton roll in the vestibule between the teeth and the cheek (Fig. 28-15A). This procedure moves the adjacent soft tissues away from the tooth and provides a cushion on which the tip of the evacuator is placed to prevent impingement on the gingival tissue (Fig. 28-15C). Usually, the assistant will place the cotton roll just before the operative procedure is to begin.

The evacuator tip is held by the right hand in a palm and thumb grasp with the thumb directed away from the patient's mouth (Fig. 28-15B). This grasp is recommended to prevent fatigue in the fingers when pressure is required to retract the cheek or depress the tongue. The left hand is free to exchange instruments or to manipulate the multipurpose syringe. The evacuator tip is positioned just posterior (when possible) to the tooth to be prepared. By placing the tip first it retracts the cheek to provide the necessary access for the operator to position the mirror and handpiece. The disadvantage of placing the tip after the operator begins cutting is that vision and access are reduced to a minimum.

For the most part, the standard tip with the beveled end is utilized for both the maxillary and mandibular teeth; however, tips with a tissue-retracting flange are available and prove useful when tongue or cheek retraction presents a problem. As stated previously, the assistant should position the evacuating tip before the operator enters the mouth with the handpiece and mouth mirror. Once the operation is begun, the assistant should not attempt to move the tip, particularly while the operator is cutting tooth structure. Periodically, during the cutting operation, the operator will pause to examine the cavity, change burs, obtain a clean mirror, or reposition the handpiece. At this time the assistant should evacuate the material (water and debris) which has collected in the floor of the mouth. This movement can usually be made in 2 or 3 seconds and the tip returned to its original position without any interruption in the procedure.

The position for placement of the evacuating tip depends on the area to be operated upon. On the left posterior areas, both maxillary and mandibular, the tip is positioned adjacent to, or preferably just posterior to, the tooth to be prepared and should rest on a cotton roll previously placed in the vestibule (Fig. 28-15D). On the mandibular right teeth, the tip is placed to the lingual surface of the tooth. In the mandibular arch, a large cotton roll is placed between the teeth and tongue. On the right side, this provides a rest for the tip as well as to help hold the tongue aside (Fig. 28-15E). When the operative site is in the maxillary right arch, the assistant must be extremely cautious not to rest the tip on the delicate palatal tissue. When the anterior teeth are to be operated upon, a cotton roll is placed in the vestibule regardless of the direction of approach the dentist might choose. Usually, the tip is positioned next to the tooth surface opposite the approach of the handpiece.

When operating on the maxillary teeth, the operator uses the mouth mirror for visibility and light reflection. The assistant should direct a stream of air onto the mirror surface to keep it free of moisture and debris, permitting continu-

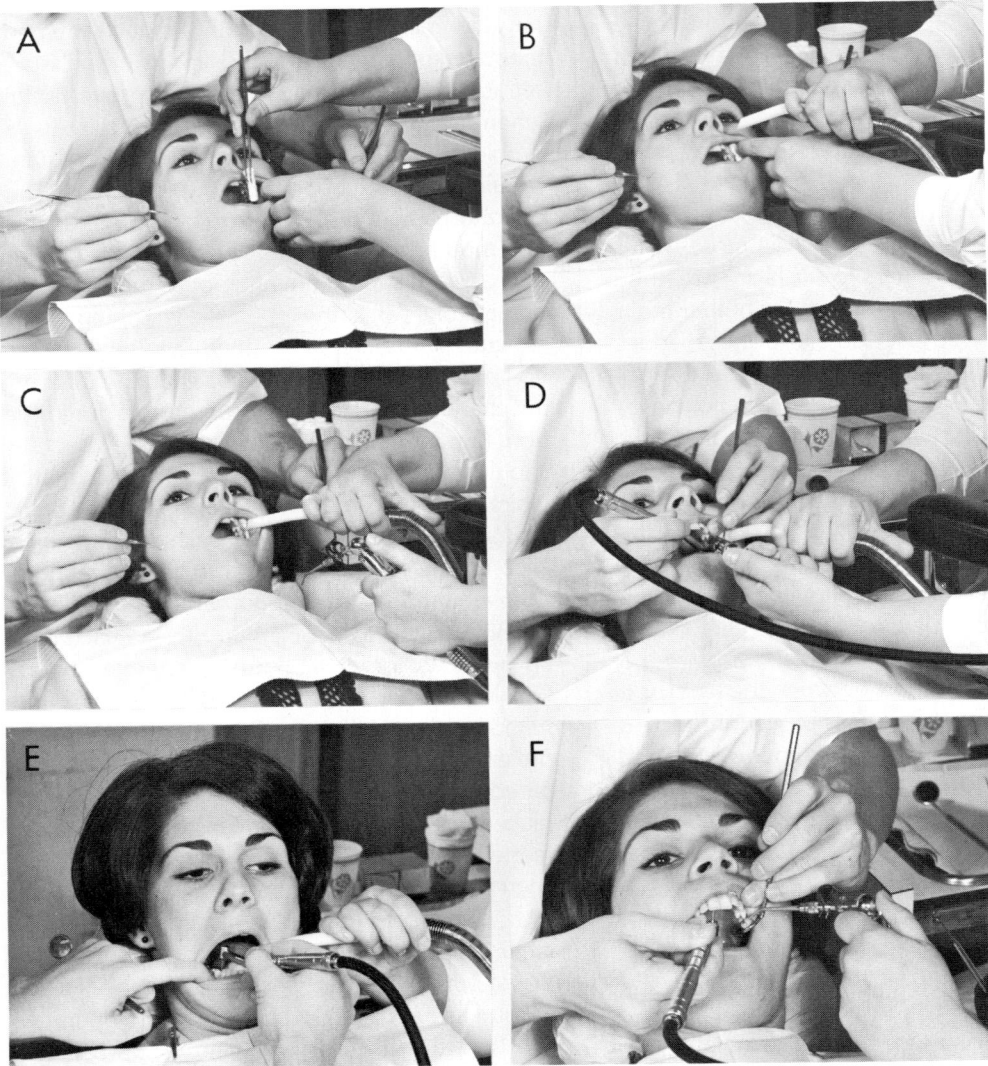

Figure 28-15 | Use of oral evacuator. A. Assistant positioning cotton roll. B. Proper grasp of evacuator tip. C. Evacuator tip retracting lip and cheek and positioned on cotton roll. D. Proper position for maxillary left. E. Proper position for mandibular right. F. Air tip directed onto mirror surface.

ous operation with maximum visibility. To be completely effective the tip of the air nozzle should be placed very close to the mirror surface (Fig. 28-15F) and the flow of air should be forceful enough to prevent accumulation of moisture and debris.

The above technique describes using the evacuator when the teeth have not been isolated with the rubber dam. Obviously, when the rubber dam is in place, the lips, cheek, and adjacent soft tissue are somewhat retracted. However, the assistant must continue to be cautious when positioning the evacuator tip to prevent soft-tissue injury under the rubber dam.

INSTRUMENT EXCHANGE

It is important that the operator and assistant have and practice a definite technique for the exchange of instruments (Fig. 28-16). Only when the pattern of exchange is standardized will the operating team eliminate confusion in chairside procedures.

First, it should be emphasized that the setup should be arranged in an orderly fashion. Usually, instruments are placed in the setup from left to right, in the sequence in which they are to be used, and they are returned to their original position following use. The major advantage of returning each instrument to its proper place is ease of locating a particular instrument in the event it must be reused. By being totally familiar with operative procedures, the auxiliary will be able to decide when the operator has no further need for some individual instruments. Rather than returning these instruments to the setup, they may be placed to one side out of the work area.

The dentist also has a part in helping to keep the instrument setup in an orderly manner. Should it be necessary to reach to the setup (this should not be necessary as long as the assistant is at the chairside), the dentist has the same responsibility of returning instruments to their proper place. The dentist contributes more significantly in two other ways: (1) by standardizing procedures and (2) by working in a systematic manner. When the dentist operates in this manner, the assistant easily anticipates the next step eliminating constant verbal instructions from the operator. Also, this kind of team effort allows the operator to concentrate vision on the operating site rather than the setup or dental unit. Ideally, the assistant should observe the tooth being operated upon and at the same time anticipate the needs of the operator in such a manner that the sequence of the operation is not interrupted.

The exchange of instruments usually takes place in a zone approximately 12 in^2 in front of the patient's mouth and at chin level. Obviously the exchange should not be directly over the patient's face. When both the operator and the assistant are familiar with the mutual area of exchange, delay and confusion in passing instruments are eliminated.

Once the patient is seated and the operator is ready to begin, the assistant will pass an explorer and a mirror. The signal for this procedure is when the dentist's hands are positioned in the exchange zone. This procedure of first passing the mirror and explorer should be standard operating procedure in order for the operator to examine the tooth (teeth) to be operated on. This is a necessary procedure to determine that conditions concerning the treatment plan have not changed since it was formulated.

In any pattern of instrument exchange, there should be a signal from the operator when an instrument needs to be discarded. The alert assistant will not need a verbal command to make the exchange but will constantly be ready when the exchange sign from the operator occurs. The usual instruction (sign language) for exchange is when the operator directs the handle of the instrument toward the assistant. When this type of movement begins, the assistant moves a hand into the exchange zone and receives the instrument by grasping the handle. The assistant may retrieve the instrument with either hand. At the time of release, the operator maintains hand position in such a manner that the next instrument can be received in the pen grasp so that it is ready to use when placed in the patient's mouth. When no other duties are required of the assistant, the exchange may take place with the assistant using one hand to receive and the other to pass the next instrument. However, an effective exchange procedure involves the left hand of the assistant, leaving the right hand to hold the evacuator or for other duties required at the time. Using this method, the little finger of the assis-

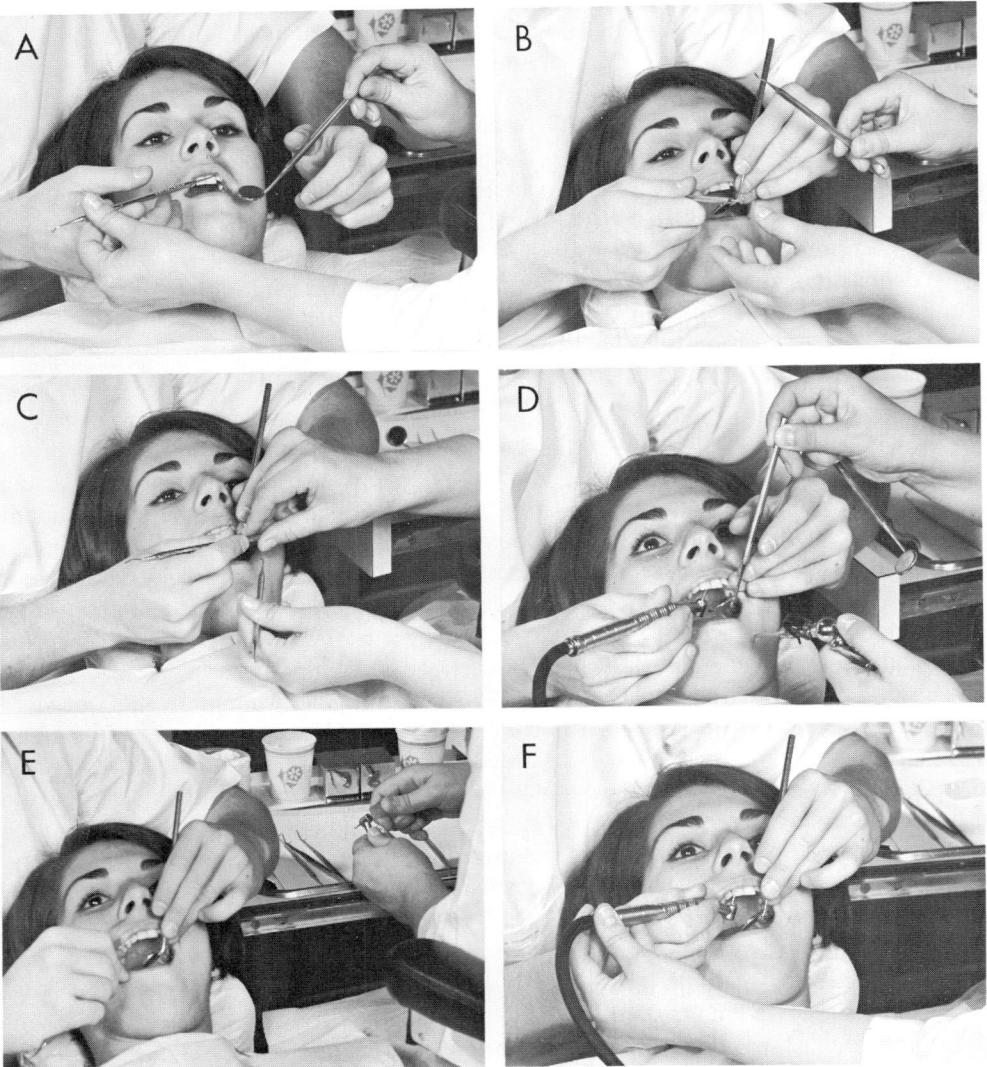

Figure 28-16 | Instrument exchange. A. Assistant passing mirror and explorer. B. Instrument exchange in progress. C. Exchange completed. D. Assistant positioning clean mirror. Note that operator has not moved rest finger. E. Assistant changing bur in handpiece while operator uses hand instrument. F. Assistant positioning handpiece in operator's hand.

tant's left hand retrieves while the thumb and forefinger hold the instrument to be delivered. This is easily accomplished by a rotation of the hand once the little finger has received the instrument being discarded (Fig. 28-17).

Most instruments used in operative dentistry are held in a pen grasp, and the hand position of the operator will indicate to the assistant how the instrument should be passed. When the operator wishes to use the palm and thumb grasp, the in-

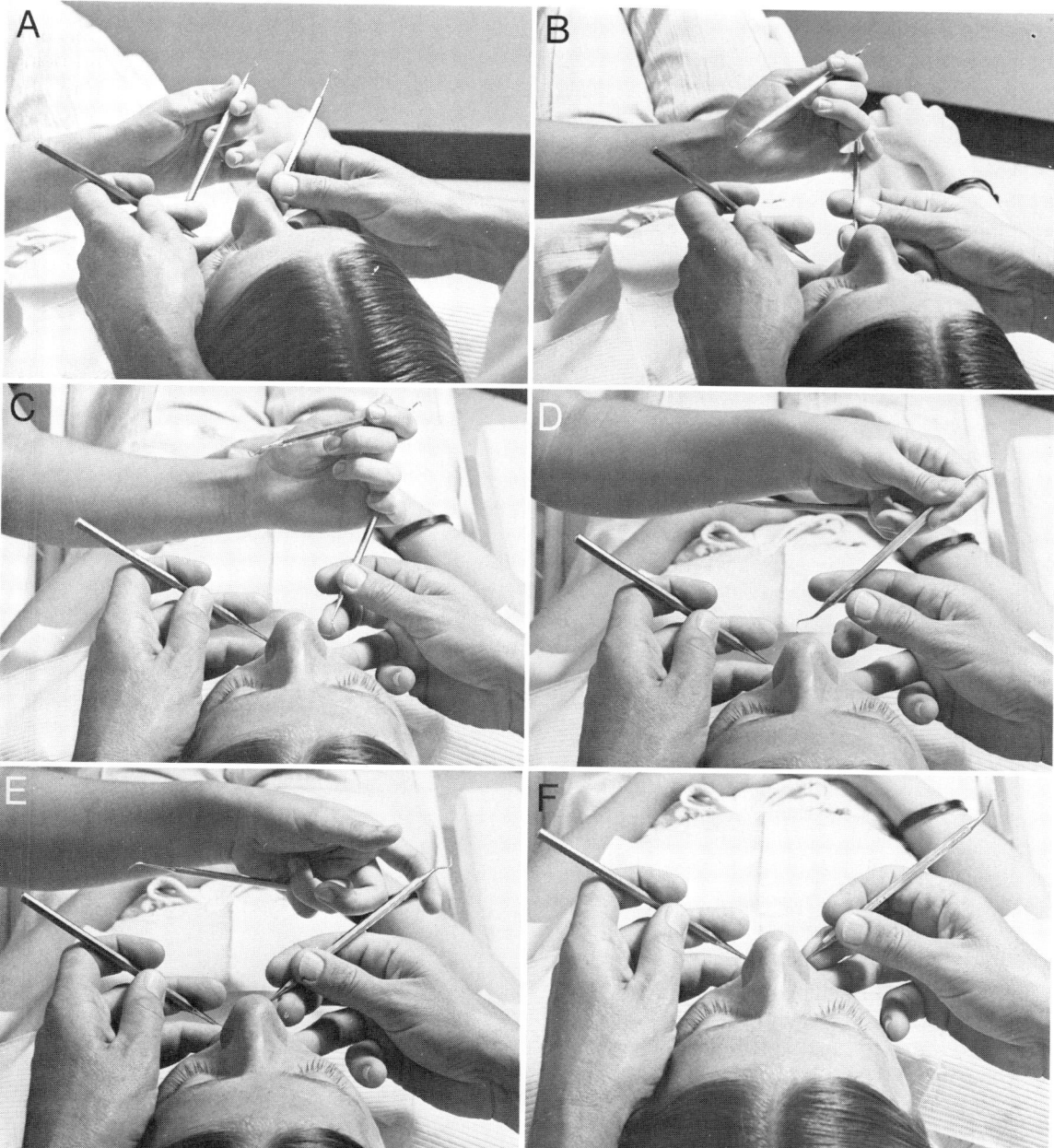

Figure 28-17 | Instrument exchange. A. Ready position. Note parallelism of both instruments. B. Little finger ready to grasp instrument to be retrieved. C. Instrument being removed from operator's grasp. D. Second instrument being placed in operator's hand. E. Second instrument released by assistant. F. Exchange completed.

strument will be correctly placed for use when the operator's hand is positioned in a palm open (and facing up) position. When the instrument is placed in the operator's hand ready to use either in the pen grasp or the palm and thumb position, it is not necessary for the instrument to be rotated or twirled into the work position.

During the greater part of most operative procedures the operator holds a mirror for indirect vision and to reflect light. The alert assistant will place two or more mirrors in the setup and will exchange an unclean mirror for a clean one without interfering with the operation. Obviously, the assistant should make no attempt to exchange the mirror while the operator is using the handpiece unless a signal for exchange is made. The appropriate time is when the bur is removed from the tooth. The reflecting surface of the clean mirror should be placed in the same position as the soiled one was prior to the exchange.

The exchange of all instruments is done with firm, deliberate movements to give both the operator and the assistant the feeling of confidence and to eliminate lost time and motion.

The exchange of handpiece burs can also be a team effort in that the operator holds the handpiece in the area of exchange and the assistant removes and replaces the bur. Should the operator use a different instrument between bur exchanges, the assistant changes the bur outside the exchange zone, usually over the tray setup.

Patients become aware of efficiency in the dental office, particularly during operative procedures. A sure, practical method of instrument exchange is one way to show efficiency and promote the patient's confidence in the operating team.

GENERAL OFFICE DUTIES

Traditionally, the dental assistant has done more than assist at the chair. This includes being efficient at the chairside, as well as being able to perform the business office duties, accomplishing some laboratory procedures, and being a good housekeeper. Offices vary from the one-assistant office to those which employ two or more assistants (chairside and roving), a hygienist, a laboratory technician, and an office or business secretary. Regardless of the number of employees, certain duties which are general in nature, but still related to the function of the office, must be performed at the beginning of each workday. When more than one assistant is employed, these duties are usually shared. All specific nonprofessional duties plus chairside performance are expected from the one auxiliary if no others are employed.

Early Morning Routine

Usually, all personnel arrive at the office 15 to 30 minutes earlier than the dentist during which time the office is prepared to receive patients. Most dentists employ professional janitorial services which clean the office after working hours. Even with this kind of service, the early morning routine should include a general "tidy-up" of the entire office. The following items are necessary each day before the first patient is scheduled to arrive:

1. Survey the entire office to determine that all areas are clean.
2. Turn on all electrical equipment normally turned off at night. This allows time for the heating elements in the multipurpose syringe to warm, for the sterilizer to heat, and for the air compressor to function.
3. Check and set the thermostat for proper temperature and humidity control as governed by the outside weather conditions.
4. Prepare and post in the operatory a patient list for the day. Such a schedule should include the patient's name, the time for the appointment, and the type of service to be accomplished. Such a list is extremely helpful for the operator to plan the day. Patients' charts for the day should be placed in the operatory.

5. Inspect the darkroom. Process all films exposed the previous day. These radiographs should be placed in suitable mounts and labeled with the patient's name, chart number, and date. Change the solutions as required.
6. Stock the operatory with expendable supplies, such as cotton rolls, bracket-table covers, towels, and sponges, to prevent interruptions during chairside procedures. The assistant should maintain a supply of materials in the operatory and reorder as necessary to maintain the stock.
7. Sterilize any instruments remaining from the last appointment of the previous day and return them to their proper place, either on the prepared trays or in the instrument cabinet.

After this early morning routine is completed, there should be very little need for this kind of activity during the remainder of the day.

Preparation for First Patient

Certain procedures are necessary to prepare the operatory for the first patient of the day, and the same procedures will be repeated between all patients. When two assistants are available, one may act as the full-time chairside assistant while the roving assistant does all preparations for receiving and dismissing patients. Preparation for the first patient should include the following items:

1. Refer to the patient's chart or to the patient list for the day to determine what dental operation is to be performed and obtain the proper tray setup from the tray storage area. Place the tray on the mobile cabinet or the tray arm.
2. Prepare the anesthetic syringe for the area to be injected and place it on the setup.
3. Position the patient's chair in its lowest position. Move the operating light and any unit attachments out of the way to permit the patient to be seated without difficulty.
4. Place the foot controller in the proper position for the dentist.
5. Place the patient's radiographs on the x-ray viewer and set the patient's record nearby, open to the examination and treatment chart.

Before the patient is escorted to the operatory, the assistant should sit in the dental chair and look over the area to make sure everything is in readiness for the day. Personal items for patient use are placed after the patient is seated.

Seating the Patient

Upon arrival, the patient is escorted to the operatory by the chairside or roving assistant and seated. The assistant should adjust the chair to make the patient as comfortable as possible and in such a position that the operator and assistant may approach the patient most conveniently for the procedure to be performed. Contour chairs are easily adjusted, usually by depressing one or more switches, which lowers the backrest and at the same time raises the footboard. Because of full-length body support, comfort offered the patient is superior to that of conventional chairs.

The conventional dental chair is so constructed that the headrest, arms, back support, and footrest are movable so that the chair may be adjusted to accommodate patients of varying sizes. As the patient is seated and leans back in the chair, the assistant should raise or lower the backrest to position it for support of the lumbar region. Next, the headrest is adjusted so that the neck muscles are not in a strained position. The chair is then tilted backward to place the patient in the most convenient operating position. Conventional chairs may be used for sit-down dentistry, but the contour chair is recommended because of superior patient comfort (Fig. 28-18).

In most instances, the assistant can place the patient in one of three chair positions from which the operator may make minor adjustments as required for access and comfort. These positions are:

1. *Upright position.* A very slight backward tilt to the chair or backrest positions the patient as required

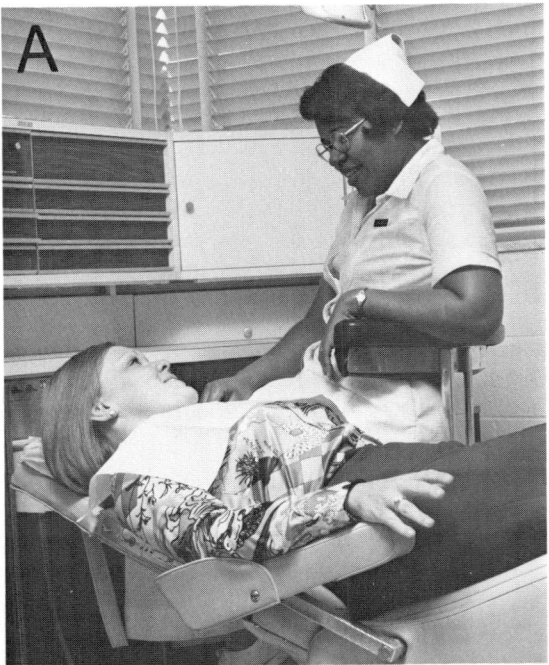

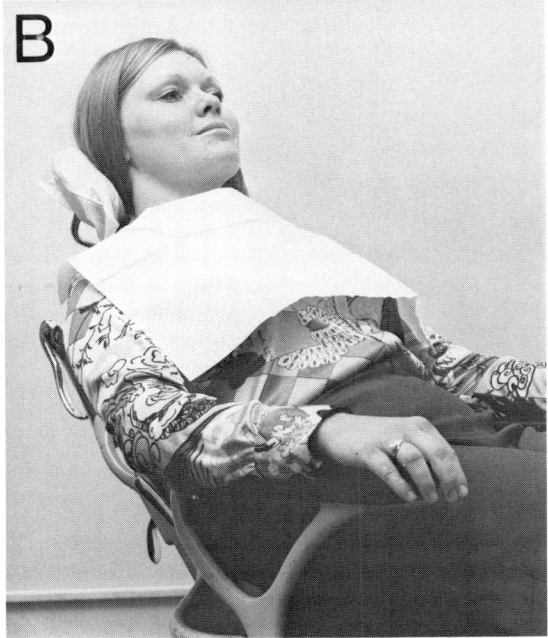

Figure 28-18 | Seating the patient. A. Patient seated in a contour chair. B. Patient seated in a conventional chair.

for exposing radiographs, taking impressions, and for some surgical procedures (Fig. 28-19A).
2. *Fully reclined position.* With slight adjustments from this position the operator is afforded access to the entire maxillary arch and to the mandibular left segment from a right-rear approach (Fig. 28-19B).
3. *Intermediate position.* When the backrest is positioned at a 45 degree angle, the operator may approach the patient from a right-front position for access to the mandibular right teeth (Fig. 28-19C).

Before the operator is ready to begin, the height of the patient's chair must be adjusted, depending on the height of the seated dentist. Also important in sit-down dentistry is the assistant's position. The assistant's operating chair should be adjusted to a position 4 to 6 in higher than the operator. When work is done from this correct position, tension and fatigue are reduced.

Preparing Patient for Treatment

After the patient is seated and the chair adjusted, the operating light is moved into position, adjusted for maximum illumination, and turned off. After hand washing, the assistant proceeds with placing personal items as needed for the operative procedure. The following list of procedures, always executed in the patient's presence, should be added assurances to the patient that cleanliness is supreme in the office:

1. Place a fresh towel over the patient's chest and clip with a napkin chain, or tie in place a plastic apron. The plastic apron may be preferred by some dentists because of the additional protection it affords to the patient's clothes.
2. Provide women patients a tissue to remove lipstick.
3. Have available a sanitary paper cup. When a full-time chairside assistant is utilized, expert use of the oral evacuator reduces the need for a paper cup for rinsing. Provide another paper cup in the setup to serve as a waste receiver.
4. Unwrap a sterile air tip and saliva ejector and place them in position.
5. Inform the dentist that everything is in readiness.

6. Finally, the assistant turns on the operating light, sits, positions the mobile cabinet, and is ready to pass the mirror and explorer as soon as the operator is ready to begin.

Assisting at the Chair

When the dentist first enters the operatory, everything should be in readiness so that work may be started immediately after greeting the patient. The dentist is productive only while working at the chair, and the activities of the dental assistant should be coordinated with the operator's efforts to make difficult operations easier for both the patient and the dentist. This kind of effort will increase productivity and improve the quality of dental care.

The successful assistant will relieve the dentist of, or assist in, as many tasks as possible. The major responsibility is to coordinate activities in the field of operation with those outside the field of operation which are necessary to the procedure the dentist is performing. This type of coordination prevents interruption of the procedure. To do this, the assistant must pay attention to the field of operation as much as possible to *anticipate* the requirements of the dentist and must be adept at quickly moving to and from the setup without interfering with the operative procedure.

Specific chairside duties related to the various operations will be discussed when individual operative procedures are discussed.

Dismissing the Patient

Patients first form their image of the dental office and its personnel when they arrive at the office. Equally important is the final impression the patient forms when leaving the office because this impression will last until the next visit.

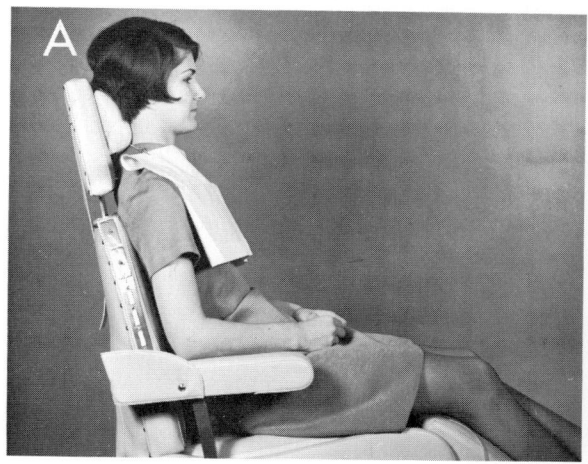

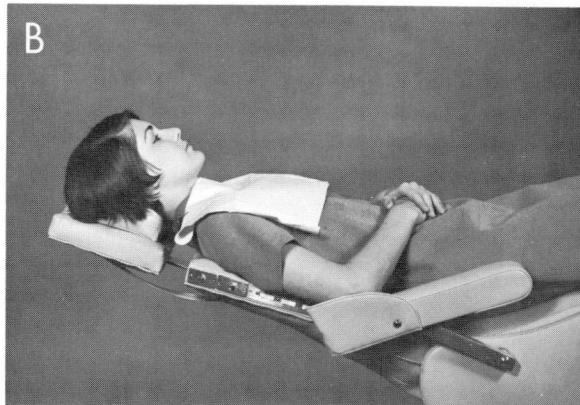

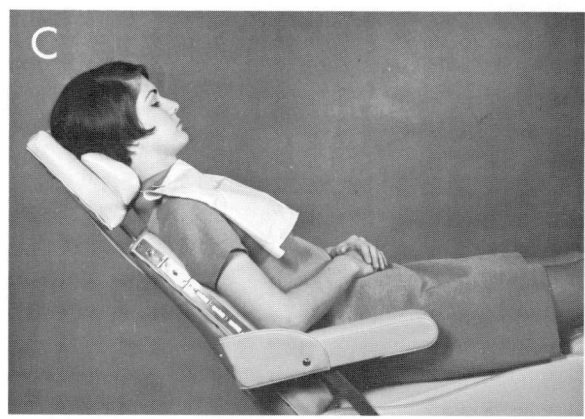

Figure 28-19 | Patient positions. A. Upright position. B. Fully reclined position. C. Intermediate position.

When the treatment procedure has been completed, the dentist may give the patient postoperative care instructions and leave the operatory. Either the chairside assistant or the roving assistant will dismiss the patient. The procedure to follow may be summarized as follows:

1. Raise the backrest of the chair to the upright position and lift the armrest.
2. Remove the napkin.
3. Assist patient in rising from the chair.
4. Hand the patient any personal items, such as purses, eyeglasses, and wraps removed in the operatory.
5. Invite women patients to use the powder room or provide a large hand mirror so that they may replace lipstick and adjust their hairdo.
6. Escort the patient to the business office to make appointments or to complete such business as might be necessary.

The assistant should immediately return to the operatory to clean up and prepare for the next patient. A routine should be developed to ensure that *no trace of the previous operation remains when the next patient is brought into the room.* Cleaning and preparing the operatory is the responsibility of the roving assistant while the dentist and the chairside assistant are treating another patient in a second operatory. The following routine is essential each time a patient is dismissed:

1. Discard the used napkin, paper cup, and any other disposable items.
2. Gather all instruments and burs and scrub with a stiff brush, soap, and water. Rinse completely and prepare them for sterilization either in the autoclave, dry-heat oven, or in cold disinfecting solutions.
3. Return to the unit and wipe the handpieces, multipurpose syringe, bracket table (if one is present on the unit) or the tray stand, handles of the operating light, and arms of the chair with a suitable disinfectant. Finally, clean the cuspidor (if one is present).
4. Run water through the evacuator and saliva-ejector hoses. Sterilize the evacuator tip and saliva ejector.

When the above procedures have been accomplished, prepare for the next patient by following the same routine as described in previous sections. Because the duties necessary to prepare, treat, dismiss, and again prepare for the patient must be repeated often during the day, it is essential that a fixed routine be followed for proper utilization of time.

End-of-Day Responsibilities

When an operatory has been used for the last appointment of the day, duties required after dismissal of the patient are accomplished followed by as much preparation as possible for the following day:

1. Clean and lubricate all handpieces.
2. Turn off all electrical equipment (units, sterilizers, lab equipment, x-ray machines, dryers, and lights.) Cut off all gas and water outlets.
3. Return all sterilized instruments to their proper place.
4. Restock the operatories with expendable materials and supplies.
5. Reorder items to maintain a minimum stock level.
6. Box and prepare for mailing items to be sent to the commercial laboratory.
7. Return all patient records to the business office.
8. Set the thermostat for night or weekend temperatures.
9. Turn off all lights except the night light and lock the doors.

CHAIRSIDE DUTIES IN OPERATIVE DENTISTRY

In the general practice of dentistry a major portion of the assistant's chairside duties are related to operative dentistry. The following material is presented to aid the chairside assistant in becoming efficient and effective in the various operative dentistry procedures. When these instructions are mastered they are easily applied to chairside duties necessary in the other divisions of dentistry.

Oral Examination and Charting

The assistant's role in oral examination and charting will vary from one dental office to another. Regardless of the extent of the assistant's responsibilities, they are significant to all the preliminary procedures accomplished for the patient prior to the actual beginning of treatment (see also Chap. 17).

The setup for examination and charting (Fig. 28-20) should include:

1. Front-surface mouth mirror
2. Explorer
3. Operating pliers
4. Periodontal probe
5. Saliva ejector and air tip
6. Cotton rolls
7. Dental floss
8. Paper cup
9. Articulating paper
10. Tongue blade
11. Red and blue pencil
12. Patient's chart and radiographs

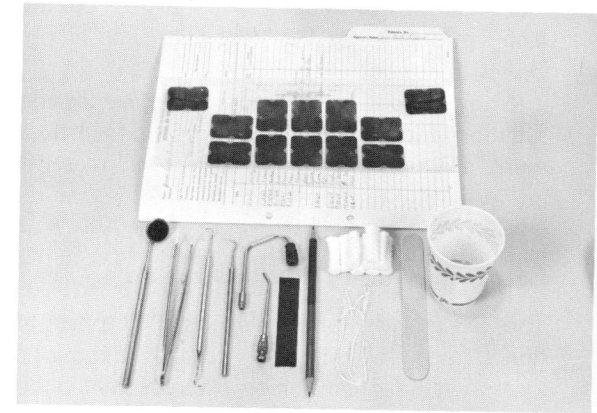

Figure 28-20 | Setup for examination and charting.

When the patient has been seated, the assistant should confirm that the information and health questionnaires have been properly completed by the patient and should inquire about omissions of required information. Specifically, be certain the patient has indicated a reason (chief complaint) for seeking dental treatment. Additional questions may be asked by the dentist when more information is needed. The knowledgeable assistant will only record information which is pertinent to the diagnosis and valuable in formulating a treatment plan.

When the dentist is ready to begin the oral examination, pass a tongue blade to retract the lips and cheek and depress the tongue. At this time the dentist will inspect the oral cavity for possible infectious lesions before touching the soft tissues. When this procedure has been accomplished, receive the tongue blade and pass the mirror and explorer.

Now, the assistant should assist the dentist in examination of the teeth. Cotton rolls should be placed to isolate the teeth. The assistant should do this, after which the teeth should be dried with the air syringe. A stream of air should be directed on the mirror surface to prevent fogging. As the dentist examines the teeth the assistant should record all the necessary information, being careful to record the proper entry in the correct place. During the examination the assistant must also pass and receive other instruments as required, plus use the air syringe and record the facts concerning the teeth.

While the electric pulp tester is not usually placed in a setup for examination and charting, it should be readily available for use when required. The assistant should assemble the pulp tester, assist in its use, and record the results.

Treatment Planning and Case Presentation

Often, the dentist will plan the course of treatment for the patient during those times when patients are not scheduled. The assistant should provide the patient's chart, radiographs, study models, and any other preliminary record obtained and assist by recording the proposed outline of treatment.

When the patient returns to the office for consultation and discussion of the proposed treatment, the assistant should see that all materials are available for the dentist.

Local Anesthetic Administration

The dental assistant's responsibility prior to, during, and following the administration of a local anesthetic cannot be underestimated because many successful practices are the result of an injection routine which is performed with little or no discomfort to the patient.

Prior to the injection procedure, the dental assistant prepares the syringe, usually while making the setup or obtaining the prearranged tray. When the patient has already been seated, the syringe should be prepared behind the patient. Reference to the patient's chart to note the intended treatment permits the assistant to select the proper needle for the injection, and, in many instances, to choose the correct anesthetic solution based on previous treatment procedures. Should some physical disorder be noted on the medical history, consultation with the dentist is required. While the assistant is preparing the syringe, reassuring conversation will often relieve the nervous patient.

When the operator is ready to administer the anesthetic, the assistant should pass to the operator a sterile gauze sponge to dry the injection site. While the operator is drying the injection site, the assistant picks up the cotton-tipped applicator which has been dipped in topical anesthetic ointment. The operator will exchange the gauze sponge for the applicator and apply the topical anesthetic. During the short waiting time for the topical anesthetic to become effective the assistant picks up the prepared syringe, loosens (but does not remove) the needle cover, and positions it so that when placed in the operator's hand the rubber stopper may be viewed by the operator during the procedure to judge the rate of injection. The syringe is passed to the operator in front of and just below the patient's chin. Once the operator has possession of the syringe the needle cover is removed with the right hand while the left hand and arm are positioned over the patient to guard against any sudden upward movement of the patient's arms. Figure 28-21 illustrates some of the assistant's responsibilities in local anesthetic procedures.

After the injection has been completed, the assistant receives the syringe, replaces the needle cover, and places the anesthetic setup aside. The assistant or operator, or both, should remain with the patient to watch for complications. The assistant should be prepared to administer first aid for syncope (fainting), which is the most frequent postinjection complication.

To eliminate the waiting period for the topical anesthetic to act, many auxiliaries will position the cotton-tipped applicator as soon as the patient is seated so that the injection site is already anesthetized when the dentist arrives in the operatory. The alert assistant will consult the patient's records for the teeth to be operated and will place the topical anesthetic on the appropriate injection site.

Moisture Control

The control of moisture in operative dentistry is extremely important because those restorations which are contaminated while being inserted into the cavity preparation are weakened and will not provide the best possible service to the patient. Different operative procedures require varying degrees of dryness, varying from short periods of dryness to absolute dryness for extended lengths of time.

Absorbents

Procedures such as examinations, polishing, and cementing of inlays and crowns require dryness, but for short periods of time. Cotton rolls and sponges when used in conjunction with the saliva ejector (Fig. 28-22) provide satisfactory

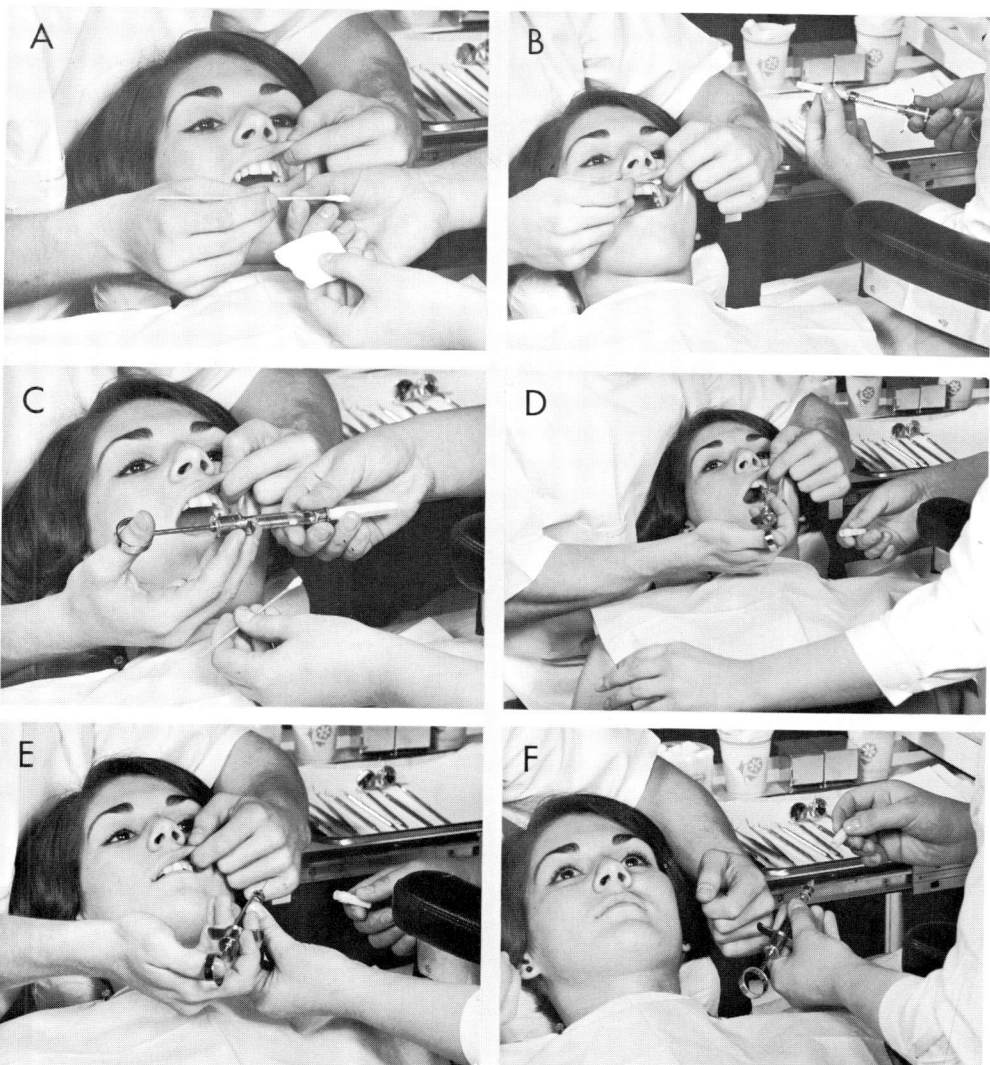

Figure 28-21 | Assisting in administration of local anesthetic. A. Operator receiving cotton-tipped applicator. B. Operator applying topical anesthetic; assistant loosening protective cover over needle. C. Assistant passing syringe. D. Assistant's left hand and arm positioned over patient during injection procedure. E. Assistant receiving syringe. F. Assistant replacing needle cover.

dryness for periods up to 10 minutes, particularly when the assistant changes them periodically. The assistant should change cotton rolls before they become completely saturated with saliva by first retracting the lips or cheek with the forefinger of the left hand. Then, the wet cotton roll is removed with the operating pliers, discarded in the waste receiver, and a dry one placed. In addition, the oral evacuator may be used from time to time to clear the mouth of saliva not removed

Chapter Twenty-Eight | Operative Dentistry | 581

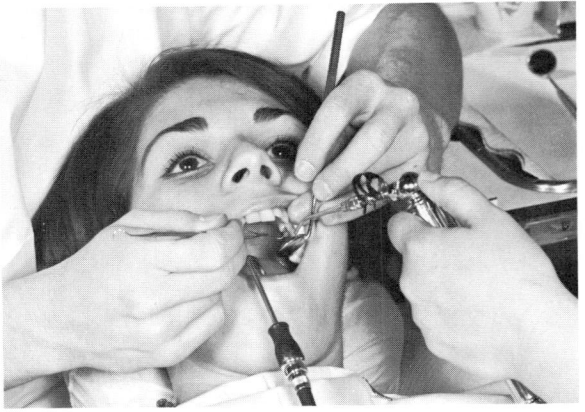

Figure 28-22 | Short periods of dryness are obtained using cotton rolls in conjunction with the saliva ejector.

by the saliva ejector. When the assistant is efficient in changing cotton rolls and in using the air syringe and oral evacuator, dryness can be maintained in the operative field to permit the operator to work without interruption.

Rubber Dam

When the situation demands maximum dryness, the rubber dam, which completely eliminates saliva from the field of operation, is used (Fig. 28-23). Usually, the rubber dam can be applied to the teeth in 3 to 5 minutes, the time necessary to obtain profound anesthesia following an injection. The advantages of the rubber dam are:

1. It provides a clean, dry, operating field.
2. It provides protection to the patient and the operating team.
3. It provides conditions for improved properties of all dental materials.
4. It mildly retracts the lips, tongue, and gingiva.
5. It is an economic aid to the office.
6. It creates conditions that promote dental service of the highest quality.

Because these advantages are a real asset to the practice of operative dentistry, the dental assistant should be efficient in assisting with the application and removal of the rubber dam.

Figure 28-23 | Rubber dam in position.

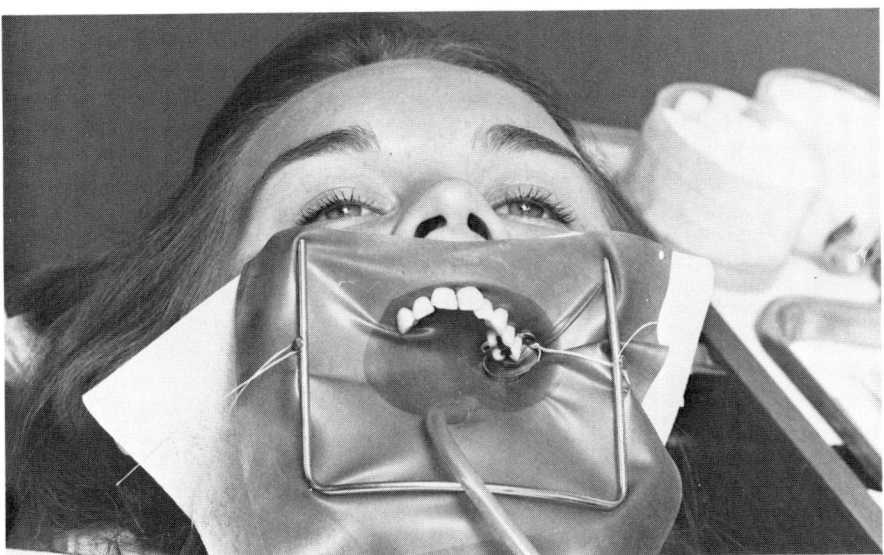

Materials and Instruments

The materials and instruments required for the use of the rubber dam may be placed on each prepared tray or may occupy a special place in an instrument drawer in the mobile cabinet to be removed and positioned on the cabinet top for those procedures which require its use (Fig. 28-24). The materials and instruments necessary are:

1. *Rubber dam material.* Both light and dark rubber dam material are available in rolls or in ready-cut squares (5 × 5 or 6 × 6 in) and may be ordered in one of five thicknesses: thin (0.006 in), medium (0.008 in), heavy (0.010 in), extra heavy (0.012 in), and special heavy (0.014 in). The dark dam is preferred for better contrast and the heavier thicknesses are recommended because they are less likely to tear and are more effective in retracting the soft tissue. Purchase dam material in small quantities as it deteriorates with age.
2. *Rubber dam holder.* The holder serves to maintain the position of the rubber dam and to hold it securely in place. Holders of various types are available but the Young's holder is perhaps the most convenient to use.
3. *Rubber dam clamp.* The clamp is used to anchor the dam and is usually placed on the most posterior tooth to be isolated. Some clamps are primarily designed to retract the gingival tissue and are used in addition to the anchor clamp.
4. *Rubber dam punch.* The punch is used to cut holes in the dam material. It is a precision instrument having a rotating disc with six holes of varying sizes and a sharp plunger.
5. *Rubber dam clamp forceps.* The clamp forceps hold the clamp during its placement and removal. It is so designed that when the handles are tightened the jaws of the clamp are opened to facilitate its passage over the crown portion of the tooth.
6. *Rubber dam napkin.* A napkin of soft, absorbent material is placed between the rubber dam and the patient's skin to act as a cushion, prevent contact of rubber, absorb saliva at the corners of the mouth, and provide a method of wiping the patient's mouth when the dam is removed.
7. *Lubricant.* A suitable lubricant is applied to both sides of the dam in the area of the punched holes to aid the passing of the dam through the tooth contacts. Also, the patient's lips and particularly the corners of the mouth should be lubricated to prevent irritation.
8. *Modeling compound.* Softened modeling compound is applied to the clamp to secure its position and prevent movement.

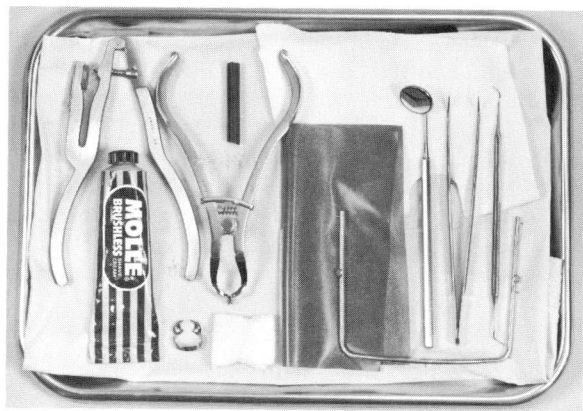

Figure 28-24 | Setup for rubber dam application.

Positioning the Holes in the Rubber Dam

For the most part, the successful application of the rubber dam depends on the proper size and position of the holes. Holes that are too large result in leakage around the teeth while small holes may tear when stretched over the teeth. The plate on the punch usually has six holes of varying sizes. Use the largest hole for molar teeth that are to be clamped. In general, the three smaller holes are used for incisors, canines, and premolars, and the larger holes for the molars.

The following rules will aid the assistant in positioning the holes to ensure successful application of the dam each time it is used:

1. A sufficient number of teeth should be isolated to permit the best possible access and visibility for

both the operator and the assistant. A good rule to follow is to isolate to the canine of the opposite arch from the operating site. This establishes a routine in which the operator and the assistant will know that the most forward tooth to be isolated will always be the same. In addition, the isolated anterior teeth provide adequate finger rests for the operator. Isolating the number of teeth as described above is best, but a minimum of three teeth should always be isolated except in endodontic therapy when only the involved tooth is isolated.
2. Punch the holes so that the distance from one hole to the next is equal to the distance from the center of one tooth to the center of the adjacent teeth, measured at the level of the gingival tissue. This will in most situations approximate one-quarter in.
3. When the maxillary teeth are to be isolated, punch the holes for the central incisors first, and locate these holes approximately 1 in from the superior border of the dam. This provides sufficient dam material to cover the patient's upper lip. This distance must be increased if the patient has a moustache or may have to be decreased if the patient's upper lip is very thin. The remaining holes are positioned following the arch form, with adjustments being made for missing or malposed teeth (Fig. 28-25).
4. When the mandibular teeth are to be isolated, the first hole to be punched is for the tooth to receive the clamp. This procedure is necessary to provide sufficient dam material to come from behind the clamped tooth and to position the superior edge of the dam over the upper lip. To locate the hole position for the mandibular first molar mentally divide the dam into equal top and bottom halves and into three vertical sections and punch the hole where the vertical line (left or right) crosses the horizontal dividing line (Fig. 28-26A). The remaining holes are then punched to correspond to the arch form. When teeth other than the first molar are to serve as the anchor tooth, adjustment must be made to properly locate the position of the hole. Study of Fig. 28-26 will indicate the hole position as required for other teeth in the mandibular arch.
5. When a Class V cavity is to be prepared using a cervical clamp, the hole for the tooth should be punched facial to the arch form to compensate for extension (stretching) of the dam (Fig. 28-27).
6. Hole sizes should become smaller as thinner dam is used because thin dam will stretch more.

Applying the Rubber Dam

The application of the rubber dam can be a well-executed team effort when the assistant makes every action sequential to the efforts of the dentist (Fig. 28-28). Briefly, the duties of the assistant should follow a routine such as:

1. Pass a length of dental floss to the operator to test the contacts.
2. Punch holes for the area to be isolated (this may be done during preparation procedures for the appointment).
3. Pass clamp forceps to operator to ascertain proper fit of clamp.
4. Lubricate dam.
5. Hold dam in position to permit operator to pass bow of clamp through anchor hole.

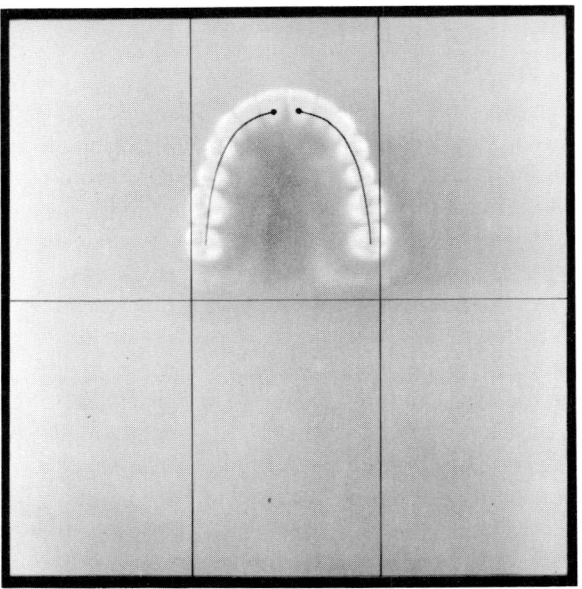

Figure 28-25 | Hole position for maxillary central incisors. (From Sturdevant, Barton, and Brauer (eds.), The Art and Science of Operative Dentistry, copyright 1968 by McGraw-Hill, Inc. Used by permission of McGraw-Hill Book Company.)

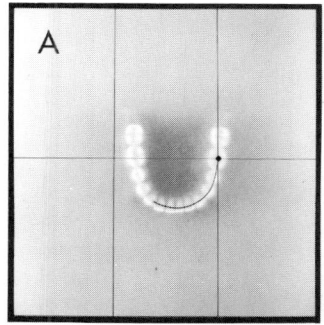 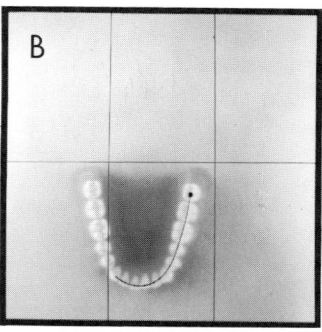 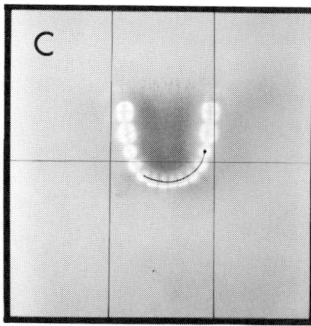

Figure 28-26 | Hole position for mandibular anchor teeth. A. First molar. B. Third molar. C. Second premolar. (*From Sturdevant, Barton, and Brauer (eds.), The Art and Science of Operative Dentistry, copyright 1968 by McGraw-Hill, Inc. Used with permission of McGraw-Hill Book Company.*)

6. While operator positions clamp, obtain napkin, and place in position at the proper time.
7. Hold frame in position and secure the dam on the patient's left side while operator attaches the dam on the right side.
8. Attach tieback to left side of frame, pass behind the patient's neck for the operator to adjust, and tie to right side of frame.
9. Heat and temper the end of a stick of compound and hold it in the exchange zone. The operator will pinch off a sufficient amount to secure the clamp to the anchor tooth.
10. As the operator begins to stretch the dam over the remaining teeth, assist by passing dental floss through those contacts which are tight.
11. Direct a stream of air on each tooth as the operator inverts the edge of the dam into the gingival crevice.
12. Cut a small hole in the dam just lingual to the mandibular incisors and position the saliva ejector.

The student is encouraged to study Fig. 28-28 to note the duties the assistant usually performs in the application of the dam.

Removing the Rubber Dam

Before the rubber dam is removed the assistant should use the oral evacuator and water syringe

Figure 28-27 | Hole position for tooth to receive a Class V restoration is punched facial to the arch form. (*From Sturdevant, Barton, and Brauer (eds.), The Art and Science of Operative Dentistry, copyright 1968 by McGraw-Hill, Inc. Used with permission of McGraw-Hill Book Company.*)

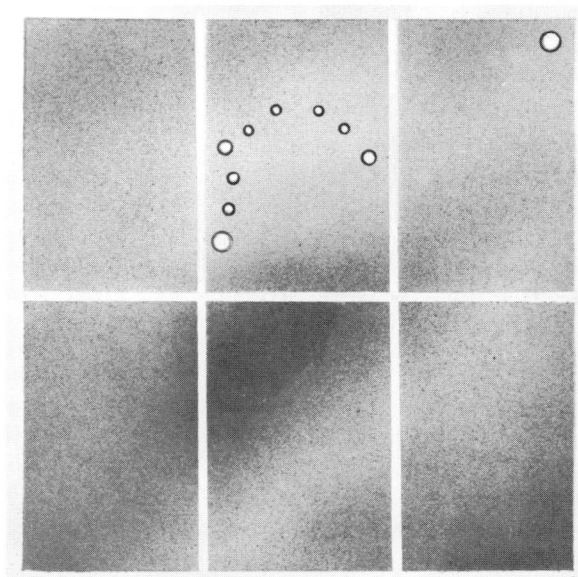

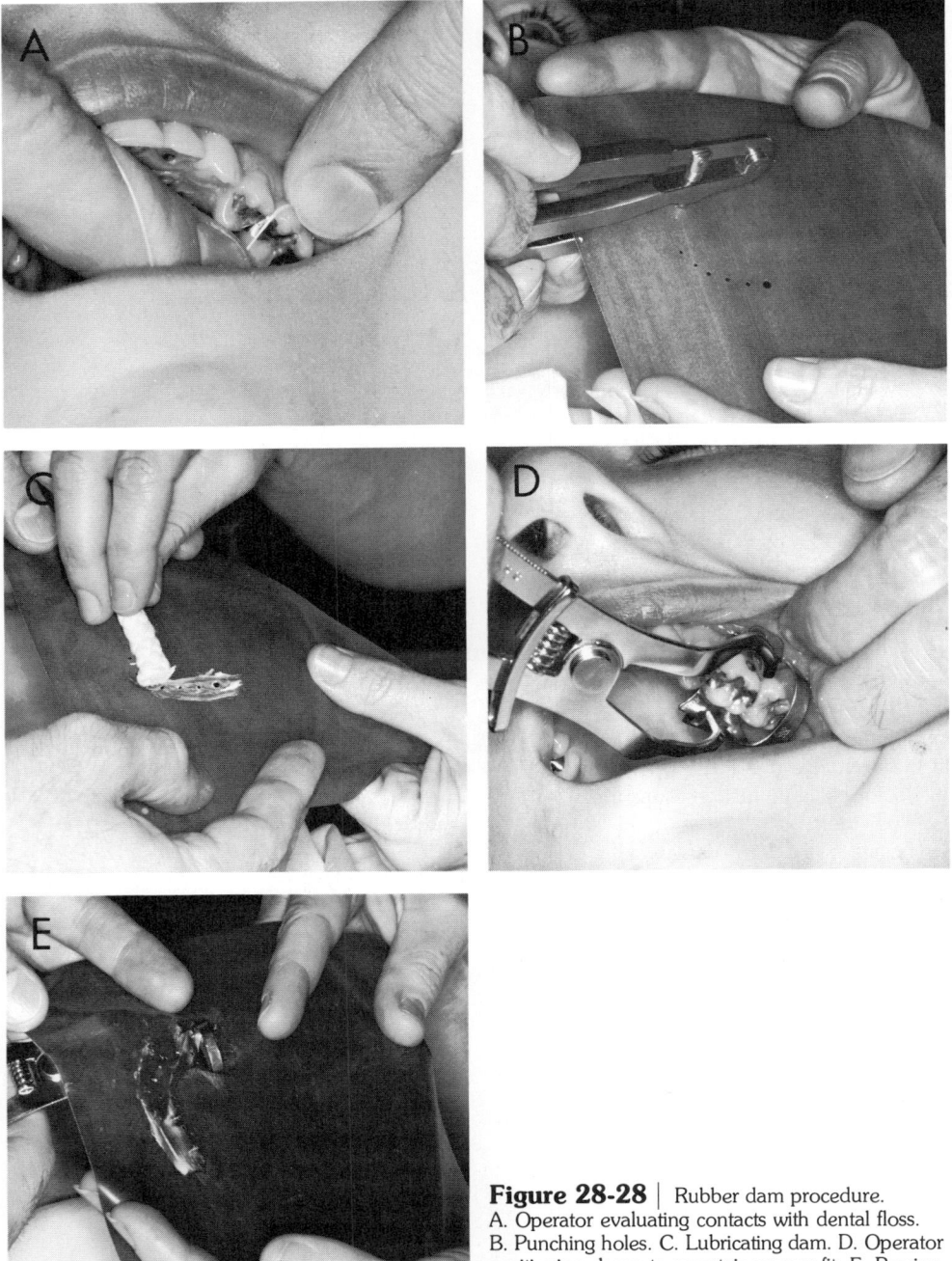

Figure 28-28 | Rubber dam procedure. A. Operator evaluating contacts with dental floss. B. Punching holes. C. Lubricating dam. D. Operator positioning clamp to ascertain proper fit. E. Passing bow of clamp through hole punched for anchor tooth.

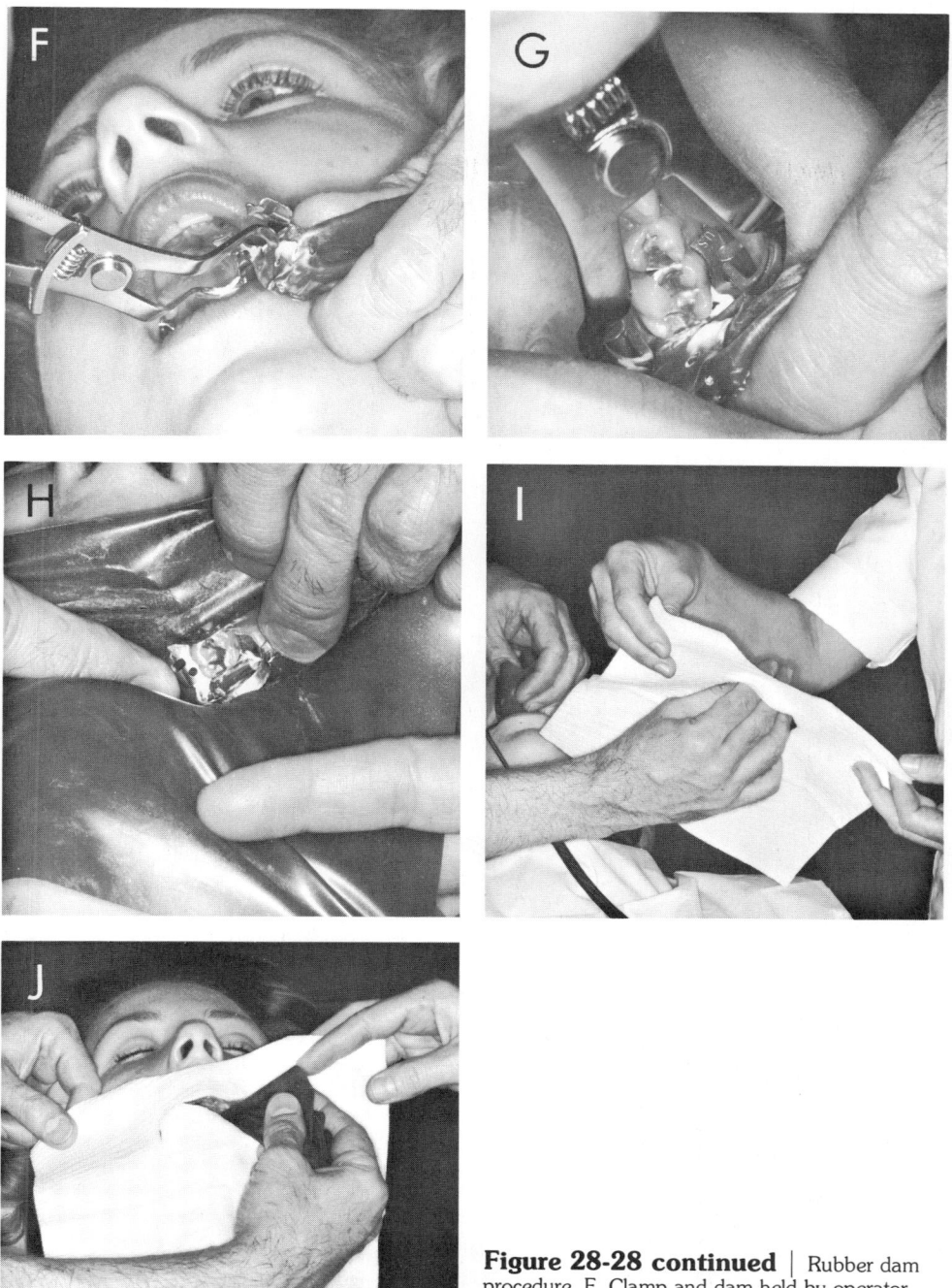

Figure 28-28 continued | Rubber dam procedure. F. Clamp and dam held by operator prior to positioning clamp. G. Positioning clamp on anchor tooth. H. Operator moving dam under wings of clamp. I. Operator receiving napkin. J. Assistant and operator positioning napkin.

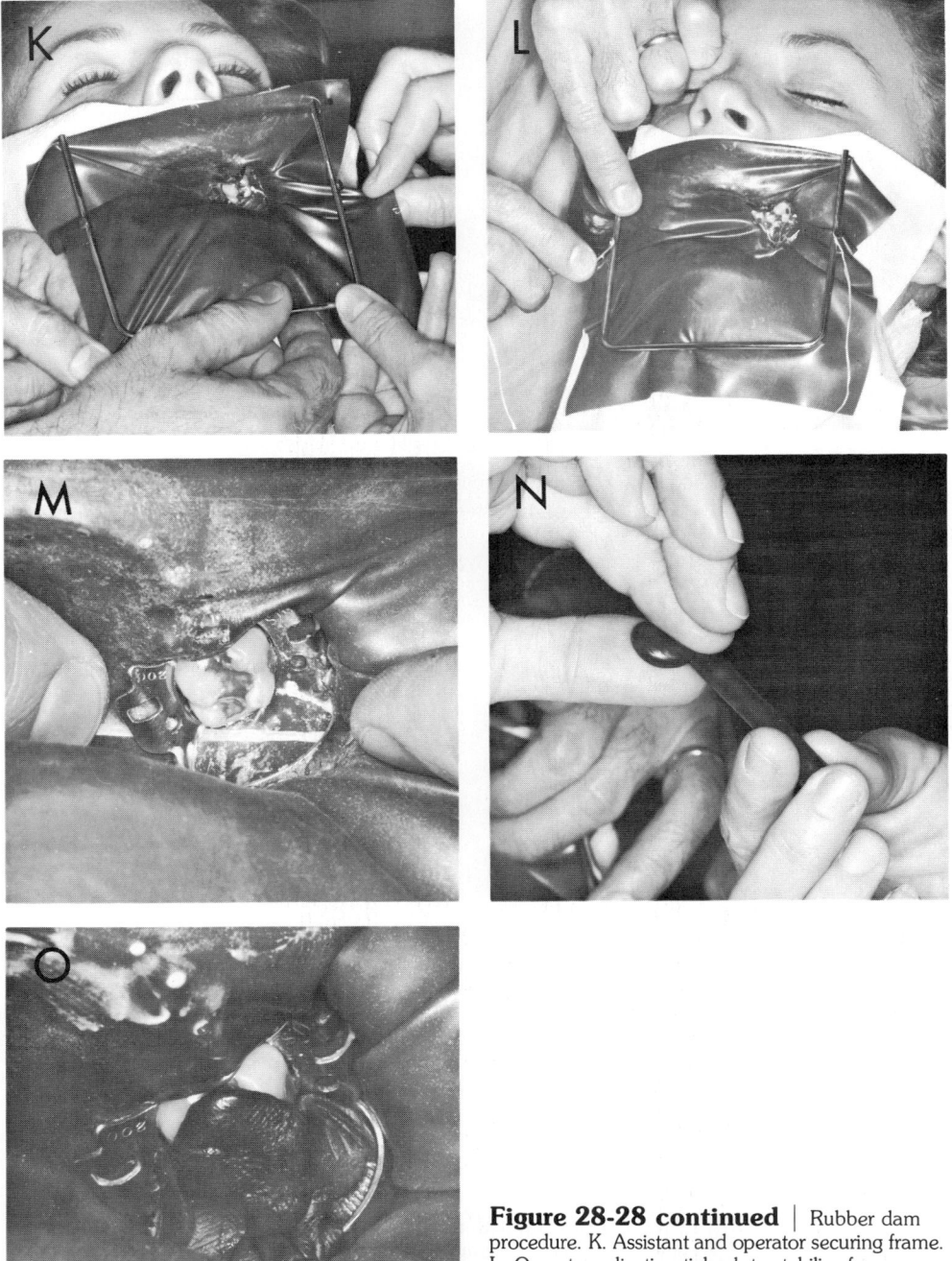

Figure 28-28 continued | Rubber dam procedure. K. Assistant and operator securing frame. L. Operator adjusting tieback to stabilize frame. M. Operator passing dam behind anchor tooth with aid of dental tape. N. Operator receiving heated compound. O. Clamp securely stabilized with compound.

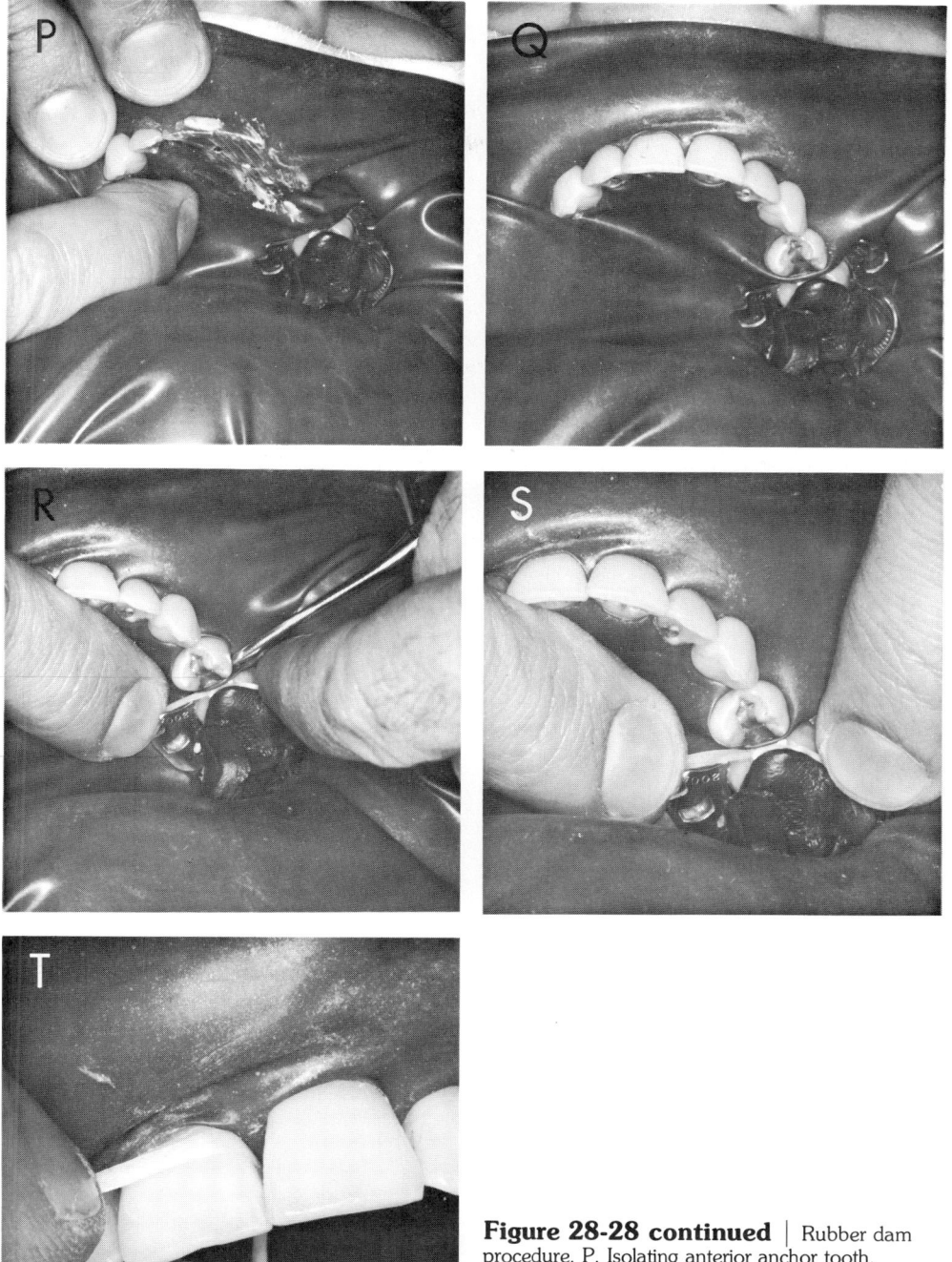

Figure 28-28 continued | Rubber dam procedure. P. Isolating anterior anchor tooth. Q. Isolation complete except between anchor tooth and premolar. R. Assistant separating teeth while operator passes rubber dam through tight contact. S. Operator completing isolation. T. Inverting interproximal dam.

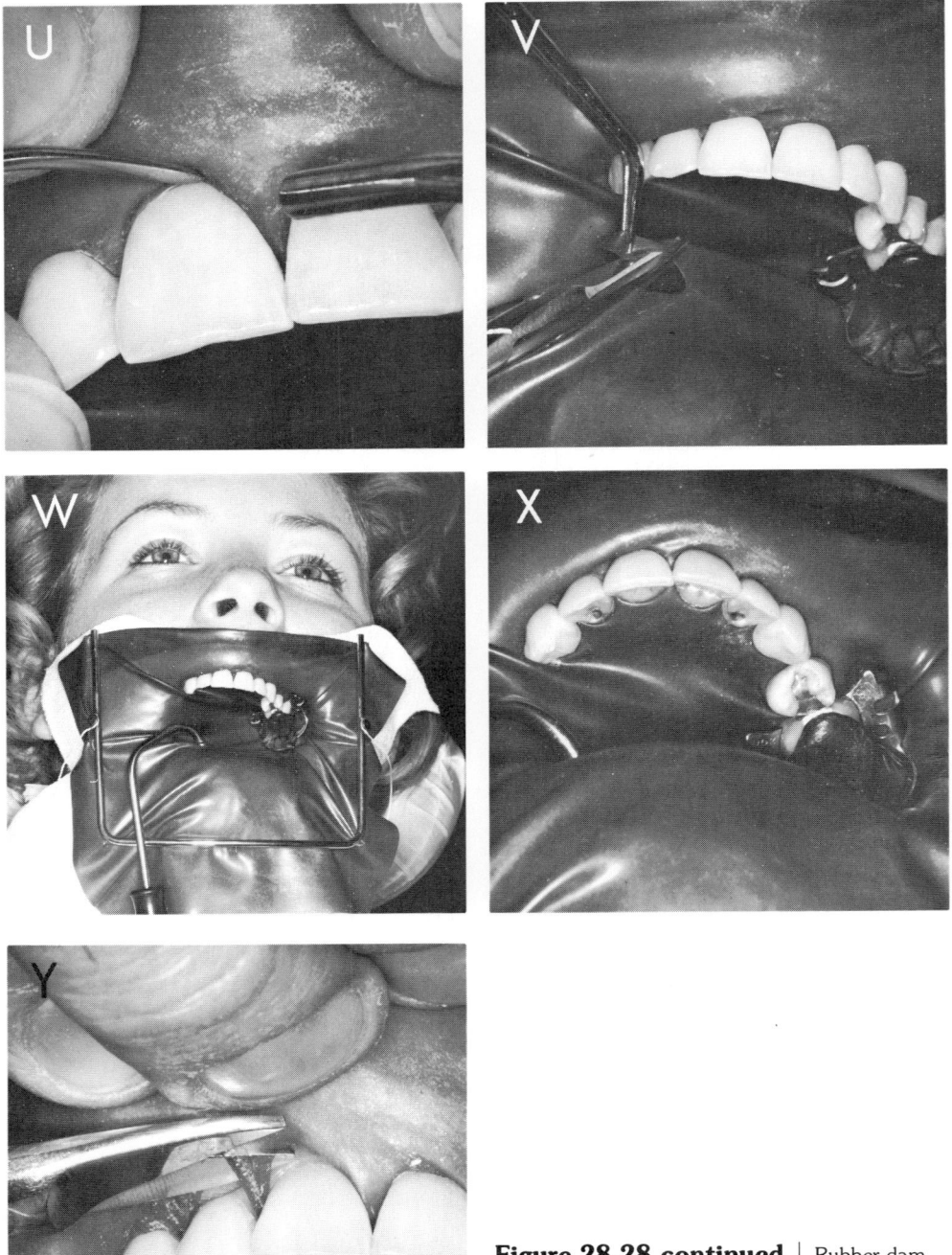

Figure 28-28 continued | Rubber dam procedure. U. Completing seal about tooth by inverting facial areas. V. Cutting hole lingual to mandibular incisors to receive saliva ejector. W. Completed rubber dam. X. Incisal view of completed rubber dam. Y. Cutting interproximal septa in preparation for removal of rubber dam.

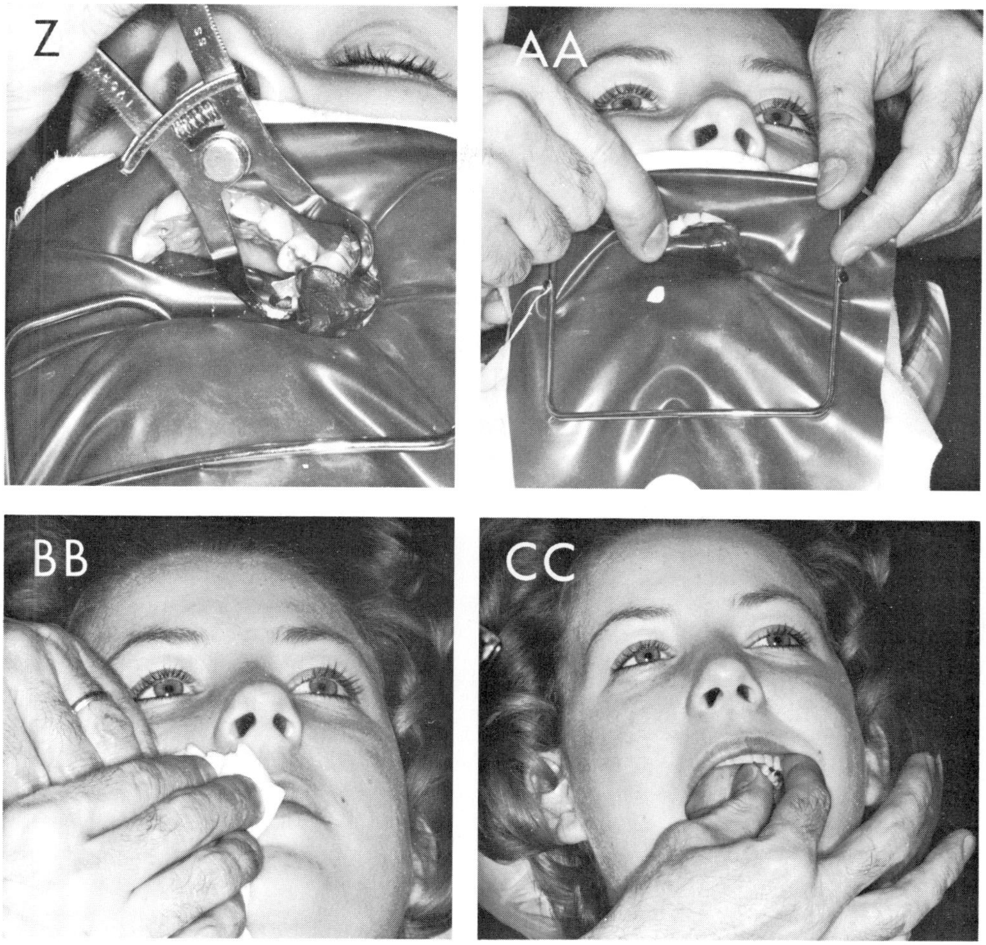

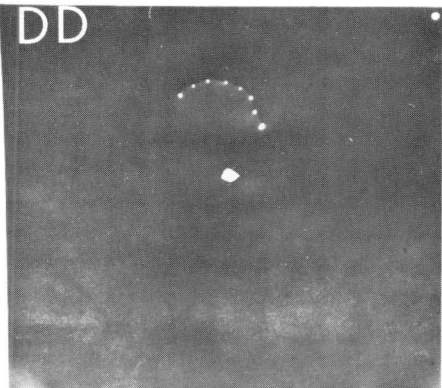

Figure 28-28 continued | Rubber dam procedure. Z. Removing clamp. AA. Removing frame and rubber dam. BB. Wiping patient's mouth with napkin. CC. Massaging tissue around clamped tooth. DD. Rubber dam placed over light background to inspect for missing segments. (*From Sturdevant, Barton, and Brauer (eds.), The Art and Science of Operative Dentistry, copyright 1968 by McGraw-Hill, Inc. Used with permission of McGraw-Hill Book Company.*)

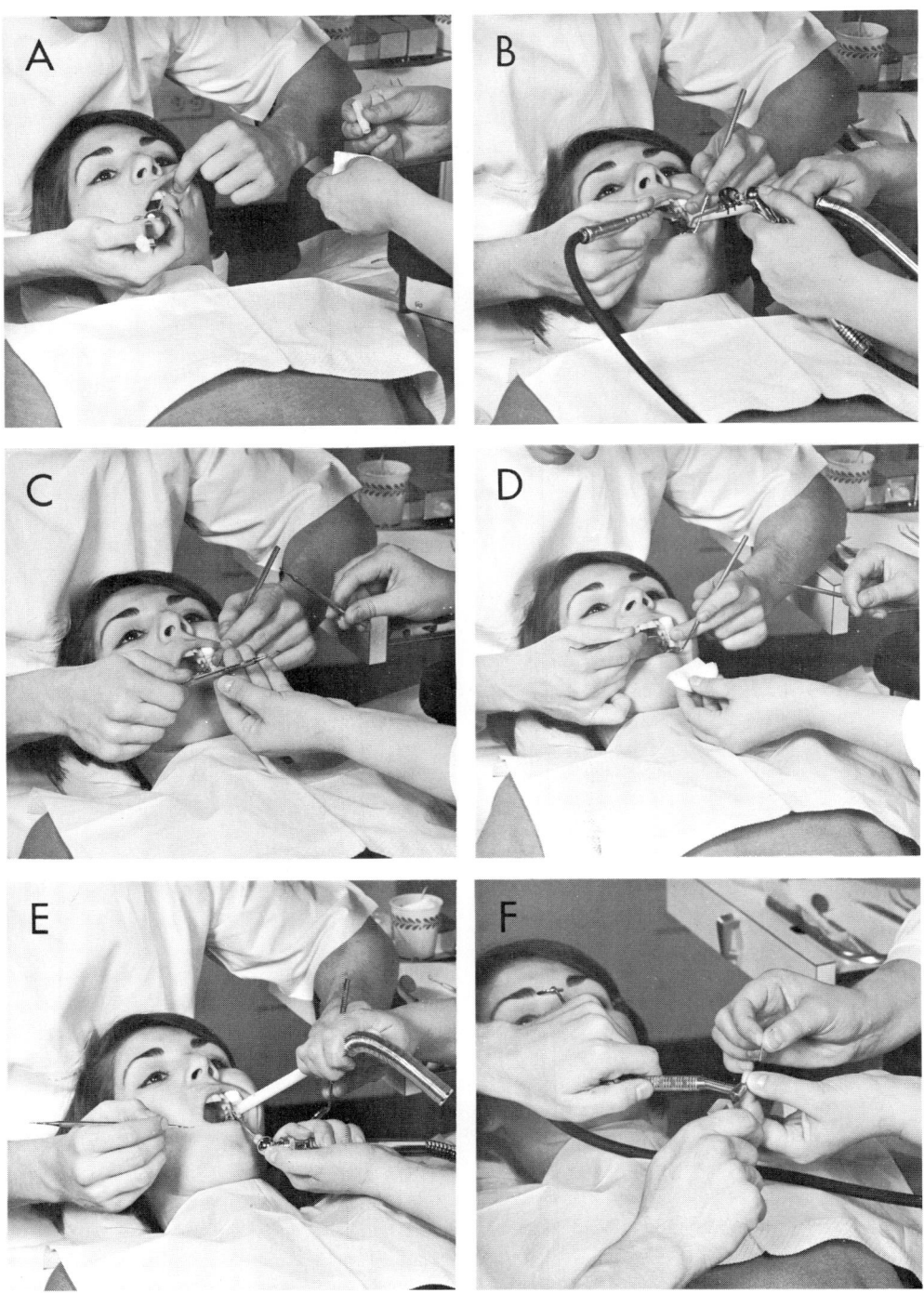

to flush out all debris that may have collected during the procedure. Again in brief form, the following duties are required of the assistant during the removal of the rubber dam:

1. Pass the operator a pair of small scissors to cut each septum of rubber to free the dam from the interproximal spaces. The assistant should place a finger behind the dam and pull the septa facially for access. An alternate method is for the assistant to cut the septa as the operator pulls them away from the interproximal spaces.
2. Pass the clamp forceps immediately after the operator releases the dam from the anterior anchor.
3. Undo the tieback while the operator is positioning the forceps and removing the clamp.
4. Receive the forceps and, as the operator removes the frame and dam, wipe the patient's mouth with the napkin.
5. Flush the operative site, using the evacuator and water syringe.
6. Inspect the dam to determine that no small portions of rubber remain between the teeth.

Some operators do not isolate the teeth until the cavity preparation is almost completed. However, earlier application provides increased access and visibility and makes the use of the oral evacuator more convenient.

Cavity Preparation

At no time is the assistant more helpful to the dentist than in the procedures incident to cavity preparation (Fig. 28-29). It is during cavity preparation procedures that the assistant is truly the dentist's "second pair of hands." The assistant's duties include everything that does not require the special talents and skills of the dentist. Ideally the assistant should be so familiar with the order of the procedure that the dentist's attention need not be interrupted to wait for materials or instruments or to give instructions to the assistant. One of the essential prerequisites is that the assistant anticipate the needs of the operator. The value of this has already been discussed, but it should be reemphasized that it is the basis for skillful chairside assisting.

In preparing for a given procedure, the assistant will obtain a setup, after first consulting the patient's chart to ascertain the type of procedure to be accomplished. In almost every situation the assistant can have in readiness all instruments and materials that will be necessary to complete the cavity preparation and restoration, thus preventing any absence from the chair once the operator begins work. When the assistant has properly prepared the armamentarium, time required to complete the procedure is significantly reduced. Also, the patient will be more comfortable because the operation will be smooth and efficient.

The following duties are performed by the assistant during cavity preparation and with minor modifications are repeated for the various types of preparations:

1. Assist in the administration of the local anesthetic.
2. Assist in the application of the rubber dam if the operator wishes to prepare teeth with the dam in place. Many operators prepare the tooth without the dam except for retention form and final finishing, which are completed with the dam in place.
3. If the rubber dam is not being used, isolate the teeth by placing a cotton roll in the vestibule. Recall that this procedure retracts the lips and cheek away from the teeth and provides a cushion for the evacuator tip.
4. Pass the handpiece and mirror to the operator. The alert assistant will already have placed the correct bur in the handpiece.
5. Position the evacuator tip and, as the operator begins the preparation, direct air from the multipurpose syringe across the mirror surface to keep it clear of moisture during the cutting procedure.
6. Periodically, as the operator stops the handpiece,

Figure 28-29 | Assistant's duties during cavity preparation. A. Assisting in local anesthetic administration. B. Use of oral evacuator. C. Instrument exchange. D. Assisting in removal of caries. E. Washing and drying operative site. F. Bur exchange.

suction the floor of the mouth to remove any accumulated water and debris not removed during the cutting procedures.
7. Many cavity preparations cannot be completed entirely with burs. Whenever a hand cutting instrument is required, the operator will indicate the name of the instrument a few seconds before it is needed, allowing sufficient time for the assistant to obtain it from the setup. With experience, the assistant will be able to anticipate when the next instrument is required and will have it ready to pass at the proper time. The extent to which this can be practiced also depends on the operator. It is necessary that each procedure for a given operation be standardized and followed routinely. When exceptions are necessary, verbal instructions must be given to the assistant in advance. Receive the handpiece and pass the specified hand instrument. While the operator uses this instrument, change the bur in the handpiece if procedures dictate a bur change at this point. The assistant now holds the handpiece in readiness to return it to the operator when the signal for exchange is made.
8. Removal of decay (a step in cavity preparation) may be accomplished using round burs or spoon excavators, or both. When the operator chooses to use a spoon excavator, the assistant should hold a 2 by 2 gauze sponge near the exchange area to wipe the debris from the working end of the instrument.
9. Continue to make any required instrument exchanges until the cavity preparation is completed.
10. During the preparation of the tooth the operator may wish to thoroughly inspect progress. This is best done when the tooth is clean and dry. Without removing the evacuator tip, wash the cavity preparation and adjacent tooth structure and immediately dry the area using the air syringe. One tooth or several may be rapidly dried using the air syringe and the oral evacuator.
11. Bur changes are usually made on request by the operator. As previously stated, the assistant changes the bur while the operator uses a hand instrument. However, at any point in the procedure, a bur change may be necessary at a time when the operator is using the handpiece. Pass the chucking tool to the operator and remove the bur from the handpiece when the chucking mechanism is loosened. Insert the next bur and hold it by the cutting portion until the operator tightens the chuck. Receive the chucking tool.

Caries Control

In teeth with extensive caries in which the condition of the pulp is in question and/or when the patient complains of discomfort (pain), a procedure known as *caries control* is indicated to determine the relative prognosis of the pulp and the type of restoration material best suited to properly restore the tooth. Caries control should be performed only when the tooth (teeth) is isolated with the rubber dam to prevent contamination of the pulp in the event it is exposed. The following assistant duties are required in caries control:

1. Assist in the administration of the local anesthetic.
2. Assist in the placement of the rubber dam.
3. Assist in those steps of cavity preparation which are necessary to remove unsupported enamel to gain access to the carious areas. The assistant's duties are similar to those in any normal cavity preparation, namely, using the evacuator and multipurpose syringe, keeping the area free of debris, washing and drying the tooth, and instrument and bur exchange.
4. Assist the operator during the removal of the caries by passing spoon excavators or the handpiece with a round bur in position. Initially, the bulk of the decay may be removed with a spoon excavator. At the proper time receive the spoon and pass the handpiece. Remember to use the 2 by 2 in gauze sponge to clean the spoon as the operator removes it from the mouth. When the handpiece is used, occasionally direct a short blast of air into the cavity to remove the debris that collects within the excavation. Pass the explorer when the operator returns the handpiece. As the excavation is examined to determine the completeness of the decay removal, be prepared to exchange the explorer for the handpiece (or spoon) should additional tooth structure removal be necessary.
5. Assist in the placement of necessary medicaments, cement bases, and temporary restorative materials

to restore the tooth. Usually, where caries control is performed, the tooth is restored with a suitable temporary filling material until the prognosis of the pulp is determined. Several months' service can be expected from this type of temporary restoration.

Placement of Cavity Liners and Cement Bases

Most operators use some type of cavity liner or cement base, or both, in almost all cavity preparations. Primarily, liners and bases are used for protection of the pulp and to aid the pulp in recovering from irritation resulting from cavity preparation. The following guidelines will aid the dental assistant in determining the types of materials to be placed in the setup. When a pulp is exposed, the exposure site is covered with a calcium hydroxide–containing material, followed by a second material to provide a thickness of material to withstand forces incident to insertion of the restorative material. Deep excavations not involving a pulp exposure require the use of a zinc oxide–eugenol material and may be overlayed with zinc phosphate cement. Shallow excavations may require only the zinc oxide–eugenol cement. A cavity varnish is normally placed in all cavity preparations after cement bases have been placed to prevent marginal leakage and to reduce thermal shock to the pulp.

Liners and cement bases are placed following the completion of the cavity, just prior to insertion of the restorative material. The following information should aid the assistant in becoming effective in this phase of operative dentistry:

1. As the operator completes the cavity preparation, instructions on the type of cement base required will permit the assistant to mix and have it ready. The alert assistant, after having learned the operator's technique, will automatically prepare the mix at the proper time and move it to the exchange zone as the operator receives the instrument used to apply the cement. Most cements are best applied when the instrument is wiped clean between each

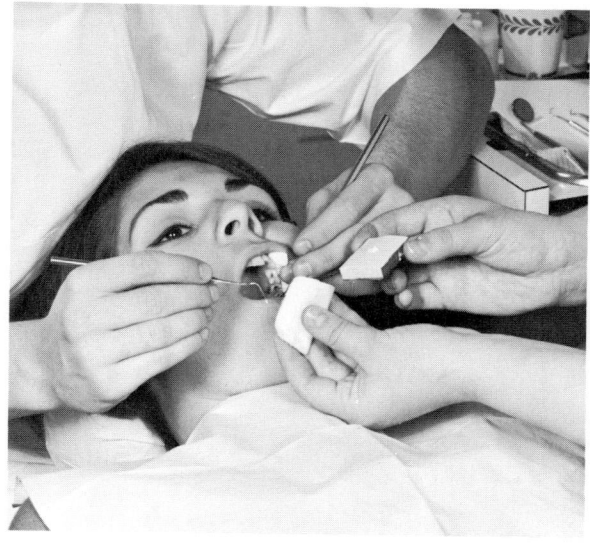

Figure 28-30 | Assisting in placement of cement bases.

small increment. Hold a gauze sponge in the exchange zone and quickly wipe the end of the instrument as the operator moves toward the cement mix (Fig. 28-30).
2. When more than one type of cement must be used, do not mix the second until the first has completely set so that application of the second cement does not disturb the first. Any waiting time can be used to obtain instruments or materials for the next step (i.e., matrix retainer, wedges).
3. If the operator inadvertently gets cement on the cavity walls outside the excavation, be prepared to pass instruments for removal of this cement.
4. Liners (cavity varnish) are applied to the preparation via a small cotton pellet. The cotton pellet is held by cotton pliers and dipped in the varnish just sufficiently to wet the pellet. Pass the cotton pliers to the operator. If the cavity preparation is small, the operator may need the explorer to move the cotton pellet throughout the preparation.

Amalgam Restorations

The restoration of teeth, regardless of the type of restorative material to be used, involves certain

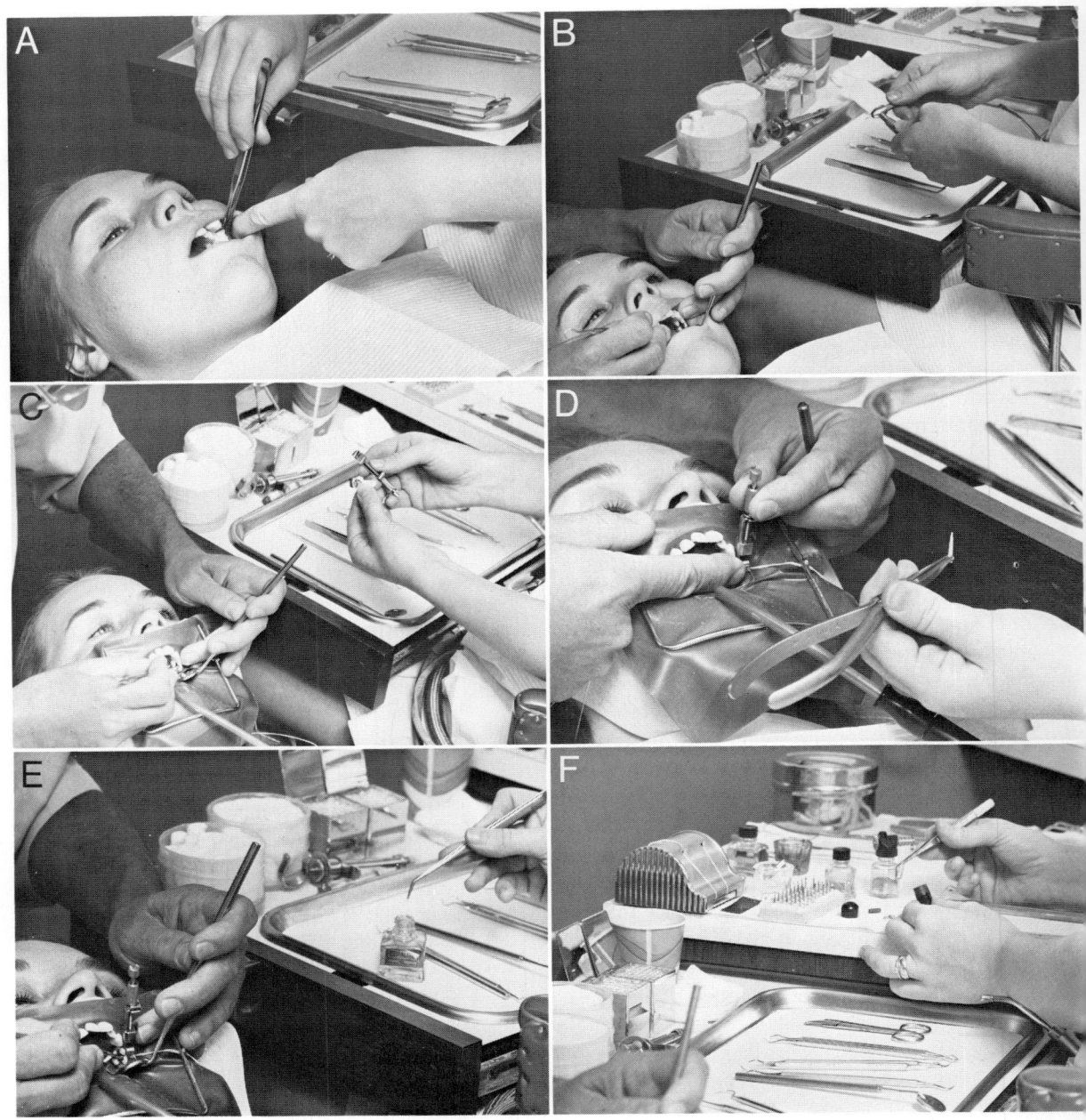

Figure 28-31 | Assisting in amalgam restoration. A. Placing cotton roll. B. Changing bur. C. Preparing matrix retainer and band. D. Passing wedge held in pliers. E. Preparing cavity varnish. F. Preparing to triturate amalgam alloy.

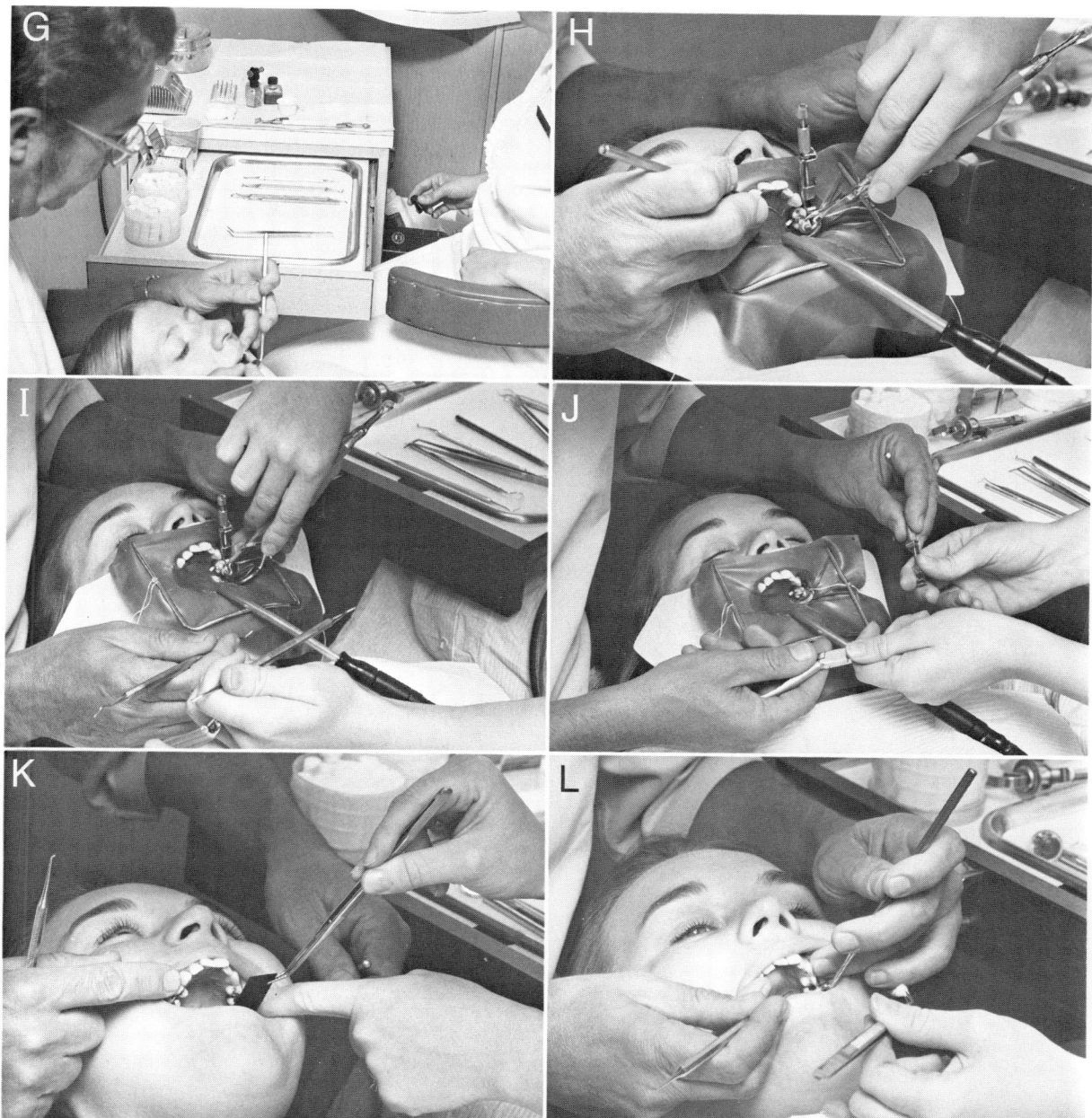

Figure 28-31 | Assisting in amalgam restoration. G. Placing capsule in triturator. H. Placing alloy in cavity preparation. I. Condenser exchange. J. Receiving matrix retainer, passing pliers. K. Placing articulating paper. L. Cotton pellet in operating pliers, ready to receive carver.

responsibilities of the assistant. Previous sections have described those chairside duties required of the assistant in the administration of the local anesthetic, cavity preparation, rubber dam placement, and insertion of liners and bases. The following sequence of responsibilities is necessary for the assistant to properly assist the operator in completing an amalgam restoration (Fig. 28-31):

1. During the final cutting steps in cavity preparation, the assistant should note if a matrix band is to be used. With some experience, the assistant will be able to observe the occlusogingival height of the preparation and select a band of proper size. The band is positioned in the retainer at a time when the assistant's attention may be directed away from the field of operation.
2. Assist in the final step of cavity preparation (cleansing the preparation). From this point to the completion of the restoration the attention of the assistant is especially critical in that each step in the procedure must be rapidly anticipated in order to have the necessary materials ready at the proper time. More instruments are needed to place the restoration than to prepare the tooth; therefore, more instrument exchanges are necessary, and they occur more rapidly than in cavity preparation.
3. When the cavity preparation is cleaned, pass the matrix retainer.
4. While the operator positions the retainer and band, obtain from the setup a wedge and place it in the serrated-tip pliers. Position the pliers (with the handles directed toward the operator) to rapidly place them in the operator's hand.
5. Pass the pliers and, as the operator places the wedge, prepare a small cotton pellet and wet it with varnish. The cotton pellet can be made in advance when the setup is prepared and will be ready when required.
6. Receive the serrated-tip pliers and pass the operating pliers with the cotton pellet in position. Receive the operating pliers and pass the explorer. Many operators prefer to move the pellet throughout the preparation with the explorer.
7. While the operator applies the varnish, load the mixing capsule with alloy and mercury. This may be accomplished earlier in the procedure provided the capsule is stored so that the mercury does not contact the alloy. Many dentists use precapsulated alloy, and the capsules must be activated prior to trituration to release the mercury into the mixing chamber.
8. Receive the operating pliers and pass a suitable burnishing instrument for final adjustment to the contact areas.
9. Triturate the alloy and mercury while the operator completes the adjustments to the contacts.
10. Receive the burnishing instrument and pass the first condensing instrument.
11. Load the amalgam carrier and place the amalgam alloy in the cavity preparation. Always begin the placement by inserting the first increment into the proximal boxing. Usually the operator will indicate thereafter the area of the cavity preparation in which the next portion is to be placed. During the condensing procedure the operator will indicate when a change in condensers is needed. The experienced assistant will know when a change is needed by observing the stage of completion and will move to exchange condensers at the proper time. Continue to insert the alloy and make the exchange of condensers as required.
12. When the last increment of alloy has been placed in the preparation, discard the carrier and obtain the explorer. The explorer is followed with a carving instrument. Hold the evacuator tip adjacent to the tooth to remove the shavings from the carving procedure. Observe when the occlusal carving is near completion and obtain the serrated-tip pliers.
13. Receive the carver and pass the pliers. Receive the pliers and wedge(s).
14. Hold left hand in position to receive the matrix retainer and have pliers in position to pass. Pass the pliers as retainer is received.
15. Receive the pliers and matrix band. Pass the explorer. The operator may require the carver for additional shaping of the restoration.
16. Receive the explorer or carver and assist in removal of the rubber dam. Wash the patient's mouth using the oral evacuator and water syringe.
17. Pass a carver to the operator and place articulating paper between the teeth. Be careful to hold the paper in such a position that the beaks of the

operating pliers are not positioned between the teeth as the patient closes. The operator will instruct the patient on which jaw movements to make. The operator will adjust the occlusion as necessary. The sequence of the assistant placing the articulating paper and the operator adjusting the restoration is repeated until the proper occlusion is obtained.

18. Receive the carver and pass a wet cotton pellet held in the operating pliers. The operator will smooth the newly inserted restoration.
19. Using the water syringe and evacuator tip remove all alloy shavings resulting from the occlusal adjustment.
20. Be certain the patient understands the operator's postoperative instructions. Repeat them if necessary.

When all amalgam restorations have been placed, the patient is appointed for polishing. When the patient is seated, clothing should be protected from the polishing agents by draping the patient with a plastic apron. Chairside assisting associated with polishing amalgam restorations is not different from other procedures in that a definite routine is also followed to accomplish the polishing in the most efficient manner.

1. Pass a mirror and the straight handpiece with the proper size round finishing bur. Some operators prefer to use the finishing burs in the air-turbine handpiece.
2. When the operator completes the surfacing with the finishing burs, remove the bur from the handpiece and position the prophylaxis angle on the straight handpiece while the operator maintains the position of the handpiece in the exchange zone. A tapered bristle brush should have been placed in the prophylaxis angle when the setup was prepared.
3. Hold the pumice paste in the exchange area for easy access by the operator.
4. Wash the pumice paste from the teeth when the operator completes this step.
5. Replace the bristle brush with a rubber cup and hold the polishing agent near the patient's mouth.
6. Wash all traces of polishing agents from the patient's mouth using the evacuator tip and the water syringe.
7. Patients appreciate the opportunity to see the completed restorations. Pass a hand mirror to the patient. Dry the teeth as the operator shows the restorations to the patient.

Matrices for Amalgam Restorations

When one or both of the proximal surfaces of posterior teeth have been included in the cavity preparation, it is necessary to apply a matrix to the tooth to restore the proximal contour and contact. Various commercial matrices are available, or the matrix may be custom-made for the individual tooth. The latter matrix is usually compound-supported and provides more of the essential qualities of a good matrix. Regardless of the type of matrix, certain requirements are essential for the proper restoration of the tooth. The matrix should be rigid, provide proper interproximal contour and contact, and be easy to apply and remove. Also, when properly wedged, it should prevent gingival overhangs.

It is often the responsibility of the auxiliary to prepare the matrix for application to the tooth and in many instances (depending on state's dental laws) to position and wedge the matrix.

Universal matrix The Universal matrix retainer (Tofflemire) is a very popular type used on two- or three-surface cavity preparations. Depending on the type of design (straight or contra-angled) (Fig. 28-32) the matrix may be positioned on the facial or lingual side of the tooth. Usually, the retainer is positioned on the facial surface for convenience (Fig. 28-33).

During the final stages of tooth preparation, the auxiliary will observe the size and extent of the cavity and select the proper band for positioning in the retainer. Bands of various widths are available, and a band must be selected which is slightly wider than the total occlusogingival width of the preparation. When the cavity preparation is such that one of the proximal portions is

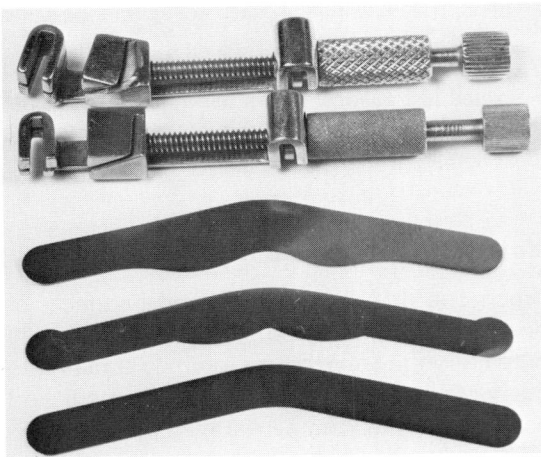

Figure 28-32 | Straight and contra-angled Universal retainers with a selection of bands.

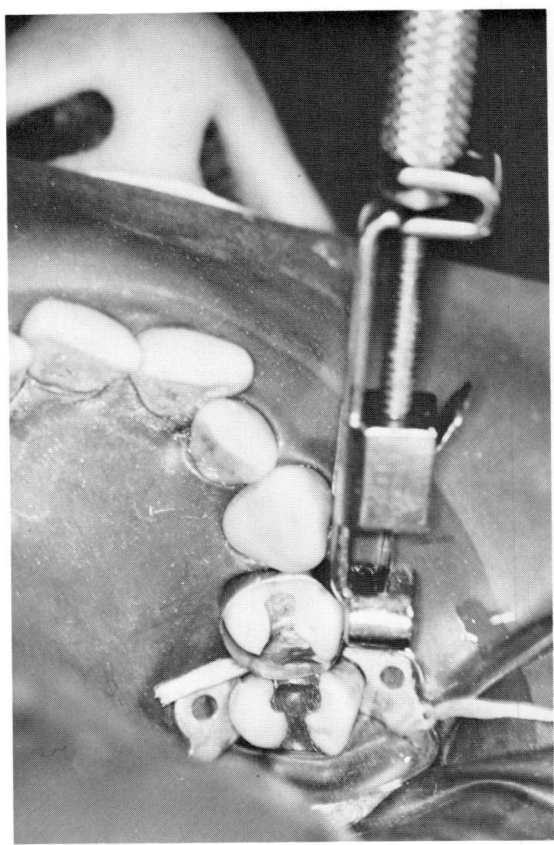

Figure 28-33 | Universal retainer positioned on facial of maxillary left teeth.

deeper gingivally than the other, some alteration to the band is usually required. Figure 28-34 illustrates how a band may be shortened on one side to permit the opposite side to extend further into the gingival crevice.

When the proper band has been selected, it must be contoured by burnishing the areas of the band which provide proximal contour and contact. This is accomplished by placing the band on a paper pad and rubbing with a large ball-burnisher until a convexity appears as shown in Fig. 28-35. Heavy pressure with the burnisher is necessary to properly reshape the band. Experience will dictate just how much pressure is required.

After burnishing, the band is ready to be placed in the retainer.

1. Holding the retainer in one hand, turn the larger of the two round, serrated nuts until the locking vise is about one-quarter in from the end of the retainer (Fig. 28-36A).
2. While holding the large nut, turn the smaller nut in a counterclockwise motion until the spindle can no longer be seen in the slot of the locking vise (Fig. 28-36B). The retainer is now ready to receive the band.
3. Fold the burnished band end to end. Notice that one circumference of the loop is smaller than the other (Fig. 28-36C). The smaller circumference is always positioned toward the gingival aspect of the cavity preparation. This is necessary to draw the band tightly around the tooth, because the gingival circumference of the tooth is less than the occlusal dimension. Place the band in the retainer by first sliding the occlusal edges of the band into the proper guide channel while in the same motion positioning the ends of the band in the slot of the locking vise. (*Note:* The slotted side of the end of

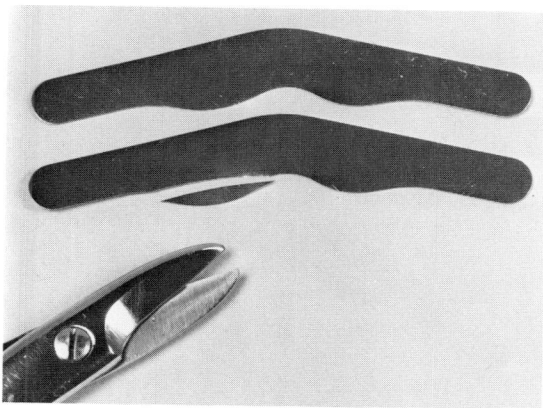

Figure 28-34 | Alteration of molar band.

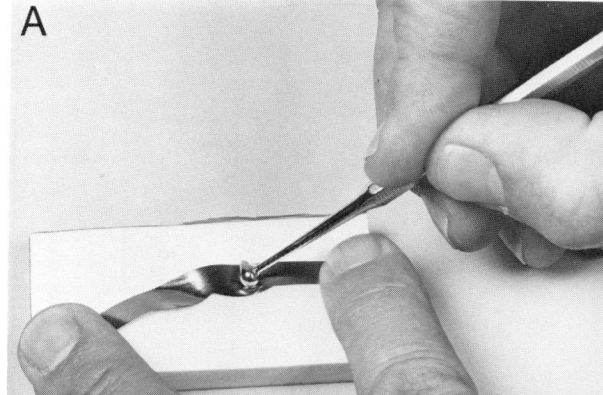

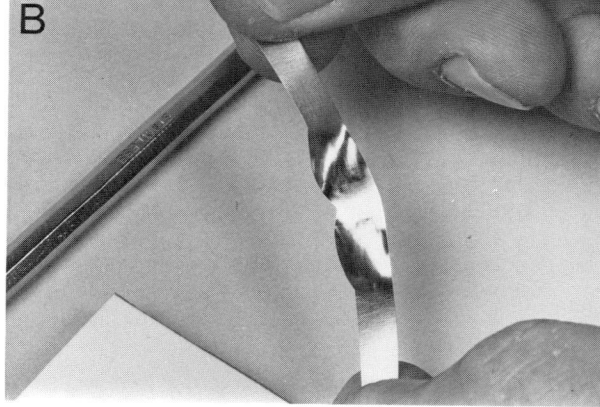

Figure 28-35 | Burnishing band. A. Burnishing band with large burnisher over paper pad. B. Properly burnished band.

the retainer is always positioned in a gingival direction to permit removal of the retainer in an occlusal direction.)

4. Next, turn the small nut in a clockwise motion until the spindle presses against the band. This locks the band in the retainer. The band and retainer are now ready to be placed on the tooth (Fig. 28-36D).
5. Position the band loop over the tooth. Adjust the size of the loop to approximate the size of the tooth. By turning the larger of the serrated nuts the band loop is made smaller or larger as required to fit the prepared tooth. Move the band in a gingival direction until the edge of the band is positioned in the gingival crevice. It may be necessary to reduce the size of the loop as the band is moved in a gingival direction to prevent trapping the gingival tissue between the band and the gingival margin of the preparation.
6. When the band is properly positioned in the gingival crevice, turn the large nut in a clockwise motion to tighten the band securely around the tooth (Fig. 28-36E).
7. The gingival portion of the band must be wedged against the unprepared tooth. Wedging provides slight separation which compensates for the thickness of the band material to ensure a tight contact upon removal of the band. Also, wedging should be tight enough to prevent alloy from escaping between the gingival margin of the preparation and the band. Should this occur because of improper wedge placement, gingival excesses occur which are commonly referred to as "overhangs." A suitable wedge is usually obtained by breaking off approximately one-half in of a round toothpick. The wedge is picked up and held in the tips of the no. 110 serrated-tip pliers. Insert the wedge, pointed tip first, from the facial or lingual embrasure, in such a manner that the wedge is gingival to the gingival margin of the cavity preparation (Fig. 28-36F). When the wedge is of proper size, reasonable pressure will result in the contact of the wedge against the adjacent tooth, ensuring that the

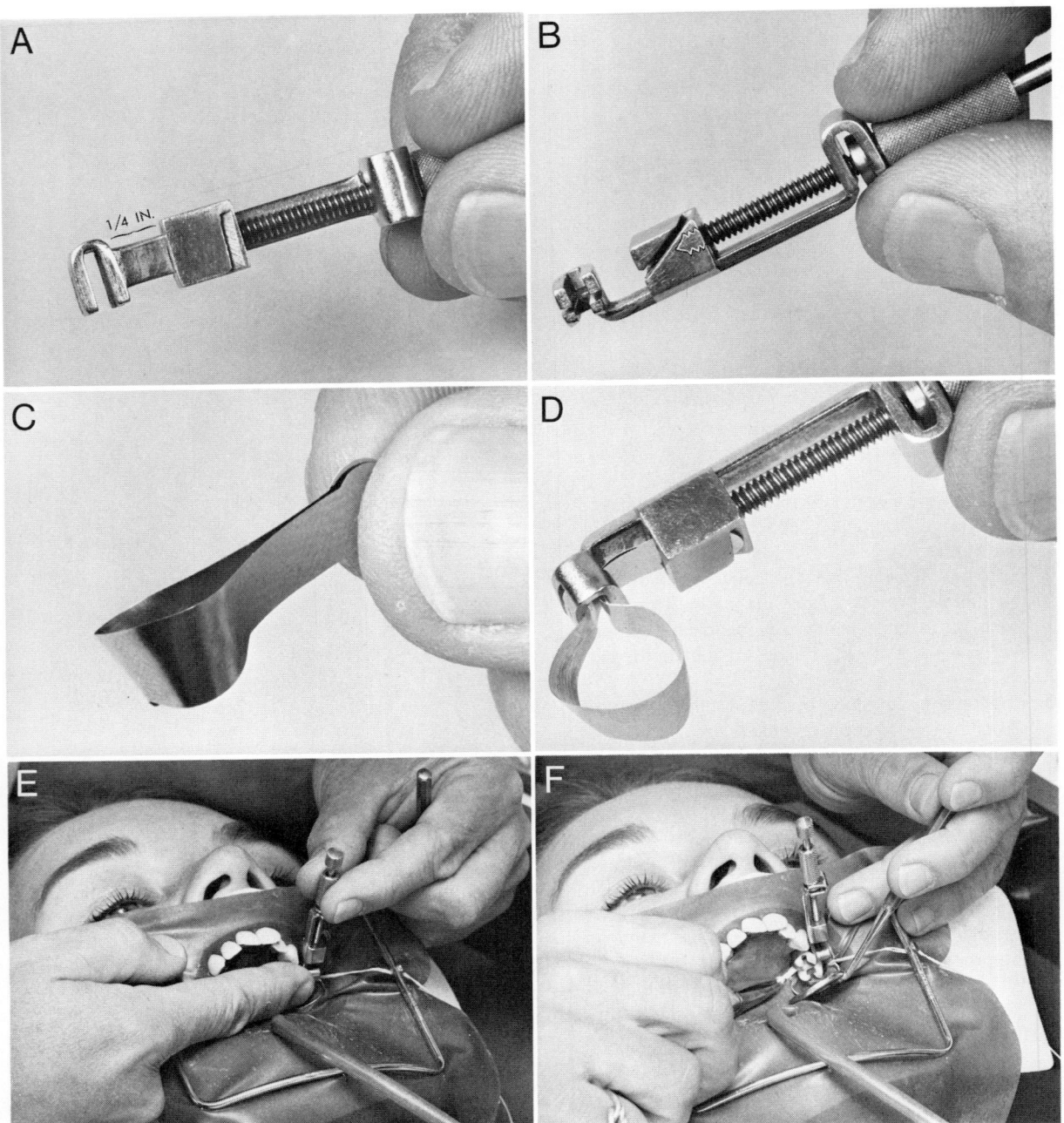

Figure 28-36 | Preparing and positioning Universal retainer. A. Locking device one-quarter in from end of retainer. B. Spindle retracted from slot in locking device. C. Folded band ready for placement in retainer. D. Band and retainer properly assembled. E. Band being tightened around tooth. F. Insertion of wedge.

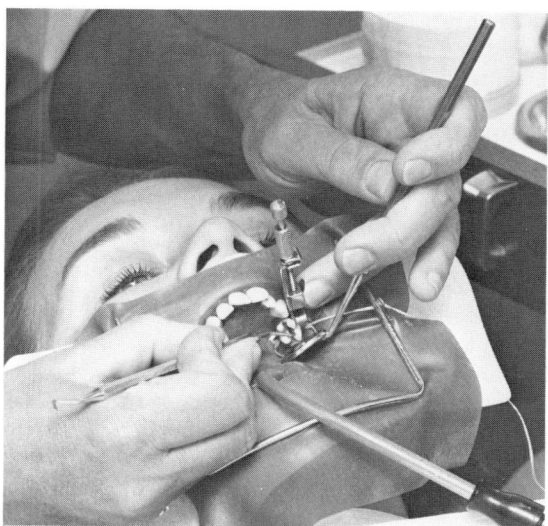

Figure 28-37 | Contact and contour of band being adjusted with 15-8-14 spoon.

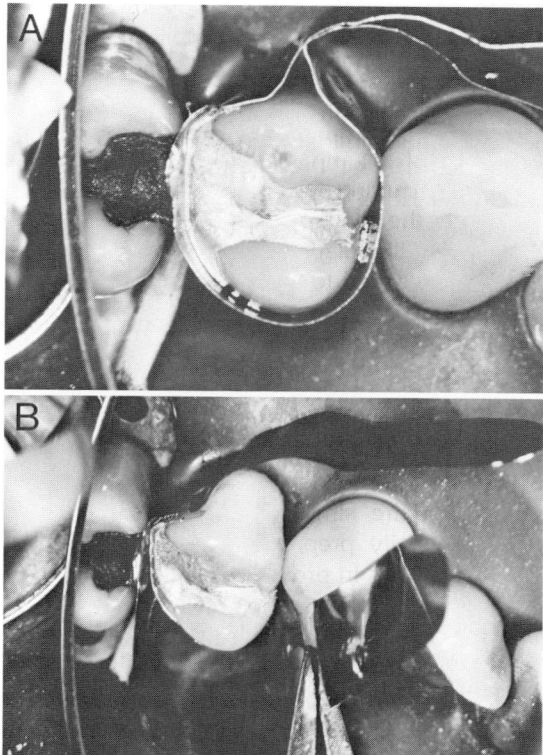

Figure 28-38 | Retainer and band removal. A. Initial carving and retainer removed. B. One side of band being removed with pliers.

band is pressed tightly against the gingival margin of the preparation. It is extremely important that no part of the wedge be occlusal to the gingival margin of the preparation. Should this occur, an abnormal contour in the proximal surface would be created.

8. Next, observe the size and level of the contact area by noticing how the band contacts the adjacent tooth. Should adjustment be required to broaden the contact in size or to change the occlusogingival level of the contact, burnishing with the back side of a 15-8-14 spoon excavator will suffice to make minor adjustments (Fig. 28-37). When major adjustments are required, the band and retainer should be removed from the tooth and the band returned to the paper pad for additional burnishing.

9. Insertion of the alloy and carving procedures are accomplished as described elsewhere in this chapter. To remove the retainer, first loosen the small serrated nut (turn in a counterclockwise motion) until the spindle is no longer in contact with the band. When this has been accomplished, remove the retainer from the band by moving it in an occlusal direction (Fig. 28-38A). Remove the wedges with the no. 110 pliers. The band is next removed by grasping one end of the band with the no. 110 pliers and moving the band lingually with a slight occlusal motion until the band is free of the contact (Fig. 28-38B). Follow this with removal of the band from the other contact using the same linguoocclusal motion. When the band has been removed, final carving procedures may be completed.

Gold Inlay Restorations

Completion of gold inlay restorations requires two appointments, one for cavity preparation, impression, and placement of a temporary restoration, and a second for cementation of the restoration. Between these two appointments laboratory procedures must be accomplished to build the inlays. Usually, the order of procedure is cavity preparation, impression of the preparation, placement of a temporary restoration, pouring the model, carving the inlay pattern, investing and casting the inlay, polishing the inlay, and cementation of the inlay. In some offices, the assistant may be asked to accomplish certain of the laboratory procedures, but the primary responsibility is to provide chairside assistance.

Cavity Preparation

The chairside procedures related to inlay cavity preparation are similar in scope to those of amalgam cavity preparation. There are some basic differences in procedure which will be discussed in the following guidelines for effective chairside assisting in gold inlay procedures. Prior to the operator beginning cavity preparation the assistant should have obtained or prepared the proper setup and materials necessary to complete cavity preparation, obtain necessary impressions, and place the temporary restoration. When the operative site has been properly anesthetized, the following routine is required of the assistant:

1. Assist in cavity preparation as previously described. When the operator has progressed to the primary cavity preparation stage (preparation essentially completed except for beveling and placement of retention grooves), pass the operator the explorer or a small plastic instrument, whichever is preferred, to place the gingival retraction cord. First, be certain that the teeth are clean and the area is isolated with dry cotton rolls. Pass a length of gingival retraction cord (string) via the operating pliers. With practice, the assistant may place the cord in the proximal boxing in position for the operator to begin its placement into the gingival crevice. (Note: The gingival retraction cord is necessary at this point in the preparation procedure to retract the gingiva away from the tooth to permit the subgingival margination to be accomplished without unnecessary damage to the soft tissues. The retraction cord remains in the crevice for 3 to 5 minutes.)
2. As the operator completes the placement of the string the bur in the handpiece is replaced with a flame-shaped diamond stone. Also, the materials necessary for the impression may be arranged during this time if they were not prepared prior to the beginning of the procedure. The materials for impression procedures may be prepared by the second assistant if one is employed, thereby permitting the chairside assistant to devote full attention to chairside duties.
3. Many operators utilize the time during the wait for gingival retraction to occur to remove the remaining decay (that which has extended beyond the normal pulpal and axial wall position) and to place cement bases. Should this be the operator's standard routine, the assistant should assist in decay removal as described in a previous section.
4. Pass the handpiece to the operator. Remove the retraction cord systematically from one proximal boxing to another as the operator marginates the preparation. When the cavity preparation is completed, wash the tooth and the mouth free of debris.

Impression of the Preparation

An impression of the prepared tooth is necessary when the operator prefers to make the inlay indirectly. Because most operators use the indirect method of obtaining the wax pattern the procedure for the rubber impression is presented. Accurate impressions can be obtained only when the teeth are dry. Isolate the prepared teeth (preferably the entire quadrant) with cotton rolls and place the saliva ejector. When the teeth have been dried, assist the operator in again placing the gingival retraction cord. The hemostatic agent incorporated in the cord helps to stop any gingival hemorrhage stimulated during the margination procedure. During the 3- to 5-minute wait before the impression can be made, arrange the setup for the impression (Fig. 28-39). This may already have been arranged by the second assistant or arranged prior to seating the patient. The setup should include: syringe and tip, a paper funnel for loading the syringe, a tray, two mixing pads, two spatulas, "heavy" and "injection" types of rubber, and any additional hemostatic agents used in conjunction with the retraction cord. The following procedure is necessary for the assistant to properly prepare for and assist in rubber impression procedures:

1. Apply one or two coats of rubber adhesive cement to the tray, allowing sufficient drying time. When stock polystyrene trays are used, the assistant is urged to prepare a number of these trays with the adhesive in advance, thereby assuring an adequate supply of trays ready for use. No disadvantage has been found in applying the adhesive days in advance of using the tray.
2. Remove a sheet of paper from one of the mixing pads and fold it into a funnel as shown in Fig. 28-40. The funnel is used to load the syringe with the "injection" material. The assistant should prepare a supply of these funnels in advance. It is embarrassing to the assistant to have the rubber material on the mixing pads only to discover the funnel is not ready.
3. Assemble the syringe by unscrewing the hub, placing a plastic tip over the end of the barrel, and repositioning the hub. Adjust the fit of the Teflon washer on the end of the piston to permit the piston to move through the barrel with about the same finger pressure as is customarily applied to the anesthetic syringe. Remove the piston and place the syringe aside for the present.
4. Proper proportioning, handling, and mixing of the rubber materials are covered in Chap. 11. Usually the assistant will mix the tray rubber and load the tray, while the dentist mixes the injection-type rubber and loads the syringe, or vice versa. When a second assistant is available to mix, the operator may remain at the chairside to maintain dryness of the area.
5. Pass a mirror to the operator. The syringe is passed with the tip properly directed so that the operator does not have to rotate it to begin the injection procedure.
6. Obtain the operating pliers and carefully remove the gingival retraction cord. The operator will follow by injecting the rubber into the gingival crevice. When more than one tooth is to be impressed, the assistant should endeavor to remove the retraction cords on a second tooth while the operator injects about the first. The procedure is repeated until all prepared teeth have been covered.
7. When the last retraction cord has been removed, discard the operating pliers and prepare to pass the tray to the operator. Receive the syringe and pass the tray. Position the tray so that the operator grasps the handle rather than the body of the tray.
8. Most operators prefer to place a small amount of injection-type rubber in the mouth to test for the proper set. The assistant retracts the patient's lip or cheek and drys one or two teeth, and injects a small amount of rubber into the facial embrasure. The lip is then allowed to cover this material; later, it is retracted and the rubber is tested periodically to ascertain set. This procedure is necessary because the tray usually covers all the injection-type material and testing for set is impossible.
9. During the wait for the impression material to set, heat in an open flame the end of a stick of inlay wax.
10. Receive the impression tray when the operator has removed it from the mouth and pass the softened inlay wax.
11. The operator will insert the softened wax into the preparations and instruct the patient to close the teeth together and make certain movements to obtain a wax occlusal registration (wax bite). While the wax registration is being obtained, mix

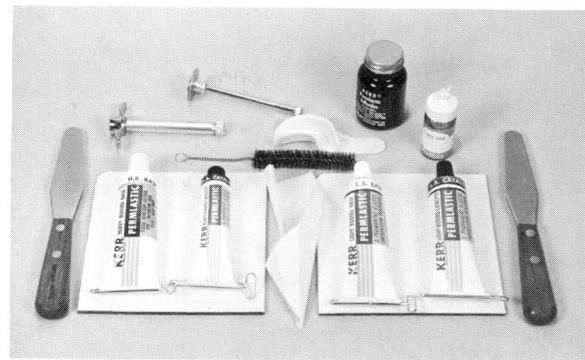

Figure 28-39 | Setup for rubber-base impression.

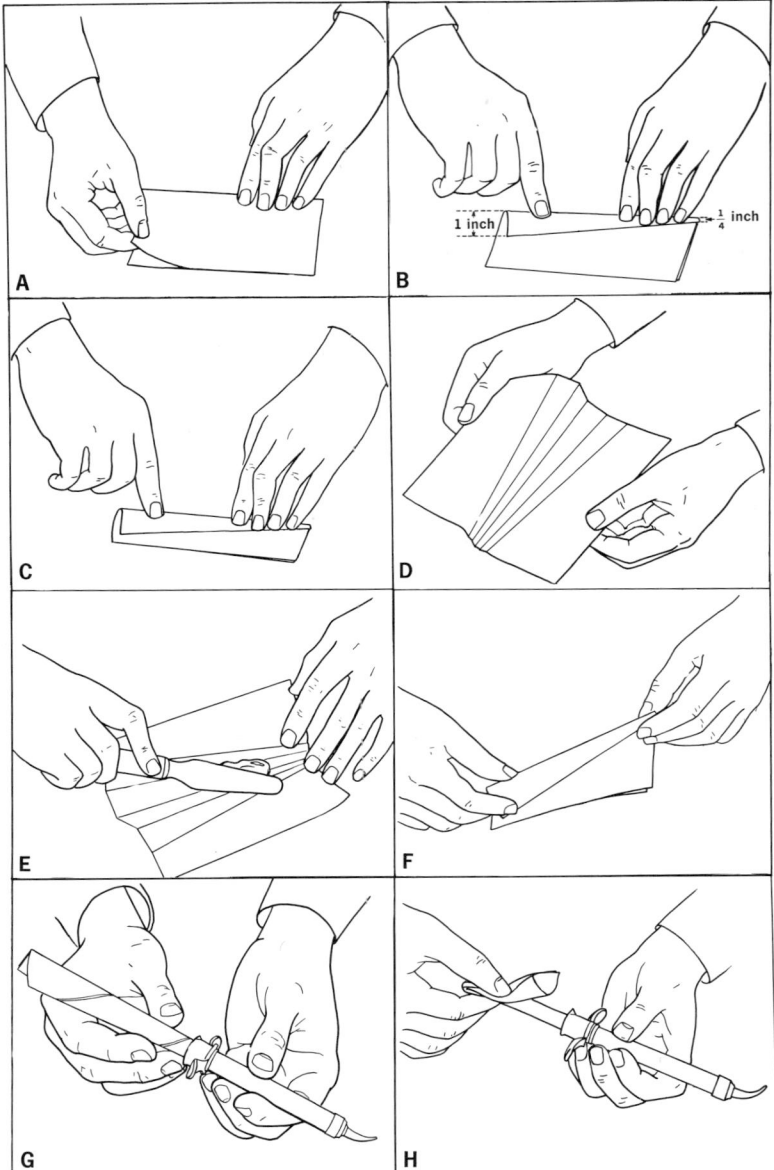

Figure 28-40 | Preparing paper funnel and loading syringe.

a small amount of fast-set plaster and load a suitable tray to complete the functional core. A suitable tray for the plaster is the metal or plastic trays on which artificial teeth are mounted. Pass the tray to the operator for placement over the wax and adjacent teeth which is held in position until the plaster has set.

12. Clean the mixing spatulas and syringe after the impression material has set or when convenient at a later time. Gauze sponges (2 by 2 in) soaked

in 70 percent ethyl alcohol are ideal for wiping clean the spatulas. Manufacturer's instructions should be followed for procedures necessary to clean the syringe.

Placement of Temporary Restoration

One of several methods can be used to produce resin temporary restorations or one of several temporary restorative materials can be mixed for insertion into the tooth. Whichever method the operator prefers, the dental assistant should be prepared to assist in the preparation of and insertion of the various materials. The various cements and temporary restorations require different lengths of time to prepare. It is evident that proper timing by the assistant will avoid unnecessary delays for the operator while materials are being prepared.

When temporary restorations have been placed, the assistant should be certain the patient understands instructions as to necessary precautions before being dismissed.

Pouring Models, Carving, Investing, Casting, and Polishing Inlays

In some dental offices the dental assistant may have certain responsibilities related to laboratory procedures required to construct gold inlays. However, the full-time chairside assistant's major responsibility is at the chairside and those laboratory procedures accomplished in the office are usually delegated to the second or roving assistant.

Cementation of the Inlay

When the laboratory fabrication of the inlay is completed, the patient returns for cementation. The following duties are required of the assistant during the cementation appointment (Fig. 28-41).

1. Prepare the proper setup for cementation procedures.
2. Seat the patient and assist in administration of the local anesthetic. During the wait for onset of anesthesia, remove the inlay(s) from the die and be certain no particles of die stone remain on the cavity side of the inlay.
3. Assist in the removal of the temporary restoration and clean the cavity by using the oral evacuator and the water syringe.
4. Place a cotton roll(s) and dry the tooth.
5. Pass the inlay. Because of its small size it is best to place the inlay in the palm of the hand and let the operator pick it up rather than trying to pass such a small item.
6. While the operator positions the inlay in the tooth, prepare to pass a rubber wheel held in the operating pliers. The rubber wheel is placed between the teeth, and the patient is instructed to close firmly to seat the inlay in the cavity preparation. The experienced assistant may place the rubber wheel between the teeth rather than passing it to the operator. Exercise care to position the wheel so that the beaks of the pliers are out of the way.
7. While the operator evaluates the contact, contour, margins, and occlusion, obtain those instruments the operator may require to finish the margins and adjust the contacts and occlusion. When the occlusion is to be evaluated, place articulating paper between the patient's teeth. At this time, the operator will instruct the patient in those movements of the mandible necessary to evaluate the occlusion. As the operator instructs the patient to open, remove the articulating paper by grasping it with the operating pliers. When occlusal adjustments are necessary, pass the handpiece with a small, pointed Carborundum stone in place. As the operator adjusts the inlay, use the evacuator to remove all shavings or grindings.
8. When the inlay has been properly fitted, pass the operator such instruments as may be required to remove it from the tooth. Place the tip of the index finger over the occlusal surface of the tooth to prevent the inlay from dropping unexpectedly from the cavity preparation. It is quite possible that the inlay could be swallowed very easily when the patient is seated in a reclined position.
9. Dry the inlay; change the cotton roll and redry the tooth in preparation for cementation.
10. Assist in placement of any required cement bases and cavity varnish.

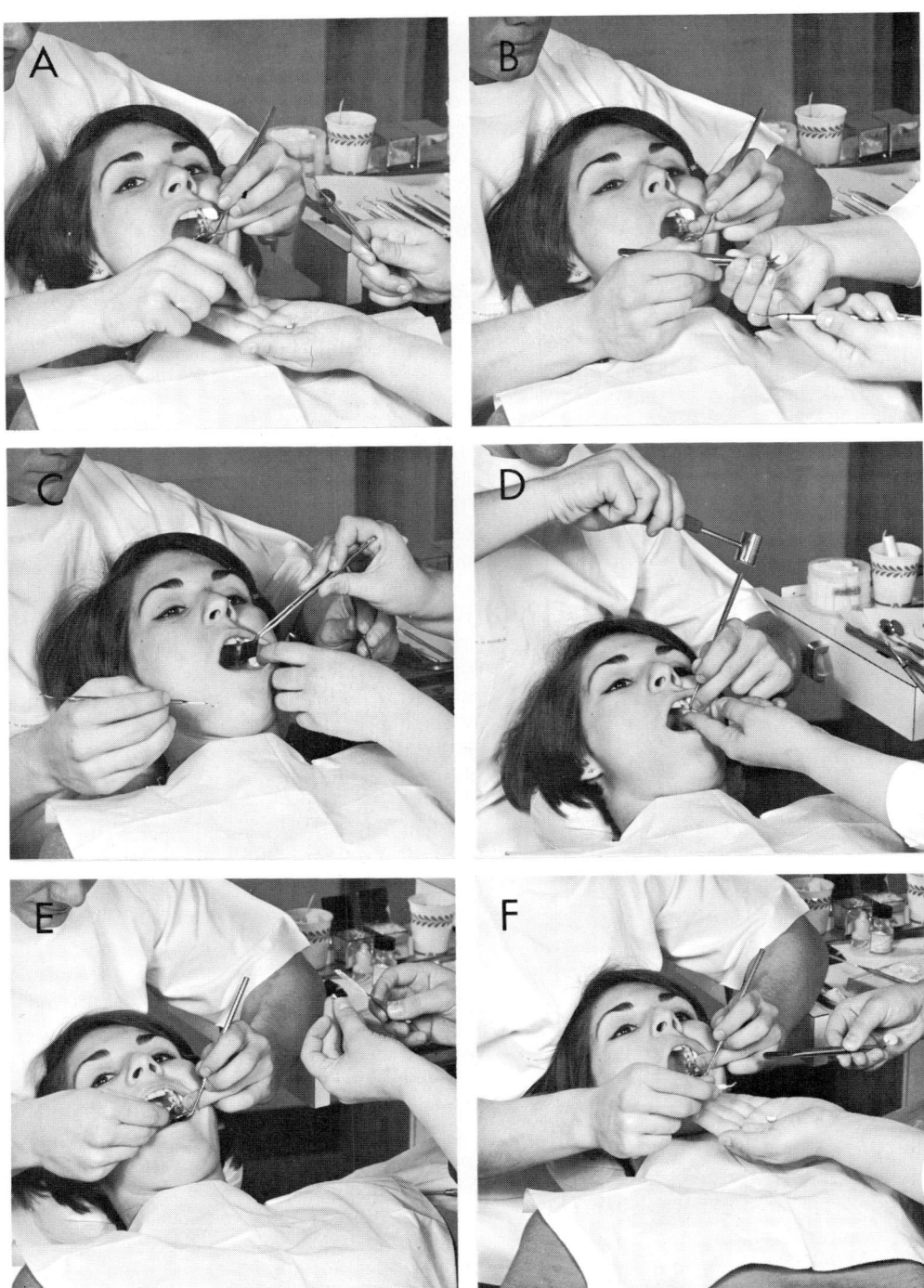

11. Mix the cement, load a jiffy tube, and pass it to the operator. Cover the cavity side of the inlay with cement while the operator applies cement to the cavity preparation.
12. Place the inlay on the end of the glass slab and hold the slab in the exchange area.
13. Receive the jiffy tube and, as soon as the operator picks up the inlay, prepare to pass a ball burnisher which the operator will use to seat the inlay.
14. When the operator has seated the inlay, place the rubber wheel between the teeth as the patient is instructed to close firmly. This procedure assures final seating of the inlay.
15. Maintain dryness until the cement has set.
16. Pass the mirror and explorer. Position the evacuator tip to remove the cement as the operator loosens it from the tooth.
17. Pass a length of dental floss for the operator to clear the contacts of cement.
18. Wash the area free of all cement particles.
19. Dismiss the patient.

Removal of Cement

The removal of excess, set cement around inlays, crowns, and bridges may be the responsibility of the auxiliary depending on the various state dental practice laws.

Several different types of cement are available for final cementation for cast restorations, porcelain crowns, and fixed bridges; however, zinc phosphate cement is probably the most universally used. Removal of any zinc phosphate cement should not be commenced until the cement is completely set. When the explorer tip will no longer make an indentation in the cement surface, a final set has occurred.

It is usually most convenient to remove that cement which has collected in the facial and

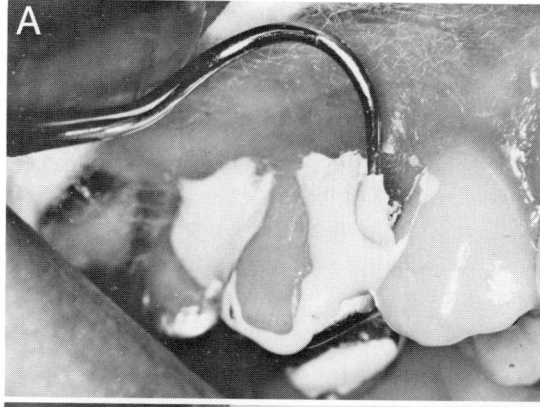

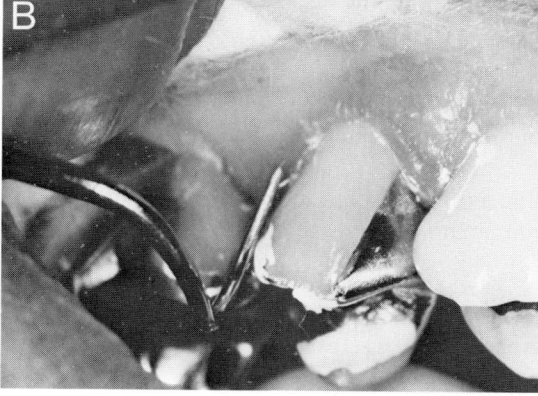

Figure 28-42 | Cement removal. A. Explorer used to remove cement from facial embrasure. B. Side of explorer used on facial surface for cement removal.

Figure 28-41 | Assisting in inlay cementation. A. Passing inlay in open palm. B. Passing Burlew wheel held in operating pliers. C. Placing articulating paper. D. Finger position during removal of inlay. E. Covering inlay with cement while operator coats cavity preparation. F. Hand position for receiving jiffy tube and passing inlay.

lingual embrasures as the first step. This is done by sliding the tip of the explorer under the edge of the cement adjacent to the tooth and moving the explorer in an occlusal direction (Fig. 28-42A). Caution must be exercised not to penetrate the soft tissue when positioning the explorer tip. Careful placement of the explorer with a good finger rest should prevent soft-tissue trauma. Follow this procedure in all the embrasures which require cement removal. Next, the side of the explorer tip may be used on the facial and lingual surfaces of the tooth to loosen any remaining cement (Fig. 28-42B). The explorer or a small ball-burnisher may be used to rub the occlusal surface of the tooth to facilitate removal of cement from the occlusal anatomy of the tooth restoration.

The above procedure will not remove cement in and just below the contact area. Using a length of dental floss with proper finger rests, pass the floss through the contacts. Once the floss has been moved gingival to the contact, pull it either facially or lingually. This motion will help remove cement from the interproximal gingival crevices.

Next, isolate the teeth with cotton rolls and dry the area. A strong stream of air directed into the gingival crevice will help remove small remaining fragments of cement. Any remaining cement which has not been loosened may be seen easily and removed with the explorer tip.

Using the oral evacuator and the water syringe the mouth is completely rinsed to remove any remaining particles of cement.

Silicate Cement and Self-curing Resin Restorations

An important facet in silicate cement and resin restorations is the selection of the proper shade. It is necessary that the shade be selected before the teeth are permitted to dry as a result of isolation with cotton rolls or the rubber dam because dryness results in the tooth becoming lighter in color. A convenient time to select the shade is during the wait for onset of anesthesia.

Assisting in the preparation of the cavity to receive either silicate cement or resin materials is similar to that required for other types of preparations. Also, both materials may require the application of a matrix prior to insertion.

As in other restorative procedures, the assistant mixes the filling material and assists in its placement and in finishing and polishing procedures.

The proper technique of preparing and handling both silicate cement and the self-curing resins is discussed in Chap. 12. Application of previously described chairside duties and a knowledge of the preparation and handling of these materials should permit the assistant to be effective at the chairside when these materials are to be used.

Composite Resin Restorations

Composite resin materials (Fig. 28-43) are available in a variety of forms: a paste-paste system, a powder-liquid system, premeasured capsulated systems, and an ultraviolet light–activated paste system. Usually, the dentist will select a particular brand based on personal choice of the working qualities. It is important that the assistant read and follow the manufacturer's directions on mixing as instructions may vary with different products.

Most of the composite resins are composed of an organic resin matrix and a filler of inorganic ceramic substances. In order for the filler particles to bond to the resin matrix (which improves the physical properties) the filler particles must be surface treated. Completed composite resin restorations are somewhat rough, which makes them susceptible to staining. Most manufacturers supply a glazing material which is applied over the surface of the composite material which provides an initial smoother surface.

Depending on the manufacturer, color systems vary. Some brands offer several color selections while others are supplied in a universal shade. Universal shades may be altered by the addition of lighter, darker, or opaque additives. When the patient presents with a difficult shading problem, test mixes of various combinations may be necessary which can be used as shade guides before a final color is selected.

Chairside assisting procedures for composite resin restorations are similar to those for silicate cement and/or self-curing resin restorations. It is the auxiliary's responsibility to properly prepare instruments and materials, to assist during the

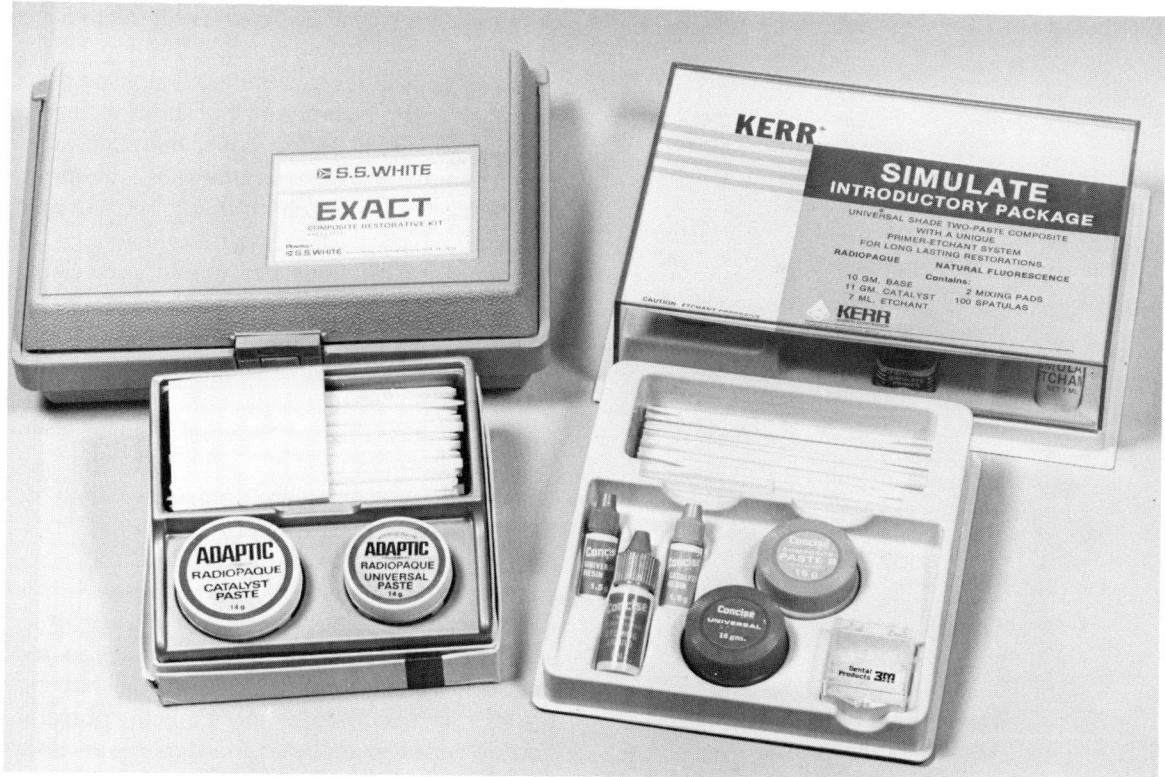

Figure 28-43 | Composite resin materials.

procedure, and to clean the operatory following completion of the restoration.

Acid-Etching Procedures

Improved retention of self-curing resins and composite resins may be obtained by acid-etching the enamel portion of cavity preparations with a 30 to 50 percent solution of phosphoric acid. Phosphoric acid is applied to the enamel surface of the cavity preparation with a small cotton pellet and allowed to be in contact with the enamel for a period of 1 to 2 minutes. The area is then thoroughly washed with water and dried. The etched enamel surface when dried has a ground-glass appearance because of slight dissolution of the surface enamel which leaves microscopic voids.

It is extremely important when washing an acid-treated tooth that the patient's eyes be closed and/or protected. The use of the oral evacuator to suction away the solution is highly recommended to prevent splashing toward the patient's face and eyes.

When self-curing resin is applied to this etched surface, the resin invades the surface voids and irregularities and, when allowed to cure, provides a mechanical bond. This type of surface union between the restorative material and the enamel not only improves the retention qualities

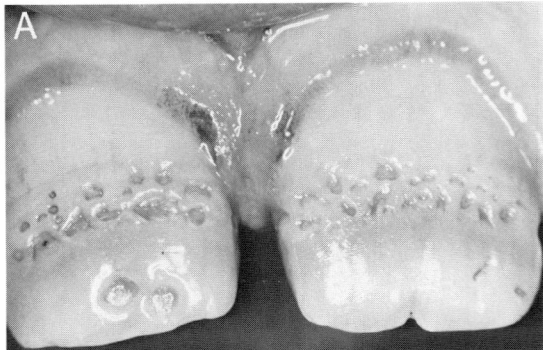
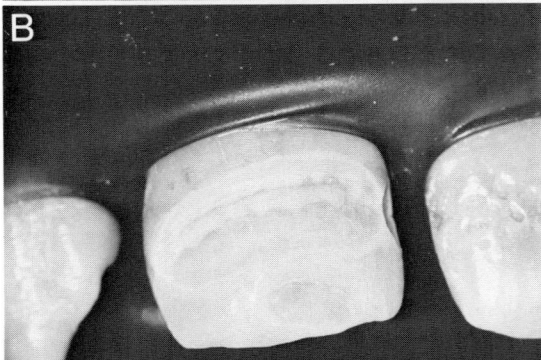
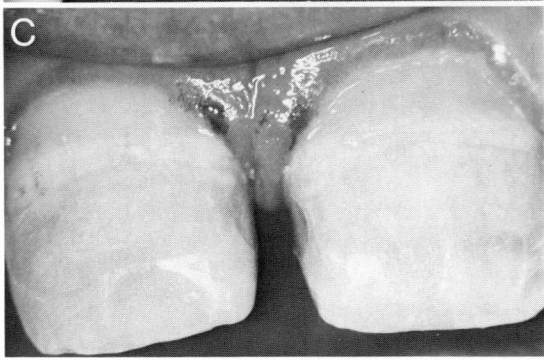

Figure 28-44 | Composite resin restoration. A. Preoperative condition of tooth. B. Cavity preparation and acid-etching of enamel. C. Completed restoration.

composite resin is to be used as the restorative material. Immediately preceding the application of the composite resin, a coating of unfilled resin is applied to the etched surface. This is the same material which is used to cover the restoration upon completion of contouring and finishing. The unfilled resin penetrates the surface irregularities to which the filled resin is applied.

Because of the improved retention available through the use of enamel etching, cavity preparation in certain situations may deviate from the conventional type of preparation with butt joints and undercut retention areas. Developmental defects, areas of enamel staining, fractured incisal corners of anterior teeth, and eroded/abraded areas are particularly ideal for the modified type of tooth preparation. An example of conservative tooth reduction, acid-etching, and restoration with a composite resin is illustrated in Fig. 28-44. Notice how the enamel surrounding the defect has been prepared (shallow, dished-out, and extended well beyond the enamel defect). Also, notice that the preparation does not extend into the dentin and does not have the conventional 90-degree cavosurface margin. Inclusion of a moderate amount of enamel beyond the defect provided a large surface area of enamel to be etched which greatly increased the retention without severe preparation into the tooth. This type of conservative tooth preparation and restoration provides the dentist an opportunity to restore many teeth which previously required a more radical reduction of the tooth and restoration with gold inlays or full crowns.

Insertion of Materials

Insertion of self-curing resin and composite resins into cavity preparations (particularly those with limited access) can be effectively and efficiently accomplished using a syringe which utilizes a disposable plastic tip. The materials are mixed as recommended by the manufacturer and then loaded into the plastic tip which is

but provides a smoother cavity margin, which also improves the esthetics of the restoration. Because of the improved enamel-restorative union less marginal leakage is likely to occur.

The same acid-etch procedure is used when

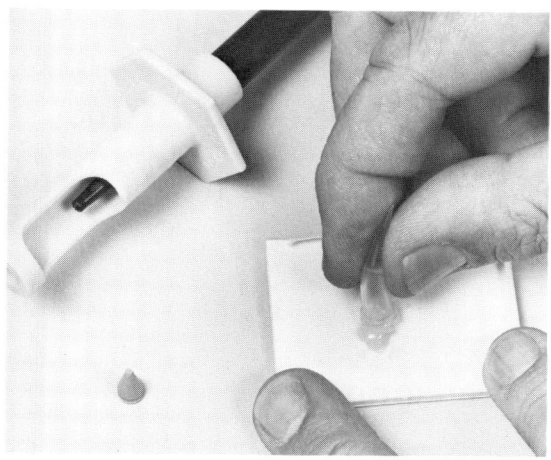

Figure 28-45 | Loading disposable plastic tip with composite resin.

immediately placed in position in the syringe and passed to the operator.

Because of the fluid consistency of the self-curing resin, it may be poured directly from the mixing vessel into the plastic tip. The plastic tip is closed with its accompanying stopper before positioning in the syringe.

The plastic tip may be loaded with composite resin by holding the tip as illustrated in Fig. 28-45 and "cookie-cutting" the material in several motions which should remove all the mixed material from the paper pad. Again, the stopper must be placed in the plastic tip before positioning in the syringe.

Because this syringe method provides relatively easy insertion of both materials into cavity preparations, most dentists will fill more than one cavity preparation with a single mix.

The insertion of the ultraviolet light–activated system requires preparation of materials and equipment by the auxiliary. The sealant must be activated at the beginning of the work day to obtain proper viscosity, and a new bottle must be prepared each day the material is to be used. The ultraviolet light must be turned on at least 10 minutes prior to its anticipated use to obtain adequate light intensity for proper polymerization of the material. When the light is not in use in the mouth, it should be returned to its proper position in the console to prevent heat buildup in the lamp. At the completion of the procedure, the light is allowed to cool before the cover is replaced over the console.

Gold Foil Restorations

Gold foil restorations involve assisting procedures not unlike those required for other restorative materials and the assistant must provide chairside assistance in the preparation, insertion, and polishing of the restoration.

The most important role the assistant plays in gold foil procedures is in the insertion of the material. At the proper time, usually near the completion of the cavity preparation, the foil should be placed on the annealing tray. When the cavity preparation is ready to fill, the foil is transferred from the tray to the cavity via a gold foil carrier. This is accomplished in such a manner that the operator's attention need not be diverted from the condensation procedure as it is a meticulous operation. The alert assistant will observe the condensation procedure and place the next piece of foil in the cavity preparation at the proper time and in such a manner that it is placed against the previously condensed foil. It should be held in position until the operator secures it by condensation against that foil already in the preparation.

Following condensation procedures, the foil is polished with the rubber dam in place. This helps to protect the soft tissue and also to prevent damage to the tooth structure gingival to the restoration.

When the restoration has been polished, the dam is removed, and the area is washed as is done in other procedures.

29

Gene A. Holland
Fixed Prosthodontics

INTRODUCTION

Prosthodontics is that branch of dental art and science pertaining to the restoration and maintenance of oral functions by the replacement of missing teeth and structures by artificial devices (Boucher, 1963). *Fixed prosthodontics* is the art and science of restoring and maintaining oral function by the replacement of missing teeth (bridges) or crown portions of teeth (crowns) by artificial materials which are firmly attached (cemented) to remaining natural tooth structure.

Current concepts and methods for the prevention and control of dental diseases have resulted in a decrease in the incidence of loss of permanent teeth. However, the need and demand for fixed prosthodontic services remain for several reasons (1) primary preventive or control measures have not proved to be 100 percent effective; (2) traumatic injuries continue to result in fracture and even loss of teeth; (3) permanent teeth are oftentimes congenitally missing or malformed; (4) cosmetics, particularly from the patient's standpoint, often demands restoration of anterior teeth; (5) fixed prostheses are indicated in many instances as a means of stabilizing periodontally weakened teeth by "splinting" the involved teeth; and (6) fixed prostheses (both crowns and bridges) are indicated in some instances to assist in the retention and stabilization of removable partial dentures.

As is true with regard to other dental services, the dental assistant should be familiar with the scope of fixed prosthodontics and understand the basic clinical procedures associated with the development of fixed prostheses. This chapter is intended to introduce the assistant to the more common types of crowns and bridges and to describe those clinical procedures fundamental to the development of such restorations. The assistant's general responsibilities in these procedures are identified and emphasized as they relate to specific fixed prosthodontic techniques. Details of chairside assisting in techniques common to fixed prosthodontic and other restorative procedures (e.g., gold inlays) have purposefully been excluded since these are described in Chap. 28, Operative Dentistry.

THE FIXED BRIDGE

A "fixed bridge" is a restoration (prosthesis) which replaces one or more missing teeth and gains its support through fixation (cementation) to remaining natural teeth. Its primary purpose as a restoration is to maintain the integrity of the dental arches. Secondary functions of the fixed bridge include the restoration of masticatory efficiency and, in some situations, the restoration or improvement of cosmetics. Regardless of its extent (in terms of length or number of teeth involved), the fixed bridge contains three basic parts: *retainers, pontics,* and *connectors.* The supporting teeth (*abutments*), although not to be considered as part of the bridge proper, constitute a fourth critical feature of the prosthesis clinically (Fig. 29-1).

Abutments

By definition, an *abutment* is a remaining natural tooth used for the support or anchorage of a fixed or removable prosthesis (Hickey, Boucher, and Hughes, 1968).

As a general rule, a fixed bridge should be supported by at least two abutments, one on either end of the edentulous space. However, there are instances in which a single abutment might be adequate support for the replacement of a missing tooth. Probably the most common example would be the use of a maxillary canine as an abutment for the replacement of the missing lateral incisor. On the other hand, clinical conditions sometimes indicate the use of more than two remaining teeth as abutments to support the prosthesis.

As a part of diagnosis and treatment planning, the dentist *must* consider several factors when selecting abutment support for a fixed bridge. Among the more critical factors are:

1. The number and position of the teeth to be replaced
2. The number and position of available abutment teeth
3. The relative mobility of potential abutment teeth
4. Direction and magnitude of occlusal stresses which are potential to the prosthesis and abutments

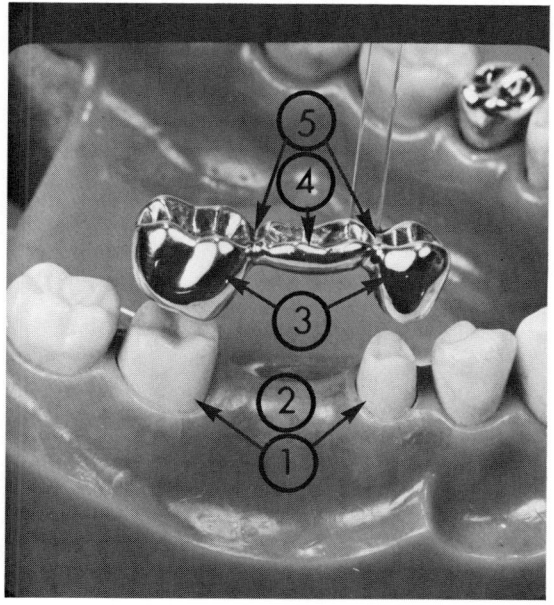

Figure 29-1 | Dental bridge. (1) Abutment teeth; (2) residual alveolar ridge; (3) retainers (full-gold crown); (4) pontic; (5) connectors.

Retainers

A *retainer* is that part of a fixed bridge that unites the abutment tooth with the suspended portion of the bridge. In other words, a retainer is a cast restoration which is cemented to the abutment tooth and "fixes" the replacement tooth (pontic) firmly in position. When properly used, any one of a number of cast restorations can serve as a bridge retainer. The most common type of cast restoration used as a fixed bridge retainer is the *full crown*. Although used less frequently than the full crown, *partial crowns* (*three-quarter crowns* and *pinlays*) and *onlays* (cusp-capping inlays) can serve quite adequately as retainers under certain conditions. Whatever type of retainer is used the restoration must satisfy those criteria which are basic to any cast restoration. It must:

1. Restore form and function to the prepared abutment tooth
2. Be of a material and design such that it will resist bending or rupture under occlusal stress
3. Be retentive on the prepared abutment tooth such that it is not easily displaced nor dislodged
4. "Fit" the prepared abutment tooth such that, when cemented, the tooth is sealed against the ingress of oral fluids and microorganisms
5. Provide features of resistance form which will protect the tooth itself against fracture

As its name implies, the *full crown* is a cast restoration which covers the entire coronal (crown) portion of a tooth and extends usually to just beneath the free gingival crest (Fig. 29-2). The full crown is designed to be placed over a prepared tooth form in which all the *external* surfaces (facial, lingual, mesial, and distal axial surfaces) converge slightly toward the occlusal or incisal. The slight taper (occlusal convergence) of these walls permits the placement and removal of the crown. At the same time, minimal taper of *opposed* external walls provides the necessary retention form which inhibits the easy

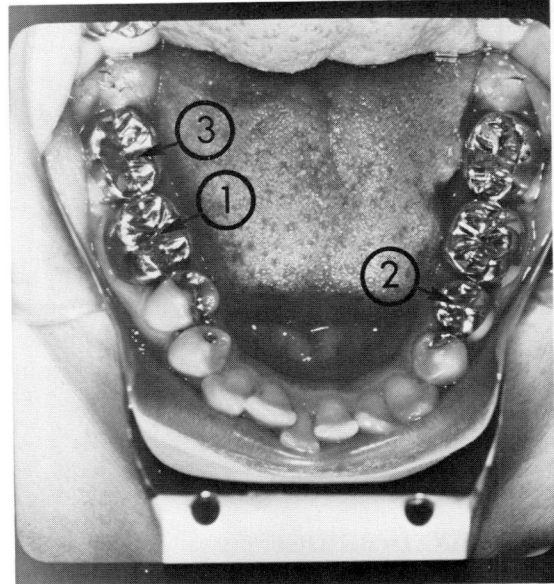

Figure 29-2 | Series of posterior cast gold restorations. (1) Full-gold crown; (2) gold onlay; (3) three-quarter crown.

Figure 29-3 | Dental bridge with partial crown retainers and porcelain faced pontics. *Canine,* pinledge retainer; *first premolar and second molar,* onlay retainers; *second premolar and first molar,* porcelain-faced pontics (note the minimal display of gold for esthetics across the incisal of the canine and facial cusps of the posterior teeth).

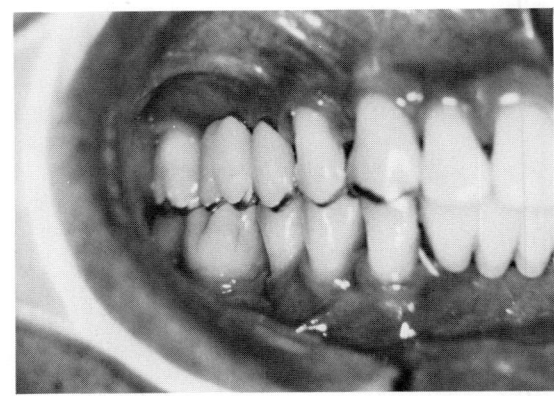

displacement of the restoration. The full crown is referred to as an *extracoronal* restoration.

The *inlay* or *onlay* is constructed to fit into a cavity preparation having internal box form as its primary means of retention. Internal walls which *diverge* slightly toward the occlusal (or incisal) provide the necessary "draw" or "draft" for placement and removal of the restoration. Opposed internal walls which are relatively parallel provide the primary retention form. The inlay or onlay is referred to as an *intracoronal* restoration.

The *three-quarter crown* is essentially an extracoronal restoration which covers three of the four axial surfaces (mesial, distal, facial or lingual, plus the occlusal or incisal) (Fig. 29-2). In most instances the facial surface of the tooth is not disturbed for esthetic reasons. Since the facial or lingual surface will not provide an opposed wall for retention, retention grooves are placed in the mesial and distal proximal surfaces. These proximal grooves (along with an occlusal or incisal groove) add internal retention form to complement that provided by the near parallelism of the prepared external walls. The three-quarter crown design thus has features of both the extracoronal and intracoronal restorations.

The *pinlay* or *pinledge* is a restoration design for anterior teeth, and is similar in its general outline to an anterior three-quarter crown (Fig. 29-3). In contrast to the three-quarter crown, the pinlay gains its retention primarily from either cast or wrought metal pins which extend into carefully prepared parallel holes in dentin.

It should be pointed out that any one of the previously described retainers can serve as individual tooth restorations where indicated.

Pontics

A *pontic* is the suspended member of a bridge, the artificial replacement for a missing tooth (Fig. 29-1). Although there are several functions of a bridge pontic, *its primary function is to maintain the integrity of the dental arches*. This is accomplished by its stabilizing effect on (1) the abutment teeth to which the bridge is attached and (2) the opposing tooth (teeth) through the restoration of proper occlusion.

Pontics are classified basically according to their relationship to the alveolar ridge (edentulous ridge) in the area of the missing tooth (teeth). A *hygienic* or *sanitary* pontic is one designed such that a space (approximately 2 mm) exists between the gingival surface of the pontic and the ridge mucosa (Fig. 29-4). The gingival surface of the hygienic pontic should be convex both faciolingually and mesiodistally so that it can be easily cleansed by the patient. In the anterior region, esthetics and phonetics oftentimes necessitate a pontic design which contacts the ridge tissue. The *tissue-contacting pontic*, likewise, should have a convex gingival surface and should provide minimum contact with the tissue (Fig. 29-5). Either design is acceptable, but the hygienic pontic is preferred whenever possible.

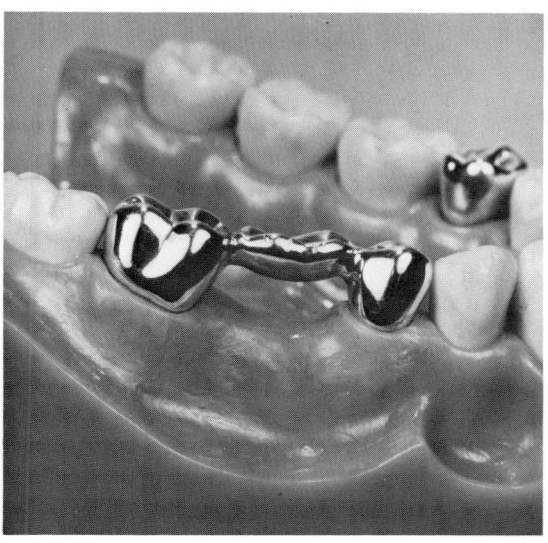

Figure 29-4 | Mandibular all-gold posterior hygienic bridge (technique example).

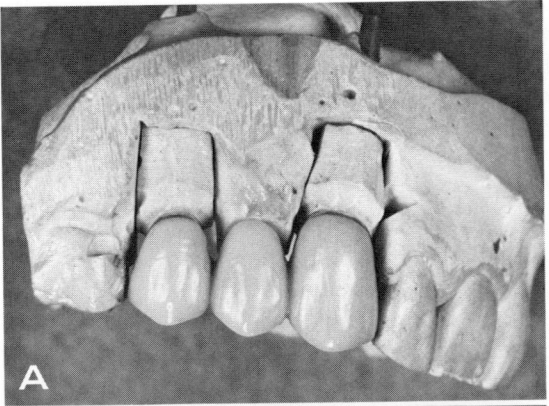
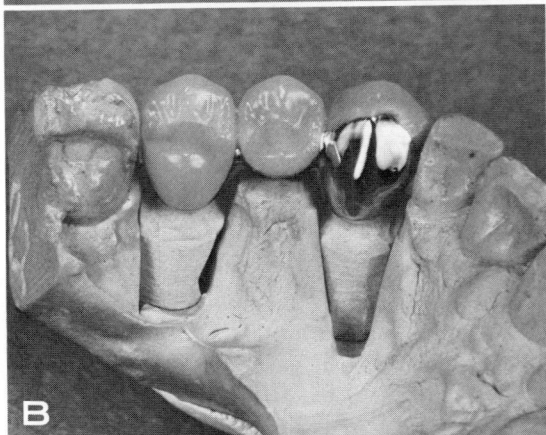
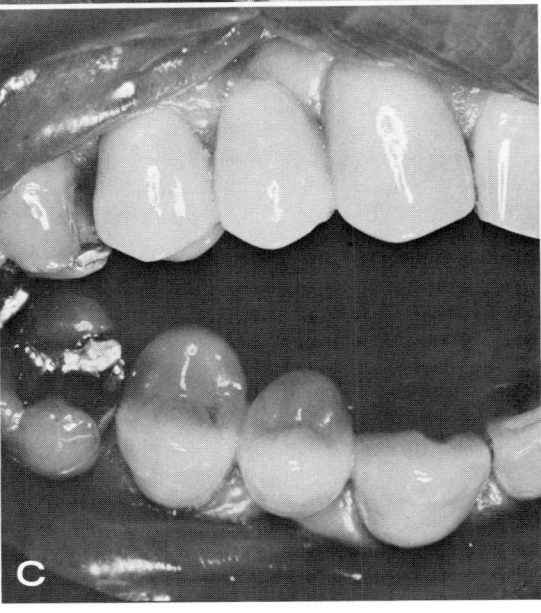

Regardless of the type of pontic used it is most important that the design permit ready accessibility for the patient to clean all surfaces of the pontic and the retainers.

Connectors

A connector is that part of a fixed bridge which unites the retainer and the pontic to form a rigid unit (Fig. 29-1). Connectors are classified as either *cast* or *soldered*. Cast connectors are developed in wax along with the retainers and pontics, and the bridge is cast as a single unit. More often than not bridge components are connected by *soldering*. This procedure requires indexing the relationship between the cast pontic(s) and retainers either from the working cast or directly from the mouth following try-in and adjustment of the individual components. Fast-setting stone or plaster or an autopolymerizing resin can be used to form a rigid index (impression) of the occlusal surfaces of the units to be soldered. The retainers and pontic(s) are then removed from the working cast (dies) or mouth (teeth) and carefully repositioned into the index. The positional relationship of the bridge components is then fixed by a high-heat investment. A soldered connector is formed by flowing gold solder, which fuses at a lower temperature than the casting alloy, into the space provided between approximating surfaces of the pontic(s) and the associated retainers. Final finishing and polishing of the prosthesis is completed following soldering of the connectors.

TYPES OF FIXED BRIDGES

Fixed bridges are generally described according to either the material used in fabrication, method

Figure 29-5 | Maxillary PFM anterior-posterior bridge with tissue-contacting pontic. A. Facial view on working cast. B. Occlusal view. C. Mirror view of bridge in mouth.

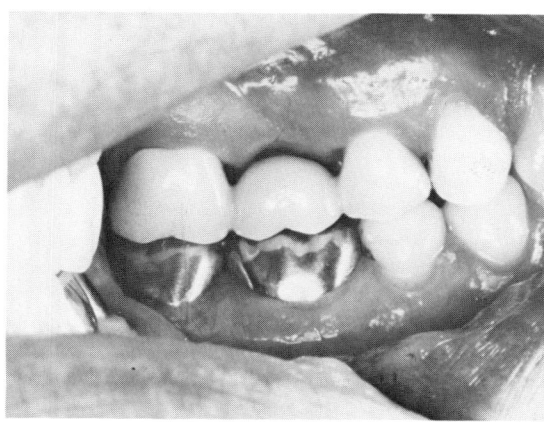

Figure 29-6 | Clinical example of maxillary PFM posterior hygienic bridge.

of construction, or the area of the mouth being restored. Examples of bridges classified according to the material or method of construction are the all-metal cast bridge (Figs. 29-1 and 29-4) and the porcelain-fused-to-metal (PFM) bridge (Figs. 29-5 and 29-6). Based on the location of the restoration in the mouth the fixed bridge is generally classified as (1) a posterior bridge which replaces a posterior tooth (Figs. 29-4 and 29-6), (2) anterior bridge which replaces an anterior tooth (Fig. 29-21G), (3) combination anterior and posterior bridge (Fig. 29-5), or (4) full-arch splint which involves restoration of all the remaining teeth (and edentulous areas) in one arch or the other (Fig. 29-7).

MATERIALS USED IN FIXED PROSTHESES

Except in situations which require the utmost in esthetics, the *cast gold* crown or bridge is the restoration of choice because of the relative simplicity involved in development of the restoration and the excellent clinical performance, both biologically and mechanically, of dental gold casting alloys. It should be pointed out, however, that numerous new alloys have recently been introduced with lower gold content than those of the conventional 65 to 75 percent gold. Casting alloys are described in Chap. 14. Where esthetics becomes a determining criterion for materials selection, tooth-colored *acrylic resins* or *porcelain* can be used as a veneering material for either single crowns or fixed bridges.

Acrylic Resin

Acrylic resins used as veneering materials for permanent restorations are generally from the polymethylmethacrylate group of resins (Fig. 29-8). These materials are generally heat-cured directly onto cast crowns or bridges in areas (primarily facial surfaces) which are readily visible clinically. Surface roughness of those areas receiving the resin serves to retain the resin on the casting. This roughness is generally provided in the form of small beads or very fine loops in the casting which provide undercuts for retention. Permanent resin-veneered restorations are quite esthetic initially, but with age the resin tends to become discolored (due to absorption of stains and oral fluids) and tends to lose surface contour because of its relatively low resistance to abrasion. Even though not so popular as it once was, acrylic resin is still preferred by some practitioners over porcelain as an esthetic veneering material. Cited advantages of resin over porcelain include (1) lower cost of material and fabrication of the restoration, (2) its compatibility with conventional casting alloys, and (3) relative ease of repair without having to remake the restoration.

Porcelain

Porcelain is one of the oldest materials used in restorative dentistry for the repair or replacement of teeth. It is used in fixed prosthodontics for the development of three types of restorations—the *porcelain jacket crown* (PJC); the *porcelain-*

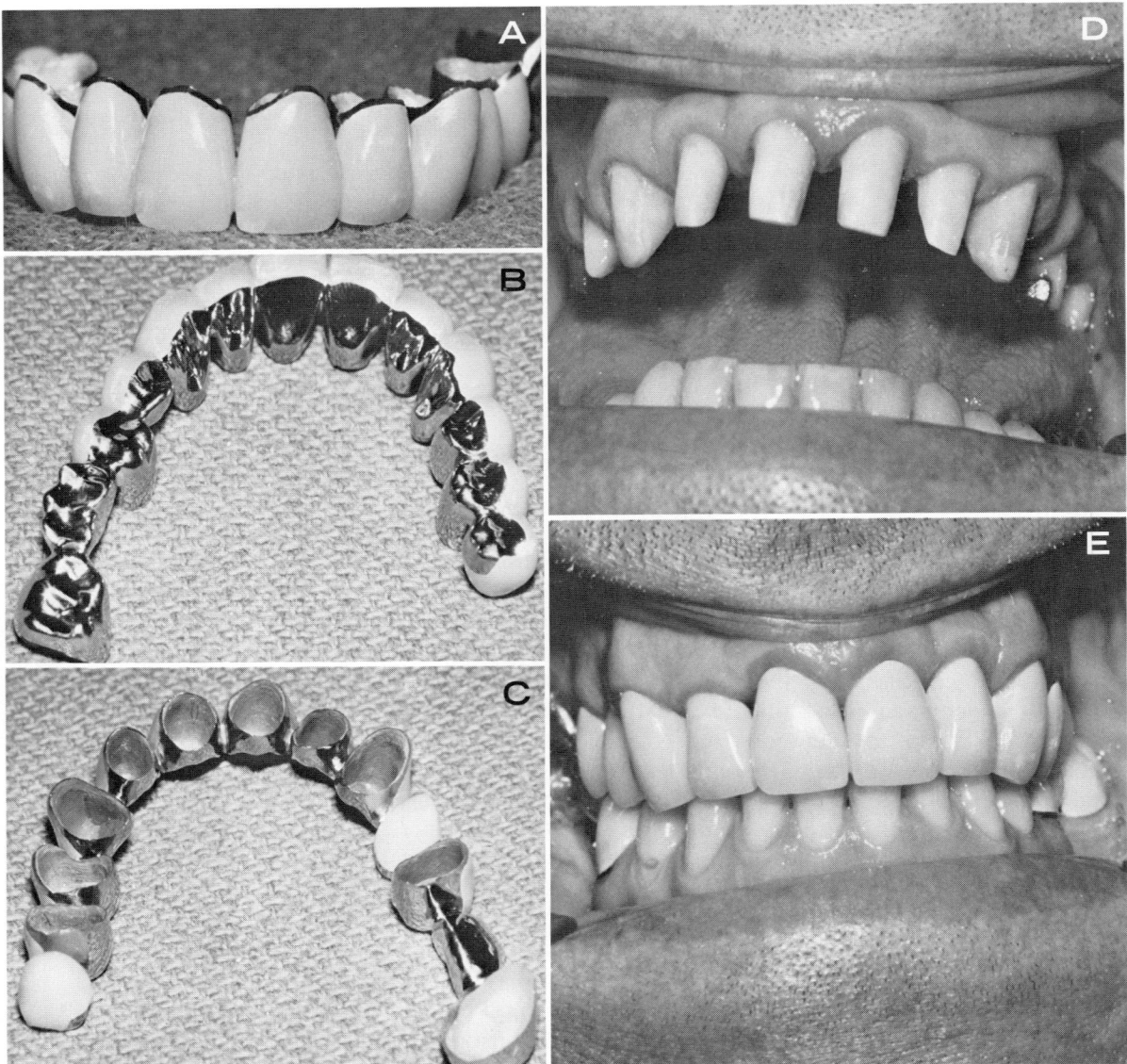

Figure 29-7 | Maxillary full-arch PFM splint. A. Facial view (note narrow gingival metal "collar"). B. Occlusal and lingual view (note metal occlusal and lingual surfaces). C. Gingival view illustrating ten retainers and three pontics. D. Tapered form of full-crown preparations. E. Splint seated.

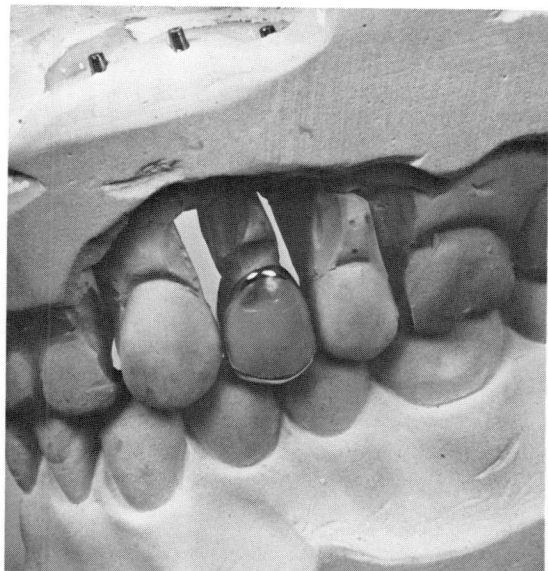

Figure 29-8 | Processed acrylic resin crown with metal coverage of facial cusp tip and gingival "collar" of metal.

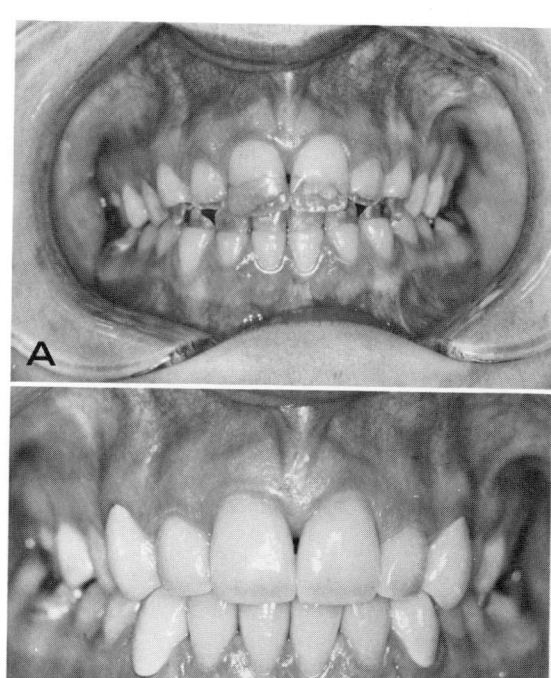

Figure 29-9 | Porcelain jacket and PFM crowns. A. Preoperative photograph illustrating enamel hypoplasia of maxillary and mandibular anterior teeth. B. PJCs on all eight incisors and PFM crowns on all four canines.

faced crown or pontic (cast gold restoration having a cemented porcelain facing); and the *porcelain-fused-to-metal (PFM) crown or bridge.*

The porcelain jacket crown (PJC) is a porcelain restoration which potentially represents the ultimate in esthetics for a single-tooth restoration (Fig. 29-9). Being all porcelain (not requiring a metal coping or substructure), the PJC can be developed with the desired contour and color for esthetics and sufficient bulk for strength with less reduction of the tooth than that required for the porcelain-faced or PFM crown. However, two factors render the PJC somewhat limited in its application as a single-tooth restoration, and porcelain alone is never indicated as a material for a fixed bridge. Matured dental porcelain is essentially a glass and, as such, is a brittle material. Although it is quite strong when subjected to compressive forces, its brittle nature makes it relatively weak when subjected to tensile or shear stresses. Since few occlusal forces are of the compressive type, particularly in the anterior region where the PJC is most often indicated, fracture of the PJC is not an uncommon occurrence. Secondly, the fit of the PJC about the tooth in the area of gingival tissues is, at best, poor in contrast to the cast metal crown which can be developed with a well-adapted "margin" (junction between restoration and tooth at the external tooth surface). Inadequacies in marginal fit of any restoration can result in recurrent decay or gingival irritation from the accumulation of microorganisms along the irregular marginal interface.

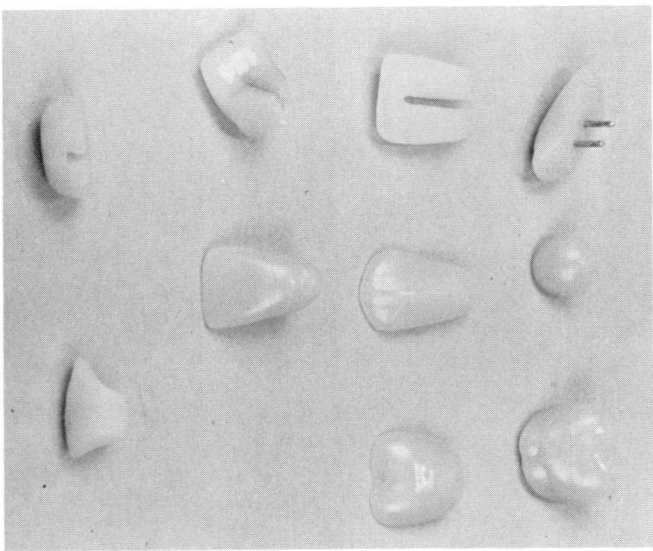

Figure 29-10 | Manufactured porcelain facings for esthetic veneers.

Porcelain facings for both anterior and posterior teeth are commercially available in a number of molds (shapes) and shades (colors) for the esthetic veneering of cast crowns or bridges (Figs. 29-3 and 29-10). Such a facing can be further adjusted by the technician (or dentist) to adapt to a particular pontic space or die of a prepared tooth (stone replica of the tooth in a working cast). Once a casting is obtained from a wax pattern (developed directly against the facing), the facing is cemented, usually with a zinc phosphate cement. A cemented porcelain facing, like the PJC, is brittle and is difficult to replace if fractured once the restoration is cemented onto the prepared teeth.

Developments in recent years have led to mechanisms by which a ceramic (porcelain) can be bonded (fused) directly to the surface of gold casting alloys. As a result, *porcelain-fused-to-metal (PFM)* has become the most popular system for esthetic fixed restorations (Figs. 29-5 to 29-7).

Glazed porcelain has long been recognized as a material with excellent esthetic potential and biologic compatability with oral structures. Being chemically bonded to a metal substructure (coping), porcelain of a PFM restoration is mechanically stronger than that of other systems (e.g., porcelain facing). This added advantage is due to the fact that occlusal forces imposed on the porcelain are transmitted into and resolved through the cast framework and underlying tooth.

The bonding of porcelain to a cast alloy is brought about primarily by a chemical reaction between metallic oxides (usually of iron, tin, and indium) which are common constituents of both the porcelain and the alloy. This reaction occurs as the maturing or fusing temperature of the porcelain is approached (about 1700°F, depending upon the particular ceramic and type furnace used to "bake" the porcelain). Specially formulated porcelains and casting alloys (containing the metallic oxides) are commercially available for the development of PFM restorations.

Basic steps in the fabrication of a PFM restora-

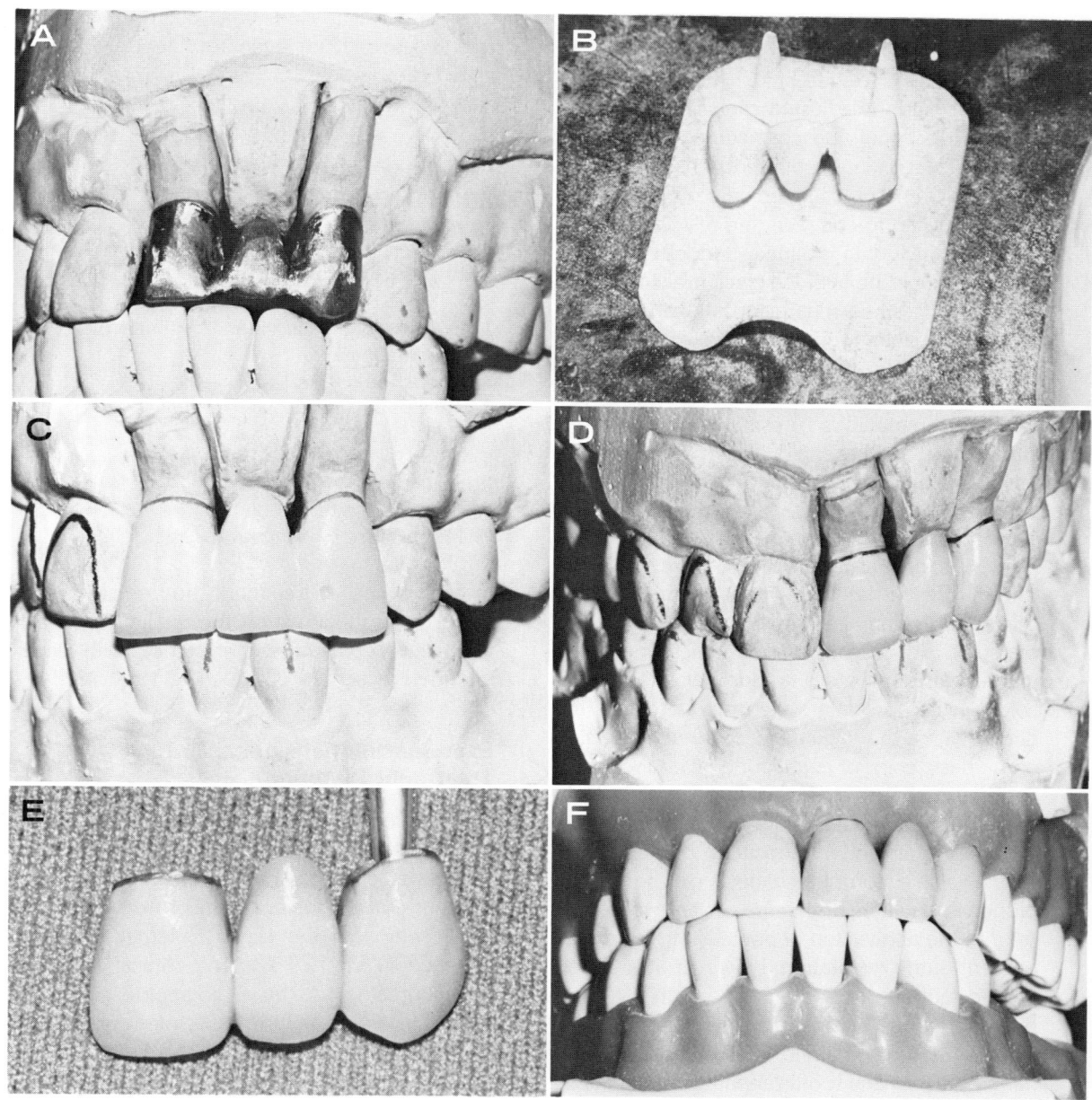

Figure 29-11 | Basic steps in development of a PFM bridge (technique example). A. Metal framework (substructure) developed from wax pattern, surfaced and ready to receive porcelain. B. Bridge on saggar tray (for placement in furnace) with thin layer of opaque porcelain baked onto the surfaces to be veneered. C. "Bisque" bake of gingival and incisal porcelain. From this point various abrasives (discs and stones) are used to contour the bridge using the articulated working cast as a guide in the development of functional and esthetic contours. D. Bridge contoured and ready for clinical try-in. E. The porcelain has been "fired" to develop a surface "glaze." F. Bridge seated.

tion are illustrated in Fig. 29-11. The dentist receives the crown or bridge from the laboratory technician in a "bisque bake" (unglazed) form. The restoration is adjusted clinically to develop desired functional and cosmetic contours, then stained* and glazed prior to insertion (Fig. 29-11E). Some practitioners rely on the laboratory technician to complete the restoration prior to try-in, including staining and glazing. This practice should be avoided since functional contouring and esthetic characterization (both contouring and staining) are most effectively accomplished clinically. It should be emphasized that the only advantage of porcelain over gold as a restorative material is its esthetic potential. The dentist, therefore, should use every option to maximize the esthetic result of any PFM restoration.

Although all dental porcelains are prepared from the same basic ingredients, there are significant differences between various brands of porcelain, particularly with regard to color, due primarily to the method of manufacturing. Each manufacturer provides a number of different colors in its porcelain system and provides the dentist with a shade guide for use in the selection of the basic color or colors for a given tooth. It is important that the shade guide used clinically in shade selection be compatible with the porcelain material to be used in fabrication of the restoration. The selection of a shade(s) can be accomplished at any time during the clinical procedures prior to the application of porcelain in the development of the restoration. However, it is preferable to make the selection as early in the treatment sequence as possible. In most instances, best results are obtained if the shade is determined prior to any tooth preparation. The assistant can be an invaluable aid to the dentist in determining shades since finite color perception is oftentimes difficult, even for the most experienced clinician.

CLINICAL FIXED PROSTHODONTICS

The fundamental clinical procedures involved in fixed prosthodontic services include:

1. Examination (diagnosis and treatment planning)
2. Tooth preparation
3. Impression making
4. Temporary (provisional) restoration of prepared teeth
5. Try-in, adjustment, and temporary cementation of restorations
6. Permanent cementation
7. Maintenance

In each phase of treatment the dental assistant has a direct influence on the quality of the service rendered and the efficiency with which treatment is carried out.

Examination (Diagnosis and Treatment Planning)

Essential to the success of any dental treatment is a thorough oral and dental examination from which the dentist can derive a diagnosis and subsequent comprehensive plan of treatment. The basic setup for the clinical examination is illustrated in Fig. 29-12. The clinical examination supplemented by radiographic evaluation should routinely include assessment of:

1. The status of individual teeth, including existing restorations
2. The periodontal status of each tooth, including tooth mobility
3. The pulpal status of questionable teeth
4. Residual ridge areas where teeth have been lost
5. The patient's occlusion. (This phase of the examination should be supplemented by study casts mounted in an adjustable articulator.)

---

* *Ceramic stains* are metallic oxides of particular color which can be added to the surface of a porcelain restoration and become infused into the surface of the porcelain during the glaze firing.

The assistant's responsibilities at the examination appointment include:

1. Preparation of the examining area including necessary materials and instruments
2. Assisting in the examination and recording information in the patient's record as related by the dentist
3. Compiling the information gathered and preparing it for the dentist to refer to in deriving a diagnosis and planning treatment
4. Cleaning the examining area in preparation for the next patient

In addition, the dental assistant might be directed to develop study casts from alginate impressions, and to mount such casts on an adjustable articulator (Fig. 29-13) for the dentist to refer to in making a diagnosis and developing a treatment plan. Definitive treatment should not be initiated until the patient fully understands and accepts the dentist's recommendation(s) for treatment. A short consultation appointment is scheduled following the examination for the dentist to discuss the patient's problem and to outline a plan of treatment. The assistant should prepare and make available all diagnostic information for the case presentation.

Tooth Preparation

As already noted the most common type of retainer used in fixed prosthodontics is the full crown. The skillful preparation of a tooth to receive such a restoration represents one of the most difficult challenges the dentist faces. The following discussion will outline the basic steps in the preparation of a tooth to receive a full crown and the assistant's role in the operation. Specific steps in tooth preparation for other types of cast restorations are similar and will, therefore, not be included.

A basic tray setup for tooth preparation is represented in Fig. 29-14. The assistant should be-

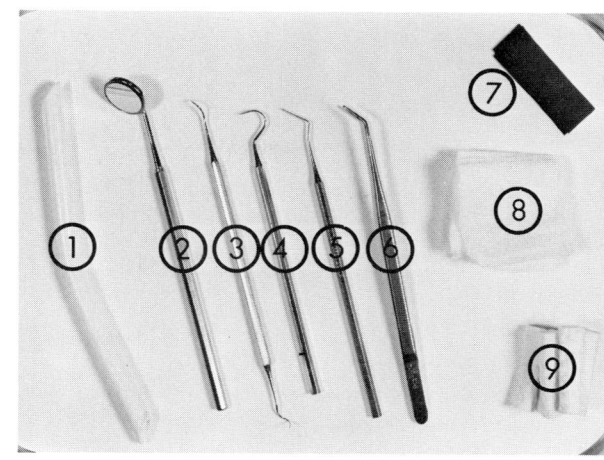

Figure 29-12 | Tray setup for clinical examination. (1) Evacuator tip, (2) front surface mouth mirror, (3) no. 2 explorer, (4) no. 23 explorer, (5) periodontal probe, (6) cotton pliers, (7) articulating paper, (8) 2 by 2 in gauze sponges, (9) cotton rolls.

come thoroughly familiar with each instrument and material illustrated and understand the use of each.

Following the administration of a local anesthetic and before tooth preparation, the dentist will make a full-arch alginate impression to serve as a mold for subsequent fabrication of a temporary crown or bridge. Tooth preparation for a full crown involves two primary steps: (1) gross preparation and (2) establishing the finish line. Gross preparation of the tooth is achieved with a suitable tapered diamond point (or carbide bur) in the turbine handpiece operated with an air-water spray to keep the tooth debrided and to dissipate heat generated during the cutting process. The assistant's responsibility is to retract either the cheek and lips or tongue and to evacuate debris during removal of tooth structure. This step is most efficiently accomplished by reduction first of the occlusal or incisal surface to decrease the length of the clinical crown, thus making the axial wall reductions easier. Reduction of the axial (F, L, M, and D) surfaces follows,

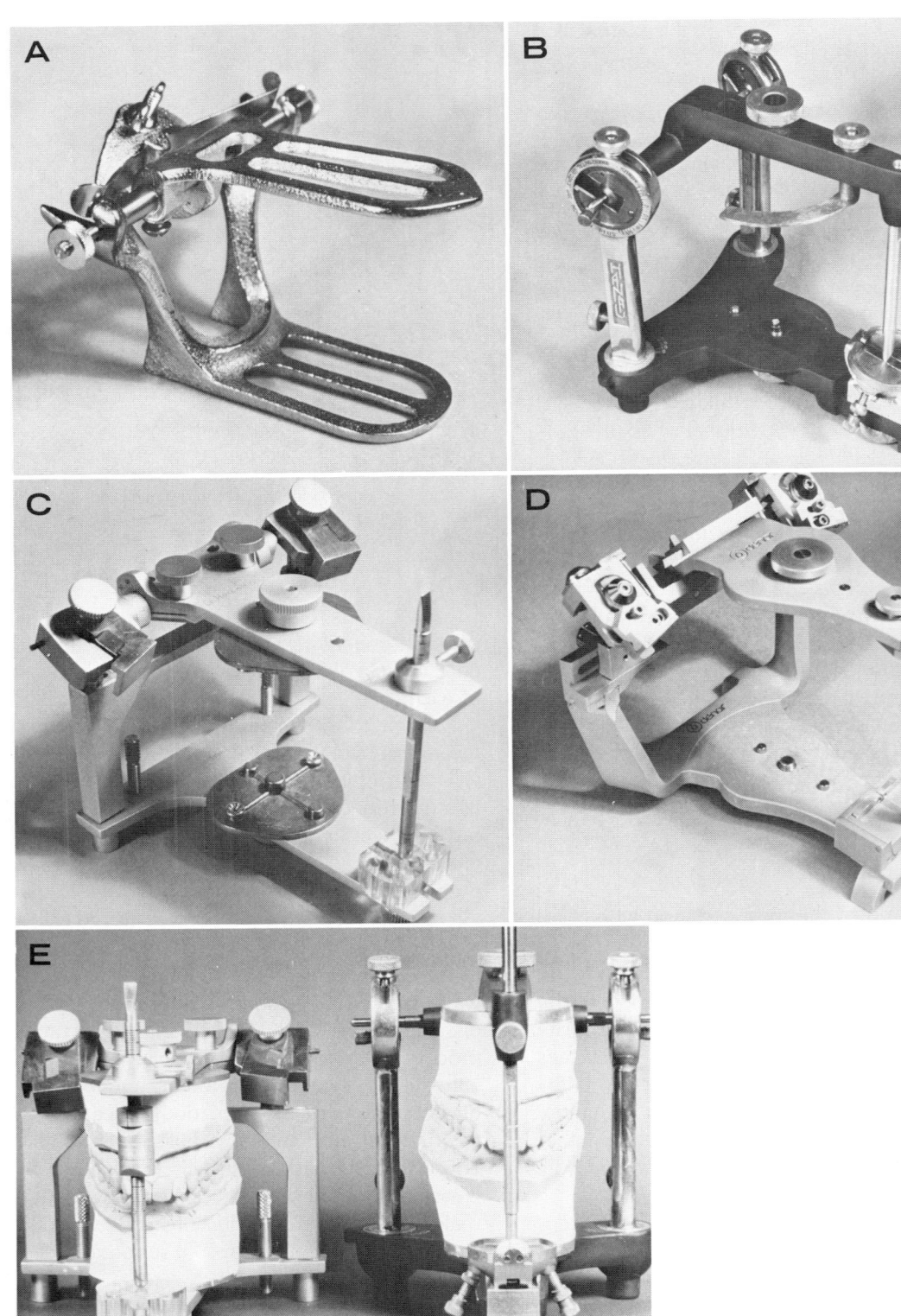

using the same instrument, with the gingival extent of such reduction terminating at the free gingival margin (Fig. 29-15A). A ledge of predetermined width (depending upon the type of full-crown retainer to be used, gold or PFM) is thus created at the free gingival margin to serve as a guide for finishing the preparation (Fig. 29-15B). The lingual fossa of an anterior tooth is best reduced with a small cylindrical diamond (Fig. 29-14B). The primary purposes of the gross preparation are to (1) remove sufficient tooth structure to provide for an adequate bulk of restorative material for strength, (2) establish draw of the preparation to allow for placement and removal of the restoration, and (3) establish relative parallelism between opposed axial walls for retention of the casting.

In developing the finish line (margin), usually beneath the free gingival margin, the dentist must be extremely careful not to abuse the supporting tissues of the tooth. Displacement of the free gingivae away from the tooth is one means of control and can be readily achieved by packing a length of tightly wound cotton cord, impregnated with an astringent to control hemorrhage, into the gingival crevice. A flat-bladed plastic filling instrument serves well for placement of the cord (Fig. 29-15D). In order to prevent the diamond instrument from "grabbing" the string during the finishing procedure and removing it from the gingival crevice, it is imperative that no loose ends of the cord be exposed. Before the last 5 to 6 mm of the string is placed into the crevice, excess length should be removed such that, when finally positioned, the two ends of the string will overlap by approximately 1 mm. The assistant should place clean cotton rolls and maintain a clean, dry field while

Figure 29-13 | Articulators used in prosthodontics. A. Nonadjustable simple hinge. B. Semiadjustable (Hanau). C. Semiadjustable (Whip-Mix). D. Fully adjustable (Denar). E. Study casts of patient mounted in two different types of semidjustable articulators. (Refer to section on articulators in Chap. 16.)

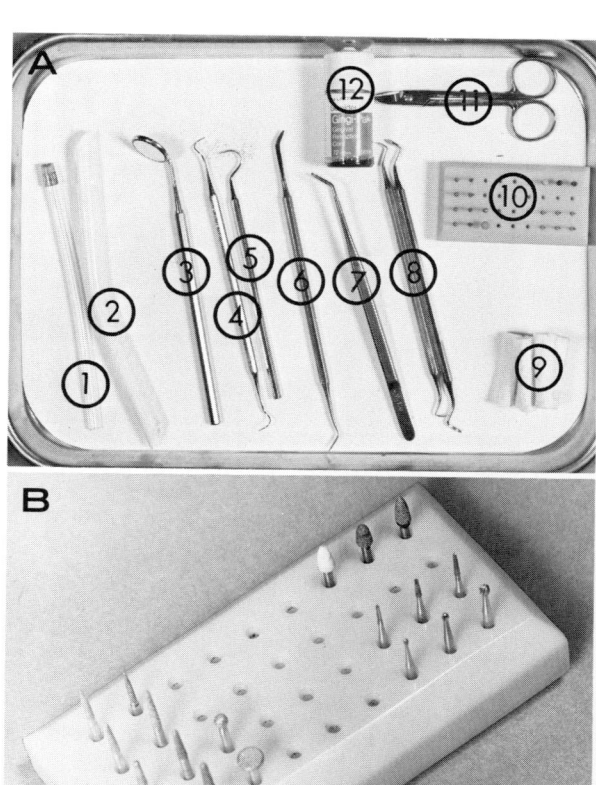

Figure 29-14 | A. Tray setup for tooth preparation, impression making, and temporization. (1) Saliva ejector tip, (2) evacuator tip, (3) front surface mouth mirror, (4) no. 2 explorer, (5) no. 23 explorer, (6) plastic filling instrument, (7) cotton pliers, (8) spoon excavators, (9) cotton rolls, (10) bur block with assorted burs, diamonds, and stones, (11) scissor, (12) gingival retraction cord. B. Bur block containing assorted carbide burs, diamond points, and abrasive stones for high-speed handpiece utilized in crown preparations.

the dentist inserts the retraction cord. While the retraction cord is in place, the preparation is completed. A flame-shaped fine-grit diamond point is used to establish the finish line (margin) about 1 mm beneath the free gingival crest (Fig.

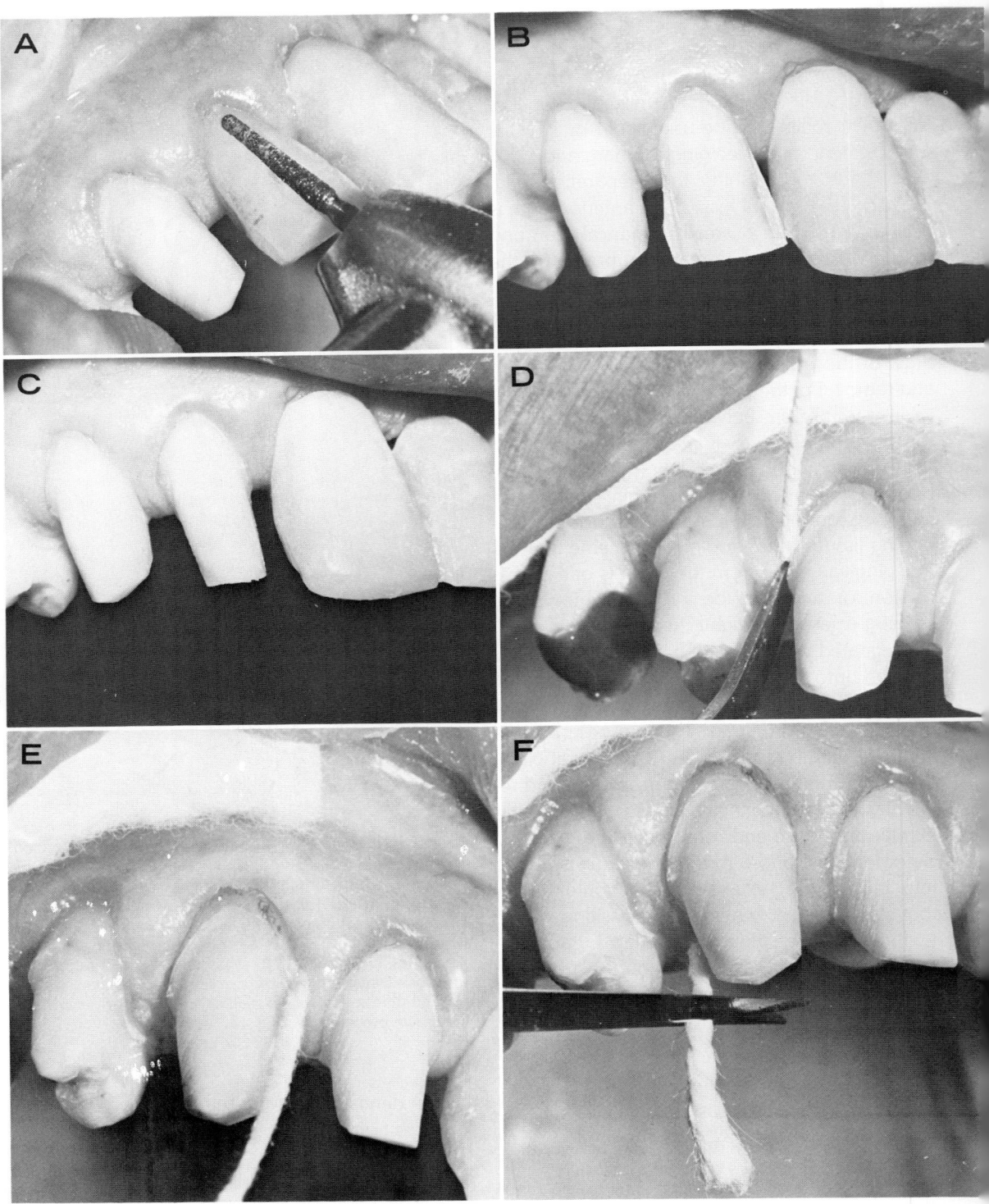

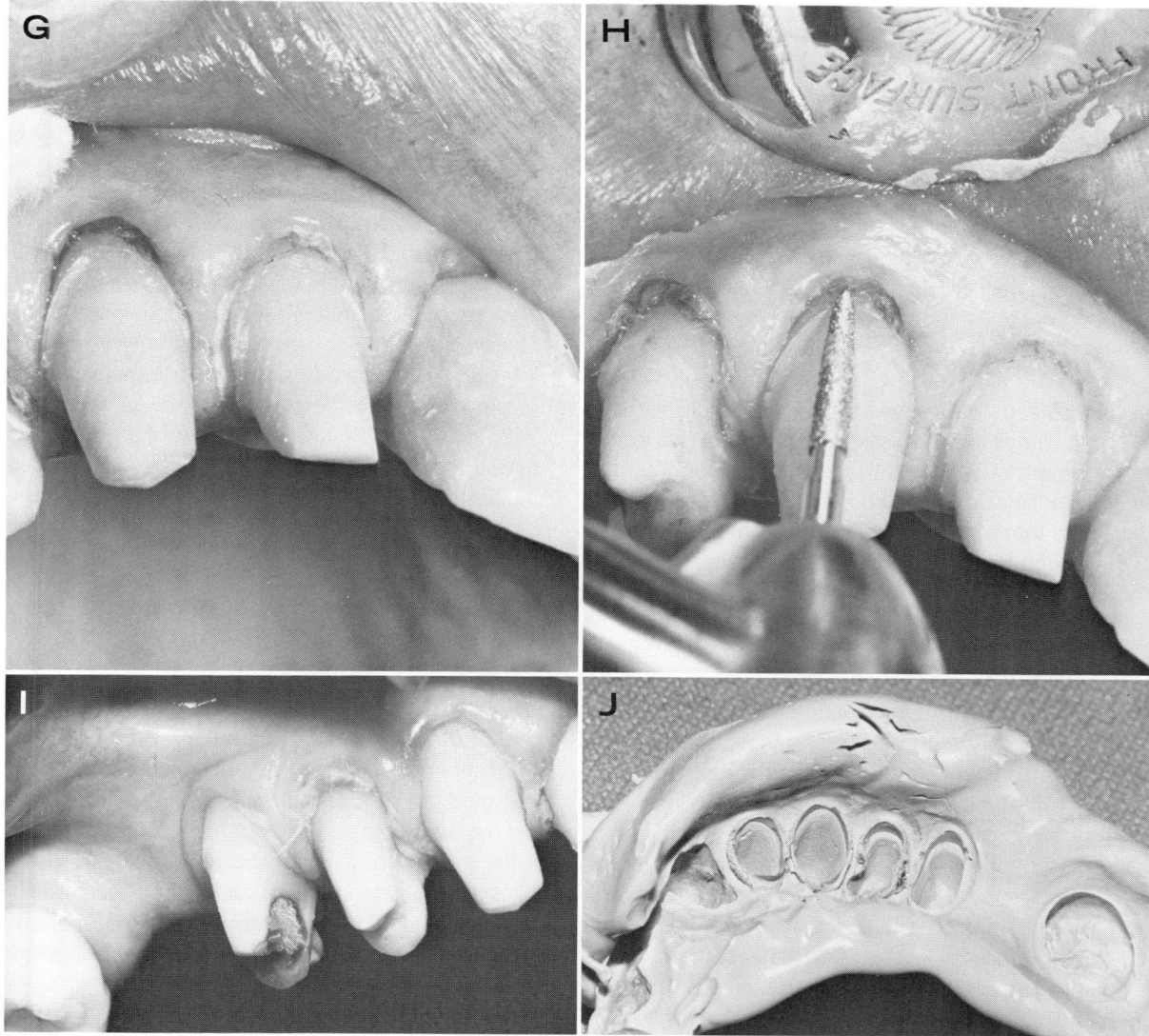

Figure 29-15 | Tooth preparation for full crown. A. Using a tapered cylindrical diamond point for "gross" reduction of facial surface following reduction of incisal. B. Facial surface reduced (lateral incisor) to provide space for restorative material and to provide incisogingival taper to the surface. C. Gross preparation of incisal and axial surfaces with "ledge" created at crest of gingivae. D. Starting placement of cord into a proximal crevice using blade of plastic filling instrument. E. Packing cord progressively about the tooth. F. Cutting off excess cord such that there is minimal overlap of the two ends of the string once it is packed into the crevice. G. The gingival area of each tooth has been isolated with retraction cord saturated with an astringent such as aluminum chloride. H. "Finishing" the preparation using a flame-shaped diamond point to establish the finish line (margin). I. Completed preparations for PFM crown retainers. J. Rubber-base impression of prepared teeth (note the definition of the facial margins of the four preparations).

29-15H and I). All line and point angles are gently rounded and the axial surfaces smoothed with the same instrument used in preparing the finish line. If the retraction cord was removed prior to or during preparation of the margin, another string is inserted to open the gingival crevice for the subsequent impression. Removal of remaining carious dentin and/or existing restorations is accomplished as described previously in Chap. 28.

Impressions of Prepared Teeth

Accuracy of dies and their relationship to each other in a working cast is essential to the development of functionally acceptable fixed restorations. Such accuracy obviously can be no greater than that of the materials and techniques used in making impressions of prepared teeth and associated oral structures.

Of the many impression materials available today, the *impression rubbers* (polysulfide, silicone, and polyether) are the most popular for routine fixed prosthodontic procedures because of their elastic properties and versatility of application. *Reversible hydrocolloid* is also an excellent elastic impression material and is preferred by some practitioners; however, it is not so versatile as the impression rubbers, and its use requires special equipment for preparation and clinical manipulation. *Impression waxes and compound,* which at one time were basic to impression techniques for full-crown preparation, have essentially been replaced by the elastic materials. Their use was (is) limited to individual tooth impressions since they are nonelastic and will not withdraw from undercuts without either fracturing or distorting permanently.

There are two basic methods for making impressions of full-crown preparations: (1) *the copper band technique* for individual tooth impressions, and (2) *the tray technique* for complete arch or quadrant impressions. When the copper band method is used, an additional impression (*coping transfer impression*) is required to develop a working cast with dies accurately related to one another and to associated unprepared teeth. Rubber base can be used with any of these techniques, while the use of reversible hydrocolloid is limited to the tray impression.

Examples of *copper band–rubber base impressions* are illustrated in Fig. 29-16. Copper bands are available in a number of different sizes (diameters) and they measure approximately $1/2$ in in occlusogingival length. Following preparation of the tooth the dentist selects a band ("tube") of the appropriate diameter which will provide $1/2$ mm of clearance between the band and the greatest dimension of the prepared tooth. The band is then carefully contoured ("festooned") at its gingival end to follow the general outline of the prepared margin about the tooth. When the margin of the preparation extends beneath the free gingival crest, care must be exercised not to permit the band to impinge on the gingival tissues during the adaptation and festooning process. The occlusal (incisal) end of the band is then closed with either softened compound or a metal washer soldered to the band. In either case, the outer surfaces of the band should be reinforced with compound to minimize the likelihood of its bending, thus distorting the impression, while being removed from the tooth (Fig. 29-16A). Retention for the impression material inside the band can be provided by (1) application of a thin coat of rubber-base adhesive or (2) roughening the band using a mounted green stone. The dental assistant should complete the preparation of the copper band beyond the stage of adaptation and festooning as described above, particularly when more than one tooth is to be impressed. The assistant also mixes the impression material, fills the band, being careful not to entrap air, and passes the band to the dentist for placement over the tooth.

A *coping transfer impression* is necessary to develop a working cast with removable dies when copper band impressions are used (Fig.

29-16J). Individual dies are first developed from the copper band impressions (Fig. 29-16C), and cast metal or acrylic resin transfer copings* are then fabricated on the dies (Fig. 29-16E). At a subsequent appointment the temporary crowns are removed, the teeth debrided, and the copings seated onto the prepared teeth (Fig. 29-16E). If two or more teeth are involved in the transfer procedure, the copings should be joined together. A length of an old bur shank and autopolymerizing acrylic resin can be used for this purpose (Fig. 29-16F). A full-arch rubber-base impression is made (Fig. 29-16G). The dental assistant's duties during the making of the impression itself include (1) isolating the area and providing a relatively dry field, (2) mixing the material and filling the impression tray, (3) assisting the dentist in retraction of soft tissues (lips and cheeks) until the tray has been seated, (4) placement of the saliva ejector after the tray has been seated.

The dies are carefully seated in the copings (firmly secured in the transfer impression) and luted in place with sticky wax (Fig. 29-16H). Dental stone is then poured into the impression to form the base of the working cast (Fig. 29-16I). Sufficient time must be allowed for the stone to set and develop its maximum properties before any attempt is made to remove the cast from the impression. After the working cast is recovered and wax removed from the dies, the cast is ready to be related to an opposing stone cast for the laboratory fabrication of the restoration. The dental assistant might be instructed in the laboratory phase of developing a working cast from a transfer impression and should, therefore, be thoroughly familiar with the technique. Other techniques utilizing impression plaster or a combination of plaster and alginate ("plaginate") for the transfer impression have been described (Murray and Sluder, 1972).

---

* A *transfer coping* is a thin rigid shell similar in design to a sewing thimble, of either acrylic resin or a cast alloy, used specifically to transfer the relationship of individual dies to each other and to other dental structures in the same arch.

When used with care, any of the techniques can result in accurate working casts. The coping transfer technique has its greatest application when multiple abutments are involved in the prosthesis (such as a full-arch splint) and the use of a tray technique is impractical.

The most accurate working casts are routinely developed from impressions using the *tray technique* with an elastic impression material, primarily because the need to transfer relationships of prepared teeth (via copings) is eliminated. Clinical success with the tray technique is dependent upon (1) proper control of supporting (gingival) tissues during tooth preparation, (2) adequate isolation and moisture control during the impression procedure, and (3) proper handling of the impression material. The chairside assistant assumes a major role throughout the procedure.

Preparation for the tray impression actually begins during tooth preparation at the stage when the gingival area is isolated with retraction cord. A properly positioned cord can serve the dual function of (1) displacing the full gingivae for completing the tooth preparation, and (2) opening the gingival crevice for the impression. If the cord was removed during (or before) development of the preparation margin, the tissue must be repacked for the impression (Fig. 29-15I). At this stage one end of the cord should protrude from the crevice so it can be easily grasped with operating pliers for removal just prior to injecting impression material into the gingival crevice. Further preparation of the mouth for the impression (following completion of all tooth preparations) includes washing the operating field and isolating the area with clean, dry cotton rolls. Procedures for mixing rubber-base materials (both tray and injection types) are described in Chap. 11. Usually the dentist or a second assistant will mix the injection material and load the syringe while the chairside assistant prepares the tray material. As the retraction cord is removed and each tooth injected individually, the chairside assistant should assist the dentist in

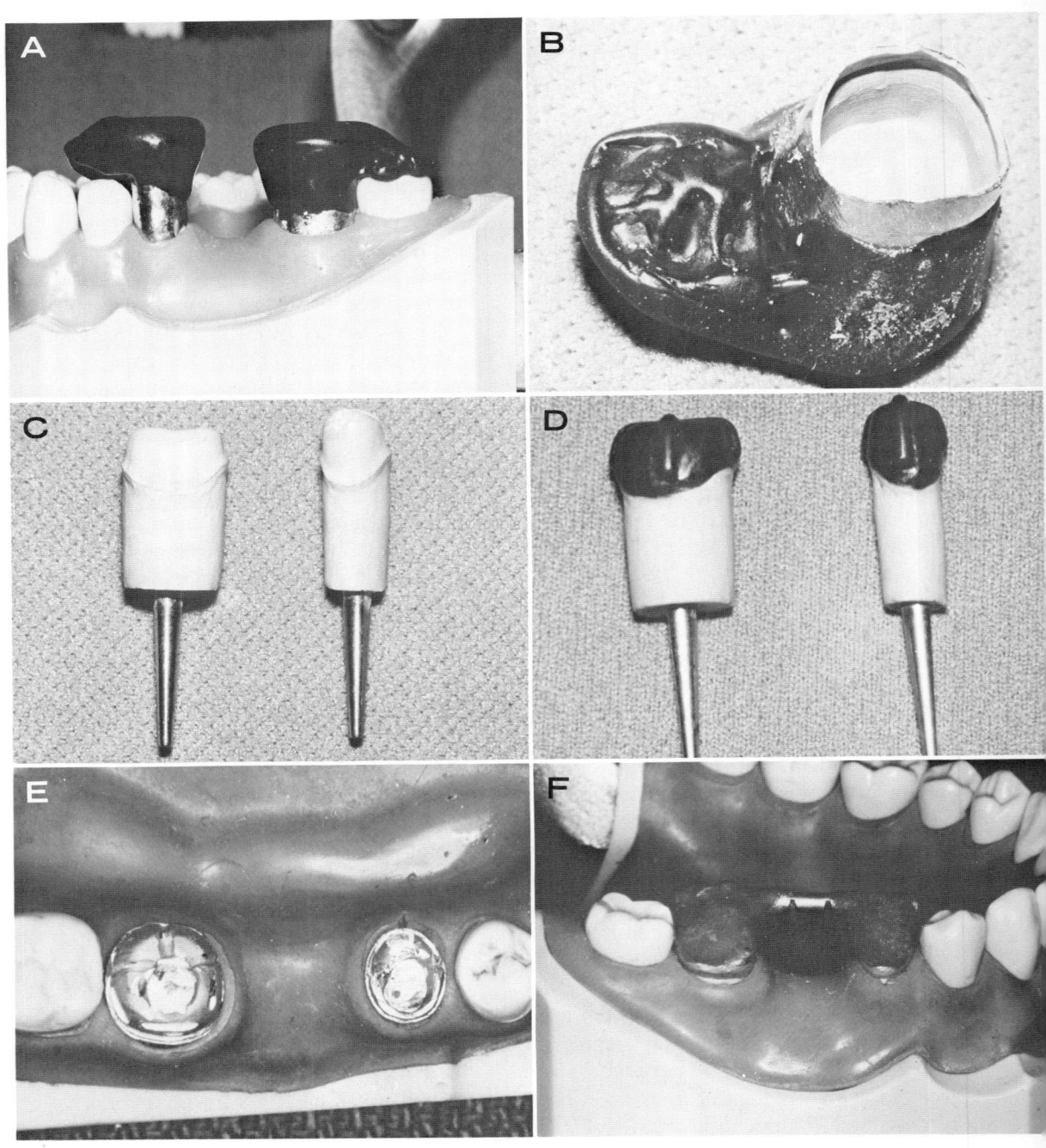

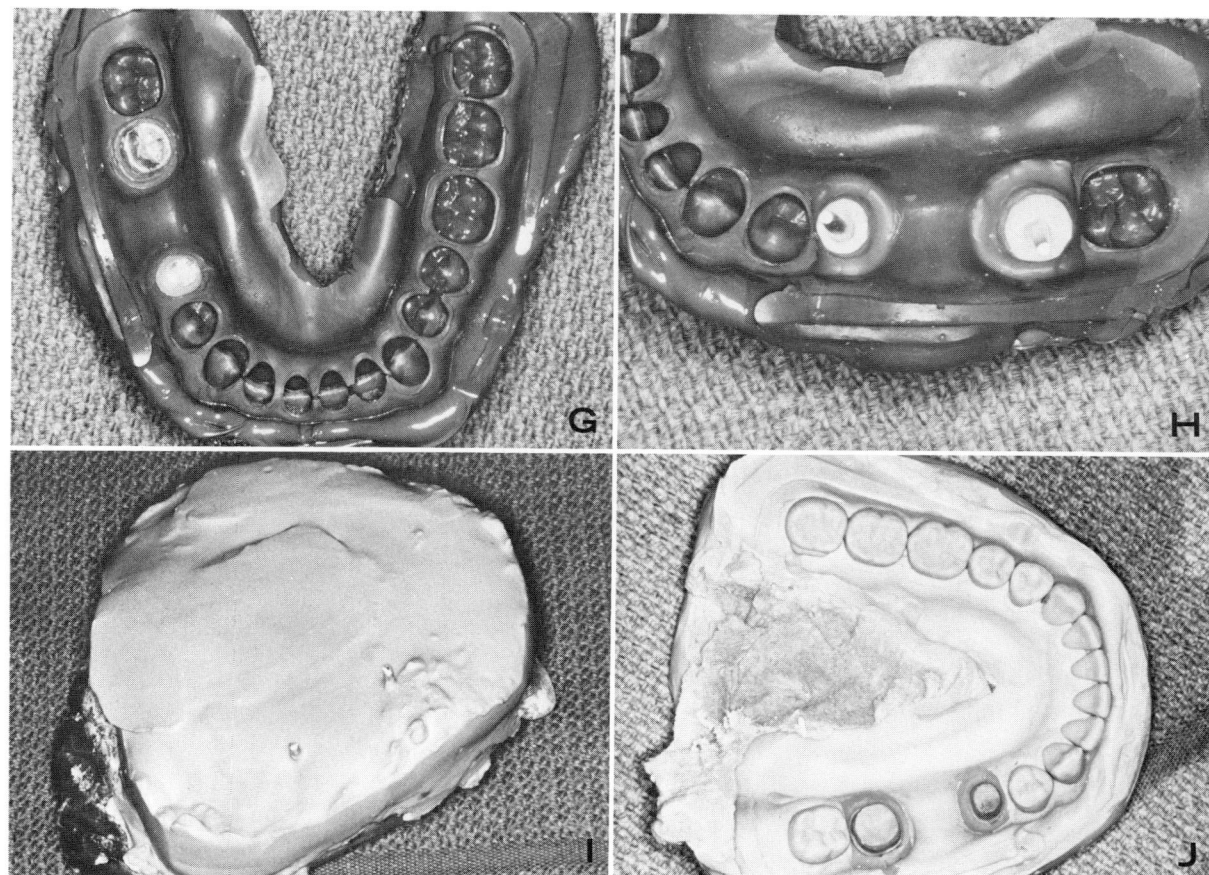

Figure 29-16 | Copper band and coping transfer impressions. A. Copper bands adapted and festooned to prepared teeth, and reinforced with impression compound (occlusal "stops" on adjacent unprepared teeth have also been provided to prevent overseating of the bands while placing the bands over the teeth for the impressions). B. Impression of the prepared tooth with minimal extension of the band beyond the prepared margin. C. Stone dies from band impressions. D. Copings ("thimbles") waxed and ready to be invested and cast. E. Cast copings seated on prepared teeth in preparation for transfer impression. F. Bur shank luted to the copings with autopolymerizing resin to stabilize their positions within the subsequent rubber-base impression. G. Transfer impression with copings firmly positioned. H. Stone dies reseated in copings and stabilized with "sticky wax" prior to pouring base of working cast. I. Base of working cast poured with dental stone leaving ends of dowel pins exposed. J. Working cast recovered from transfer impression ready to be trimmed prior to mounting in an articulator.

retraction of the lip, cheeks, and/or tongue. Once the tray has been seated, the assistant places a saliva ejector in the mouth to remove excess saliva during the polymerization of the impression material. The development of the working cast from a tray impression is described in detail elsewhere (Sturdevant, Barton, and Brauer, 1968) and will not be reviewed in this text. At times, a combination of the coping transfer and tray techniques can be used effectively when several teeth have been prepared (Fig. 29-17).

Temporary (Provisional) Restorations

Since fixed restorations routinely involve a minimum of two appointments, provisions must be made to adequately cover prepared teeth during the interim following tooth preparation while the restoration is being fabricated. In order for a temporary (provisional) crown or bridge to serve successfully it must meet the following basic requirements:

1. It should cover and seal the prepared tooth (dentin) to prevent penetration of oral fluids and bacteria which can cause the tooth to become hyperemic, and thus sensitive.
2. It should provide physiologic axial contours which are compatible with the remaining unprepared teeth and supporting tissues.
3. It should provide appropriate occlusal form and relationship to any opposed tooth or teeth.
4. It should provide appropriate proximal contact relationships with unprepared adjacent teeth to prevent drifting.
5. It should provide for esthetics in the case of anterior teeth.
6. It should be smooth and polished so as not to be irritating to the tongue, lips, cheeks, or gingival tissues.

Preformed *acrylic resin and aluminum shell* temporary crowns (Fig. 29-18) are commercially available and are quite adequate for some clinical situations, but are limited in application to

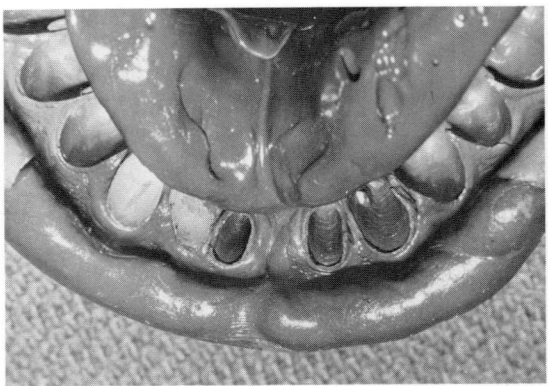

Figure 29-17 | Combination rubber-base impression involving the coping transfer technique for five prepared teeth—the mandibular left canine and lateral incisor being transferred by copings.

the temporary restoration of single-tooth preparation. A more versatile method of fabricating either temporary crowns or bridges directly in the mouth is the *preoperative alginate–acrylic resin technique* (Fig. 29-19). A full-arch alginate impression is made following the administration of local anesthetic and prior to preparation of the tooth (teeth). After completion of the tooth preparation(s) a relatively thin mix of a tooth-colored autopolymerizing acrylic resin is flowed into the impression up to the gingival line in the area to be temporized (Fig. 29-19D). (When abutment teeth for a bridge have been prepared, material can be easily removed from the preoperative impression in the edentulous space area so that a pontic can be incorporated into the temporary.) The resin in the impression is allowed to set until it reaches a "doughy" stage, evidenced by a loss of surface gloss (Fig. 29-19E). The impression is placed over the arch of teeth and the patient is asked to close on cotton rolls or folded 2 by 2 in sponges to maintain the position of the impression while the resin polymerizes (Fig. 29-19F). A small (pea-size) specimen of the resin mix is rolled between the fingers to determine when the material in the mouth has set adequately and

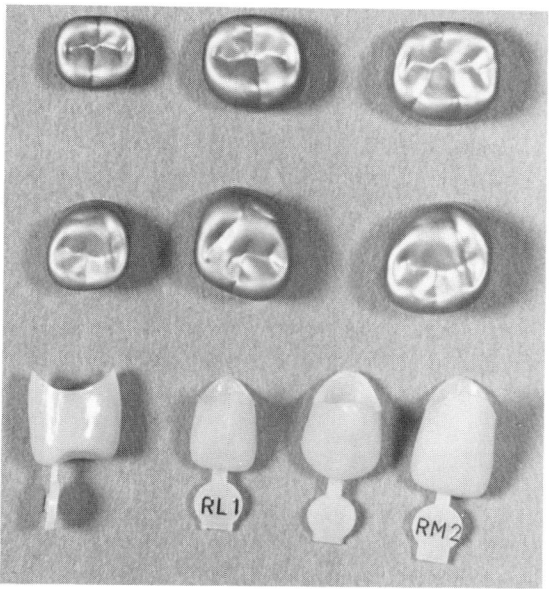

Figure 29-18 | Prefabricated individual tooth temporaries. *Top and middle rows,* aluminum "shell" temporaries for molars. *Bottom row,* acrylic resin temporaries for anterior and premolar teeth.

is ready to be removed. The resin should not be fully set when the impression is removed from the mouth because of the cold, wet environment of the alginate impression. However, removal of the temporary from the tooth (teeth) should not be attempted until the resin is hard when tested with a blunt instrument. After the alginate impression is removed, the patient should be instructed to flush the mouth several times with cool water to dissipate the heat generated during the final polymerization reaction of the resin. Usually removal of the temporary is easily accomplished by gentle prying along the resin flash on the facial and lingual surfaces using a heavy-bladed spoon excavator (Fig. 29-19G). Once trimmed, occluded, smoothed, and polished, the temporary should represent a near duplicate of the original tooth form.

A zinc oxide–eugenol temporary cement is used as a luting agent for the provisional restoration. The assistant prepares a mix of cement according to the manufacturer's directions and carefully lines the internal aspect of the temporary restoration (Fig. 29-19J). A small-bladed instrument (such as a plastic filling instrument) is best used for placing the cement to minimize excess which must later be removed from the mouth. The temporary is seated onto the prepared tooth (teeth) and evaluated for assurance that it is fully seated. Once fully set, all excess cement is removed from the crown and, particularly, from the gingival area (Fig. 29-19K). Some state laws now permit the trained dental assistant to fabricate and cement temporary restorations under the direct supervison of a dentist.

Try-In, Adjustment, and Temporary Placement of Restorations

For the try-in appointment the assistant should prepare the basic setup (Fig. 29-20) including assorted stone and burs for adjustment of the prosthesis. The temporary restoration is removed and the tooth (teeth) cleaned. Usually no anesthetic is required for the try-in.

For any fixed restoration the first step in the try-in procedure is adjustment of proximal contacts. (If the technician has exercised care in fabrication of the appliance, this and subsequent adjustments should be minimal and require but little chair time.) Proximal contacts between adjacent teeth should be positive, yet passive (nonwedging), as demonstrated by a light "snap" of dental floss as it is passed through the contact area.

If the restoration (bridge) contains a tissue-contacting pontic, the next step in the try-in is adjustment of the gingival aspect of the pontic tip such that it adapts passively to the residual ridge tissue. The pontic tip adaptation is evaluated visually, and by passing dental floss between the pontic tip and the ridge tissue. With the bridge fully seated, there should be little, if any, pressure on the residual ridge mucosa. The occlusion is evaluated and adjustments made to provide a

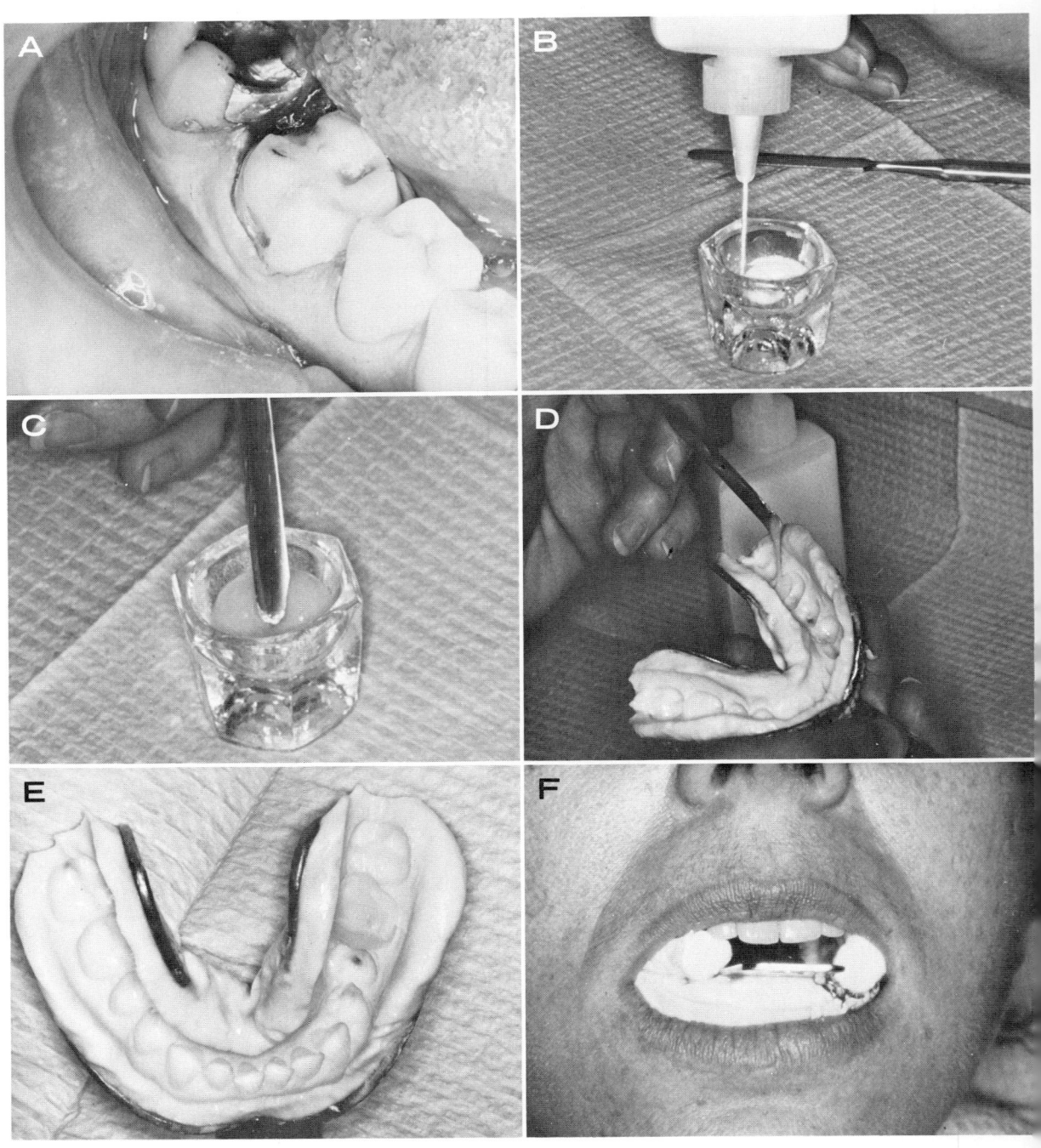

harmonious relationship between all the dental components. Articulating paper is used to mark any areas of interference between the restoration and its opposed tooth (teeth).

Final clinical adjustments of the restoration include improvements in functional and esthetic contours when necessary. The axial surfaces of the restoration must be designed so as to provide physiologic embrasure forms surrounding the proximal contact(s) and physiologic relationships to the supporting gingivae. Supplemental occlusion grooves might also need to be "carved" into the restoration to improve its masticatory efficiency. These same considerations of contours are also important factors of esthetics. Further characterization of a porcelain or PFM restoration for maximum esthetics involves the careful addition of surface stains (powdered metallic oxides) to the porcelain prior to "glazing" the restoration. Once the PFM restoration has been glazed, any exposed metal of the framework is highly polished. Likewise, for the all-metal crown or bridge, surface roughness resulting from clinical adjustment is eliminated, and the metal is highly polished prior to insertion of the restoration.

Temporary cementation of a fixed restoration is indicated in most instances primarily to (1) allow the prosthesis to "settle" and thus seat more completely with greater ease, and (2) provide a better environment than that afforded by the temporary restoration for the gingival tissues to heal, particularly when retainer margins extend into the gingival sulcus. In addition, such a routine practice offers the dentist an opportunity, prior to final cementation, to evaluate (1) the patient's overall response to the restoration, (2) the occlusion, and (3) soft-tissue response to the prosthesis, especially to tissue-contacting pontics.

An excellent material for temporary cementation is zinc oxide–eugenol (ZOE) to which has been added an equal amount of petroleum jelly to reduce the strength of the ZOE. For best results (assuming that the restoration is retentive without being cemented) only a thin liner of the temporary cement should be placed inside each retainer, and the tooth (teeth) should be dried only by wiping away visible moisture with a cotton roll or gauze sponge. It is imperative that *all* excess cement be removed from the gingival crevice before the patient is dismissed. The patient is instructed in procedures for cleaning the appliance(s), particularly if it contains a pontic or splinted retainers.

Final (Permanent) Cementation

No procedure in clinical fixed prosthodontics requires more care in its execution than does the cementation of a restoration, for at this point the quality of an otherwise excellent crown or bridge can be reduced to mediocrity or even clinical unacceptability. The operating field must be kept *clean and dry* throughout the procedure. Most patients can tolerate the minimal discomfort associated with the cementation procedure without anesthesia. However, since pain is a stimulus for salivation, it sometimes becomes necessary to anesthetize the area as an aide to maintaining a dry field.

The assistant should prepare the same basic tray setup for cementation as used for try-in and adjustment (Fig. 29-20). The dentist removes

Figure 29-19 | Fabrication of direct resin temporary using the preoperative alginate technique. A. Completed tooth preparation. B. Tooth-colored acrylic resin powder (polymer) is "sifted" into liquid (monomer) to slight excess (a minimum of ten drops of liquid should be used for each prepared tooth and fifteen drops for each pontic). C. Powder is gently stirred into liquid primarily to disperse the colorants added by the manufacturer (vigorous mixing will incorporate air into the mix and result in voids in the temporary). D. While the mix is still fluid it is poured from the spatula blade into the area of the prepared tooth in the alginate impression. Care must be used to completely fill the tooth impression without trapping air. E. Impression, with acrylic resin having reached the "doughy" stage of set, is ready to be reseated in the mouth. F. Impression seated and patient instructed to close on cotton rolls to stabilize the tray and prevent its "floating."

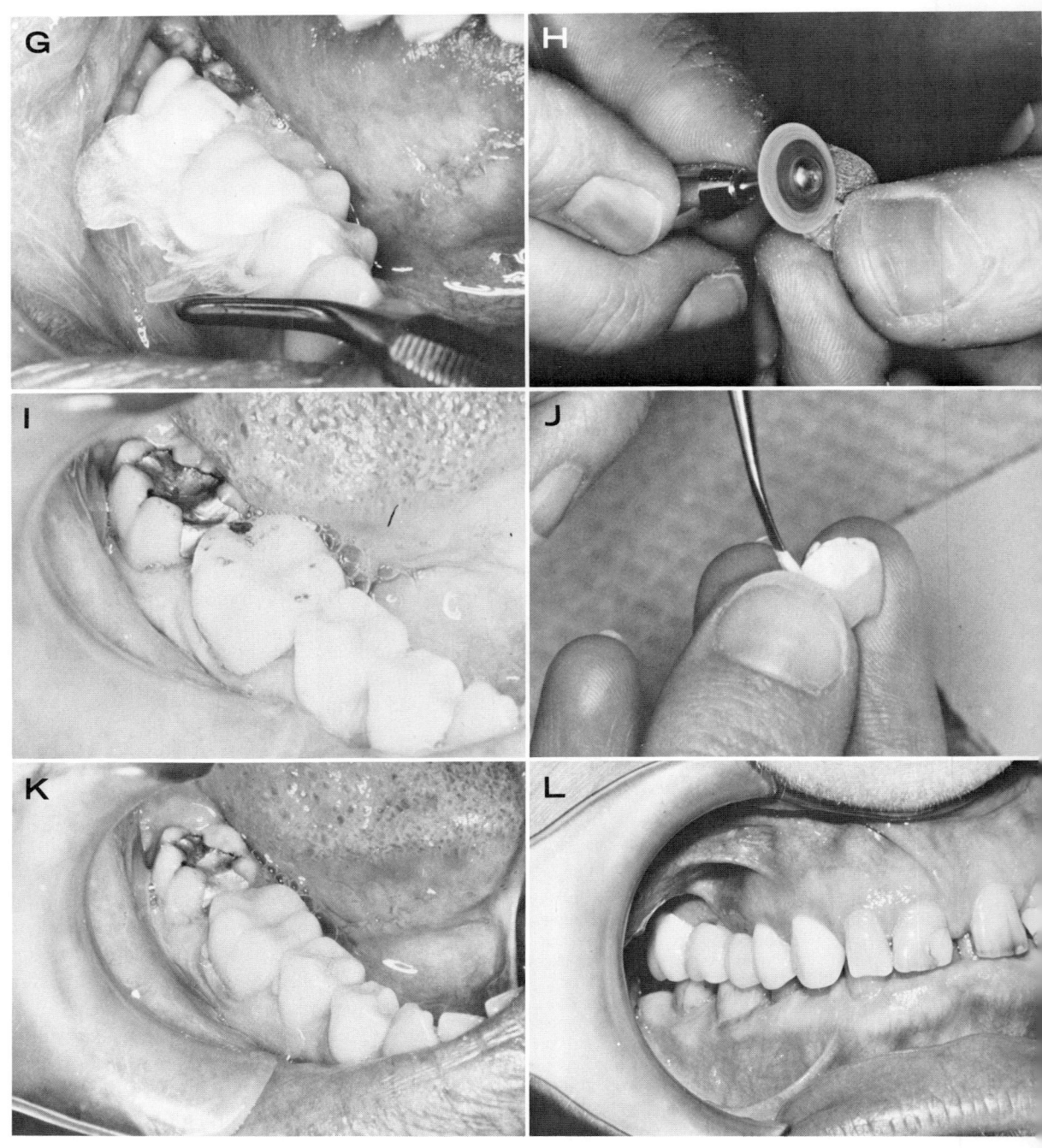

the temporarily cemented crown or bridge and proceeds to clean the prepared tooth (teeth) while the assistant cleans the prosthesis. A cotton pellet or cotton swab moistened with a grease solvent, such as xylene, can be used to remove temporary cement from the restoration. Further cleansing is best accomplished with a jet of steam if such is available. If steam is not available, the restoration should be scrubbed with warm, soapy water and a soft-bristle brush, rinsed with warm water followed by cold water, then thoroughly dried. (It is important that the restoration not be left warm since this will decrease the setting time, thus working time, of the cement.) Temporary cement can usually be removed from the prepared tooth (teeth) with an explorer or small, dry, cotton pellet followed by a spray of warm water from the air-water syringe. At times it might be necessary for the dentist to use a paste of fine pumice, carefully applied with a prophylaxis cup or brush, to remove debris from the tooth surfaces.

Zinc phosphate cement has long been recognized as an excellent permanent luting agent for cast restorations. However, it is highly acidic during the initial stages of setting due to the presence of phosphoric acid and, therefore, can be quite irritating to pulpal tissues if the cementation process is not handled properly. Some advocate coating exposed dentin of a prepared tooth with a copal varnish prior to cementing with zinc phosphate (Sturdevant, Barton, and Brauer,

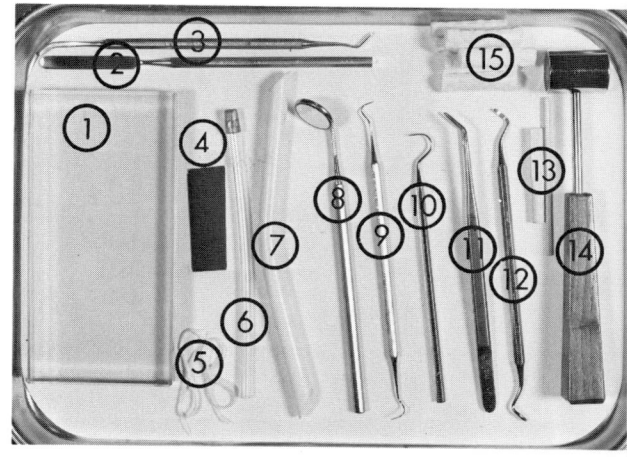

Figure 29-20 | Tray setup for try-in, adjustment, and cementation. (1) Glass mixing slab, (2) no. 324 cement spatula, (3) plastic filling instrument, (4) articulating paper, (5) dental floss, (6) saliva ejector tip, (7) evacuator tip, (8) front surface mouth mirror, (9) no. 2 explorer, (10) no. 23 explorer, (11) cotton pliers, (12) spoon excavator, (13) orangewood sticks, (14) leather-headed mallet, (15) cotton rolls.

Figure 29-19 continued G. A heavy-gauge spoon excavator can be used to remove the set acrylic temporary from the tooth. H. Trimming of gross "flash" can be accomplished with curved crown and bridge scissors; final trimming and smoothing should be done with a mounted rubber wheel. I. Once trimmed, the temporary is placed on the tooth and evaluated for proximal contacts, contours, ma. ʾinal adaptation, and occlusion (note articulating paper marks on occlusal). Following clinical adjustments, the temporary is smoothed and polished prior to cementation. J. The inside of the temporary is lined with a mix of temporary cement. K. Polished temporary cemented, and *all* excess cement removed. L. Example of a five-tooth temporary bridge fabricated using the preoperative alginate technique.

1968). Other permanent cements have recently been developed and are quite popular among some practitioners. Although demonstrated to be less irritating to the pulp tissues, the reinforced ZOE, EBA (ethoxybenzoic acid), and PCA (polycarboxylate) cements have not proven to be clinically superior to zinc phosphate as permanent cements (Dennison and Powers, 1974). Regardless of the type cement one chooses to use, it is mandatory that the assistant follow the recommended technique for dispensing and mixing the material. (Improper mixing of any cement will result in decreased physical properties of the material and might cause ultimate failure of the restoration.)

When the teeth and restoration have been properly cleaned, the cementation process can begin as illustrated in Fig. 29-21. The operating area is isolated with clean, dry, cotton rolls (Fig. 29-21A), and the teeth are dried with a gentle blast of warm air. (It must be emphasized that

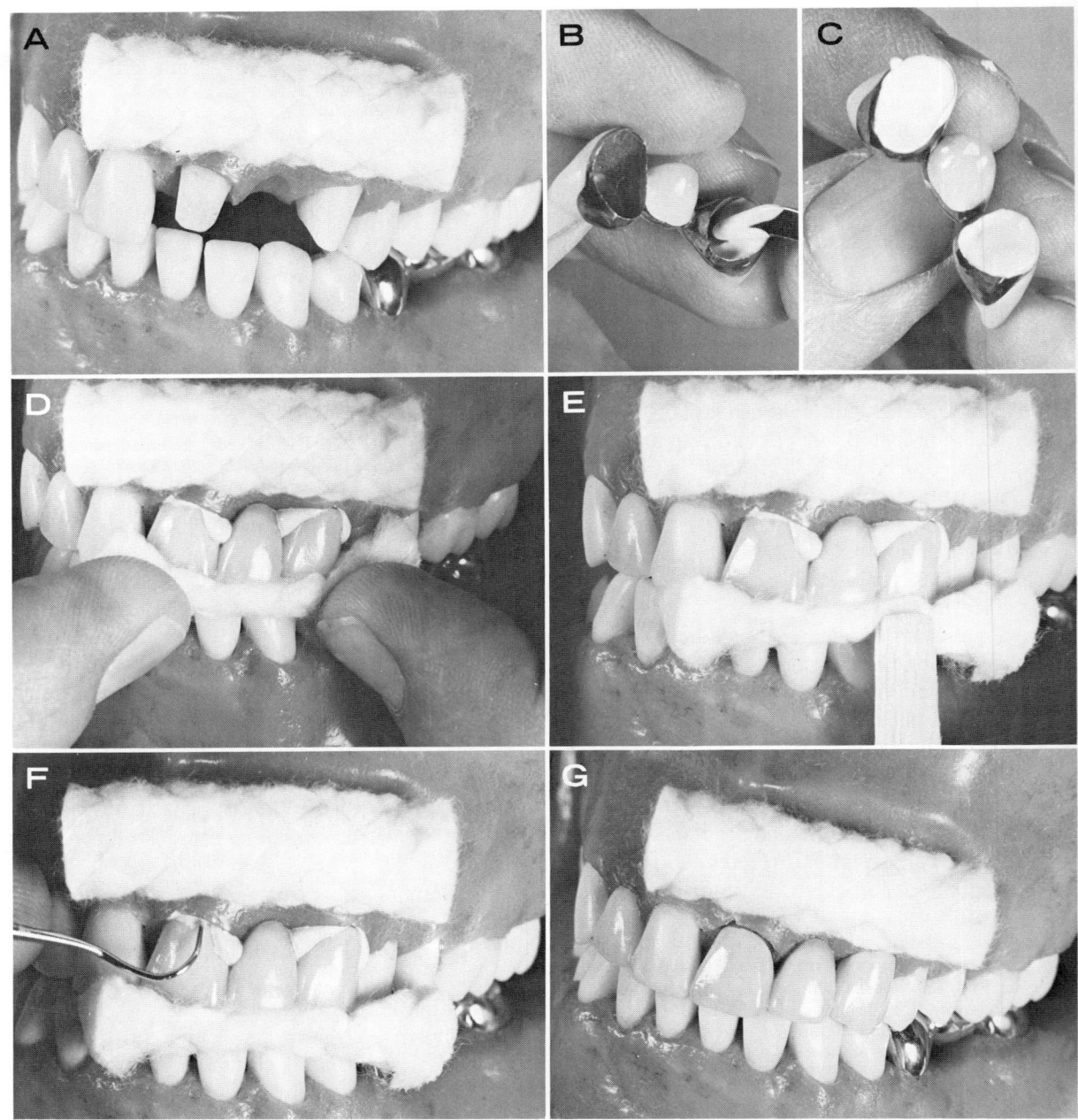

Figure 29-21 | Procedure for permanent cementation. A. Teeth cleaned and area isolated with cotton roll(s). B. Filling retainers with proper mix of cement using a plastic filling instrument. C. Retainers filled to margin with cement. D. Bridge seated initially with firm finger pressure. E. Final seating accomplished by "tapping" to place using an orangewood stick and leather headed mallet. (For posterior appliances biting pressure on an orangewood stick will usually be adequate for complete seating.) F. Exploring the gingival margins; testing for complete seating. G. Bridge cemented and *all* excess cement removed.

prolonged drying with compressed air is not necessary and is actually contraindicated since it might result in postoperative sensitivity due to dehydration of the tooth.) The assistant prepares a mix of cement having a cementing consistency as described in Chap. 12. Each retainer is carefully filled to its margin using a small instrument such as a plastic filling instrument to avoid entrapment of air in the cement (Fig. 29-21B and C). *Never attempt to apply cement to a casting with the spatula used for mixing.* The crown or bridge is carefully seated over the prepared tooth (teeth). Once it is determined that the prosthesis is going to place easily, firm finger pressure is applied to the occlusal (or incisal) surface for further expression of excess cement (Fig. 29-21D). Final seating requires rather heavy pressures which in some instances, such as with posterior units, can be attained by masticatory force. In the anterior segments, final seating is best achieved by tapping the appliance in place using an orangewood stick and leather-headed mallet (Fig. 29-21E). While the cement is still fluid, the dentist uses the tine of a sharp explorer to examine the marginal fit and to verify that the restoration is completely seated (Fig. 29-21F). The area must be maintained dry (isolated with cotton rolls) while the cement sets, and *no attempt should be made to remove excess cement until it has set to the point of being "brittle-hard."* As already pointed out relative to temporary cements, all cement must be removed from around the restoration and particularly from the gingival crevice area.

Maintenance of Fixed Prostheses

Periodic recall maintenance of a fixed prosthesis is just as critical to its success as is recall maintenance for any other dental service. Evaluation at 6-month intervals will often reveal problems which are easily and effectively corrected without jeopardy to the restoration. Such evaluation should routinely include:

1. Assessment of the periodontal condition of all teeth, including plaque accumulation
2. Examination of abutment teeth for mobility and recurrent decay
3. Examination of each retainer to determine that the cement has not "washed out"
4. Evaluation of occlusal relationships

The assistant prepares the examination tray (Fig. 29-12) for the recall appointment and assists at the chairside during the examination.

POST AND CORE RESTORATION FOR ENDODONTICALLY TREATED TEETH

Nonvital teeth which have received root canal therapy are generally "weaker," thus more prone to fracture, than vital teeth for two basic reasons. First of all, a nonvital tooth is more brittle due to the loss of its primary nutrient supply, the pulp. Secondly, access preparation into the pulp cavity is usually of such an extent that it significantly reduces the supporting dentin and enamel through the center portion of the tooth crown. In addition, most teeth requiring endodontic therapy have already had their crowns weakened by either previous restorations or the ravages of dental decay.

Adequate restoration of such endodontically treated teeth usually requires some type of foundation ("buildup") for the remaining crown and root to (1) strengthen the entire tooth through the principle of reinforcement (resistance form), and (2) provide adequate retention form to the coronal portion for subsequent placement of a cast restoration. The *cast gold post and core* is but one of a number of such foundations which can fulfill these two basic objectives (Fig. 29-22). While other types of foundations (such as pin-retained amalgam and composite buildups) can serve quite adequately in many instances, the cast post and core is generally indicated for any single rooted endo-

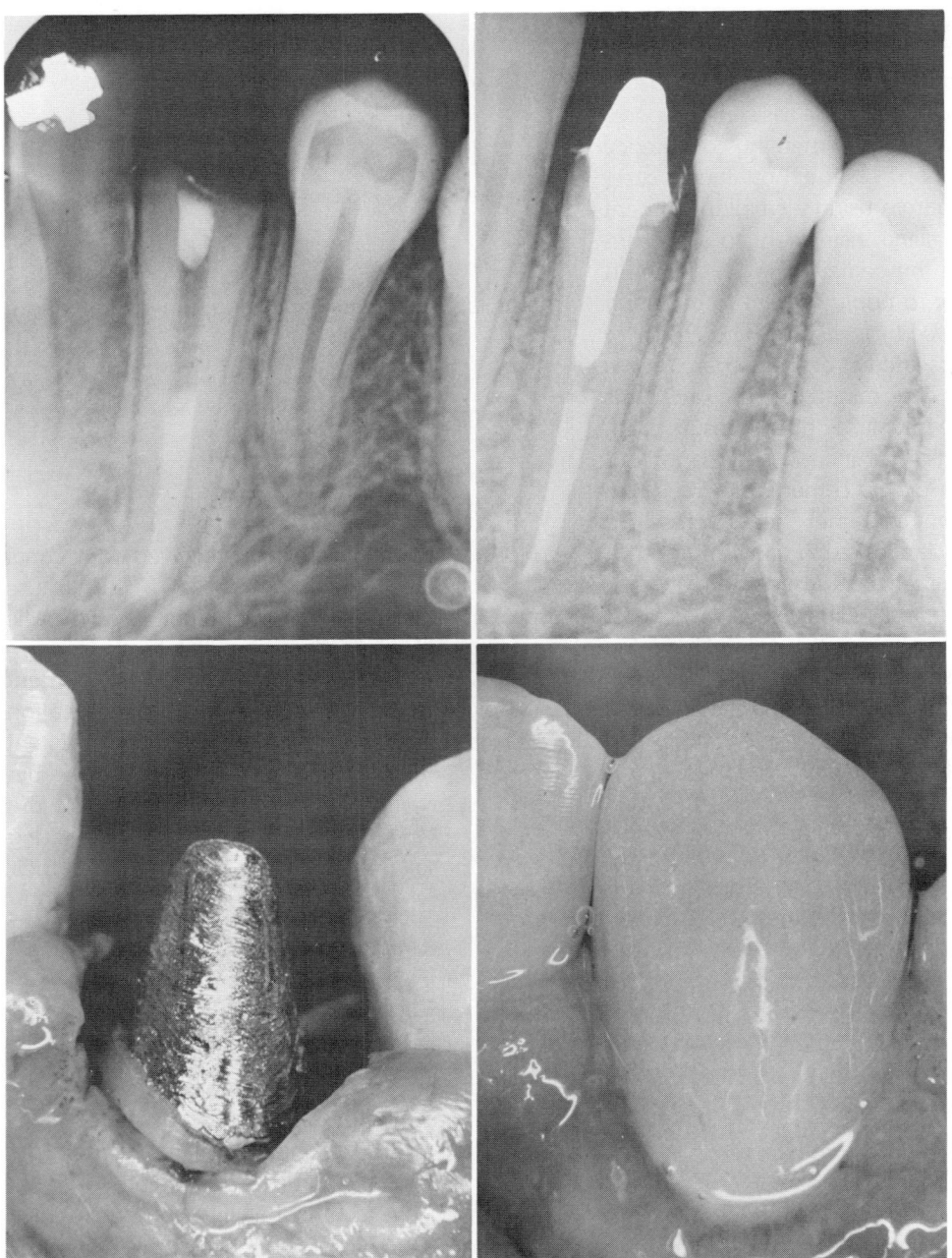

Figure 29-22 | Post and core restoration for endodontically treated tooth.
A. Preoperative radiograph. B. Radiograph of cemented post and core foundation.
C. Clinical view of post and core with tooth prepared to receive a PFM crown.
D. PFM crown cemented.

dontic tooth which, for other reasons, requires restoration. The cast post and core is definitely indicated for any single rooted endodontic tooth (and some multirooted) which is to serve as a bridge abutment.

The basic design of the cast post and core is one of a tapered rod (post) with an attached coronal portion (core) having a tapered form similar to the prepared form of a tooth which is to receive a cast crown. The post itself is developed such that it will precisely fit into the prepared root canal(s) to a depth approximately one-half to two-thirds the length of the clinical root (Fig. 29-22B) and thus provide maximum resistance against fracture of the remaining tooth. The pattern for the post and core casting can be developed *directly* in the mouth from wax and/or resin or *indirectly* on a die made from an impression of the prepared tooth.

Zinc phosphate cement is the material of choice for cementing a cast post and core, and preparation of the material is just as critical as it is for cementation of any other fixed restoration.

Instrumentation, materials, concepts, and clinical techniques in restorative dentistry are constantly changing. The material presented in this chapter is introductory and in no way intended to represent the entire scope of clinical fixed prosthodontics. Many acceptable philosophies and clinical techniques are presented in detail in the dental literature, and the interested assistant is referred to the textbooks listed in the bibliography for additional information. The clinical responsibilities of the assistant are essentially the same, however, regardless of variations in techniques employed by the dentist.

BIBLIOGRAPHY

Boucher, C. O. (ed.): *Current Clinical Dental Terminology,* 3d ed., The C. V. Mosby Company, St. Louis, 1963.

Dennison, J. B., and Powers, J. M.: "A Review of Dental Cements Used for Permanent Retention of Restorations. Part 2: Properties and Criteria for Selection," *J. Mich. Dent. Assoc.,* **56:**218–225, 1974.

Hickey, J. C., Boucher, C. O., and Hughes, G. A. (eds.): *Glossary of Prosthodontic Terms,* 3d ed., The C. V. Mosby Company, St. Louis, 1968.

Johnston, J. F., Phillips, R. W., and Dykema, R. W.: *Modern Practice in Crown and Bridge Prosthodontics,* 3d ed., W. B. Saunders Company, Philadelphia, 1971.

Murray, H. V., and Sluder, T. B.: *Dental Laboratory Technology—Fixed Restorative Techniques,* University of North Carolina, Chapel Hill, 1972.

Skinner, E. W., and Phillips, R. W.: *The Science of Dental Materials,* 7th ed., W. B. Saunders Company, Philadelphia, 1973.

Sturdevant, C. M., Barton, R. E., and Brauer, J. C. (eds.): *The Art and Science of Operative Dentistry,* McGraw-Hill Book Company, New York, 1968.

Tylman, S. D.: *Theory and Practice of Crown and Fixed Partial Prosthodontics (Bridge),* 6th ed., The C. V. Mosby Company, St. Louis, 1970.

30 David P. Dobson

Removable Prosthodontics

PSYCHOLOGY OF DENTURE PATIENTS

Patients who present themselves for complete dentures often have some type of psychologic problem; there are others who are normal individuals in every respect. Usually patients can be classified as philosophic (cooperative), apprehensive, indifferent, or unreasonable.

The cooperative patients generally are those who truly desire to have complete dentures made to improve their appearance, chewing capacity and efficiency, and general health. These patients are usually easy to please.

The apprehensive individuals might be classified as those who do not want others to know they need dentures, are afraid of wearing them, lack confidence in the dentist, and in general, are not quite sure they want treatment. A typical patient of this type is an elderly person who desires to have dentures and wishes all the wrinkles erased from his or her face. This request is almost impossible, but, nevertheless, it is demanded of the dentist by the patient on many occasions. The dental assistant is very valuable to the dentist in such cases. The assistant's reassurance and calm assistance to the patient and admiration of the results of the denture will do much to ease the patient's mind and, further, will reflect a favorable opinion of the dentist.

The indifferent patient is one who is not concerned about whether or not to wear dentures. Many times such patients are urged by their children to have their teeth replaced. Some of these patients have for many years worn their dentures only occasionally and, accordingly, are not convinced that they are required. Such patients are usually difficult to please, and they may not wear the dentures with success when they are completed.

The unreasonable patient is uncooperative and demands a denture service impossible for the dentist to deliver.

By anticipating the questions of concern which the patient might ask or the demands they might make, the dental assistant many times can prevent a misconception about dentures before it becomes fixed in the patient's mind. Patients may be more attentive to an assistant's comments than to the opinions of the dentist, as they sometimes feel that the dentist is "making excuses" for the work which has been accomplished.

The dental assistant may also be of inestimable value by personal interest and assistance to the patients who have dentures made which are inserted immediately after the remaining teeth have been extracted. Problems or questions concerning the loss of their last teeth often arise in an individual's mind. Some people associate the loss of teeth with the loss of youth and virility and, accordingly, believe that old age is approaching. Many individuals express great concern in their attitude toward age.

The cheerful assistant will prove invaluable in the management of patients. Through encouragement and favorable expressions the assistant can help inspire confidence in the patient, which may mean the difference between success and failure of the denture service.

OPERATIVE PROCEDURES FOR THE CONSTRUCTION OF COMPLETE DENTURES

First Appointment

The first appointment for the edentulous patient is usually spent by taking a panoramic radiograph and, if need be, a full-mouth series of periapical radiographs. The dentist can then determine whether there are any remaining root tips, impacted teeth, cysts, or other abnormalities of the tooth-supporting structures which may have to be removed surgically prior to new construction. The dental assistant can accomplish this task as a part of the denture treatment (see Chap. 18). At this first appointment the dentist usually will interview the patient to ascertain past denture history, which will become a part of the prognosis for the success of the dentures. Many dentists will also have a diagnostic survey sheet or card on which various items will be recorded. These materials should be in a place of convenience for the dentist's chairside use.

If a "wet reading" of the radiographs does not show any need for surgery, preliminary impressions are made at this appointment, or the dentist may wish to make the final impression with dental compound.

Treatment Relines

In many cases the patient's ridges are in a state of poor health, and the tissues are deformed because of the patient's ill-fitting dentures. The dentist then will want to do a chairside reline with a conditioning material which stays fairly soft for several days and is therefore comfortable. A reline is the resurfacing of the tissue side of a denture with the new base material to make it fit more accurately. In this case the lining material is of a temporary nature and can easily be removed. This material is a powder-liquid mix.

The dental assistant will have the following items available for this procedure:

1. Disposable plastic apron to cover the patient's clothing
2. Treatment and reline material
3. Paper mixing pad
4. Spatula, either metal or wooden
5. Acrylic burs or mandrel-mounted arbor bands for

the dentist to remove some of the tissue side of the patient's dentures
6. Small scissors and a surgical scapel to remove excess reline material

The reline material is mixed by the dental assistant according to the manufacturer's directions and can be placed on the tissue side of the dentures either by the dental assistant or by the dentist, who then seats the dentures in the patient's mouth. On removal the dental assistant may trim the excess material which has flowed over the denture edges onto the polished-surface side of the dentures. This is accomplished with the scissors and/or the surgical scapel.

This conditioning reline procedure may have to be repeated several times over a period of 2 or 3 weeks before the tissue over which the dentures will fit is fully "recovered" to a state of health.

In those cases for which treatment relines are not necessary the dentist will proceed on the first appointment with preliminary impressions or, as previously mentioned, with final compound impressions.

Preliminary Impressions with Alginate Hydrocolloid

These impressions are made with stock trays which may be perforated for the impression material's retention, or the stock tray may be made of unperforated metal with borders of rounded metal to lock the material within the tray. The dental assistant should have the following items available for this procedure:

1. Disposable plastic apron to cover the patient's clothing.
2. Impression material, alginate hydrocolloid, and water-measuring cup.
3. Rubber or plastic mixing bowl.
4. Spatula.
5. Stock upper and lower trays of several sizes. The dental assistant can become proficient in selecting the proper size by placing the patient's dentures in-

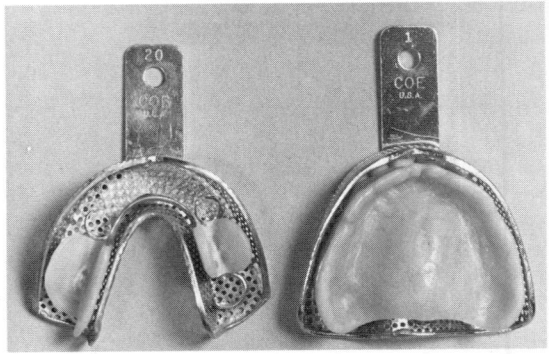

Figure 30-1 | Selecting the proper-size impression trays.

side the tray to see that the tray is large enough to cover the area of the mouth to be recorded (Fig. 30-1).
6. Utility wax ropes to modify the stock tray by adding the wax along the edges of the tray (Fig. 30-2) to make it conform more closely to the size and shape of the ridges and associated parts.

Chair Procedures

The patient is comfortably seated in the chair, and his or her present dentures are removed and placed in a container of water. Plastic or paper denture cups should be used for this procedure. Glasses and other items that may hinder the dentist's work should be laid aside for safekeeping. In the case of a female patient, disposable tissues should be available so that she may remove lipstick, which may be smeared during the impression making. A light coating of petroleum jelly should be placed by the assistant on the patient's lips and surrounding areas to facilitate the removal of any of the impression material which may remain on the face after the impression is made (Fig. 30-3).

Thirty minutes prior to their need an assortment of thoroughly scrubbed trays should be placed in a cold disinfecting solution. Immediately prior to use, the trays are removed from the

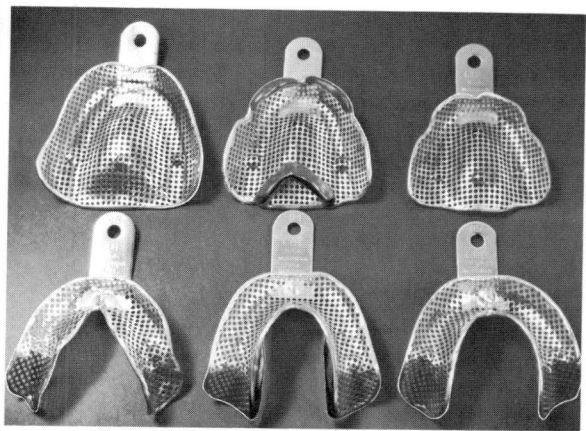

Figure 30-2 | Alginate complete denture trays. Rope wax has been added to middle trays.

Figure 30-3 | Applying petroleum jelly to patient's lips and face.

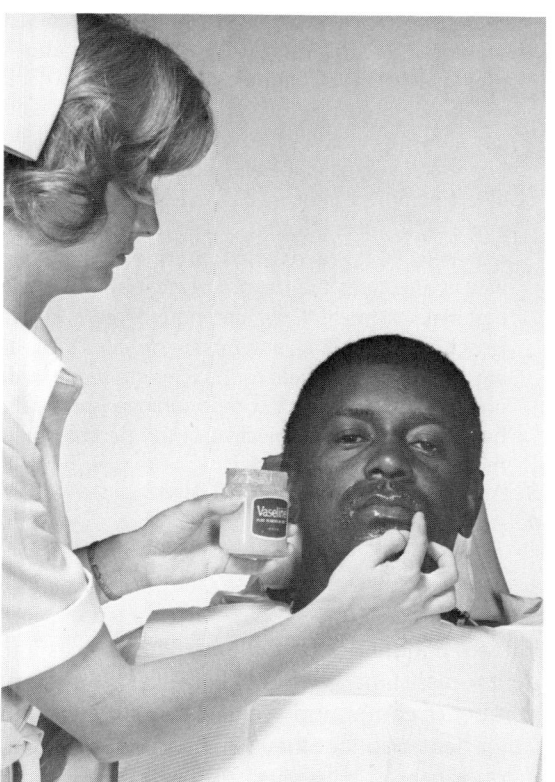

bath, washed under clean tap water, shaken to remove most of the water, and placed in a position convenient for the dentist.

Mixing of the impression material demands care and skill. The manufacturer's directions on the package must be studied and followed exactly in order to obtain good results. Water in the specified amount is placed in a dry, clean plaster bowl, and to it is added the full measure of powder. If packaged powder is used, smooth the container, and tap it edgewise on the desk to get all the powder to one end. By cutting off the upper end of the package with straight scissors, one may quickly pour the contents into the plaster bowl and be sure all of the powder has been used. Since there is an optimum mixing time, the spatula must be set to work immediately and wielded in a smoothing or wiping motion against the side of the bowl which is being revolved in the other hand.

When the allotted time is up, the creamy homogeneous mix must be rapidly loaded in the tray selected by the dentist. For the average-size mouth one mix will adequately fill the tray and supply a small excess, which may be reserved for placement in the palate or for whenever supplemental material is deemed necessary prior to the insertion of the tray. Once loaded, the material in the tray may be smoothed by a wet finger and passed, handle first, to the doctor for insertion in the mouth. Some operators prefer to have the assistant hold the bowl while the dentist loads the tray.

Alginate impression materials take a short time to set, and this gives the assistant adequate opportunity to clean and dry the bowl, the spatula, and the working area. By working efficiently, the latter items will have been cleaned in time to receive the impression. Under no circumstances should the impression by allowed to dehydrate, since this will result in a distorted cast. Either the impressions must be kept wrapped in a wet paper towel until poured or the assistant must immediately pour both impressions with plaster or a dental stone specified by the doctor.

Preliminary Impression with Dental Compound

Some dentists prefer to make the preliminary impressions by using dental compound instead of alginate hydrocolloid. For this procedure the dental assistant should have available:

1. Compound trays that are not perforated and may be made of a heavier-gauge metal. These trays come in various sizes and shapes which will fit different types of dental-arch ridges. Any complete selection of stock trays will fit all types of mouths. Trimming of the trays with files, metal shears, or grinding wheels is sometimes necessary. The edges of a tray should be smooth and even and not irritating to the patient's mouth. It is the assistant's job to see that these edges are smooth before the tray is inserted into the patient's mouth. All trays should be cleaned and sterilized before being presented to the dentist for trial in the patient's mouth.

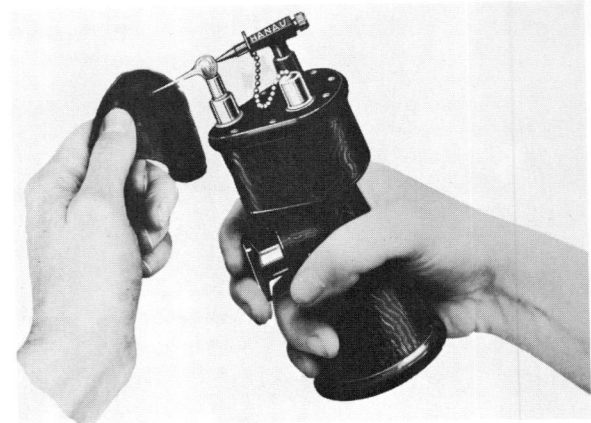

Figure 30-5 | Alcohol torch. (*Courtesy of Hanau Engineering Company, Inc.*)

Figure 30-4 | Compound adapted to impression trays in preparation for the making of maxillary and mandibular impressions. Compound heater also shown.

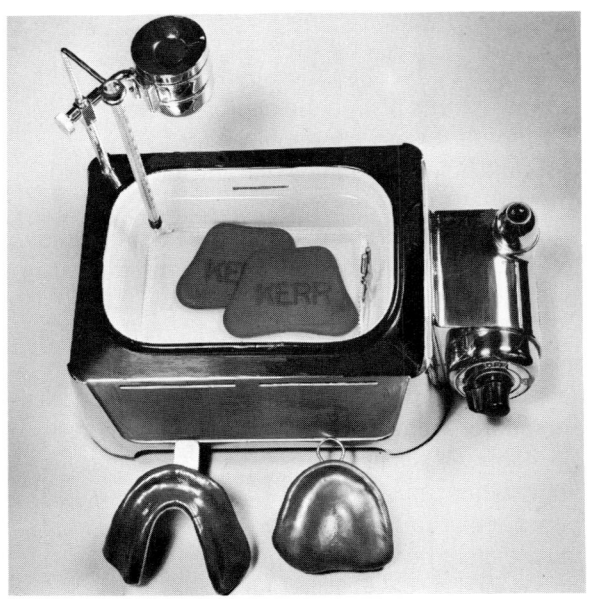

2. Impression compound, which is a material with a shellac base that is thermoplastic, that is, it becomes soft upon heating and hardens when cooled. This compound will soften slightly above mouth temperature at ranges from 110 to 130°F. It will become solid and hard at about 99°F. This permits the use of the compound in making impressions of a patient's mouth. This material also is commonly known as modeling plastic and is available in several forms. These usually consist of materials that are different in color. The color usually indicates the degree of heat at which the material will melt. Gray compound requires the least heat for melting, and next in order of increasing requirement of heat for melting are green, red, and black; that is, black compound needs the most heat to soften. The objective of the dentist determines the compound used.
3. A compound heater (Fig. 30-4).
4. An alcohol torch (Fig. 30-5).

Chair Procedures

Fifteen minutes before the patient arrives the dental assistant should place the necessary number of compound "cakes" in the compound water heater so that they will be in a plastic condition for the dentist's use. After the compound is heated sufficiently, the heater control can be set at a low, tempering heat so that the compound may be placed in the patient's mouth without discomfort. The first number on the heater switch provides the hottest water, and the third number provides the lowest temperature. Petroleum jelly may be placed on the dental assistant's fingers so that the softened compound will not stick. The compound is folded to conform to the impression trays (Fig. 30-4) and handed to the dentist, who may wish to flame the material with an alcohol torch to remove any surface wrinkles (Fig. 30-5). The compound heater should be in close proximity to the dentist, who can then temper the heated compound in the water just prior to placing the tray in the mouth.

The compound will become hard in the patient's mouth. However, the setting time can be hastened by the use of the air syringe or by the water syringe, which should be used in conjunction with the saliva ejector as an aspirator.

The impressions do not have to be wrapped in wet paper towels if they are not poured immediately as is the case with alginate hydrocolloid because there will be no change in the impression shape once it is set. The impressions are separated by placing the poured casts in the compound heater to soften the compound.

Laboratory Procedures

Pouring of Initial Impressions

A cast is a positive reproduction of a patient's denture-bearing area. It is made by pouring some gypsum product into the negative reproduction of the patient's mouth, which heretofore has been referred to as an impression. The preliminary casts, made from the alginate or compound preliminary impressions, are used to fabricate custom-made trays to make a second and more accurate impression of the patient. Although it is usually a laboratory technician's job, the dental assistant may fabricate an autopolymer tray or a shellac-base tray for the making of final impressions.

The initial impression should be washed thoroughly before the cast is poured. A thick mix of plaster should be used for the cast. The procedure for the mixing of the plaster has been covered in Chapter 10. The plaster is vibrated into the impression so that no bubbles will be produced (Fig. 30-6). It is mixed thick enough to permit piling up of the material in the impression. An impression should never be turned over when one is pouring any type of case, as gravity will tend to pull the material away from the impression and, thereby, cause an inaccurate reproduction of the patient's mouth. After the plaster is set thoroughly, it will be necessary to remove the compound impression from the preliminary cast. This is done by holding the cast

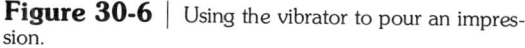

Figure 30-6 | Using the vibrator to pour an impression.

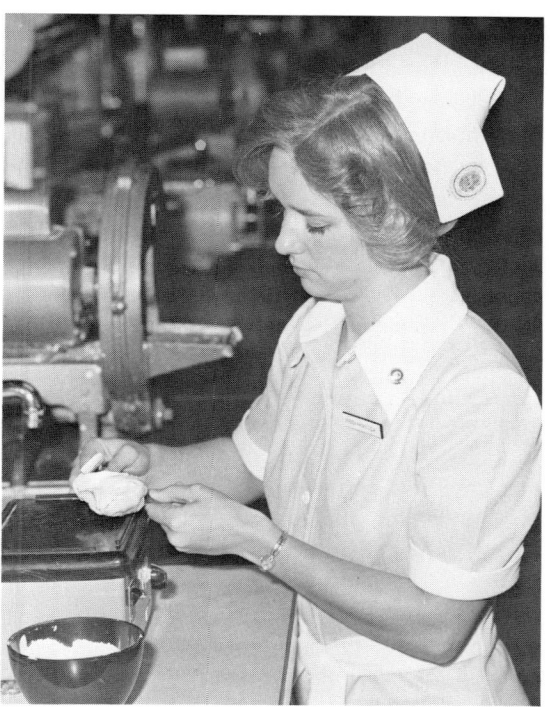

and the impression under warm water or by placing the cast in the compound water heater. The tray usually will separate from the impression compound, and then the compound may be rolled away easily from the preliminary cast. Alginate impressions are separated merely by lifting the tray off the cast. No heating is necessary because of the elasticity of the impression material. The cast should then be trimmed to the desired dimensions, care being taken not to destroy the anatomic parts (Fig. 30-7).

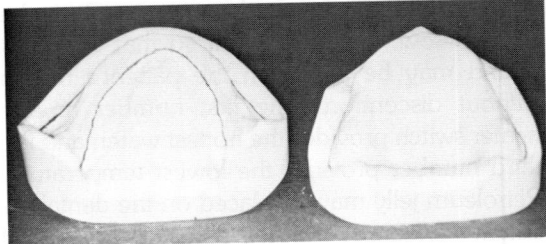

Figure 30-7 | Properly trimmed preliminary casts.

Cleaning of the Impression Trays

Usually some compound will adhere to the impression tray. This can be removed easily by wiping some petroleum jelly over the tray and by holding the tray over an open flame until the compound has softened. It then can be wiped off with a paper towel. This is the most efficient and the easiest method of cleaning compound from the trays. The same procedure may be followed in removing metallic-oxide paste from trays or instruments.

Alginate trays can be cleaned with a stiff brush and tap water. If the material is allowed to harden, there are available several types of solvents in which the trays may be soaked overnight to remove any of the impression material.

Chair Procedures for Final Compound Impressions

Although the majority of dentists use a plastic custom tray, some dentists prefer to use compound preliminary impressions as part of their technique for final impressions. No custom trays are constructed, but it requires the following additional armamentarium:

1. Sharp compound knife or a disposable blade knife such as B-P no. 6
2. Stick compound (either green or gray) and/or impression wax
3. Metallic-oxide paste

The dentist will trim the preliminary compound impression with the compound knife to reduce the excessive thickness of the borders and will usually go back to the mouth to "border mold" or "muscle trim," which is the shaping of the impression material by the manipulation or action of the tissues adjacent to the borders of an impression. Stick compound, alcohol torch, and the compound heater are used for this procedure as is the Bunsen burner.

After the border-molding procedures the final step in the impression technique calls for a thin coating inside the compound tray with a metallic-oxide paste, plaster of paris, or rubber-base impression material. This will be described in conjunction with the use of a custom-tray final impression technique.

Fabrication of Custom-made Trays

Shellac Trays

The simplest method of producing a custom-made tray is to use shellac baseplates.* Usually a shellac baseplate of double thickness is used for this, Shellac-base material will soften upon the application of heat. Care should be exercised that no melted material get on the hands, as it

---

* For detailed instruction in this and all laboratory procedures mentioned in this chapter, a manual, *Dental Laboratory Technology, Prosthodontic Techniques,* is available from the University of North Carolina Press, Box 2288, Chapel Hill, N.C., 27514.

will cause serious burns. It should not be heated enough to melt but just to soften. The cast should be soaked thoroughly in water before any of this material is applied to prevent it from sticking. After the cast has been prepared, lay the shellac tray over the cast so that it is centered properly. With a Bunsen burner or heat gun soften the center of the upper base material first (Fig. 30-8). It will then begin to flow down against the cast. As it softens, gently mold it to the palate with your fingers. Care should be taken not to stretch it thin to any great extent. A thin tray will not be very strong. Be sure to hold it until the material cools; if it is not held, the material will tend to warp and will not be accurate. Next heat around the periphery, and soften one area of the ridge portion at a time. Adapt this over the cast, hold until each section is cool, and then proceed to the next section. A shellac tray now is complete which is adapted accurately to the cast, including the periphery. Next soften the edges, and trim all excess except for 3 to 4 mm off the tray. This is accomplished by softening the edges of the tray in a flame and by trimming with a pair of scissors or laboratory shears. Next, with a flame, soften the edge and roll it back so that a roll twice the thickness of the tray is formed around the peripheral edge. Make sure that this roll is smooth with no sharp points. A file, sandpaper, or a scraper may be used to facilitate making this roll smooth. At this point the tray should be completed except for a handle, which is necessary. Take the scraps of material that have been left over, mold them into a handle, flame the bottom until it is in a softened state, and attach the piece to the anterior part of the tray. This will provide a handle to help in carrying the impression material in the tray into the patient's mouth.

For a lower tray, follow the same procedure. Soften the lingual side of the material first so that it will fall into the lingual contour of the preliminary cast. Then adapt the outside. Always be sure to hold each section against the cast until it is cooled thoroughly to prevent any warping of the material. Attach a handle to the anterior portion. The tray now should be ready to make the final impression.

Quick-Cure or Autopolymerizing Resin Trays

This is the most popular method of constructing custom trays, and while the technique is more involved, it produces a stronger and more versatile tray which can be used with all types of impression materials (Fig. 30-9).

The materials required for the construction of a custom tray are

1. Power and liquid tray material
2. Measuring devices
3. Paper cups and wooden tongue blades
4. Petroleum jelly
5. Glass slab
6. Tray former
7. Baseplate wax
8. Bunsen burner
9. Tinfoil substitute and brush
10. Wax knife and wax spatulas

An indelible-pencil tray outline is drawn on the preliminary plaster casts by the dentist to determine the borders, and a single thickness of softened wax baseplate is adapted to the casts from 2 to 3 mm short of the outline.

Tinfoil substitute is painted on the exposed plaster casts to ensure separation of the resin tray material.

The glass slab is lubricated with petroleum jelly, and the tray material is mixed according to the manufacturer's instructions. A paper cup and a wooden tongue blade are satisfactory for mixing the material.

The tray former is placed on the glass slab, and the mixed material is patted to uniform thickness. Petroleum jelly is used to lubricate the fingers to prevent the material from sticking to them. The wafer of material is carefully lifted from the slab and adapted to the cast being

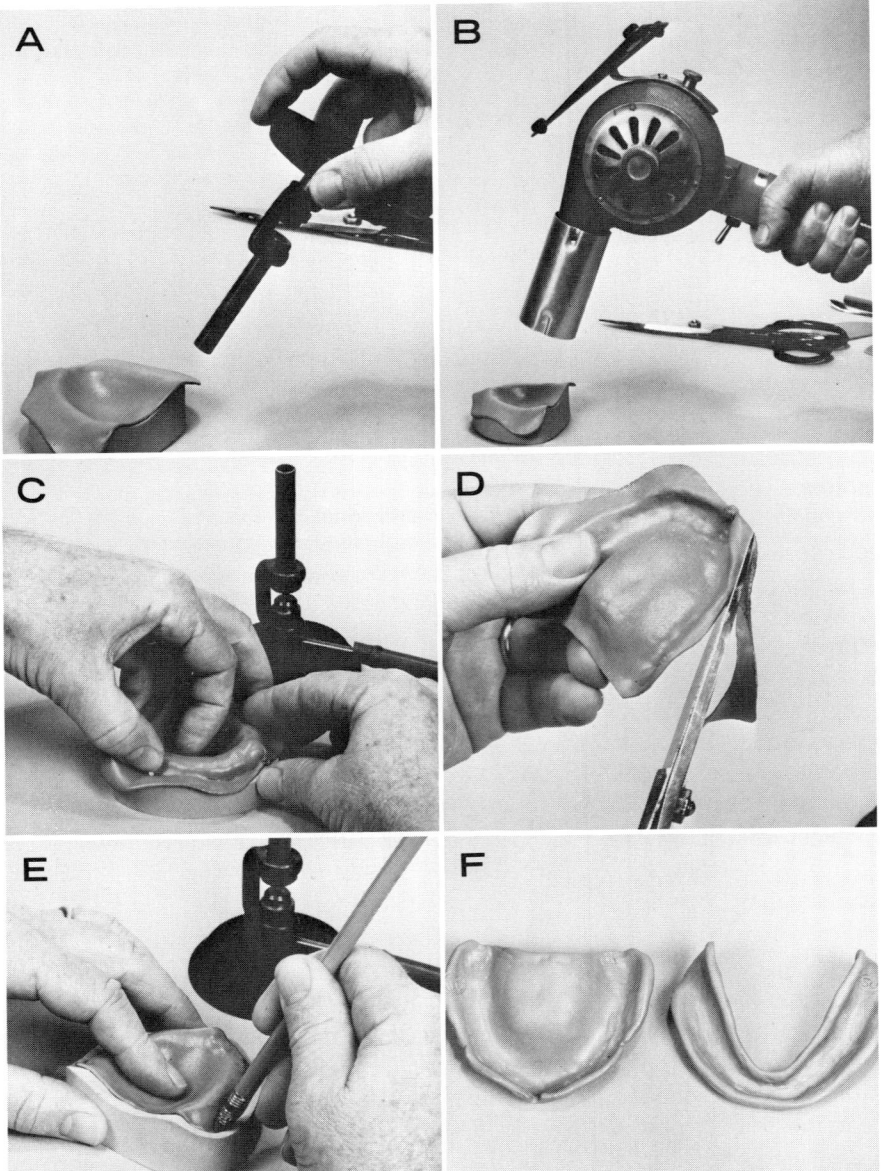

Figure 30-8 | Shellac custom trays. A. Using a Bunsen burner to soften the shellac baseplate. B. Using a heat gun in lieu of burner. C. Adapting the tray. D. Trimming the tray. E. Adapting the edges of the tray. F. Completed trays. (*From Dental Laboratory Technology, Prosthodontic Techniques,* University of North Carolina at Chapel Hill, 1968.)

careful not to create thin areas. A warm knife is used to trim the excess material to the pencil outline, and a vertical handle is constructed with the excess scrap material. Wetting the base area of the tray handle with tray material liquid will ensure a good bond for the handle. The handle must not protrude facially, and it must have a concave form so that it will be easy to grip.

The tray material will cure in about 15 minutes. Do not separate until the heat of polymerization has dissipated.

Carefully pry the trays off of the casts, but do not put them in hot water, as the wax spacer must not be disturbed. There are occasions when the casts must be broken to facilitate removal of the tray from the anatomic "undercuts." A sharp blow with the handle of a plaster spatula will accomplish this procedure.

The trays are then trimmed to the outline using a grinding stone on the lathe or with acrylic burs and stones and a straight handpiece. A ragwheel and pumice will ensure smooth, rounded borders. The completed trays are now ready to deliver to the dentist.

Final Impressions Using Custom Trays

The armamentarium is the same as for a final compound impression with the addition of acrylic burs which the dentist may use to trim the custom-tray borders if the trays need adjustment.

Border molding is accomplished in the same manner as described before by the use of stick compound which is trimmed with sharp compound knives and softened by the dentist with the alcohol torch. A compound water heater is necessary to temper the material before the tray is placed in the mouth.

Final "wash" impression: this is the last step in the final impression technique and occurs after the final border molding is done. The items needed for this procedure are an apron to protect the patient's clothes, petroleum jelly, gauze squares, a pad for mixing the metallic-oxide paste, spatula, mouth mirror, operative pliers, saliva ejector, oral evacuator, air-syringe tip, and mouthwash (Fig. 30-10).

Since the metallic-oxide pastes are the most universally used materials, their manipulation will be discussed here. When the paste is being mixed, all dry skin surfaces that will come in contact with the metallic-oxide paste should be well lubricated. Petroleum jelly is good for this purpose. The assistant should place petroleum jelly on his or her hands, including the area around and under the fingernails. Petroleum jelly also should be placed around the exterior of the patient's mouth and on the lips. Lipstick should be removed from the patient's lips before the petroleum jelly is applied. A large disposable plastic apron is used for the patient when these impressions are being made to prevent the material from coming in contact with clothing (Fig. 30-11).

Expel from each of the tubes the correct amount of the material to be used as indicated by the manufacturer. The material, once it is expelled from the tube, will begin to harden and set up. The darker material is usually the accelerator, while the other material will tend to give a longer setting time and a softer mix. From the time spatulation is begun, there is a period of 4 to 5 minutes during which the material will remain plastic. The assistant should be able to spatulate the material and load the tray for the dentist, with 1 minute for spatulation and 15 seconds for loading. The tray should be loaded in such a manner that all the surfaces are equally covered. *Do not overload the tray!* Only enough material is needed to record fine detail in an already well-adapted custom tray. Overloading will cause a dangerous gag reflex, and the material could be aspirated in the trachea if care is not used.

The patient may be rinsing with mouthwash during this procedure to reduce the saliva in the mouth. For patients with thick, ropey saliva, 2 by 2 in gauze squares may be needed for the dentist to wipe the patient's mucosa just before the tray is placed in the mouth.

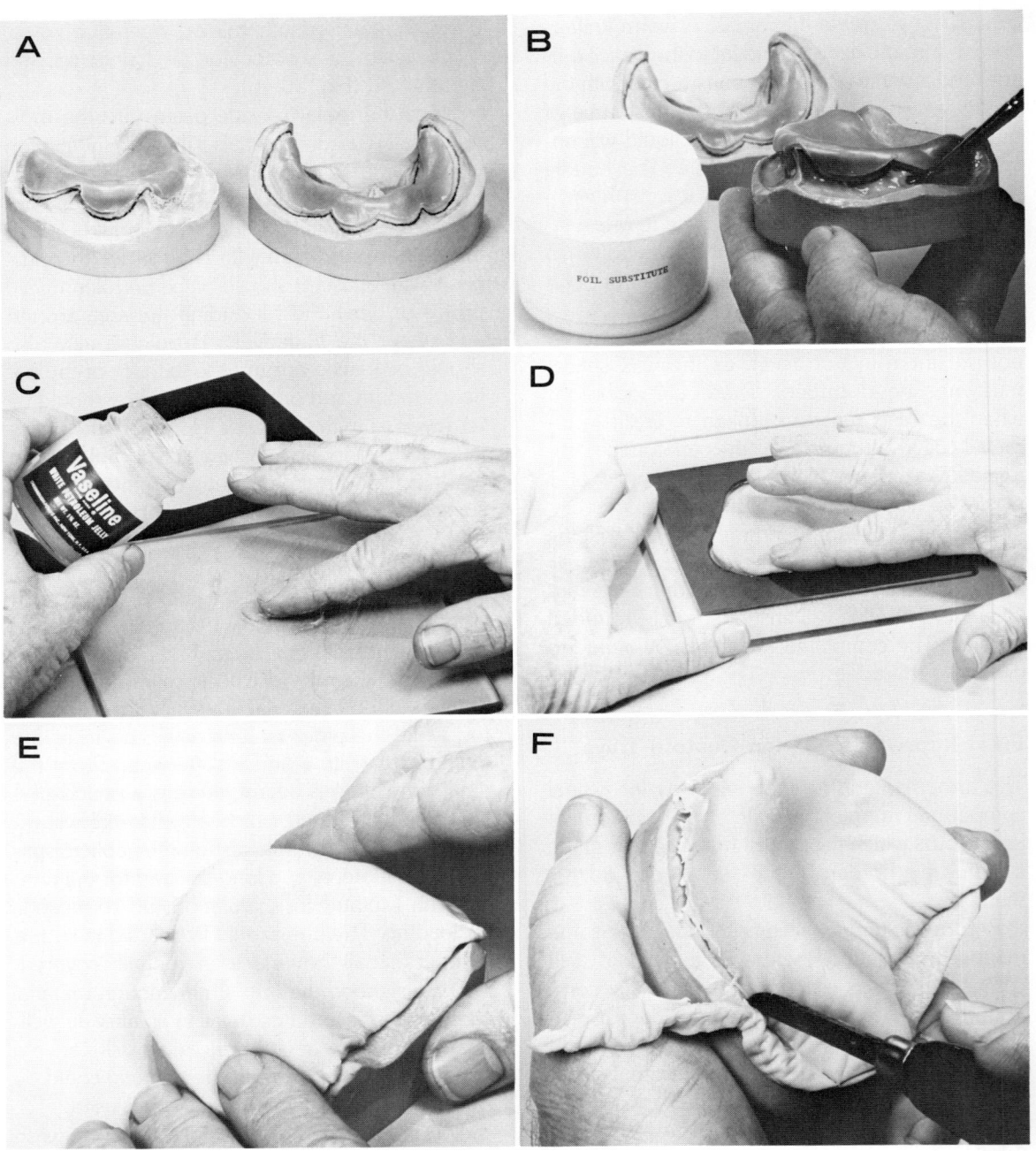

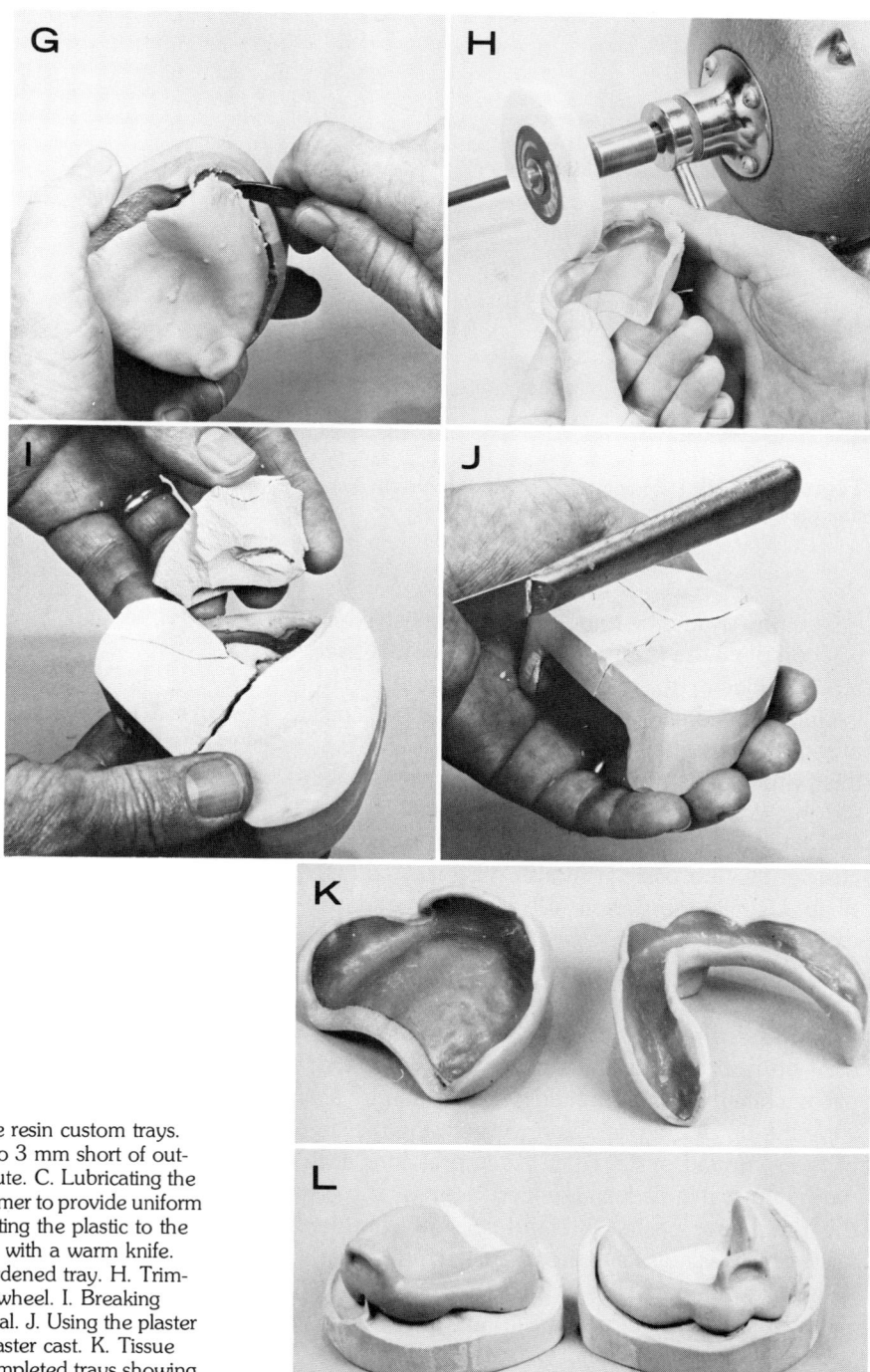

Figure 30-9 | Quick-cure resin custom trays. A. Baseplate wax adapted 2 to 3 mm short of outline. B. Applying tinfoil substitute. C. Lubricating the glass slab. D. Using the tray former to provide uniform thickness of material. E. Adapting the plastic to the cast. F. Trimming the material with a warm knife. G. Carefully removing the hardened tray. H. Trimming the tray with a grinding wheel. I. Breaking the cast to facilitate tray removal. J. Using the plaster spatula handle to crack the plaster cast. K. Tissue side of completed trays. L. Completed trays showing indented handles. (*From Dental Laboratory Technology, Prosthodontic Techniques, University of North Carolina at Chapel Hill, 1968.*)

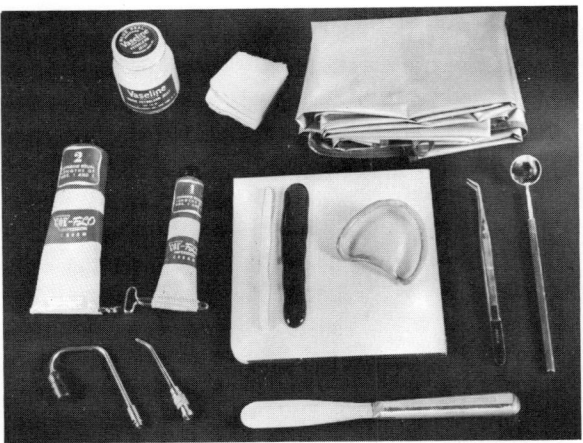

Figure 30-10 | Equipment needed for complete denture impression.

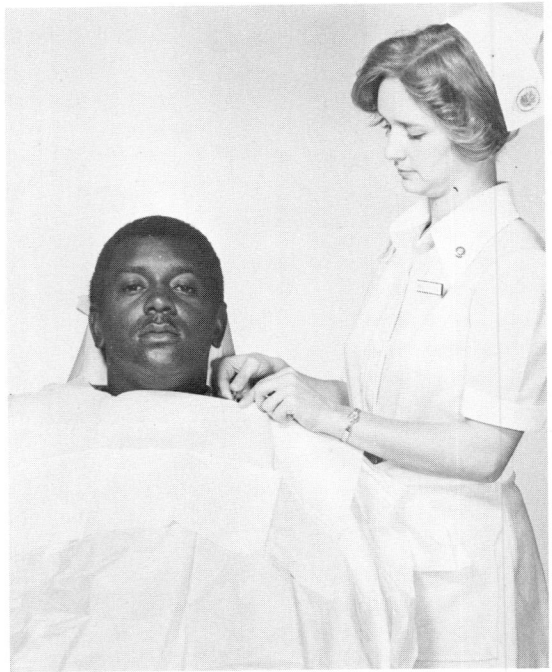

Figure 30-11 | Draping patient with a large disposable apron.

The tray should be handed to the dentist, who will complete the impression. Some dentists use a saliva ejector to keep the patient from swallowing unnecessarily and consequently causing a gag reflex. Others use the oral evacuator for this purpose. As a precaution the assistant may aid the dentist in reflecting the material which has flowed on the soft palate back onto the custom tray by using a mouth mirror or cotton swab. Usually the dentist will do this procedure while the assistant operates the oral evacuator. Prior to removing the impression any excess of hardening paste on the soft palate or on the side wall of the throat (anterior pillar of the fauces) may be removed by the dentist with operative pliers while the assistant holds a gauze square to wipe the tip of the pliers and to catch the pieces of the removed paste. After the impressions are made, the patient's face is wiped clean of any of the remaining paste. A bland solvent can be used which will dissolve the metallic-oxide paste without burning the lips or skin (Fig. 30-12).

The final impressions (wash) may be made with rubber-base material or with silicone-base materials (Fig. 28-39). After the tray is border-molded with compound, the assistant dries it with air and applies rubber-base adhesive to the inside of the tray and over the peripheries for at least 6 mm on the outer portion of the tray.

Plaster of paris is also used for the final impression by some dentists. It is mixed to a creamy consistency in a plaster bowl and placed in the custom tray for the dentist to insert in the patient's mouth. Usually a quick-set plaster is used, so the dental assistant must accomplish the procedure quickly.

At this time the dentist or assistant will ask the patient to bring any smiling snapshots or portraits taken before the natural teeth were extracted. This will provide an invaluable aid to the next appointment when teeth are selected.

The dentures are then returned to the patient

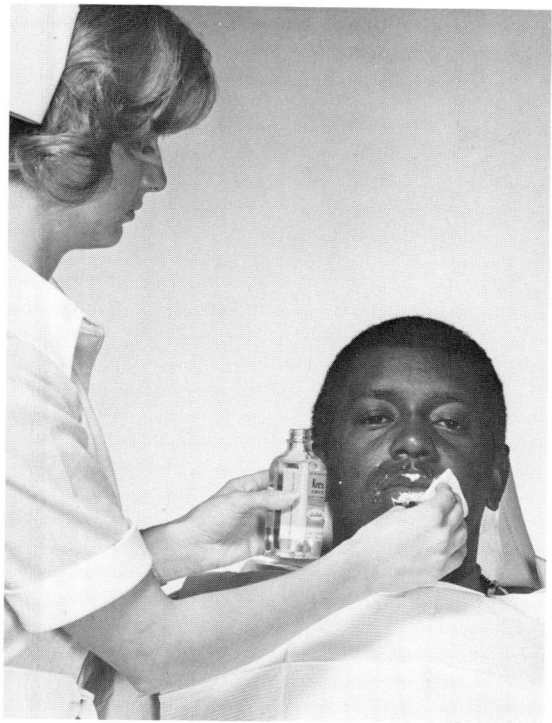

Figure 30-12 | Removing metallic-oxide paste with a bland solvent.

and the next appointment is arranged with the appointment desk.

Pouring Final Impressions for Master Casts

The final impression should be boxed before pouring to provide a neater and stronger cast. The resulting cast is called the *master cast* and is made of dental stone (Fig. 30-13).

The border areas of the impression are very important, as they form the seal which retains the dentures in place. For this reason a definite technique which differs from pouring the preliminary impressions is necessary.

Rope wax is added to the border of the impression to determine how much border will be shown in the final cast. The wax should be placed on the widest dimension of the impression border or at least 3 mm from the edge. It should be from 3 to 5 mm wide. This will create a stone border on the master cast which is called the *land*. In the case of the mandibular cast, boxing wax is added in the tongue space to prevent the poured stone from filling that area.

Plaster bases are poured after the handles are cut off of the impression trays to facilitate the later removal of the trays from the plaster.

The bases are poured so that the ridges of the impressions are parallel to the bench top, and the plaster base is trimmed even to the wax rope with a model trimmer.

Many experienced laboratory technicians pour the master cast by beading with wax rope, pouring a stiff mix of stone, and inverting the impression onto a patty of stone. Unless a dental assistant has poured many final impressions, it is better to box the impression by adding boxing wax around the rope wax. This will ensure a master cast of even proportions and proper thickness. The wax is luted carefully, and a thick mix of stone is vibrated into the impression.

After the stone is set, the wax rope and boxing wax are removed, and the plaster base is carefully separated from the tray. The cast and tray are placed in hot tap water or in a compound water bath for at least 5 minutes to soften the compound and metallic-oxide material to facilitate separation of the tray.

The land of the cast is beveled to aid in record-base construction, and the casts are adjusted on the model trimmer if necessary. The master casts are now ready for record base construction.

If the commericial laboratory is to make the master cast, the final impression should be preserved very carefully and placed in a container supplied by the laboratory. It should be sent to the laboratory immediately. The laboratory will pour the master cast and fabricate the record bases which will be returned for trial in the patient's mouth.

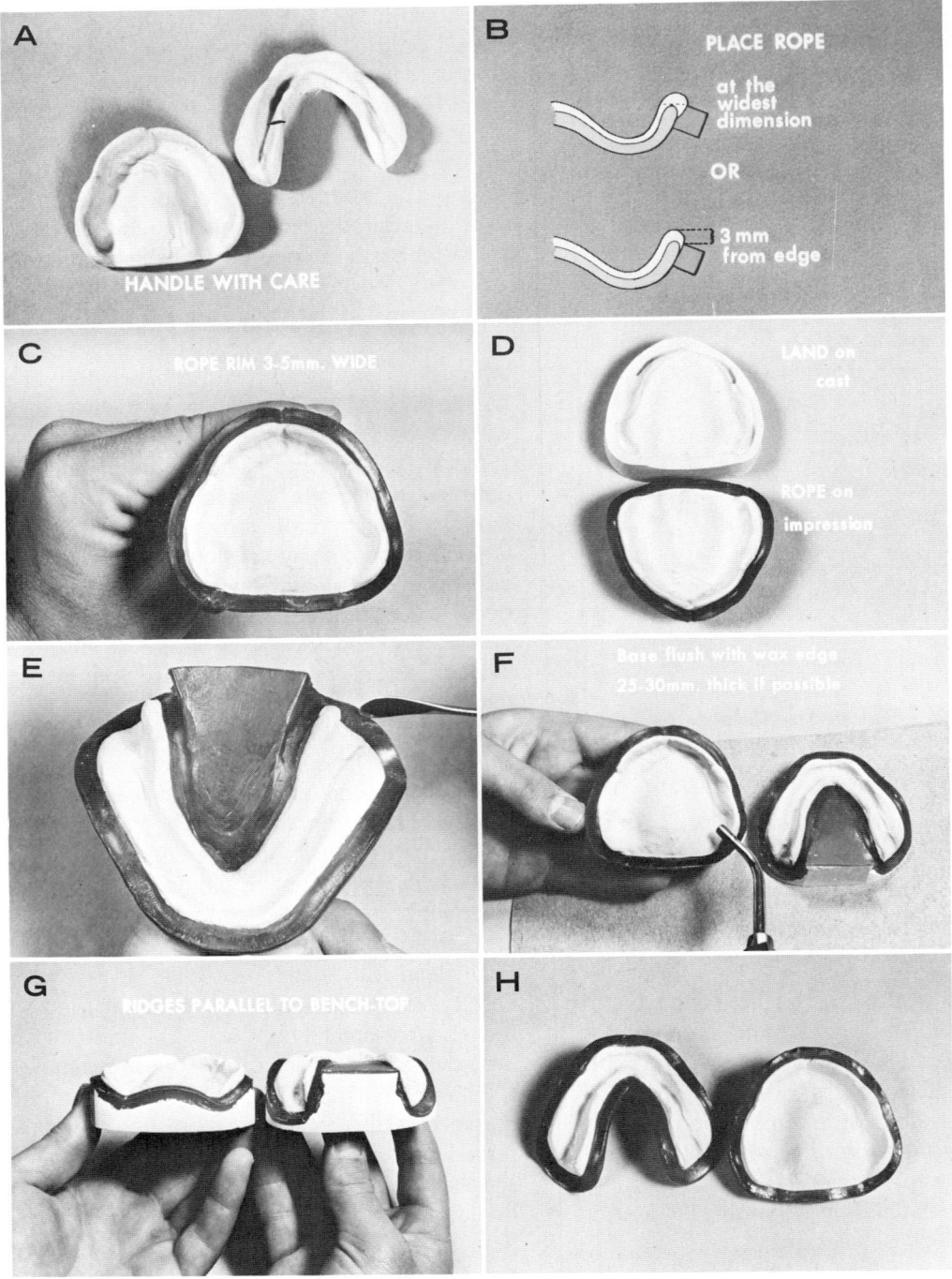

Figure 30-13 | Boxing final impressions. A. Final impressions before boxing and pouring of cast. B. Proper placement of wax rope. C. Completed wax roping of maxillary impression. D. Roped impression with its counterpart poured cast. E. Completed roping of mandibular impression. Note the need for tongue space wax addition. F. Roped impressions with plaster bases. G. Impressions with plaster bases. H. Wax beaded impressions used by commercial laboratories for final cast pouring. No boxing.

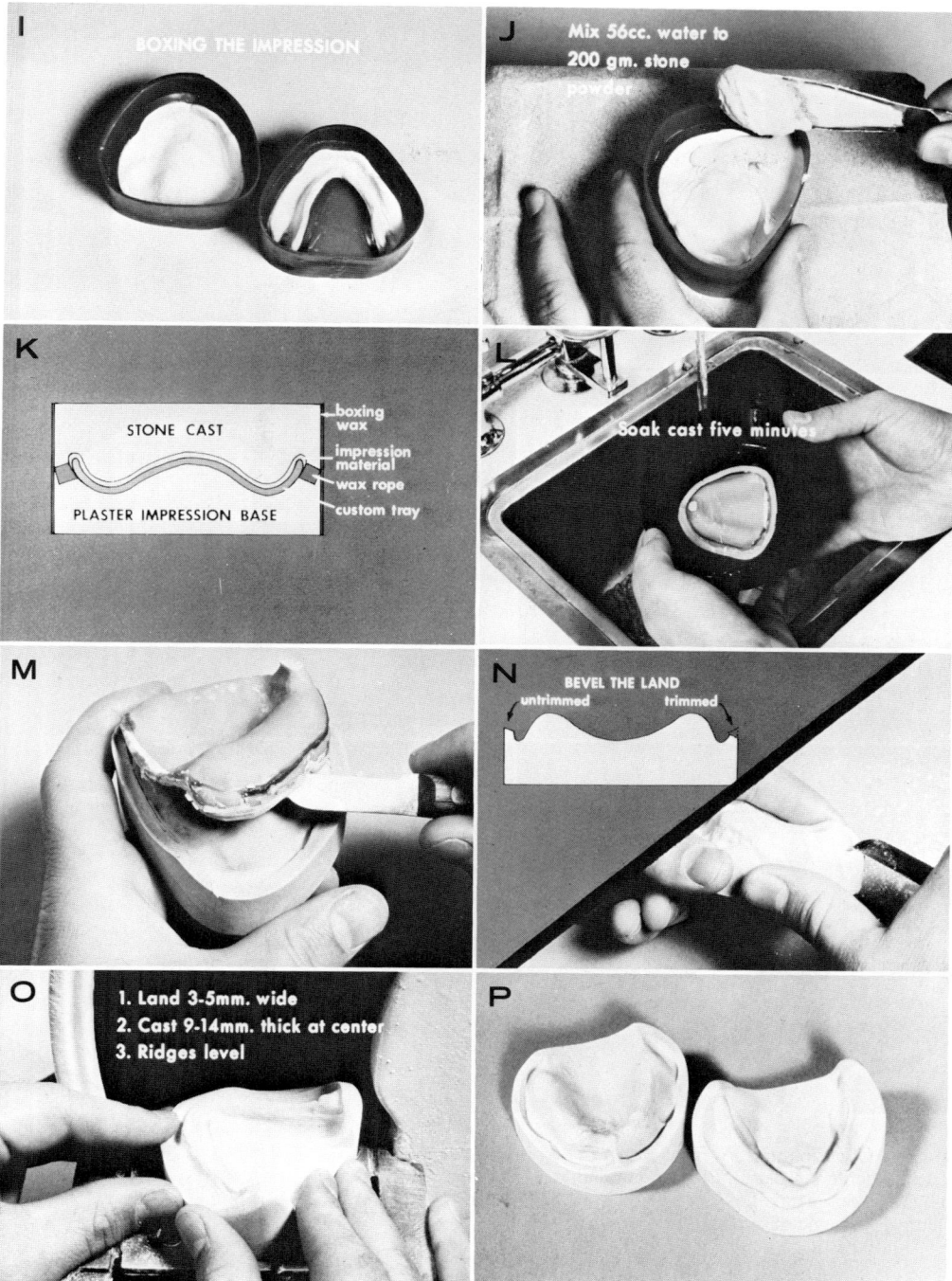

Figure 30-13 continued | I. Boxed impressions. J. Pouring the cast with a vibrator. K. Schematic drawing of poured impression and cast. L. Soaking the cast in hot water. M. Separating the softened metallic oxide and compound impression tray. N. Beveling the land of the cast. O. Trimming the casts with a model trimmer. P. Completed master casts.

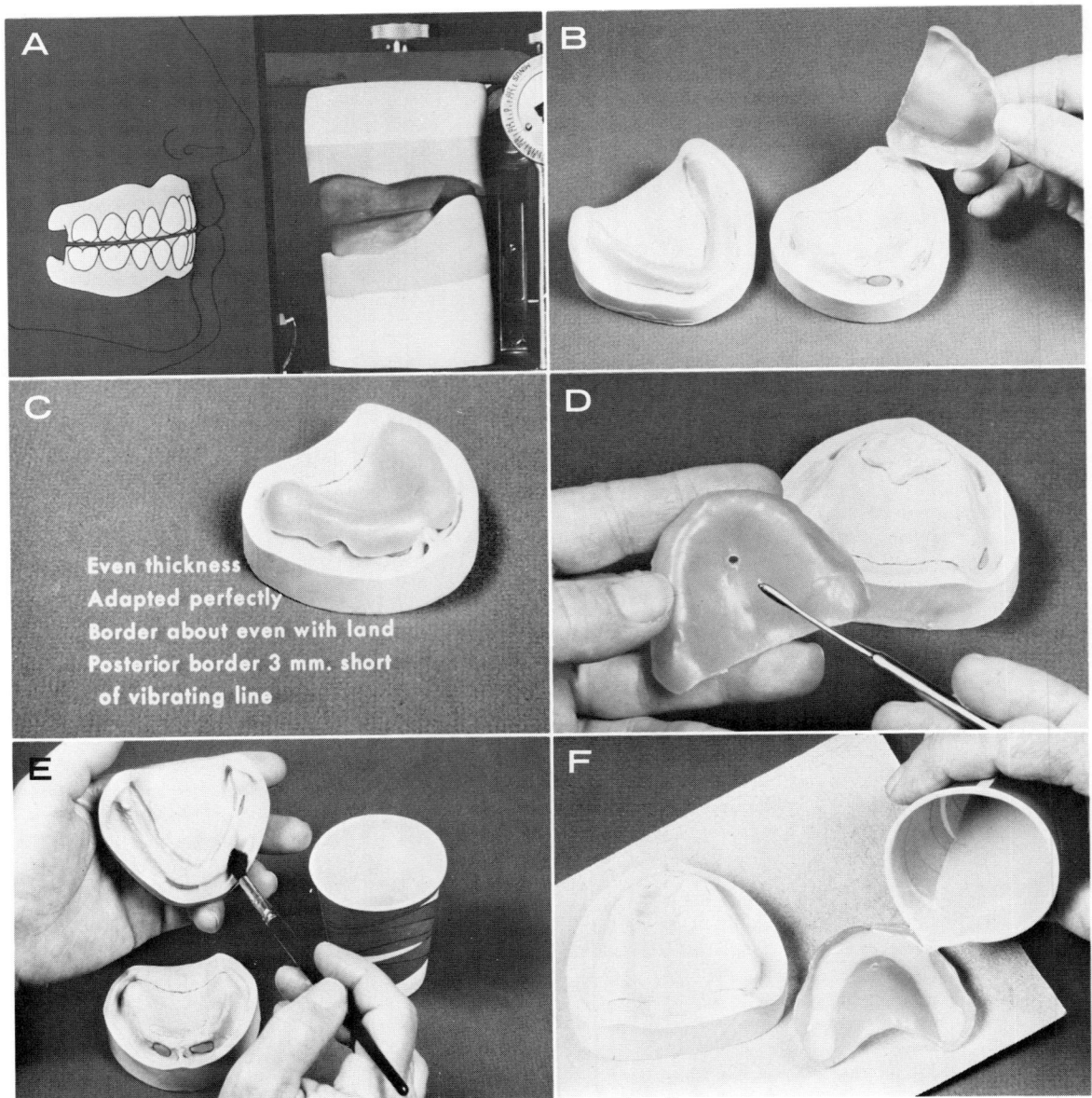

Figure 30-14 | Occlusion rims. A. Relationship of occlusion rims mounted on the articulator to the denture try-in. B. Blocked-out undercuts on a maxillary cast. C. Adapted baseplate wax matrix. D. Hole placement in wax matrix. E. Application of tinfoil substitute. F. Pouring mixed acrylic into wax matrix.

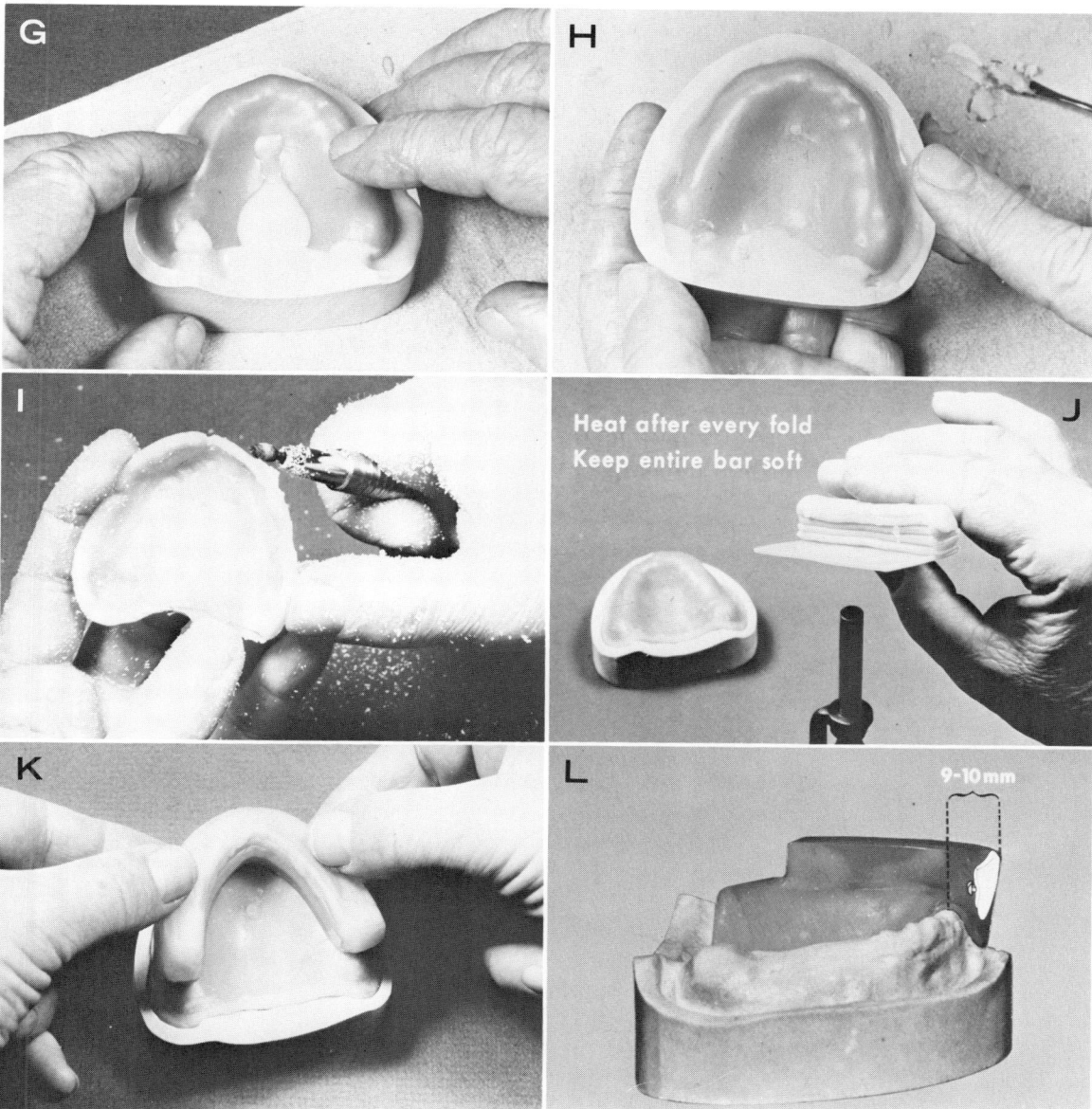

Figure 30-14 continued | G. Pressing wax matrix to make acrylic approximately 1 mm thick. H. Adapting acrylic to peripheries. I. Trimming excess resin with acrylic burs. J. Heating baseplate wax for the occlusion rims. K. Preliminary placement of wax bar. L. Facial inclination of occlusion rim.

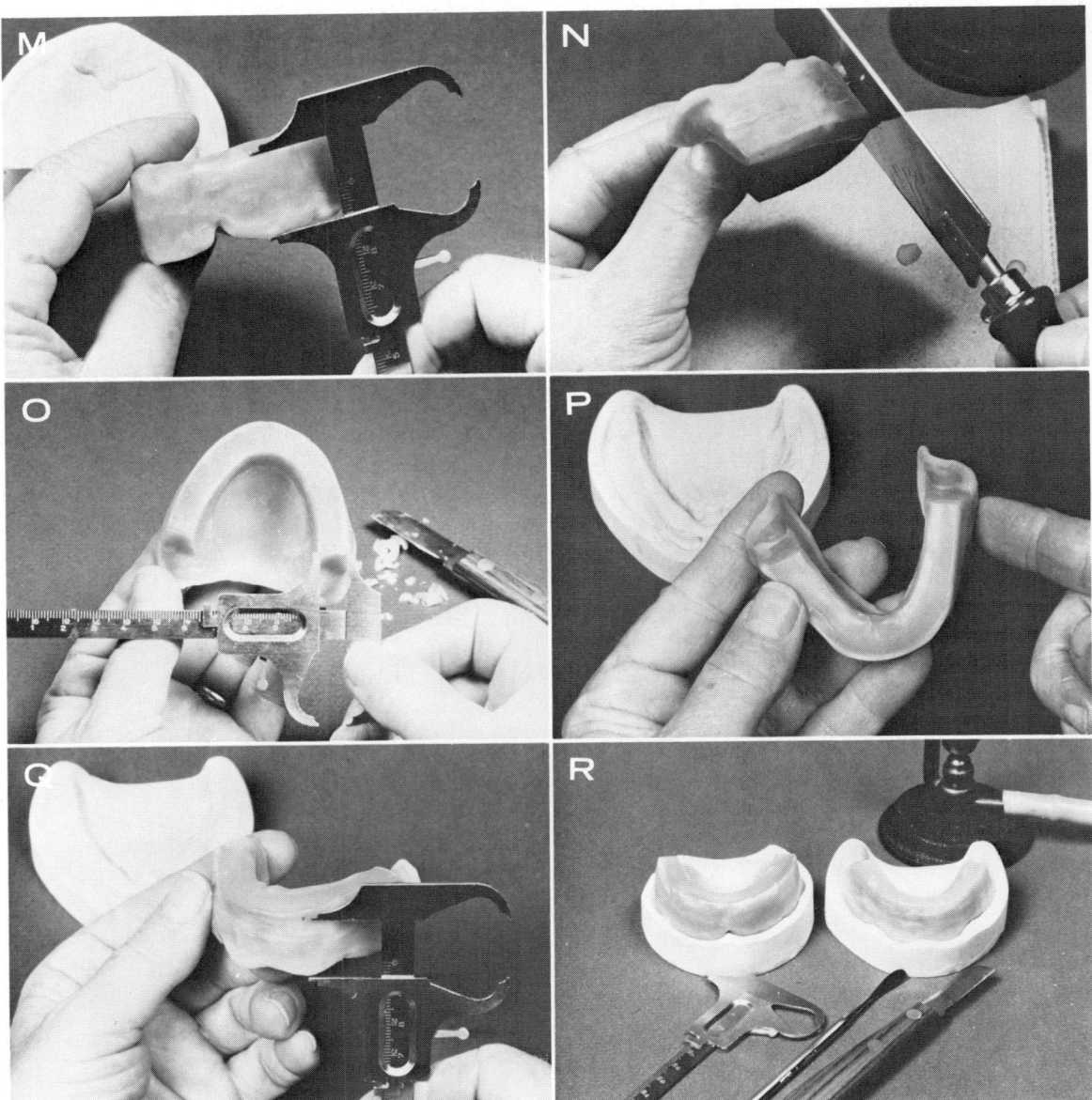

Figure 30-14 continued | M. Measuring the length of the anterior rim. N. Use of the wax melting plate to contour rims. O. This 10-mm occlusion rim does not cover tuberosities. P. Mandibular rim does not cover retromolar pads. Q. Mandibular anterior rim height is approximately 18 mm. R. Completed occlusion rims.

Fabrication of Record Bases (Occlusion Rims)

Wax record bases (also called occlusion or bite rims) are fabricated on the master casts which have been made from the final impressions. These bases are used to record and establish the correct position of the mandible to the maxilla. Later teeth will be arranged on the bases for "try-in" at a later appointment. Record bases are usually constructed by a commercial laboratory, but the dental assistant may be called upon to make them (Fig. 30-14).

The master casts have areas called undercuts which must be "blocked out" with baseplate wax before the record base is made. These areas are on the facial of the maxillary tuberosities, the papilla of the anterior ridge, and the rugae areas of the maxillary cast. The retromylohyoid and ridge crest areas of the mandibular cast are usually undercut.

The casts are soaked in water for a few minutes and a layer of baseplate wax is softened over the Bunsen burner and adapted to within 2 to 3 mm of the borders of the cast. Tinfoil substitute is painted over the exposed portions of the stone cast to prevent the acrylic stabilizing material from sticking to the cast.

A small hole is placed in the maxillary wax matrix, and a quick-cure acrylic is mixed according to the manufacturer's instructions and poured into the border areas of the cast and into the inverted wax matrix. The matrix is pressed evenly to make the acrylic approximately 1 mm thick. The acrylic excess is pressed into the border reflection areas, and the excess is trimmed by finger pressure over the sharp edge of the land. Do not allow any excess to be reflected onto the ridge slopes of the wax matrix as it will interfere later when teeth are set in the occlusion rim.

The excess resin is trimmed with suitable acrylic burs and stones so that the borders are smooth and rounded.

Wax occlusion rims are then added to the bases by heating a sheet of baseplate wax which is folded into a bar about 10 mm wide. Fold the heated wax back and forth, accordian style. Keep it heated with every fold so that it can be folded into a soft bar.

Place the softened bar on the record base and position it over the ridges with the anterior part approximately 10 mm facial to the anterior papilla.

The occlusal surface of the rim should not cover the tuberosities. Build up any concave facial areas by dripping wax or adding extra wax strips. Use wax spatulas for this procedure. The wax melting plate can provide smooth occlusal and facial surfaces. The occlusal surface will be approximately 22 mm from deepest part of the anterior border and level with the base of the cast. It should be approximately 10 mm wide.

The mandibular occlusion rim is constructed in a similar fashion being sure not to cover the retromolar pad areas with the rim. The occlusal surface should be adjusted to a height of approximately 18 mm from the deepest anterior border, and should be level with the highest point of the retromolar pad area. The width of the rim should be approximately 10 mm. Figure 30-15 shows the approximate facial and lingual contours of the maxillary and mandibular occlusion rims.

Some dentists use single-thickness shellac baseplate instead of acrylic for the record base. This is adapted to the master cast by the same method employed in adapting the double-thickness shellac for making a final impression tray.

Intermaxillary Relationship Appointment

The next step in complete denture construction is the establishment of the correct jaw relationships. This is an extremely important step, because there is no exact scientific method to record this position, and it depends a great deal on the patient's cooperation.

The dental assistant should have available for

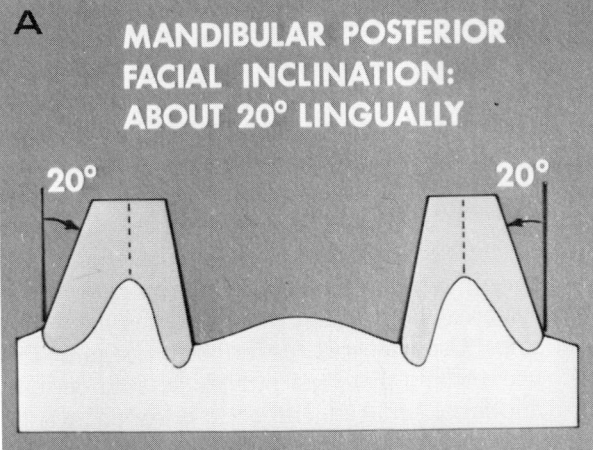
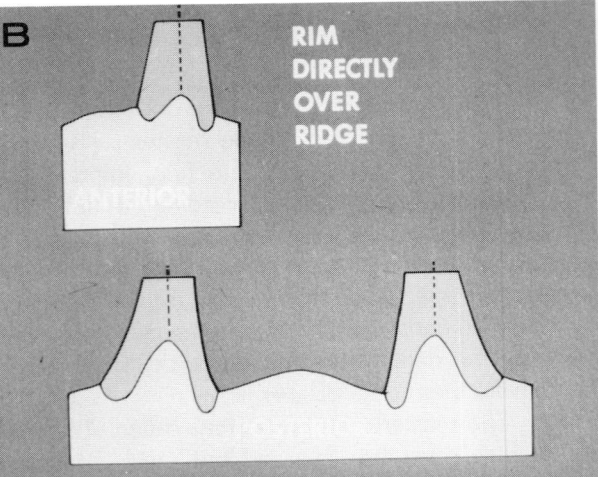
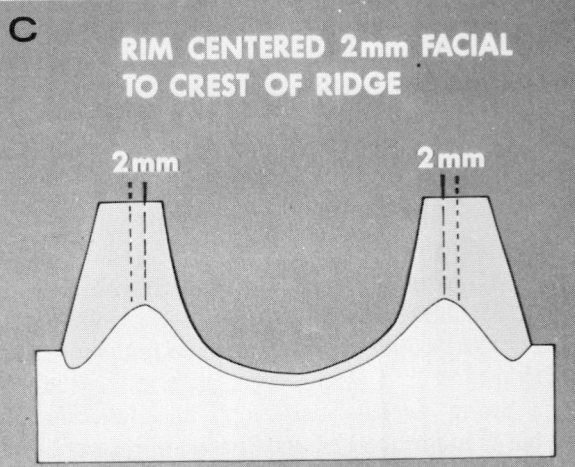
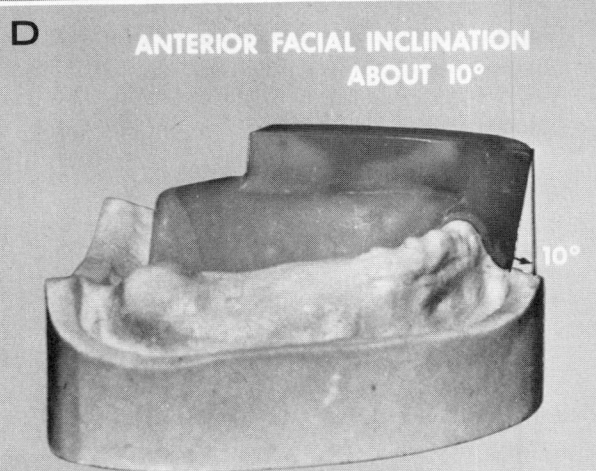
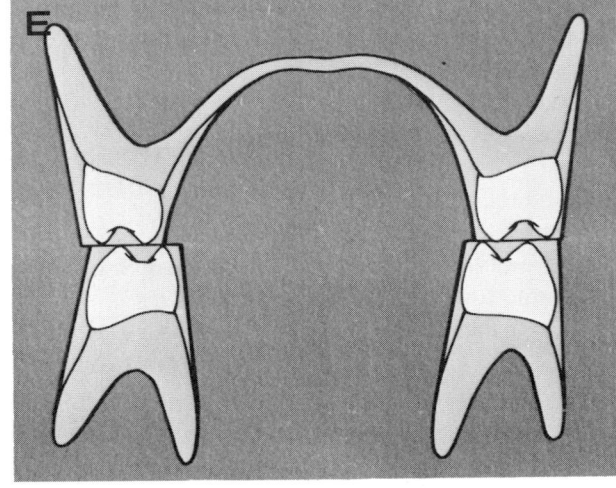

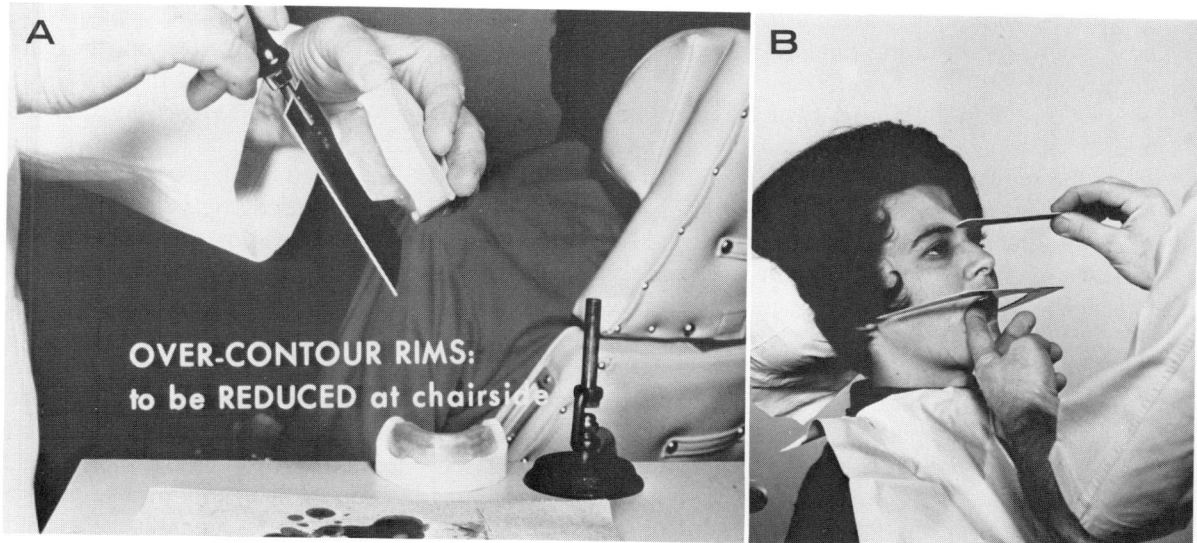

Figure 30-16 | Intermaxillary relations. A. Chairside contouring of occlusion rims. B. Use of the Fox plane guide. (*From Dental Laboratory Technology, Prosthodontic Techniques, University of North Carolina at Chapel Hill, 1968.*)

use a Bunsen burner, a wax melting plate (a flat metal plate with a handle which can be heated and used in removing wax on the occlusion rims) (Fig. 30-16A), wax spatulas of choice, a Fox plane guide (Fig. 30-16B), and some type of sharp knife. A facebow may be used at the completion of the appointment. An articulator should be available. The large wax spatula is heated by the dentist to soften the lower wax rim prior to having the patient close into the keyed upper rim at the proper position (Fig. 30-17). This is the tactile or interocclusal "check-bite" method of jaw registration.

This recording returns the mandible to the approximate position it had relative to the maxilla before all the teeth were lost. This anterior-posterior position is called *centric relation*.

Figure 30-17 | Softening the bite wax with a pooling spatula.

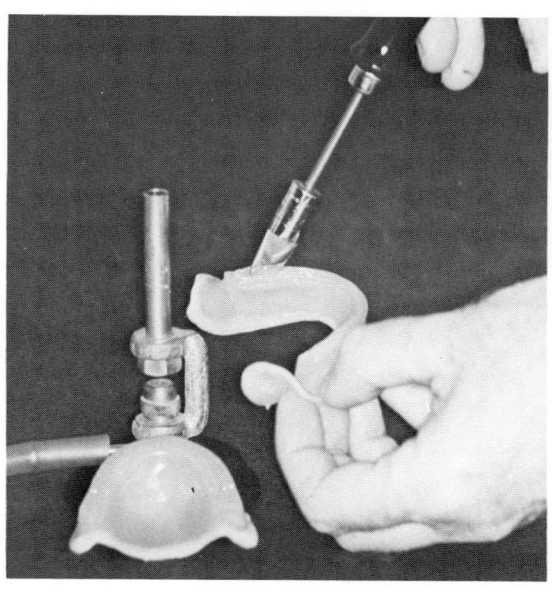

Figure 30-15 | A to E. Facial and lingual contours of maxillary and mandibular occlusion rims.

The proper vertical relation is called *occlusal vertical*. At this position the denture teeth will be fabricated.

After obtaining the proper vertical dimension and initial centric relationship, the dentist may make the transfer with a facebow. The facebow is an appliance that records the relation of the maxilla to the temporomandibular joint condyle axis. The dental assistant may assist in holding the facebow over the patient's condyles while the dentist tightens the bite fork (Fig. 30-18), or the procedure may be reversed.

Mounting the master casts to the articulator is most always accomplished by the commercial laboratory. The dental assistant may, however, be called upon to accomplish this procedure. The facebow with the maxillary cast which has been previously "keyed" with grooves cut in the base is centered on the articulator and mounted to the upper mounting ring with plaster (Fig. 30-19A). The articulator is inverted, and the mandibular cast with occlusion rim is mounted (Fig. 30-19B). No matter what type of articulator is used, be sure it is locked so that it can move only in the open and closed positions.

If a facebow is not used, this procedure is accomplished by placing the master casts into the record bases, which are then secured to the casts with sticky wax. The record bases are then related in the same keyed position recorded by the dentist, and sticky wax is applied to hold the wax rims together. Modeling clay is placed over the lower mounting ring of the articulator to support the casts (Fig. 30-20). The casts are arbitrarily positioned in the middle of the articulator. The maxillary cast is fixed to the articulator with plaster, the articulator is inverted, and the lower cast is secured with plaster.

Figure 30-18 | Dental assistant holding facebow.

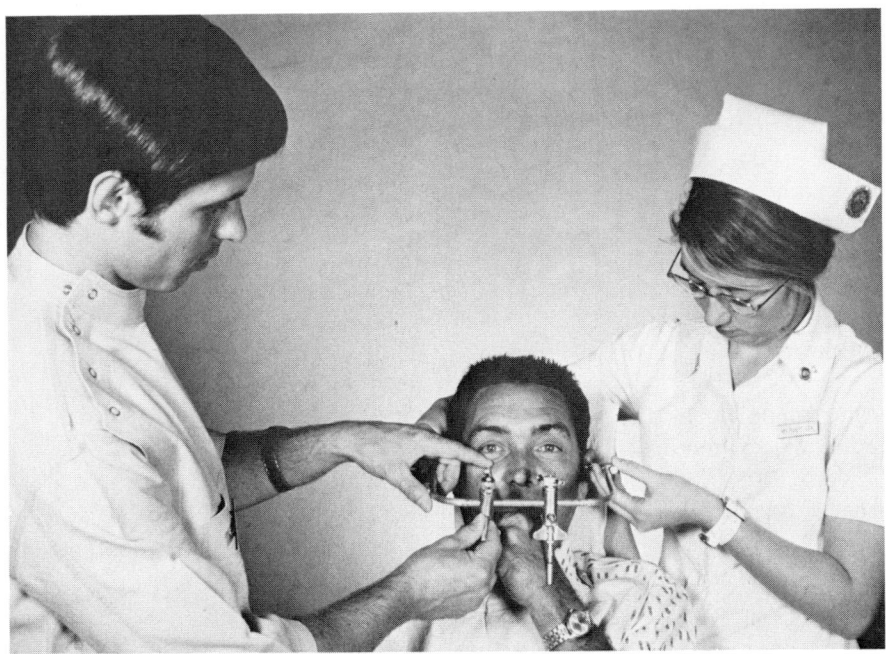

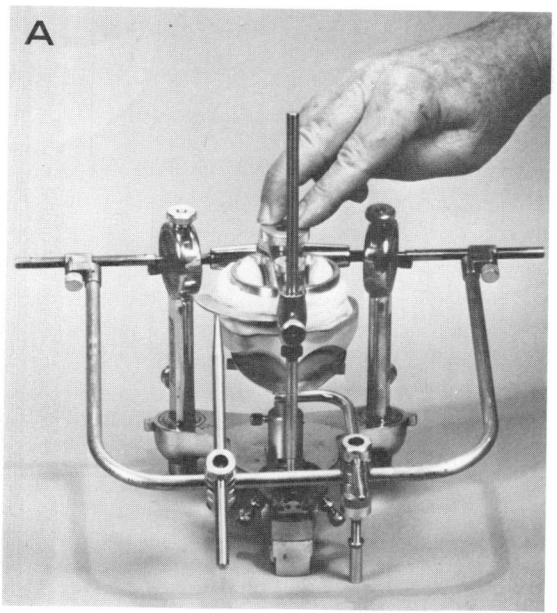

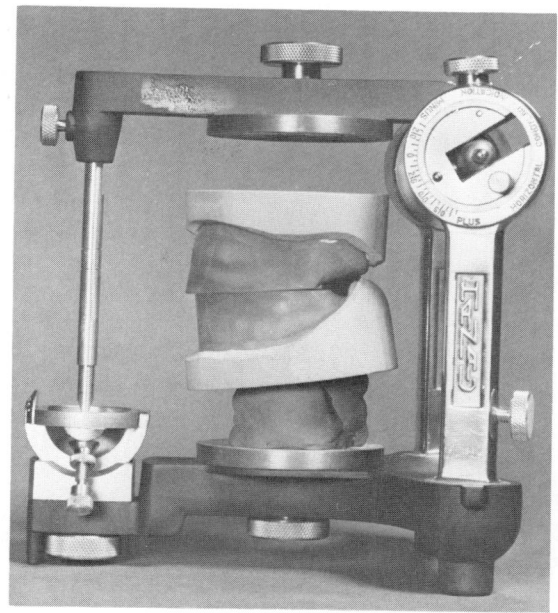

Figure 30-20 | Arbitrary placement of occlusion rims before mounting casts with plaster.

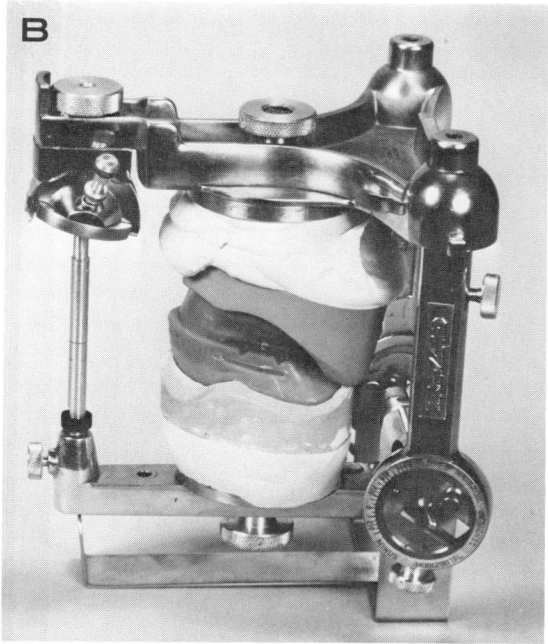

Figure 30-19 | Intermaxillary relations. A. Mounting the maxillary cast to the articulator. B. Mounting the lower cast. (*From Dental Laboratory Technology, Prosthodontic Techniques, University of North Carolina at Chapel Hill, 1968.*)

Gothic Arch Tracing

Some dentists record the centric relation position by using the graphic instead of the tactile or check-bite method. This makes use of central bearing devices which usually are arranged on the occlusion rims after a tactile record has been made. These appliances graphically record the movements of the jaw (called a gothic arch tracing). This indicates the proper relationship of the jaws and permits the accurate setting up of the artificial teeth.

There are two types of central bearing devices, intraoral and extraoral (Fig. 30-21). These appliances usually are mounted by the dentist or laboratory technician, or the dental assistant may accomplish this procedure. These devices and a plaster gun should be present at the chair. Quick-set plaster is used to lock the devices in the centric relation position (Fig. 30-22).

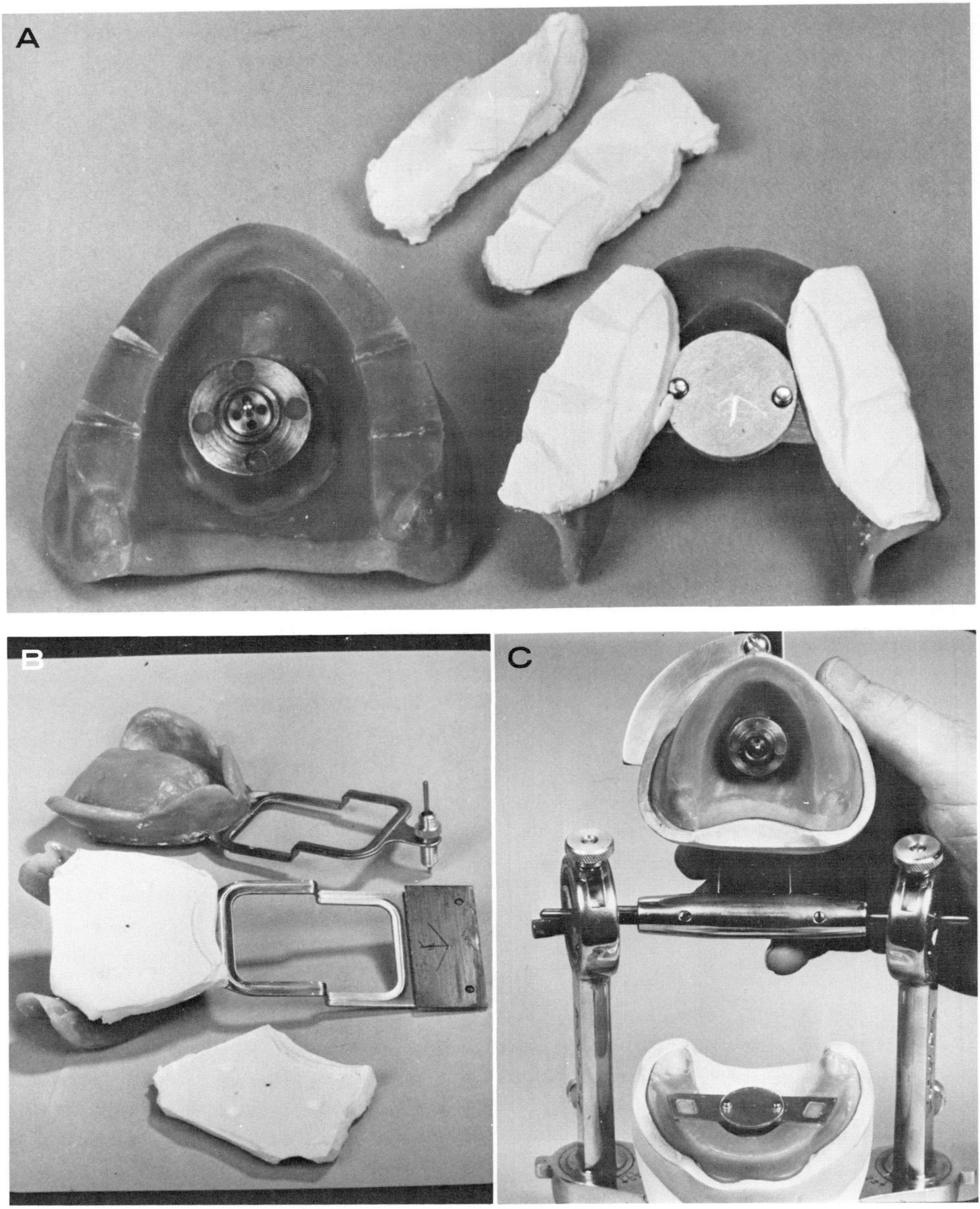

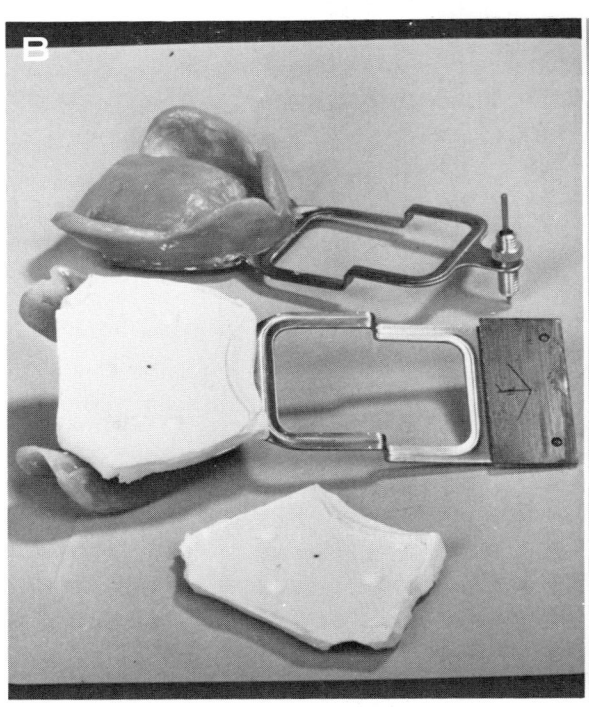
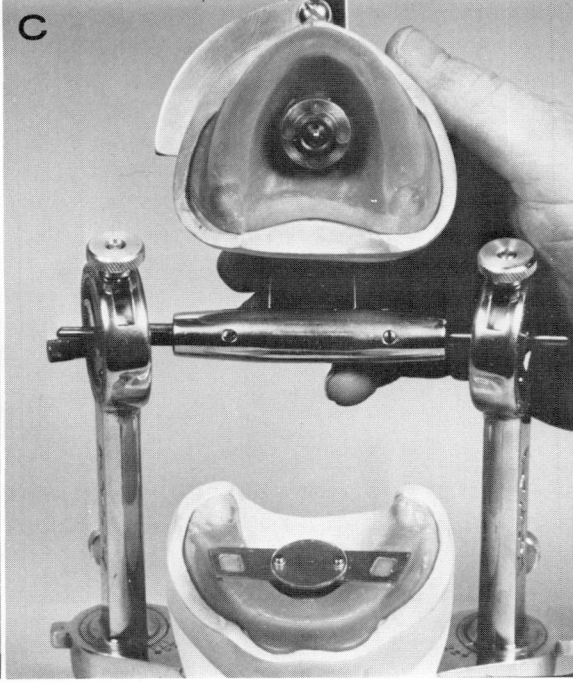

668 | The Dental Assistant | Chapter Thirty

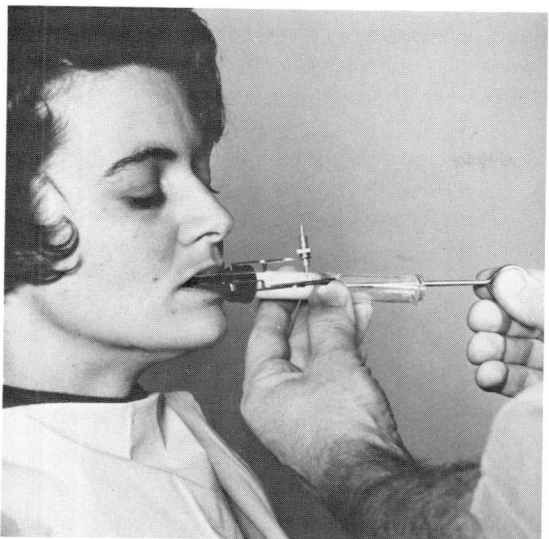

Figure 30-22 | Using plaster gun to lock tracing devices in centric relation. (*From Dental Laboratory Technology, Prosthodontic Techniques, University of North Carolina at Chapel Hill, 1968.*)

Tooth Selection

The tooth and shade selection is made at this appointment if it was not done previously. Therefore, shade guides should be available to permit the dentist to select the proper shade of tooth to be used in the artificial denture (Fig. 30-23). Frequently, the dental assistant helps in the selection of the shade, since his or her color perception may be as good as or better than that of the dentist. The selection of the mold or shape of the tooth also is made at this time. This latter selection is done by measuring the distance between the canine teeth, or where the canine teeth should be, and by making use of the mold guides that are supplied by the various manufacturers

Figure 30-21 | Gothic arch devices. A. Intraoral tracer. B. Extraoral tracer. C. Mounted intraoral tracer on articulator. (*From Dental Laboratory Technology, Prosthodontic Techniques, University of North Carolina at Chapel Hill, 1968.*)

of artificial teeth (Fig. 30-24). Previous casts of the patient's teeth are the most valuable aids in tooth selection as are old smiling photographs or snapshots. Previous periapical x-rays are also used for mold selection.

Denture teeth are made either of porcelain or plastic and are manufactured by companies throughout the United States and the world. The anterior teeth are made in many molds and sizes and in from eight to nine different shades to better harmonize with the patient's coloring. The posterior teeth vary according to cusp height (see Chap. 4 concerning natural teeth) and are commonly listed as having 0-degree cusps or monoplane occlusal surfaces, or as polyplane teeth, which include 20-, 30-, and 33-degree cusp teeth. They have the same harmonizing shade as do the anterior teeth and are manufactured in several sizes to fit the posterior arches (Fig. 30-25).

Ordering Artificial Teeth

Anterior teeth (upper and lower) by common agreement include centrals, laterals, and cuspids, six teeth in all. Hence, an order for the anterior teeth for one arch is written (1×6). An order for two sets of anterior teeth for the same arch is written (2×6). An order for one set of anterior teeth for the upper arch and one for the lower arch is written ($1 \times 6U$) and ($1 \times 6L$).

Posterior teeth (upper and lower) include the first and second bicuspids and the first and second molars, eight teeth in all. Hence, the set of eight posteriors for one arch is written (1×8); two sets for the same arch is written (2×8); and one set for both arches is written (1×16), if the mold is the same. If not, it is written ($1 \times 8U$) and ($1 \times 8L$).

An order for a complete set for one denture is not written (1×14). Rather, it is written (1×6) and (1×8). In every case the mold and shade must accompany the order.

This is the system for the numbers of teeth to be ordered; in addition to this must be listed the

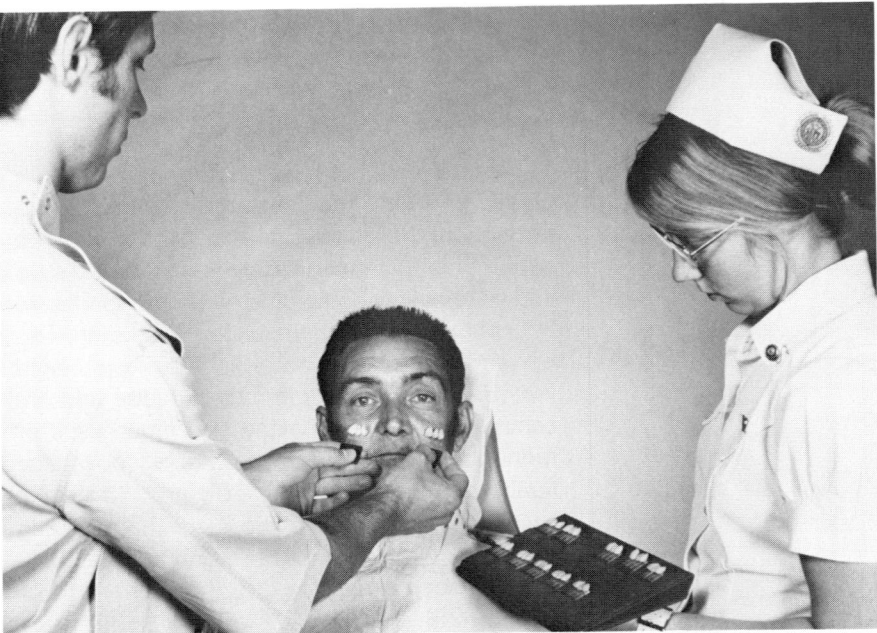

Figure 30-23 | Using guide to select tooth shade.

mold number (every manufacturer has a different mold numbering system), the shade, the manufacturer's name, and the type (porcelain or plastic and cusp height from 0, 20, 30, or 33 degrees).

The numerical value listed for posterior teeth is in most classifications the horizontal distance in millimeters from the mesial of the first bicuspid to the distal of the second molar. The letter value listed for posterior teeth indicates the vertical distance (occlusogingival) of the teeth and is usually S = Short, M = Medium, and L = Long.

Some tooth manufacturers furnish commercial laboratories with printed tooth-order information. The dentist or assistant have only to check the necessary items to complete the order. With this type of order the 1×6, 1×8 numbers need not be used (Fig. 30-26).

Once the anterior and posterior teeth have been selected, the assistant may fill out the tooth order or authorization which will then be signed by the dentist. The dentist's signature is necessary to ensure the accuracy of the order and to comply with the state law which requires this procedure.

If the assistant will become familiar with the mold charts in the dentist's office, it will be possible to order the teeth with ease.

Denture Try-in

At the next appointment the dentures are tried in the patient's mouth. These dentures for the try-in have shellac or stabilized acrylic bases with teeth set in wax. The teeth have been set in the previous wax rims by skilled laboratory technicians, and the dentist is allowed to change the

Figure 30-24 | Tooth selection. A. Using facial proportion guide to select size and mold of anterior teeth. B. Anterior tooth guide using types of manufactured teeth.

A
B
TRUBYTE Bioblend VACUUM FIRED PORCELAIN BLENDED PLASTIC
SQUARE
SQUARE TAPERING
TAPERING
11D 11G 11H 12E 12G 13E
SQUARE OVOID
31F 32B 32E 32G
21C 21D 21E 21H 22C 22E 22H 22G 24F 25G 21X 21G
42C 42F 42H 42D 42G 43D 43F 44E 45F 45H
TRUBYTE Bioblend VACUUM FIRED PORCELAIN BLENDED PLASTIC
TAPERING OVOID
OVOID
SQUARE TAPERING OVOID
52C 54F 55D 55F
62D 62G 65G
75E A84
LOWERS
C D E F H K M
O P R S U W Z
NOTE
ALL MOULDS SHOWN IN THIS MOULD GUIDE ARE ALSO AVAILABLE IN TRUBYTE BIOBLEND MULTI-BLENDED PLASTIC ANTERIORS

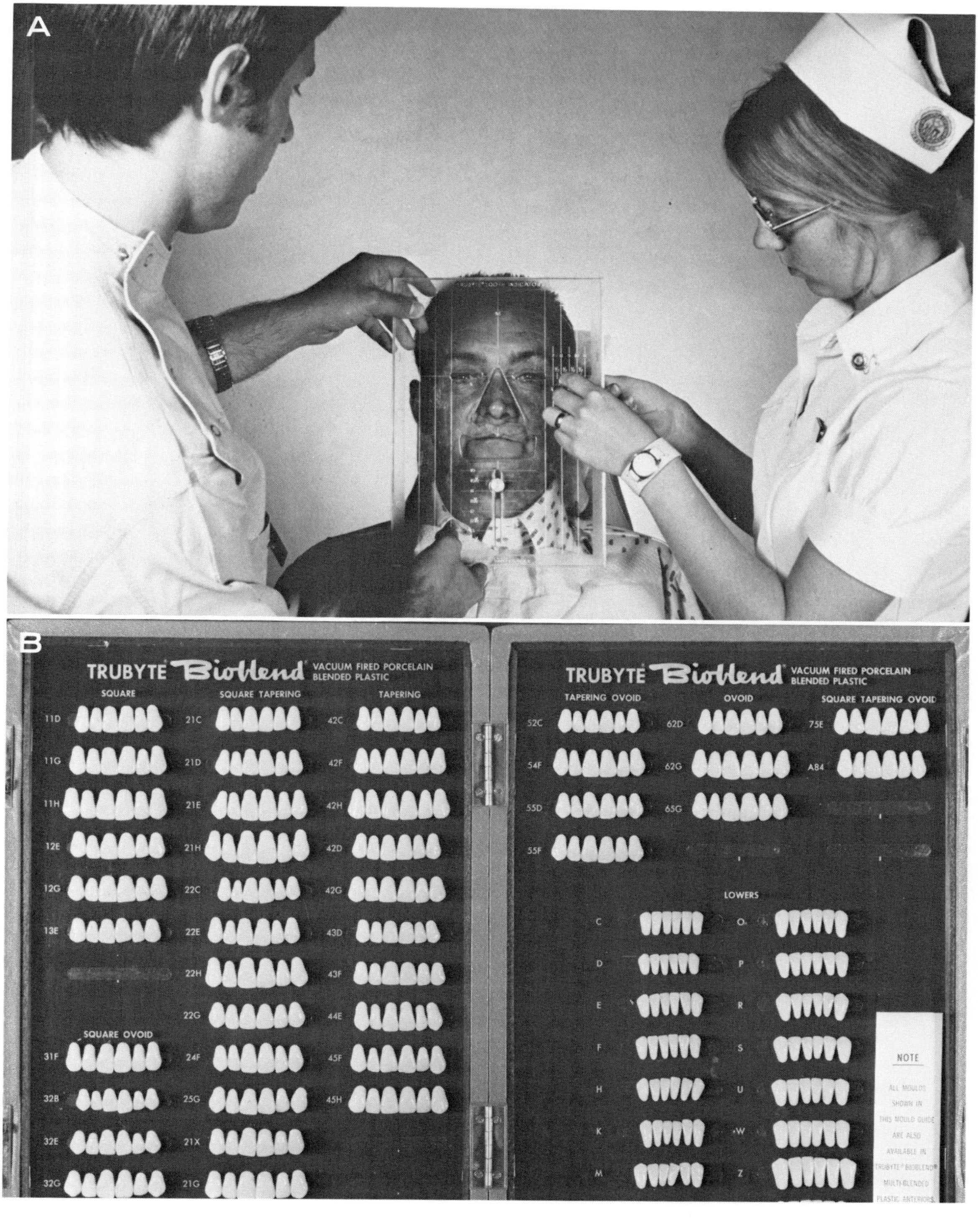

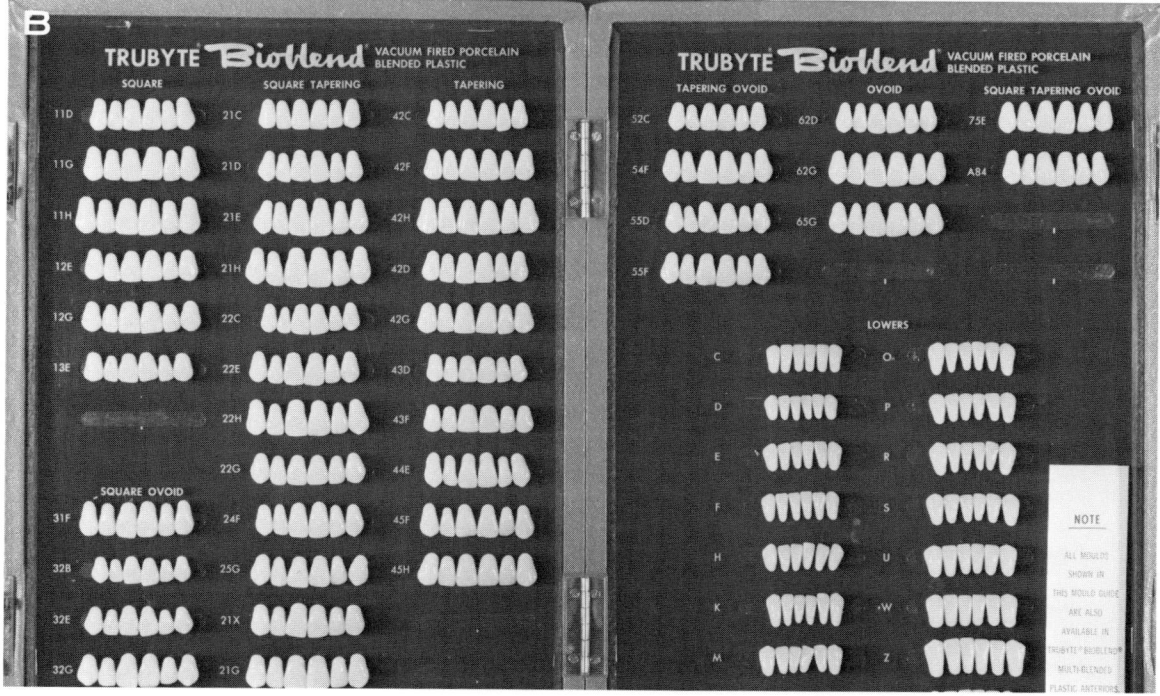

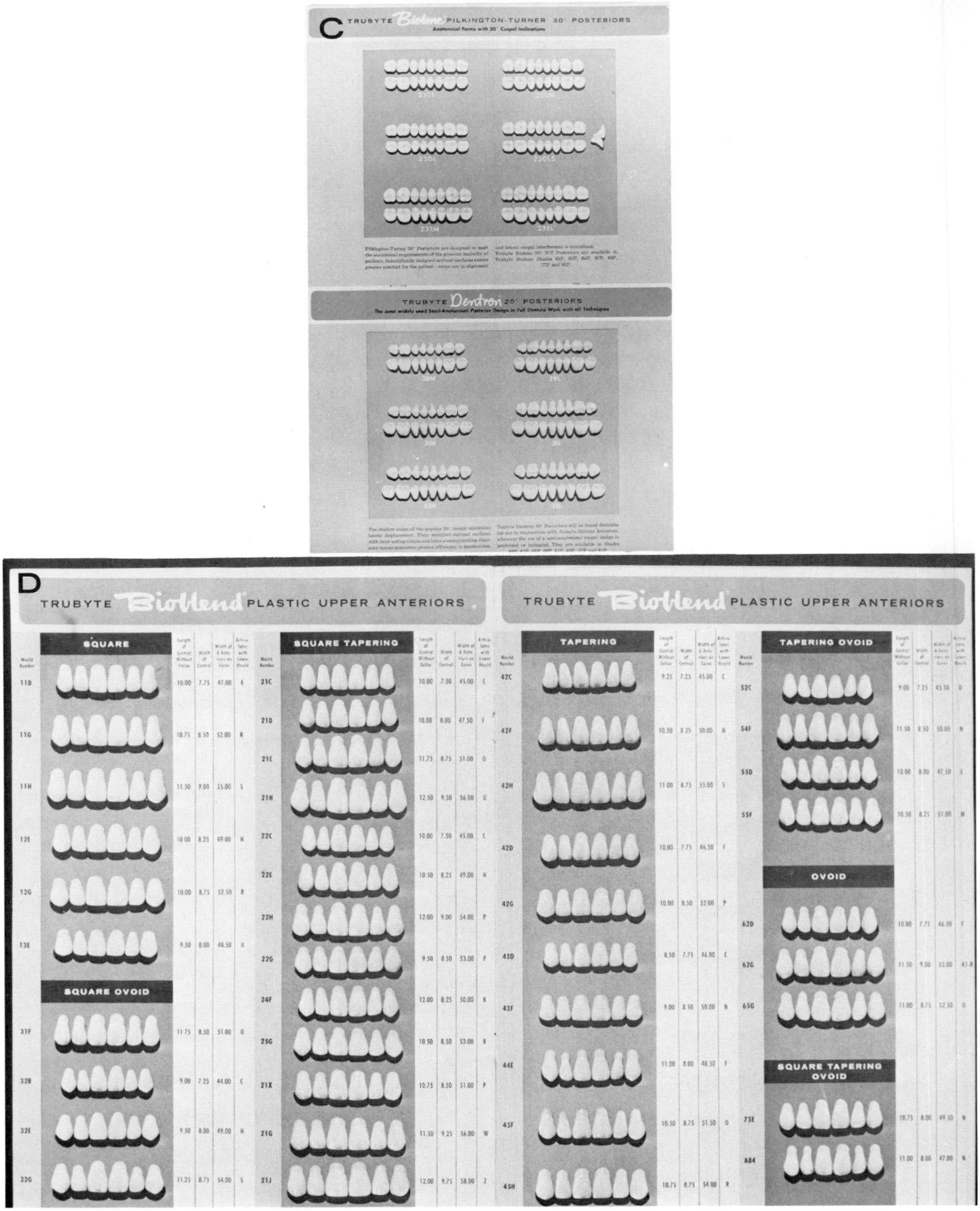

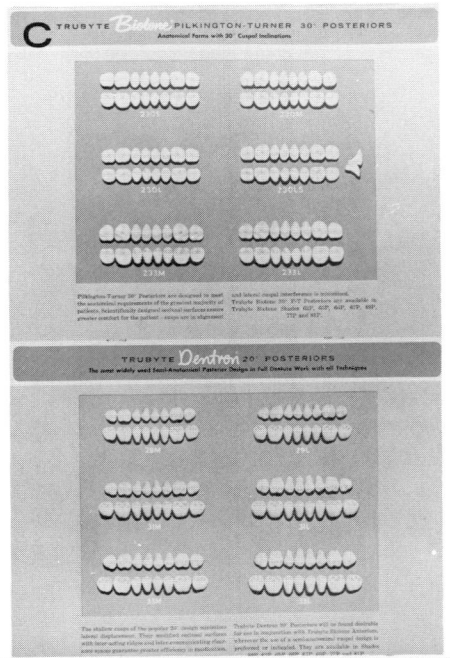

Figure 30-24 continued | C. Pictoral posterior tooth guide. D. Pictorial anterior tooth guide.

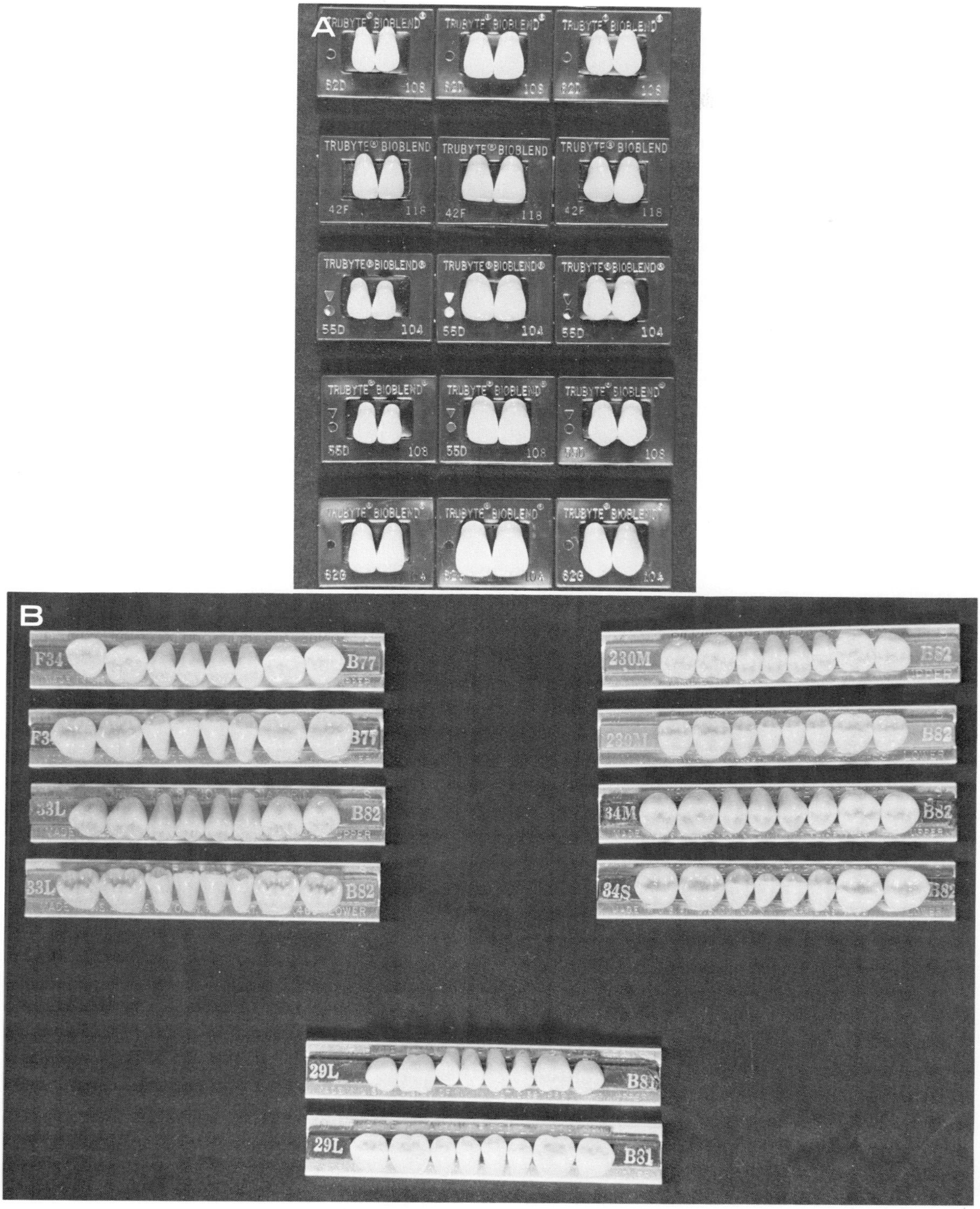

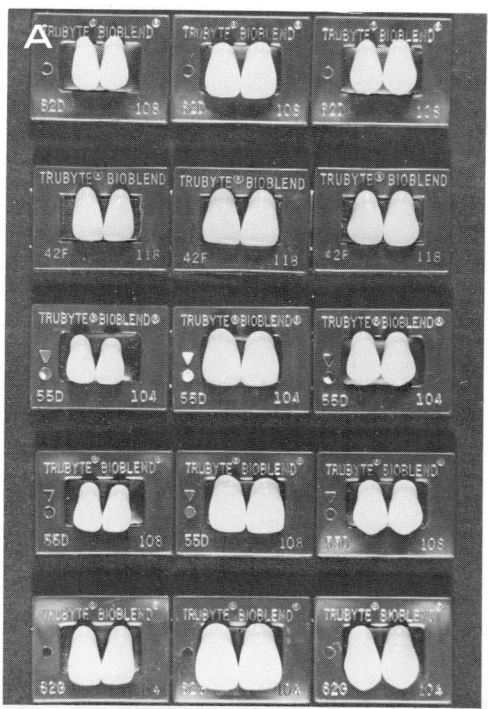

Figure 30-25 | Denture teeth. A. Maxillary anteriors. B. Maxillary and mandibular posteriors.

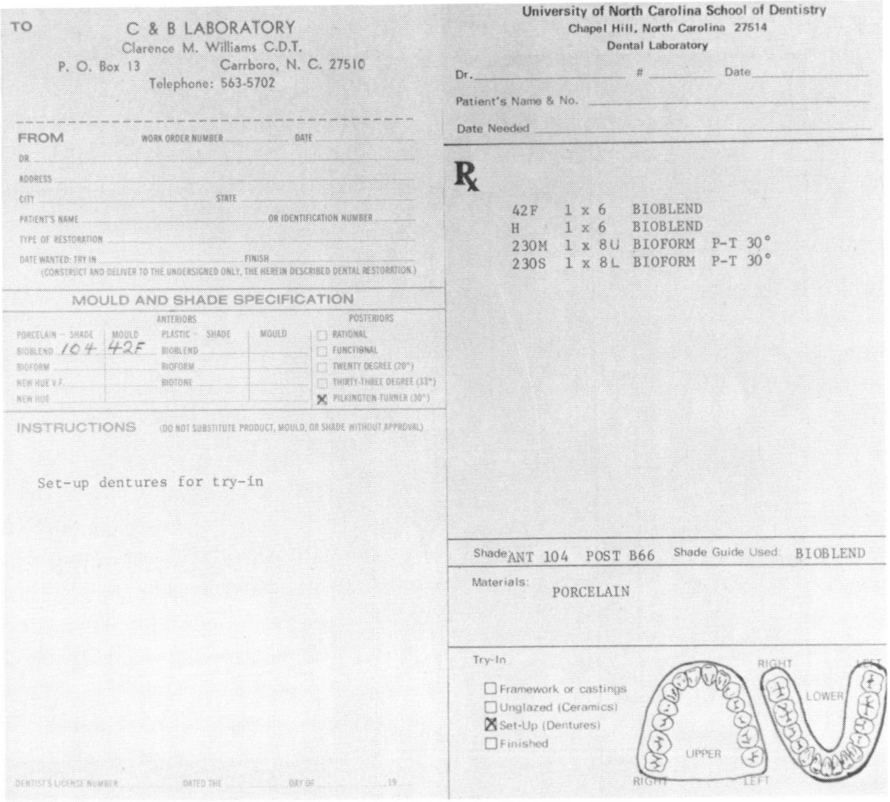

TO C & B LABORATORY
Clarence M. Williams C.D.T.
P. O. Box 13 Carrboro, N. C. 27510
Telephone: 563-5702

FROM WORK ORDER NUMBER ______ DATE ______
DR ______
ADDRESS ______
CITY ______ STATE ______
PATIENT'S NAME ______ OR IDENTIFICATION NUMBER ______
TYPE OF RESTORATION ______
DATE WANTED: TRY IN ______ FINISH ______
(CONSTRUCT AND DELIVER TO THE UNDERSIGNED ONLY, THE HEREIN DESCRIBED DENTAL RESTORATION.)

MOULD AND SHADE SPECIFICATION

ANTERIORS				POSTERIORS
PORCELAIN – SHADE	MOULD	PLASTIC – SHADE	MOULD	☐ RATIONAL
BIOBLEND 104	42F	BIOBLEND		☐ FUNCTIONAL
BIOFORM		BIOFORM		☐ TWENTY DEGREE (20°)
NEW HUE V.F.		BIOTONE		☐ THIRTY-THREE DEGREE (33°)
NEW HUE				☒ PILKINGTON-TURNER (30°)

INSTRUCTIONS (DO NOT SUBSTITUTE PRODUCT, MOULD, OR SHADE WITHOUT APPROVAL)

Set-up dentures for try-in

DENTIST'S LICENSE NUMBER ______ DATED THE ______ DAY OF ______ 19__

University of North Carolina School of Dentistry
Chapel Hill, North Carolina 27514
Dental Laboratory

Dr. ______ # ______ Date ______
Patient's Name & No. ______
Date Needed ______

℞

42F 1 x 6 BIOBLEND
H 1 x 6 BIOBLEND
230M 1 x 8U BIOFORM P-T 30°
230S 1 x 8L BIOFORM P-T 30°

Shade ANT 104 POST B66 Shade Guide Used: BIOBLEND

Materials: PORCELAIN

Try-In
☐ Framework or castings
☐ Unglazed (Ceramics)
☒ Set-Up (Dentures)
☐ Finished

Figure 30-26 | Two types of work authorizations.

arrangement of the teeth according to the patient's needs and desires.

The dental assistant should provide the following at the chair: a Bunsen burner or an equivalent, various wax spatulas, and grinding stones and discs, so that if the shape of a tooth is to be altered, it can be done quickly and conveniently. A dental assistant also may be invaluable at this appointment in reassuring a patient that the teeth look acceptable and have a pleasing effect. It is a dentist's responsibility to determine that the denture will function correctly and that the proper centric relationship has been obtained. The dental assistant can aid the dentist by giving suggestions for improvement relating to the esthetic appearance of the denture setup.

After the wax dentures have passed this test, they are sent to the laboratory where they are processed. The dental assistant may aid in the packaging process. Following their completion in the laboratory, they are returned to the dentist for delivery to the patient.

Return of Completed Dentures from Laboratory

Denture bases are usually made of acrylic plastic material. This plastic material has various prop-

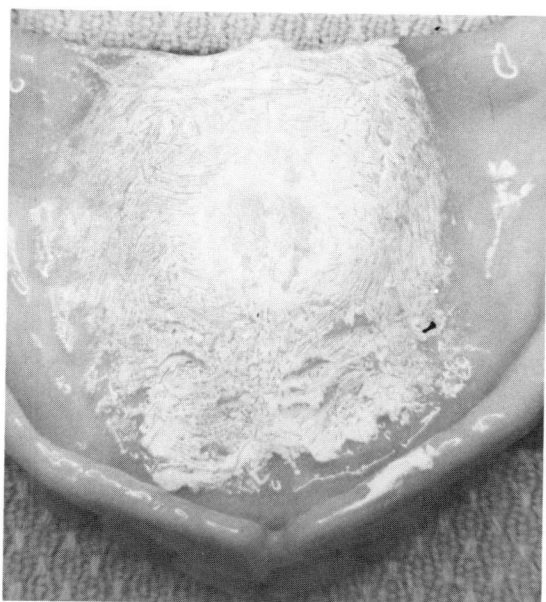

Figure 30-27 | Use of pressure-indicating paste to show need for midpalatal relief.

one when the wax dentures were tried in. It is necessary for the assistant to have available various burs and stones in the event any relief is necessary. A pressure-indicator paste should be available so that the dentist can make chairside adjustments of the base areas. This paste is applied on the tissue side of the dried dentures with a stiff brush. Excessive pressure will leave a bare spot on the denture that will show at what point pressure is being exerted (Fig. 30-27). The dentist then will relieve this area on the denture. A hand mirror also should be present for the use of the patient.

Many times the dentist will do what is called a clinical remount at the time of delivery. In anticipation of this procedure a Bunsen burner, bite wax, and suitable wax spatulas must be available. The assistant may be called upon to mount the case on the articulator using the recorded re-

Figure 30-28 | Mounting a clinical intermaxillary check-bite. (*From Dental Laboratory Technology, Prosthodontic Techniques, University of North Carolina at Chapel Hill, 1968.*)

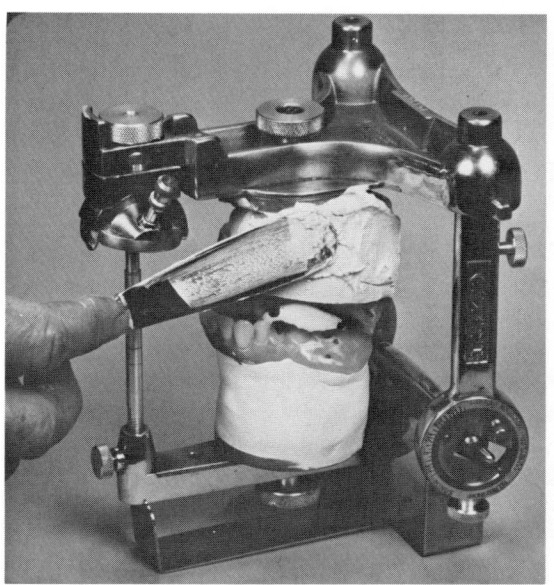

erties which demand that it be kept in water at all times. If it is not kept in water, the material will tend to shrink, distort, and not fit accurately. It is necessary that the bases be kept in the containers provided by the laboratory or in a denture cup of water at all times. A denture-base material known as styrene does not require such treatment. It is recommended, however, that any completed denture be kept in water when not worn by the patient. The patient should be instructed either by the assistant or the dentist in this procedure.

Denture Delivery to Patient

Patients usually will come to the office with a feeling of anticipation, regardless of whether or not this is their first or second experience with artificial teeth. They will be very exacting, often more so at this appointment than at the previous

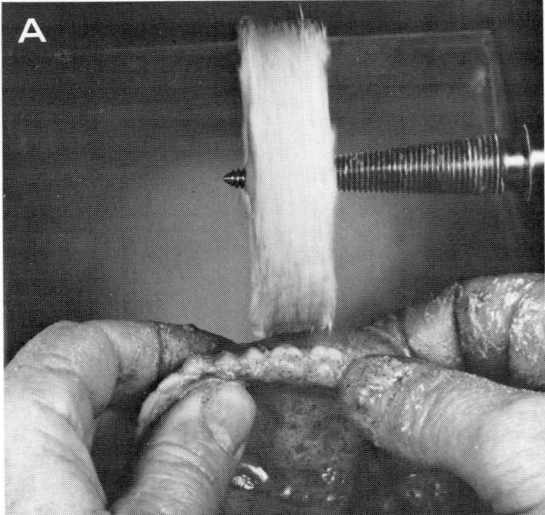

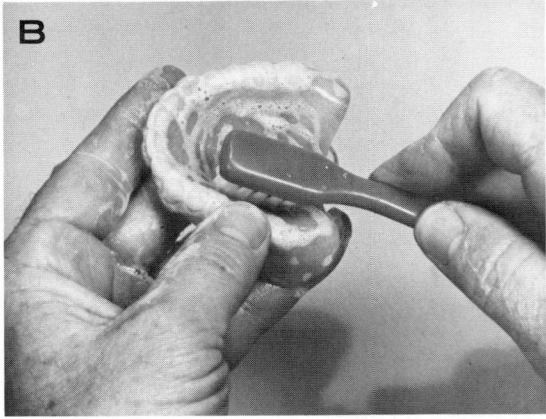

Figure 30-29 | Denture delivery. A. Repolishing adjusted denture base. B. Cleaning dentures before delivery. (*From Dental Laboratory Technology, Prosthodontic Techniques, University of North Carolina at Chapel Hill, 1968.*)

mount check-bite which has been obtained by the dentist (Fig. 30-28).

After the mounting the dentist will need articulating paper, suitable stones for the handpiece, and rubber pumice wheels in order to obtain a final refinement of the occlusion and articulation of the denture teeth. A carborundum paste is used for the final milling of the tooth surfaces.

The peripheries or edges of the dentures may be slightly altered at this time by using acrylic burs and stones. The assistant may be asked to polish these areas with a wet muslin wheel and pumice and high-shine materials. Always use the slow speed on the lathe to prevent accidentally losing your grip on the denture. The dentures are scrubbed carefully with soap and water and returned to the dentist for delivery (Fig. 30-29).

The assistant must be careful in making comments at this particular time and appointment. A few ill-chosen words may mean that the case will be a failure. Commending the dentist in the presence of the patient will help ensure the success of the dentures.

Before dismissing the patient it is a good policy to instruct the patient on the care of the dentures. A denture brush should be given to the patient along with a small booklet which describes the problems of learning to wear the dentures and the patient's home-care responsibilities. These booklets may be obtained from the American Dental Association or from other sources.

Adjustments

Usually after a denture has been inserted, a patient will develop sore spots where the denture may be overextended or pressing too hard on the tissue. These places have to be relieved by the dentist. Pressure-indicating paste and a selection of stones and burs in a convenient place will enable the dentist to reduce the spots that are causing pressure and soreness. Sometimes instead of using this paste the dentist will use an indelible pencil or disposable indelible stick to mark the sore spot. The dentures are then placed in the mouth and the indelibly marked spot will register on the tissue side of the denture. After the adjustments have been made, it will be the assistant's duty to take the denture to the laboratory where the spot which has been ground will be polished. All areas on the periphery of a denture should be polished to a high surface glaze so that there will be no chance of irritating the patient's mouth. Areas on the tissue side of the dentures may be smoothed with a soft rubber abrasive wheel but should not be polished as are the peripheries.

Complete Denture Relines

There are two types of relines for removable dentures—chairside and laboratory.

Chairside Reline

The chairside reline for treatment liners has previously been discussed, and the armamentarium and procedures are the same except for the lining material, which is a type of powder and liquid quick-set acrylic that becomes hard.

The dentist may want to relieve the dentures on the tissue side, or he or she might want to adjust the edges of the denture. For this reason acrylic burs and suitable stones should be available.

The reline material is mixed in either plastic or foil paper cups with either a metal or wooden spatula according to the manufacturer's directions. Usually the dentures are relined one at a time although some operators attempt to do both dentures at the same time. The mixed material is applied inside the dentures by the dental assistant, who must be sure that the acrylic covers all the surface which will come in contact with the denture-bearing areas of the mouth.

The dentist will seat the denture or dentures in the mouth and have the patient repeat the border-molding movements. Because of the heat generated by the self-curing acrylic, the dentures must be removed in 2 to 3 minutes to prevent an uncomfortable burn. They must then be placed in a bowl of warm water for 10 minutes to allow for further curing, or, better still, the dentures should be placed in a pressure cooker with one-half in of water in the bottom of the pan. The pressure should be 30 psi, and the time 10 minutes.

The dentures are trimmed in the usual manner in the dentist's laboratory and polished. It is well to coat the teeth and the polished-surface side of the dentures with petroleum jelly or the lubricant furnished by the manufacturer to prevent the cured material from sticking needlessly.

Laboratory Reline

This procedure is the same as the chairside reline except that the metallic-oxide paste, rubber-base, or silicone-base impression materials are used for the impression. Some dentists use one of the tissue-conditioning materials for this impression.

Once the impressions are made, the dentures are carefully packaged and sent to the laboratory for processing with the regular methyl methacrylate plastic replacing the reline material. The relined dentures are returned to the dentist and delivered in the same fashion as are new dentures.

The Immediate Denture

This type of denture is one which is constructed for insertion immediately following removal of natural teeth. The advantage of this type of complete denture is that the dentist will be able to duplicate the patient's anterior teeth in shade, mold, and position if it is desired. It is also a psychologic aid to the patient, who will never have had to be completely without teeth (even though they might be prosthetic teeth). The big disadvantage is that resorption or shrinkage will take place quite soon, necessitating an early reline.

Preliminary impressions are made in the same fashion as would be accomplished for a partial denture.

Plaster casts are poured and custom trays are constructed with quick-cure tray acrylic. A double layer of baseplate wax is adapted over the remaining anterior teeth and adjacent areas both facially and palatally (rugae area). A single layer of wax is adapted to the remaining anatomic parts of the cast, and over this is adapted the soft tray plastic material in the same manner as was described for the custom tray. The difference in this tray, besides the fact that it includes the anterior teeth, is that the wax inside the tray is removed and holes (no. 8 round burs) are drilled in the tray about one-quarter in apart for an alginate impression (Fig. 30-30). Holes are not drilled if a rubber-base material is used. The inside and edges of the rubber-base tray would be painted with adhesive, of course.

The rest of the technique for the impression is similar to that which was described previously, except for the fact that an elastic impression material is used instead of metallic-oxide paste. The dental assistant's duties therefore are the same as for the remote (no teeth remaining) denture.

Denture Repair

Denture repairs can be an extremely difficult aspect of prosthodontic service. They also can be very simple. The dentist determines the character of the service that is to be rendered by the laboratory. There is, however, one type of denture repair that frequently is required and that can be performed by the dental assistant with excellent results (Fig. 30-31). Such a repair involves replacing one or more teeth in a denture as a result of a fracture of the original teeth. The task involves four individual steps:

1. *Removal of the fractured tooth stump.* Removal of the remaining portion of the fractured tooth always is done from the lingual aspect. The object is to leave the facial undisturbed and, as a result, to maintain the esthetics originally realized. By grinding on the denture-base material around the tooth to be replaced, the stump can be removed easily.
2. *Selection of tooth shade and mold for the repair.* If the fracture was small, enough of the tooth to be replaced may remain to serve as a guide for the proper selection of its replacement. If such is not the case, the mate to the fractured tooth on the op-

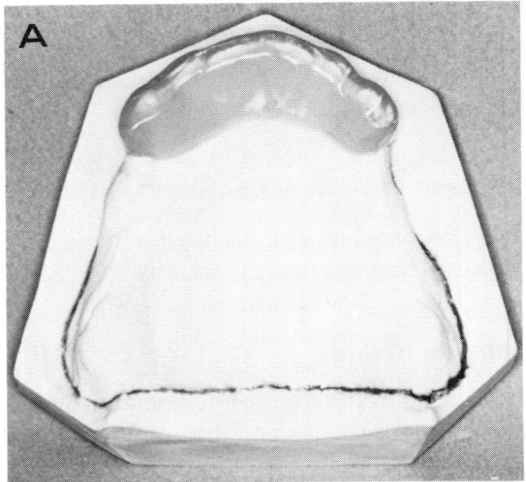

Figure 30-30 | Maxillary custom tray. A. Final layer of relief wax for immediate denture custom tray. One layer of wax is applied over relief and remaining cast to outline. B. Completed maxillary custom tray for an immediate denture impression.

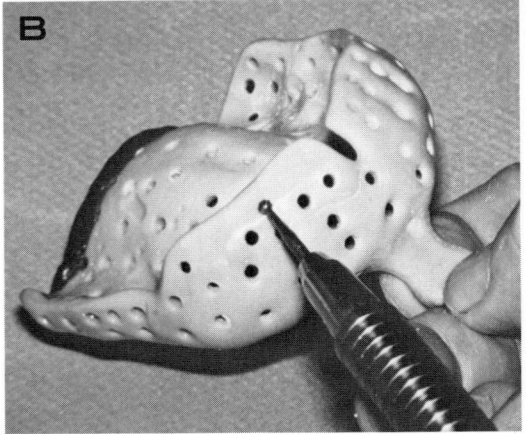

Figure 30-31 | Replacing broken denture tooth. A. Selecting tooth to be replaced. B. Prepared denture base. C. Pouring plaster matrix on positioned tooth. D. Adding quick-cure acrylic. E. Pressure pot for curing. Denture is covered with warm water. F. Replaced tooth after curing and before polishing. (*From Dental Laboratory Technology, Prosthodontic Techniques, University of North Carolina at Chapel Hill, 1968.*)

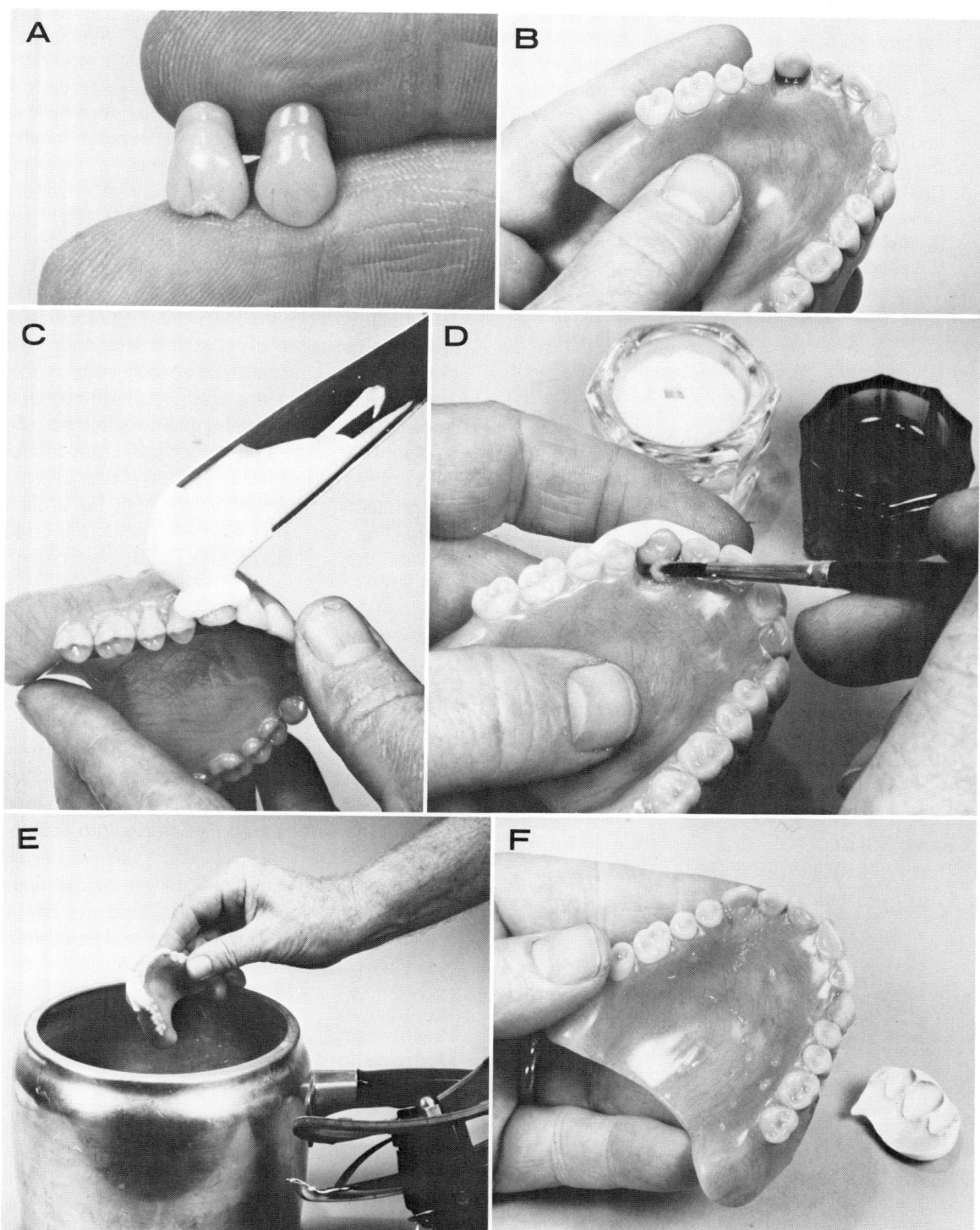

posite side of the denture is usually intact, and it is the best guide for the correct tooth selection.

If corresponding pairs are involved, by using the size of the remaining space, the shade of the remaining teeth, the shape of the patient's face, and the patient's complexion, the dentist can make the necessary tooth selection.

3. *Replacement of the tooth with a self-curing acrylic.* Once the correct tooth has been selected and ground to fit properly into the space in the denture, it is positioned and stabilized with wax. The wax is then carved, and all excess is removed.

In order to maintain this position, a plaster matrix is made by coating the labial surface in the area involved with a suitable plaster separating medium and by applying a small mass of plaster on the tooth to be replaced and on the adjacent areas. With such an index to orient the new tooth, the wax now can be removed with hot water. With a suitable brush, "bead and brush" the quick-cure acrylic in the area to be repaired after having painted the inside of the matrix with tinfoil substitute. Place the repaired denture in a pressure cooker for 10 minutes at 20 psi.

4. *Polishing the repair.* All that remains to be done on such a repair is the necessary trimming and polishing of the repaired area in order to be certain that it will cause no irritation in the patient's mouth. A satisfactory polish can be achieved in a variety of ways. Hence, it is advisable to follow the directions of your dentist. All methods essentially involve initial trimming of excess and grinding of the surface to be polished, first with a coarse abrasive, followed by an increasingly fine abrasive until the surface is smooth. If there is an old discarded denture available in the office, practice in making repairs on it will be invaluable experience.

REMOVABLE PARTIAL DENTURE PROSTHODONTICS

The first step preparatory to starting any dental operation consists of conducting a thorough examination. The assistant should comfortably seat the patient in the chair and remove and place in water any dental appliances that may be present. Glasses and other items that may hinder the dentist's work should be laid aside. Glasses are particularly hazardous and can be broken easily. The patient should be suitably draped to prevent the spilling of impression material on clothing.

Information concerning the oral cavity may be gained by two basic methods, namely, direct and indirect examination. Direct examination is fundamental; much can be learned through sight and palpation. The assistant should have on the bracket table an assortment of mouth mirrors, explorers of the dentist's choice, and tongue blades, if the latter are used. The light should be directed into the mouth and never into the patient's eyes.

Radiographic examination is an indirect method of gaining information, and the dental assistant should be prepared for such measures (see Chap. 18).

Preliminary Alginate Hydrocolloid Impressions

Generally preliminary impressions will be made following the mouth examination. These impressions usually are taken with an alginate hydrocolloidal material (Fig. 30-32). Perforated trays or trays with metal rims are necessary in order to

Figure 30-32 | Materials and equipment needed for alginate partial denture impressions.

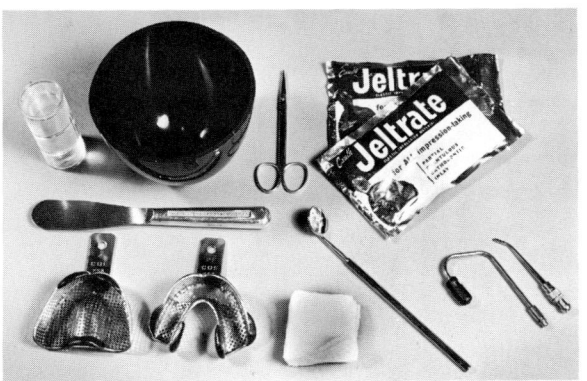

retain the material in the tray while it is being removed from the mouth. The technique and the materials used are the same as for the preliminary edentulous alginate impression.

Pouring Preliminary Casts

Pouring plaster is a simple procedure if one cardinal rule is obeyed. Always cover each area with plaster as it is reached, and push the air ahead of the plaster. Otherwise air will be trapped, and this will show as an unsightly or damaging bubble in the stone model.

If any saliva remains in the alginate impression, it must be removed by rinsing with a solution of plaster and water. The saliva will adhere to the plaster, which is then rinsed with room-temperature tap water, and the excess water is removed with compressed air. Do not completely dry out the impression.

Stone is poured by starting at one heel and letting the material flow from one tooth impression to the next in a cautious manner. Once the tooth and ridge areas are filled, the bulk of plaster may be applied rapidly to make the base of the cast. Enough material should be used to have a base of one-quarter-in thickness along the anteroposterior midline after a minimal amount of trimming.

Mandibular casts are more difficult to pour because of the open lingual area. To overcome the problem of loading this base with unwanted plaster, a block may be effectively established by filling in the lingual area with one or two wet paper hand towels or by luting a piece of baseplate wax to the lingual flange of the tray. Obviously any stone that engages the tray will have to be removed prior to separating the model from the tray, so that the time involved in preventing this condition is well spent.

Separation of the model from the impression may be simple or difficult. If it is done approximately 1 hour after pouring, the impression material still is elastic enough to slip past undercut areas. Delay finds the impression material becoming progressively firmer until it becomes extremely difficult to remove the cast, and fractured teeth may result. Further delay may also cause an etched cast surface. All the force in removing the cast must be applied in the direction of least resistance, always favoring the most friable portion of the cast, namely, the teeth.

The trimming of plaster casts is most efficiently done on a model trimmer by a sharp, clean rotary disc (Fig. 30-33). The aid for cleaning this disc is a stream of water which is directed in sufficient quantity to wash away the powdered plaster but is not of such intensity as to throw water and debris on the bench top.

All removable prosthodontic casts are trimmed in a uniform manner. Ideally the base should be one-half-in thick and parallel with the occlusal plane or ridges. The sides bordering the posterior teeth are in one plane and parallel with the facial surfaces of the posterior teeth. The latter sides (bordering the posterior teeth) should extend inward to within 3 mm of the vestibule.

Figure 30-33 | Trimming cast with a model trimmer.

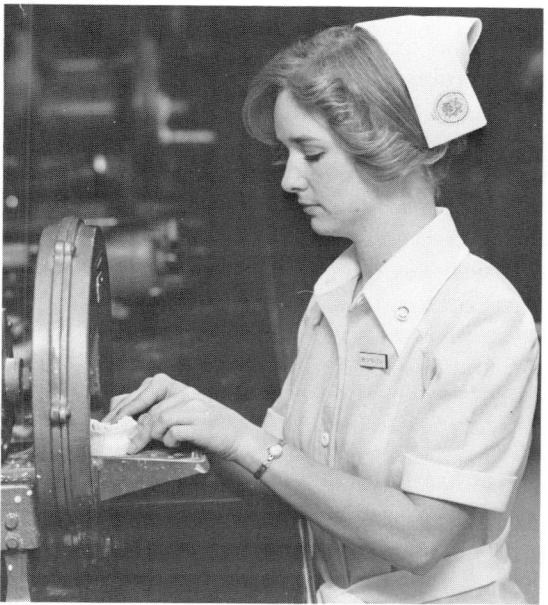

The anterior cut is rounded to parallel the curve of the anterior teeth. When sufficient teeth are present to occlude the models, they should be properly occluded and trimmed along the posterior border. The cut should stop just short of the pterygomaxillary notch. The sharp angle is then beveled off to finish the trimming. The patient's name is printed on the base of the cast with an indelible ink marker.

Mouth Preparation

By carefully studying the preliminary casts and by adding to this the knowledge gained in the initial mouth examination, the dentist is able to develop a suitable treatment plan. Many times this will involve some type of mouth preparation. Since the preparation of the mouth may be extended and varied, a plan of procedure is developed.

Sometimes bony protuberances may have to be removed surgically, crowns constructed on some of the remaining teeth, periodontic treatment accomplished, or certain extruded teeth extracted before the final impressions are made for the partial denture. This would take several additional appointments.

Construction of Trays for Final Impression

Self-curing plastic trays may be used in making a final impression if the dentist so desires. The preliminary cast is used as a backing to which the plastic material may be adapted. Two layers of baseplate wax will have to be adapted to the ridge areas in order to give the hydrocolloidal material enough bulk for strength and elasticity.

Holes are cut in the wax spacer over the occlusal or incisal surfaces of the plaster teeth which are *not* abutment teeth (the teeth which will be clasped by the partial denture). This produces stops for the tray and aids in making the final impression (Fig. 30-34).

The technique for making the tray from this point on is the same as for the tray resin immedi-

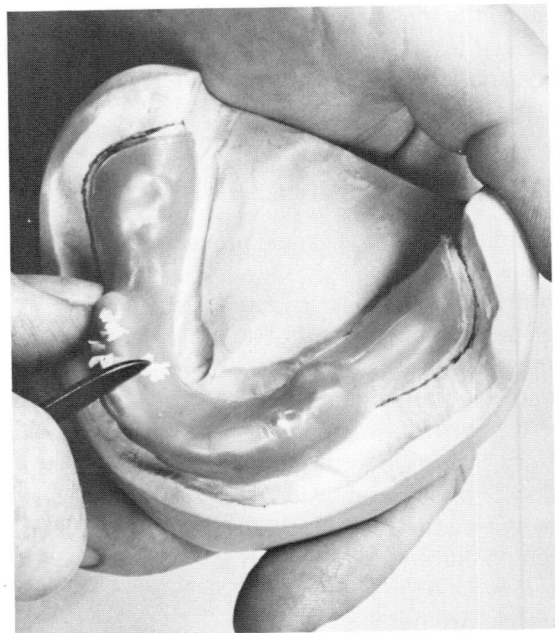

Figure 30-34 | Wax shim adaptation before custom-tray resin is applied. (*From Dental Laboratory Technology, Prosthodontic Techniques, University of North Carolina at Chapel Hill, 1968.*)

ate denture tray. Holes are placed in the tray for an alginate impression, and no holes are needed for the rubber-base impression (Fig. 30-35).

If stock trays will adequately fit the mouth, they may be used for the final alginate impression. The chair procedure would be the same, and the casts would be poured in stone.

The master stone casts and the preliminary cast with the design indicated on the cast are then sent to the laboratory along with a detailed prescription or work order. Both the dentist and the laboratory use surveyors (Fig. 30-36) to determine the denture design.

Metal Framework Insertion

When the cast metal framework is returned from the laboratory, the dentist will insert it in the patient's mouth to determine the accuracy of the fit and will make any necessary adjustments to en-

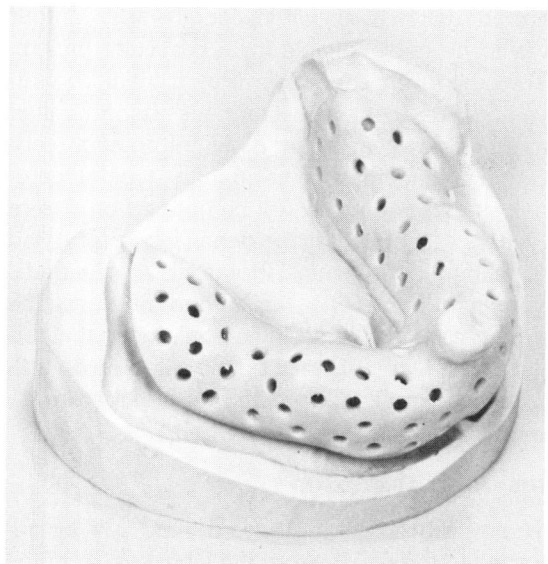

Figure 30-35 | Completed mandibular partial denture custom tray. (*From Dental Laboratory Technology, Prosthodontic Techniques, University of North Carolina at Chapel Hill, 1968.*)

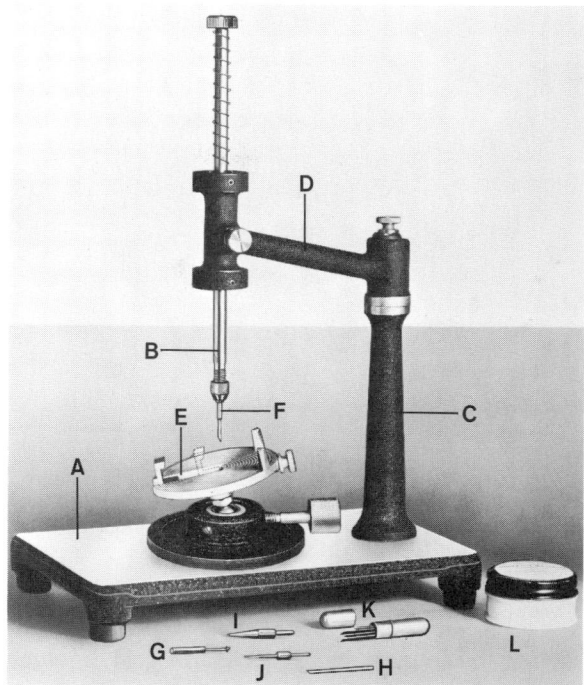

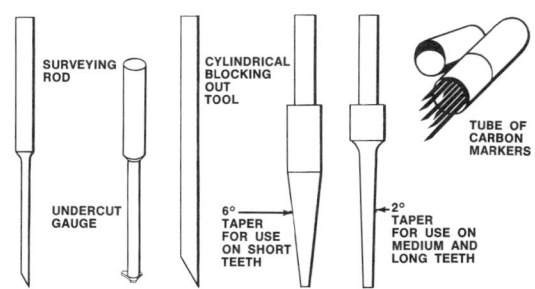

Figure 30-36 | Surveying and designing tools supplied with Wills' surveyor and designer. *Top,* Wills' surveyor and designer. A. Horizontal-plane table. B. Surveying spindle with chuck to hold tools. C. Upright post. D. Surveying arm which swings on upright post. E. "Kwikmount" base able to hold any size model; ball-and-socket joint permitting tilting in any direction. F. Surveying rod (in chuck). G. Undercut gauge. H. Cylindrical blocking-out tool. I. Six-degree taper tool for use on short teeth. J. Two-degree taper tool for use on long teeth. K. Tube of carbon markers. L. Jar of Wills' undercut filling material. *Bottom,* an enlarged view of surveying and designing tools, showing detailed construction. (*Courtesy of J. F. Jelenko and Company, Inc.*)

sure proper occlusal contacts (Fig. 30-37). For this latter operation the assistant should have an assortment of marking materials present. Carbon marking strips and occlusal marking waxes are sometimes helpful, as is some equipment for carbonizing the inside of the casting. Relieving the high spots will require the use of small stones of various shapes and sizes. Contouring pliers may be used on occasion, but an accurate impression technique can generally limit the need for such instruments. The dental assistant may be called upon to polish ground areas at this time.

An intermaxillary relationship record is next recorded. Baseplate wax and bite wax should be available. In some cases the dentist will use quick-cure acrylic to make a base on the edentulous part of the casting over which bite wax is placed to record the intermaxillary relationship (Fig. 30-38).

At this appointment the tooth shade and mold also may be determined. Thirty minutes prior to

Chapter Thirty | Removable Prosthodontics | 683

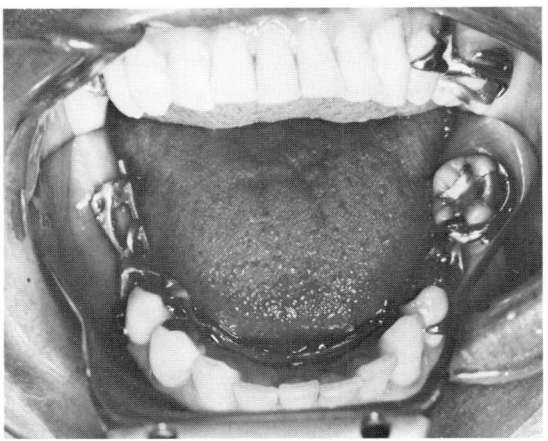

Figure 30-37 | Try-in of mandibular partial denture framework casting. (*From Dental Laboratory Technology, Prosthodontic Techniques, University of North Carolina at Chapel Hill, 1968.*)

use, the shade guide is placed in a cold disinfecting solution. Then, just before it is used, it may be removed and rinsed with cool tap water. Drying is not necessary, since the dentist will want a wet guide in order to get a more accurate shade. Mold guides are an aid in helping the dentist de-

Figure 30-38 | Bite wax attached to metal cast for intermaxillary relationship record. (*From Dental Laboratory Technology, Prosthodontic Techniques, University of North Carolina at Chapel Hill, 1968.*)

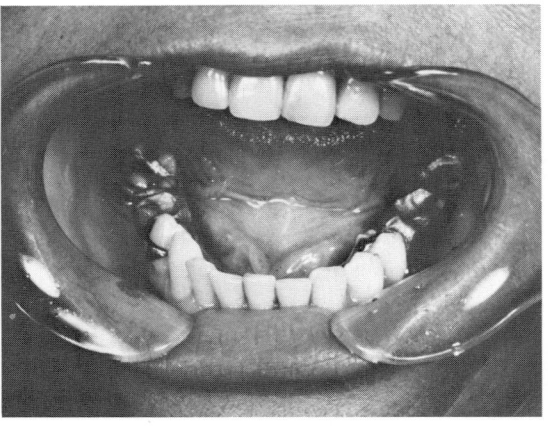

termine what tooth width, length, and contour would be most suitable for a particular patient. To assist in the tooth selection, it would be advantageous to have a complete assortment of mold guides near at hand. All information concerning the teeth, such as quantity, type of material, shade, and mold, will be entered on a form (generally supplied by the dental laboratory) and submitted to the dental laboratory with the metal framework and bite registration fitted to the master cast. The opposing cast also is sent at this time. The two casts may be mounted on an articulator before it is submitted to the laboratory.

Insertion of Wax-up

The prosthesis in the waxed state will be returned to the dentist from the laboratory for final appraisal. For the clinical try-in the only equipment necessary would be a wax spatula for the dentist and a hand mirror for the patient. Vertical dimension will be checked and frequently a slight modification in the position of the teeth may be made before sending the appliance back to the laboratory for final processing.

Equilibration

Upon the presentation of the completed partial denture to the patient, a certain amount of occlusal equilibration may be needed. The dentist can accomplish this by using one of the many occlusal marking devices and preparing the bracket table accordingly. The offending occlusal areas will be reduced with stones of convenient size and shape.

Adjustment Appointment

Usually one or two appointments are necessary to adjust the partial denture to its optimum efficiency. Pressure-indicating paste and indelible sticks are used to adjust pressure areas. Suitable stones and rubber polishing wheels should be available.

After completing adjustment grinding, the

dentist may ask the assistant to polish the appliance.

Polishing an Appliance

A laboratory procedure that may be assigned to the dental assistant is that of polishing. Acrylic polishing has been discussed in the full-denture technique; therefore, metal polishing will be presented here briefly. Since the chrome-cobalt alloys are difficult to polish, they should be completed by the commercial laboratory. Gold, however, can be made very brilliant with a minimum of effort. While gross polishing will not be required of the dental assistant, small areas of polishing after a denture is relieved may be necessary. A fine stone is used first to remove any of the gross scratches. This is followed with some medium-grit rubber wheels. These wheels, which are impregnated with an abrasive, do a very fine job of cutting. Next, a finer rubber abrasive wheel is used. If rag wheels are used with wet pumice and high-shine polishing materials, two considerations are important. (1) Rag wheels generally are used for one type of abrasive, and they must be changed when a different polishing agent is used. (2) These wheels are prone to tear the partial denture from your grasp while polishing. Therefore, a tight grip must be maintained on the appliance, and clasps should be guarded with the fingers and thumbs.

In summary, it should be emphasized that there are a host of methods by which a satisfactory partial denture can be constructed. To be of paramount value, the assistant must learn the dentist's preferences, be familiar with the sequence of steps, and act as a liaison between the office, patient, and commerical laboratory.

Appendix

Comparative Values of Apothecaries' and Metric Liquid Measures

Minims	Cubic centimeters	Flui-drachms	Cubic centimeters	Fluid-ounces	Cubic centimeters
1	0.06	1	3.70	1	29.57
2	0.12	2	7.39	2	59.15
3	0.19	3	11.09	3	88.72
4	0.25	4	14.79	4	118.29
5	0.31	5	18.48	5	147.87
6	0.37	6	22.18	6	177.44
7	0.43	7	25.88	7	207.01
8	0.49			8	236.58
9	0.55			9	266.16
10	0.62			10	295.73
11	0.68			11	325.30
12	0.74			12	354.88
13	0.80			13	384.45
14	0.86			14	414.02
15	0.92			15	443.59
16	0.99			16	473.17
17	1.05			17	502.74
18	1.11			18	532.31
19	1.17			19	561.89
20	1.23			20	591.46
25	1.54			21	621.03
30	1.85			22	650.60
35	2.16			23	680.18
40	2.46			24	709.75
45	2.77			25	739.32
50	3.08			26	768.90
55	3.39			27	798.47
				28	828.04
				29	857.61
				30	887.19
				31	916.76
				32	946.33
				48	1419.49
				56	1656.08
				64	1892.66
				72	2129.25
				80	2365.83
				96	2839.00
				112	3312.16
				128	3785.32

Tables of Weights and Measures

Table for Converting Apothecaries' Weights into Metric Weights

Grains	Grams	Grains	Grams	Grains	Grams	Grains	Grams
1/50	0.00130	18	1.166	50	3.240	82	5.314
1/32	0.00202	19	1.231	51	3.305	83	5.378
1/20	0.00324	20	1.296	52	3.370	84	5.443
1/18	0.00360	21	1.361	53	3.434	85	5.508
1/16	0.00405	22	1.426	54	3.499	86	5.573
1/15	0.00432	23	1.490	55	3.564	87	5.638
1/12	0.00540	24	1.555	56	3.629	88	5.702
1/10	0.00648	25	1.620	57	3.694	89	5.767
1/8	0.00810	26	1.685	58	3.758	90	5.832
1/6	0.01080	27	1.749	59	3.823	91	5.897
1/5	0.01296	28	1.814	60	3.888	92	5.962
1/4	0.01620	29	1.879	61	3.953	93	6.026
1/3	0.02160	30	1.944	62	4.018	94	6.091
1/2	0.03240	31	2.009	63	4.082	95	6.156
3/4	0.04860	32	2.074	64	4.147	96	6.221
1	0.0648	33	2.138	65	4.212	97	6.286
2	0.1296	34	2.203	66	4.277	98	6.350
3	0.1944	35	2.268	67	4.342	99	6.415
4	0.2592	36	2.333	68	4.406	100	6.480
5	0.3240	37	2.398	69	4.471	120	7.776
6	0.3888	38	2.462	70	4.536	150	9.720
7	0.4536	39	2.527	71	4.601	180	11.664
8	0.5184	40	2.592	72	4.666	200	12.958
9	0.5832	41	2.657	73	4.730	480	31.103
10	0.6480	42	2.722	74	4.795	500	32.396
11	0.7128	43	2.786	75	4.860	600	38.875
12	0.7776	44	2.851	76	4.925	700	45.354
13	0.8424	45	2.916	77	4.990	800	51.833
14	0.9072	46	2.981	78	5.054	900	58.313
15	0.9720	47	3.046	79	5.119	960	62.207
16	1.037	48	3.110	80	5.184	1000	64.799
17	1.102	49	3.175	81	5.249		

Metric Linear Measure

	Meter	U.S. inches	Feet	Yards	Miles
Millimeter =	.001 =	.03937 =	.00328		
Centimeter =	.01 =	.3937 =	.03280		
Decimeter =	.1 =	3.937 =	.32808 =	.10936	
Meter =	1. =	39.37 =	3.2808 =	1.0936	
Decameter =	10. =		= 32.808	= 10.936	
Hectometer =	100. =		= 328.08	= 109.36	= .062137
Kilometer =	1000. =		= 3280.8	= 1093.6	= .62137

Troy Weight

1 pound = 22.816 cubic inches of distilled water at 62°F

Grains gr	Pennyweights dwt	Ounces oz	Pounds lb
24 =	1		
480 =	20 =	1	
5760 =	240 =	12 =	1

Apothecaries' Weight

Grains gr	Scruples ℈	Drachms ʒ	Ounces ℥	Pounds lb
20 =	1			
60 =	3 =	1		
480 =	24 =	8 =	1	
5760 =	288 =	96 =	12 =	1

Apothecaries' Measure

Minims ♏	Fluidrachms fʒ	Fluidounces f℥	Pints O.	Gallon C.
60 =	1			
480 =	8 =	1		
7680 =	128 =	16 =	1	
61440 =	1024 =	128 =	8 =	1

Metric Weights

1 gram = 1 cubic centimeter of distilled water at 4°C

	Grams		Grains		Av. Ounces
Milligram =	0.001 =	0.01543			
Centigram =	0.01 =	0.15432			
Decigram =	0.1 =	1.54324			
Gram =	1. =	15.43248 =			.03528
Decagram =	10. =			=	.3528
Hectogram =	100. =			=	3.52758
Kilogram =	1000. =			=	35.2758

Table for Converting Metric Weights into Apothecaries' Weights

Grams	Exact equivalents in grains	Grams	Exact equivalents in grains
0.01	0.1543	12.0	185.189
0.02	0.3086	13.0	200.621
0.03	0.4630	14.0	216.054
0.04	0.6173	15.0	231.486
0.05	0.7716	16.0	246.918
0.06	0.9259	17.0	262.351
0.07	1.0803	18.0	277.783
0.08	1.2346	19.0	293.216
0.09	1.3889	20.0	308.648
0.1	1.543	21.0	324.080
0.2	3.086	22.0	339.513
0.3	4.630	23.0	354.945
0.4	6.173	24.0	370.378
0.5	7.716	25.0	385.810
0.6	9.259	26.0	401.242
0.7	10.803	27.0	416.674
0.8	12.346	28.0	432.107
0.9	13.889	29.0	447.538
1.0	15.432	30.0	462.971
2.0	30.865	31.0	478.403
3.0	46.297	32.0	493.835
4.0	61.730	40.0	617.294
5.0	77.162	45.0	694.456
6.0	92.594	50.0	771.618
7.0	108.027	60.0	925.942
8.0	123.459	70.0	1080.265
9.0	138.892	80.0	1234.589
10.0	154.324	90.0	1388.912
11.0	169.756	100.0	1543.236

Avoirdupois Weight

1 pound = 1.2153 pounds troy

Grains gr	Drachms dr	Ounces oz	Pounds lb
27.34375 =	1		
437.5 =	16 =	1	
7000 =	256 =	16 =	1

Comparative Values of Metric, Liquid, and Apothecaries' Measures

Cubic centimeters	Fluid-ounces	Cubic centimeters	Flui-drachms	Cubic centimeters	Minims
30	1.01	5	1.35	0.05	0.81
50	1.69	6	1.62	0.07	1.14
75	2.54	7	1.89	0.09	1.46
100	3.38	8	2.17	1	16.23
200	6.76	9	2.43	2	32.5
300	10.15	10	2.71	3	48.7
400	13.53	25	6.76	4	64.9
473	16.00				
500	16.91				
600	20.29				
700	23.67				
800	27.05				
900	30.43				
1000	33.82				

Comparative Values of Standard and Metric Measures of Length

Inches	Centimeters	Inches	Millimeters
1	2.54	1/25	1.00
2	5.08	1/12	2.12
3	7.62	1/8	3.18
4	10.16	1/4	6.35
5	12.70	1/3	8.47
6	15.24	1/2	12.70
7	17.78	5/8	15.88
8	20.32	2/3	16.93
9	22.86	3/4	19.05
10	25.40	5/6	21.16
11	27.94	7/8	22.22
12	30.48	11/12	23.28

Comparative Values of Avoirdupois and Metric Weights

Av. Ounces	Grams	Av. Pounds	Grams
1/16	1.772	1	453.59
1/8	3.544	2	907.18
1/4	7.088	2.2	1000.00
1/2	14.175	3	1360.78
1	28.350	4	1814.37
2	56.699	5	2267.96
3	85.049	6	2721.55
4	113.398	7	3175.15
5	141.748	8	3628.74
6	170.097	9	4082.33
7	198.447	10	4535.92
8	226.796		
9	255.146		
10	283.495		
11	311.845		
12	340.194		
13	368.544		
14	396.893		
15	425.243		

Metric Doses with Approximate Apothecary Equivalents

The approximate dose equivalents in the following table represent the quantities that would be prescribed, under identical conditions, by physicians trained, respectively, in the metric or in the apothecary system of weights and measures.

When prepared dosage forms such as tablets, capsules, pills, etc., are prescribed in the metric system, the pharmacist may dispense the corresponding approximate equivalent in the apothecary system, and vice versa. However, this does not authorize the alternative use of the approximate dose equivalents given below for specific quantities on a prescription that requires compounding, nor in converting a pharmaceutical formula from one system of weights or measures to the other system; for such purposes exact equivalents must be used.

Liquid measures		*Weights*			
Metric, ml	*Approximate apothecary equivalents*	*Metric*	*Approximate apothecary equivalents*	*Metric*	*Approximate apothecary equivalents*
1000	1 quart	30 g	1 ounce	50 mg	3/4 grain
750	1 1/2 pints	15 g	4 drachms	40 mg	2/3 grain
500	1 pint	10 g	2 1/2 drachms	30 mg	1/2 grain
250	8 fluidounces	7.5 g	2 drachms	25 mg	3/8 grain
200	7 fluidounces	6 g	90 grains	20 mg	1/3 grain
100	3 1/2 fluidounces	5 g	75 grains	15 mg	1/4 grain
50	1 3/4 fluidounces	4 g	60 grains	12 mg	1/5 grain
30	1 fluidounce		(1 drachm)	10 mg	1/6 grain
15	1/2 fluidounce	3 g	45 grains	8 mg	1/8 grain
	(4 fluidrachms)	2 g	30 grains	6 mg	1/10 grain
10	2 1/2 fluidrachms		(1/2 drachm)	5 mg	1/12 grain
8	2 fluidrachms	1.5 g	22 grains	4 mg	1/15 grain
5	75 minims	1 g	15 grains	3 mg	1/20 grain
	(1 1/4 fluidrachms)	0.75 g	12 grains	2 mg	1/30 grain
4	1 fluidrachm	0.6 g	10 grains	1.5 mg	1/40 grain
3	45 minims	0.5 g	7 1/2 grains	1.2 mg	1/50 grain
2	30 minims	0.45 g	7 grains	1 mg	1/60 grain
1	15 minims	0.4 g	6 grains	0.8 mg	1/80 grain
0.75	12 minims	0.3 g	5 grains	0.6 mg	1/100 grain
0.6	10 minims	0.25 g	4 grains	0.5 mg	1/120 grain
0.5	8 minims	0.2 g	3 grains	0.4 mg	1/150 grain
0.3	5 minims	0.15 g	2 1/2 grains	0.3 mg	1/200 grain
0.25	4 minims	0.12 g	2 grains	0.25 mg	1/250 grain
0.2	3 minims	0.1 g	1 1/2 grains	0.2 mg	1/300 grain
0.1	1 1/2 minims	75 mg	1 1/4 grains	0.15 mg	1/400 grain
0.06	1 minim	60 mg	1 grain	0.1 mg	1/600 grain

Source: *Blakiston's Gould Medical Dictionary*, 3d ed., McGraw-Hill Book Company, New York, 1972.

Table of the More Common Latin or Greek Terms and Abbreviations Used in Prescription Writing

Term of abbreviation	Latin or Greek	Translation
āā, aa	ana	of each
a.c.	ante cibum	before meals
ad	ad	to, up to
ad lib.	ad libitum	at pleasure
alternis horis	alternis horis	every other hour
ante	ante	before
aq.	aqua	water
aq. dest.	aqua destillata	distilled water
b.i.d.	bis in die, bis in dies	twice daily
bis	bis	twice
c̄, c	cum	with
caps.	capsula	a capsule
chart.	charta	a paper
collyr.	collyrium	an eyewash
divid.	divide	divide (thou)
d.t.d. No. iv	dentur tales doses No. iv	let four such doses be given
elix.	elixir	an elixir
enem.	enema	an enema
et	et	and
fldxt.	fluidextractum	fluidextract
ft.	fac; fiat; fiant	make (thou); let it be made; let them be made
ft. chart. vi	fiant chartulae vi	let six powders be made
ft. pulv. et div. in char. xii	fiat pulvis et divide in chartulas xii; *or,* fiat pulvis in chartulas xii dividenda	let twelve powders be made
gtt.	gutta(e)	drop(s)
H.	hora	an hour
hor. som., H.S.	hora somni	at bedtime
in d.	in dies	from day to day, daily
inf.	infusum	an infusion
inject.	injectio	an injection
inter	inter	between
lin.	linimentum	a liniment
liq.	liquor	a solution
lot.	lotio	a lotion
M.	misce	mix (thou)
m.	minimum	a minim
min.	minimum	a minim
mist.	mistura	a mixture
no.	numero, numerus	number
noctis	noctis	of the night
non	non	not
non rep.	non repetatur	do not repeat
O.D.	oculus dexter	the right eye
O.L.	oculus laevus	the left eye
omn. hor.	omni hora	every hour
omni nocte	omni nocte	every night
p.c.	post cibos; post cibum	after eating; after food
pil.	pilula(e)	pill(s)

Appendix | 691

Common Latin or Greek Terms (continued)

Term of abbreviation	Latin or Greek	Translation
p.r.n.	pro re nata	as occasion arises, occasionally
pulv.	pulvis; pulveres; pulveratus	powder; powders; powdered
q.h.	quaque hora	each hour, every hour
q. 2 h.	quaque secunda hora	every 2 hours
q.i.d.	quater in die	4 times a day
q.s.	quantum sufficit; quantum sufficiat; quantum satis	a sufficient quantity; as much as is sufficient
S.	signa; signetur	write (thou); let it be written; label (thou)
S.A.	secundum artem	according to art
sig.	signa; signetur	write (thou); let it be written; label (thou)
sine	sine	without
sol.	solutio	a solution
sp.	spiritus	spirit
ss, s̄s̄	semis	a half
suppos.	suppositorium	a suppository
syr.	syrupus	syrup
tabel.	tabella (dim. of *tabula*, a table)	a lozenge
talis	talis	such; like this
t.d.	ter die	3 times a day
t.i.d.	ter in die	3 times a day
tinct.	tinctura	a tincture
tr.	tinctura	a tincture
ung.	unguentum	an ointment
ut. dict.	ut dictum	as directed

Source: *Blakiston's Gould Medical Dictionary*, 3d ed., McGraw-Hill Book Company, New York, 1972.

Table of Thermometric Equivalents
Centigrade to Fahrenheit Scales

$$9/5 \; C° + 32 = F°$$

C°	F°	C°	F°	C°	F°	C°	F°	C°	F°
−20	−4.0	21	69.8	61	141.8	101	213.8	141	285.8
−19	−2.2	22	71.6	62	143.6	102	215.6	142	287.6
−18	−0.4	23	73.4	63	145.4	103	217.4	143	289.4
−17	1.4	24	75.2	64	147.2	104	219.2	144	291.2
−16	3.2	25	77.	65	149.	105	221.	145	293.
−15	5.	26	78.8	66	150.8	106	222.8	146	294.8
−14	6.8	27	80.6	67	152.6	107	224.6	147	296.6
−13	8.6	28	82.4	68	154.4	108	226.4	148	298.4
−12	10.4	29	84.2	69	156.2	109	228.2	149	300.2
−11	12.2	30	86.	70	158.	110	230.	150	302.
−10	14.	31	87.8	71	159.8	111	231.8	151	303.8
−9	15.8	32	89.6	72	161.6	112	233.6	152	305.6
−8	17.6	33	91.4	73	163.4	113	235.4	153	307.4
−7	19.4	34	93.2	74	165.2	114	237.2	154	309.2
−6	21.2	35	95.	75	167.	115	239.	155	311.
−5	23.	36	96.8	76	168.8	116	240.8	156	312.8
−4	24.8	37	98.6	77	170.6	117	242.6	157	314.6
−3	26.6	38	100.4	78	172.4	118	244.4	158	316.4
−2	28.4	39	102.2	79	174.2	119	246.2	159	318.2
−1	30.2	40	104.	80	176.	120	248.	160	320.
0	32.	41	105.8	81	177.8	121	249.8	161	321.8
1	33.8	42	107.6	82	179.6	122	251.6	162	323.6
2	35.6	43	109.4	83	181.4	123	253.4	163	325.4
3	37.4	44	111.2	84	183.2	124	255.2	164	327.2
4	39.2	45	113.	85	185.	125	257.	165	329.
5	41.	46	114.8	86	186.8	126	258.8	166	330.8
6	42.8	47	116.6	87	188.6	127	260.6	167	332.6
7	44.6	48	118.4	88	190.4	128	262.4	168	334.4
8	46.4	49	120.2	89	192.2	129	264.2	169	336.2
9	48.2	50	122.	90	194.	130	266.	170	338.
10	50.	51	123.8	91	195.8	131	267.8	171	339.8
11	51.8	52	125.6	92	197.6	132	269.6	172	341.6
12	53.6	53	127.4	93	199.4	133	271.4	173	343.4
13	55.4	54	129.2	94	201.2	134	273.2	174	345.2
14	57.2	55	131.	95	203.	135	275.	175	347.
15	59.	56	132.8	96	204.8	136	276.8	176	348.8
16	60.8	57	134.6	97	206.6	137	278.6	177	350.6
17	62.6	58	136.4	98	208.4	138	280.4	178	352.4
18	64.4	59	138.2	99	210.2	139	282.2	179	354.2
19	66.2	60	140.	100	212.	140	284.	180	356.
20	68.								

Source: Courtesy of *The Pharmacopeia of the United States of America.*

Table of Thermometric Equivalents
Fahrenheit to Centigrade Scales

$$(F° - 32) \times 5/9 = C°$$

F°	C°	F°	C°	F°	C°	F°	C°	F°	C°
0	−17.78	51	10.56	101	38.33	151	66.11	201	93.89
1	−17.22	52	11.11	102	38.89	152	66.67	202	94.44
2	−16.67	53	11.67	103	39.44	153	67.22	203	95.
3	−16.11	54	12.22	104	40.	154	67.78	204	95.56
4	−15.56	55	12.78	105	40.56	155	68.33	205	96.11
5	−15.	56	13.33	106	41.11	156	68.89	206	96.67
6	−14.44	57	13.89	107	41.67	157	69.44	207	97.22
7	−13.89	58	14.44	108	42.22	158	70.	208	97.78
8	−13.33	59	15.	109	42.78	159	70.56	209	98.33
9	−12.78	60	15.56	110	43.33	160	71.11	210	98.89
10	−12.22	61	16.11	111	43.89	161	71.67	211	99.44
11	−11.67	62	16.67	112	44.44	162	72.22	212	100.
12	−11.11	63	17.22	113	45.	163	72.78	213	100.56
13	−10.56	64	17.78	114	45.56	164	73.33	214	101.11
14	−10.	65	18.33	115	46.11	165	73.89	215	101.67
15	−9.44	66	18.89	116	46.67	166	74.44	216	102.22
16	−8.89	67	19.44	117	47.22	167	75.	217	102.78
17	−8.33	68	20.	118	47.78	168	75.56	218	103.33
18	−7.78	69	20.56	119	48.33	169	76.11	219	103.89
19	−7.22	70	21.11	120	48.89	170	76.67	220	104.44
20	−6.67	71	21.67	121	49.44	171	77.22	221	105.
21	−6.11	72	22.22	122	50.	172	77.78	222	105.56
22	−5.56	73	22.78	123	50.56	173	78.33	223	106.11
23	−5.	74	23.33	124	51.11	174	78.89	224	106.67
24	−4.44	75	23.89	125	51.67	175	79.44	225	107.22
25	−3.89	76	24.44	126	52.22	176	80.	226	107.78
26	−3.33	77	25.	127	52.78	177	80.56	227	108.33
27	−2.78	78	25.56	128	53.33	178	81.11	228	108.89
28	−2.22	79	26.11	129	53.89	179	81.67	229	109.44
29	−1.67	80	26.67	130	54.44	180	82.22	230	110.
30	−1.11	81	27.22	131	55.	181	82.78	231	110.56
31	−0.56	82	27.78	132	55.56	182	83.33	232	111.11
32	0.	83	28.33	133	56.11	183	83.89	233	111.67
33	0.56	84	28.89	134	56.67	184	84.44	234	112.22
34	1.11	85	29.44	135	57.22	185	85.	235	112.78
35	1.67	86	30.	136	57.78	186	85.56	236	113.33
36	2.22	87	30.56	137	58.33	187	86.11	237	113.89
37	2.78	88	31.11	138	58.89	188	86.67	238	114.44
38	3.33	89	31.67	139	59.44	189	87.22	239	115.
39	3.89	90	32.22	140	60.	190	87.78	240	115.56
40	4.44	91	32.78	141	60.56	191	88.33	241	116.11
41	5.	92	33.33	142	61.11	192	88.89	242	116.67
42	5.56	93	33.89	143	61.67	193	89.44	243	117.22
43	6.11	94	34.44	144	62.22	194	90.	244	117.78
44	6.67	95	35.	145	62.78	195	90.56	245	118.33
45	7.22	96	35.56	146	63.33	196	91.11	246	118.89
46	7.78	97	36.11	147	63.89	197	91.67	247	119.44
47	8.33	98	36.67	148	64.44	198	92.22	248	120.
48	8.89	99	37.22	149	65.	199	92.78	249	120.56
49	9.44	100	37.78	150	65.56	200	93.33	250	121.11
50	10.								

Source: Courtesy of The Pharmacopeia of the United States of America.

METRIC CONVERSION FACTORS
APPROXIMATE CONVERSIONS TO METRIC MEASURES

Symbol	When you know	Multiply by	To find	Symbol
Length				
in	inches	*2.5	centimeters	cm
ft	feet	30	centimeters	cm
yd	yards	0.9	meters	m
mi	miles	1.6	kilometers	km
Area				
in^2	square inches	6.5	square centimeters	cm^2
ft^2	square feet	0.09	square meters	m^2
yd^2	square yards	0.8	square meters	m^2
mi^2	square miles	2.6	square kilometers	km^2
	acres	0.4	hectares	ha
Mass (weight)				
oz	ounces	28	grams	g
lb	pounds	0.45	kilograms	kg
	short tons (2000 lb)	0.9	tonnes	t
Volume				
tsp	teaspoons	5	milliliters	ml
Tbsp	tablespoons	15	milliliters	ml
fl oz	fluid ounces	30	milliliters	ml
c	cups	0.24	liters	l
pt	pints	0.47	liters	l
qt	quarts	0.95	liters	l
gal	gallons	3.8	liters	l
ft^3	cubic feet	0.03	cubic meters	m^3
yd^3	cubic yards	0.76	cubic meters	m^3
Temperature (exact)				
°F	Fahrenheit temperature	5/9 (after subtracting 32)	Celsius temperature	°C

```
°F    32              98.6                          212
-40   0    40   80    120    160    200
-40  -20   0    20   40   60    80   100
°C                    37                            °C
```

Symbol	When you know	Multiply by	To find	Symbol
Length				
mm	millimeters	0.04	inches	in
cm	centimeters	0.4	inches	in
m	meters	3.3	feet	ft
m	meters	1.1	yards	yd
km	kilometers	0.6	miles	mi
Area				
cm^2	square centimeters	0.16	square inches	in^2
m^2	square meters	1.2	square yards	yd^2
km^2	square kilometers	0.4	square miles	mi^2
ha	hectares (10,000 m^2)	2.5	acres	
Mass (weight)				
g	grams	0.035	ounces	oz
kg	kilograms	2.2	pounds	lb
t	tonnes (1000 kg)	1.1	short tons	
Volume				
ml	milliliters	0.03	fluid ounces	fl oz
l	liters	2.1	pints	pt
l	liters	1.06	quarts	qt
l	liters	0.26	gallons	gal
m^3	cubic meters	35	cubic feet	ft^3
m^3	cubic meters	1.3	cubic yards	yd^3
Temperature (exact)				
°C	Celsius temperature	9/5 (then add 32)	Fahrenheit temperature	°F

SOURCE: U.S. Department of Commerce, *Metric Conversion Factors*, National Bureau of Standards Letter Circular 1051, July 1973.

*1 in = 2.54 cm (exactly). For other exact conversions and more detailed tables, see NBS Misc. Publ. 286, Units of Weights and Measures, Price $2.25, SD Catalog No. C13.10: 286.

Hidden Sugars

Breads

Hamburger bun	4 tsp
Hot dog bun	3½ tsp
White bread	3 tsp

Candies

Chewing gum	½ tsp
Chocolate bar	7 tsp
Mints	3 tsp
Fudge (1 piece)	4 tsp
Gum drops (4)	8 tsp
Hard candy	5 tsp
Marshmallow	1½ tsp
Breath mint	⅓ tsp

Cereals

Presweetened cereals have a sugar content ranging from 33 to 50%. *Read labels.*

Crackers

The sucrose content of crackers range from a low of 0.3% to a high of 14.8% (graham crackers). *Read labels.*

Dairy products

Chocolate milk	9 tsp
Cocoa (6 oz)	5 tsp
Ice cream (½ cup)	5½ tsp
Ice cream soda	5 tsp
Ice cream sundae	7 tsp
Ice cream plus sugar cone	7 tsp
Milk shake	8 tsp
Sherbert	6 tsp

Desserts

Angel food cake	7 tsp
Apple pie a la mode	13½ tsp
Cherry pie	12 tsp
Chocolate cake	10 tsp
Chocolate chip cookie	2 tsp
Coconut macaroon	6 tsp
Cream pie	8 tsp
Cupcake, iced	6 tsp
Custard	2 tsp
Donut, glazed	6 tsp
Donut, plain	3 tsp
Fruit gelatin	4½ tsp
Jelly roll	4 tsp
Lemon pie	7 tsp
Pumpkin pie	7 tsp
Rice pudding	5 tsp

Fruits and juices: canned

Apple sauce	4 tsp
Fruit cocktail	5 tsp
Peaches with syrup	1¾ tsp
Stewed, sweetened fruits	4 tsp
Sweetened juices (6 oz)	4 tsp
Orange juice, sweetened	2 tsp

Miscellaneous: antacid tablets, vitamins, etc.

Antacid tablets contain as much as 56.5% sugar. Other products manufactured for relief of digestive disorders contain as little as 0.08% sugar. *Read labels.*

Some vitamin tablets are flavored or have their sale aimed at specific segments of the population. These may contain as much as 47.6% sugar.

Read the labels on miscellaneous products such as mayonnaise, peanut butter, instant breakfasts, chocolate drinks, canned products (fruits, vegetables, or meats), and prepared foods. Many of them contain more than 50% sugar.

Preserves, jellies and topings

Apple butter	3½ tsp
Chocolate sauce	4 tsp
Honey	3 tsp
Marmalade	3½ tsp
Peach butter	1 tsp
Strawberry preserves	4 tsp
Jelly	3 tsp

Soft drinks

Some soft drinks are sweetened with sugar substitutes. The more popular carbonated and noncarbonated brands, when sweetened with sugar, contain from 8.4 to 2.5% sugar.

Syrups

Maple	5 tsp
Molasses	3½ tsp

Snack Foods for Health

High protein	Fruit-vegetables	Drinks	Breads-cereals
Beef or beef sticks Bologna Canned meats Cheese, all types, sliced, dips, or spreads Chicken Corned beef Eggs, boiled Ham Meatballs Nuts Oysters Pastrami Pizza, individual Salami Salmon Sardines Sausages, pork, Vienna Shrimp Smoked sliced beef Spreadables Tuna Turkey	Any fresh fruit in season Apples Bananas Blueberries Grapes Oranges Peaches Pears Pineapples, fresh, sliced Plums Strawberries Carrots Cauliflower bits Celery Cucumbers, sliced Green peppers, sliced Olives Tomatoes, cherry	Coffee, sucrose substitute Grape juice, fresh Grapefruit juice, fresh Milk Orange juice, fresh Sugarless soft drinks, carbonated and noncarbonated, all flavors Tea, sucrose substitute Tomato juice V-8 juice	Bread sticks Cheese Curls Cheese Tid-Bits Chee-tos Cheez-its Corn chips Corn curls Doritos, several flavors Melba toast Popcorn Potato chips Potato sticks Pretzels Rounds (bacon, garlic, onion, salty rye, sesame) Ry-King, several flavors Ry-Krisp, several flavors Tacos Triscuits Wheat Thins

Vitamin A Food Content

The recommended daily allowance (RDA) of vitamin A is 5000 IU. The below listed foods *contain vitamin A in the amounts noted when 100 g (approximately 3.5 oz) is consumed.*

Food	IU	Food	IU	Food	IU
Apricots, canned	1800	Endive	3300	Pimentos	2300
dried, uncooked	10,900	Fruit salad, canned	470	Pizza with cheese	630
nectar	950	Grapefruit, pink	440	Plums, purple	1200
raw	2700	white	0	Prunes, cooked	760
Asparagus, canned	500–800	Grapefruit juice	(negligible)	uncooked	2170
fresh, cooked, drained	900	Halibut	6680	Prune juice	460
Beans, snap, cooked	540	Ice cream	450–650	Pumpkin, canned	6400
Beef pot pie	820	Kale	9000	Rutabagas	550
Beef stew	980	Kidneys, beef	1150	Salad dressing, Russian	690
Beet greens	5000–6000	Kumquat	600	Sausage, liver	6250
Bread stuffing	650	Lettuce, iceberg	330	Soup, chicken vegetable	880
Broccoli	2000–2500	looseleaf	1900	minestrone	960
Brussel sprouts	570	romaine	1900	tomato	460
Butter	3300	Liver	17,000–53,000	vegetable	1200
Cabbage (white mustard)	3100	Mackerel	500	vegetable beef	1100
Carrots	10,500	Mango	4800	Soybean	660
Chard, Swiss	5500	Margarine	3300	Spaghetti and meatballs in	
Cheese, American, blue, camembert, cheddar, cream, limburger, parmesan, roquefort, Swiss	1100	Muskmelons, cantaloupe	3400	tomato sauce	640
		honeydew	0	Spanish rice	660
		Mustard greens	6000	Spinach	8100
		Nectarines	1650	Squash, winter	1000–6000
Cherries, red sour	700–1000	Okra	500	Swamp cabbage	6300
Chicken, fried	820	Olives, green	300	Sweet potatoes	5000–12,000
Chicken giblets	5750	ripe	0	Swordfish	1750
Chicken pot pie	910	Onions, bulb and top	2000	Tangerine	420
Chili powder	65,000	bulb only	0	Tomatoes	900
Chives, raw	5800	Oysters, fried	440	Tomato, catsup	1400
Collards	7000–9000	Papaya	1750	puree	1600
Cookie, ladyfinger	650	Parsley	8500	Tomato juice	800
Corn, sweet	400	Peaches	650–1330	Turkey pot pie	900–1300
Cornmeal	510	Peas	610	Turnip greens	6300
Cowpeas	1400	Peas and carrots	9300	Vegetables, mixed	5000
Crab	2170	Peppers, hot chili	770	Watercress	4900
Cream	480–1540	red	21,600	Watermelon	590
Cream substitutes	520–960	Peppers, sweet, raw	420	Welsh rarebit	530
Cress	7000–9000	sweet red, raw	4500	Whitefish	2200
Dandelion greens	11,000–14,000	Pie, cherry, peach, pumpkin, sweet potato	440–2400	White sauce	320–570
Eggs	1200				

Food Vitamin C Content

The recommended daily allowance of vitamin C is 45 mg per day. The below listed foods *contain vitamin C in the amounts listed* (in mg) *when 100 g (approximately 3.5 oz) are consumed.*

Food	mg	Food	mg	Food	mg
Apricots, dehydrated uncooked	15	Leeks	17	Pineapple, raw	17
Asparagus, canned	15	Lemon	53	Pineapple juice 3:1	12
cooked	26	Lemon and peel	77	Pineapple and grapefruit juice	16
Avocado	15	Lemon juice, canned	42	Pineapple and orange juice	16
Beans, lima, cooked	17	fresh	46	Potato, baked in skin	20
Beans, snap, cooked, little water	12	Lemon peel	129	boiled in skin	16
Beans, wax, cooked, little water	13	Lemonade, diluted 1:4	7	chips	16
Beet greens, boiled, drained	15	Lettuce, crisphead	6	french fried	21
Blueberries, raw	14	looseleaf	18	fried from raw	19
Broccoli, cooked, boiled, drained	90	romaine	18	mashed	10
frozen, boiled, drained	57	Lime	37	salad	10
Brussel sprouts, boiled, drained	87	Lime juice	21	scalloped	10
frozen, boiled, drained	80	Limeade, diluted 1:4	2	sticks	40
Cabbage, cooked	30	Liver, beef, cooked	27	Prickly pear	22
raw	47	calf, cooked	37	Quinces, raw	15
Cauliflower, cooked, boiled, drained	55	chicken, cooked	16	Radishes	26
		hog, cooked	22	Raspberries, black	18
		lamb, cooked	36	red	25
frozen, boiled, drained	41	Lobster salad	18	Roe	18
raw	78	Loganberries, canned (juice)	12	Rutabaga, raw	43
Chard, cooked	16	raw	24	cooked	26
raw	32	Mango	35	Sauerkraut, canned	14
Chives, raw	56	Muskmelon, cantaloupe	33	juice	18
Coleslaw	29	casaba	13	Soybean, cooked	17
Collards, cooked	76	honeydew	23	raw	29
frozen, cooked	33	Mustard greens, cooked	48	Rice, spanish	15
Cow/black-eye peas, boiled, drained	17	frozen, cooked	20	Spinach, canned	14
		raw	97	cooked	28
Cranberry-orange relish	18	Mustard spinach, cooked	65	frozen	19
Cress, cooked	30	raw	130	Squash, most varieties, cooked	9–13
raw	69	Nectarines	13	Strawberries, frozen	55
Currants, black, raw	200	Okra, cooked	20	raw	59
white and red, raw	41	frozen, cooked	12	Swamp cabbage, cooked	16
Dandelion greens, cooked	18	raw	31	Sweet potatoes, baked in skin	22
raw	35	Onion, green	32	boiled in skin	17
Elderberries, raw	36	Orange	45–71	candied	10
Garlic, raw	15	Orange juice, canned	40	canned	8
Gooseberries, canned	10	fresh	37–61	Tangerine	31
raw	33	frozen, diluted 3:1	45	Tangerine juice, fresh	22
Grape juice drink	16	Orange peel	136	frozen 3:1	27
Grapefruit, canned	30	Oysters, Pacific & Western, raw	30	Tomato, canned	17
raw	40	Eastern	0	catsup	15
Grapefruit juice, fresh	40	Papaya	56	chili sauce	16
Grapefruit and orange juice	34	Parsley	172	cooked	24
frozen, diluted 3:1	41	Parsnips, raw	16	juice	16
Guavas, raw	242	Peas, green, cooked	14	puree	33
Guava strawberry	37	Peas, sweet, cooked	8	raw	23
Kale, cooked	60–90	Peppers, chili sauce	68	Turnips, boiled, drained	22
		hot chili, canned	68	raw	36
raw	130	raw	235	Turnip greens, cooked, drained	50–70
Kohlrabi, cooked	43	sweet	100	raw	139
raw	66	Pie, strawberry	25	Watercress	79
Kumquat	36	Pimentos	95		

Calcium Needs per Day, 1300–1400 mg through Teen Years; 800 mg Adults*

The following foods contain 100 mg or more of Ca in 100 g (3.5 oz) portions.

Food	mg	Food	mg	Food	mg
Almonds	235	Cream, light coffee	102	Orange peel	161
Baby food cereal	750–800	Cupcakes	161	Oysters	152
Baking powder	1000–6000	Custard	112	Pancakes	100
Beans, mung	118	Dandelion greens	140	Parsley	203
pinto	135	Egg yolk	141	Pistachio nuts	131
Beef, creamed	105	Figs, dried	126	Pizza with cheese	127
Beets	100	Filberts	209	Potatoes with cheese	127
Biscuits	120	Fish flour	1000–6000	Pudding	117
Bread, wheat	105	Gingerbread	100	Rennin dessert	122
white	112	Herring	147	Rice pudding	100
Bread pudding	122	Ice cream, 10% fat	146	Rolls, whole wheat	106
Bread stuffing	124	Ice cream, 12% fat	123	Salmon	175
Broccoli	100	Ice cream cones	156	Sardines	400
Buttermilk	121	Ice milk	156	Scallops	115
Cake, angel food	108	Kale	150	Sesame seeds	110
white	100	Lemon peel	134	Shrimp, canned	115
Candy, caramel	140	Macaroni and cheese	181	Smelt	350
milk chocolate	228	Mackerel	280	Spinach	100
Cheeses	200–1140	Milk	130	Tapioca pudding	105
Chocolate syrup	127	Milk, condensed/evaporated	260	Turnips	180
Chocolate, hot	275	Molasses	300	Waffles	120
Collards	180	Muffins	104	Watercress	151
Cookies, butter	126	Muffins, bran	142	Welsh rarebit	250
Cornbread	110	corn	110	White sauce	115
Crackers and cheese	336	Mustard	130	Yoghurt	115
Crackers, graham	113	Mustard greens	138		
Cream, half and half	108	Olives, ripe	106		

* Ca input from sources less than 100 mg/100 g of input can probably be estimated as 250 mg. This means that 550–1150 mg must come from these listed sources.

Glossary

ab·nor′mal 1. Not normal or usual. 2. Deviating from the normal in structure, form, or position; not conforming with the general or natural rule. See *resorption*.

a·bra′sion Mechanical wear of teeth from excessive function or abnormal causes. Improper brushing may cause notching or grooving of the teeth.

ab′scess A localized pus formation in any part of the body.

ab·sorp′tion The process of sucking up, taking in, and assimilating certain substances, as fluids and other suitable matter, by the skin, mucous membranes, blood vessels, or lymphatics.

a·but′ment A tooth used to support or stabilize one end of a prosthetic appliance, such as a dental bridge.

ac·cel′er·a″tor A device or chemical that causes a moving object or a chemical reaction to go faster; any agent or part that quickens the speed of a function. *v.* **accelerate**.

ac·count′ A formal record of the debits and credits of the person or persons named at the head of a ledger, usually showing a balance.

ac·cre′tion An accumulation of foreign matter, as tartar on a surface of a tooth or decayed matter within a cavity.

ac″i·do′sis A condition caused by a reduction of the blood components that neutralize acids in the blood.

ac″i·du′ric Able to grow in an acid medium; said of bacteria.

ac·quired′ Developed as a result of environment, use, or disuse, as acquired character. See acquired *immunity*.

a·cryl′ic One of a group of synthetic thermoplastic substances resembling clear glass, but lighter in weight, which permit passage of ultraviolet rays, used in making dental prostheses and temporary artificial eyes. Lucite and Plexiglas are commercial forms.

    autopolymerizing a. A plastic material having two aspects, a powder and a liquid, which, when mixed together (like plaster), form

701

a mass that can be molded and will then harden without further external stimuli.

a·cute′ Having a rapid onset, a short, severe course, and pronounced symptoms; not chronic.

ADA American Dental Association.

ADAA American Dental Assistants Association.

ADHA American Dental Hygienists Association.

ad·sorp′tion 1. The power possessed by certain substances of taking up fluids, apart from capillary attraction. 2. The attraction and concentration on a hard surface of molecules of a substance, such as a gas or a liquid, by adhesion.

ad′ver·tis″ing The business of preparing, publishing, and circulating advertisements.

a′er·obe A microorganism that requires free atmospheric oxygen for the maintenance of life.

a′er·o·sol″ized Atomized particles suspended in air.

ag·glu′tin·in An antibody occurring in a normal or immune serum which, when added to a suspension of its homologous particulate antigen, causes the antigen elements to adhere to one another, forming clumps.

air′way A respiratory passage.

al′co·hol A colorless, volatile, highly inflammable liquid which is a product of the distillation of fermented grains, fruits, and starches.

al′gin·ate A salt of alginic acid extracted from marine kelp; an essential component of elastic impression materials.

al′ka·li Any of a class of compounds which react with acids to form salts, turn red litmus blue, saponify fats, and form soluble carbonates.

al′ka·line 1. Containing more hydroxyl than hydrogen ions. 2. Having the qualities of, or pertaining to, an alkali.

al′ka·loid Any naturally occurring basic organic nitrogenous compound, usually of plant origin.

al′ler·gy Altered reaction capacity to a specific substance which will cause no such reaction in the nonsensitive.

al′loy The product of the fusion of two or more metals. In dentistry, a silver alloy is used to combine with mercury to produce an amalgam for restoration of destroyed tooth structure.

al·ve′o·lar Pertaining to an alveolus.
   a. bone The bone of the jaw immediately surrounding and supporting the roots of the teeth.

al″ve·o·lec′to·my Surgical removal of part of the alveolar bone of the upper or lower jaw.

al·ve′o·lus The bony cavity or socket in which the root of a tooth is held by the periodontal ligament.

a·mal′gam An alloy of mercury with any other metal.
   a. carrier An instrument for carrying and introducing amalgam into the prepared cavity of a tooth.
   a. condenser An instrument for condensing or compressing freshly mixed amalgam into a prepared cavity in a tooth.
   dental a. A compound of a basal alloy of silver and tin with mercury, used for restoring teeth. Copper and zinc are usually added as modifying metals to the basal alloy.

a·mal′gam·ate To unite a metal or an alloy with mercury.

a·mel′o·blast An enamel cell; one of the columnar cells of the enamel organ which helps in forming dental enamel.

a·mi′no ac′id (a·mee′no, am′i·no) Any of a large group of organic compounds with the basic formula NH_2—R—COOH. From amino acids the body resynthesizes its proteins. Ten of them are considered essential to life: arginine, histidine, isoleucine, leucine, lysine, methionine, phenylalanine, threonine, tryptophan, and valine.

am′me·ter An instrument for measuring the amperage of an electric current.

am·ne′sic Pertaining to loss of memory or inability to recall experiences.

a·mor′phous Having no definite form; shapeless.

a·mor′phous sol′id A solid in which unit particles (atoms or molecules) do not take a definite and regular position in relation to one another.

am′pul, am′pule A small glass container capable of being hermetically sealed, intended to preserve its contents in a sterile condition; used principally for hypodermic solutions.

an·a′er·obe A microorganism that will grow in the absence of molecular oxygen. Exposure to air for any length of time will usually destroy these microorganisms.

an″al·ge′si·a Insensibility to pain without loss of consciousness. *adj.* **analgesic.**

an″al·ge′sic A remedy for relieving pain.

an″a·phy·lax′is A severe hypersensitive state produced by injecting an antigen into a person or animal who is already sensitive to the antigen; usually accompanied by spasms of smooth muscle, increased glandular secretions, and varying degrees of shock.

a·nat′o·my The science of the structure of organisms and the relation of their parts.

   dental a. The science of the structure of the external and internal forms of teeth and their surrounding structures.

a·ne′mi·a A significant reduction below normal in the number of red blood cells per cubic millimeter, in the hemoglobin concentration, and in the volume of packed red cells per 100 ml of blood, resulting in a decrease in the oxygen-carrying capacity of a given volume of blood.

an″es·the′si·a Loss of sensation.

   block a. Anesthesia produced by injecting an anesthetic solution into the nerve trunks supplying the operative field, called **regional block,** or by infiltrating close to the nerves, called **infiltration block,** or by a wall of anesthetic solution injected about the field, called **field block.** In all these methods the nerve conduction is blocked, and painful impulses fail to reach the brain.

   general a. Loss of sensation with loss of consciousness.

   infiltration a. That induced by the injecion of the anesthetic solution directly into the tissues that are to be anesthetized.

   local a. Anesthesia limited to a local area.

   regional a. Local anesthesia.

an″es·the″si·ol′o·gy The art and science of administering local and general anesthetics to produce the various types of anesthesia.

an″es·thet′ic A drug which produces local or general loss of sensation and sometimes of consciousness.

   general a. An agent which produces general anesthesia either by injection or by inhalation.

   local a. A drug which, when topically applied or injected into the tissues, causes local insensibility to pain.

an·gi′na 1. Any disease marked by attacks of choking or suffocation, particularly an affection of the throat. 2. A spasmodic, cramplike pain or attack.

an′gle The degree of divergence of two lines or planes that meet at a point; the space between two such lines.

Angle's classification A classification of occlusion based on the mesiodistal (anteroposterior) relationship of the upper and lower jaws.

ang′strom A unit of length equal to 10^{-8} cm (one hundred-millionth of a centimeter); used for measuring wavelengths, as of visible light, x-rays, and radium radiation.

an′ky·lo′sis Stiffness or fixation of a joint; also, bony union of a tooth to its aveolus.

an·neal′ To temper; to apply a regulated process of heating and subsequent cooling to glass or metal to render it less brittle and more workable.

an·neal′ing of gold foil See *degassing.*

an·neal′or A device used to anneal metal, glass, or wax.

an′ode The positively charged component of an x-ray tube containing a target area made of tungsten.

an″o·don′ti·a Lack of teeth.

a·nom′a·ly 1. Any deviation from the usual. 2. Any organ or part existing in an abnormal form, structure, or location.

an″ox·e′mi·a A lack of oxygen in the blood resulting from insufficient aeration due to high elevation, low partial pressure of oxygen in anesthesia, cardiac failure, or strangling.

an·ox′i·a Inadequate supply of oxygen; also, the disturbance of bodily functions resulting from a deficiency of oxygen.

an·tag′o·nist 1. Any agent that opposes, resists, or neutralizes the action of another agent. 2. A tooth in the upper jaw that articulates with a tooth in the lower jaw, or vice versa.

antecubital fossa The depression in front of the elbow.

an·te′ri·or Situated in front of or in the forward part.

an″ti·bi·ot′ic 1. Tending to destroy life. 2. Of or pertaining to an antibiotic.

an″ti·bi·ot′ic The extract of any of certain microorganisms used to destroy other disease-producing organisms.

an″ti·bod″y One of a class of substances produced by the animal body to destroy some specific antigen.

an″ti·co·ag′u·lant 1. Opposed to or preventing coagulation. 2. Of or pertaining to an anticoagulant.

an″ti·co·ag′u·lant A substance, as a drug, used to prevent or to dissolve blood clots.

an′ti·dote An agent that prevents or counteracts the action of a poison or a drug.

an″ti·emet′ic Pertaining to the prevention of nausea and vomiting.

an′ti·flux Material added to minerals or metals to prevent or to limit fusion.

an′ti·gen Any substance which, when introduced into the animal body, stimulates the production of antibodies or reacts with them.

an″ti·py·ret′ic An agent, as a drug, used to reduce fever.

an″ti·ra·chit′ic Of or pertaining to an antirachitic.

an″ti·ra·chit′ic An agent for the prevention or cure of rickets.

an″ti·sep′tic Checking or preventing decay and putrefaction.

an″ti·sep′tic Any of a large group of organic and inorganic compounds that stops or inhibits the growth of bacteria without necessarily killing them, thus checking putrefaction.

an″ti·si·al′a·gogue, an″ti·si·al′a·gog A drug or other agent that prevents or checks the flow of saliva.

an″ti·tox′in 1. A substance, elaborated in the body, capable of neutralizing a given toxin (bacterial, plant, or animal toxin). 2. One of the class of specific antibodies.

a′pex The terminal end of the root of a tooth. *adj.* **apical.**

api″co·ec′to·my Removal of the apex of a tooth root.

ap′o·plex″y The symptom complex resulting from hemorrhage into or upon the brain, or from embolism or thrombosis of the cerebral vessels, characterized chiefly by paralysis of one side of the body and unconsciousness.

ap·plied′ psy·chol′o·gy That branch of psychology which emphasizes practical rather than theoretical objectives. It includes medical, industrial, educational, clinical, and similar branches of psychology.

ap·pren′tice·ship The learning of a trade or art by serving under a master or expert; also, the length of time during which an apprentice serves.

arch wire In *orthodontics*, the main wire framework which is attached to bands and passes around the entire dental arch, either on the lingual surface or facial surface or on both, and which serves as the frame of attachment for finger springs.

ar″ma·men·tar′i·um All the books, journals, medicines, instruments, and laboratory and therapeutic equipment possessed by a dentist, physician, or surgeon to assist in the practice of their professions.

Armed For′ces The United States Army, Navy, Air Force, and Marines.

ar″o·mat′ic Having a spicy odor; characterized by a fragrant, spicy taste and odor, as cinnamon or ginger.

ar·tic′u·late To bring the teeth in one arch into proper position with the teeth in another arch.

ar·tic′u·la″tor An instrument for holding casts of the jaws or teeth in proper relation during various steps of artificial denture construction. It may be adjusted so as to duplicate the mandibular movements of the patient.

ar″ti·fi′cial teeth A denture or bridgework; dental prosthesis. Artificial teeth are composed of two materials; porcelain or plastic. The former is a hard, baked vitreous material with specific properties. The latter is a less hard, more resilient material with different characteristic indicated uses.

a·sep′sis Exclusion of microorganisms.

a·sep′tic Free of microorganisms.

a·sep′tic tech·nique′ The modern method of sterilizing an operating area and instruments, so that ideally no bacteria are present.

as·phyx′i·a Unconsciousness due to suffocation or interference of any kind with oxygenation of the blood.

as′pi·rate 1. Act of sucking up or sucking in; inspiration; imbibition. 2. Act of using the aspirator. 3. Method of withdrawing fluids and gases from a cavity, usually by forced air.

as′pi·ra″tor A negative-pressure apparatus for withdrawing liquids from cavities.

as′pir·in Acetylsalicylic acid, a mild analgesic.

as·trin′gent An agent that causes contraction of organic tissue or arrests bleeding or diarrhea.

at′om The smallest particle of an element capable of existing individually or in combination with one or more atoms of the same or another element. It consists of a dense inner core or nucleus, made up of neutrons and protons, with electrons vibrating in a relatively empty surrounding space.

at′o·py A form of allergy occurring only in the human species and subject to hereditary influence. Hay fever and asthma are examples.

at′ro·phy A reduction in size of an organ or cell which had previously reached mature size.

at·tri′tion (a·trish′un) Normal wear on teeth; thus, the wearing away of tooth enamel by mastication is called **attrition of enamel.**

audioanalgesia The use of sound to allay pain produced by dental operations.

au′to·clave An apparatus for sterilizing objects by steam heat at high pressure.

au′to·clave To sterilize in an autoclave.

aux·il′ia·ry Supporting; helping; assisting.

aux·il′ia·ry per·son·nel′ Personnel such as the dental assistant, dental hygienist, or dental laboratory technician. Also called *paradental personnel.*

ax′i·al (ak′se·al) Pertaining to the long axis of a tooth.

ax′is A real or imaginary line passing through a body or a part, as the vertical axis of a tooth.

ba·cil′lus Any member of a large group of aerobic rod-shaped microorganisms of the genus *Bacillus.* Plural: *bacilli.*

back′ing A piece of metal, usually gold, that backs up an artificial bridge or tooth and to which the tooth is soldered or otherwise attached.

back or′der A memorandum for an item or items not supplied on an order for supplies.

bac″te·re′mi·a The presence of bacteria in the bloodstream.

bac·te′ri·al spore The reproductive cell of some bacteria, which is capable of living through dry periods or adverse conditions.

bac·te′ri·cide A substance, such as a drug, that destroys bacteria.

bac·te″ri·ol′o·gy The science and study of bacteria.

bac·te″ri·o·stat′ic An agent that inhibits or stops the growth of bacteria.

bac·te′ri·um 1. Any of a very large group of unicellular vegetable microorganisms. A relatively small group is pathogenic, while most are nonpathogenic. Plural: *bacteria.* 2. A member of the genus *Bacterium.*

bake In *fixed prosthodontics,* to fire in a furnace a porcelain restoration.
  biscuit b. The initial firing of a porcelain restoration.
  glaze b. The final firing of a porcelain restoration.

band In *orthodontics,* a metallic attachment that surrounds and is cemented on the tooth, used to anchor arch wires to the teeth.

bar·bit′u·rate One of a large group of drugs used as sedatives or hypnotics.

base A protective material, such as a cement, placed over the pulpal area of the tooth (pulp not exposed) to reduce irritation and thermal shock to the pulp.

base′·plate, rec′ ord base A temporary form to represent the base of a denture which is used for making maxillomandibular (jaw) relation records and for the arrangement of teeth.

bell′-crowned Pertaining or referring to a tooth crown which is largest at the occlusal surface and tapers to the gum, usually used on incisors and bicuspids.

be·nign′ Not endangering life or health; not malignant.

bi·cus′pid Having two cusps, as bicuspid teeth; a premolar.

bi′fur·cate Forked; divided into two branches.

bile A very bitter alkaline greenish-yellow to golden-brown fluid, secreted by the liver and poured into the duodenum. Functionally, it aids in the digestion and absorption of fats, in the alkalinization of the intestines, and in the prevention of putrefaction.

bind′er One of the ingredients of investment materials used in laboratory procedures; namely, plaster of paris or dental stone.

bi′op·sy The excision, during life, of tissue to establish the diagnosis by means of a microscopic examination of the excised piece.

bis′que See *biscuit bake.*

bite A plastic impression of the relationship of the upper and lower teeth in occlusion.
  closed b. A condition in which the upper teeth close too far over the lower teeth when the jaws are closed tightly together. The lower anterior teeth usually bite into the roof of the patient's mouth.
  cross b. One in which the jaws can be in normal relation when closed, but the buccal cusps of the upper molars bite inside the buccal cusps of the lower molars.
  open b. A condition in which the upper and lower incisors do not occlude.

bite fork A forklike metal piece used with a facebow to transfer a wax rim to an articulator from the mouth in proper relationship.

bite rims A device consisting of upper and lower bite rims together to measure and record the vertical distance between the two jaws. It also records the horizontal space relationship between the jaws. The rims establish where the teeth of an artificial denture are to be placed, and eventually they may be used as the base to support these teeth. The base of the rims is made of acrylic or shellac-base material properly constructed, and upon it a mass of wax is placed and contoured to specific dimensions.

brack′et In *orthodontics,* an attachment which is either welded or soldered to a band (except a molar band) and which is the means by which arch wires are secured to bands.

brack′et table The movable operating table mounted on the dental operating unit on which are arranged the instruments and materials used in dental treatment procedures.

bridge A partial denture; bridgework.

fixed b. One which is permanently attached to its abutments.

removable b. One which, though held firmly in place, may be removed by the wearer.

removable fixed b. One which may be removed, without mutilation of any of its parts, by the dentist but not by the patient.

bridge′work″ An appliance made of artificial crowns of teeth to replace missing natural teeth. Such crowns are connected to natural teeth or roots for anchorage by means of a bridge.

broach *In dentistry,* a delicate, tapered flexible steel instrument having a spring temper; various styles are used for removing the dental pulp and for opening, enlarging, and treating the root canals.

bruise An injury, usually caused by a blow, in which the skin is not broken but in which there is bleeding under the skin surface and into the tissue.

brush Toothbrush, tooth-cleaning brush.

brux′ism The unconscious habit of gnashing or grinding the teeth, often limited to the sleeping period but sometimes occurring during mental or physical concentration or strain.

buc′cal Pertaining to the cheek. The buccal surface of a tooth is the surface next to the cheek.

buc′cal tube *In orthodontics,* an attachment which is either welded or soldered to a molar band and is the means by which the ends of the labial or lingual arch wire are secured to molar bands.

buck slip A memorandum of services or operation performed and charges for a particular visit of a patient, which is transcribed to the permanent records.

buf′fer A substance that, when added to a solution, causes resistance to any change of hydrogen-ion concentration when either an acid or alkali is added.

bur *In dentistry,* a cutting instrument with a rounded, pointed, cylindrical, or ovoid head having numerous blades, and operated usually in the handpiece of the dental engine for excavating carious dentin and for other purposes.

bur′nish·er A steel instrument with a ball or rounded smooth, working point which is used to burnish (adapt) margins of gold restorations and to aid in the placement of some plastic filling materials.

cal·car′e·ous 1. Pertaining to limestone. 2. Having a chalky appearance or consistency. 3. Containing calcium.

cal″ci·fi·ca′tion The deposit of calcareous matter within the tissues of the body.

cal′cine To drive off animal matter and volatile chemical constituents from inorganic compounds by heat.

cal′cu·lus A hard calcareous concretion deposited on the surface of the crown or root of a tooth; tartar.

salivary c. Calcareous deposits in the duct of a salivary gland or on the surfaces of the teeth and which originate from the salivary secretion.

serumal c. Calcareous deposits formed about the teeth by exudation from diseased gums.

cal′o·rie, cal′o·ry One of two recognized units of heat used especially to express the heat- or energy-producing content of foods.

great c. The amount of heat required to raise the temperature of 1 kg of water 1°C.

small c. The amount of heat required to raise the temperature of 1 g of water 1°C.

ca·nal′ Any tubular and relatively narrow passage or channel; a duct.

can′cer Any malignant tumor.

cap A substance or structure designed to cover the exposed pulp of a tooth. *v.* **cap.**

cap′i·ta′tion A uniform payment payable on a per capita basis; one basis for grant monies.

cap′sule A gelatinous sticky polysaccharide

surrounding certain bacteria. It often helps to protect the bacteria from destruction and to make them more invasive.

car'at A twenty-fourth part, used to express the proportion of gold in an alloy.

car·bol'ic ac'id Phenol.

Carborundum A registered trademark for silicon carbide, a substance of extreme hardness used as an abrasive.

Carborundum stones and wheels Small stones and wheels made of Carborundum, used in dentistry for grinding and polishing teeth and restorations.

car"ci·no'ma A type of cancer.

car'di·ac Pertaining to the heart.

ca'ri·es (kair'eez) A molecular death of bone or teeth, corresponding to ulceration in the soft tissues. *adj.* **carious.**
  c. of the teeth. A localized, progressive molecular disintegration of the teeth, beginning with the solution of the enamel by lactic and pyruvic acids. The acids break down and remove the inorganic constituents of the enamel and dentin, and the unsupported organic matrix is gradually removed, leaving the so-called *cavity of decay*.
  interproximal c. Caries on the surfaces of teeth in contact with each other.

car'io·gen'ic Conducive to the development of dental caries.

car'o·tene A red, orange, or yellow hydrocarbon belonging to the group of carotenoids. It is synthesized by many plants and is the precursor of vitamin A.

Carpule Trademark for a glass cartridge containing a sterile solution of a drug, as for local anesthetic, which is loaded into a specially contrived syringe and is ready for hypodermic injection.

car'ri·er A normal person or one convalescing from an infectious disease who shows no signs or symptoms of the disease, but who harbors and eliminates the microorganism and so spreads the disease.

case his'to·ry Information obtained from a patient and others, regarding the past history of the case, which will aid in diagnosis and treatment of dental and medical conditions.

cas·sette' A holder for a roentgenographic film or plate.

cast A positive reproduction of the form of the tissues of the upper or lower arch.
  transfer c. One which has dies of abutment teeth incorporated into it.

cast To form a substance, as molten metal or a plastic, into a particular shape by pouring or injecting into a mold.

cat'a·lyst A substance that speeds up a chemical reaction by its presence but does not, itself, change.

cath'ode The negatively charged component of an x-ray tube which contains a filament wire coil made of tungsten.

caus'tic A substance capable of burning or destroying tissue.

cav'i·ty The lesion produced by dental caries.
  incipient interproximal c. One that is just beginning to form on the contacting surface of a tooth.

cav'i·ty lin'er A substance that is placed on the walls of a cavity prior to insertion of a restoration.

cc Abbreviation for cubic centimeter.

CDA Certified Dental Assistant; one who has met the formal requirements for certification.

Cel'lu·loid strip A thin strip of Celluloid used to compress silicate restorations into dental cavities.

ce·ment' In dentistry, an adhesive filling material used for cementing bridges, crowns, and inlays. It is used also as a temporary filling material in certain instances.
  acrylic resin c. A type of autopolymerizing acrylic which is used as a restorative material.
  copper phosphate c. Zinc phosphate cement to which copper oxide has been added; this is thought to impart germicidal qualities to the cement.
  silicate c. A cement commonly employed to fill cavities in the anterior teeth, made of

powdered kaolin, quartz, lime, and magnesia mixed with liquid phosphoric acid.

zinc phosphate c. The cement commonly employed to seal the gold inlays and crowns into place on the teeth and as a base under metallic restorations.

zinc oxide–eugenol c. A sedative cement used as a temporary filling or as a base under restorations, where sedative treatment of the tooth is indicated.

ce·men'to·blast The type of tissue cell that takes part in the formation of cementum.

ce·men'tum The layer of bone deposited on the root of a tooth.

cen'ti·grade Graduated into 100 equal divisions or degrees. Abbreviated, C. (Also, Celsius).

c. thermometer A thermometer graduated to read 0° at the freezing point of water and 100° at the boiling point of water. To convert Fahrenheit to centigrade, the formula is $C = {}^5/_9(F - 32)$. See *Fahrenheit*.

cen'ti·me"ter, cen'ti·me"tre The hundredth part of a meter, equal to 0.3937 (or about $^2/_5$) inch. Abbreviated, cm.

cubic c. The one one-thousandth part of a liter, roughly equivalent to $^1/_{28}$ ounce. Abbreviated, cc.

cen'tric Pertaining to or describing the relationship of the lower jaw (mandible) to the upper jaw (maxilla) when all associated muscles are in balance. This relationship is observed by the dentist to aid in correct placement of the artificial teeth of one denture in relation to the other.

ceph'a·lo·gram" A radiographic headplate.

ceph"a·lo·met'ric Pertaining to measurement of the head.

cer'vi·cal Pertaining to the neck or cervix of a tooth.

cer'vi·cal an'chor·age In orthodontics, a strap of elastic tape with wire hooks that fits around the back of the patient's neck and is used where a force from outside the mouth is desirable in order to move teeth distally.

chan'cre The lesion formed at the site of primary inoculation: usually an ulcer. The term generally refers to the initial lesion of syphilis, although it may be used for the primary focus of certain other diseases.

chei·li'tis (kigh·li'tis) Inflammation of the lips.

chei·lo'sis A disorder of the lips, usually caused by a vitamin deficiency.

chem"o·ther'a·py Prevention or treatment of infective diseases by chemicals which act as antiseptics within the body, without producing serious toxic effects on the patient.

chlor'o·phyll The green coloring matter of plants. In the presence of light it makes carbohydrates, such as starches, from carbon dioxide and water. It is used in the treatment of some infections and as a deodorant.

chron'ic Of long duration; long-continued; not acute.

chron"o·log'ic According to the order of time.

chron"o·log'ic age The actual age of a person in time, counting from the date of birth.

cin'gu·lum The lingual lobe of an incisor tooth which is located in the cervical third of the lingual surface; a bandlike enamel ridge rising crownwise from the cervix and often accentuated to a blunt point or a rudimentary cusp.

cleft pal'ate A congenital defect due to failure of fusion of embryonic facial processes, resulting in a fissure through the palate. This may be *complete*, extending through both hard and soft palates into the nose, or any degree of *incomplete*, or *partial*, cleft.

cle'oid Clawlike; the name given excavating and carving instruments having this type of blade.

clin'ic A place, usually connected with a hospital or medical or dental school, where outpatients can receive treatment.

closed bite See under *bite*.

clot A semisolid coagulum of blood or lymph.

clot To coagulate.

co·ag'u·late A curdle; a clot.

co·ag′u·late To cause to change from a fluid state to a compact, jellylike mass; to solidify.

co·ag′u·lum A clot; a coagulated mass.

coc′cus A round or spherical bacterium whose greatest diameter is not more than twice its shortest. Plural: *cocci*.

co′de·ine A white crystalline alkaloid of opium, used as a narcotic and for relief of pain.

co·he′sion The attractive force between the same kind of molecules, that is, the force which holds the molecules of a substance together.

coil spring *In orthodontics*, a small wire spring wrapped around the main arch wire which is used as a force either to pull teeth together or to push them apart.

col′li·ma″tor A lead ring located in the cone of an x-ray machine which limits the size of the beam of radiation.

col′loid A state of subdivision of matter in which the individual particles are of submicroscopic size and consist either of single large molecules or aggregates of smaller molecules. The dimension of a colloid particle, arbitrarily fixed, is between 1 and 100 millimicrons. Colloids do not actually dissolve but remain suspended in a suitable gas, liquid, or solid.

   hydrophilic c. One capable of combining with, or attracting to it, water to form a stable dispersion.

   hydrophobic c. One incapable of combining with, or attracting to it, water.

col·lo′qui·al Of or pertaining to conversation and informal speech; not literary.

col′o·ny A mass or group of microorganisms in a culture, derived from a single cell. A colony may develop from a single bacterium in 18 hours.

co′ma Profound unconsciousness from which the patient cannot be aroused.

com·mer′cial den′tal lab′o·ra·tor″ies Dental laboratories operated elsewhere than in a dental office, usually as a private enterprise.

com′pen·sate To make good a defect; to counterbalance; to make an equal return to.

com·po′nent den′tal so·ci′e·ty A district dental society, recognized by a state dental society.

com′pound A resinous waxlike material, capable of being molded when heated and used in many ways in dental procedures.

com·pres′sive strength The greatest compression force that can be applied to a material before its rupture.

con·cre′tion 1. *In dentistry*, a deposit on the surface of a tooth. 2. A calculus.

con″den·sa′tion *In dentistry*, the packing of a restorative material into the prepared cavity of a tooth.

con·duc′tor A body or substance that transmits heat, electricity, light, or sound. Gold is a good conductor of heat or cold.

con′dyle Any rounded eminence such as occurs in the joints of many of the bones.

con′dy·loid Resembling a condyle or knuckle.

cone *In radiology*, a conical or tubular device, made of various materials, and attached to the head of the x-ray machine in the path of radiation, which serves as an aid in the determination of the correct angulation of the primary beam of radiation and the proper target-film distance. It also, when made of metal, aids in controlling the size of the beam of radiation.

con·gen′i·tal Existing before or at birth.

con·nec′tor That part of a dental bridge which connects the pontic to the retainer, and which may be rigid or nonrigid.

con·stit′u·ent so·ci′e·ty A state dental society, recognized by the American Dental Association.

con·sult′ant A consulting physician or dentist; specifically, one called in on a given case, by the attending dentist, to give counsel.

con″sul·ta′tion A deliberation between two or more dentists or physicians concerning the diagnosis and the proper method of treatment of a case.

con′tact a′re·a The area of a tooth's surface that touches another.

con·tam′i-nate To make impure as by contact or pollution; to infect with bacteria.

con′tract A written agreement between two or more parties.

con′trast The distinction between the light and dark shadows on a radiograph.

con·vul′sion An involuntary general paroxysm of muscular contraction. It is either *tonic* (without relaxation) or *clonic* (having alternate contractions of opposite groups of muscles).

cool′ant A stream of water or air or an air and water spray, directed on rotary tooth-cutting instruments, to keep the tooth and instrument from overheating and to keep the instrument free of debris.

co′ping A thin metal covering or cap over a tooth prepared for a restoration; a thimble.

   index or **transfer c.** A guide, usually made of plaster, used to reposition teeth, casts, or parts in their original positions and relationships.

cop′y·right″ The exclusive legal right to make and sell a certain book, picture, or device.

co·ro′nal Pertaining to the crown of a tooth.

cor′o·noid Like a beak; as the coronoid process of the mandible.

cor·rode′ To eat or be eaten away; to rust.

cor·ro′sion Process of corroding or the resulting condition.

cor·ro′sive A substance that destroys organic tissue either by direct chemical means or by causing inflammation and suppuration.

cot′ton rolls Small rolls of absorbent cotton used in dentistry to isolate an area in the mouth and thus to prevent saliva from coming in contact with that area. They are manufactured in various lengths and sizes.

C.P. Chemically pure.

cra′ni·al cav′i·ty The space within the skull that contains the brain, its membranes, and blood vessels.

cra′ni·um The part of the skull that contains the brain, its membranes, and vessels.

cross bite See under *bite*.

crown The top part of anything; any structure like a crown.

   artificial c. A cap of metal, plastic, or porcelain processed to cover that portion of the tooth which projects beyond the gum line.

   c. of a tooth That part covered with enamel.

   full-veneer c. A dental restoration that covers in its entirety that part of a tooth exposed to the oral environment.

   three-quarter c., partial-veneer c. A dental restoration that covers all of a tooth exposed to the oral environment except the labial or buccal surface.

crys′tal A colorless, transparent mineral.

crys′tal·line sol′id A solid that has unit particles (atoms or molecules) which take a regular, homogenous, spatial arrangement, called **space lattice.**

cu′bic cen′ti·me″ter The one one-thousandth part of a liter. Abbreviated, cc.

cul′ture The growth of microorganisms on artificial media; also, a group of microorganisms grown in an artificial medium.

   c. medium A substance used for cultivating bacteria. Culture media are either liquid or solid, bouillon and milk being the important liquid media, and gelatin, agar, blood serum, and potato the principal solid media.

   pure c. A growth of bacteria that contains only one species of bacteria; a culture of a single microorganism.

cu·rette′ An instrument, shaped like a spoon or scoop, for scraping away exuberant or dead tissue.

cu·rette′ To scrape with a curette.

cusp A pointed or rounded eminence on or near the masticating surface of a tooth.

   c. of Carabelli The fifth cusp of the upper first permanent molar.

cus′pid A cuspid tooth; a canine tooth; a tooth having one point or cusp.

cu·ta′ne·ous Pertaining to the skin.

cy″a·no′sis A bluish tinge in the color of mucous membrane and skin, due to the presence of excessive amounts of reduced hemoglobin in the capillaries, less frequently to the presence of methemoglobin. *adj.* **cy·a·not′ic.**

cy″clo·pro′pane A colorless gas used as a general anesthetic. It produces rapid and deep anesthesia; it is inflammable and should, therefore, be guarded from contact with a flame or electric spark.

cyst A sac with a distinct wall, containing fluid or other material. It may be a normal or a pathologic structure.

cy·tol′o·gy The subdivision of biology which deals with cells.

dam Rubber dam; a thin sheet of rubber used to isolate individual teeth from the oral environment during dental treatment procedures.

dark′room The room in a dental office where x-ray and photographic films are processed.

DAU Program A training program designed to teach the dentist and the auxiliary to work together with maximum efficiency.

D.D.S. Doctor of Dental Surgery.

DEA United States Department of Justice, Drug Enforcement Administration.

de·bris′ Soft foreign material loosely attached to the surface of a tooth, as the refuse from the drilling of a cavity.

de·cal″ci·fi·ca′tion The withdrawal or removal by acid of the mineral salts of bone or other calcified substance.

de·cid′u·ous Falling off or shed at maturity. Said of the primary dentition.

de·gass′ing The process of driving off impurities from the surface of gold foil by the use of heat; also called *annealing*.

de·lir′i·um A condition of mental excitement, confusion, and clouded sensorium, usually with hallucinations, illusions, and delusions; precipitated by toxic factors in diseases or drugs.

den′si·ty The closeness and compactness of any space distribution.

den′tal Pertaining to the teeth.

den′tal arch The parabolic curve formed by the cutting edges and masticating surfaces of the teeth.

den′tal disc A thin circular piece of paper or other material, such as metal, covered with an abrasive; used for polishing or cutting teeth and restorations.

den′tal floss A fine string used to aid the mechanical cleaning of the interproximal surfaces of the teeth.

den′tal hy′gi·en·ist One who is licensed by law to clean and polish teeth and to instruct in the fundamentals of oral hygiene.

den′tal lab′o·ra·to″ry tech·ni′cian A person trained to perform certain mechanical operations that are necessary in preparing dental appliances and restorations for placement in the mouth.

den′tal pulp The soft vascular tissue that fills the pulp chamber and the root canals of a tooth and that is responsible for its vitality. It consists of connective tissue, blood vessels, and nerves.

den′tal stone An abrasive wheel or mounted point or sphere used for cutting or grinding teeth, fillings, or prosthetic restorations.

den′tal strip A thin cloth, paper, or metal strip, one surface of which has bonded to it an abrasive material, used in cutting or polishing the surfaces of teeth or fillings.

den′tal u′nit A piece of equipment (unit) having lines for water, gas, air, and electricity, an attached cuspidor (bowl with running water), light (designed to reflect light into patient's mouth), and a motor with an extension arm which the dentist uses for various operative procedures.

den′ti·frice A substance, as a paste or a powder, used in the mechanical cleaning of the teeth.

den′tin The calcified tissue that forms the major part of a tooth. Dentin is related to bone but differs from it in the absence of included cells. It is covered by the enamel over the crown of the tooth, by the cementum over the roots, and itself surrounds the pulp chamber and root canals which contain the dental pulp.

den′tist·ry The profession that is concerned with the prevention, diagnosis, and treatment of diseases of the teeth and adjacent tissues, and the restoration of missing dental and oral structures.

operative d. The phase or branch of dentistry that is concerned with the preservation of the natural teeth and their supporting structures and with the restoration of lost tooth structure to a state of normal function and aesthetics.

preventive d. The phase or branch of dentistry dealing with prevention of dental diseases by prophylactic and educational methods.

prosthetic d. The phase or branch of dentistry which deals with the replacement of missing teeth or oral tissues by artificial means. Syn., *prosthodontics.*

den·ti′tion 1. The process of teething; the eruption of the teeth through the alveolar ridge. 2. The character and arrangement of the teeth of an individual.

den′to·le′gal Pertaining to dental jurisprudence.

den′ture The natural or artificial teeth of an individual considered as a unit.

artificial d. A complete artificial replacement of either the upper or the lower teeth.

full d. A replacement of the complete dental equipment of either jaw.

immediate full d. A denture so constructed as to permit some natural teeth to remain in the mouth during its fabrication. When the remaining teeth are removed, the denture is inserted. Hence, the patient is never without teeth of some kind.

den′ture flange That portion of an impression or denture which surrounds the edge and is in contact with the tissues.

der″ma·ti′tis An inflammation of the skin.

der″ma·to′sis Any disease of the skin.

de·ter′gent A drug, compound, or solution used for cleansing wounds or ulcers.

di″a·be′tes A disease characterized by the habitual discharge of an excessive quantity of urine and by excessive thirst; used without qualification, the word means *diabetes mellitus.*

d. mellitus An inheritable, constitutional disease of unknown cause, characterized by the failure of the body tissues to oxidize carbohydrate at a normal rate. It manifests itself in an excess of sugar in the blood, presence of sugar in the urine, and in more advanced stages, acidosis and coma, with symptoms of intense thirst and hunger, weakness, and loss of weight.

di·ag·nose′ To determine the nature of a disease.

di″ag·no′sis The art or the act of determining the nature of a disease; also, the decision reached.

di″ag·nos′tic Pertaining to or serving as evidence in diagnosis.

di″a·pho·ret′ic An agent that increases the secretion of sweat.

di″a·stol′ic Pertaining to the dilatation phase of the cardiac cycle.

die An exact reproduction in metal of any object or cast.

inlay d. An exact reproduction of a prepared tooth in high-strength dental stone or metal.

di′et The customary daily allowance of food and drink taken by any person; also, food and drink prescribed, as to kind and amount, for therapeutic or other purposes.

dig′i·tal Pertaining to the fingers.

dip″lo·coc′cus A micrococcus that occurs in groups of two.

disc′oid Rounded; the name given excavating and carving instruments having this type of blade.

dis·ease′ An illness or sickness; a disturbance

in function or structure of any organ or part of the body.

acute d. One marked by rapid onset and short course.

chronic d. One that is slow in its course and of long duration.

dis"in·fect'ant An agent that destroys or inhibits the microorganisms causing disease.

dis"in·fec'tion The destruction or removal of pathogenic organisms, especially by means of chemical substances.

dis"lo·ca'tion The displacement of one or more bones of a joint or of any organ from the original normal position.

dis'tal Away from the median line, following the curve of the dental arch.

dis"to·clu'sion Occlusion of the teeth in which the mesiobuccal cusp of the upper first molar interdigitates between the lower second bicuspid and the lower first molar.

ditched Said of deficient margins of dental restorations.

di"u·ret'ic An agent that increases the volume of urine.

D.M.D. Doctor of Dental Medicine.

dor'sum 1. The back. 2. Said of the top, or exposed surface, of the tongue.

do·sim'e·ter *In radiology,* an instrument for measuring, usually by ionization methods, exposure to x-rays or to radioactive emanations.

draft See *draw.*

dram A unit of weight equal to one-eighth of an apothecary's ounce or 60 grains: also spelled *drachm.*

draw The taper or divergence of the walls of a tooth preparation for a restoration which is to be cemented; the feature which permits the seating or withdrawal of the restoration.

drug Any substance used as a medicine.

duct A tube or channel, especially one that serves for the passage of excretions or secretions.

duc'tile Capable of being hammered out thin or drawn out into a wire, as gold or copper.

dys·cra'si·a An abnormal state of the body.

blood d. A morbid state of the blood, usually of permanent character.

dysp·ne'a Difficult or labored breathing.

ec"chy·mo'sis Bleeding into the subcutaneous tissues. It is marked by a purple discoloration of the skin, the color gradually changing to brown, green, and yellow.

e·de'ma An excessive accumulation of fluid in the tissue spaces, sometimes called *dropsy.*

e·dem'a·tous Having or characterized by edema.

e·den'tu·lous Without teeth.

ef·fu'sion A pouring out of fluid, either serous, bloody, or purulent, from its natural vessels into other spaces.

e·las'tic lim'it The greatest load that can be applied to a material and have the material return to its original shape when the force is released.

e·las'tics *In orthodontics,* rubber bands used for exerting forces between upper and lower arches or within the same arch to close spaces.

el'e·va'tor An instrument for elevating or lifting a part, or for extracting the roots of teeth.

elon Monomethyl paramidophenol sulfate, used in a solution for developing x-ray film.

em'bo·lus A bit of matter foreign to the bloodstream—it may be a blood clot, air, cancer or other tissue cells, fat, cardiac vegetations, clumps of bacteria, or a foreign body, such as a needle or bullet—that either gains entrance to the circulation of the individual's body or is carried by the bloodstream until it lodges in an artery and obstructs it, causing an **embolism.**

em·bra'sure The space between the sloping proximal surfaces of the teeth. The opening may be toward the cheek (*facial*), toward the lips (*labial*), or toward the tongue (*lingual*).

em"bry·on'ic Of or pertaining to or like an embryo; undeveloped.

e·mol'li·ent A substance used externally to soften the skin.

em·pir′ic, em·pir′i·cal 1. Based on practical observation and not on scientific reasoning or education. 2. In the practice of medicine, reliving solely on experience and not on scientific training and reasoning; charlatanic.

e·mul′sion *In radiology,* a gelatin suspension of silver halide salts; the x-ray–sensitive material which is applied to the cellulose acetate film in the manufacture of x-ray films.

en·am′el The vitreous substance of the crowns of the teeth.

en′do·crine glands Ductless glands that secrete hormones directly into the bloodstream. The adrenals, the thyroid, and the pituitary are among those classified as endocrine glands.

en″do·don′tics That branch of dentistry which deals with the diagnosis and treatment of diseases of the dental pulp and periapical tissues.

en″do·the′li·um The simple squamous epithelium that lines the heart, blood vessels, and lymph vessels.

en″do·tox′in A poisonous product, or toxin, released on the destruction of a bacterial cell. It is heat-stable, generalized in its effect on the animal body, and elicits poor antibody response.

en′gine belt A continuous cord used to transmit motion from the dental engine to the dental handpiece.

en·rich′ment The adding back to foods of nutrients that have been lost in processing of the food, such as vitamin B to grain flours.

en·vi′ron·ment Those external conditions which surround, act upon, and influence an organism or its parts.

en′zyme A catalytic substance formed by living cells and having a specific action in promoting a chemical change.

e′o·sin A bacteriologic stain used for staining specimens for microscopic study.

ep′i·lep″sy A disorder of the central nervous system, characterized by recurring explosive nerve-cell discharges and manifested by transient episodes of unconsciousness or psychic dysfunction, with or without convulsive movements.

ep″i·the′li·um A tissue composed of cells with a minimum of intercellular substance. The outer layer of the skin is composed of epithelium.

ep′o·nym A term, or word, that is formed or derived from the name of a person known or assumed to be the first, or from one who is prominently, connected with anything, as a disease, symptom complex, theory, or invention. A practice which is discouraged by the Principles of Ethics of the American Dental Association.

ep·u′lis Any solitary tumorlike lesion developing from the periosteum of the maxilla or mandible, appearing clinically as a circumscribed swelling beneath the gum.

e″qui·li′brate To be in balance; to balance.

e″qui·li·bra′tion The achievement or maintenance of equilibrium, as of pressure.

  occlusal e. The modification of occlusal form by grinding for equalizing occlusal stress, producing simultaneous occlusal contacts, or harmonizing cuspal relations.

e″qui·lib′ri·um Perfect balance. That condition which is made possible by complete synchronization and harmony between all vital factors.

e·rep′sin An enzyme mixture produced in the intestines that converts proteins to amino acids.

e·ro′sion A localized, progressive decalcification of enamel and dentin, notably on the labial and buccal surfaces of the teeth, causing a hollow or shallow cavity the bottom of which is hard and smooth; probably due to chemical action.

e·rup′tion The act of breaking out, appearing, or becoming visible; the appearance of a tooth through the gums.

er″y·the′ma Abnormal redness of the skin, sometimes occurring in patches.

es·thet′ic pertaining to the senses; also, pertaining to beauty.

es·thet'ics The science of beauty and fine taste.

es·thet'ic try-in Trial fitting of artificial teeth for appearance. When the selected teeth are mounted in wax in a fashion deemed to provide the patient with a definite appearance, the patient is recalled, and these temporarily arranged teeth are placed in the mouth, to ascertain to what extent the desired objectives have been realized. If no changes are needed, the processing of the denture will be initiated. Frequently, however, changes are made to enhance the appearance of the patient before the processing is started.

e'ther A highly volatile, colorless, and inflammable liquid used in dentistry as an anesthetic agent. It is also called **ethyl oxide,** although the United States Pharmacopeia recognizes as **ethyl oxide** a less pure form of the substance for use as a solvent.

eth'i·cal Having to do with standards of right and wrong.

eth'ics A system of moral principles and ideals of human behavior.

    dental e. The principles of professional conduct; duties dentists owe to themselves, their colleagues, their patients, and their fellow human beings.

eth'yl chlo'ride A colorless, inflammable liquid used as a spray for local anesthesia of short duration.

eth'yl·ene A colorless gas of slightly sweet ordor and taste; used as an inhalation anesthetic. A preparation containing not less than 98 percent per volume is used by inhalation for producing surgical anesthesia.

e"ti·ol'o·gy The science or study of the causes of disease and the mode of their operation: not synonymous with cause of disease but often loosely so used.

eu'ge·nol A colorless or pale-yellow liquid having a clove odor and spicy, pungent taste; obtained from clove oil and other sources.

ex·am"i·na'tion Inspection or investigation, especially as a means of diagnosing disease, qualified according to the methods employed, as a physical examination.

ex·fo"li·a'tion A peeling and shedding of a horny layer of skin or of a tooth.

    normal e. time The time at which a primary tooth is expected to become loose and fall out of the child's mouth.

ex"o·don'ti·a, ex"o·don'tics The art and science of the extraction of teeth.

ex"o·don'ti·a sponge A square of folded gauze used to remove blood, mucus, and debris in dental surgery.

ex"os·to'ses Bony outgrowths from the surface of a bone, as localized enlargements of outer cortical plate of maxilla and mandible. Singular: *exostosis.* See also *torus.*

ex"o·ther'mic A substance formed with the liberation of heat.

ex"o·tox'in A toxin that is given off by a living microorganism and can afterward be obtained in bacteria-free filtrates without death or disintegration of the microorganisms. The toxin is readily changed by heat, usually affects a specific tissue, and causes production of large numbers of antibodies.

ex·pec"to·ra'tion The act of spitting.

ex'pert tes'ti·mo"ny 1. A statement or affirmation of fact, as before a court, by a specialist or person of authority on the subject. 2. The act of testifying by a specialist or person of authority.

ex"pi·ra'tion The act of breathing out. *v.* **expire.**

ex·plor'er A hand instrument with a sharp fine tine or tines, used when making an examination of the teeth or dental restorations; a probe.

ex·trac'tion of a tooth The surgical removal of a tooth from the alveolus.

ex·trem'i·ties The arms, hands, legs, and feet.

ex·u'ber·ant Pertaining to or characterized by excessive proliferation or growth of a tissue, as a granulation tissue.

eye'tooth" A canine tooth of the upper jaw.

face′bow 1. A caliper-like device that is used to record the relationship to the maxillae to the temporomandibular joint. 2. A caliper-like device that is used to record the relationship of the jaws to the temporomandibular joint and to orient the casts in this same relationship to the opening axis of an articulator.

fac′ing A manufactured porcelain piece that simulates the facial surface of a natural tooth.

Fahr′en·heit scale The series of graduations on the **Fahrenheit thermometer** upon which the freezing point of water is 32° and the boiling point is 212°. Abbreviated, F. To convert centigrade to Fahrenheit, the formula is $F = 9/5 C + 32$. See *centigrade*.

faint A state of weakness or unconsciousness due to circulatory failure; a swoon.

F.D. & C. An abbreviation for *food, drug,* and *cosmetic,* indicating federal acceptance in accordance with the Food, Drug, and Cosmetic Act.

felt cones and wheels Cones and wheels made of felt, for use on the dental laboratory lathe for polishing various dental appliances.

fes·toon′ Carvings in the base material of an artificial denture, simulating contours of the natural tissues which are being replaced by the denture.

fi′bro·blasts Connective tissue cells found in fibrous tissue, fundamental to all healing processes.

fi·bro′ma A benign tumor composed primarily of white fibrous connective tissue.

fill′ing 1. The material used in closing cavities in carious teeth. 2. The process of inserting, condensing, shaping, and finishing a filling. The term *restoration* and its variants are the preferred terms.

film badge A pack of appropriate film and filters used to determine the amount of radiation exposure to an individual who is occupied within the area of radiation.

fil′ter In *radiology,* a metal disc placed in the path of the x-ray beam, to absorb the undesirable and less penetrating rays.

fil·tra′tion In *radiology,* the effect obtained by the placing of a filter or filters in the path of radiation.

    inherent f. Filtration of the useful beam of radiation due to the window of the x-ray tube and any permanent tube enclosure.

    total f. The sum of the inherent filtration and any added filtration.

fin′ger spring In *orthodontics,* a small wire attachment soldered to the main arch wire which acts as a spring force to move teeth.

fin′ish·ing strip A thin strip of linen-like material with an abrasive incorporated on one side, used to finish fillings and polish interproximal areas of the teeth.

fins Surface roughness of castings due to cracks in the casting mold.

fis′sure A groove or cleft; a fault in the enamel of a tooth caused by imperfect union.

fis′tu·la A narrow tube or canal formed by incomplete closure, as of an abscess, wound, disease process, or (congenitally) a part, usually transmitting some fluid, either pus or the secretions or contents of some organ.

fla·gel′lum A whiplike process: the organ of locomotion of sperm cells and of certain bacteria. Plural: *flagella.*

flask A metal case for containing plaster or stone, in which a denture is placed for processing.

floss A waxed or unwaxed silk or nylon thread, used to clean the interproximal surfaces of the teeth. It may also be used as a ligature to secure a rubber dam to the teeth.

flu″o·ri·da′tion The addition of fluorides to the water supply of a community as an aid in the control of dental caries.

flu′o·ride A salt of hydrofluoric acid. Fluorides, in drinking water, are effective in resisting tooth decay.

flu′o·ro·scope An instrument used for examining the form and motion of the internal structures of the body by means of x-rays.

flux Material added to minerals or metals to promote fusion.

fo'cus The point where rays of light or heat meet, appear to meet, or should meet after being bent by a lens or curved mirror. The principal site of a disease, from which the infection spreads into the circulation and thus throughout the body, is called the **focus of infection.** *adj.* **focal.**

foil A thin sheet of metal, especially gold or tin, used for filling teeth or in dental laboratory work.

fo·ra'men A hole, perforation, or opening, especially in a bone. Plural: *foramens, foramina.*
   mental f. The aperture in the body of the mandible, usually between the two bicuspid teeth, through which pass the mental vessels and nerve.

for'ceps A surgical instrument with two opposing blades or limbs, controlled by handles or by direct pressure on the blades.
   dental f. Any of a variety of forceps adapted for the extraction of teeth.

for"ti·fi·ca'tion The addition of more nutrients to a food than are usually found in the food, such as vitamin D to milk.

fos'sa A depression or pit; specifically, a round or angular depression in the surface of a tooth. Plural: *fossae.*

frac'ture The breaking of a bone or cartilage.

fre·nec"to'my Surgical removal of a frenum.

fre'num A fold of integument or mucous membrane that checks or limits the movements of any organ.
   labial f. The fold of tissue that connects the lip with the gingiva at a point normally in the median line.
   lingual f. The fold of tissue that connects the tongue to the gingiva and the floor of the mouth in the median line.

fun'gus A low form of plant life which includes mushrooms, toadstools, and molds; many are pathogenic for human beings, such as *Candida albicans,* which causes oral and systemic candidiasis (thrush). Plural: *fungi.*

fur'ca The area between the roots of multirooted teeth.

fu'sion The process of melting; the act of uniting or cohering.

g, Gm Abbreviation for gram.

gas The vaporous or airlike state of matter. A fluid that distributes itself uniformaly throughout any space in which it is placed, regardless of its quantity.

gas"tro·in·tes'ti·nal Pertaining to the stomach and intestinal tract.

gel A colloidal system comprising a solid and a liquid phase, which exists as a solid or semi-solid mass.

ge·ner'ic drug Nonproprietary, as of a drug not registered or protected by a trademark.

ge·net'ic Produced by genes; pertaining to the phenomena of heredity and variation; inheritance.

ger"mi·ci'cal Capable of destroying germs.

ger'mi·cide An agent, as a drug or a spray, that destroys germs or bacteria. See also *bactericide.*

ger"o·don'tics The practice of dentistry as it pertains to aged patients.

gin'gi·va That part of the gum which surrounds the tooth and lies close to the crest of the alveolar ridge.
   free g. That portion of the gingiva about the neck of the tooth which is not closely opposed to or attached to the tooth surface. Plural: *gingivae.*

gin'gi·val Of or pertaining to the soft tissues that invest a tooth.
   g. crevice The narrow opening or sulcus between the circumferential soft tissue of the gum and the tooth.
   g. papillae Extensions or projections of gum tissue in the interproximal areas between the teeth.

gin"gi·vec'to·my Excision of a portion of the gingiva to reduce sulcular pockets.

gin"gi·vi·tis Inflammation of the gingiva.

gin'gi·vo·plas"ty The surgical recontouring or reshaping of the gingiva for the achievement of physiologic form.

gin″gi·vo·sto″ma·ti′tis Inflammation of the oral mucosa generally and including the gingival mucosa.

gland A cell, tissue, or organ that elaborates and discharges a substance which is used elsewhere in the body (secretion) or which is eliminated (excretion).

glos·si′tis Inflammation of the tongue.

gom·pho′sis A form of articulation in which a conical process is held by a socket, as a tooth in its supporting bone.

goth′ic arch tracing The graphic registration of jaw movements which indicate the proper relationship of the jaws to permit the accurate setting up of artificial teeth.

gram A unit of weight in the metric system. Abbreviated, g.

gram′-neg′a·tive Remaining unstained by the Gram method for staining bacteria. Microorganisms that are decolored by alcohol or acetone and are red when stained by Gram's method are said to be *gram-negative*.

gram′-pos′i·tive Holding the dye after being stained by the Gram method. Those microorganisms which remain purple when stained by Gram's method and are not decolored by alcohol or acetone are said to be *gram-positive*.

gran″u·la′tion tis′sue Young new connective tissue; the mixture of newly formed capillaries and fibroblasts in connection with inflammation, especially of exudative character, representing the early stages of healing.

gran″u·lo′ma *In dentistry,* a small mass of granulation tissue containing bacterial deposits found on the root of a tooth, or in an edentulous area of the jaw after the removal of a tooth.

groove 1. An elongated depression, as in the surface of a tooth. 2. That portion of a cast which corresponds to the periphery of the impression.

gum The mucous membrane and underlying connective tissue covering the alveolar processes and the necks of erupted teeth. See also *gingiva*.

gut′ta-per′cha The coagulated latex of several Malayan trees, used as a temporary filling material.

gyp′sum Native calcium sulfate, $CaSO_4 \cdot 2H_2O$, which, when deprived of the major portion of its water of crystallization, constitutes plaster of paris.

hal′ide A binary salt in which a halogen serves as anion.

hal′o·gen Any one of the nonmetallic elements chlorine, iodine, bromine, and fluorine.

hand′piece *In dentistry,* an instrument designed to hold burs, stones, and other dental instruments and appliances to permit various operative procedures via slow or high speeds. The straight Doriot handpiece for long-shanked burs and the contra-angle type for short-shanked burs are two examples of handpieces.

hard′ness The resistance of a surface to indentation.

hare′lip″ A cleft, or clefts, in the upper lip, so called from its resemblance to a hare's lip.

height of con′tour The most prominent portion of the axial surface of a tooth in an occlusogingival or incisogingival direction.

hemi″sec′tion The division of the crown and separation of the roots of a tooth for the removal of the diseased or affected part to accomplish endodontic therapy.

he″mo·glo′bin The respiratory pigment of the red blood cells. It is a readily crystallizable protein consisting of hematin and globin and has the reversible property of combining with the releasing oxygen.

hem′or·rhage An escape of blood from the vessels, either through intact walls or by flow through ruptured walls.

he′mo·stat An agent or instrument that arrests the flow of blood.

he″mo·stat′ic Arresting hemorrhage.

he″mo·stat′ic An agent that arrests hemorrhage.

he′red·i·tary Genetically transmitted or capable of being genetically transmitted from parent to offspring.

HMO Health Maintenance Organization.

ho″·mo·ge′ne·ous Having the same nature or qualities; of uniform character in all parts. **Homogeneity** means identity or similarity of structure or kind.

hor′mone A specific chemical product of an organ or of certain cells of an organ, transported by the blood or other body fluids, and having a specific regulatory effect upon cells remote from its origin. Insulin and thyroxin are typical hormones.

host The organic body upon which or in which parasites live.

Hutch′in·son's teeth The notched or pegged teeth seen in patients with congenital syphilis.

hy′dra·ted Combined with water to form a hydrate.

hy·drau·li′cit·y Ability of a cement to harden under water.

Hydrocal A trademark for certain high-strength cements made by superheating gypsum with steam: suitable for molding purposes.

hy″dro·col′loid Any colloidal material wherein water is the dispersion medium. See hydrophilic *colloid*.

 irreversible h. A colloidal solution that changes to a gel by chemical reaction and which cannot be reversed to the liquid condition; e.g., alginate-base impression material.

 reversible h. A colloidal solution that changes to a gel upon cooling and back again to a liquid solution upon heating; e.g., agar-base impression material.

hy″dro·qui·none′ Para-dihydroxybenzene, used in a solution for developing x-ray film.

hy′giene The science that treats of the laws of health and the methods of their observation.

hy′gi·en·ist One who specializes in hygiene.

hy″gro·scop′ic set′ting ex·pan′sion That expansion which occurs in a mix of a gypsum product and water when water, in addition to the mixing water, is allowed to contact the mix during the period of initial set.

hy″per·ce″men·to′sis Excessive formation of cementum.

hy″per·gly·ce′mi·a Excess of sugar in the blood.

hy″per·ker″a·to′sis Retention of the cells of the horny layer of the skin, usually associated with hypertrophy or hyperplasia of the granular and prickle-cell layers.

hy″per·ki·net′ic Pertaining to excessive movement.

hy″per·pla′si·a An excessive formation of tissue; an increase in the size of a tissue or organ due to an increase in the number of cells.

hy″per·sen′si·tive Abnormally sensitive or susceptible, as to the action of allergens.

hy″per·ten′sion Excessive tension, usually synonymous with high blood pressure.

hy·per′tro·phy An increase in size of an organ, independent of natural growth, due to enlargement or multiplication of its constituent cells. It usually connotes accompanying increase in functional capacity.

hyp·not′ic 1. Inducing sleep. 2. Pertaining to hypnotism.

hyp·not′ic 1. A remedy that causes sleep. 2. One who is susceptible to hypnotism; one who is hypnotized.

hy′po Sodium thiosulfate, a constituent of x-ray-film fixing solution.

hy″po·der′mic 1. Pertaining to the region beneath the skin. 2. Placed or introduced beneath the skin.

hy″po·der′mic 1. Injection under the skin. 2. Syringe used in hypodermic injection.

hy″po·gly·ce′mi·a The condition produced by a low level of glucose in the blood.

hy″po·pla′si·a A defective development of any tissue.

hys·te′ri·a A psychoneurotic disorder, characterized by extreme emotionalism involving disturbances of the psychic, sensory, motor, vasomotor, and visceral functions. Frequently a result of repression of conflicts from the conscious mind.

id″i·syn′cra·sy 1. Any special or peculiar characteristic or temperament by which a person differs from other persons. 2. A peculiarity of constitution that makes an individual react differently from most persons to drugs or treatments.

im″bi·bi′tion A process of sorption of water by a gel which is lacking in water content.

im·mune′ Not susceptible; protected from attack; especially, exempt from an attack of a disease.

im·mu′ni·ty The condition of a living organism whereby it resists and overcomes infection.

   acquired i. That obtained by a living organism as the result of active or passive immunity.

   active i. That possessed by an organism as the result of disease or unrecognized infection, or that induced by immunization with bacteria or products of bacterial growth.

   natural i. That which is inborn, either from the mother or the race.

   passive i. 1. That conferred through the parenteral injection of antibodies prepared in the lower animals or other human beings. This gives immediate protection but is effective for only a few months. 2. That acquired by the child in utero by the placental transfer of antibodies from the mother.

im·mu″no·log′ic 1. Of or pertaining to immunity. 2. Forming an immunity.

im″mu·nol′o·gy The science and study of immunity, its characteristics, and the methods by which it is developed.

im·pres′sion A mold, usually of a jaw or its parts, from which a cast is made. Materials employed commonly include plaster of paris, wax mixtures, hydrocolloids, and rubber-like compounds.

   plaginate i. A relationship impression taken in a combination of quick-set plaster and alginate.

   relationship i. One taken to establish the relationship of abutment teeth.

im·pres′sion trays Metal or plastic trays used to contain and hold the impression material while taking an impression.

in·ci′sal Cutting; pertaining to the cutting edges of incisor and cuspid teeth.

in·ci′sor A cutting tooth; one of the four front teeth of either jaw.

in′cu·ba″tor A laboratory cabinet with controlled temperature for the cultivation of bacteria or for facilitating biologic tests.

in′dex See *coping*.

indicator tape A type of heat-sensitive tape used to seal or to identify sterilized packets of instruments and materials; the tape changes color when subjected to sterilization.

in″di·rect′ trans·mis′sion Method of transmission of disease from one individual to another through contaminated materials or objects such as urine, stools, food, and drinking glasses.

in′du·ra·ted Hardened.

in·fec′tion 1. The implantation of an infective agent; also, the microorganism or bacteria implanted. 2. The communication of disease from one person to another or from one part of the body to another.

in·fe′ri·or Lower.

in″fra·or′bit·al Beneath or below the floor of the orbit.

in·ha′lant 1. One who inhales. 2. That which is inhaled, as a medicine.

in·ha′lant Of or related to a drug used for inhaling.

in·her′ent Innate; natural to the organism.

in·i′tial cen′tric A centric determination made by the dentist, usually without the use of mechanical aids, that is fairly accurate and is commonly utilized in the final process of establishing true centric. See centric *occlusion*.

in·lay″ A dental restoration shaped to the form of a cavity and then inserted and secured with cement.

in″or·gan′ic Not organic; not produced by animal or vegetable organisms.

in″spi·ra′tion The act of breathing in.

in′su·la″tor Any nonconducting material used to prevent loss or transference of heat, sound, or electricity.

in′te·gra″ted Unified into a single whole.

in″ter·cusp′ing The correct occlusion of the cusps of the teeth of one jaw with the corresponding depression in the occlusal surfaces of the teeth in the opposite jaw.

in″ter·den′tal Located or placed between the teeth.

   i. papilla The free gingiva that lies between two teeth.

in″ter·dig″i·ta′tion *In dentistry,* in closure of the posterior teeth, the striking of the cusps of one denture fairly into the occluding sulci of the other denture. *v.* **interdigitate.**

in″ter·prox′i·mal Between the proximal surfaces of two adjacent teeth.

in″tra·mus′cu·lar Within the substance of a muscle, as an intramuscular injection. Abbreviated, I.M., i.m.

in″tra·ve′nous Within or into a vein, as an intravenous injection. Abbreviated, I.V., i.v.

in·unc′tion 1. The act of rubbing an oily or fatty substance into the skin. 2. The substance used.

in·vest′ *In dentistry* to embed a pattern or appliance in a refractory material for the purpose of making a casting or to carry out a soldering procedure.

in·vest′ment A sheath; a covering; specifically, a plaster-like material in which inlays, crowns, and dentures are enclosed during casting and soldering.

i″on·i·za′tion Electrolytic dissociation; the production of ions.

ir·ra″di·a′tion Exposure to radiation of varying wavelengths, such as infrared, ultraviolet, roentgen rays, or gamma rays.

I.V. Intravenous; a route of drug administration.

ju″ris·pru′dence The science of law, its interpretation and application.

ju′ve·nile Pertaining to youth or childhood; young, immature.

kil′o·gram A unit of mass and weight, being 1000 grams or 2.2046 pounds avoirdupois. Abbreviated, kg.

kVp Kilovolt peak.

la′bi·al Of or pertaining to the lips; toward the lips.

lab′o·ra·to″ry A place fitted up for experimental work; a room in a dental office or an independent business where prosthetic and other operative services or techniques are performed on models or instruments.

lab′o·ra·to″ry stone A substance similar to plaster of paris, used to produce casts from impressions in the dental laboratory. Casts made from stone are harder than those made from ordinary laboratory plaster.

lac″er·a′tion 1. A tear. 2. The act of tearing or lacerating.

lac·ta′tion 1. The period during which the child is nourished from the breast. 2. The formation or secretion of milk.

la′i·ty Nonprofessional people, as distinguished from those in any professional group.

lam′i·nar Arranged in layers.

lan′cet A small, pointed surgical knife.

land a′re·a That portion of a cast which is outside that of the impression of the mouth.

lan′o·lin Hydrous wool fat, used as a vehicle for medicines that are to be applied to the skin.

le′sion Any alteration of the structure of a tissue or of functional capacity due to injury or disease.

leu·ke′mi·a A disease of the blood-forming organs characterized by uncontrolled proliferation of the leukocytes.

leu′ko·cyte One of the colorless, more-or-less amoeboid cells of the blood, having a nucleus and cytoplasm; a white blood cell.

leu″ko·pla′ki·a A disease or condition characterized by a whitish thickening of the mucous membrane.

lig′a·ment A band of flexible, tough, dense white fibrous connective tissue connecting the articular ends of the bones and sometimes enveloping them in a capsule.

lig′a·ture wire *In orthodontics,* a fine wire used to tie the main arch wire into the brackets on the bands or to the teeth.

lin′e·ar Of, pertaining to, or in a line; made of lines; long and narrow.

lin′gual (ling′gwal) Of or pertaining to the tongue; toward the tongue; on the tongue side.

   l. bar A metal bar fitting to the tongue side of the lower anterior incisors and attached to the denture base (saddle) of a lower partial denture.

lin′i·ment An oily solution of medicaments to be applied to the skin by gentle friction.

lo′cal Restricted to or pertaining to one spot or part; not general.

lute To seal.

mac′ro·tooth An unusually large tooth.

ma·laise′ A general feeling of illness, discomfort, or uneasiness.

ma′lar Pertaining to the cheek or to the cheekbone.

ma·lig′nant Threatening life, as cancer; bad.

mal″e·a·bil′i·ty The quality or state of being malleable.

mal′le·a·ble Capable of being beaten or rolled into thin sheets without being broken.

mal″oc·clu′sion Any deviation from normal occlusion of the teeth, usually associated with abnormal developmental growth of the jaws.

mal·prac′tice Criminal neglect or improper medical or surgical treatment of a patient through carelessness, ignorance, or intent.

man′di·ble The lower jawbone.

man·dib′u·lar Pertaining to the mandible.

man′drel A shank or spindle designed to fit a dental engine handpiece for the purpose of carrying a revolving instrument.

mar′gin The boundary or edge of a surface.

mar′gin·al ridge A ridge or elevation of enamel forming the margin of a surface of a tooth; specifically, one on the mesial or distal borders of the lingual surfaces of anterior teeth and the occlusal surface of posterior teeth.

mas′ti·cate To chew.

mas″ti·ca′tion The act of chewing.

ma·te′ri·a al′ba A soft cheeselike white deposit on the necks of teeth and adjacent gums, made up of epithelial cells, leukocytes, bacteria, and molds.

ma·te′ri·a med′i·ca That branch of medical science which deals with the sources and preparations of substances used in medicine.

ma′trix 1. A mold. 2. *In dentistry,* any material that is used to supply a missing wall of a cavity in order to retain a filling material while in a plastic state.

   m. retainer A mechanical device to hold the matrix in place.

mat″u·ra′tion The process of bringing or of coming to full development.

ma·tu′ri·ty Full development; ripeness.

max·il′la The bone of the skull that supports the upper teeth. Commonly, the term is used to denote the upper jaw with its teeth, when present, and associated soft tissues. Plural: *maxillae.*

max′il·lar″y Pertaining to the maxilla.

max′i·mum The greatest possible degree or amount of anything; the greatest actual effect; the highest point attainable.

me′di·an Situated or placed in the middle of the body or in the middle of a part of the body.

me·dic′a·ment A substance such as a medicine or liniment.

med′i·cine 1. Any substance used for treating disease. 2. The science of treating disease; the healing art.

me′di·um *In bacteriology,* a substance used for the cultivation of bacteria; a culture. Plural: *media.*

mel′a·nin A group of black or dark brown pigments which occur in the skin and mucous membranes, normally and abnormally.

melt′ing (hot) plate A square flat piece of metal with a handle that, after it has been heated, is used to melt wax from the occlusal surface of the wax rims.

men′o·pause The physiologic cessation of menstruation, usually between the forty-fifth and fiftieth years. Also called *climacteric.*

men′tal Of or pertaining to the mind.

men′tal Of or pertaining to the chin.
   m. foramen See under *foramen.*

mer′cu·ry A shining, silver-white, liquid, volatile, metallic element; quicksilver: used in dentistry to mix with silver alloy to form an amalgam for filling cavities in teeth.

me′si·al Toward the median line following the curve of the dental arch.

me″si·o·clu′sion Occlusion of the teeth in which the mesiobuccal cusp of the upper first molar interdigitates between the lower first and second molars.

me·tab′o·lism The phenomena of synthesizing foodstuffs into complex tissue elements and complex substances into simple ones in the production of energy.
   basal m. The minimum amount of energy expenditure necessary to maintain cellular activity when the body is at complete rest in a warm atmosphere 12 to 18 hours after the intake of food.

met′al A chemical element that ionizes positively in solution.

met′al·loid A chemical element such as carbon, silicon, and boron that does not ionize positively in solution but that has many characteristics of metals under certain circumstances.

met·as′ta·sis The transfer of disease from a primary site to a distant one by dissemination of the causative agent or cells through the blood vessels or lymph channels.

mi′ca A heat-resistant silicate mineral occurring in the form of thin, shining, transparent scales.

mi′crobe A microorganism; fungus, bacterium, or virus.

mi″cro·bi·ol′o·gy The study of microscopic forms of life that includes fungi, bacteria, and viruses.

mi′cron The one-thousandth part of a millimeter, or the one-millionth part of a meter. Symbol, μ.

mi″cro·scop′ic Visible only with the aid of the microscope.

mi′cro·tooth An unusually small tooth.

mil″li·am′me·ter A gauge or ammeter that records electric current in milliamperes.

mil′li·li′ter The one-thousandth part of a liter, for all practical purposes equivalent to a cubic centimeter. Abbreviated, ml.

mil′li·me″ter One one-thousandth of a meter. Abbreviated, mm.

min′er·al An inorganic compound occurring in nature, which is neither plant nor animal.

ml Abbreviation for milliliter.

mm Abbreviation for millimeter.

mod′el A reproduction in plaster or metal of any object, as a tooth or the dental arch, made by pouring the material into an impression taken from that object. See also *cast.*
   m. trimmer Mechanical device for shaping the base of a model or cast.

mod′u·lar Sectional. A term applied to a design of cabinetry in the dental operatory, consisting of individual components adaptable to different functional combinations or arrangements.

mo′lar A grinding tooth; a grinder.

mold Any of those fungi which form slimy or cottony growth on foodstuffs, leather, etc.

mold 1. A hollow form in which anything is shaped or cast. 2. The form or shape of an artificial tooth or bridge facing.

mold guide A set of artificial teeth, demonstrating available variations in the shape and size of the teeth of a given manufacture, to enable the dentist to choose a desired form.

mol'e·cule 1. A minute mass of matter. 2. The smallest quantity into which a substance can be divided and retain its characteristic properties; the smallest quantity that can exist in a free state. *adj.* **molecular.**

mon'i·tor·ing *In radiology,* the periodic or continuous evaluation of the radiation dose received by a person.

mon'o·mer The liquid that is used in mixing acrylic resin cement and denture-base material.

Monsel's solution Ferric subsulfate solution, used to control hemorrhage.

mor·bid'i·ty The quality or state of being diseased.

mor·phol'o·gy The branch of biology that deals with structure and form. It includes the anatomy, histology, and cytology of the organism at any stage of its life history.

mor'tar and pes'tle *In dentistry,* a small ground-glass bowl and matching rod used to triturate silver alloy and mercury to produce amalgam.

mot'tled en·am'el A dappled condition of the enamel of the teeth caused by the ingestion of too high a concentration of fluorides during the formative period; **chronic dental fluorosis.**

mounts Supports, backings, or settings on or in which something is to be mounted or fixed, as radiographic mounts.

mouth mir'ror A small mirror attached to a removable handle, used to reflect light and observe surfaces of the teeth.

mu"co·cu·ta'ne·ous Pertaining to a mucous membrane and the skin and to the line where these join.

mu"co·gin'gi·val Pertaining to the gingiva and adjacent reflected oral mucosa.

mu·co'sa A mucous membrane, such as lines the entire oral cavity.

mu'cous Relating to mucus; secreting mucus, as mucous gland; depending on the presence of mucus.

mu'cus The viscid liquid secreted by mucous glands.

mul'ti·ple-root'ed having more than one root.

mu"ri·at'ic ac'id An old term for hydrochloric acid, HCl.

NADL National Association of Dental Laboratories.

nar·cot'ic Producing stupor.

nar·cot'ic 1. A drug, such as opium, chloral, or cannabis, that produces stupor, complete insensibility, or sleep. There are three main groups: the opium group which produces sleep, the belladonna group which produces illusions and delirium, and the alcohol group which produces exhilaration and sleep. 2. An individual addicted to the use of narcotics.

na'sal Pertaining to the nose.

Nasmyth's mem'brane The transitory remnants of the enamel organ and oral epithelium covering the enamel of the tooth after eruption.

na'tal Native; associated with one's birth.

nau'se·a A feeling of sickness at the stomach with aversion to food and an inclination to vomit.

ne·cro'sis The pathologic death of a cell or group of cells in contact with living cells.

ne·crot'ic Relating to necrosis.

nee'dle A sharp-pointed steel instrument of various shapes, sizes, and edges, used for puncturing or for sewing tissue.

   hypodermic n. A hollow needle, used with a hypodermic syringe for injecting liquids into tissues.

   suture n. A curved needle with an eye for carrying suture material, used for suturing or closing incisions.

neg'a·tive 1. Denying; contradicting; opposing. 2. Not indicating a suspected disease or condition, as a negative test.

ne"o·na'tal Pertaining to the newborn; a term applied to infants up to 2 or 3 days of age.

ne'o·plasm Any new growth; a tumor.

neu·ro·lep"tic an"al·ge'sia A state of altered consciousness produced by a combination of one or more tranquilizer-type drugs with an analgesic, allowing painless surgery to be carried out on a wakeful subject.

neut′ro·clu″sion Occlusion of the teeth in which the mesiobuccal cusp of the upper first molar interdigitates with the buccal groove of the lower first molar.

N.F. Abbreviation for National Formulary.

NHSC National Health Service Corps.

nib The working face or end of a condensing instrument.

ni′tro·gen A gaseous element; a colorless, odorless, tasteless gas that forms about 77 percent of the air by weight.

ni′trog′en·ous Containing nitrogen.

ni′trous ox′ide *In dentistry,* a colorless gas, used as a general anesthetic for the performance of uncomplicated operations; also called *laughing gas* and *nitrogen monoxide.*

N.N.R. Abbreviation for *New and Nonofficial Remedies,* a book describing articles, such as drugs, that have been approved by the Council on Pharmacy and Chemistry of the American Medical Association.

no′men·cla″ture Terminology; a system of distinctive names used in the classification of any science or art.

nu′cle·us The differentiated central protoplasm of a cell; its trophic center.

nu·tri′tion The utilization of what is eaten in providing growth, maintenance, and repair of tissues and energy requirements.

oc·clude′ To close; specifically, to close so that the cusps of the posterior teeth fit together.

oc·clu′sal Of or pertaining to occlusion.

  o. surface The surface of occlusal contact; the chewing or grinding surface of a tooth.

oc·clu′sion 1. A closing or shutting up. 2. The state of being closed or shut. 3. The full meeting or contact in a position of rest of the masticating surfaces of the upper and lower teeth: erroneously called *articulation.*

  centric o. The relation of the incisal edges and the inclined planes of the teeth when the jaws are closed in the position of rest.

o″don·tal′gia Toothache.

o·don′to·blast One of the cells covering the dental papilla or dental pulp and responsible for dentin formation.

o″don·to′ma A tumor that develops from one or more parts of a tooth germ. The resulting tissue may be soft or calcified, or a mixture of both.

o″don·to·path′ic Conducive to the development of dental disease.

o·pac′i·ty The condition of being impervious to light.

o·paque′ Not transparent; not letting light through.

open bite See under *bite.*

op″er·a′tion Anything done or performed, especially with instruments; a surgical procedure.

op′er·a·tor″y An operating or treatment room in a dental office.

oph″thal·mol′o·gist One skilled or specializing in the science of the anatomy, physiology, and diseases of the eye.

o′pi·um The dried juice from unripe capsules of the poppy; a narcotic. It contains a number of alkaloids of which morphine is the most important.

op′so·nin A substance, occurring in blood serum, which is necessary to prepare bacteria for phagocytosis. It occurs normally and may be increased by immunization.

op′ti·mum The temperature or other conditions at which vital processes are carried on with the greatest activity.

o′ral Pertaining to the mouth.

  o. cavity The cavity of the mouth.

  o. hygiene The laws of health as applied to the mouth.

  o. pathology That branch of pathology dealing especially with the oral cavity.

  o. surgery That branch of surgery dealing with operative procedures as related to the teeth and jaws.

or'bit The bony cavity containing the eye.

or·gan'ic Having, pertaining to, or characterized by organs; pertaining to living substances; affecting the structure of organs.

oro·phar'ynx The upper part of the throat seen through the oral cavity.

or"tho·don·tics The branch of dentistry that deals with malocclusion; the prevention and correction of irregularities of the teeth and dental arches.

   preventive o. The application of any dental procedures that are necessary to maintain the health of the teeth and surrounding tissues and to maintain normal occlusion.

os·mo'sis The passage of a solvent through a membrane from a dilute solution to a more concentrated one.

os'te·o·clasts" Giant multinucleated cells capable of destroying bone.

os"te·o·ma·la'ci·a Osteoporosis resulting from lowered calcium absorption from the intestine, due usually to vitamin D deficiency.

os"te·o·po·ro'sis An enlargement of the spaces of bone whereby a porous appearance is produced. The loss of bony substance results in brittleness or softness of the bones.

o'ver·head" ex·pense' Expense incurred in running a business or an office, such as for lights, water, heat, rent, and office help.

ox"i·da'tion The process of combining with oxygen.

ox"i·di'zing a'gent A substance that produces oxidation.

ox'y·gen A colorless, tasteless, odorless gas, constituting one-fifth of the atmosphere, eight-ninths of water, and about one-half of the crust of the globe; it supports combustion and is essential to life of animals.

P.A.C. *In psychology,* parent ego state, adult ego state, child ego state.

pal'a·tal Of or pertaining to the roof of the mouth.

pal'ate The roof of the mouth.

pal'a·tine Of or pertaining to the palate.

pal'li·a·tive treat'ment Treatment that relieves pain or prevents a condition from becoming worse, but which does not cure it.

pal'lor Paleness, especially of the skin and mucous membranes.

pal·pa'tion *In diagnosis,* examination of a body part by fingers or hand to determine its characteristics or condition.

pan'o·ram'ic A term applied to any one of several techniques for making an x-ray picture of all the teeth and contiguous structures on a single film.

pap"il·lo'ma A neoplastic growth of surface epithelium, clinically having a white, warty-like appearance.

par"a·den'tal per·son·nel' Auxiliary personnel.

pa·ral'y·sis Loss of muscle function or of sensation, caused by injury to nerves or by destruction of neurons.

par"a·med'i·cal per·son·nel' Auxiliary personnel.

pa·rot'id Situated near the ear, as the parotid gland.

pa·ru'lis Abscess of the gum; incorrectly, gumboil.

pat'ent A legal grant to a person by which that person alone is allowed to make, use, or sell an invention for a certain number of years.

path"o·gen'e·sis The course of development of disease, including the sequence of processes or events from inception to the characteristic lesion or disease.

path"o·gen'ic Disease-producing; able to produce disease.

pa·thol'o·gy That branch of biologic science which deals with the nature of disease, through study of its causes, its process, and its effects, together with the associated alterations of structure and function.

pe"do·don'tics That branch of dentistry which deals with the teeth and oral conditions of children.

pel·la'gra A deficiency disease marked by eruption on the skin, a nervous condition, and sometimes insanity, caused by an improper diet, niacin deficiency, and incomplete proteins.

pen′ny·weight″ A weight of 24 grains.

per·cus′sion *In diagnosis,* the light tapping of a tooth with an instrument to identify periapical tenderness.

per′fo·rate To pierce with holes.

per″i·ap′i·cal Surrounding the apex of a tooth.

per″i·cor′o·nal Pertaining to the tissue or area immediately surrounding the crown of a tooth.

per″i·cor″o·ni′tis Inflammation of the tissue surrounding the coronal portion of the tooth, usually a partially erupted third molar.

per″i·o·don′tal Surrounding a tooth, as the periodontal membrane.

p. ligament The connective tissue between the root of a tooth and the bone of the alveolar process, or extending from the root into the gingiva. Radiographically it appears as a dark thin line around the circumference of the tooth root.

per″i·o·don′tics That branch of dentistry which deals with the prevention and treatment of diseases of the bone and soft tissues surrounding the teeth.

per″i·o·don·ti′tis Inflammation of the periodontium.

per″i·o·don′ti·um The investing and supporting tissues surrounding a tooth; namely, the periodontal ligament (membrane), the gingiva, and the alveolar bone.

per″i·o·don·to′sis Degenerative destruction of the investing and supporting tissues surrounding a tooth, characterized by noninflammatory degeneration of connective tissue of the periodontal ligament.

per″i·os′te·um The tough fibrous membrane that surrounds and adheres to all surfaces of bones except the articular extremities and certain points of attachment for tendons or ligaments where cartilage takes its place.

pe·riph′er·al Pertaining to the circumference or external surface of anything.

per′ma·nent Lasting; fixed; enduring, as permanent teeth.

pet′ty cash A cash fund maintained for the purchase of miscellaneous low-cost items where the ordinary use of checks is impracticable.

PFM A restoration that consists of porcelain fused to metal.

pH Hydrogen-ion concentration. The numerical expression of relative acidity or alkalinity of a solution; above 7 is alkaline; below 7, acid.

phag″o·cy·to′sis The engulfing of bacteria or other antigens by certain cells.

phar″ma·col′o·gy The science of the nature and properties of drugs, particularly their actions.

phar″ma·co·pe′ia, phar″ma·co·poe′ia A collection of formulas and methods for the preparation of drugs; especially, a book of such formulas recognized as a standard, as the United States Pharmacopeia or the British Pharmacopoeia.

phe′nol (fee′nole) A product of coal tar that is caustic in action and serves as a powerful antiseptic, disinfectant, germicide, and poison; carbolic acid.

p. coefficient A figure representing the relative strength of an antiseptic, as compared with phenol acting on the same organism and for the same length of time.

pho·net′ics The science dealing with the mode of production of speech sounds.

phys′i·cal 1. Pertaining to nature; pertaining to the body of material things. 2. Pertaining to physics.

phy·si′cian A doctor of medicine; a person authorized to practice medicine.

phys″i·o·log′ic Pertaining to physiology or to the natural and normal functions of the body and its organs and parts.

p. age The age of an individual as evidenced by functional development, irrespective of chronologic age.

phys″i·ol′o·gy The science that treats of the functions of living organisms or their parts.

dental p. The study of the normal function of the teeth and their supporting structures.

pick'le *In metal work,* a bath, as of acid, to cleanse the surface of castings.

pick'ling The process of heating and acid treating a metal casting in order to remove oxides and impurities acquired during the casting process.

pit An indentation; a depression.

pla'gin·ate A combined plaster and alginate impression material used in coping transfer procedures.

plaque A patch.
   dental p. The bacterial plaque that forms on the crowns of teeth.

plashy Colloquial for wet or sloppy.

plas'ter Specifically, plaster of paris, which, when mixed with water in the proper ratio and in a prescribed fashion, forms a soft mass. It will remain in this state for a definite time during which it can be placed in a variety of molds. Subsequently, it hardens in the mold to produce a copy, or a cast, of the original from which the mold was made.
   p. of par'is Calcined gypsum or calcium sulfate, used for making molds, impressions, and casts.

plas'tic Capable of being molded; hence, pliable.

plas'ti·ciz"er A substance incorporated in an organic formulation or substances to maintain it in a plastic condition.

ple"o·mor'phic Having many shapes, varying in shape and size.

plex'us A network, chiefly of interlacing nerves or blood vessels.

pli'ers Small tong-jawed pincers or tweezers, used for bending metals or holding small objects.
   contouring p. Pincers used for shaping and molding, as dental crowns, bands, or matrices.
   cotton p. Small pincers used for placing cotton pellets in cavities or applying medicaments to areas in the oral cavity.

plug'ger A condenser. Any instrument used for condensing amalgam or gold foil.

pneu·mat'ic Pertaining to gas or air; moved or worked by the pressure of air.

p.o. Per oral; by mouth.

pol'y·mer The powder that is used in mixing acrylic resin cement and denture base material.

pol'y·mer·ize To change (by union of two or more molecules of the same kind) into another compound having the same elements in the same proportion but with a higher molecular weight and different physical properties.

pol"y·neu·ri'tis Simultaneous involvement of several nerves, due to poisons or diseases.

pon'tic That portion of a dental bridge which replaces the missing tooth or teeth.

por'ce·lain restoration A term sometimes used for silicate restoration or cement.

po'si·tion·er *In orthodontics,* a device worn over the teeth to maintain their positions after treatment.

postdam The area of an upper artificial denture base which is built up in order to create a pressure along the junction of the hard and soft palates to aid in the retention of the denture.

pos·te'ri·or Situated behind or toward the rear.
   p. palatal seal The postdam.

post·na'tal Occurring after birth.

post·op"er·a·tive Occurring after an operation; following closely upon an operation.

prac'tice The routine application of the principles of medicine or dentistry to the diagnosis and treatment of disease.

pre·cede' To come before.

pre"ma·ture' Occurring before the proper time; too soon.

pre·mo·lar One of the two teeth between the canine and the first molar in each quadrant of the adult human dentition; a bicuspid. The premolars replace the deciduous molars.

pre·na'tal Occurring before birth.

pre·scribe' To recommend the use of a certain remedy; to direct the dosage, preparation, and dispensing of a drug or remedy, usually in writing.

pre·scrip'tion Written instructions designating the preparation and use of substances to be administered.

pri'mary beam The radiation emanating directly from the focal spot of the target of an x-ray tube and which, for the most part, emerges through the opening of the tube housing directly behind the pointer cone.

primate spaces In the primary dentition, spaces mesial to maxillary cuspids and distal to mandibular cuspids.

pri'vate prac'tice Practice, such as rendering dental treatment or service, without public (governmental) control or ownership.

pro·ce'dure A particular course or mode of action.

proc'ess A prominence or outgrowth, as the alveolar process.
   alveolar p. 1. The border of the maxilla in which the alveoli, or bony sockets of the upper teeth, are embedded. 2. The border of the mandible in which the alveoli of the lower teeth are embedded.

pro·fes'sion An occupation requiring specialized education, such as law, dentistry, medicine, teaching, or the ministry.

pro·gnath'ic Anterior deviation of the mandible; "juttjawed."

pro·lif'er·a'tion A multiplying, as by cellular division; an increase.

pro"phy·lac'tic o"don·tot'o·my The technique of opening and filling structural imperfections of the enamel to prevent dental caries.

pro"phy·lax'is Prevention of disease; measures preventing the development or spread of disease. *adj.* and *n.* **prophylactic.**
   dental p. The control of dental and oral diseases by preventive measures, especially the mechanical cleansing of the teeth.

proprietary drug A drug, the manufacture of which is limited or controlled by an owner because of a patent, copyright, or secrecy as regards its constitution or manufacture.

pros'the·sis 1. Replacement or substitution. 2. An artificial substitute for a missing part, as a denture, a hand, an eye, etc. Plural: *prostheses.*
   dental p. A denture, crown, or bridgework that replaces missing teeth.

pros·thet'ic Pertaining to prosthesis.

pros·tho·don'tics That branch of dentistry which deals with the replacement of missing teeth or oral tissues by artificial means, such as crowns, bridges, and artificial dentures.

pro·tec'tive bar'ri·er Barrier of attenuating materials used to reduce radiation exposure to all persons in the area except the subject.

pro'to·plasm The viscid material constituting the essential substance of living cells, upon which all the vital functions of nutrition, secretion, growth, reproduction, irritability, and motility depend.

pro·vid'er In third-party payment plans, the dentist or dental group delivering dental care.

prox'i·mal Nearest to the body, or to the median line of the body, or to a point considered as the center of a system. *In dentistry,* the **proximal surface** of a tooth is that surface next to the adjacent tooth.

psi Pounds per square inch.

psy·che (sigh'kee) The mind or self as a functional entity, serving to adjust the total organism to the needs or demands of the environment.

psy'chic Pertaining to the mind or psyche.

psy"cho·gen'ic Originating in the mind.

psy·chol'o·gy The science that deals with the functions of the mind.

pty'a·lin (tie'a·lin) An enzyme, found in the saliva, that converts starch to dextrin, maltose, and glucose.

pub'lic health den'tis·try Dentistry concerned with the dental health of the people.

pulp The soft part in the interior of an organ, as the pulp of a tooth. *adj.* **pulpal.**
   p. capping A protective material, such as dental cement or metal foil, placed over an exposed portion of the pulp of a tooth in a deep-seated cavity or fractured tooth.

p. stone A hard, calcified nodule found in the pulp of a tooth.

pulp·ect′o·my The complete removal of the dental pulp, vital or partially vital, from the pulp chamber and root canals; sometimes called *extirpation of the pulp*.

pulp·i′tis Inflammation of the dental pulp.

pulp·ot′o·my An operation by which the bulbous or crown portion of a dental pulp is removed.

pum′ice A substance of volcanic origin, used in powdered form as a polishing material.

pus A semifluid creamy-yellow or greenish yellow product of inflammation, composed mainly of leukocytes and serum.

py·e′mi·a A disease due to the presence of pyogenic microorganisms in the blood and the formation, wherever these organisms lodge, of abscesses.

py″o·gen′ic Of or pertaining to the formation of pus.

py″or·rhe′a A purulent discharge; especially, progressive inflammatory and degenerative changes in the periodontium, usually characterized by purulent discharge from the alveoli of the teeth. The term is more colloquial than scientific.

q.s. An abbreviation for *quantum sufficit* meaning *as much as suffices*.

quack A pretender to medical or dental skill.

ques″tion·naire′ A list of questions designed for compiling information on a specific subject and for a specific purpose.

ra·chit′ic Affected with, resembling, or produced by rickets.

ra″di·a′tion *In physics,* the emission and propagation of energy through space or through a material medium in a form having certain characteristics of waves, including the energy commonly described as electromagnetic and that of sound; usually, electromagnetic radiation, classified, according to frequency, as Hertzian, infrared, visible, ultraviolet, x-ray, and gamma ray; also, by extension, such corpuscular emissions as alpha and beta particles and cosmic rays.

    primary beam of r. See *primary radiation*.

    primary r. The original *radiation* as defined above.

    scattered r. Radiation that, during passage through matter, has been deviated in direction. It may also have been modified by a decrease in energy.

    secondary r. Radiation emitted by any irradiated material.

    useful beam of r. See *useful beam*.

ra′di·o·ac·tiv′i·ty A property of certain substances, such as radium, of spontaneously emitting radiant energy that can penetrate most matter that is opaque to ordinary light rays.

ra′di·o·graph″ An x-ray photograph. Also called *radiograph*.

ra″di·ol′o·gy That branch of medicine which deals with radioactive substances, x-rays, and other ionizing radiations and with their utilization in the diagnosis and treatment of disease.

ra″di·o·lu′cent Pertaining to or designating a tissue or material that is partly or wholly nonresistant to the passage of x-rays.

ra″di·o·paque′ Pertaining to or designating a tissue or material that is resistant to the passage of x-rays.

ra′mus A branch, as of an artery, bone, nerve, or vein; the ascending branch at each end of the lower jawbone. Plural: *rami*.

RDA Recommended Daily Dietary Allowance, Food and Nutrition Board, National Academy of Sciences–National Research Council.

ream′er *In endodontics,* an instrument used to clean and enlarge root canals.

re·cep′tion·ist The employed person who receives or greets patients, obtains routine information for them, and usually performs other duties of the business office.

re·cep′tion room The room of the dental office where patients are received; also called *waiting room,* which term may be bad usage from a psychologic viewpoint.

rec'ord An official document for the preservation of information. Information may be recorded in writing, or it may be in the form of photographs, x-ray pictures, or study models.

re·cov'er·y room The room of a dental office where patients may lie down to recover from temporary illness or to recover from the effects of an anesthetic.

re·duc'tion *In radiology,* the removal of some of the oxidized silver from a developed x-ray film so as to produce a less intense image.

re'flex An involuntary, invariable, adaptive response to a stimulus.

re·frac'to·ry Any of various materials highly resistant to the action of great heat, as fire clay, graphite, or casting investments.

re"ha·bil"i·ta'tion The rendering of a physically or mentally handicapped person fit to engage in a remunerative occupation.

rem Radiation equivalent in human beings; the unit of relative biologic effectiveness (RBE) dose.

re·sorp'tion Removal by absorption. In dentistry, **abnormal resorption** refers especially to the manner in which the roots of primary teeth do not become shorter at the normal time.
   internal r. That resorption which occurs within the body of the tooth as a result of abnormal pulpal activity.

res"pi·ra'tion The act or function of breathing; the act by which air is drawn in and expelled from the lungs, including inspiration and expiration.

res"to·ra'tion The process of replacing a lost tooth or part, or the diseased portion of one, by artificial means; also, the filling, crown, bridge, or denture designed to restore proper dental function.

re·sus'ci·tate To restore to life from apparent death; to prevent asphyxial death by artificial respiration.

re·tain'er A dental appliance that fits a prepared abutment tooth and supports a dental bridge; any device that holds teeth in position after an orthodontic operation.

re·tard'er A device or chemical that slows down a moving object or a chemical reaction; any agent or part that slows the speed of a function.

ret"ro·gnath'ic Posterior deviation of the mandible; weak-appearing chin.

rick'ets A disease of childhood due to vitamin D deficiency, manifested by improper growth and development of the long bones of the body and breastbone.

ridge An extended elevation or crest.
   alveolar r. The ridge left after resorption of the alveolar process in an edentulous jaw.
   re·sid'u·al r. The healed alveolar ridge devoid of natural teeth.

roent'gen·o·gram" A roentgen-ray photograph. Also called *x-ray picture. Radiograph* is the preferred term.

roent"gen·ol'o·gy The branch of medical science which deals with the diagnostic and therapeutic application of roentgen rays. Also called *radiology.*

roent'gen ray The radiant energy of short wavelengths discovered by Röntgen, and named *x-rays* by him.

roent'gen-ray der"ma·ti'tis An inflammation of the skin due to prolonged exposure to roentgen rays.

root *In dentistry,* that part of the tooth which is covered with cementum and which normally is invested in the alveolar bone and gingiva.

rouge Ferric oxide, a red powder used for polishing metal. It may be used in compressed cake form.

rpm Abbreviation for revolutions per minute.

rub'ber dam A thin sheet of rubber or latex used to isolate and keep dry and clean one or more teeth during dental operations.

ru'gae A series of mucosal ridges which occur on the anterior portion of the hard palate.

sac'cha·ride A compound of a base with sugar.

sad'dle A partial denture base, made of metal

or other denture-base material, that fits over the soft-tissue ridge where natural teeth have been extracted.

safelight A light used in the darkroom from which all rays that would damage or alter photographic film have been filtered out.

sa·ggar (sah'ger) A tray made of a refractory material (e.g., fireclay) to carry condensed porcelain into a furnace for firing.

sag'it·tal plane A plane that bisects a bilaterally symmetrical body; the median plane.

sa'line Saltlike; a solution of solium chloride (salt).

san"i·tar'y 1. Hygienic. 2. Pertaining to health.

sap'ro·phyte A usually nonpathogenic organism that lives on dead or decaying organic matter.

sar·co'ma A type of cancer.

sca'ler An instrument for removing calcareous or other deposits from the surfaces of teeth.

scur'vy A nutritional disorder caused by deficiency of vitamin C, characterized by extreme weakness, spongy gums, looseness of the teeth, and a tendency to develop hemorrhages under the skin and from the mucous membranes.

sec'ond·ar·y ra"di·a'tion See radiation.

se·cre'tion 1. The act of secreting or forming, from materials furnished by the blood, a certain substance that is either eliminated from the body (excretion) or used by the body in carrying on special functions. 2. The substance secreted.

se·da'tion 1. A state of lessened functional activity; specifically, such a state produced by sedatives. 2. The production of a state of lessened functional activity.

sed'a·tive An agent that quiets activity.

se'nile Pertaining to, caused by, or characteristic of old age or the infirmities of old age. n. **senility.**

sen·so'ri·um A center for sensations, especially the part of the brain that receives and combines impressions conveyed to the individual centers of sensation.

sep'a·rat"ing wire In orthodontics, a soft wire tied around the contact area of two adjacent teeth and twisted tightly, thereby creating a force that moves teeth apart.

sep"ti·ce'mi·a A systemic disease caused by microorganisms and their toxic products in the bloodstream.

se·que'la An abnormal condition following, or a complication of, a disease. Plural: *sequelae.*

se'rous 1. Pertaining to, characterized by, or resembling serum. 2. Producing or containing serum.

set'ting ex·pan'sion That expansion of a mix of a gypsum material and water which occurs normally when it sets.

set'ting time The time required for a mix of a gypsum material and water or a plastic material to set into a solid mass.

 final s. t. The time required for a mix of a gypsum material and water to acquire such strength that pressure from the edge of the fingernail can cause little or no indentation of the surface of the specimen.

 initial s. t. The time required for a mix of a gypsum material and water to lose its gloss.

shade guide A series of mounted teeth which is supplied by a manufacturer to illustrate various shades of artificial teeth, used in selecting the shade of tooth most suitable for a particular patient.

shel·lac'-base ma·te'ri·al A thermoplastic material used as a tray material and as a base for wax bite rims, supplied in sheet form by a manufacturer. A piece, softened by heating, is adapted to a cast, trimmed, and then chilled to form a custom-built tray.

shock A combination of symptoms resulting from injury; a derangement of many functions, basically of the circulatory and nervous systems. It is characterized by signs such as pallor, clamminess of the skin, diminished blood pressure, and weak and rapid pulse.

shoul'der In dentistry, a type of gingival margination for a dental restoration, basically a butt joint.

si·al′a·gogue, si·al′a·gog A drug or other agent that produces a flow of saliva.

sig′moid Shaped like the letter S.

sign A mark or objective evidence; in a restricted sense, a physical manifestation of disease.

   vital s. E.g., blood pressure, pulse, respiratory rate, and body temperature.

silicone Any of a class of synthetic polymers having the composition of a polyorganosiloxane. *In dentistry,* synthetic combinations of a hydrocarbon and silicon. When the material is cured, it forms a rubber-like mass.

so′di·um flu′o·ride A chemical that reduces tooth decay when placed in drinking water in quantities not exceeding 1 part per million or when applied to the clean surfaces of children's teeth.

sol·der To join by solder.

sol″u·bil′i·ty The extent to which a substance dissolves in a liquid to produce a solution.

so·lu′tion A liquid containing at least one dissolved substance.

space main·tain′er A mechanical or prosthetic device to prevent the drifting of teeth in an area where there has been premature loss of a tooth or teeth.

spasm A sudden, involuntary muscular contraction.

spat′u·la A flexible, blunt blade used for mixing or spreading.

spat·u·la′tion The act of using a spatula, as in mixing or spreading.

spe′cial·ist One who limits a practice to certain diseases, to the diseases of a single organ or class, or to a certain type of therapy.

spe′cial·ty The branch of medicine or dentistry pursued by a specialist, as oral surgery or orthodontics.

sphyg″mo·ma·nom′e·ter An instrument for measuring the arterial blood pressure.

spi′ro·chete (spy′ro·keet) Any of an order of spiral or coiled microorganisms that are the causative agents of many diseases. These organisms are gram-negative and propel themselves by bending or coiling. They are easily destroyed.

split fee The division of a consultant's fee between the referring doctor and the consultant. An unethical and practically obsolete practice.

spore A reproductive cell of protozoan, bacterium, or higher plant. There is usually a thick cell wall enabling the cell to survive in adverse environments.

sprain A wrenching of a joint, producing a stretching or laceration of the ligaments.

sprue An attachment of metal or wax to a wax pattern. It is invested with the pattern and, following removal, provides the path and direction of molten metal to the mold in casting.

squa′mous Flat and scale-shaped.

stand′ard Anything taken as a basis of comparison; a model; a rule.

Staph″y·lo·coc′cus A genus of gram-positive cocci that grow in groups resembling clusters of grapes.

state′ment An abstract of an account, as one rendered to show the balance due.

steel Iron chemically combined with a certain proportion of carbon. It holds an intermediate position between white cast iron and wrought iron, partaking of the most valuable qualities of both.

   stainless s. A steel that contains elements such as nickel and/or chromium; it does not tarnish on exposure and is extensively used in the manufacture of high-grade cutlery.

ster′ile 1. Not fertile; not capable of reproducing. 2. Free from germs.

ster″i·li·za′tion The removal or destruction of all forms of life. Substances may be sterilized by the use of physical or chemical agents, heat being the most important.

ster′i·lize To render sterile or free from bacteria. The autoclave is one of the most effective means of sterilizing instruments.

ster′i·liz′er An apparatus, a chemical, or a physical agent used in the process of sterilization.

steth′o·scope An instrument for listening to sounds arising within the body.

stim′u·lus An agent that produces increased mental or bodily activity; an excitant or irritant.

stip′pled Having an irregularity of surface due to small nodules and depressions which give the appearance of stippled paper.

sto″ma·ti′tis Inflammation of the soft tissues of the mouth.

Strep″to·coc′cus A genus of gram-positive cocci that form long chains.

stud′y mod′el A reproduction of an organ or a part, as in plaster, clay, wax, stone, or metal, used as an aid in diagnosis and in planning treatment for certain conditions; study cast.

stu′por The condition of being partly conscious or sensible; a condition of insensibility. *adj.* **stuporous.**

styp′tic An agent that checks bleeding by causing contraction of the blood vessels.

sub″gin′gi·val Adjacent to and underneath the free gingiva.

sub·jec′tive symp′toms The complaints or feelings mentioned by a patient when describing a disease or illness.

sub·lin′gual 1. Lying beneath the tongue. 2. Pertaining to the parts lying beneath the tongue.

sub·max′il·lar″y Lying beneath the mandible or lower maxilla.

sub″mu·co′sa The layer of fibrous connective tissue beneath a mucous membrane.

suc″ce·da′ne·ous Pertaining to something which follows after, as a permanent tooth that replaces a primary or deciduous tooth.

su′crose A sugar, $C_{12}H_{22}O_{11}$, used as a food and a sweetening agent.

su″per·fi′cial Confined to or pertaining to the surface.

su′per·heat″ To increase or cause to increase temperature above that of saturated steam.

su·pe′ri·or *In anatomy,* higher; denoting the upper of two parts.

sur′geon One who practices surgery. The term implies the possession of a medical degree and license and is used irrespective of the field or limitation of practice.

su′ture 1. *In anatomy,* a line of junction or closure between bones. 2. *In surgery,* fine threadlike material used to close a wound.

su′ture To sew up or close a wound.

sym·path″o·mi·met′ic Having the power to cause physiologic changes similar to those produced by action of the sympathetic nervous system.

symp′tom The phenomena of disease which lead to complaints on the part of a patient; subjective signs in contrast to signs which are objective.

syn′co·pe (sing′ko·pee) A swooning or fainting; a temporary suspension of consciousness due to cerebral anemia.

syn·er′e·sis A process of losing fluid by a gel which is not in contact with moisture.

syn′er·gist A remedy, drug, or other agent that aids the action of another.

syn′the·sis *In chemistry,* the processes and operations necessary to build up a compound.

syn·thet′ic Made by artificial means.

  s. porcelain Silicate cement.

syr′inge An apparatus of metal, glass, or plastic material, consisting of a nozzle, a barrel, and a plunger or a rubber bulb; used to inject a liquid into a cavity or under the skin.

sys′tem 1. A methodical arrangement. 2. A combination of parts into a whole, as the digestive system, the nervous system. 3. The body as a whole.

sys·tem′ic Pertaining to the entire body as distinguished from any of its individual parts.

sys·tol′ic Pertaining to the contraction phase of the cardiac cycle.

tar′get-film dis′tance The distance from the point of emanation of x-rays (target of the anode) to the film to be exposed.

tar′tar A concretion that is deposited on the surfaces of the teeth; technically, salivary calculus. Its composition varies, but in the main it consists of calcium carbonate, calcium phosphate, mucin, disorganized organic matter, and bacterial debris, with other compounds present.

TEAM Training in Expanded Auxiliary Management Program.

tech·nique′ (tek·neek′) The method of procedure in operations or manipulations of any kind.

tem′po·rar″y stop′ping A waxlike material inserted temporarily into prepared cavities in the teeth.

tem″po·ro·man·dib′u·lar Pertaining to the temporal bone and the mandible.

ten′sile strength A resistance of a material to longitudinal stress without breaking.

ter″mi·nol′o·gy Nomenclature; a system of technical names or terms.

test An examination or trial.

tet′a·ny A disease characterized by intermittent, bilateral, painful tonic spasms of the muscles, common in children and young adults. It is due to abnormal calcium metabolism, occuring in deficiencies of parathyroid secretion, alkalosis, vitamin D deficiency, and after extirpation of the parathyroid glands.

ther″a·peu′tic Having to do with the treatment or curing of disease; curative.

ther′a·py Treatment; specifically, the treatment of disease.

  rational t. The treatment of a disease after its cause is determined.

ther′mal ex·pan′sion That expansion of an investment material or wax which occurs as a result of subjection of the material to heat.

ther″mo·plas′tic Capable of becoming soft and being molded when heated and of becoming hard again when cooled.

ther″mo·set′ A term applied to those materials in which a chemical change takes place when cured under heat and pressure.

throm′bin 1. An enzyme elaborated in shed blood that induces clotting. 2. A gray-white powder obtained by special chemical treatment of blood and beef lung.

throm·bo′sis The process by which a thrombus is formed.

throm′bus A clot of blood formed within the heart or blood vessels, due usually to a slowing of the circulation or to alteration of the blood or vessel walls.

thy′roid One of the endocrine glands, lying in front of the trachea and consisting of two lateral lobes connected centrally by an isthmus.

tinc′ture An alcoholic or hydroalcoholic solution of a medical substance.

tin′ foil″ A very thin sheet of tin.

todd′ler·hood″ The period of a child's development between the ages of 15 months and 2½ years.

tol′er·ance The ability of enduring or being less responsive to the influence of a drug, particularly when acquired by continued use.

tone The normal state of tension of a part or of the body. *adj.* **tonic.**

ton′ic An agent or drug that produces, restores, or maintains the normal tone of an organ or of the patient generally.

tooth One of the calcified organs supported by the alveolar processes and gums of both jaws, serving to masticate food, aid speech, and influence facial contour. Each tooth consists of (1) a main mass of dentin surrounding a pulp cavity which contains the dental pulp with its nerves and vessels, (2) a crown covered by enamel, (3) a root, and (4) a neck, the junction of crown and root. Plural: *teeth.*

  canine t. One with a conical crown situated between the lateral incisor and the first premolar in each quadrant of the jaws.

  deciduous teeth The twenty primary or first teeth; those replaced by permanent teeth. There are eight incisors, four canines, and eight molars.

  denture teeth Artificial teeth made of baked porcelain or plastic that are used in artificial dentures.

  impacted t. A tooth that for one reason or another cannot erupt.

locked t. Any tooth (or teeth) in one arch that is biting inside the teeth of the other arch when the jaws are closed normally.

milk teeth The deciduous teeth.

missing t. An absent tooth; specifically, one that failed to develop in the dental arch.

nonvital t. One whose pulp has been removed or has degenerated.

peg t. A conical-shaped tooth usually formed in the anterior part of the dental arch. In most instances it is an irregularly formed upper permanent lateral incisor.

primary t. One of the deciduous teeth.

supernumerary t. An extra tooth; an additional one to the number normal to a given area of the dental arch.

unerupted t. One that has not come through the gum tissue into the mouth but is evident on x-ray examination.

vital t. One in which the nerve and blood supply is intact.

wisdom t. The third molar tooth.

young permanent t. A tooth of the second dentition that has erupted through the gum tissue but whose root development is not complete.

tooth′brush″ A brush with a slender handle, usually of a plastic material, for cleaning the teeth and stimulating the gums.

tooth-clean′ing brush A small-bristle brush that can be operated in a dental handpiece for the purpose of cleaning and polishing the teeth.

tooth fac′ing A porcelain or plastic reproduction of the outer surface of a tooth. It is reinforced by gold to restore the full form of the tooth.

top′i·cal Pertaining to a definite place or locality; local, as a topical anesthetic.

to′rus A hard, localized, bony enlargement of the outer plate of a bone. Plural: *tori*. See also *exostoseis*.

t. palatinus A torus which occurs in the midline of the hard palate.

t. mandibularis A torus which occurs on the lingual side of the lower jaw, usually in the bicuspid region.

tour′ni·quet Any apparatus for controlling hemorrhage from, or circulation in, a limb or part of the body, where direct pressure can be brought upon the blood vessels by means of straps, cords, rubber tubes, or pads. Tourniquets are made in a multiplicity of forms, from the simplest emergency adaptation of a handkerchief or piece of clothing wound about the limb and tightened with a stick, to elaborate instruments where pressure is made by means of screws acting upon metal pads or where a rubber hose encircling the limb is distended with air by means of a pump.

tox′ic Pertaining to a poison or toxin.

tox·ic′i·ty (tock·sis′i·tee) 1. The quality of being poisonous. 2. The kind and amount of poison or toxin produced by a microorganism.

tox′in A poisonous product of animal or vegetable cells that, on injection into animals or human beings, causes the formation of antibodies. The most important toxins are those produced by bacteria. See also *antitoxin*.

tra′che·a (tray′kee·uh) The windpipe; the cartilaginous and membranous tube extending from the lower part of the larynx to its division into the two bronchi.

tra″che·ot′o·my The operation of cutting into the trachea.

transfer See *coping*.

trans·fu′sion A transfer of blood into the veins.

tran′sient Passing with time; not lasting or enduring.

trans″il·lu″mi·na′tion 1. The act of causing light to show through an organ or part as a means of diagnosis. 2. The inspection of an organ or part by means of a strong light made to pass through certain areas.

trau′ma A wound or injury. *adj.* **traumatic.**

trau′ma·tize To wound or injure.

tray 1. A flat, shallow vessel of glass, hard

rubber, or metal, for holding instruments during a surgical operation. 2. The vessel by which impression material is carried to the mouth to produce an impression or mold. It may be made of metal or other material such as shellac-base material or autopolymerizing acrylic.

treat'ment The means employed in effecting the cure of disease; the management of disease or of diseased patients.

trit"u·ra'tion In dentistry, the mixing of silver alloy with mercury to produce an amalgam. v. **triturate.**

tu"ber·os'i·ty A protuberance on a bone.

ul'cer A lesion or sore of a cutaneous or mucous surface with an inflamed base.

ul"tra·son'ic In excess of the speed of sound. A vibrating motion of 0.001 inch up to 25,000/second.

un·con'scious Insensible; in a state lacking conscious awareness.

unc'tion The act of anointing or smearing with an ointment or an oil; also, an ointment.

un·guen'tum An ointment.

USDHEW United States Department of Health, Education, and Welfare.

use'ful beam The primary beam of radiation that passes through the aperture of the x-ray tube and the pointer cone.

U.S.P. Abbreviation for the United States Pharmacopeia.

vac'cine Any organism used for preventive inoculation against a specific disease.

va'por A gas, especially the gaseous form of a substance that at ordinary temperatures is liquid or solid.

var'nish A resinous solution with a volatile solvent or vehicle, such as oil, alcohol, ether, or chloroform, that, when spread upon a surface, dries quickly and leaves a firm glossy film.

   cavity v. One used to line cavities in teeth prior to placement of restorations to protect their pulps from thermal shock.

vas"o·con·stric'tor Causing a constriction of the blood vessels.

vas"o·con·stric'tor A nerve or a drug that causes constriction of the blood vessels.

vas"o·di·la'tor Pertaining to the relaxation of the smooth muscle of the vascular system.

vas"o·di·la'tor Any agent producing dilation of blood vessels.

vault Space formed by the arch of the hard palate.

ven'i·punc"ture The surgical puncture of a vein.

ves'i·cle A small sac or bladder containing fluid; also, a small skin blister.

vir'u·lence The disease-producing power of a microorganism; malignancy; infectiousness.

vir'u·lent Capable of causing infection or disease.

vi'rus One of a group of pathogenic agents smaller than the accepted bacterial forms, some being visible by ordinary microscopic examination; others, also known as ultraviruses, are beyond this range. In each virus disease they are represented by particles of fairly constant size. Among the well-known virus diseases of human beings are rabies, poliomyelitis, encephalitis, smallpox, chickenpox, common cold influenza, measles, yellow fever, and mumps. The virus diseases of animals and plants are also numerous.

vi'ta·min One of a group of organic compounds present in variable minute quantities in natural foodstuffs, required for the normal growth and maintenance of the life of animals, including human beings, who, as a rule, are unable to synthesize these compounds.

vol'a·til·ize" To change into vapor; to evaporate.

volt'me"ter An instrument for measuring voltage or electromotive force.

vul'can·ite A type of rubber that was the first nonmetallic denture base material.

wax Any substance, of plant, animal, or mineral origin, consisting of a mixture of one or more of the following constituents: high molecular weight fatty acids, high molecular weight monohydric alcohols, esters of the fatty acids and alcohols, and solid hydrocarbons. There are a variety of commercial waxes available, each varying in its composition and each created to perform a specific function. All become soft and workable when heated, the degree of heat needed varying with the wax.
  baseplate w. A prepared wax used in making artificial dentures.
  casting w. A prepared wax used to wax up a pattern for casting the metal framework for a partial denture.
  inlay w. A prepared wax used to prepare patterns for inlays, bridges, and crowns.
  utility w. A prepared wax which is tacky but pliable at room temperatures.
weld To unite and consolidate, as masses of a cohesive substance, especially metal, such as gold, in the building of a restoration.
with·hold′ing Holding back; specifically, holding back a part of a salary for tax or other purposes.
work′ing time That period of time permissible from the start of the mixing of a plastic or gypsum material that it is subject to manipulation.
wrought Produced or shaped by mechanical force.

x-ray de·vel′op·er A chemical for developing x-ray radiographs.
x′ray film Film for making a radiograph.
x′ray film hang′er A mechanical device to hold an x-ray film during processing.
x′-ray fix′er A solution of sodium hyposulfite used as a fixing agent in processing x-ray films; sometimes called *hypo*.
x′ray pic′ture A radiograph.

zinc oxide ZnO. Occurs as a fine, amorphous, white or yellowish white powder; insoluble in water and alcohol; dissolves in dilute acids. Used in *dentistry* in combination with other agents as a sedative cement or temporary filling material; also in impression pastes.
ZOE Zinc oxide and eugenol; combined to make temporary, sedative restorations; also used as a cavity base and root canal sealer.
zo″o·gle′a Microorganisms which are embedded in a jelly-like matrix formed as the result of their metabolic activities.
zo·ol′o·gy The study of animals.

Index

AADS (American Association of Dental Schools), 136, 141, 142
Abcesses, 158–159
   illustrated, 486
Absorbent paper points used in pulp canal, 475–476
   illustrated, 476
Absorbents for moisture control, 581–582
   illustrated, 582
Abutments, illustrated, 615
Accepted Dental Therapeutics (Council on Dental Therapeutics), 169, 176
Accreditation of education programs, 16
Acellular cementum, 111
Acetaminophen, 176
Acid-etching procedures, 611–613
   illustrated, 612
Acid-forming bacteria (*see* Lactobacillis)
Acriflavine, 178
Acrylic resins (*see* Synthetic resin materials)
Acrylics, self-curing, 610
Action of drugs, 175–179
   age and, 172
Acute necrotizing ulcerative gingivitis (*see* Vincent's disease)
ADA (*see* American Dental Association)
ADA News, 15
ADAA (*see* American Dental Assistants Association)
Addition, polymerization as, 212
ADHA (American Dental Hygienists Association), 22–24, 32
Adjustments:
   for clinical fixed prostheses, 635–637
   for complete dentures, 676–677
   occlusal, 491–492
      illustrated, 492
   for partial dentures, 684–685
Administration, 38–49
   appointment control in, 44–49
      illustrated, 45, 47, 48
      (*See also* Appointments)
   handling of telephone in, 41–44
      illustrated, 42
   office manual for, 39–40
   role of office managers and business assistants in, 40
   (*See also* Records)
Adolescents, orthodontics for, 540
Adrenalin (epinephrine), 178, 179
Adult ego state (A), 64

Adults:
   attitudes of, toward dentistry, 69
   orthodontics for, 540–541
Age, effects of, on drug action, 172
Agriculture, U.S. Department of, 413
Air compressors, care of, 281
Air syringes, 278–279
   illustrated, 279
Air-water syringes, sterilization of, 149
Alabama, University of, 18
Alban's test, 384
Alcohol (*see* Ethyl alcohol)
Alcohol torch, illustrated, 648
Alginate-acrylic resin technique, 634–636
   illustrated, 636
Alginate hydrocolloid impressions (irreversible hydrocolloids), 203–205
   for complete dentures, illustrated, 646, 647
   illustrated, 204
   for partial dentures, 680–681
      illustrated, 681
Allergies to drugs, 172, 177
Alloys, 239–240
   illustrated, 239, 245
   (*See also specific alloys*)
Allport, G. W., 63
Alterations of universal retainer bands, 600–601
   illustrated, 601
Alum, 177
Aluminum filtration as radiation protection, 348
Aluminum shells, temporary, 634–635
   illustrated, 635
Alveolar bone, 83–84, 115–116
   illustrated, 85, 115
Amalgam carriers, 305–306
   illustrated, 306
Amalgam condensers (pluggers):
   for condensed gold, 309–310
      illustrated, 310
   illustrated, 305
   sterilization of, 148
Amalgam matrix retainers, 306–308
   illustrated, 308
Amalgam tatoos, 164
Amalgams, 234–243
   amalgamation, 238
   care of instruments, illustrated, 305–307

Amalgams:
   carving of, 305
      illustrated, 243
   chairside duties in restoration of, 595–603
      illustrated, 596, 597, 600–603
   composition of, 237–238
   illustrated, 234, 235
   manipulation of, 239–243
      illustrated, 240–243
   properties of, 236–237
   table, 237
   retention forms for, 562–563
      illustrated, 562
   (*See also* Silver amalgams)
Ameloblastomas, 162–163
Ameloblasts, 108
American Academy of Pedodontics, 502
American Association of Dental Examiners, 14
American Association of Dental Schools (AADS), 136, 141, 142
American Board of Orthodontics, 6
American Board of Pedodontics, 502
American Council on Education, 17
American Dental Assistants Association (ADAA), 14–16, 30, 32
   Certifying Board, 14–16
   Education Committee, 14
American Dental Association (ADA), 9, 53, 70, 208, 375, 378, 394
   Board of Trustees, 375
   Bureau of Economic Research and Statistics, 11, 68, 72
   Commission on Accreditation of Dental and Dental Auxiliary Educational Programs, 16
   Council on Dental Education (*see* Council on Dental Education)
   Council on Dental Materials and Devices, 184, 235
   Council on Dental Therapeutics, 14, 169, 379
   Council on Judicial Procedure, 32
   dental laboratory technicians and, 24
   dentifrice classification and, 392
   endodontics and, 467
   expanded functions and, 17, 18, 20
   House of Delegates (*see* House of Delegates)
   Principles of Ethics of, 31–36

American Dental Association(ADA):
  standards of: for amalgams, 239
    for dental cements, 218–219, 224
    for dental materials, 184
  water fluoridation and, 155
American Dental Hygienists Association (ADHA), 22–24, 32
American Journal of Dental Science, The, 3
American Psychological Association, 62
American Society of Dental Surgeons, 3
American Society for the Promotion of Dentistry for Children, 502
Ames, L. B., 509, 511, 512
Amino acids, 403
Ammonia, aromatic spirits of, 179
Amputations, root, 497
Amyl nitrite, 179
Anacin, 176
Analgesia, 452–453
  equipment used in, 286–287
    illustrated, 287, 453
  neuroleptic, 454
Analgesics, 176
Anaphylactic shock, treatment of, 435–437
Anatomic portion of models, 193
Anchor teeth, mandibular, rubber dam hole position for, illustrated, 585
Anesthesia, 5, 445–453
  anatomy, psychology, and physiology of pain and, 446–448
    illustrated, 447, 448
  defined, 448
  general, 447–448
  history of, 445–446
  local (*see* Local anesthesia)
Anesthetic test, 471
Angle, E. H., 531
Angle formers, illustrated, 298
Angles (instruments), sterilization of, 148–149
Angles of teeth, 89–90, 555–556
  illustrated, 556
  (*See also* Line angles; Malocclusion; Occlusion)
Animals as sources of drugs, 169
Anlage, 108
Annealing (degassing) trays, 309
Anodes of x-ray generating tubes, 344
Anodontia, defined, 155
Anterior teeth:
  caries in, illustrated, 156
  embrasures of, illustrated, 93
  guides for selection of artifical, illustrated, 671–673
  line and point angles on, illustrated, 90
  mandibular and maxillary anatomic form and relationship of pulp cavity to hard structure of, illustrated, 94, 95
  prefabricated, illustrated, 635
Antibiotics, 177
Antiflux, use of, in soldering, 256
Antiseptic(s), 150, 178
  term, defined, 137
ANUG (*see* Vincent's disease)
Aperture of x-ray generating tube, 344
Aphthous stomatitis, 131–132
Aphthous ulcers (canker sores), illustrated, 159

Apollonia, Saint, 3
Appliances, orthodontic, 541–544, 551
  illustrated, 541–543
Applied psychology:
  defined, 62
  dental assistants and, 77–79
Appointment books:
  recording appointments in, 46–48
    illustrated, 47, 48
  selection and preparation of, 44–45
    illustrated, 45
Appointment calls, 42–43
Appointments:
  adjustment (*see* Adjustments)
  control of, 44–49
    illustrated, 45, 47, 48
  to establish proper intermaxillary relationship for complete dentures, 663–667
    illustrated, 665–667
  orthodontic, 551
  pedodontic consultation, 515–517
  reminder calls for, 43–44
  treatment-plan, 76–77
  try-in, 635–637, 670, 674
  (*See also* First appointments)
Apposition stage of tooth development, 153
Arch(es):
  bronchial, defined, 156
  gothic arch tracing, 667–669
    illustrated, 668, 669
  lingual, illustrated, 541
  (*See also* Edentulous arches)
Arch wires, 542
Armamentarium:
  for local anesthesia, 451–452
    illustrated, 449, 452
  for periapical surgery, illustrated, 479
  (*See also* Equipment; Instruments)
Arnim, Sumpter, 127
Arrested caries, defined, 157
Art portion of models, 193
Arteries, blood supply to teeth and, illustrated, 93
Articulated models, trimming of, illustrated, 195
Articulators:
  care of, 316–317
    illustrated, 316
  used in prosthodontics, illustrated, 626
Artifical teeth:
  ordering and selection of, 669–674, 678
    illustrated, 670–674
  prefabricated, illustrated, 635
Asepsis, 137
  in oral surgery, 458–461
    illustrated, 121, 458, 459, 461
Asgar, K., 267
Aspirin, 175
  burns cause by, illustrated, 165
Astringents, 177
Atrophy, tissue, 152
Attitudes toward dentistry, 68–72
  table, 70
Attrition stage of tooth development, 153
Ausculation, recording blood pressure by, defined, 522
Autoclaving, sterilization by, 142–143
  illustrated, 142

Automatic processing of films, 352
  illustrated, 354
Auxiliary personnel, 7
  growth of, 11
  (*See also* specific auxiliary personnel)

Bacilli (rods), illustrated, 118
Back-order notices, illustrated, 57
Bacteria (*see* Cross-infections; Infections; Microbiology; *and specific bacteria*)
Bacterial endocarditis, 124
Bacterionema species (bacteria), 125
Bacteriostatic chemicals, defined, 137
Bacteroides species (bacteria), 122
Baird, K. M., 18
Baker, Benjamin R., 61–80, 501–526
Baldwin, K. H., 441
Balinsky, B., 73
Baltimore College of Dental Surgery, 3
Bands:
  orthodontic, 542
    illustrated, 257
  retainer, illustrated, 600, 601, 603
Barbital, 175
Barbiturates, 175, 179
Barton, Roger E., 197–233, 244–259, 273–319, 634, 639
Base-formers, illustrated, 193
Base materials for dentures, 212–213
Baseplate waxes, 209–210
  illustrated, 210
Bass technique of toothbrushing, illustrated, 389
Bead application technique (brush application technique), 230–232
Becks, Herman, 377, 400
Beeswax, 211
Bell, G. D., 64, 67
Bell, W. H., 422
Bell development stage of teeth, illustrated, 108, 109
Benign neoplasms, 161–162
  illustrated, 162
Benzalkonium chloride (Zephiran chloride), 178
Berlove, I. J., 431, 441
Berman, D. L., 422
Berne, E., 63, 64
Betadin, 178
Bibby, B. G., 400
Bicuspids (premolars):
  bitewing of, illustrated, 369
  functions of, 89
  prefabricated, illustrated, 635
  relative position of, illustrated, 103
  (*See also* Mandibular bicuspids; Maxillary bicuspids)
Billing, 51
Binders in casting investments, 261
Biology, radiation, 346–347
Biopsies in diagnosis of oral lesions, 163
Bisecting-angle technique 356–363
  illustrated, 356–362
Bite:
  closed and open, 532–533
    illustrated, 332, 537
  intermaxillary check-bite, illustrated, 675

Bite rims, illustrated, 210
Black, Greene Vardiman, 4, 377
Blood pressure, taking of, 326-338
　illustrated, 327
　as preventive measure, 422-423
　　illustrated, 423, 424
Blood supply to teeth, illustrated, 93
Blue Cross and Blue Shield, 11
Boiling water, sterilization with, 146-147
Bone implants, 496
Bones:
　alveolar, 83-84, 115-116
　　illustrated, 85, 115
　oral cavity, 81-84
　　illustrated, 82-84
　(See also entries beginning with elements os-, oste-, osteo-)
Borrelia, 125
Boucher, C. O., 614, 615
Boxing method of pouring, 191
Boxing waxes, illustrated, 210, 211
Bracket tables, 280
Brackets, 542
Branchial arch, defined, 156
Brauer, J. C., 505, 517, 518, 521, 634, 639
Bread-cereal group (food group), 413
Brearley, L. J., 17
Bremmer, M. D. K., 5, 167
Broaches used in pulp canal, 473
　illustrated, 475
Brown, W. E., 504
Bruises, treatment of, 443
Brush application technique (bead application technique), 230-232
Buccal mucosa, 112-113
　aspirin burn of, illustrated, 165
　hyperkeratosis of, illustrated, 160
Buccal tubes, 543
Bufferin, 176
Bulk application technique (flow application technique), 230-232
　illustrated, 231, 232
Bulk buying, advantages of, illustrated, 56
Buonocore, M. G., 525
Burbank, Luther, 501
Burger, R., 73
Burket, L. W., 507
Burnishers, 305
Burnishing of retainer bands, 600-601
　illustrated, 601
Burs:
　illustrated, 294
　shanks of, illustrated, 293
　sterilization of, 148
Business assistants, functions of, 40

C (Child ego state), 64
Caffeine, 179
Cake compounds, illustrated, 201
Calcification stage of tooth development, 153
Calcium, 406-407
　RDAs for, table, 409
　sources of, 411, 700
　table, 406
Calcium hydroxide paste, 178

Calcium hydroxide paste:
　in pedodontic pulp therapy, 519, 520
　for pulp filling, illustrated, 478
Calhoon, R. P., 66, 73
Callahan, J. D., 69, 508-509, 512
Camahan, C. W., 27, 30
Cancer (*see* Neoplasms)
Candidiasis (moniliasis), 132
Canines (*see* Mandibular canines; Maxillary canines)
Canker sores (aphthous ulcers), illustrated, 159
Cap stage of tooth development, 107-108
　illustrated, 107
Capping:
　cusp-capping inlays, 616-617
　　illustrated, 616
　pulp, 478, 519-520
Carat of gold alloys, 250
Carbohydrates:
　dental disease and, 401-402
　RDAs for, table, 408
Carborundum as polishing agent, 258
Carcinomas, 153, 162-163
　illustrated, 163
Card-index inventory control, 56-57
　illustrated, 57
Cardiac emergencies, treatment of, 438
Care:
　general, of patients, 422-428
　　illustrated, 423-426
　of instruments and equipment, 273-319
　　air compressors, 281
　　amalgam instruments, illustrated, 305-307
　　analgesic apparatus, 286-287
　　　illustrated, 287
　　dental chairs, 281-282
　　　illustrated, 281
　　dental units, 275-280
　　　illustrated, 274-277
　　explorers and pliers, 302-303, 307
　　　illustrated, 303, 309
　　glass slabs and burnishers, 304-305
　　　illustrated, 304
　　hand cutting instruments, illustrated, 296-300
　　handpieces (and handpiece equipment), 289-296
　　　illustrated, 289-295
　　hydrocolloid conditioners, 287-288
　　instruments used with condensed gold, 309-310
　　　illustrated, 310
　　mirrors, 300-302
　　　illustrated, 302
　　operating stools, illustrated, 282, 283
　　oral evacuating machines, 284-285
　　　illustrated, 285
　　plastic instruments and spatulas, 302-304
　　　illustrated, 303, 304
　　prophylaxis and periodontal instruments, 300-301
　　　illustrated, 301
　　prosthodontic and laboratory equipment, 316-319
　　　illustrated, 316-318

Care:
　of instruments and equipment: reamers and files, 307
　　rubber dam equipment, 311-312
　　　illustrated, 312
　　sterilization and disinfection equipment, 312
　　surgical equipment, 288
　　syringes, 310-311
　　　illustrated, 311
　　ultrasonic units, 286-287
　　　illustrated, 287
　　ultraviolet activator light, 285-286
　　　illustrated, 286
　　x-ray units, 288-289
　　　illustrated, 288
　postoperative, 498
　(*See also* Dental care)
Caries:
　activity tests for, 384-385
　in anterior teeth, illustrated, 156
　arrested, defined, 157
　assistant's duties in control of, 594-595
　illustrated, 156-157
　microbiology of, 128-131
　　illustrated, 131
　operative dentistry and, 552-555
　　illustrated, 553
　　preventive recurrence of, as objective in operative dentistry, 554-555
　　(*See also* Operative dentistry)
　removal of carious dentin, 563-564
　Vipeholm study on, 400
　(*See also* Cavities)
Carving:
　of amalgams, 305
　　illustrated, 243
　of gold inlays, 607
Cascara, 178-179
Cassidy, R. J., 382
Cast gold post and core restorations, 641-643
　illustrated, 642
Casting gold alloys, 251-253
　illustrated, 245
Casting investments, 260-272
　composition of, 260-262
　defective, 270-271
　finishing of, 271-272
　of gold inlays, 607
　procedures used, 262-270
　　illustrated, 263-270
Casting waxes (sheet waxes; shape waxes), 209-210
　illustrated, 210
Casts (models):
　defined, 197
　of edentulous maxillary arch, illustrated, 198
　made with gypsum products (*see* Gypsum products, study models made of)
　pouring of final impressions into master, for complete dentures, 657-659
　　illustrated, 658-659
　preliminary, for partial dentures, 681-682
　　illustrated, 681
　records of, 50
　stone, illustrated, 186

742 / Index

Casts (models):
　trimming of: illustrated, 195
　　trimmers used, illustrated, 318
　(See also Casting investments; Impressions)
Cathodes of x-ray generating tubes, 344
Cavities:
　classification of, 556–558
　　illustrated, 556, 557
　preparation of: chairside duties in, 592–594
　　for gold inlay restorations, 604–607
　　　illustrated, 605, 606
　　illustrated, 392
　defined, 555
　designs for, 558–561
　　illustrated, 559–561
　steps in, 560–564
　　illustrated, 562, 563
　walls of, defined, 555
　(See also Pit and fissure cavities)
Cavitron, illustrated, 491
Cavity line (cavity varnishes), 595
Cavosurface margin, illustrated, 556
Cellular cementum, 111
Cement(s), 215–229
　copper phosphate, 222
　　table, 216
　resin and polycarboxylate, 228–229, 639
　　table, 216
　silicate (see Silicate cement)
　zinc oxide–eugenol [see Zinc oxide–eugenol (ZOE) paste cement]
　zinc phosphate (see Zinc phosphate cement)
　zinc silicophosphate, 228
　　table, 216
Cement bases, placement of, illustrated, 595
Cementation:
　of gold inlays, 607–610
　　illustrated, 608, 609
　in prosthodontics: final, 637–641
　　illustrated, 639, 640
Cementoblasts, 111, 115
Cementocytes, 111
Cementum, 111–112
　illustrated, 112
Center for Disease Control, 10
Central bearing devices, extraoral and intraoral, 667–668
　illustrated, 668
Central incisors:
　deciduous: bell stage of development of, illustrated, 108
　　illustrated, 109
　　pits and groove defects in, illustrated, 154
　(See also Mandibular incisors, central; Maxillary incisors, central)
Central nervous system (CNS), drugs affecting, 176–177
Centric intermaxillary relation of complete dentures:
　defined, 665
　locking tracing devices, illustrated, 669
Cephalometrics, 545–550
　illustrated, 548, 549
Ceramic stains, 624
Certification:
　of dental assistants, 13–14

Certification:
　of dental laboratory technicians, 24–25
Certified Dental Assistant (CDA) 14, 15
Certified Dental Technician (CDT), 25
Certified Dental Technician Examination, 25
Certifying Board (ADAA), 14–16
Chairside duties:
　in complete denture construction: for final compound impressions, 650
　　illustrated, 665, 666
　in taking impressions with alginate hydrocolloid, 646–647
　　illustrated, 647
　in denture relines, 677
　in operative dentistry, 577–613
　　in acid-etching procedures, 611–613
　　　illustrated, 612
　　in amalgam restorations, 595–603
　　　illustrated, 596, 597, 600–603
　　in caries control, 594–595
　　in cavities preparation (see Cavities, preparation of)
　　in composite resin restorations, 610–613
　　　illustrated, 611–613
　　in gold foil restorations, 613
　　in gold inlay restorations, 603–610
　　　illustrated, 605, 606, 608, 609
　　in local anesthetic administration, 580–581
　　　illustrated, 581
　　in moisture control, 581–593
　　　illustrated, 582–591
　　in oral examination and charting, illustrated, 579
　　in placement of cavity liners and cement bases, illustrated, 595
　　in silicate cement and self-curing resin restorations, 610
　　in treatment planning and care presentation, 579–580
　in orthodontics, 545–546
　　instrument preparation, illustrated, 546–547
Chalk as polishing agent, 259
Charter's technique of toothbrushing, 390–391
　illustrated, 391
Charts:
　dental, illustrated, 336
　diagnosis and treatment entered on, 50
　operative dentistry, illustrated, 479
　of patient's oral condition, 425–426
　　illustrated, 426
　pedodontic, illustrated, 511
　periodontic, 487
　　illustrated, 488
Check-bite, intermaxillary mounting of, illustrated, 675
Check-bite method of jaw registration, illustrated, 665
Cheeks, examination of, 330–331
　illustrated, 331
Chemical corrosion, defined, 257
Chemical injuries to teeth, 165
Chemical modifiers, 261
Chemicals, bacteriostatic, defined, 137
Chicago Research Study Club, 377

Child ego state (C), 64
Children:
　attitudes of, toward dentistry, 69
　(See also Pedodontics)
Chirurgien Dentiste, Le (Fauchard), 3, 166–167
Chisels, illustrated, 299
Chlordiazepoxide hydrochloride, 176
Chue, P. W. Y., 423
Cieszynski, 357
Cinotti, W. R., 62, 63, 65, 68, 77
Circulatory difficulties, treatment of, 437–438
Civil law, 27
Clamps, 582
　illustrated, 311
　sterilization of, 148
Clark, W. E., 445
Class attitudes toward dentistry, 70–71
　table, 70
Class 1 cavities, 558
Class II cavities, 558
Class III cavities, 558
Class IV cavities, 558
Class V cavities, 558
Class VI cavities, 558
Cleaning:
　of castings, 269–270
　of cavities, 564
　of impression trays, 650
　(See also Sterilization)
Cleft palate, 2, 155–156
Cleoid edge of spoon excavators, 298
Clinical fixed prosthodontics, 624–641
　examination for, 624–626
　　illustrated, 625, 626
　final cementation in, 637–641
　　illustrated, 639, 640
　maintenance of prostheses, 641
　temporary restorations in, 634–636
　　illustrated, 635, 636
　tooth preparation for, 625–630
　　illustrated, 627–629
　impressions of, 630–634
　　illustrated, 632–634
　try-in, adjustment and temporary placement of restorations in, 635–637
　　illustrated, 639
Closed bite, 533
　illustrated, 532
Clostridium botulinum, 122
Clostridium tetani, 122
Clostridium welchii, 122
Clothing, control of cross-infections and, 138–139
Cloves, oil of, 179
Cocci, defined, 118
Codeine, 175–176
Coil springs, 543
Cold disinfection method, 142
Cold germs, 123
Cold sterilization, 142
Cole, W. H., 433
Collimation, use of proper, as radiation protection, 348
Coma, diabetic, 439
Commercial dental laboratories (see Laboratories)

Commission on Accreditation of Dental and Dental Auxiliary Educational Programs (ADA), 16
Committee on the National Formulary, 168
Common law (unwritten law), 27
Communication, importance of, 39
Community health centers, dental care in, 13
Compilation of Facts Related to the Teaching of Expanded Functions, A (Council on Dental Education), 18
Complementary transactions between dentists and patients, illustrated, 75
Complete dentures:
  construction of: adjustments of dentures, 676–677
    custom trays for (see Custom impression trays)
    delivery of dentures, illustrated, 675–676
    final impressions (see Final impressions, for complete dentures)
    first appointment for, 645
    gothic arch tracing for, 667–669
      illustrated, 668, 669
    intermaxillary relationship in, 663–667
      illustrated, 665–667
    laboratory procedures in, illustrated, 649, 650
    ordering and selecting artificial teeth, 669–670
      illustrated, 670–674
    preliminary impressions (see Preliminary impressions, for complete dentures)
    record bases for (see Occlusion rims)
    try-in of dentures, 670, 674
  immediate, 677–678
    illustrated, 678
  relines of, 645–646, 677
  repair of, 678–680
    illustrated, 679
Complex cavities, 556–557
  illustrated, 556
Complications with local anesthesia, 452
Composite resin restorations:
  chairside duties in, 610–613
    illustrated, 611–613
  materials used in, 232–233
Composition:
  of amalgams, 237–238
  of casting investments, 260–262
  of pattern waxes, 208
  of resin cements, 228
  of silicate cements, 223
  of zinc oxide–eugenol cements, 215–216
  of zinc phosphate cements, 217
Composition of Foods: Agriculture Handbook No. 8 (Department of Agriculture), 413
Compound cavities, 556–557
  illustrated, 556
Condensation:
  of amalgams, 241–243
    illustrated, 242
  polymerization as form of, 212
Condensed gold, 248–249
  care of equipment used with, 309–310
    illustrated, 310
  illustrated, 249

Condensers (see Amalgam condensers)
Cone compounds, illustrated, 201
Cone-socket handles of mirrors, 301
Cones, long, lead-lined, open, use of, as radiation protection, 348
Conn, R. D., 428, 429
Connecticut Dental Hygienists Association, 22
Connective tissues, 107
Connectors in bridges, 618
Consent, defined, 30
Contact area (contact point) of teeth, 90
  illustrated, 104
Contours of teeth, 103–104
  illustrated, 103
Contra-angled universal matrices, 599–600
  illustrated, 600
Contracts between patients and dentists, 27–29
Contributory negligence, defined, 30
Controlled Substances Act, 175
Convenience forms in cavity preparation, illustrated, 563
Conventional handpieces, illustrated, 289, 290
Coolant equipment, 292
Coping transfer impressions, 630–634
  illustrated, 632–634
Copper in gold alloys, 250
Copper band-rubber base impressions, 630
  illustrated, 632–633
Copper heat radiator of x-ray generating tube, 344
Copper phosphate cement, 222
  table, 216
Copper sulfate, 177
Corrosion of gold alloys, 256–257
Costs, dental, 11–12
Cotton pliers (operating pliers; tweezers), 302–303
  illustrated, 303
Council of the American Pharmaceutical Association, 168
Council on Dental Education (ADA), 14
  dental hygienists and, 22
  dental laboratory technicians and, 26
  expanded functions and, 17, 20
  pedodontics and, 501–502
Council on Dental Laboratory Relations, 24, 26
Council on Dental Materials and Devices (ADA), 184, 235
Council on Dental Therapeutics (ADA), 141, 169, 379
Council on Education, 16
Council on Judicial Procedure (ADA), 32
Council on Post-Secondary Education, 16
Countra-angles, sterilization of, 148–149
County health departments, dental practice in, 7
Craig, R. A., 261
Craig, R. G., 238
Crawford, James J., 117–150
Credit form, illustrated, 59
Creep, defined, 236
Criminal law, 27
Cross-infections, 137–149
  control of, 135–136, 138–149

Cross-infections:
  control of: clothing and personal hygiene in, 138–139
    by dispensing clean and sterile items, illustrated, 141
    hand washing and, illustrated, 139
    by surface disinfection, 139–141
      illustrated, 140
    (See also Instruments, sterilization of)
  defined, 135
Crossed transactions between dentists and patients, illustrated, 75
Crowns (see Full crowns; Partial crowns; Porcelain-faced crowns; Porcelain-fused-to-metal crowns)
Crystal structure of dental materials, illustrated, 182
Cubic centimeter, 173
Cultures, root canal, 477–478
Curettage, gingival, illustrated, 494
Curettes, 300–301
  illustrated, 301
  periodontic, illustrated, 490
  sterilization of, 148
Cusp-capping inlays (intracoronal restorations; onlays), 615–617
  illustrated, 616
Cuspidors, care of, 277
Cuspids:
  characteristics of, 92
  illustrated, 100
  functions of, 89
  mandibular, illustrated, 162
Custom impression trays, 650–657
  for complete dentures: fabrication of, 650–653
    illustrated, 651, 654–655
    final impressions using, 653–657
      illustrated, 656, 657
    maxillary trays, illustrated, 678
  for partial dentures, illustrated, 682, 683
  sterilization of, 148
Cuttle as polishing agent, 258
Cysts, 159
Cytology in diagnosis of oral lesions, 163–164
  illustrated, 164

Darkroom, illustrated, 350–355
Darvon, 176
DAU program (Dental Auxiliary Utilization program), 16
DEA (Drug Enforcement Administration, 174
Dead man switch of x-ray machine, 345
Dead tract, 111
  illustrated, 113
Deciduous central incisors:
  bell stage of development of, illustrated, 108
  illustrated, 109
Deciduous dentition (see Primary dentition)
Deciduous mandibular incisors, cap stage of development of, illustrated, 107
Degassing of gold, 247–248
  illustrated, 248
Degassing (annealing) trays, 309
Degeneration of tissue as response to injuries, 152
Delayed eruption, 155

Delta Dental Plan, 11, 50, 53
Demeritt, W. W., 513
Demerol, 175–176
Dennison, J. B., 639
Dental assistants:
  expanded function of, 16–22
    experimental programs in, 18
    legal provisions for, 19–22
      illustrated, 19, 21
    rationale behind, 16–18
    teaching of, 18, 20
  role of, 2, 11
    (See also Chairside duties)
  status of, 13–15
Dental Auxiliary Utilization (DAU) program, 16
Dental cabinets, mobile,
  illustrated, 568
Dental care:
  delivery of, 12–13
  philosophy of, 375, 384
  (See also Care)
Dental chair, 281–282
  illustrated, 281
  positioning of, for operative dentistry, 575–577
    illustrated, 576, 577
  (See also Chairside duties)
Dental compound, impressions for complete dentures with, illustrated, 648, 649
Dental Cosmos, 22
Dental disease:
  etiology of, illustrated, 387
  as infection and multifactorial process, illustrated, 376
  prevention of, 379–380
    (See also Preventive dentistry)
  role of carbohydrates in, 401–402
  (See also specific types of dental disease)
Dental Dispensary (Tufts University, Boston, Mass.), 502
Dental engine (and foot controller), 279–280
Dental examinations, 332–337
  illustrated, 333, 334, 336, 337
Dental floss, 390–392
  illustrated, 391, 392
  threaders and holders of, 393–395
    illustrated, 394, 395
Dental Hygiene Aptitude Test, 23
Dental Hygiene Council, 22
Dental hygienists, 11
  role of, 7
  status of, 22–24
Dental lamina, illustrated, 107
Dental materials, 181–184
  base materials for dentures, 212–213
  for pulpotomy, 478–479
  standards for, 184
  structure and properties of, 182–184
    illustrated, 182
    mechanical properties, table, 183
    thermal properties, table, 184
  used in composite resin restorations, 610–613
    illustrated, 611, 613
  used in prosthodontics, 619–624
    illustrated, 621–623
  (See also specific dental materials)

Dental operatory cabinet, 282–284
  hand cutting instruments in, illustrated, 296–300
  illustrated, 283, 284
Dental personnel, statistics on, 11
Dental profession, 1–13
  areas of practice of, 5–9
  dental-care delivery and, 12–13
  dental hygienists in (see Dental hygienists)
  ethics in, 30–36
  history of, 3–5
  jurisprudence and, 27–30
  laboratory technicians in (see Laboratory technicians)
  role of dental assistants in, 2, 11
    (See also Dental assistants)
  status of, 9–13
Dental psychology, 72–76
Dental tissues:
  composition and classification of, 106–107
  examination of, 465
  reactions of, to injuries, 151–153
  (See also Mature dental tissues)
Dental units, 275–280
  types of, illustrated, 274–277
Dentifrices, 391–393
  illustrated, 393
Dentin, 90–91
  hereditary opalescent, 155
  illustrated, 85, 113
  interglobular, 110
  pulpitis and secondary, 158
  removal of carious, 563–564
Dentin wall, illustrated, 556
Dentinal fibers, 110
Dentists:
  responsibilities of, in orthodontic procedures, 551
  statistics on number of, 11
  transactions between patients and, illustrated, 75
  (See also Dental profession)
Dentition (see Permanent dentition; Primary dentition; Teeth)
Denture patients, psychology of, 644–645
Dentures:
  base materials for, 212–213
  liners for, 213
  repairs of, 213–214
  sterilization of, 148
  (See also Complete dentures; Partial dentures)
Depressants, 175–176
Developing tank, 350–351
  illustrated, 350
Developmental anomalies, 153–156
  illustrated, 154, 155
Diabetes mellitus, treatment of, in emergency situations, 438–439
Diabetic coma, 439
Diagnosis, 320–340
  of anaphylactic shock, 435–437
  of cardiac emergencies, 438
  of circulatory difficulties, 437
  of dislocated mandible, 440
  endodontic, 467–471
    equipment used in, illustrated, 468–471
  of epileptic seizures, 439

Diagnosis:
  examination and (see Examinations)
  of hemorrhages from lacerations, 441
  of neurogenic shock, 434–435
    illustrated, 437
  of oral lesions, 163–164
    illustrated, 164
  orthodontic, 530–538
    illustrated, 531–537
  patient history and, 321–326
    sample questionnaires, illustrated, 322, 324
  of respiratory difficulty, 430
  uses of diagnostic findings, 339–340
Diamond as polishing agent, 258
Diamond instruments, illustrated, 295
Diarthroidal joints, 83
Diazepam, 176
Dictionary of Psychological and Psychoanalytical Terms, 63
Die, defined, 197
Diet:
  diet prescription, 417–419
    illustrated, 418
  evaluation of, 397, 412–417
    Diet Evaluation Summary, illustrated, 410
    food intake diary, illustrated, 412
  orthodontics and, 550
  (See also Nutrition)
Diet Evaluation Summary, illustrated, 410
Differentiation stage of tooth development, 153
Dimensional stability of gypsum products, 188–189
Discoid-cleoid instruments, 299–300
  illustrated, 299
Discoid edge of spoon excavators, 298
Discs, 295–296
  illustrated, 295
Disinfectants:
  used in root canal therapy, 476
  (See also specific disinfectants)
Disinfection:
  to avoid posttreatment infections, 149–150
  care of equipment used in, 312
  defined, 137
  of instruments, 147
  sterilization vs., 141–142
Dislocations, 443–444
  mandibular, 440–441
    illustrated, 441
Dismissal of operative dentistry patients, 577–578
Displacing elevators, 460
  illustrated, 462
Disposable items, handling of, 148
Distal contact in maintenance of tooth position, 102–103
Distance, effects of, on film image, 346
Distocclusion (Angle Class II), illustrated, 531, 532, 534, 535
Dobson, David P., 644–685
Dosages, drug, 175–179
Double pour method (inverted method), 191–193
  illustrated, 192, 193

Index / 745

Drives, internal and learned, 65–66
Drug Enforcement Administration (DEA), 174
Drugs:
  administration of, 170–172
    assistant's role in, 455–456
    routes of, for analgesics, 455
  antibiotic, 177
  antiseptic, 178
  astringent, styptic, hemostatic, and vasoconstrictor, 177–178
  combinations of, for analgesic purposes, 454–455
  conditions modifying action of, 172–173
  depressant, 175–176
  emergency, 179, 430
  general anesthetic, 448
  important actions of, 173
  local anesthetic, 449–450
    table, 450
  for office use, 178–179
  prescriptions for, 174–175
  responsibility and standards related to, 167–169
    illustrated, 168
  sedative, 453–454
  sources of, 169–170
  stimulant, 176–177
  weights and measures in preparation of, 172–173
Dry-heat sterilization, 143–144
  illustrated, 143
Ductility of metals, defined, 245
Dyes, action of, 178

Earl, Ethel M., 38–60
Eastman Dispensary, 22
EBA (ethoxybenzoic acid), 639
Ebers, George, 3
Economic Opportunity, Office of (OEO), 13
Economic Research and Statistics, Bureau of (ADA), 11, 68, 72
Ectoderm, defined, 107
Edentulous arches:
  maxillary, impression and model of, illustrated, 198
  wax impression of, illustrated, 211
Education:
  of dental assistants, 13–14
  of dental hygienists, 23–24
Education, Office of, 16
Educational programs:
  accreditation of, 16
  advanced placement in, 26
Ego states, 63–64
Elastic impression materials, 202–207
  illustrated, 202–204, 206
Elastics, orthodontic, 543
Electric handpieces, illustrated, 292
Electric pulp test, equipment used in, illustrated, 468–469
Electric toothbrushes, 393
Electrolytic (electrochemical) corrosion of metals, 257
Electromagnetic radiation, 342–343
  illustrated, 242
Embrasures, 90

Embrasures:
  form of, and maintenance of tooth position, illustrated, 104
  illustrated, 93
Emergencies:
  armamentarium for dealing with, 428–430
    illustrated, 429, 431
  drugs for, 179
  measures for preventing, 421–428
    illustrated, 423–426
  preparedness for, 428
  treatment of, 430–444
    anaphylactic shock, 435–437
    cardiac emergencies, 438
    circulatory difficulties, 437–438
    diabetes mellitus, 438–439
    dislocation of mandible, 440–441
      illustrated, 441
    epileptic seizures, 439–440
      illustrated, 440
    eye injuries, 441–442
      illustrated, 442
    falls and resulting injuries, 442–444
    hemorrhages from lacerations, 441
    methods of resuscitation, 431–436
      illustrated, 432–436
    neurogenic shock, 434–435
      illustrated, 437
    respiratory difficulties, 430–431
Emery as polishing agent, 258
Employer's Quarterly Federal Tax Return, 54
Enamel, 90
  cross section of, illustrated, 111
  at dentinoenamel junction, illustrated, 112
  hypoplasia of, 152–154
    illustrated, 154
  illustrated, 85
  in mature dental tissues, 109–112
    illustrated, 110–112
  mottled, 154–155
    illustrated, 155
Enamel hatchet, 298
  illustrated, 299
Enamel organ, 107–108
  illustrated, 107
Enamel spindles, 110
  illustrated, 111, 112
Enamel tufts, 109–111
  illustrated, 111
Enamel wall, 564
  illustrated, 556
Encyclopedia Britannica, 30
Endocarditis, bacterial, 124
Endoderms, defined, 107
Endodontics, 467–481
  defined, 5
  diagnosis in, 467–471
    equipment used in, illustrated, 468–471
  periapical surgery in, 479–481
    illustrated, 479
  post and core restorations in, 641–643
    illustrated, 642
  pulp capping, illustrated, 478
  pulpotomy, 478–479
  root canal therapy in, 471–478
    illustrated, 472–477
Endosteum, 116

Energy, carbohydrates as major source of, 401
English, A. C., 63
English, H. B., 63
English, S. O., 65
Environmental Protection Agency (EPA), 145
Epidemics, microbes responsible for, 124
Epidermoid carcinomas (squamous cell carcinomas), 162–163
  illustrated, 163
Epinephrine (adrenalin), 178–179
Epithelial attachment, illustrated, 114
Epithelial tissues, 106–107
Epulis, illustrated, 162
Equilibration of partial dentures, 684
Equipment:
  for analgesia, 286–287
    illustrated, 287, 453
  care of (*see* Care, of instruments and equipment)
  for complete denture impressions, illustrated, 656
  darkroom, illustrated, 350–352
  for drug administration, 455
  emergency, 429
    illustrated, 431
  endodontic diagnostic, illustrated, 468–471
  for impressions of prepared tooth for gold inlay restorations, 604–606
    illustrated, 605, 606
  for mixing and handling gypsum products, illustrated, 185, 189–191
  for preparation of partial dentures, 682–683
    illustrated, 683
  for preparation of wax patterns, illustrated, 208
  pulpotomy, 478–479
  storage of, 60
  used for alginate denture impressions, illustrated, 680
  (*See also* Instruments)
Erosion, illustrated, 157
Eruption stage of tooth development, 153, 155
Essential amino acids, 403
Esthetics in operative dentistry, 555
Ethics of dental profession, 30–36
Ethoxybenzoic acid (EBA), 639
Ethyl alcohol:
  action of, 179
  used in root canal therapy, 476
Ethylene oxide sterilization, illustrated, 146
Etiologic agent of disease, defined, 120
Eutectic alloys, defined, 245
Examinations:
  for clinical fixed prostheses, 624–626
    illustrated, 625, 626
  diagnosis and, 326–337
    dental examination, 332–337
      illustrated, 333, 334, 336, 337
    physical examination, 326–332
      illustrated, 327–332
  histopathologic, 465
  orthodontic, 534
  periodontic, illustrated, 487, 489
Excavators, illustrated, 298

Excisional biopsy, defined, 163
Expansion:
   of casting investments, 261–262
   of gypsum products, 188
Expendable supplies, control of, 55–56
   illustrated, 56
Expense records, 51, 53
Explorers, 302–303
   illustrated, 303
   sterilization of, 148
   used in endodontic diagnosis, illustrated, 468
Express contract, defined, 28
External pterygoid, 85
   illustrated, 87
Extraoral central bearing devices, 667–668
   illustrated, 668
Extraoral films, 349
   orthodontic, 536–537
   illustrated, 529
Eye injuries, 441–442
   illustrated, 442

Face examination, illustrated, 328
Facial muscles and maintenance of tooth position, 102
Facial surface (labial surface) of teeth, 90
   path of food over, illustrated, 103
   universal retainers on, illustrated, 600
Fairhurst, C. W., 271
Family history of patients, 325–326
Fats (nutritional), 402–403
Fauchard, Pierre, 3, 166
FDA (Food and Drug Administration), 167, 379, 413
Federal health plan, 53–54
Federal programs, 10–11
   influence of, on pedodontic care, 504
Federal services, dental practice in, 7
Federal Trade Commission (FTC), 167
Fees, 30
   collection of, 51
   with third-party payment plans and prepaid dental care, 52–53
      illustrated, 52
   fee-shopper calls, 43
Ferric bisulfate (Monsel's salt), 177
Fibroblasts, illustrated, 112, 113
Fibromas, defined, 162
Filaments, defined, 118
Files (instruments), 299–300
   endodontic, 307
      illustrated, 300
   periodontic, 300–301
      illustrated, 301
   used in pulp canal, 474–475
      illustrated, 475
Fillings, root canal, 478
   instruments used for, 477
Film holders, 363–364
   illustrated, 358
   use of, as radiation protection, 348
Film image, effects of technique and distance on, 346
Film racks, 351–352
   illustrated, 352

Films:
   high-speed, 348
   intraoral and extraoral, 349
   processing of, 351–355
      illustrated, 353–355
Final impressions:
   for complete dentures, 650
      pouring into master casts, 657–659
         illustrated, 658–659
      using custom impression trays, 653–657
         illustrated, 656, 657
   for partial dentures, illustrated, 682, 683
Financial records of patients, 50
Finger springs, 543
   illustrated, 541
Finishing:
   of amalgams, 243
   of castings, 271–272
   of gold alloys, 257–259
      illustrated, 258, 259
   (*See also* specific finishing procedure)
First aid, 420–421
   general considerations on, 421
   (*See also* Emergencies)
First appointment(s):
   for complete dentures, 645
   pedodontic, 513–515
      illustrated, 515
Fistulae, defined, 158
Fixed prosthodontics, 614–643
   clinical (*see* Clinical fixed prosthodontics)
   defined, 614
   fixed bridges, illustrated, 615–620
      types of, 618–620
         illustrated, 615, 617–620, 640
      materials used in, 619–624
         illustrated, 621–623
Flagg, Josiah, 3, 4
Floss (*see* Dental floss)
Flow application technique (bulk application technique), 230–232
   illustrated, 231, 232
Floxite mirrors, 395
Floxite reflectors, 385
   illustrated, 387
Fluorides, 5, 179, 377–379, 406–408
   mottled enamel, 155
   systemic, 377–378
   table, 408
   topical, 378–379
   treatment with, 395–396
Flux, use of, during soldering operation, 256
Focal infections, defined, 159
Focal spot of x-ray generating tube, 344
Focusing cup of x-ray generating tube, 344
Fogel, H. R., 520
Fones, Alfred C., 22
Food:
   path of, over facial surface of mandibular molars, illustrated, 103
   (*See also* Diet; Nutrition)
Food, Drug, and Cosmetic Act, 167–169
Food and Drug Administration (FDA), 167, 379, 413
Food and Nutrition Board (National Academy of Sciences-National Research Council), 409
Food groups, 411–413

Forceps, 311–312, 460, 583
   illustrated, 312, 461
Formaldehyde-alcohol vapor pressure sterilization, 141–145
   illustrated, 144, 145
Formocresol pulpotomy, 520
Forsyth Infirmary, 22
Fortification with vitamin D, defined, 405
Fractured permanent teeth, pedodontic procedures for, 523–525
   illustrated, 524
Fractures, treatment of, 442–443
Framework of partial dentures, 682–684
   illustrated, 684
Frankel, S. N., 520
Free gingivae, illustrated, 114
Free-gingival grafts, 494
French, N., 378
Frenectomies, 494–496
FTC (Federal Trade Commission), 167
Full crowns (extracoronal restorations), 616–617
   illustrated, 616
   tooth preparation for, illustrated, 628–629
Fusion temperature of gold alloys, 251
Fusion welding, described, 256
Fusobacterium, 125

Galagan, D. J., 503
Galvanic current, corrosion caused by, 257
Garn, R., 64, 67, 73
Garnet as polishing agent, 258–259
   illustrated, 259
Gelatin sponges, 178
General anesthesia, 447–448
General care of patients as preventive measure, 422–428
   illustrated, 423–426
General information and health questionnaire, illustrated, 423
General practice, 5
Genetic factors in etiology of orthodontics, 528–529
   illustrated, 529
Gentian violet, 178
Geographic tongue (wandering rash), illustrated, 160
Germicides, 137
Gillmore needles, illustrated, 188
Gingivae, 113–114
   illustrated, 114
   normal, illustrated, 483
   normal melanin pigmentation of, illustrated, 164
Gingival margin trimmers, 298–299
   illustrated, 299
Gingival sulcus, illustrated, 114
Gingivectomies, 494
Gingivitis:
   illustrated, 483, 484
   microbiology of, 124–127
      illustrated, 126
   (*See also* Vincent's disease)
Gingivoplasties, 494–496
   illustrated, 495
Glands, 87–88

Glands:
  illustrated, 88
  lymph, 329
Glass slabs, 304–305
  illustrated, 304
Glutaraldehyde, 147
Glyceryl trinitrate, 179
Gnarled enamel, defined, 109
Gold, 246–250
  condensed (see Condensed gold)
  removing impurities from, 247–248
    illustrated, 248
  types of, 246–247
    illustrated, 247
Gold alloys, 250–259
  carat, fineness, and troy weight of, 250
  general effects of constituents of, 250–251
  illustrated, 250, 254, 257–259
Gold foil, 246
  restorations with, 613
  retention form for, illustrated, 563
Gold inlay restorations, chairside duties in, 603–610
  illustrated, 605, 606, 608, 609
Gomphosis, defined, 84
Gothic arch tracing, 667–669
  illustrated, 668, 669
Grafts, free-gingival, 494
Grain (gr), 173
Grainger, R. M. 130
Grainger test, 384–385
Gram (g), 173
Granulation tissue, described, 152
Granulomas, 159
  pyogenic, illustrated, 161
Greene, J. C., 10, 11
Grieder, A., 62, 63, 65, 68, 77
Grossman, L. I., 519
Ground sections of teeth, 109–110
  illustrated, 110
Group practice, 12–13
Guerini, V., 5
Guide to Dental Materials and Devices (ADA), 184, 216
Guides to selection of artificial teeth, illustrated, 671–673
Gumma, defined, 161
Gustafson, B. E., 376
Gustafsson, R., 400
Gypsum products, 184–196
  expansion of, 188
    illustrated, 185
  setting reaction of, 186
  setting time of, 187–188
  strength, surface hardness, and dimensional stability of, 188–189
  study models made of, 190–196
    impressions, 190–191
      illustrated, 192
      (See also Impressions)
    polishing and identifying, 196
    pouring procedures, 191–193
      illustrated, 192, 193
    trimming procedures, 193–196
      illustrated, 194–196
  technique for using, illustrated, 189–191
  types of, 185–187
    illustrated, 186, 187

Hagen, J. O., 433
Hammons, P. E., 17, 18
Hand cutting instruments, illustrated, 296–300
Hand sharpening of instruments, 313–316
  illustrated, 314–316
Hand washing, control of cross-infections with, illustrated, 139
Handpieces (and handpiece equipment):
  care of, 289–296
    illustrated, 289–295
  disinfection of, 149
Haney, R., 66
Hanke, M. T., 377, 400
Hard palate, examination of, 330–331
  illustrated, 331
Hard soldering gold alloys, 255
Hardness of gypsum products, 188–189
Harelip, 155–156
Harper, R. A., 62, 64, 65
Harris, Chapin A., 3
Harris, T. A., 63, 64
Haversian system, 115
Hayden, Horace H., 3
Head examination, illustrated, 328
Health, Education, and Welfare, Department of (HEW), 10, 20, 167
Health departments, dental practice in, 7
Health Maintenance Organizations (HMOs), 13
Health plans, 53–54
Heat-hardened alloys, 245, 251
Heat test, 469
  illustrated, 471
Heavy (or tray) type of high viscosity of rubber materials, 205
Heimlich, H. J., 434
Heimlich maneuver as resuscitation method, 433–435
  illustrated, 434, 435
Hemisections, root, 497
Hemophilus influenzae, 123
Hemorrhages from lacerations, treatment of, 441
Hemostatics, 177
Hepatitis A (see Viral hepatitis)
Hepatitis B (serum hepatitis), 133, 136
Hereditary opalescent dentin, 155
Herpes simplex (Herpes labialis), 131, 159–160
  illustrated, 160
HEW (Department of Health, Education, and Welfare), 10, 20, 167
Hickey, J. C., 615
Hidden Persuaders, The (Packard), 67
Hierarchy of needs, 66, 380
  illustrated, 381
High-speed films, use of, as radiation protection, 348
High-speed handpieces, 290–291
  illustrated, 291
High-temperature casting gold alloys, 252–253
Hippocrates, 3
Histology (see Dental tissues)
Histopathologic examinations following surgery, 465

HMOs (health maintenance organizations), 13
Hoe excavators, illustrated, 298
Hogeboom, F. E., 502
Holding instruments for condensed gold, 309–310
  illustrated, 310
Holland, Gene A., 614–643
Hollinshead, B. S., 17, 22, 24
Hooley, J. R., 428, 429
Horney, K., 64
Hospitals, surgery performed in, 460
Hot bead sterilizers, 144
Hot oil, sterilization with, 146
House of Delegates (ADA), 14
  ADA *Principles of Ethics* and, 35n.
  definition of oral surgery and, 457
  dental laboratory technicians and, 24, 25
  expanded functions and, 17, 20
Housekeeping, 427–428
Howard, W. W., 30
Hughes, G. A., 615
Hullihen, Simon P., 457
Hunter, Grover C., Jr., 151–165, 482–500
Hunter College (New York City), 22
Hurme, V. O., 510
Hutchinson's teeth, illustrated, 154
Hwang-ti, 3
Hydrochloric acid, 476
Hydrocolloid conditioners, 287–288
  illustrated, 203
Hydrocolloids:
  illustrated, 202, 203
  irreversible (see Alginate hydrocolloid impressions)
  reversible, 630
Hydrogen peroxide, 179
Hydroxyzine hydrochloride, 176
Hygiene:
  gingivitis and, 484
  personal, in control of cross-infections, 138–139
  (See also: Disinfection; Sterilization)
Hygienic (sanitary) pontics, illustrated, 617
Hygroscopic expansion method (low-heat technique), 261
  illustrated, 267
Hyperkeratosis (leukoplakia; smoker's patches), illustrated, 160
Hyperplasia of tissue as response to injuries, 152–153
Hypertrophy of tissue as response to injuries, 152–153
Hypoplasia of tissue as response to injury, 152

Ice test, 469–470
  illustrated, 470
Ideal occlusion (normal occlusion), illustrated, 531
I-Em-Hetep, 3
Ilg, F. L., 509, 511, 512
Implants, bone, 496
Implied contracts, defined, 28–29
Impression trays:
  for complete dentures: cleaning of, 650

Impression trays:
    for complete dentures: illustrated, 646–648
        (See also Custom impression trays, for complete dentures)
        illustrated, 202, 204, 206
    for partial dentures, illustrated, 682, 683
    sterilization of, 148
Impressions (reverse reproductions):
    defined, 197
    final (see Final impressions)
    gypsum, 190–192
        illustrated, 192
    illustrated, 198
    materials for, 197–207
        desirable properties in, 197–198
        elastic, 202–207
            illustrated, 202–204, 206
        plastic, 200–201
            illustrated, 201
        rigid, 198–200
            illustrated, 200
    preliminary (see Preliminary impressions)
    of prepared teeth: for fixed prosthodontics, 630–634
        illustrated, 632–634
        for gold inlay restorations, 604–607
            illustrated, 605, 606
    wax, 630
        illustrated, 211
    (See also Models; and specific types of impressions)
Improperly-fitting castings, 271
Improved stones, general properties of, 185–187
    illustrated, 187
Incisional biopsy, defined, 163
Incisors:
    coverage for fractured, illustrated, 524
    functions of, 89
    lateral, illustrated, 162
    relative position of, illustrated, 103
    (See also Mandibular incisors; Maxillary incisors; Permanent incisors)
Income records, 51
Incomplete castings as defective, 271
Indian Health Service, 10
Indiana University School of Dentistry, 514
Indications for general anesthesia, 448
Indigenous bacteria (normal flora of bacteria), 122–123
Infection(s):
    dental disease as, 376
    (See also Cross-infections)
Inflammation and repair of tissues, 151–152
Information forms, 49
Inhalation, drug administration by, 171
Inhibitors of polymerization, 212
Initiation stage of tooth development, 153
Initiators of polymerization, 212
Injections:
    drug administration by, 171–172
    sites for local anesthesia, 450–451
        illustrated, 447, 448
Injuries:
    eye, 441–442
        illustrated, 442
    radiation, 165

Injuries:
    resulting from falls, 442–444
    tissue response to, 152–153
Inlays:
    cusp-capping, 616–617
        illustrated, 616
    retention form for, illustrated, 562
    (See also Gold inlay restorations)
Instruments:
    care of (see Care, of instruments and equipment)
    for emergencies, 429–430
        illustrated, 431
    exchange of, in operative dentistry, 571–574, 592–593
        illustrated, 572, 573, 592
    moisture control, illustrated, 583
    orthodontic, preparation of, illustrated, 546–547
    periodontic, 300–301
        illustrated, 301, 487
        sharpening of, 487, 489–490
            illustrated, 490
        surgical, illustrated, 493
        ultrasonic, 490–491
            illustrated, 491
    prosthodontic, 624–625
        illustrated, 625, 627, 639
    sharpening of, 312–316
        illustrated, 313–315
        of periodontic instruments, 489–490
            illustrated, 490
    sterilization of, 141–149
        acceptable methods of, 142–143
        with boiling water and hot oil, 146–147
        cleaning and preparation of, 147–148
            illustrated, 148
        disinfection vs., 141–142
        by dry heat, 143–144
            illustrated, 143
        of endodontic instruments, 469, 472–473, 475
            illustrated, 480
        with ethylene oxide, illustrated, 146
        with formaldehyde-alcohol vapor pressure sterilizers, 144–145
            illustrated, 145
        of hand cutting instruments, illustrated, 300
        with hot heat and salt sterilizers, 144
        test of sterilizers, illustrated, 145
    surgical, 458–463
        illustrated, 458, 459, 462–464
        preparation and sterilization of, 466
    used in root canal therapy, illustrated, 472–477
    (See also Equipment; and specific instruments)
Insulin shock, 438–439
Insurance company dental health plans, 53
Insurance coverage, 11
Interarticular disc (meniscus), 83–84
    illustrated, 84
Intercuspal relation, maintenance of tooth position and, 101–103
    illustrated, 103
Interdental stimulators, 392–394
    illustrated, 394
Interglobular dentin, 110

Intermaxillary check-bite, mounting of, illustrated, 675
Intermaxillary relationship:
    of complete dentures, 663–667
        illustrated, 665–667
    of partial dentures, 683–684
        illustrated, 684
Intermaxillary suture (median palative suture), 81–83
    illustrated, 82, 83
Internal defects of castings, 271
Internal drives (primary innate drives), 65–66
Internal pterygoid, 85
    illustrated, 87
Internal Revenue Service (IRS), 54
Internal wall of crowns, 617
Interval timers, illustrated, 351
Interviewing techniques used in diet evaluation, 413, 414
Intracoronal restorations (cusp-capping inlays; onlays), 616–617
    illustrated, 616
Intramuscular injections, 171–172
Intraoral central bearing devices, 667–668
    illustrated, 668
Intraoral films, 349, 535–536
Intraoral structures, examination of, illustrated, 329–332
Intraoral x-rays (see X-rays, intraoral)
Intravenous injections, 172
Inunction, drug administration by, 171
Inventory control, 55–57
    illustrated, 56, 57
Inverted method (double pour method), 191–193
    illustrated, 192, 193
Investments (see Casting investments)
Invoice, illustrated, 60
Iodine:
    as antiseptic, 178
    as nutrient, 408–410
        RDAs for, table, 409
        table, 406
Irby, W. B., 441
Iron, 408–410
    RDAs for, table, 409
    sources of, 411, 413
    table, 406
Irradiation injuries to teeth, 165
Irreversible hydrocolloids (see Alginate hydrocolloid impressions)
IRS (Internal Revenue Service), 54

Jamison, H. C., 17, 18
Jaws, nerve anatomy of, 446–448
    illustrated, 447, 448
Jay, Philip, 129, 377
Jerge, C. R., 12, 13
Johnson, Charles Nelson, 32
Jordan, Evangeline, 502
Journal of the American Dental Association, 184, 235
Juvenile periodontitis (periodontosis), 484

Kahn test for syphilis, 132
Keyes, Paul, 376, 378
Kilovoltage (kVp), effects of, on film image, 346

Index / 749

Kinney, W. B., 435
Kirk, E. C., 22
Knives, illustrated, 299
Knoedler, D. J., 18
Koch, C. R. E., 5
Koch, Robert, 120
Kozak, S. F., 271
Kruger, G. W., 429

Labial surface (facial surface) of teeth, 90
Laboratories:
  construction of complete dentures in, illustrated, 649, 650
  denture relines done in, 677
  importance of, 8–9
Laboratory equipment, care of, 317–319
  illustrated, 317, 318
Laboratory technicians, 11, 24–26
  role of, 7
Lacerations, treatment of hemorrhages from, 441
Lactobacillis, 134
  caries and, 129–130
  tests for, 130–131
  illustrated, 131
Lactobacillus acidophilus, illustrated, 120
Lamellae:
  defined, 109
  illustrated, 110, 111
Lamina dura, 115
Laminia propria, illustrated, 114
Land, defined, 657
Laskin, D. M., 437, 439
Lateral incisors, illustrated, 162
  (See also Mandibular incisors, lateral; Maxillary incisors, lateral)
Lateral sliding flaps (pedicle grafts), 494
Laxatives, 178–179
Lead aprons, use of, as radiation protection, 348
Learned drives (secondary drives), 66
Leeuwenhoek, Antonj van, 118
Legal provisions for expanded functions, 19–22
  illustrated, 19, 21
Legal Provisions on Expanded Functions for Dental Hygienists and Assistants (HEW), 20
Leinferder, Karl F., 206–272
Leptotsichia buccalis, 125
Leukemia, gingivitis and, 484
Leukoplasia (hyperkeratosis; smoker's patches), illustrated, 260
Lever elevators, 460
  illustrated, 462
Librium, 176
Lichen planus, 161
Ligature wires, 543
Light (or syringe) type of low viscosity of rubber materials, 205
Lindahl, R. L., 520, 523
Line angles of teeth:
  illustrated, 90, 556
  mesiolabial and mesiolabioincisal, illustrated, 90, 91
Liners:
  cavity, 597
  denture, 213

Lingual arch, illustrated, 541
Lining mucosa, 113
  of cheeks, examination of, 330–331
    illustrated, 331
  of lips, examination of, illustrated, 330
Lip examination, illustrated, 329, 330
Lipids, 402–403
Lister, Joseph, 121
Liter (liquid measure), 173
Local anesthesia, 448–452
  illustrated, 449, 452
  in operative dentistry, 580–581, 592–593
    illustrated, 581, 592
  table, 450
Local health departments, dental practice in, 7
Local health plan, 53–54
Localized shrinkage porosity of castings, 271
Loe, Harold, 125
Long, Crawford W., 167, 445, 446
Lost wax process, 260
Low-heat technique (hygroscopic expansion method), 261
  illustrated, 267
Lubricants for moisture control, 583
Ludwick, W. E., 18
Lupton, Cecil R., 166–180, 445–466
Lymph glands, examination of, illustrated, 329

McBride, W. C., 501
McCarthy, F. M., 420, 422, 438
McCaslin, A. J., 504
McFall, Walter T., Jr., 106–116
Magnesium, RDAs for, table, 409
Mahler, D. B., 267
Major adult orthodontics, 541
Malleability of metals, defined, 245
Malocclusion, 530–537
  classification of, illustrated, 531–537
  defined, 97
  prevalence of, 2
Malpractice, 29–30
Maltz, M., 63
Mandibles:
  dislocation of, 440–441
    illustrated, 441
  illustrated, 82–84
Mandibular bicuspids (premolars):
  bisecting-angle technique used with, illustrated, 362
  characteristics of, 94
    illustrated, 101
  paralleling technique used with, 368
Mandibular canines:
  lateral bisecting-angle technique used with, 361
  paralleling technique used with, illustrated, 367
Mandibular cuspids, illustrated, 162
Mandibular foramina, 83
  illustrated, 84
Mandibular incisors:
  bisecting-angle technique used with, 361
  central: paralleling technique used with, illustrated, 367
  screwdriver-shaped, illustrated, 154
  characteristics of, 91–92

Mandibular incisors:
  characteristics of: illustrated, 100
  deciduous, cap stage of development of, illustrated, 107
  lateral: bisecting-angle technique used with, 361
  paralleling technique used with, illustrated, 367
Mandibular molars:
  bisecting-angle technique used with, illustrated, 362
  characteristics of, 95–96
    illustrated, 102
  paralleling technique used with, 368
  path of food over facial surface of, illustrated, 103
Mandibular occlusion rims, illustrated, 664
Mandibular partial dentures, illustrated, 684
Mandibular teeth:
  anchor, rubber dam hole position for, illustrated, 585
  anterior, anatomic form and relationship of pulp cavity to hard structure of, illustrated, 95
  illustrated, 97
  posterior, guide for selection of artificial, illustrated, 673
Manipulation:
  of amalgams, 239–243
    illustrated, 240–243
  of casting investments, 262
  of pattern waxes, 209
  of polycarboxylate cement, 229
  of synthetic resin materials, 213
Marchand, Louis, 73
Marks, S. C., 508, 524
Maslow, Abraham, 66, 380–381
Masseter, 85
  illustrated, 86
Massler, M., 153, 156, 507
Master casts, pouring of final impressions into, for complete dentures, 657–659
  illustrated, 658–659
Master on-off switch of dental units, 276–277
Mastication muscles, 84–87
  illustrated, 86, 87
Masticatory mucosa, 113
Mat gold, illustrated, 247
Materials (see Dental materials)
Matrices for amalgam restorations, 599–603
  illustrated, 600–603
Matteson, Stephen R., 341–374
Mature dental tissues, 109–113
  cementum of, 111
    illustrated, 112
  dentin in, 110–112
    illustrated, 112, 113
    (See also Dentin)
  enamel in, 109–112
    illustrated, 110–112
    (See also Enamel)
  pulp in, 91, 111–113
    illustrated, 85, 113
Maxillae, 81–83
  illustrated, 82–83
Maxillary arch, impression of edentulous, illustrated, 198

Maxillary bicuspids (premolars):
  bisecting-angle technique used with, 360
  characteristics of, 91
    illustrated, 101
  paralleling technique used with, illustrated, 366
Maxillary canines:
  bisecting-angle technique used with, 359
  paralleling technique used with, illustrated, 365
Maxillary incisors:
  central: bisecting-angle technique used with, illustrated, 359
    paralleling technique used with, illustrated, 365
    rubber dam hole position for, illustrated, 584
    screwdriver-shaped, illustrated, 154
  characteristics of, 91
    illustrated, 100
  lateral: bisecting angle-technique used with, illustrated, 359
    paralleling technique used with, illustrated, 365
Maxillary molars:
  bisecting-angle technique used with, 360
  characteristics of, 94–95
    illustrated, 102
  paralleling technique used with, illustrated, 366
Maxillary occlusion rims, illustrated, 664
Maxillary teeth:
  anatomic form and relationship of pulp cavity to hard structure of, illustrated, 94
  guide for selection of artifical, illustrated, 673
  illustrated, 96
  left, universal retainers on facial surface of, illustrated, 600
Maximum inventory list, illustrated, 56
Measures and weights in drug preparations, 172–173
Meat group (food group), 411
Mechanical amalgam mixing, 240–241, 306–307
  illustrated, 240, 307
Mechanical properties of dental materials, table, 183
Mechanical sharpening of instruments, illustrated, 313
Median palatine cysts, 159
Median palatine sutures (intermaxillary sutures), 81–83
  illustrated, 82–83
Medicaid, 10, 50, 54
Medical history of patients, 325, 423–424
  illustrated, 424
  records of, 49–50
Medicaments:
  used in root canal therapy, 475–476
  (See also Drugs)
Medicare, 50, 54
Melanin pigmentation of gingivae, illustrated, 164
Melting range of alloys, 245
Meniscus (interarticular disc), 83–84
  illustrated, 84
Mental foramina, illustrated, 82, 83

Mercury in alloys, 239–240
  illustrated, 239
Meredith, H. V., 507
Merrill, S. A., 525
Mesial contact in maintenance of tooth position, 102–103
Mesial surface of teeth, 90
Mesiocclusion (Angle Class III), illustrated, 531, 536
Mesiolabial line angle of teeth (mesiofacial line angle), illustrated, 90, 91
Mesiolabioincisal (mesiofacioincisal) angle of teeth, 90
Mesoderm, defined, 107
Metabolism, regulation of, 408
Metal framework of partial dentures, 682–684
  illustrated, 684
Metal trays (see Trays)
Metallic oxide impression paste, 199–200
  illustrated, 200
Metalloids, general characteristics of, 245
Metals:
  characteristics of, 244, 245
  corrosion of, 257
  porcelain-fused-to-metal crowns, 618–624
    illustrated, 618–621, 623
  (See also specific metal)
Metaphen tincture:
  action of, 178
  used in endodontics, 472, 478
Meter, defined, 173
Microbiology, 117–134
  bacterial groups of clinical importance in, 121–124
  of caries, 128–131
    illustrated, 131
  fundamentals and history of, 118–121
  of gingivitis and periodontitis, 124–127
    illustrated, 126
  of oral and related infections, 131–132
    illustrated, 132
  phase contrast microscopy of plaque bacteria, 127–128
    illustrated, 128
  scope of, 118
  viruses, 132–133
Microscopy (see Phase contrast microscopy)
Midpalatal relief, pressure-indicating parts to show, illustrated, 675
Milk group (food group), 411
Millamperage (MA), effects of, on film image, 346
Miller, W. D., 125, 376–377, 400
Milliliter, defined, 173
Minerals, 406–409
  RDAs for, table, 409
  as sources of drugs, 169
  tables, 406, 408
Minimum inventory list, illustrated, 56
Minor orthodontics for adults, 540–541
Mirrors, 300–302
  Floxite, 395
  illustrated, 302
  sterilization of, 148
  used in endodontic diagnosis, illustrated, 468
Mixed dentition, 509–512

Mixed dentition:
  illustrated, 99, 511
Mixing:
  of amalgams, illustrated, 240–241
  of zinc oxide–eugenol cement, 216–217
    illustrated, 217
  of zinc phosphate cement, 219–224
Mixing spatulas, care of, 302–304
  illustrated, 304
Mixing valves, 351
Mobile dental cabinets, illustrated, 568
Mobility test, 470–471
Modeling compound, 583
Models (see Casts)
Moisture control in operative dentistry, chairside duties in, 581–593
  illustrated, 582–591
Molars:
  bitewing of, illustrated, 369
  functions of, 89
  ground section of, illustrated, 113
  illustrated, 113
  mulberry, 154
  prefabricated, illustrated, 635
  relative position of, illustrated, 103
  (See also Mandibular molars; Maxillary molars)
Mold, defined, 197
Moniliasis (candidiasis), 132
Monitoring:
  of drugged patients, 455–456
  preoperative, of patients undergoing surgery, 461–462
Monomer, defined, 211
Monsel's salt (Ferric bisulfate), 177
Morphine, action and dosage of, 175–176
Morr, D. V., 24, 25
Mortars and pestles used in mixing amalgams, 240–241
  illustrated, 240
Morton, William T. G., 5
Motivation, 65–68
  role of, in preventive dentistry, 380–382
    illustrated, 381
Mottled enamel, 154–155
  illustrated, 155
Mounting of films, 353–355
  illustrated, 355
Mouth administration (p.o.) of drugs, 171
Mouth preparation for partial dentures, 682
Mouth-to-mouth breathing, 431–433
  illustrated, 432–433
Mouthwashes, 393
Moyer, R. E., 508, 510
Mucogingival problems, illustrated, 485
Mucogingival surgery, 494–496
Mucosa, 84
  illustrated, 85
  (See also Buccal mucosa; Lining mucosa; Masticatory mucosa)
Mucous patches, described, 161
Mulberry molars, described, 154
Multifactorial process, dental disease as, illustrated, 376
Multiple-surface cavities, prepartion designs for, 559–561
  illustrated, 561
Murray, H. V., 631

Index / 751

Muscles:
  facial, and maintenance of tooth position, 102
  mastication, 84–87
    illustrated, 86, 87
  tissues of, 107
Mycobacterium tuberculosis, 123
Myers, B. A., 13
Myren, R. A., 30

NADL (National Association of Dental Laboratories), 24–26
Narcotics, 175–176
National Academy of Sciences-National Research Council, 409
National Association of Dental Laboratories (NADL), 24–26
National Board of Certification (NBC), Recognized Graduate Program, 25
National Center for Health Statistics, 1
National Committee on Radiation Protection, 349
National Formulary (Committee on the National Formulary), 168
National Health Service Corps (NHSC), 10
NBC (see National Board of Certification)
Neck examination, illustrated, 328, 329
Necrotic ulcerative gingivitis (NUG; trench mouth), 131
  illustrated, 132
Needs, hierarchy of, 66, 380–381
  illustrated, 381
Neisseria meningitidis, 123
Neisseria species, 125
Nelson, Robert M., 527–551
Neoplasms, 153
  benign, 161–162
    illustrated, 162
  defined, 153
  odontogenic, 162–163
Nerves:
  anatomy of tooth and jaw, 446–448
    illustrated, 447, 448
  supply of, to teeth, illustrated, 94
  tissues of, 107
Neurogenic shock, treatment of, 434–435
  illustrated, 437
Neuroleptic analgesia, 454
New York Times, The (newspaper), 9, 11
Newman, Irene, 22
NHSC (National Health Service Corps), 10
Nitrous oxide machine (and mask), illustrated, 453
Nizel, A., 399, 400, 413
Nonessential dietary amino acids, 403
Nonexpendable supplies, control of, 57
Nonremovable appliances, orthodontic, 542–544
  illustrated, 543
Normal flora of bacteria (indigenous bacteria), 122–123
Normal occlusion (ideal occlusion), illustrated, 531
North Carolina, University of, 15, 514
Northwestern University Dental School, 4
Nutrition, 399–403
  defined, 400
  dental disease and carbohydrate, 401

Nutrition:
  in etiology of orthodontic problems, 529
  food groups, 411–413
  gingivitis and, 484
  lipid, 402–403
  (See also Diet; Minerals, Proteins; Recommended Daily Dietary Allowances; Vitamins)

O'Brien, W. J., 267
Occlusal adjustments, 491–492
  illustrated, 492
Occlusal contact, maintenance of tooth position and, 101
  illustrated, 102
Occlusal form, maintenance of tooth position and, 104–105
Occlusal sealing, 525
Occlusal-surface cavities, preparation of, for silver amalgams, 558–559
  illustrated, 559
Occlusal technique, 373–374
  illustrated, 370, 371
Occlusal trauma, defined, 483
Occlusal vertical intermaxillary relation, 666
Occlusion, 97–101
  defined, 530–531
  illustrated, 531
  of primary dentition, 507–508
Occlusion rims (record bases):
  arbitrary placement of, illustrated, 667
  fabrication of, 661–664
    illustrated, 660–662, 664
  maxillary and mandibular, illustrated, 664
  sterilization of, 148
Odbert, H. S., 63
Odontoblasts, 108
  illustrated, 112, 113
  role of, in degeneration of tissue, 152
Odontogenic neoplasms, 162–163
Odontomas, illustrated, 163
OEO (Office of Economic Opportunity), 13
Office duties in operative dentistry, 574–578
  illustrated, 576–577
Office managers, functions of, 40
Office manual, 39–40
Official Drugs, 169
Oil of cloves, 179
O'Leary, T. J., 385
One-surface cavities, preparation designs for, 558–560
  illustrated, 559, 560
Onlays (cusp-capping inlays; intracoronal restorations), 616–617
  illustrated, 616
Open bites, 532–533
  illustrated, 537
Open panel defined, 13
Operating environment, 427
Operating light, 278–279
  illustrated, 279
Operating pliers (cotton pliers; tweezers), 302–303
  illustrated, 303
Operating stools, illustrated, 282, 283
Operative dentistry, 552–613
  caries and, 552–554
    illustrated, 553

Operative dentistry:
  (See also Caries)
  chairside duties in (see Chairside duties, in operative dentistry)
  defined, 553
  dental team in, 564–568
    illustrated, 565–568
  exchange of instruments in, 571–574, 592–593
    illustrated, 572, 573, 592
  objectives of, 554–555
  office duties in, 574–578
    illustrated, 576, 577
  pedodontic, 517–519
    illustrated, 518
  terminology of, 555–556
    illustrated, 556
  use of oral evacuators in, 568–571
    illustrated, 570
Oral antiseptics, 150
Oral evacuators, 284–285, 568–571
  illustrated, 285, 570
Oral exfoliative cytology (see Cytology)
Oral express contracts, defined, 28
Oral lesions:
  biopsies and cytology in diagnosis of, 163–164
    illustrated, 164
  illustrated, 159–162
Oral pathology, defined, 5
Oral physiotherapy, 387–388
  techniques of, 395
Oral pigmentation, 163–165
  illustrated, 164
Ordering of supplies, 57–58
Ordinary hatchet excavators, illustrated, 298
Orland, F. J., 121, 129, 376
Oropharyngeal airway tube, illustrated, 431
Oropharynx, examination of, illustrated, 332
Orthodontic wires (and bands), 542
  illustrated, 257
Orthodontics, 527–551
  for adolescents, 540
  for adults, 540–541
  appliances used in, 541–544
    illustrated, 541–543
  cephalometrics and, 545–550
    illustrated, 548, 549
  defined, 5
  diagnosis in, 530–538
    illustrated, 531–537
  duties of assistants in, 544–545
  etiology of, 528–530
    illustrated, 529
  preventive, 538–540
    illustrated, 539
  responsibilities in, 550–551
Osler, Sir William, 400
Osseous defects, surgical correction of, illustrated, 496, 497
Ostectomies, 496
Osteoblasts in periodontal ligament, 115
Osteoclasts, role of, 158
Osteomyelitis, defined, 158
Osteoplasties, illustrated, 496
Outline forms, establishing, in cavity preparation, 560–561
Overberger, James E., 181–196, 234–243

Ownership of prostheses, 30
Oxidized cellulose, 178
Oxygen inhalation, 179

Packard, Vance, 67
Packing list, illustrated, 58
Pain control (see Analgesia; Anesthesia; Sedation)
Palate:
　cleft, 2, 155–156
　examination of, 330–331
　　illustrated, 331
　pressure-indicating paste to show mid-palatal relief, illustrated, 675
Palladium in gold alloys, 251
Palpation in endodontic diagnosis, 470
Palpatory systolic pressure, defined, 423
Panoramic radiology, 372–374
　illustrated, 372, 373
Paper points, absorbent, used in pulp canal, 475–476
　illustrated, 476
Papillomas, defined, 162
Paralleling technique, 363–371
　illustrated, 363–368
Parent ego state (P), 64
Parents, responsibilities of, in orthodontic procedures, 550–551
Parfitt, G. J., 390
Parks, A. L., 30
Parotid gland, 87
　illustrated, 88
Partial crowns (three-quarter crowns; pinlays), 616–617
　illustrated, 616
Partial dentures, 680–685
　illustrated, 680–684
　impressions for, illustrated, 680
Parulis, defined, 158
Paste-liquid application technique, 233
Paste-paste application technique, 233
Pasteur, Louis, 119–121
Pathogen, defined, 122
Pathologic conditions, action of drugs on, 173
Pathology, defined, 151
Pathology laboratories, 9
Patient history, 321–326
　medical, 325, 423–424
　　illustrated, 424
　records of, 49–50
　for orthodontic procedures, 534
　sample questionnaires for, illustrated, 322, 324
Pattern waxes, 208–209
　illustrated, 208
　(See also Wax patterns)
Payments, 11–12
Payroll, records of, 54
PCA cement (polycarboxylate cement), 228–229, 639
　table, 216
Pedicle grafts, 494
Pedodontics, 501–526
　defined, 5, 502–503
　history of, 502
　need and demand for, 503–504
　procedures followed in, 512–525
　　consultation appointments, 515–517

Pedodontics:
　procedures followed in: first appointment, 513–515
　　illustrated, 515
　for fractured permanent teeth, 523–525
　　illustrated, 524
　in occlusal sealing, 525
　in operative dentistry, 517–519
　　illustrated, 518
　prosthetics, 520–523
　　illustrated, 521–523
　pulp therapy in, 519–520
　for 6-to-12-year-old children, 509–512
　　illustrated, 511
　for 2-to-6-year-old children, 508–509
　(See also Primary dentition)
Pelton, W. J., 1, 2
Penicillin, 177
Penny test, 351
Percussion test, 469–470
Periapical abcesses (root-end abcesses), 158
Periapical cysts, 159
Periapical granulomas, 159
Periapical surgery, 479–481
　illustrated, 479
Periodontal disease (see Periodontitis)
Periodontal ligament, 114–115
　illustrated, 114
Periodontal membrane, 83–85
　illustrated, 85
Periodontics, 482–500
　conditions treated in, 482–486
　　illustrated, 483–486
　defined, 6
　examination and charting in, illustrated, 487–489
　initial preparation in, 487
　　response to, illustrated, 490
　instruments used in (see Instruments, periodontic)
　occlusal adjustment in, 491–492
　　illustrated, 492
　recall maintenance needed in, 499
　surgery in (see Surgery, periodontic)
Periodontitis (periodontal disease; pyorrhea), 482–485
　bacteriology of, 124–127
　　illustrated, 126
　illustrated, 483, 484
　statistics on, 1
Periodontium:
　examination of, 332–334
　　illustrated, 333, 334
　(See also Alveolar bone; Cementum; Gingivae; Periodontal ligament)
Periosteum, 116
Peristalsis, defined, 401
Permanent dentition, 88
　eruption of, table, 92
　illustrated, 99
　pedodontic procedures for fractured permanent teeth, 523–525
　illustrated, 524
Permanent incisors:
　developing, illustrated, 109
　ground section of, illustrated, 110
Personal hygiene in control of cross-infections, 138–139
Personality development, 63–64

Pestles and mortars used in mixing of amalgams, 240–241
　illustrated, 240
Peyton, F. A., 261, 267
PFM crowns (see Porcelain-fused-to-metal crowns)
Phagocytosis, defined, 152
Pharmacists, 9
Pharmacology:
　historical perspective on development of, 167
　(See also Drugs)
Phase contrast microscopy:
　of plaque bacteria, 127–128
　　illustrated, 128
　in preventive dentistry, 387
Phenobarbital, 175
Phenol compounds, 179
Phillips, R. W., 236, 271
Phosphorus, 406–407
　RDAs for, table, 409
　table, 406
Photographs:
　orthodontic, 537–538
　periodontic, 499
　records of, 50
Physical examinations, 326–332
　illustrated, 327–332
Physical properties of pattern waxes, 208–209
Physician's Desk Reference (Medical Economics), 169
Physics of radiation, 342–344
　illustrated, 342, 343
Physiotherapy, periodontic postsurgical, 498–499
Pickling of castings, 269–270
Pigmentation, oral, 163–165
　illustrated, 164
Pinlays (pinledges), 616–617
　illustrated, 616
Pit and fissure cavities:
　defined, 156
　illustrated, 557
PJC (porcelain jacket crowns), 619
　illustrated, 621
Plak-Lite, 396–397
　illustrated, 397
Plants as sources of drugs, 169
Plaque, 123, 376
　bacteria causing, 125
　　accumulative changes in, illustrated, 126
　phase contrast microscopy of, 127–128
　　illustrated, 128
　control of, 379
　mechanical devices for removal of, 393
　　illustrated, 395
　recognition of, 394–395
　role of sucrose in formation of, 402
Plaque index, 385–386
　illustrated, 386
Plaster:
　general properties of, 185
　　illustrated, 186
　orthodontic plaster models, 537
　of paris, 198–199
Plastic evacuator tips, 148
Plastic impression materials, 200–201

Plastic impression materials:
  illustrated, 201
Plastic instruments, care of, 302–304
  illustrated, 303
Plastic trays (see Trays)
Platinum in gold alloys, 251
Pliers:
  care of, 302–303, 307
    illustrated, 303, 309
  sterilization of, 147
  used in endodontic diagnosis, illustrated, 468
Pluggers (see Amalgam condensers)
Point angles of teeth, illustrated, 90, 556
Policies and Guidelines for the Training of Dental Auxiliaries (ADA Council on Dental Education), 26
Polishing:
  of amalgams, 243
  of casting, 271–272
  of gold alloys, 257–259
    illustrated, 258, 259
  of gold inlays, 607
  of partial dentures, 685
  of repairs on dentures, 680
Polycarboxylate cement (PCA cement), 228–229, 639
  table, 216
Polymer, defined, 211
Polymerization, 211–212
Polymerizing impression trays (quick-cure resin impression trays), 652–655
  illustrated, 654–655
Polyps, pulp, illustrated, 158
Pontics (see Porcelain-faced crowns)
Porcelain used in prosthodontics, 619, 621–624
  illustrated, 621–623
Porcelain-faced crowns (pontics), 620–621
  illustrated, 617, 618
Porcelain-fused-to-metal crowns (PFM crowns), 618–624
  illustrated, 618–621, 623
  restorations of, 637
Porcelain jacket crowns (PJC crowns), 619
  illustrated, 621
Porosity:
  of casting gold alloys, 253
  of castings, 271
Post and core restorations, 641–643
  illustrated, 642
Posterior teeth:
  anatomic form and relationship of pulp cavity to hard structure of, illustrated, 94, 95
  embrasures of, illustrated, 93
  guide for selection of artificial, illustrated, 672, 673
  line and point angles on, illustrated, 91
Postoperative care, 498
Postoperative instructions, 465–466, 498–499
  postoperative instruction card, illustrated, 465
Posttreatment infections, 136, 149–150
Pouring:
  of final impressions into master casts for complete dentures, 657–659
    illustrated, 658–659
  of gold inlay models, 607

Pouring:
  methods of, 191–193
    illustrated, 192, 193
  of preliminary casts for partial dentures, 681–682
    illustrated, 681
  of preliminary impressions for complete dentures, 649–650
    illustrated, 649
Powder-liquid application technique, 233
Powder-water ration in casting investments, 262
Powdered gold, 247
Powers, J. M., 639
Prefabricated teeth (see Artificial teeth)
Preliminary casts for partial dentures, pouring of, 681–682
  illustrated, 681
Preliminary impressions:
  for complete dentures: with dental compound, illustrated, 648, 649
    pouring of, 649–650
      illustrated, 649
    preliminary alginate hydrocolloids, illustrated, 646, 647
    properly trimmed, illustrated, 650
  for partial dentures, 680–681
    illustrated, 680
Premedication, 427
Premolars (see Bicuspids)
Preoperative alginate-acrylic resin technique, 634–636
  illustrated, 636
Prepayment programs, 11–12
Prescription(s):
  diet, 417–419
    illustrated, 418
  form and content of, 174–175
Press roll technique of toothbrushing, 389–390
  illustrated, 390
Pressure-indicating paste to show need for midpalatal relief, illustrated, 675
Pressure release test, 471
Pressure welding, 256
Prevention of emergencies, 421–428
  illustrated, 423–426
Preventive dentistry, 375–398
  defined, 375
  developing program of, 380–382
  history of, 376–377
  instructing patients in, 382
  plaque control in, 379
  role of fluorides (see Fluorides)
  step-by-step plan for, 383–398
    adjuncts to teeth cleaning, 391–394
    segment 1 of, 383–388
      illustrated, 386, 387
    segment 2, 394–396
    segment 3, 396–397
      illustrated, 397
    toothbrushing, illustrated, 388–391
    use of dental floss, 390–392
      illustrated, 391, 392
Preventive orthodontics, 538–540
  illustrated, 540
Primary dentition (deciduous dentition), 88, 504–508
  eruption of, 506–507

Primary dentition (deciduous dentition):
  approximate eruption times.
    illustrated, 96
    table, 92
  illustrated, 98, 505–507
  importance of, 505–506
  occlusion of, 507–508
Primary innate drives (internal drives), 65–66
Primary radiation, defined, 347
Primate spaces, defined, 508
Prinz, H., 5, 167
Processing waxes, 210–211
  illustrated, 213
Profession, defined, 30
Proliferation stage of tooth development, 153
Properties:
  of metals, 245, 246
  of synthetic resins, 212–213
Prophylaxis angles, sterilization of, 148–149
Prophylaxis brushes, sterilization of, 148
Prophylaxis cups, sterilization of, 148
Prophylaxis instruments, 300–301
  illustrated, 301
Prostheses, ownership of, 30
  (See also specific kinds of prostheses)
Prosthodontics:
  care of equipment, 316–317
    illustrated, 316
  defined, 6, 614
  pedodontic, 520–523
    illustrated, 521–523
  removable (see Denture patients; Dentures)
  (See also Fixed prosthodontics)
Proteins, 403
  RDAs for, table, 408
  source of, 411
Prothero, D. H., 18
Psychology:
  defined, 61–62
  dental, 72–76
  of denture patients, 644–645
  historical development of, 62–63
  and physiology of pain, 446–447
  in treatment-plan appointments, 76–77
Pterygoid, internal, 85
  illustrated, 87
Public health dentistry, defined, 6
Public Health Service, 7, 10, 155
Pucket, H. C., 502
Puestow, C. G., 433
Pulp, 91, 111–113
  illustrated, 85, 93–95, 113
Pulp canal, 473–475
  illustrated, 475
Pulp capping, 478, 519–520
Pulp cavity, opening of, 472–474
  illustrated, 473, 474
Pulp polyps, illustrated, 158
Pulp stones, 152
Pulp test, electric, illustrated, 468–469
Pulp therapy, pedodontic, 519–520
Pulpectomy, 520
Pulpitis, 157–158
  illustrated, 158
Pulpotomy, 478–479, 520
Pulse, taking of, 326–327
  illustrated, 327

754 / Index

Pumice as polishing agent, illustrated, 258
Punches, 311–312, 583
　illustrated, 312
Purdy, E. G., 18
Pure gold (see Gold)
Pyogenic granulomas, illustrated, 161
Pyorrhea (see Periodontitis)

Questionaires, 321–324
　illustrated, 322, 324
Quick-cure resin impression trays (autopolymerizing impression trays), 652–655
　illustrated, 654–655

Radiation, 342–349
　injuries from, 165
　physics of, 342–344
　　illustrated, 342, 343
　protection from, 347–349
　radiation biology, 346–347
Radiographs (see X-rays)
Radiology:
　darkroom, illustrated, 350–355
　films used in (see Films)
　intraoral technique of (see X-rays, intraoral)
　operation of x-ray machine, 344–346
　　illustrated, 345
　panoramic, 372–374
　　illustrated, 372, 373
　photochemistry and, 349–350
　role and practice of, 341–342
　(See also Radiation; X-rays)
Rash, wandering, illustrated, 160
RDAs (see Recommended Daily Dietary Allowances)
Reamers:
　care of, 307
　used in pulp canal, 473–475
　　illustrated, 475
Recall appointments, 48–49
Reception of supplies, illustrated, 58–60
Receptionists, orthodontic assistants as, 544
Recession, 485–486
Recommended Daily Dietary Allowances (RDAs), 408–411
　diet prescription fulfilling, 417
　　illustrated, 410
　table, 409
Record bases (see Occlusion rims)
Records, 49–54
　of administered drugs, 456
　of appointments, 46–48
　　illustrated, 47, 48
　of diagnostic data, 340
　income, expense and disbursement, 51, 53
　keeping of, 50–51
　of medication and patient's reaction to it, 170–171
　orthodontic, 534
　　radiographic, 535–537
　　taking, 544–545
　tax and payroll, 54
　(See also Charts; Patient history)
Rectal administration of drugs, 171
Red-flag tag inventory control, illustrated, 56, 57

Reflectors, Floxite, 385
　illustrated, 387
Refractory material in casting investments, 261
Relines, denture, 645–646, 677
Remelting of casting gold alloys, 253
Reminder calls, 43–44
Removable orthodontic appliances, illustrated, 542
Removable prosthodontics (see Denture patients; Dentures)
Repairs of dentures, 213–214
　of complete dentures, 678–680
　　illustrated, 679
Reparative dentin, 111
Reppert, H. C., 72
"Requirements for an Accredited Dental Laboratory Technology Education Program," 24
"Requirements for an Accredited Program in Dental Assisting," 14
"Requirements for Approval of a Certification Board for Dental Assistants," 14
Resin cement, 228–233
　restorations with, 229–233
　　illustrated, 230–232
　　table, 216
　(See also Synthetic resin materials)
Resistance forms, obtaining, in preparation of cavities, 56
Resnick, N., 14, 15
Respiratory difficulties, treatment of, 430–431
Restorations:
　of clinical fixed prostheses: placement of, 635–637
　　illustrated, 639
　　temporary, 634–636
　extracoronal (see Full crowns)
　intracoronal, 616–617
　　illustrated, 616
　post and core, 641–643
　　illustrated, 642
　with resins, 229–233
　　illustrated, 230–232
　　table, 216
　(See also Operative dentistry)
Resuscitation methods, 431–436
　illustrated, 432–436
Retainers, 615–617
　amalgam matrix, 306–308
　　illustrated, 308
　on facial surface of maxillary teeth, illustrated, 600
　illustrated, 615, 616
Retention forms:
　illustrated, 562
　obtaining, in cavity preparation, 561–563
Retention grooves, 562–563
　illustrated, 562
Retention locks, illustrated, 562
Reverse reproductions (see Impressions)
Reversible hydrocolloids, 630
Rheumatic fever (rheumatic heart disease), 124
Richardson, Richard E., 1–37, 320–340
Riggs, John M., 5
Rigid impression materials, 198–200
　illustrated, 200

Robinson, J. B., 5, 167
Robinson, P. A., 22
Roetgen, Wilhelm von, 342
Root canal therapy, 471–478
　illustrated, 472–477
Root-end abcesses (periapical abcesses), 158
Roots, amputation and hemisection of, 497
Rose, T. A., 504
Rosenblum F. N., 17
Rosin in zinc oxide-eugenol cement, 216
Rotary cutting instruments, 292–296
　illustrated, 293–295
Rouge as polishing agent, 259
Routine data in patient history, defined, 323
Rowley, M. E., 14
Rubber dam clamp forceps, 311–312, 460, 583
　illustrated, 312, 461
Rubber dam clamps (see Clamps)
Rubber dam equipment, care of, 311–312
　illustrated, 311
Rubber dam holders, 311–312, 583
　illustrated, 312
Rubber dam napkins, 583
Rubber dam punches (see Punches)
Rubber dams, 471–473
　illustrated, 472–473
　in moisture control: application of, 584–591
　　illustrated, 585–591
　　illustrated, 582
　positioning holes in, 583–585
　　illustrated, 584, 585
　removal of, 585, 593
Rubber impression materials, 205–207
　illustrated, 206
Rubber items, sterilization of, 148
Rubber wheel used in endodontic diagnosis, illustrated, 468
Ruch, Floyd, L., 63, 65, 66
Rule of law, defined, 27
Ryge, G., 271

S-shaped dentinal tubules, illustrated, 112
Safelight in darkroom, 351
Saliva ejectors, 277–278
　illustrated, 278
Salivary glands, 86–88
　illustrated, 88
Salt sterilizers, 144
Salzmann, J. A., 507, 510
Samer, H., 30
Sand as polishing agent, 258
Sanitary pontics (hygienic pontics), illustrated 617
Sarcomas, 153, 162
Scalers, 300–301
　illustrated, 301
Scatter radiation (secondary radiation), 347–348
Schnoebelen, E. O., 18
Schour, I., 153, 507
Sclerotic dentin, 110
Scrub technique of toothbrushing, 390
Sealants, occlusal, 525
Secobarbital, 175
Secondary dentin, pulpitis and, 158
Secondary drives (learned drives), 66

Secondary radiation (scatter radiation), 347–348
Secondary teeth
 (see Permanent dentition)
Security measures in drug storage, 456
Sedation, 453–455
Selective Service Act, 6
Self-curing acrylics, 680
Self-curing resins:
 facial-surface cavity preparation for, illustrated, 560
 restorations with, 610
 retention forms for, 563
Self-evaluation, 396–397
 at home, 397
Self-examination methods, 385–386
Separating wires, 543
Sepsis, defined, 137
 (See also Cross-infections; Infections)
Serum hepatitis (hepatitis B), 133, 136
Serum test for syphilis (STS), 132
Setting reaction:
 of amalgams, 238
 of casting investments, 261
 of gypsum products, 186–188
 of resin cements, 228
 of rubber impression materials, 205
 of silicate cements, 224–225
 of zinc phosphate cements, 218–219
Shadow casting, principles of, 354–356
Shadowgram, defined, 354
Shaffer, J. I., 72
Shankle, R. Jack, 81–105, 467–481
Shannon, Ira, 378
Shape waxes (sheet waxes, casting waxes), 209–210
 illustrated, 210
Sharpening of instruments, 312–316
 illustrated, 313–316
 periodontic, 487, 489–490
 illustrated, 490
Sheet waxes (casting waxes; shape waxes), 209–210
 illustrated, 210
Shellac impression trays, 651–652
 illustrated, 651
Sheppard, G. A., 427
Shiere, F. R., 520
Shock, 434–439
 anaphylactic, 435–437
 insulin, 438–439
 neurogenic, 434–435
 illustrated, 435
Shrinkage of casting gold alloys, 253
Silicate cement, 222–228
 composition of, 223
 general characteristics of, 223–224
 mixing and placement of, 225—228
 illustrated, 225—227
 restorations with, 610
 retention form for, 563
 setting time of, 224–225
 table, 216
Silver in gold alloys, 250
Silver amalgams:
 preparation of occlusal-surface cavities for, 558–559
 illustrated, 559
 used in pedodontics, illustrated, 519

Simple cavities, 556–557
 illustrated, 556
Sim's test, 384
Skin tests, 124
Sluder, T. B., 631
Smoker's patches (hyperkeratosis; leukoplasia), illustrated, 160
Smooth-surface cavities:
 defined, 156
 illustrated, 557
Snap-A-Ray (film holder), illustrated, 358
Snyder's test, 384
Social history of patients, 325–326
Social Security Act, Title XIX of (Medicaid), 10, 11, 50, 54
Socioeconomic factors of pedodontic care, 504
Sockwell, C. L., 524, 525
Sodium benzoate, 179
Sodium hypochlorite, 476
Soft palate, examination of, 330–331
 illustrated, 331
Soggnaes, R. F., 1
Soldering:
 of bridge components, 618
 of gold alloys, 254–256
Solid solution, illustrated, 245
Solo practice, 12
Solutions used in root canal therapy, 475–476
Southard, Juliette A., 13
Space lattice, defined, 244
Spatulas, care of, 302–304
 illustrated, 303, 304
Specialty practice, 5–6
Sphygmomanometer, illustrated, 424
Spock, Benjamin, 507
Spoon excavators, illustrated, 298
Spores, 120
 illustrated, 118
Sprains, treatment of, 443
Spruing of wax patterns, illustrated, 264, 265
Squamous cell carcinomas (epidermoid carcinomas), 162–163
 illustrated, 163
Squamous epithelial cells, abnormal, illustrated, 164
Stabe film holders, 363–364
 illustrated, 364
Staff meetings, 39–40
Stains, 624
Stanmeyer, William R., 375–419
Staphylococci, illustrated, 118
Staphylococcus albus, 123
Staphylococcus aureus, 123
Starkey, P., 520, 523
State Board of Dentistry, 20
State health departments, dental practice in, 7
"Statement on Expanded Function Dental Auxiliary Utilization and Education" (ADA), 20–22
Status Seekers, The (Packard), 67
Steam autoclave-dry-heat sterilizer combination, illustrated, 142
Stephan, R. M., 377, 400
Sterile items, dispensation of, illustrated, 141
Sterilization, 135–137
 care of sterilization equipment, 312
 defined, 136–137

Sterilization:
 (See also Cross-infections, control of; Instruments, sterilization of)
Stethoscope, illustrated, 424
Stick compounds, illustrated, 201
Sticky waxes, 210
Stimulants, 176–177
Stimuli, pain, 446–447
Stippling, defined, 114
Stomatitis, aphthous, 131–132
Stone casts, illustrated, 186
Stones, 294–295
 general properties of, 185
 illustrated, 186, 294
 improved, 185–187
 illustrated, 187
 sterilization of, 148
Storage of supplies and equipment, 60
Straight universal matrices, 599–600
 illustrated, 600
Streptococci, 129
 illustrated, 118
Streptococcus fecalis, 129
Streptococcus mutans, 129–131, 402
Streptococcus pneumoniae, 123
Streptococcus pyogenes, 124
Streptococcus sanguis, 125, 129
Streptococcus viridans, 124
Strickland, William D., 552–613
Stripes of Retzius, 109–111
 illustrated, 110, 111
STS (serum test for syphilis), 132
Sturdevant, C. M., 634, 639
Styptics, 177
Sublingual administration of drugs, 171
Sublingual gland, 87–88
 illustrated, 88
Submaxillary gland, 87–88
 illustrated, 88
Subsurface porosity of castings, 271
Sucrose, role of, in formation of plaque, 402
Sulfuric acid, 476
Sullens, R. H., 14
Summers, F. W., 513, 514, 516
Supplies:
 control of, 54–60
 illustrated, 56–60
 periodontic, 499
Supply companies, 8
Support services, 7–8
Surface defects of castings, 271–272
Surfaces, scrubbing of, illustrated, 140
Surgery, 457–466
 asepsis and, 458–461
 illustrated, 458, 459, 461
 defined, 5
 orthodontic, 541
 periodontic, 492–500
 illustrated, 493–498
 postoperative procedures, 464–466
 postoperative instruction card, illustrated, 465
 preoperative plan, 460–463
 illustrated, 462, 463
 procedures for, 462–464
 illustrated, 464
 surgical equipment, 288
Surgical instruments (see Instruments, surgical)

756 / Index

"Survey of Dentistry" (1961; ADA), 22, 24
Surveying and designing tools for construction of partial dentures, 682–683
  illustrated, 683
Sutures, 461
  median palatine, 81–83
    illustrated, 82–83
Synthetic drugs, 169–170
Synthetic resin materials, 211–214
  illustrated, 212
  preoperative alginate-acrylic resin technique, 634–636
    illustrated, 636
  in prosthodontics, 619
    illustrated, 621
  for temporary shells, 634–635
    illustrated, 635
  quick-cure resin impression trays, 652–655
    illustrated, 654–655
  (See also Self-curing resins)
Syphilis, 132, 161
Syphilitic chancre, 161
Syringe (or light) type of low viscosity of rubber materials, 205
Syringes:
  air, 278–279
    illustrated, 279
  air-water, 149
  care of, 310–311
    illustrated, 311
  for injecting rubber-base impression materials, illustrated, 206
  water, 278–279
    illustrated, 279
Systemic factors in etiology of orthodontics, 529–530
Systemic fluorides, 377–378

Tannic acid, 177–178
Tarnish on gold alloys, 256–257
Tatoos, amalgam, 164
Tawney, R. H., 30
Tax records, 54
Taylor, J. A. 3, 5, 22
Teaching of expanded functions, 18, 20
TEAM (Training in Expanded Auxiliary Management) program, 16
Teeth, 87–96
  development of: chronology, illustrated, 98–99
    illustrated, 107–109
  differentiating characteristics between, 91–96
    illustrated, 100–102
  eruption of, 91
    illustrated, 96–98
    table, 92
  examination of, 330, 334–337
    illustrated, 331, 336, 337
  facial aspects of, illustrated, 102
  functions of, 88–89
  injuries to: illustrated, 165
    tissue responses to, 152–153
  maintenance of position of, 101–105
    illustrated, 103, 104
  nerve anatomy of, 446–448
    illustrated, 447, 448

Teeth:
  physiology of pain and anatomy of, 446–448
    illustrated, 447, 448
  structures of, 90–91
    illustrated, 93–96, 98
  supporting, 83–86
    illustrated, 86
  supporting tissues of, 113–116
    illustrated, 114, 115
  surfaces and landmarks of, 89–90
  (See also Permanent dentition; Primary dentition; specific teeth; and under dental)
Telephone, handling of, 41–44
  illustrated, 42
Temporal muscle of mastication, 85–86
  illustrated, 86
Temporary crowns, acrylic resin and aluminum, 634
  illustrated, 635
Temporary gold inlay restorations, 607
Temporomandibular joints, 82–84
  examination of, illustrated, 328
  illustrated, 83, 84
Test(s):
  for acid-forming bacteria, 130–131
    illustrated, 131
  anesthetic, 471
  caries activity, 384–385
  electric pulp, illustrated, 468–469
  heat, 469
    illustrated, 471
  ice, 469–470
    illustrated, 470
  instrument-sharpness, 316
  Kahn, 132
  lactobacilli, 130–131
    illustrated, 131
  mobility, 470–471
  penny, 351
  percussion, 469–470
  pressure-release and transillumination, 471
  skin, 124
  STS, 132
  Wassermann, 132
Thermal expansion method (high-heat technique) of casting investments, 262
Thermal injuries to teeth, 165
Thermal properties of dental materials, table, 184
Thermometer used in darkroom, 351
Three-quarter crowns (pinlays; partial crowns), 616–617
  illustrated, 616
Thrombin, 178
Thyroid gland, examination of, illustrated, 329
Thyroxine in regulation of metabolism, 408
Tin oxide as polishing agent, 259
Tissue-contacting pontics, 617–618
  illustrated, 618
Tolerance, drug, 172
Tongue examination, illustrated, 331, 332
Tooth buds (tooth germs), development of, 107–108
Tooth-cleaning techniques, 387–388

Tooth-colored restorative materials, facial-surface cavity preparation for, 559–560
  illustrated, 560
Tooth contours, restoring proper, as objective of operative dentistry, 555
Tooth decay:
  prevalence of, 2
    among children, 503
  statistics on, 1
  (See also specific forms of tooth decay)
Tooth loss, statistics on, 1
Toothbrushes, 388–389
  electric, 393
  illustrated, 388
Toothbrushing, illustrated, 388–391
Topical fluorides, 378–379
Tracheotomies, 434
  illustrated, 436
Training:
  of dental hygienists, 23–24
  of dental laboratory technicians, 24–25
Training in Expanded Auxiliary Management (TEAM) program, 16
Tranquilizers, 176
Transfer impressions, 630–634
  illustrated, 632–634
Transfer registrations, plaster of paris for, 199
Transillumination test, 471
Traumatic injuries to teeth, 165
Tray technique of impressions, 630
  illustrated, 634
Tray (or heavy) type of high viscosity of rubber materials, 205
Trays:
  annealing, 309
  (See also Impression trays)
Treatment:
  based on diagnostic findings, 339–340
  of emergencies (see Emergencies, treatment of)
  records of, 50
Treatment-plan appointments, 76–77
Trench mouth (see Vincent's disease)
Treponema, 125
Trimmers:
  gingival margin, 298–299
    illustrated, 299
  model, illustrated, 318
Trimming:
  of articulated models, illustrated, 195
  of models, 193–196
    illustrated, 194–196
  of partial denture casts, illustrated, 681
Tripoli as polishing agent, 258–259
Troy weight of gold alloys, 250
Try-in appointments, 635–637, 670, 674
Tumors (see Neoplasms)
Tweezers (operating pliers; cotton pliers), 302–303
  illustrated, 303
Tylenol, 176
Type I casting gold alloys, 252
Type II casting gold alloys, 252
Type III casting gold alloys, 252
Type IV casting gold alloys, 252

Ulcers, aphthous, illustrated, 159
Ultrasonic periodontic instruments, 490–491

Ultrasonic periodontic instruments:
  illustrated, 491
Ultrasonic units, 286–287
  illustrated, 287
Ultraspeed handpieces, 291–292
  illustrated, 291
Ultraviolet activator lights, 285–286
  illustrated, 286
Undercut waxes, 210
Unfilled resin restorative materials, 230–232
  illustrated, 231, 232
United States Air Force, dental practice in, 6–7
United States Army, dental practice in, 6–7
United States Navy, dental practice in, 6–7
United States Pharmacopeia, 168, 169, 173
Universal matrices for amalgam restorations, 599–603
  illustrated, 600–603
University of North Carolina School of Dentistry, 514
Unwritten law (common law), 27
Updegrave, W. J., 72
Utility waxes, 210

Valium, 176
Varnishes, cavity, 595
Vasoconstrictors, 177
VDRL (test for syphilis), 132
Vegetable-fruit group, 411, 413
Veterans Administration, 7
Vibrators used in pouring of impressions, illustrated, 649
Vincent's disease (acute necrotizing ulcerative disease; ANUG; trench mouth):
  illustrated, 486
  microorganisms associated with, illustrated, 132
Vipeholm dental-caries study, 400
Viral hepatitis (hepatitis A), 132–133, 136
  treating patients suspected of, 149
Virulence of bacteria, defined, 122
Viscosity of rubber materials, 205
Vistaril, 176
Visual examinations, 468
Vitamin A, 403–405
  RDAs for, table, 408
  sources of, 411, 413
  table, 404
Vitamin B complex, 404–406
  RDAs for, table, 409
  sources of, 411, 413
  table, 404
Vitamin C, 406
  RDAs for, table, 409
  sources of, 411, 413
  table, 404
Vitamin D, 404–405
  RDAs for, table, 408
  sources of, 411
  table, 404
Vitamin E, 405

Vitamin E:
  RDAs for, table, 408
  table, 404
Vitamin K, 405
  table, 404

Wandering rash (geographic tongue), illustrated, 160
Want lists, 57
  illustrated, 57
Wassermann test for syphilis, 132
Water irrigation devices, 392
Water/powder ratio in casting investments, 262
Water syringes, 278
  illustrated, 279
Wax patterns for casting investments, 262–264
  illustrated, 263, 264
  investing of, 265–267
    illustrated, 266
  spruing of, illustrated, 264, 265
  wax elimination, 267–268
    illustrated, 267
Wax spatulas, illustrated, 208
Wax-up, insertion of, in partial dentures, 684
Waxes, 207–211
  baseplate, 209
    illustrated, 210
  casting, 209–210
    illustrated, 210
  classification and uses of, table, 207
  pattern, 208–209
    illustrated, 208
  (*See also* Wax patterns)
Webster, W. P., 428–430, 434, 438, 440
Webster's New Twentieth Century Dictionary, 62
Weight, effects of, on drug action, 172
Weights and measures in drug preparations, 172–173
Weinberger, B. F., 167
Welding of gold alloys, 256
  illustrated, 257
Wells, Horace, 5, 167, 445, 446
Wheeler, H. L., 22
Wheeler, R. C., 103
Wheeler-Lea Act, 167
White casting gold alloys, 252
White decay, described, 156
Wilson, L. L., 18
Wires:
  arch, 542
  ligature and separating, 543
  orthodontic, illustrated, 257
Wood, Matthew T., 420–444
Work area for operative dentistry, 567–568
  illustrated, 567
Work position for dental team in operative dentistry, 565–657
  illustrated, 566, 567
World Health Organization (WHO), 2, 146, 377

World Health Organization (WHO):
  Expert Committee on Auxiliary Dental Personnel of, 16–17
Written express contracts, defined, 28
Written law, 27
Wrought gold alloys, 253–254
  illustrated, 254

X-ray units, 288–289
  illustrated, 288
  operating of, 344–346
    illustrated, 345
X-rays, 425
  in endodontics, 468
  with first pedodontic appointment, 514–515
    illustrated, 515
  generation of, 343–344
    illustrated, 343
  intraoral, 355–273
    bisecting-angle technique of, 356–363
      illustrated, 356–362
    bitewing technique of, 371–372
      illustrated, 369
    occlusal techniques of, 373–374
      illustrated, 370–371
    paralleling technique of, 363–371
      illustrated, 363–368
    principles of shadow casting in, 354–356
  records of, 50, 535–537

Zephiran chloride (benzalkonium chloride), 178
Zinc:
  in gold alloys, 251
  nutritional, RDAs for, table, 409
Zinc acetate in zinc oxide-eugenol cement, 216
Zinc oxide:
  in operative dentistry, 595
  in pedodontic pulp capping, 519
  used in endodontics, 478
Zinc oxide–eugenol (ZOE) paste cement, 199, 215–217, 637, 639
  in endodontics, 478
  illustrated, 217
  in operative dentistry, 595
  in pedodontic pulp capping, 519
  table, 216
Zinc phosphate cement, 217–222, 639, 643
  composition of, 217
  control of setting of, 218–219
  general characteristics of, 217–218
  mixing of, illustrated, 219–224
  uses of, table, 216
Zinc silicophosphate cement, 228
  table, 216
ZOE [*see* Zinc oxide–eugenol (ZOE) paste cement]
Zone of Weil, 112–113
  illustrated, 113

DECIDUOUS DENTITION

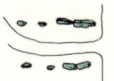 5 months in utero

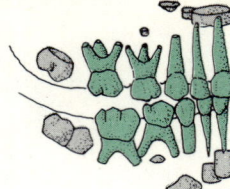 2 years (±6 mos.)

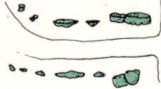 7 months in utero

PRENATAL

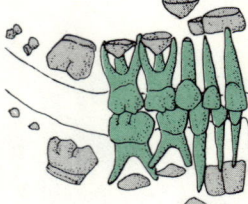 3 years (±6 mos.)

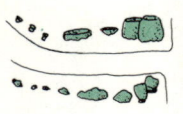 Birth

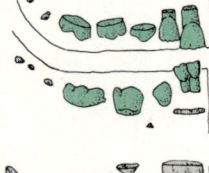 6 mos. (±2 mos.)

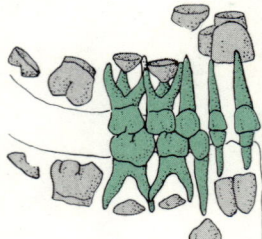 4 years (±9 mos.)

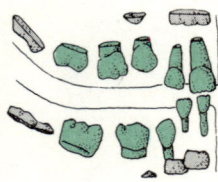 9 mos. (±2 mos.)

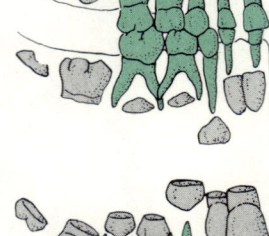 5 years (±9 mos.)

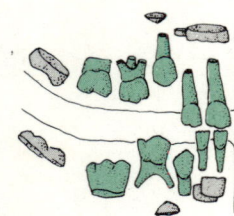 1 year (±3 mos.)

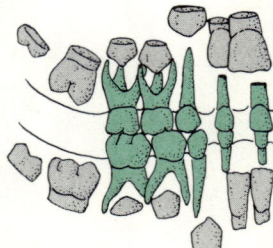 6 years (±9 mos.)

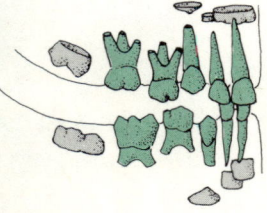 18 mos. (±3 mos.)

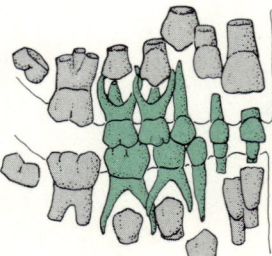

INFANCY

EARLY CHILDHOOD (PRE-SCHOOL AGE)